AF413069

LUNG INJURY

LUNG BIOLOGY IN HEALTH AND DISEASE

Executive Editor

Claude Lenfant

Former Director, National Heart, Lung, and Blood Institute
National Institutes of Health
Bethesda, Maryland

*The opinions expressed in these volumes do not necessarily represent
the views of the National Institutes of Health.*

LUNG INJURY

Mechanisms, Pathophysiology, and Therapy

Edited by

Senior Editor
Robert H. Notter
University of Rochester
Rochester, New York, U.S.A.

Jacob N. Finkelstein
University of Rochester
Rochester, New York, U.S.A.

Bruce A. Holm
State University of New York at Buffalo
Buffalo, New York, U.S.A.

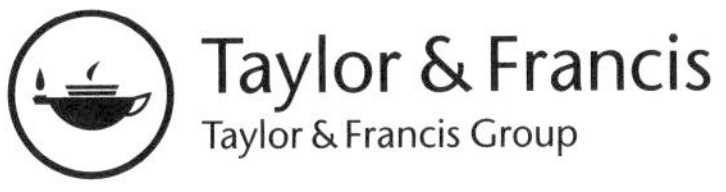

Taylor & Francis
Taylor & Francis Group

Boca Raton London New York Singapore

Published in 2005 by
Taylor & Francis Group
6000 Broken Sound Parkway NW, Suite 300
Boca Raton, FL 33487-2742

International Standard Book Number-10: 0-8247-5793-9 (Hardcover)
International Standard Book Number-13: 978-0-8247-5793-9 (Hardcover)

Library of Congress Cataloging-in-Publication Data

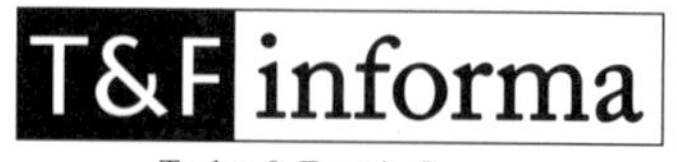

**Visit the Taylor & Francis Web site at
http://www.taylorandfrancis.com**

Introduction

Lung injury is a very broad clinical entity that may result from both endogeneous and exogeneous factors. Much credit must be given to Ashbaugh et al. who introduced the term Acute Respiratory Distress Syndrome (ARDS) in 1967.[*] Initially, this condition was defined by the widespread pulmonary infiltrate seen on chest X-rays, hypoxia and poor pulmonary compliance. Clinicians and health officials soon discovered the high prevalence and mortality of this condition resulting from a multifaceted etiology.

Over the last 30 years, a large number of studies have been conducted to attempt to uncover the pathogenesis of ARDS and to develop effective treatments. From this very intense work, the extreme complexity of this syndrome became apparent, but it was also discovered that many of the pathogenic pathways relevant to ARDS were also features, albeit with variations, of other conditions resulting either from an acute lung injury like ARDS or from a chronic disorder such as pulmonary fibrosis. Thus, the term "lung injury" became preferred to explain the similarity of the cellular and subcellular manifestations resulting from pathologies of different origin.

This volume titled *Lung Injury: Mechanisms, Pathophysiology, and Therapy* and edited by Drs. Robert H. Notter, Jacob N. Finkelstein, and

---

[*] Ashbaugh DG, Bigelow DP, Petty TL and Levine BE. Acute respiratory disease in adults. *Lancet.* 1967; 2:320–323.

Bruce A. Holm gives the reader a panoramic—indeed, unique—description of lung injury. Most volumes addressing lung injury focus almost exclusively on one cause of lung injury. This monograph presents the most current knowledge of the mechanisms of lung injury as well as therapeutic options which are derived from the mechanistic determinants. Its very valuable feature is the construct of each chapter, which leads the reader to a set of research questions that hopefully will stimulate both researchers and clinicians.

Since its inception, the series of monographs *Lung Biology in Health and Disease* has included several volumes on diseases causing lung injury. In a way, this new volume is an "integration" of all the previous monographs. Undoubtedly, readers will be challenged.

I deeply appreciate the work of the editors and authors to develop this monograph and I am grateful to them for the opportunity to include it in the series.

Claude Leufant, M.D.
Gaithersburg, Maryland

Preface

This book attempts the challenging task of providing an integrated synopsis of basic concepts, topical review, and clinical therapies relevant for pulmonary inflammation and acute and chronic lung injury. Individual chapters have been written separately, but the authors and editors have made a conscious effort to integrate coverage and emphasize connections between different areas of lung injury research and applied therapeutics. Coverage in each chapter typically proceeds from general principles and concepts to specific discussion and review of current research perspectives. The direct complementarity between mechanistic basic science understanding and clinical therapies is a major area of focus. In particular, current and evolving treatments for clinical lung injury in the latter part of the book are presented in the context of basic science understanding and research perspectives developed in preceding chapters. The editors and chapter authors hope very much that the book will prove useful to a broad audience of basic biomedical researchers and physician-scientists working in pulmonary biology, toxicology, and pulmonology, as well as to physicians-in-training and graduate students interested in learning about lung injury and its important clinical consequences.

Robert H. Notter
Jacob N. Finkelstein
Bruce A. Holm

Contributors

Tiina M. Asikainen   Hospital for Children and Adolescents, University of Helsinki, Helsinki, Finland, and National Jewish Medical and Research Center, Denver, Colorado, U.S.A.

William S. Beckett   Departments of Medicine and Environmental Medicine, Lung Biology and Disease Program, University of Rochester School of Medicine, Rochester, New York, U.S.A.

John A. Belperio   Department of Medicine, Division of Pulmonary and Critical Care Medicine, UCLA School of Medicine, Los Angeles, California, U.S.A.

Peter B. Bitterman   Department of Medicine, University of Minnesota, School of Medicine, Minneapolis, Minnesota, U.S.A.

Stephen M. Black   Department of Biomedical and Pharmaceutical Sciences, The University of Montana, Missoula, Montana, U.S.A.

Mahesh Bommaraju   Department of Pediatrics, State University of New York (SUNY) at Buffalo, The Women & Children's Hospital of Buffalo, Buffalo, New York, U.S.A.

Arnold R. Brody   Department of Pathology and Laboratory Medicine, Tulane University Health Sciences Center, New Orleans, Louisiana, U.S.A.

Patricia R. Chess   Departments of Pediatrics and Environmental Medicine, University of Rochester, Rochester, New York, U.S.A.

Ian Copland   Department of Laboratory Medicine and Pathology, Lung Biology Research Programme, Hospital for Sick Children Research Institute, University of Toronto, Toronto, Ontario, Canada

Daniel L. Costa   Pulmonary Toxicology Branch, Experimental Toxicology Division, National Health and Environmental Research Laboratory, Research Triangle Park, North Carolina, U.S.A.

Carl T. D'Angio   Department of Pediatrics and Environmental Medicine, University of Rochester School of Medicine, Rochester, New York, U.S.A.

Ian C. Davis   Department of Anesthesiology, University of Alabama at Birmingham, Birmingham, Alabama, U.S.A.

C. C. Dos Santos   Department of Critical Care Medicine, St. Michael's Hospital and Interdepartmental Division of Critical Care, Department of Medicine, University of Toronto, Toronto, Ontario, Canada

Jeffrey R. Fineman   Department of Pediatrics and Cardiovascular Research Institute, University of California, San Francisco, California, U.S.A.

Jacob N. Finkelstein   Departments of Pediatrics and Environmental Medicine, University of Rochester, Rochester, New York, U.S.A.

J. Gauldie   Department of Pathology and Molecular Medicine, McMaster University, Hamilton, Ontario, Canada

Adam Giangreco   Department of Environmental and Occupational Health, University of Pittsburgh, Pittsburgh, Pennsylvania, U.S.A.

M. Hitt   Department of Oncology, Cross Cancer Institute, Edmondton, Alberta, Canada

Bruce A. Holm   Departments of Pediatrics and Obstetrics and Gynecology, State University of New York (SUNY) at Buffalo, Buffalo, New York, U.S.A.

Julia Kaufman   Departments of Medicine and Environmental Medicine, Lung Biology and Disease Program, University of Rochester School of Medicine, Rochester, New York, U.S.A.

Michael P. Keane   Department of Medicine, Division of Pulmonary and Critical Care Medicine, UCLA School of Medicine, Los Angeles, California, U.S.A.

Paul R. Knight   Departments of Anesthesiology and Microbiology, State University of New York (SUNY) at Buffalo, Buffalo, New York, U.S.A.

M. Kolb   Department of Pathology and Molecular Medicine, McMaster University, Hamilton, Ontario, Canada

Vasanth H. Kumar   Department of Pediatrics, State University of New York (SUNY) at Buffalo, The Women & Children's Hospital of Buffalo, Buffalo, New York, U.S.A.

Satyan Lakshminrusimha   Department of Pediatrics, State University of New York (SUNY) at Buffalo, The Women & Children's Hospital of Buffalo, Buffalo, New York, U.S.A.

John D. Lang   Department of Anesthesiology, University of Alabama at Birmingham, Birmingham, Alabama, U.S.A.

Joseph A. Lasky   Department of Medicine, Tulane University Health Sciences Center, New Orleans, Louisiana, U.S.A.

Christine Martey   Departments of Medicine and Environmental Medicine, Lung Biology and Disease Program, University of Rochester School of Medicine, Rochester, New York, U.S.A.

Sadis Matalon   Departments of Anesthesiology, University of Alabama at Birmingham, Birmingham, Alabama, U.S.A.

Frederick C. Morin, III   Department of Pediatrics, State University of New York (SUNY) at Buffalo, The Women & Children's Hospital of Buffalo, Buffalo, New York, U.S.A.

Robert H. Notter   Departments of Pediatrics and Environmental Medicine, University of Rochester, Rochester, New York, U.S.A.

Michael A. O'Reilly   Departments of Pediatrics and Environmental Medicine, University of Rochester, Rochester, New York, U.S.A.

Luis A. Ortiz   Department of Environmental and Occupational Health, University of Pittsburgh, Pittsburgh, Pennsylvania, U.S.A.

David Perlman   Department of Medicine, University of Minnesota, School of Medicine, Minneapolis, Minnesota, U.S.A.

Richard Phipps   Departments of Medicine and Environmental Medicine, Lung Biology and Disease Program, University of Rochester School of Medicine, Rochester, New York, U.S.A.

Martin Post   Departments of Pediatrics, Physiology, and Laboratory Medicine and Pathology, Lung Biology Research Programme, Hospital for Sick Children Research Institute, University of Toronto, Toronto, Ontario, Canada

Gloria S. Pryhuber   Departments of Pediatrics and Environmental Medicine, University of Rochester School of Medicine, Rochester, New York, U.S.A.

Susan D. Reynolds   Department of Environmental and Occupational Health, University of Pittsburgh, Pittsburgh, Pennsylvania, U.S.A.

Alexandre T. Rotta   Department of Anesthesiology, State University of New York (SUNY) at Buffalo, Buffalo, New York, U.S.A.

Rita M. Ryan   Department of Pediatrics, State University of New York (SUNY) at Buffalo, The Women & Children's Hospital of Buffalo, Buffalo, New York, U.S.A.

P. J. Sime   Departments of Medicine and Environmental Medicine, Lung Biology and Disease Program, University of Rochester School of Medicine, Rochester, New York, U.S.A.

A. S. Slutsky   Department of Critical Care Medicine, St. Michael's Hospital and Interdepartmental Division of Critical Care, Department of Medicine, University of Toronto, Toronto, Ontario, Canada

Robert M. Strieter   Department of Pathology and Laboratory Medicine, UCLA School of Medicine, Los Angeles, California, U.S.A.

Barry R. Stripp   Department of Environmental and Occupational Health, University of Pittsburgh, Pittsburgh, Pennsylvania, U.S.A.

Keith Tanswell   Departments of Pediatrics and Physiology, Lung Biology Research Programme, Hospital for Sick Children Research Institute, University of Toronto, Toronto, Ontario, Canada

Thomas H. Thatcher   Departments of Medicine and Environmental Medicine, Lung Biology and Disease Program, University of Rochester School of Medicine, Rochester, New York, U.S.A.

Zhengdong Wang   Department of Pediatrics, University of Rochester, Rochester, New York, U.S.A.

Stephen Wedgwood   Department of Pediatrics, Northwestern University Medical School, Chicago, Illinois, U.S.A.

Christine H. Wendt   Department of Medicine, University of Minnesota, School of Medicine, Minneapolis, Minnesota, U.S.A.

Carl W. White   National Jewish Medical and Research Center, Denver, Colorado, U.S.A.

R. J. White   Department of Medicine (Division of Pulmonary and Critical Care Medicine), University of Rochester School of Medicine, Rochester, New York, U.S.A.

Contents

1

Introduction to Lung Injury

ROBERT H. NOTTER, JACOB N. FINKELSTEIN, and BRUCE A. HOLM

Departments of Pediatrics and Environmental Medicine, University of Rochester, Rochester, New York, U.S.A., and Departments of Pediatrics and Obstetrics and Gynecology, State University of New York (SUNY) at Buffalo, Buffalo, New York, U.S.A.

I. Overview

To physicians and basic biomedical scientists, the term "injury" implies more than simply cuts, abrasions, fractures, or other readily apparent forms of trauma. Rather, injury is used in a broader context to denote damage to organs, cells, and tissues at the molecular, biochemical, or physiological level. One of the most widely studied areas in pulmonary biology over the past several decades involves lung injury and the fundamental mechanisms that contribute to it. The structural and functional integrity of the pulmonary vasculature, alveoli, airways, and interstitium are essential for life. This book addresses the mechanistic pathophysiology of acute and chronic lung injury, including both basic concepts and current research perspectives. Also emphasized is the translation of emerging basic science understanding to improve the range and effectiveness of clinical therapies for injury-related pulmonary diseases in infants, children, and adults.

The pulmonary system is particularly sensitive to injury. The lungs are directly and continuously exposed to the environment via the airways, and face a spectrum of potential inhalation hazards from which other organs are shielded. The pulmonary alveoli and airways in mammals comprise a surface area of approximately 1 m^2 per kilogram of body weight that is at risk for injury or alteration from external agents. The broad extent and fragile nature of the pulmonary capillary network similarly makes the lungs sensitive to injury from the vascular side. With each systolic contraction of the heart, the lungs receive a volumetric blood flow equal to that of the remainder of the body. This blood flow is distributed through a vascular network with a huge capillary cross-sectional area, which facilitates gas exchange and broadly distributes nutrients within the lungs. However, the extensive pulmonary microcirculatory blood flow can have detrimental consequences if it carries substances that are toxic or injurious. The thin-walled pulmonary capillaries are sensitive to permeability damage and high-molecular-weight edema is common in many forms of acute lung injury. Clinically important respiratory deficits arise from any process or combination of processes that compromise a significant portion of the pulmonary vasculature, airways, or alveoli. Thus, acute and chronic lung injury are frequent contributors to pulmonary disease in infants, children, and adults.

Injury to the lungs interacts with ongoing growth and development. Like the majority of organs, the lungs continue to develop and grow post-natally as well as prenatally. Many of the cellular and molecular processes and pathways active in normal lung development and growth are recapitulated during injury and repair. In the absence of injury, or with effective repair, the lungs are a highly efficient organ system for gas exchange. However, if inflammatory lung injury is severe or progressive, or if repair of injury is abnormally regulated so that normal growth and development are compromised, serious consequences to the organism occur. The regulation and interaction of growth, development, inflammation, and repair are highly active areas of current pulmonary research. The proper balance of these processes is necessary for normally functioning lungs with adequate host defense capabilities. How the lungs accomplish this, or fail to do so, in response to various injury stresses is a major focus of this book.

II. Acute Lung Injury

Lung injury occurs through a cascade of processes beginning with an acute insult and an associated acute innate inflammatory response. Acute pulmonary injury then either resolves or progresses to persistent chronic pathology involving abnormal remodeling and tissue repair.[a] The pathophy-

---

[a] The terms "acute" and "chronic" are qualitative only. Acute lung injury commonly occurs over timescales of minutes to days following exposure to an initiating agent or condition, while chronic lung injury may involve pathology persisting for weeks to years depending on the specific injury stimulus and the animal species.

siology of acute inflammatory lung injury is complex in its features, mechanisms, and regulation. The lungs contain a large number of functionally specific cell types that can potentially be affected during injury, as well as an extensive interstitial matrix to support the airways, alveoli, and vasculature. Table 1 notes some of the many pathological features and processes that may be associated with acute pulmonary injury.

One common aspect of the pathology of acute lung injury is damage to the cells of the alveolocapillary membrane (type I and type II alveolar epithelial cells and capillary endothelial cells) with a loss of barrier integrity. If endothelial permeability alone is increased, the resultant high-molecular-weight edema may be confined to the interstitium. However, if epithelial permeability is also compromised, edema can be distributed throughout the alveoli and interstitium even if lymphatics remain functional. Another important pathophysiological feature of acute lung injury is inflammation. The innate pulmonary inflammatory response is complex, involving the recruitment and activation of circulating leukocytes as well as participation by resident lung cells. Moreover, an almost bewildering number of inflammatory mediators, factors, and transduction and regulatory pathways are involved in acute pulmonary inflammation and injury.[b] Examples of inflammatory mediators and factors relevant for acute lung injury are given in Table 2. Basic research described in the following chapters has provided important information on the activities and interactions of inflammatory mediators, and has allowed several helpful categorizations to be developed. Subgroups of cytokines can be viewed as having pro-inflammatory, anti-inflammatory, or down-modulatory activity, or as appearing early or late in the inflammatory response. Also, chemotactic cytokines (chemokines) can be grouped in C, CC, and CXC families to help to correlate their cellular effects (Chapter 4). The activities and responses of cytokines can also be better understood by categorizing their production by specific cell types or subsets of cells. For example, $CD4^+$ lymphocytes (T-helper cells), which play crucial roles in cell-mediated adaptive immune responses, can be divided into functional subsets as Th1 (T-helper-1) cells and Th2 (T-helper-2) cells that produce cytokines with diverse or opposing regulatory or cellular activities. Th1 cells secrete interleukin (IL)-2, interferon-γ (IFN-γ) and tumor necrosis factor α and β (TNFα, TNFβ), while Th2 cells secrete IL-4, IL-5, IL-6, IL-9, IL-10, IL-13, and TNFα. Th1 type immune responses tend to be more important in intracellular host defense against viruses and microorganisms and in delayed hypersensitivity reactions including transplant rejection, while Th2 type immunity and secreted cytokines are more involved in antibody and allergic responses. Selected considerations

---

[b] For reviews of inflammatory mediators relevant for acute inflammatory lung injury see, for example, Refs. 1–13.

Table 1 Selected Aspects of the Complex Pathology of Acute Inflammatory Lung Injury

Leukocyte recruitment and/oractivation
Activation of resident pulmonary leukocytes
  including alveolar and interstitial macrophages
Recruitment and activation of circulating
  neutrophils, macrophages, and lymphocytes

Alveolar epithelial celldamage/alteration
Alveolar type I cell injury and death
Alveolar type II cell injury and/orhyperplasia
Increased permeability of alveolar epithelial barrier
Impaired surfactant synthesis, secretion, recycling
Abnormal nonsurfactant type II cell function

Lung surfactant dysfunction/inactivation
Biophysical inactivation by endogenous inhibitors
Chemical degradation by lytic enzymes, oxidants
Altered alveolar surfactant aggregate subtypes

Pulmonary interstitial injury
Less prominent in acute vs. chronic injury
Early inflammation-induced changes in fibroblasts
Early changes in extracellularmatrix

Inflammatory mediators/factors produced
Multiple mediators/factors produced by leukocytes,
  alveolar epithelial cells, airway cells, and interstitial cells
Reactive oxygen/nitrogen species, proteases,
  phospholipases generated and antioxidants depleted

Microvascular dysfunction
Injury to capillary endothelial cells resulting in
  increased microvascular permeability
Interstitial and alveolar edema
Perivascular inflammation
Hypoxic vasoconstriction; ventilation/perfusion mismatching

Airway injury
Injury to Clara cells, other airway epithelial cells
Injury to airway smooth muscle cells
Small airway inflammation, collapse, or spasm

Coagulation abnormalities
Disseminated intravascular coagulation
Micro- and macropulmonary emboli
Inhibition of fibrinolysis

The multifaceted pathology of acute inflammatory lung injury typically occurs over a timescale of minutes to days following an initiating event. Severe acute pulmonary injury is associated with acute respiratory failure and ALI/ARDS as discussed in the text and detailed in subsequent chapters.

Table 2 Selected Mediators, Receptors, and Chemical Factors Important in Acute Inflammatory Lung Injury

Cytokines/growth factors
EGF
G-CSF
GM-CSF
INF-γ
IL-1β, 4, 9 (pro-inflammatory)
IL-6, 10 (anti-inflammatory)
KGF
TGF$_\alpha$
TGF$_\beta$
TNF$_\alpha$
VEGF

Reactive oxygen/nitrogen species
Free radicals — Nonradicals
Hydroxyl ($^\bullet$OH) — Peroxynitrite (ONO$_2{}^-$)
Peroxyl (RO$^\bullet{}_2$) — Alkyl peroxynitrite (ROONO)
Alkoxyl (RO$^\bullet$) — Hydrogen peroxide (H$_2$O$_2$)
Hydroperoxyl (HO$^\bullet{}_2$) — Hydroperoxide (ROOH)
Superoxide (O$^\bullet{}_2{}^-$)
Nitric oxide (NO$^\bullet$)

Antioxidants
Enzymes — Nonenzymes
Catalase — Ascorbate
GSH peroxidases — GSH
SODs — α-Tocopherol
Uric acid

Chemotactic cytokines (chemokines)
ENA-78   MIP-1
GRO   RANTES
IL-8, MIP-2
IP-10
MCP-1

Membrane receptors/ligands/adhesion molecules
CD14 (LPS receptor) — LPS binding protein
CD40/CD40-ligand — L-selectins (eg, CD62-L)
Glucocorticoid receptors — VCAM-1, ICAM-1
β_1-Integrins (e.g., $\alpha_v\beta_1$) — β_2-Integrins (e.g., CD11a,b/CD18)

(Continued)

Table 2 Selected Mediators, Receptors, and Chemical Factors Important in Acute Inflammatory Lung Injury (*Continued*)

Transcription factor families	*Other mediators/compounds*	
AP-1(fos, jun)	CBG	HSPs
C/EBP (e.g., NF-IL-6)	CCSP	Lactate
HSF	Complement (and fragments)	LPS
IκB	Ecosinoids	Neuropeptides
NFκB	Leukotrienes	NOSs
	PGs (E,F,I families)	PAF
	Thromboxanes	PAF-AcH

The tabulated mediators and factors are examples only. Inflammatory mediators important in acute lung injury are detailed further in Chapters 3 and 4. CBG: corticosteroid binding globulin; CCSP: clara cell secretory protein; C/EBP: cyclic AMP/enhancer binding protein; EGF: epidermal growth factor; ENA-78:epithelial cell-derived neutrophil activator 78; G-CSF: granulocyte-colony stimulating factor (CSF); GM-CSF: granulocyte macrophage-CSF; GRO: growth related oncogene; GSH: glutathione; HSF: heat shock transcription factor; HSPs: heat shock proteins; ICAM-1: intercellular adhesion molecule-1; IFN: interferon; IL (interleukin); LPS: lipopolysaccharide; KGF: keratinocyte growth factor; MCP: monocyte chemoattractant protein; MIP: macrophage inflammatory chemokine; NF: nuclear factor; NOSs: nitric oxide synthetases; PAF: platelet activating factor; PAF-AcH: PAF-acetylhydrolase; PGs: prostaglandins; RANTES: regulated on activation normal T expressed and secreted; SODs: superoxide dismutases; TGF: transforming growth factor; TNF: tumor necrosis factor; VCAM-1: vascular cell adhesion molecule-1; VEGF: vascular-endothelial growth factor.

Source: Compiled by Notter (63) from Refs. 3, 5–9, 28, 29, 64–80.

Table 3 Considerations Involved in Assessing the Activities and Interactions of Individual Inflammatory Mediators During Lung Injury

---

Biochemical characteristics
Cytokine family membership (e.g., C, CC, CXC families of chemokines, etc)
Primary cell receptor(s) or receptor family including specific binding behavior
Species specificity (e.g., human vs. mouse differences in cytokine
   nomenclature, structure, etc.)

Cell-specific production
By resident pulmonary epithelial, endothelial, interstitial cells
By resident pulmonary leukocytes vs. recruited leukocytes
By specific subgroups of leukocytes (e.g., T-helper cells producing Th1
   and Th2 cytokines)

Timing and patterns of mediator production and release
Biological distribution (e.g., local vs. systemic concentration; intracellular
   vs. extracellular concentration)
Timing of production/release relative to other mediators (e.g., early vs. late)
Level and timecourse of production/release in relation to other mediators

Activity characteristics
Overall category of activity (e.g., proinflammatory vs. anti-inflammatory
   or down-modulatory)
Direct effects on primary target cells and tissues
Indirect effects in modulating the expression/production/release of other
   mediators with diverse actions
Signal transduction pathways involved in direct/indirect activities

---

Although the subdivisions in the table are arbitrary and selected, they emphasize the multifaceted and interdependent nature of the pulmonary inflammatory response. The production and activities of individual inflammatory mediators not only need to be understood and characterized at the biochemical, cellular, and molecular levels as a function of time, but also must be viewed in terms of interactions with other mediators having additional effects on cells and tissues.

important in assessing the activities and interactions of inflammatory mediators in lung injury are summarized in Table 3.

Acute tissue injury and inflammation contribute to the pathophysiology of a variety of pulmonary diseases. However, the medical consequences of acute pulmonary injury are frequently defined symptomatically as syndromes: clinical acute lung injury (ALI) or the acute respiratory distress syndrome (ARDS) (Chapter 3). The syndromes of ALI/ARDS can occur in patients of all ages, and arise from multiple etiologies that cause direct or indirect lung injury including sepsis, gastric aspiration, pulmonary infection, hypovolemic shock, chest trauma, head injury, long-bone fractures, near-drowning, closed space burn injuries, smoke inhalation, radiation, hyperoxia, and many others (e.g., Refs. 1, 14–20). Although multiorgan pathology is often present in ALI/ARDS, these syndromes are diagnosed by criteria relating to acute respiratory failure (1). By definition, all patients with ARDS also have ALI, which requires a less severe level of impairment of gas exchange (1). The incidence of ALI/ARDS has been variably reported to be 50,000–150,000 cases per year in the United States, with high associated mortality and morbidity (1,14,17,21–26). A recent analysis by Goss et al. (27) has estimated that the actual incidence of clinical ALI in the United States is even higher at 22–64 cases per 100,000 persons per year. In addition to involving severe acute respiratory failure, ALI/ARDS can also progress to a "fibroproliferative" phase of disease that involves chronic lung injury with tissue remodeling and the initiation of fibrosis (15,18–20).

III. Chronic Lung Injury

Chronic injury is closely linked to abnormalities of tissue repair, i.e., the set of responses from cells intended to counteract and recover from trauma or other pathological alteration. Aberrant repair typically occurs in association with persistent inflammation and tissue damage, and is ultimately apparent as scarring or fibrosis. By necessity, chronic injury includes effects from cellular and subcellular processes initiated earlier during acute injury. On average, the more severe the acute injury, the higher the risk for persistent chronic injury. However, this correspondence is not exact. Some patients who develop severe chronic fibrogenic lung injury may have modest or minimal apparent levels of acute injury. Conversely, patients with substantial acute pulmonary injury do not always develop severe chronic injury. Mechanisms of chronic fibrogenic lung injury are detailed in later chapters and reviewed in Refs. 28–39.

Selected features of chronic lung injury are summarized in Table 4. The pulmonary interstitium is generally prominently affected, and becomes thickened with increased numbers of fibroblasts and increased deposition of collagen and other connective tissue components. Chronic lung injury can also involve an early alveolitis, with activated macrophages, lymphocytes, neutrophils, or eosinophils causing inflammation-induced damage to the alveolar epithelium. Intra-alveolar fibrosis and thickening of the alveolar epithelial wall may also occur. A variety of mediators and factors produced by inflammatory leukocytes and pulmonary endothelial, epithelial, and interstitial cells are thought to participate in the development and progression of fibrogenic chronic lung injury (see Table 5 for selected examples). In addition to the mediators and factors in Table 5, many of those given earlier as being involved in acute pulmonary injury in Table 2 are also relevant for tissue remodeling, repair, and chronic injury. As in the case of acute injury, specific signaling pathways and regulatory processes important in chronic lung injury and repair are active current areas of research investigation.

Table 4 Selected Aspects of the Pathology of Fibrogenic Chronic Lung Injury

General connective tissue repair/remodeling
Proliferation and migration of fibroblasts
Microvascular regeneration and repair
Deposition of extracellular matrix
Maturation/organization of fibrous tissue

Fibrosing alveolitis
Persistent alveolar and peri-alveolar inflammation
Alveolar accumulation of inflammation-induced products
Consolidation and fibrosis of intra-alveolar material
Re-epithelialization of intra-alveolar material

Chronic endothelial injury
Endothelial cell injury, alteration, or death
Abnormal mediator production by endothelium
Fenestrated endothelium with increased permeability
Disrupted and thickened endothelial basement membranes

Interstitial injury
Damage to fibroblasts and other interstitial cells
Production of abnormal collagen bundles, types
Abnormal matrix production (e.g., fibronectin, laminin)
Abnormal new vessel formation (abnormal angiogenesis)
Interstitial fibrosis and scarring

Alveolar epithelial injury/alteration
Injury/death of alveolar type I epithelial cells
Proliferation/alteration of alveolar type II cells
Thickening of alveolar epithelial wall
Loss of functional gas exchange units
Abnormal surfactant metabolism, recycling

Fibrogenic airway injury
Injury or altered number of bronchiolar epithelial cells
Proliferation/depletion of other airway lining cells
Abnormal airway wall remodeling and peri-airway fibrosis
Reduced airway function

Chronic injury typically becomes apparent over a prolonged timescale (e.g., weeks to months) after an initiating event. Chronic lung injury often involves prominent elements of abnormal tissue remodeling and repair following a progressive acute inflammatory injury, but chronic fibrogenic pathology can also occur without substantial apparent acute inflammation and injury.

Table 5 Selected Factors and Enzymes Involved in Tissue Repair, Wound Healing, and Chronic Lung Injury

Growth factors
Fibroblast migration (e.g., PDGF, EGF, FGFs, TGFβ, TNFα)
Fibroblast proliferation (e.g., PDGF, EGF, FGFs, TNFα)
Angiogenesis (e.g., VEGFs, angioproteins, FGFs)
Collagen synthesis and/or secretion (e.g., CTGF, PDGF, EGF,FGFs,
   TGFβ, TNFα)

Matrix-modifying enzyme families
Metalloproteinases (e.g., gelatinases A,B)
TIMP's (e.g., TIMP1-4)
Collagenases (e.g., collagenase-1)

Selected additional compounds/factors

Collagens	Fibronectin
Angiotensinogen/angiotensin II	Procoagulant TF
PGs (e.g., PGE_2)	PAI-1, PAI-2
Surfactant proteins (e.g., SP-A/D)	Endothelin-1
Leukotrienes (e.g., B4)	Cell adhesion molecules (e.g., ICAMs, VCAMs)

Many of the mediators, factors, and signaling molecules listed earlier as important in acute lung injury in Table 2 also play roles in chronic injury. Details on the pathophysiology of chronic lung injury and the mediators involved are given in Chapters 5 and 6. CTGF: connective tissue growth factor; EGF: epidermal growth factor; FGF: fibroblast growth factor; ICAMs: intercellular adhesion molecules; PAI: plasminogen activator inhibitor; PDGF: platelet-derived growth factor; PGs: prostaglandins; procoagulant TF: procoagulant tissue factor; TGF: transforming growth factor; TIMPs: tissue inhibitor of metalloproteinases; TNF: tumor necrosis factor; VCAMs: vascular cell adhesion molecules; VEGF: vascular-endothelial growth factor.
Source: Factors compiled from Refs. 28–39.

A number of important clinical respiratory diseases involve chronic injury. One example of this is the fibroproliferative pathology of late phase ALI/ARDS, as noted earlier. The interstitial lung diseases, also called the restrictive lung diseases, are perhaps the most important clinical manifestations of fibrogenic lung injury (15,18–20). These diseases comprise a heterogeneous group including idiopathic pulmonary fibrosis (IPF), pneumoconiosis from environmental or occupational inhalation exposure, sarcoidosis, pulmonary manifestations of collagen vascular diseases (e.g., scleroderma, lupus erythematosus, dermatoid arthritis), fibrosis in association with radiation and hypersensitivity pneumonitis, drug-induced fibrosis, and a number of others. Although classed as interstitial diseases, many of these disorders also incorporate a fibrosing alveolitis or related intra-alveolar component of pathology. Chronic obstructive lung diseases like emphysema, chronic bronchitis and bronchiolitis, and bronchiectasis in association with cystic fibrosis or persistent pulmonary infection also have elements of chronic injury, but fibrosis is generally less prominent than in the interstitial lung diseases.

Interstitial lung diseases vary significantly in the details of their pathology and clinical course, but all share characteristic signs and symptoms. Functionally, the lungs have decreased compliance ($\Delta V/\Delta P$) and require increased expansion pressures. Pulmonary function testing indicates near-proportional reductions in vital capacity (VC) and the fraction of expired volume in one second $(FEV)_1$, leading to little change in the $(FEV)_1/VC$ ratio. Patients typically have dyspnea, which may progress to hypoxemia with a chronic need for supplemental oxygen. Chest radiographs may show a hazy "ground glass" appearance in early alveolitis, but later disease is typified by changes associated with interstitial thickening (15,18–20). IPF is detailed in later chapters as an important example of chronic interstitial lung disease (also see Refs. 29, 31–42, for review). Idiopathic pulmonary fibrosis has an incidence of approximately 7/100,000 in women and 10/100,000 in men, and primarily occurs in individuals over the age of 50 (31,34,40–42), Respiratory deficits are progressive, and the five year survival of patients with a firm diagnosis of IPF is only about 30% (36).

Diseases involving chronic lung injury occur not only in adults, but also in infants and children. One important example of chronic lung disease in premature infants is bronchopulmonary dysplasia (BPD). This condition was first defined in 1967 by Northway et al. (43) as a requirement for supplemental oxygen at 28 days of life in premature infants treated with mechanical ventilation for hyaline membrane disease (the neonatal respiratory distress syndrome, RDS). Alternatives to the original definition have since been proposed as surfactant therapy and other medical advances have improved the survival of premature infants, and new patterns of neonatal chronic lung disease (CLD) have emerged. The majority of very premature infants with birth weights of 500–1000 g now survive, and a substantial percentage require some supplemental oxygen at 28 days of life. In many of these very premature infants, there is no clear connection between their chronic need for oxygen at 28 days and the incidence and severity of earlier acute RDS, indicating that developmental phenomena may be important in the underlying pathophysiology (44,45). A common current definition for BPD or CLD in premature infants is a requirement at 36 weeks corrected gestational age (postmenstrual age) for supplemental oxygen or ventilation either in the hospital or after discharge home (44,46). The incidence of BPD (CLD) in premature infants is inversely proportional to birth weight, but specific incidence numbers can vary significantly depending on patient demographics, diagnostic criteria, ventilation methods, and other variables (e.g., Refs. 44,45,47,48).

IV. Therapeutic Approaches for Diseases Involving Lung Injury

The translation of basic research understanding to improve the clinical treatment of injury-related pulmonary diseases is an important focus of coverage in this book. The multifaceted pathophysiology of lung injury offers many potential therapeutic targets. Patients with injury-associated respiratory failure currently receive sophisticated mechanical respiratory support with a variety of different ventilator modalities (conventional, high-frequency oscillatory, or jet ventilation) and ventilation strategies to minimize ventilator-induced lung injury (Chapter 13). Antibiotics and anti-viral agents are administered if underlying infection is present, and multiorgan failure is also addressed by specific therapies as needed. Additional therapeutic targets in the pathophysiology of clinical lung injury include inflammation, oxidant injury (Chapter 7), vascular dysfunction (Chapter 8), and surfactant dysfunction (Chapter 9). Examples of newer agents for mitigating inflammatory lung injury based on current scientific understanding include anti-inflammatory antibodies, receptors, and receptor antagonists; inhaled nitric oxide and other vasoactive drugs; exogenous surfactants; antioxidant agents; and potentially gene therapy agents (Chapters 14–19). Additional agents and interventions targeting specific aspects of acute and chronic lung injury are continuing to become available at a rapid rate through ongoing basic research on inflammation and lung injury and through new medical technology.*

V. Summary of Coverage and Chapter Organization

Coverage in this book is designed to provide current research perspectives about lung injury and its therapy while also emphasizing basic conceptual principles. Each chapter begins with an *Overview* that outlines the topics and concepts covered, and ends with a *Summary* that recapitulates selected important scientific and conceptual points. Each also contains topical literature citations and review, integrated with material on fundamental concepts, principles, and mechanistic pathways. Discussion is augmented as much as possible with specific examples drawn from the literature. The material presented is by necessity selective, and exhaustive coverage of all biological and medical topics relevant for cell and tissue injury, growth, and development has not been attempted. In this sense, coverage here is

---

* Examples of review articles providing information on therapeutic agents and ventilation strategies for lung injury with or without associated sepsis include Refs. (3,9,10,12,13,17,30–32,39,49–62).

a stepping off point intended to be supplemented elsewhere based on individual priorities and interests.

The initial third of the book focuses on the etiologies, pathophysiology, and mediators involved in acute and chronic lung injury. Chapter 2 covers general concepts of lung development and growth, which occur postnatally as well as prenatally and interact with lung injury and repair. Chapter 3 introduces basic concepts of acute pulmonary inflammation and related cells and mediators, with an emphasis on the mechanistic pathophysiology of clinical ALI and ARDS. Chapter 4 provides further coverage of important mediators involved in the acute innate pulmonary inflammatory response, particularly early response cytokines and families of chemokines that recruit and activate leukocytes. Chapters 5 and 6 provide analogous coverage on chronic lung injury, including its basic pathophysiology and clinical importance, plus selected mediators important in fibroproliferation and fibrosis.

The middle third of the book begins with chapters on three important aspects of lung injury pathophysiology, i.e., reactive oxygen/nitrogen species, vascular dysfunction, and surfactant dysfunction. Chapter 7 discusses reactive oxygen and nitrogen species and their importance in lung injury, along with related pulmonary antioxidant defenses. Chapter 8 covers the pulmonary vasculature and the mechanisms that contribute to vascular dysfunction during lung injury. Chapter 9 covers pulmonary surfactant and its activity in normal and injured lungs, with an emphasis on mechanisms of surfactant dysfunction that contribute to ALI/ARDS and related respiratory failure. The next three chapters detail experimental models used in studying lung injury mechanisms and in developing and testing potential therapeutic agents and interventions. Chapter 10 gives an overview of cell and animal models in lung injury research, while Chapter 11 provides details on the highly important topic of genetically modified mouse models of lung injury and repair. In addition, Chapter 12 examines specific methods and animal models used in the important area of inhalation toxicology.

The final third of the book focuses on current and future therapies for injury-related pulmonary diseases in the context of basic science understanding and perspectives in earlier chapters. Consistent with the multifaceted pathophysiology of acute and chronic lung injury, a spectrum of agents and interventions are relevant for treating these conditions. Chapter 13 covers ventilation therapies and strategies that form an essential component of therapy for all forms of respiratory failure. Chapter 14 examines agents targeting over-exuberant inflammation in the pathology of lung injury. Chapter 15 discusses exogenous surfactants and their potential utility in the therapy of clinical ALI and ARDS in infants, children, and adults. Chapter 16 describes antioxidant therapies that target important oxidant-induced pathology during lung injury. Chapter 17 details vasoactive agents and their use in treating reactive vasoconstriction and other aspects of vascular dysfunction in injury-induced respiratory failure. Chapter 18 examines the topical area of gene-based interventions against lung disease and injury that may lead to important new clinical therapies in the future. Chapter 19 describes the rationale and utility of combination therapies for lung injury, where several agents or interventions are used concurrently to target multiple aspects of pathophysiology. This chapter also details important considerations that impact clinical trial evaluations of combination therapies for lung injury. Finally, Chapter 20 summarizes selected perspectives on on-going lung injury research, including the importance of newer approaches that integrate genomics, proteomics, bioinformatics, and systems biology in defining mechanisms and suggesting new therapeutic strategies. Continuing advances in mechanistic understanding about acute and chronic lung injury through basic research are essential for the future development of more optimal clinical therapies for a broad spectrum of injury-related respiratory diseases.

References

1. Bernard GR, Artigas A, Brigham KL, Carlet J, Falke K, Hudson L, Lamy M, Legall JR, Morris A, Spragg R. The American–European Consensus Conference on ARDS: definitions, mechanisms, relevant outcomes, and clinical trial coordination. Am J Respir Crit Care Med 1994; 149:818–824.
2. Luce JM. Acute lung injury and the acute respiratory distress syndrome. Crit Care Med 1998; 26:369–376.
3. Karima R, Matsumoto S, Higashi H, Matsushima K. The molecular pathogenesis of endotoxin shock and organ failure. Mol Med Today 1999; 5:123–132.
4. Rinaldo JE, Rogers RM. Adult respiratory distress syndrome, changing concepts of lung injury and repair. N Engl J Med 1982; 15:900–909.
5. Meduri GU. The role of host defense response in the progression and outcome of ARDS: pathophysiological correlations and response to glucocorticoid treatment. Eur Respir J 1996; 9:2650–2670.
6. Chabot F, Mitchell JA, Gutteridge JMC, Evans TW. Reactive oxygen species in acute lung injury. Eur Respir J 1998; 11:745–757.
7. Hack CE, Aarden LA, Thijs LG. Role of cytokines in sepsis. Adv Immunol 1997; 66:101–195.
8. Sweet M, Hume D. Endotoxin signal transduction in macrophages. J Leukoc Biol 1996; 60:8–26.
9. Sessler C, Bloomfield G, Fowler A. Current concepts of sepsis and acute lung injury. Clin Chest Med 1996; 17:213–235.
10. Artigas A, Bernard GR, Carlet J, Dreyfuss D, Gattinoni L, Hudson L, Lamy M, Marini JJ, Matthay MA, Pinsky MR, Spragg R, Suter PM, and Consensus Committee. The American-European consensus conference on ARDS, Part 2: ventilatory, pharmacologic, supportive therapy, study design strategies and issues related to recovery and remodeling. Intensive Care Med 1998; 24:378–398.
11. Hinshaw LB. Sepsis/septic shock: participation of the microcirculation: an abbreviated review. Crit Care Med 1996; 24:1072–1078.

12. Temmesfeld-Wollbruck B, Walmrath D, Grimminger F, Seeger W. Prevention and therapy of the adult respiratory distress syndrome. Lung 1995; 173:139–164.

13. Kollef MH, Schuster DP. The acute respiratory distress syndrome. N Engl J Med 1995; 332:27–37.

14. Rubenfeld GD. Epidemiology of acute lung injury. Crit Care Med 2003; 31(suppl):S276–S284.

15. Cotran RS, Kumar V, Collins T. Robbins Pathologic Basis of Disease 6th ed. Philadelphia: W.B. Saunders, 1999.

16. Taussig LM, Landau LI, Le Souef PN, Morgan WJ, Martinez FD, Sly PDE. Pediatric Respiratory Medicine. St. Louis: Mosby, 1999.

17. Ware LB, Matthay MA. The acute respiratory distress syndrome. N Engl J Med 2000; 342:1334–1348.

18. Fishman AP, Elias JA, Fishman JA, Gripp MA, Kaiser LR, Senior RM. Fishman's Pulmonary Diseases and Disorders. 3rd ed. New York: McGraw-Hill, 1998.

19. Braunwald E, Fauci AS, Kasper DL, Hauser SL, Longo DL, Jameson JL, eds. Harrison's Principles of Internal Medicine. 15th ed. New York: McGraw-Hill, 2001.

20. Murray JF, Nadel JA, Mason RJ, Boushey HA. Textbook of Respiratory Medicine 3rd ed. New York: W. B. Saunders, 2000.

21. Villar J, Slutsky AS. The incidence of the adult respiratory distress syndrome. Am Rev Respir Dis 1989; 140:814–816.

22. Hudson LD, Milberg JA, Anardi D, Maunder RJ. Clinical risks for development of the acute respiratory distress syndrome. Am J Respir Crit Care Med 1995; 151:293–301.

23. Milberg JA, Davis DR, Steinberg KP, Hudson LD. Improved survival of patients with acute respiratory distress syndrome. JAMA 1995; 273:306–309.

24. Krafft P, Fridrich P, Pernerstorfer T, Fitzgerald RD, Koc D, Schneider B, Hammerle AF, Steltzer H. The acute respiratory distress syndrome; definitions, severity, and clinical outcome. An analysis of 101 clinical investigations. Intensive Care Med 1996; 22:519–529.

25. Hyers TM. Prediction of survival and mortality in patients with the adult respiratory distress syndrome. New Horizons 1993; 1:466–470.

26. Doyle RL, Szaflarski N, Modin GW, Wiener-Kronish JP, Matthay MA. Identification of patients with acute lung injury: predictors of mortality. Am J Respir Crit Care Med 1995; 152:1818–1824.

27. Goss CH, Brower RG, Hudson LD, Rubenfeld GD. ARDS Network. Incidence of acute lung injury in the United States. Crit Care Med 2003; 31: 1607–1611.

28. Zhang K, Phan SH. Cytokines and pulmonary fibrosis. Biol Signals 1996; 5: 232–239.

29. Ward PA, Hunninghake GW. Lung inflammation and fibrosis. Am J Respir Crit Care Med 1998; 157(suppl):S123–S129.

30. Berthiaume Y, Lesur O, Dagenais A. Treatment of adult respiratory distress syndrome: plea for rescue therapy of the alveolar epithelium. Thorax 1999; 54: 150–160.

31. Selman M, King TEJ, Pardo A. Idiopathic pulmonary fibrosis: prevailing and evolving hypotheses about its pathogenesis and implications for therapy. Ann Intern Med 2001; 134:136–151.

32. American Thoracic Society, European Respiratory Society, and American College of Chest Physicians. Idiopathic pulmonary fibrosis: diagnosis and treatment. International consensus statement. Am J Respir Crit Care Med 2000; 161:646–664.

33. Keogh BA, Crystal RG. Alveolitits: the key to the interstitial lung disorders. Thorax 1982; 37:1–10.

34. Crystal RG, Bitterman PB, Rennard SI, Hance AJ, Keogh BA. Interstitial lung diseases of unknown cause: disorders characterized by chronic inflammation of the lower respiratory tract. N Engl J Med 1984; 310:235–244.

35. Wolff G, Crystal RG. Biology of pulmonary fibrosis. In: Crystal RG, West JB, Weibel ER, Barnes PJ eds. The Lung: Scientific Foundations. 2nd ed. Philadelphia: Lippincott-Raven Publishers, 1997:2509–2524.

36. Strieter RM. Mechanisms of pulmonary fibrosis. Chest 2001; 120(suppl): 77S–85S.

37. Katzenstein AL, Myers JL. Idiopathic pulmonary fibrosis: clinical relevance of pathologic classification. Am J Respir Crit Care Med 1998; 157:1301–1315.

38. Finkelstein JN, Horowitz S, Sinkin RA, Ryan RM. Cellular and molecular responses to lung injury in relation to induction of tissue repair and fibrosis. Clin Perinatol 1992; 19:603–620.

39. Sime PJ, O'Reilly KMA. Fibrosis of the lung and other tissues: new concepts in pathogenesis and treatment. Clin Immunol 2001; 99:308–319.

40. Coultas DB, Zumwalt RE, Black WC, Sobonya RE. The epidemiology of interstitial lung disease. Am J Respir Crit Care Med 1994; 150:967–972.

41. Mannino DM, Etzel RA, Parrish RG. Pulmonary fibrosis deaths in the United States, 1979–1991. An analysis of multiple-cause mortality data. Am J Respir Crit Care Med 1996; 153:1548–1552.

42. Schwartz DA, Helmers RA, Galvin JR, van Fossen DS, Frees KL, Dayton CS, et al. Determinants of survival in idiopathic pulmonary fibrosis. Am J Respir Crit Care Med 1994; 149:450–454.

43. Northway WHJ, Rosan RC, Porter DY. Pulmonary disease following respirator therapy of hyaline membrane disease. N Engl J Med 1967; 276:357–368.

44. Hansen T, Corbet A. Chronic lung disease. In: Taeusch HW, Ballard RA eds. Avery's Diseases of the Newborn. 7th ed. Philadelphia: W.B. Saunders Company, 1998:634–647.

45. Kotecha S, Silverman M. Chronic respiratory complications of prematurity. In: Taussig LM, Landau LI, eds. Pediatric Respiratory Medicine. St. Louis: C. V. Mosby, 1999:488–521.

46. Shennan AT, Dunn MS, Ohlsson A, Lennox K, Hoskins EM. Abnormal pulmonary outcomes in premature infants: prediction from oxygen requirement in the neonatal period. Pediatrics 1988; 82:527–532.

47. Zimmerman JJ, Farrell PM. Advances and issues in bronchopulmonary dysplasia. Curr Prob Pediatr 1994; 24:159–170.

48. Bancalari E. Neonatal chronic lung disease. In:Fanaroff AA, Martin RJ, eds. Neonatal Perinatal Medicine. St. Louis: Mosby, 1997:1074–1089.

49. Hudson LD. New therapies for ARDS. Chest 1995; 108(suppl):79S–91S.
50. Fulkerson WJ, Macintyre N, Stamler J, Crapo JD. Pathogenesis and treatment of the adult respiratory distress syndrome. Arch Intern Med 1996; 156:29–38.
51. Paulson T, Spear R, Peterson B. New concepts in the treatment of children with acute respiratory failure. J Pediatr 1995; 127:163–175.
52. Ring J, Stidham G. Novel therapies for acute respiratory failure. Pediatr Clin North Am 1994; 41:1325–1363.
53. Weikert LF, Bernard GR. Pharmacology of sepsis. Clin Chest Med 1996; 17: 289–305.
54. Thompson BT. Glucocorticoids and acute lung injury. Crit Care Med 2003; 31(suppl):S253–S257.
55. Steinbrook R. How best to ventilate? Trial design and patient safety in studies of the acute respiratory distress syndrome. N Engl J Med 2003; 348: 1393–1401.
56. Sokol J, Jacobs SE, Bohn D. Inhaled nitric oxide for acute hypoxemic respiratory failure in children and adults (update of Cochrane Database Syst Rev 2000; (4):CD002787; PMID: 11034763). Cochrane Database Syst Rev 2003; (1):CD002787.
57. Laterre PF, Wittebole X, Dhainaut JF. Anticoagulant therapy in acute lung injury. Crit Care Med 2003; 31(suppl):S329–S336.
58. Lewis JF, Brackenbury A. Role of exogenous surfactant in acute lung injury. Crit Care Med 2003; 31(suppl):S324–S328.
59. Kaisers U, Busch T, Deja M, Donaubauer B, Falke KJ. Selective pulmonary vasodilation in acute respiratory distress syndrome. Crit Care Med 2003; 31(suppl):S337–S342.
60. Derdak S. High-frequency oscillatory ventilation for acute respiratory distress syndrome in adult patients. Crit Care Med 2003; 31(suppl):S317–S323.
61. Marraro G. Innovative practices of ventilatory support with pediatric patients. Pediatr Crit Care Med 2003; 4:8–20.
62. Notter RH, Apostolakos M, Holm BA, Willson D, Wang Z, Finkelstein JN, Hyde RW. Surfactant therapy and its potential use with other agents in term infants, children and adults with acute lung injury. Perspectives Neonatol 2000; 1(4):4–20.
63. Notter RH. Lung surfactants: Basic Science and Clinical Applications. New York: Marcel Dekker, 2000.
64. Nakos G, Kitsiouli EI, Tsangaris I, Lekka ME. Bronchoalveolar lavage fluid characteristics of early intermediate and late phases of ARDS. Intensive Care Med 1998; 24:296–303.
65. Meduri GU, Headley S, Tolley E, Shelby M, Stentz F, Postlewaite A. Plasma and BAL cytokine response to corticosteroid rescue treatment in late ARDS. Chest 1995; 108:1315–1325.
66. Headley AS, Tolley E, Meduri GU. Infections and the inflammatory response in acute respiratory distress syndrome. Chest 1997; 111:1306–1321.
67. Goodman, RB, Strieter RM, Martin DP, Steinberg KP, Milberg JA, Maunder RJ, Kunkel SL, Walz A, Hudson LD, Martin TR. Inflammatory cytokines in patients with persistence of the acute respiratory distress syndrome. Am J Respir Crit Care Med 1996; 154:602–611.

68. Baughman RP, Gunther KL, Rashkin MC, Keeton DA, Pattishall EN. Changes in the inflammatory response of the lung during acute respiratory distress syndrome: prognostic indicators. Am J Respir Crit Care Med 1996; 154:76–81.

69. Lucas R, Lou J, Morel DR, Ricou B, Suter PM, Grau GE. TNF receptors in the microvascular pathology of acute respiratory distress syndrome and cerebral malaria. J Leukoc Biol 1997; 61:551–558.

70. Chollet-Martin S, Jourdain B, Gibert C, Elbim C, Chastre J, Gougerot-Pocidalo MA. Interactions between neutrophils and cytokines in blood and alveolar spaces during ARDS. Am J Respir Crit Care Med 1996; 153:594–601.

71. Armstrong L, Millar AB. Relative production of tumour necrosis factor α and interleukin 10 in adult respiratory distress syndrome. Thorax 1997; 52: 442–446.

72. Parsons P, Gillesis M, Moore E, Moore F, Worthen G. Neutrophil response to endotoxin in the adult respiratory distress syndrome: role of CD14. Am J Respir Cell Mol Biol 1995; 13:152–160.

73. Douzinas EE, Tsidemiadou PD, Pitaridis MT, Andrianakis I, Bobota-Chloraki A, Katsouyanni K, Sfyras D, Malagari K, Roussos C. The regional production of cytokines and lactate in sepsis-related multiple organ failure. Am J Respir Crit Care Med 1997; 155:53–59.

74. Matute-Bello G, Liles WC, Radella F. Neutrophil apoptosis in the acute respiratory distress syndrome. Am J Respir Crit Care Med 1997; 156: 1969–1977.

75. Goodman ER, Kleinstein E, Fusco AM, Quinlan DP, Lavery R, Livingstone DH, Deitch EA, Hauser CJ. Role of interleukin 8 in the genesis of acute respiratory distress syndrome through an effect on neutrophil apoptosis. Arch Surg 1998; 13:1234–1239.

76. Pugin J, Ricou B, Steinberg KP, Suter PM, Martin TR. Proinflammatory activity in bronchoalveolar lavage fluids from patients with ARDS, a prominent role for interleukin-1. Am J Respir Crit Care Med 1996; 153:1850–1856.

77. Sempowski G, Chess P, Phipps R. CD40 is a functional activation antigen and B7-independent T cell costimulatory molecule in normal human lung fibroblasts. J Immunol 1997; 158:4670–4677.

78. Adawi A, Zhang Y, Baggs R, Finkelstein J, Phipps R. Disruption of the CD40–CD40 ligand system prevents an oxygen-induced respiratory distress syndrome. Am J Pathol 1998; 152:651–657.

79. Jorens PG, Sibille Y, Goulding NJ, van Overveld FJ, Herman AG, Bossaert L, DeBacker WA, Lauwerys R, Flower RJ, Bernard A. Potential role of Clara cell protein, and endogenous phospholipase A_2 inhibitor, in acute lung injury. Eur Respir J 1995; 8:1643–1653.

80. Charafeddine L, D'Angio CT, Richards JL, Stripp BR, Finkelstein JN, Orlowski CC, LoMonaco MB, Paxhia A, Ryan RM. Hyperoxia increases keratinocyte growth factor mRNA expression in neonatal rabbit lung. Am J Physiol 1999; 20:L105–L113.

2

Principles of Lung Development, Growth, and Repair

IAN COPLAND, KEITH TANSWELL, and MARTIN POST

Departments of Pediatrics, Physiology, and Laboratory Medicine and Pathology, Lung Biology Research Programme, Hospital for Sick Children Research Institute, University of Toronto, Toronto, Ontario, Canada

I. Overview

This chapter presents basic principles and current perspectives on lung development, growth, and repair. Processes of injury described in subsequent chapters must be viewed in the context of these factors. Throughout life, the lungs are a dynamic organ system that attempts to adapt to stress and to repair injury to cells and tissue. Depending on the circumstances, these processes of adaptation and repair can mitigate pulmonary damage or exacerbate the progression of injury. Many of the phenomena occurring during pulmonary adaptation and repair recapitulate those involved in growth and development. This chapter introduces basic elements of lung structure, embryology, and cellular specification, including the effects of key transcription factors, growth factors, and physical forces. Coverage includes fundamental information on alveolarization, the growth of gas exchange tissue, and the pulmonary capillary bed. A description of relevant congenital abnormalities that lead to pulmonary hypoplasia is also provided. Concepts of pulmonary remodeling and repair pertinent to both prenatal and postnatal events are introduced, and their relevance and importance for specific aspects of acute and chronic lung injury are then detailed further in following chapters.

II. Introduction

Lung development can be subdivided into five stages:

1. Embryonic* period—development of major airways
2. Pseudoglandular period—development of airways to terminal bronchioles
3. Canalicular period—development of the acinus and vascularization
4. Terminal sac (saccular) period—subdivision of saccules by secondary crests
5. Alveolar period—the appearance of alveoli

Although the morphological changes associated with lung evelopment are well characterized, the body of information regarding the molecular mechanisms that determine cellular fate, pattern formation, and growth during lung development are less clear. A better understanding of the molecular basis of pulmonary development will aid in understanding the etiology of relatively common foregut malformations (such as tracheoesophageal fistula and esophageal atresia) and less common congenital anomalies (such as tracheal stenosis, unilateral and bilateral lung agenesis, and alveolar–capillary dysplasia). Lung hypoplasia represents another common pulmonary malformation. Conditions that lead to pulmonary hypoplasia include premature rupture of the membranes (<20 weeks' gestation), severe oligohydramnios, and congenital diaphragmatic hernia. It is well known that premature infants are more susceptible to the development of chronic lung disease than their full-term counterparts and this may reflect a fundamental difference in the ability of the developing lung to undergo an efficient and controlled repair process. Ideally, the repair processes should mimic ontogeny since the use of different processes for repair than those used in normal morphogenesis would require a greater repertoire of genetic regulatory programs. In order to understand repair processes within the lungs, it is essential first to understand the physiology of normal lung development, including that of the early lung. This chapter summarizes current thoughts about lung development, growth, and repair.

---

* The early stage of development of a complex organism is called the embryo; the following stage persisting through birth is called the fetus. More quantitative definitions of these terms are obviously species specific. In humans, the developing organism is generally designated the embryo for the first 8 weeks of gestation (20% of term = 40 weeks).

III. Lung Organogenesis

The endodermal germ layer gives rise to several organs, including the thyroid, trachea, lungs, esophagus, stomach, liver, pancreas, and intestines. Initially, all cells within the epithelial compartment of the lung anlage are equipotential, but they become diversified as they proliferate and differentiate to develop different airway structures. Thus, epithelial cells in the early lung bud receive information on their position relative to other cells to ensure a proper distribution and pattern of differentiation along the proximo-distal axis of the airways. In humans at 4–5 weeks' gestation, the first indication of lung formation is the appearance of a midventral groove in the single foregut tube just posterior of the pharynx. In the next two weeks, the groove, known as the lanryngotracheal groove, deepens and finally constricts, thereby dividing the foregut tube into a ventral trachea and dorsal esophagus (1). This process is modified in the mouse and rat as their respiratory systems develop from paired endodermal buds in the ventral half of the primitive foregut, just anterior to the developing stomach at 9.5 and 10 days of gestation, respectively. At the end of the embryonic stage, the tracheal outgrowth elongates caudally and bifurcates to form two bronchial lung buds. In both rodents and human, the primary bronchi continue to grow into the splanchnic mesenchyme. During the pseudoglandular stage (day 52 to the end of 16 weeks of human gestation), a hierarchical pattern is apparent in the developing lung, the prospective conductive airways have been formed, and the acinar limits can be recognized. In the pseudoglandular phase the primitive airway epithelium starts to differentiate and neuroendocrine, ciliated and goblet cells appear while mesenchymal cells have begun to form cartilage and smooth muscle cells (2). At 8 weeks, fetal breathing movements (FBMs) can be identified (3). In the subsequent canalicular stage (17–26 weeks of gestation) there is vascularization of the lung, the airway branching pattern is completed and the prospective gas-exchange region starts to develop. During this period of development, respiratory bronchioli appear, interstitial tissue decreases, and the differentiation of the cuboidal epithelium into type I and type II cells signals the start of surfactant production (4). In the saccular (terminal sac) phase (24–36 weeks to term), the growth of the pulmonary parenchyma, the thinning of the connective tissue between the airspaces, and the further maturation of the surfactant system are the most important steps towards ex utero life. At birth, although functional, the lung is structurally still in an immature condition. Alveoli, the gas-exchange units of the adult lung, are practically missing. The airspaces present are smooth-walled transitory ducts and saccules with primitive septa that are thick and contain a double capillary network. During the alveolar stage (36 weeks to term and at least 36 months postnatal), alveoli are formed through a septation process that greatly increases the gas exchange surface area (3).

A. Mesenchymal–Epithelial Interactions

Branching of the lung buds is controlled by epithelial–mesenchymal tissue interactions. The mesenchymal component dictates the branching pattern of the epithelium and the inductive capacity of the mesenchyme is organ and species specific (5–8). Branching appears also to be regulated by positional information along the anteroposterior axis of the lung as proximal (trachea and main bronchi) and distal (lung bud) mesenchyme differ in their ability to support epithelial branching morphogenesis (7). Forces within the epithelial cells themselves alter cell and tissue shape to produce branch points. While much has been learned about developmental interactions between mesenchyme and committed lung endoderm, little is known about the molecular mechanisms that initially pattern endoderm to respiratory fate. It is likely that positional cues comprising transcription factors and morphogens play a role in specifying the morphogenetic progenitor field of the lung along the gut axis. Lung branching is likely determined by similar molecular cues regulating the precise regional-restricted pattern of expression of a gene during development (Fig. 1). Positional cues can also arise from cell–cell and cell–matrix interactions (9).

B. Proliferation During Lung Development

Fetal lung morphogenesis involves major structural changes, which are associated with cell proliferation (reviewed in Ref. 10). Lung cell proliferation is mainly confined to morphogenetically active regions that shift from central to peripheral tubules during development. The rate of proliferation of both epithelial and mesenchymal cells decreases during development, but the decline is unequal. The proportion of dividing cells which are epithelial increases initially during fetal development, but declines dramatically near term (11–13). Studies with isolated fetal lung epithelial cells have confirmed this growth pattern (14). The decline in epithelial mitotic activity is associated with an increase in cellular differentiation (15). The proportion of dividing cells, which are of mesenchymal origin (endothelial cells and fibroblasts) decreases in the initial stages of lung development, but increases sharply at the canalicular phase of development due to capillary growth. Growth of fibroblasts progressively declines during late fetal life (16). Capillary formation continues at a rapid rate during late fetal life and, consequently, mesenchymal cells are the major dividing cell type near term (11–13). These developmental differences in proliferation rates between epithelial and mesenchymal cells are also reflected in the ratio of the total numbers of epithelial cells to mesenchymal cells. The ratio increases from 1:4 at the pseudoglandular stage of development to 1:1 at the late canalicular stage before decreasing again at term (11).

Phase	Morphology	Events	Factors	
Embryonic		- Respiratory foregut specification - Separation trachea and esophagus - Formation left and right main airways	Gli2/Gli3 Foxa2 Foxf1 Foxj1 Pitx2	Shh Ttf1 Fgf10 FgfR-IIIb RAR
Pseudoglandular		-Development of tracheabronchial tree - Neuroendocrine, ciliated and globet cells appear - Cartilage and smooth muscle cells begin to form	Shh Gli2 Ttf1 Hoxb Gata-6	FGF1,7,10 Tgfβ2,3 Mash1 Hes1
Cannulicular		- Formation of prospective acinus - Vascularization - Type I and type II cells appear	Ttf1 Gata-6 Foxa1,2 Pod-1	BMP4 Vegf Foxj1a Foxf1
Saccular		- Subdivision of terminal bronchioles into saccules by primary septa - Thinning of interstitium - Maturation of surfactant system	Hif2α Fgf7 Fgf9 Fgf18 Vegf	
Alveolar		- Formation of alveoli by septation of alveolar airsacs - Thinning intraalveolar septa - Microvascular matuaration	PdgfA/PdgfRα Ttf1 Foxf1 VitA RAR/RXR FgfR3/FgfR4	

Figure 1   Transcription, growth, and other factors influencing lung development.

C. Transcription Factors and Lung Development

It is evident that foregut endoderm differentiation must be associated with the temporally and spatially restricted expression of distinct organ- and cell-selective genes along the foregut axis. This selective gene expression is determined by interactions between multiple regulatory proteins including transcription factors. Some transcription factors are ubiquitous and needed for transcription of a number of genes while others are required for tissue and cell-specific gene expression. Important transcription factors implicated in specifying the morphogenetic progenitor field of the lung along the foregut axis are hepatocyte nuclear factor-3β (Hnf3β/Foxfa2) (17–21), *Hox* genes (22,23), Gli genes (24), and the thyroid transcription factor-1 [Ttf1] or Nkx2.1(25–27). Several of the transcription factors regulating early lung bud formation are also involved in esophageal–tracheal separation as well as left–right asymmetry development, including Ttf1, Gli, Foxj1a (Hhf4) (28), and Pitx2 (29–31). A complex mixture of transcription factors that include the Hox, Fox, and Nkx families guides subsequent lung bud branching. Other transcription factors implicated in lung branching are Gata-6 (32–35) and N-myc (36–39).

As branching proceeds, numerous different cell phenotypes are formed along the anterior–posterior axis of the developing epithelial tubules and associated mesenchymal components, each with different morphologies and patterns of gene expression. Over the last decade several transcription factors involved in epithelial morphogenic patterning in the lung have been identified, including basic helix–loop–helix transcription factors such as Mash-1 (40), Hes-1 (41), and pod-1 (42). Transcription factors such as Gata-6 (32,34,35), Foxa2 (43–46), Nkx2.1 (25,26,46), and Foxfj1 (28,47,48) also influence lung epithelial specification. Recently, loss of Hif-2α has been shown to cause fatal respiratory distress in neonatal mice due to insufficient surfactant production. This is clinically relevant, since insufficient surfactant production is a common complication of preterm delivery (49).

D. Morphogens and Lung Development

In several developing systems, including invertebrates such as *Drosophila* and the nematode *Caenorhabditis elegans* as well as nonmammalian and mammalian vertebrates, positional information can be patterned along morphogen gradients (50). Morphogens are defined as molecules that diffuse away from their source and give positional information to surrounding cells based on their local concentration. Small differences in morphogen concentration may lead to dramatic alterations in gene expression resulting in cells closer to the source of the morphogen having a different phenotype than that of cells more distant from the source of the morphogen. The establishment of gradients likely involves a local source of the morphogen stimulating adjacent cells, which then become sources of new inducing signals that carry positional information to more distant cells (50–52). Members of the hedgehog (Hh) and fibroblast growth factor (Fgf) families have been identified as putative morphogens involved in embryonic lung development.

The secreted signaling molecule sonic hedgehog (shh), a vertebrate homolog of Drosophila hedgehog (hh), is highly expressed in epithelia at numerous sites of epithelial–mesenchymal interactions, including lung (53,54). Mice lacking Shh die before birth and display multiple developmental defects including a very severe pulmonary branching defect (55).

Mice overexpressing Shh in the respiratory epithelium using the SP-C promoter die shortly after birth and have abundance of mesenchyme and no functional alveoli (56). Mammalian *Gli* genes have been implicated in mammalian Shh signaling (57). Three Gli genes have been described in mice: Gli1, Gli2, and Gli3, all of which are expressed in early pulmonary mesenchyme (58). Genetic analyses have shown the importance of Gli genes for lung development (24,59). For example, mice lacking both Gli2 and Gli3 have no lung, trachea, or esophagus and die early in gestation (24). The downstream target genes for Gli in vertebrates are unknown. In *Drosophila*, there is substantial evidence to suggest that *hedgehog* regulates the expression of *Wingless* (Wg) (60). The *Wg*-type (wnt) gene family encodes a group of proteins, now numbering over 19, which are implicated in intercellular signalling in several organs. Many wnt genes are expressed in the lung (61). In vertebrates, Wnt7b has been found to regulate Shh in presumptive dental ectoderm (62), and when disrupted Wnt7b null mice exhibit perinatal death due to lung hypoplasia (63), which is similar to that seen in the shh deficient mouse (55). Overexpression of Shh in fetal lung epithelium, which resulted in abnormal lung development, did not affect the level and distribution of Wnt2 mRNA expression (56). In contrast, targeted disruption of Wnt5a gene in the mouse produces a similar lung phenotype as that of the SPC-Shh overexpressing mouse (56), and is accompanied by a 36% and 94% increase in Shh and ptc expression, respectively (64). This suggests that Wnt7b, Wnt5a may actually function upstream of Shh, but the precise functional relationship between Wnt and Shh signalling in the lung remains to be established.

The importance of Fgf signaling in lung development has been demonstrated by blocking FgfR signaling. Although all four FgfRs are expressed in the lung (65), a splice variant of the FgfR2-FgfR2-IIIb appears to be important for early lung development. The FgfR2-IIIb splice variant is expressed in lung bud epithelium (66,67). Mice that overexpress a dominant-negative FgfR2-IIIb splice variant in distal lung epithelium show a severe pulmonary defect with only the formation of the trachea and two main bronchi, but without any lateral branches (68). A targeted mutation of FgfR2 resulted in an early lethal phenotype due to placental insufficiency (69,70). To overcome this early lethality and allow lung development to be analyzed, FgfR2$^{-/-}$ chimeras were created (67). In these mice, only a trachea was formed without any further pulmonary branching (67). In contrast, a null mutation of either FgfR3 or FgfR4 caused no obvious embryonic lung defects (71). The precise ligands mediating the Fgf signalling by these receptors are not completely known. Transcripts for Fgf1, Fgf2, Fgf7, Fgf9, Fgf10, and Fgf18 have been found in the developing lung (65,72,73). Studies using animal models have shown a crucial role for Fgf10 in early lung bud outgrowth. Fgf10 is dynamically expressed in the distal mesenchyme adjacent to the primitive lung buds (74). Similar to its receptor, FgfR2-IIIB, Fgf10 deficient mice die at birth due to a severe pulmonary defect. They display complete lung agenesis, i.e., lung development has stopped after the formation of the trachea (75,76). In part, Fgf10 expression in the lung is regulated by T-box genes (77), specifically Tbx4 (78). Fgf7 is expressed in the mesenchyme and ectopic expression of Fgf7 in vivo (79,80) or its addition to lung explants in vitro (81–84) influences lung branching morphogenesis and pulmonary cell differentiation. Fgf9 is expressed in the pulmonary mesothelium and epithelium at early development and later only in the mesothelium (72). Ablation of Fgf9 signalling resulted in severe lung hypoplasia and immediate postnatal death (72). Fgf18 is expressed in the mesenchyme but its expression pattern is different from Fgf9 and Fgf10 (85). Conditional ectopic expression of Fgf18 in epithelial cells led to proximalization of the developing lung (73).

E. Growth Factors and Lung Development

There are several ways in which growth factors may reach a responsive cell. They may be synthesized elsewhere and be blood borne in an endocrine fashion. Alternatively, they may be synthesized locally by one cell type and passively diffuse to act on a different cell type in a paracrine fashion, or target the originating cell in an autocrine loop. More recently recognized modes of growth factor transfer are two juxtacrine mechanisms. Direct transfer can occur through gap junctions at cell-to-cell contacts, which are under oncogene control (86) and may be hormonally activated (87). The second juxtacrine mechanism involves the presentation of a membrane-bound proform of a growth factor on one cell to an appropriate receptor on an adjacent cell (88). Candidate inductive peptide growth factors involved in lung development include epidermal (Egf), insulin-like (Igf), fibroblast (Fgfs), platelet-derived (Pdgf), hepatocyte (Hgf), transforming (Tgf)-Betas, vascular endothelial (Vegf), and bone morphogenic proteins (Bmps), all of which exert inductive or permissive influences on lung development based on gain and loss of function experiments using embryonic lung organ culture, transgenic mice, and null mutant mice (68,84,89–99). Mechanistically, there are three major signal transduction pathways by which growth factor binding to cells influences cellular function. In the first pathway growth factors binding to plasma membrane receptors act through G-proteins to cause a phospholipase C-mediated generation of diacylglycerol (DAG) and inositol triphosphate (IP$_3$). Together, DAG and IP$_3$ activate protein kinase C (PKC), which can then phosphorylate various cellular proteins responsible for cell cycle control (100). Secondly, growth factors like fibroblast growth factors (Fgfs) may bind to their membrane protein tyrosine kinase receptor to activate a PKC, which is an integral part of the receptor complex (101). The third pathway involves a growth factor-mediated increase in intracellular cyclic AMP (cAMP), which may be either stimulatory or inhibitory through effects on protein kinases or via cAMP-responsive elements in the promoters of various genes (102).

F. Vitamins and Lung Development

Retinoic acid (RA) plays a crucial role during development and is involved in the developmental process of almost every organ (103). Both a deficiency and an excess of RA cause congenital defects during human development in a variety of organs (104). Mechanistically, RA exerts its effects via the RAR and RXR receptors (105), which act as transcriptional regulators. The RAR family has three isoforms: RARα, β, and γ. All three RARα isoforms are activated by both all-trans RA and 9-cis RA, whereas the three isoforms from the RXR family: RXRα, β, γ are only activated by 9-cis RA (105). Because of redundancy, mice deficient in only one receptor isoform develop normally (106–108). Compound mutants, on the other hand, do show defects similar to the congenital malformations observed in fetal vitamin A deficiency (VAD) (109). Specifically, $RAR\alpha^{-/-}\beta2^{-/-}$ double mutant mice die soon after birth with agenesis of the left lung and hypoplasia of the right lung (110). Lung hypoplasia was also reported in $RAR\alpha1^{-/-}\beta^{-/-}$ and $RXR\alpha^{-/-}RAR\alpha^{-/-}$ double mutants (111). Thus, RA can be seen as a critical mediator of lung development.

Besides vitamin A's effects, several other vitamins have the potential to influence lung development. In the rat, at the end of pregnancy (days 20–21), alveolar type II cells (ATII) bear vitamin D receptors and responded to the hormone by synthesizing and releasing disaturated phosphatidylcholine, a necessary component for surfactant production. Fetal lung fibroblasts do not express the vitamin D receptor; however, they can convert vitamin D into its active form, indicating that vitamin D is another local mediator of epithelial–mesenchymal cell interactions in the developing rat lung (112). By day 2 postpartum, ATII cells no longer express the vitamin D receptor suggesting that vitamin D may be a very important mediator in preparing the lung for the transition from in utero to ex utero existence (112). By adult life, ATII cells respond to the active form of vitamin D by an increase in DNA synthesis, which is not seen in fetal or early postnatal cells (113).

G. Physical Factors and Lung Growth

A variety of physical factors influence normal fetal lung growth. These include the volumes of lung and amniotic fluid (114–118), available space for the lung in the thorax (119–122), and fetal respiration (123,124). The importance of lung fluid volume in fetal lung growth has been clearly demonstrated. Distension of the lung by tracheal ligation to prevent lung fluid efflux, stimulates lung growth (115), potentially mediated by mitogen activated protein kinases (125). Conversely, tracheal drainage inhibits lung growth (115), probably by diminishing the distending fluid pressure. In the human fetus, obstruction of the trachea and bronchus has been associated with lung hyperplasia (116). Although in vivo experiments demonstrate a relationship between lung fluid and normal fetal lung growth, its direct influence on embryonic lung growth was demonstrated in vitro by restricting lung liquid secretion by blockage of transepithelial (Cl^-) transport in cultured lung explants (126). This resulted in smaller lungs, but did not affect branching.

Experimental introduction of oligohydramnios by amniotic drainage (127–129), nephrectomy (130), or obstructive uropathy (131) reduces lung growth of fetal animals, while restoring normal amniotic fluid volume, after drainage, reverses changes in lung weight (128). Tracheal ligation reverses the pulmonary hypoplasias associated with fetal nephrectomy (130). Clinically, lack of amniotic fluid (oligohydramnios) has been associated with lung hypoplasia (118,131).

Decreased thoracic space available for lung growth, as a result of diaphragmatic hernia (120,122), congenital cystic adenomatoid malformation (132), and thoracic abnormalities (133), are all associated with lung hypoplasia. Interestingly, prenatal tracheal ligation accelerates lung growth and reverses the effect of pulmonary hypoplasia in experimental models of congenital diaphragmatic hernias (134–137). Uterine and thoracic constraints may also restrict fetal respiration. The reduced distension of the lung caused by diminished fetal respiration may then lead to hypoplasia. Several lines of evidence suggest that normal lung growth is affected by intermittent stretch caused by FBM. The FBMs do not appear to stimulate fetal lung growth through changes in pulmonary blood flow (138), but rather affect lung growth by causing regional changes in lung fluid volume, which transiently increase or decrease distending pressures during fetal respiration (114). Disruption of the intermittent distension of the lung by spinal cord section (123), or phrenectomy (139), results in diminished lung growth. A complementary finding is that when lungs of myogenin null mice, which cannot produce FBMs in utero, are compared to the lungs of normal mice there is a significant decrease in lung:-body weight ratio and lung total DNA of these animals at various gestational ages (140). These decreases were not only associated with a decrease in lung cell proliferation, but also with an increase in apoptosis (140). Therefore, it appears that proper FBM are not only necessary for proper lung growth through proliferation, but also necessary for lung growth through cell survival.

The mechanisms through which lung cells convert a physical response into biochemical signals for intracellular signal transduction are not yet delineated. Within the lung, there are a variety of mechanisms by which physical forces are perceived and these mechanisms dictate whether the response is transcriptional, post-translational, or a combination of both. Among the mechanisms, stress-activated ion channels and extracellular matrix–integrin–cytoskeletal pathways have received the most attention (141,142). Numerous in vitro systems have been developed to investigate mechanotransduction and some have been adapted to simulate FBMs. It has been reported that fetal lung cells increase their proliferation when exposed to an intermittent stretch, which mimic FBMs (143). In addition, intermittently stretched fetal lung cells increase their elastin, fibronectin, and surfactant protein C production but decrease their collagen production (144). In premature lung cells, both intra- and extracellular calcium modulate strain-induced proliferative activity. The rapid entry of calcium (<1 min) through a gadolinium-sensitive pathway, presumably an activated ion channel, contributed to strain-induced PKC activation and proliferative activity (145). Intracellular concentrations of both IP_3 and DAG were dramatically increased after a short period of strain associated with the activation of phospholipase C (145). The specific activity of PKC increased 5–7 fold shortly after strain and remained elevated throughout a 48-hr period of intermittent strain. PKC inhibitors blocked strain-induced DNA synthesis (146). Activation of protein tyrosine kinases seems to be an upstream event of the PKC–phospholipase C pathway (147). Stretch-induced prostacyclin (148) and cAMP (148,149) synthesis increased in cells from premature rat lung exposed to a relatively high amplitude strain. In contrast, when fetal lung epithelial cells were subjected to a continuous stretch, proliferation decreased while programmed cell death (apoptosis) increased (150). These differences in response to different types of stretch at a specific gestational age may be particularly relevant for the prematurely born infant, whose lung is still immature, and are at greater risk of developing chronic lung disease (CLD).

H. Vascularization During Lung Growth

The lungs are composed of a complex network of airways and vessels. Although much has been learned regarding the mechanisms controlling lung bud formation and airway branching, the mechanisms involved in vascular formation during lung development remain obscure. Even in the early stages of lung development vascular connections are well established, with the development of the central bronchial arteries during the embryonic period. During the pseudoglandular phase, the disappearance of the central bronchial arteries occurs with the development of new bronchial arteries. In the canalicular phase the distal circulation develops, which connects with proximal pulmonary resistance arteries and veins. In the saccular phase capillaries are evident around the saccules and in the alveolar phase the development of the vasculature is completed with the formation of single capillary networks (151). In mice, vascular development in the lung can be identified by three features: (1) central sprouting or angiogenesis for up to approximately seven generations (counting the artery to each lung as first generation); (2) the formation of peripheral lakes by vasculogenesis; and (3) the development of communications between the central and peripheral systems (152). Alveolar capillary dysplasia is a rare cause of neonatal pulmonary hypertension characterized by developmental abnormalities in the pulmonary vasculature (153–155). In humans, lung hypoplasia has been found to be associated with decreased pulmonary arterial flow (156), and experimental evidence suggests that pulmonary arterial ligation decreases lung growth by reducing lung fluid production (156–158).

Genetic analyses have demonstrated that cell–extracellular matrix interactions, cell–cell interactions, and growth/transcription factors can influence pulmonary vascular development. Specifically, members of the Vegf family (159–161), the angiopoietin family (162–164), and members of the ephrin family (165) have all been implicated in controlling vascularization of the pulmonary system. Endothelial monocyte-activating polypeptide (EMAP) II, an antiangiogenic factor identified in tumor vascular development, shows a dynamic expression pattern during lung development. Its expression is low during embryonic mouse lung development and localizes to the submyoepithelial area, but in late gestation EMAPII expression becomes prominent around the large vessels (166).

IV. Postnatal Development and Growth of the Lung

A sequence of events is well established for the fifth and final stage of lung development, the alveolar period, which in human is initiated in utero, but continues up to approximately 8 years. At birth, immature airspaces appear as smooth-walled transitory ducts and saccules with primitive type septa that are thick and contain a double capillary network. During alveolarization (see Fig. 2), alveoli develop in a centripetal manner initially from saccules, then on respiratory bronchioles and, from 4 years onwards on terminal bronchioles (167). Most knowledge about postnatal lung development has been obtained from animal studies, in particular the rat (3,168). Postnatal lung growth in rats can be divided into four stages. Initially a phase of expansion (birth–4 days) occurs, during which lung growth lags behind the increase in body weight and lungs enlarge primarily by expansion. This is succeeded by a phase of tissue proliferation (day 4–12) where the saccule is subdivided by numerous secondary crests that develop in the saccular wall and result in the formation of alveoli. In this phase, proliferation occurs in both epithelial and mesenchymal cell populations. Interstitial fibroblasts actively proliferate early in this phase, but then slow down. Epithelial cell division in this period occurs on septal buds and walls. Both

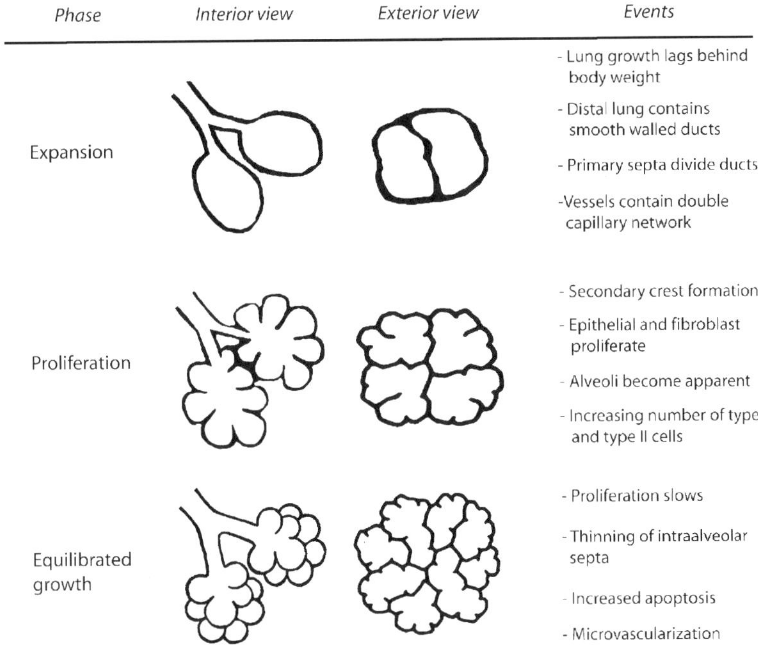

Figure 2   Schematic representation of alveologenesis.

alveolar epithelial cell populations, type I and type II cells, increase during this growth period, however, only alveolar epithelial type II cells proliferate (10,12), indicating that the alveolar type I cell population arises from type II cells. During this stage, the rate of lung growth exceeds the rate of body growth and there is a rapid increase in alveolar surface area.

Following this proliferative expansion, the rate of cellular multiplication and formation of alveoli is markedly diminished and the lung grows mainly by cellular enlargement, dilatation, and modification of pre-existing structures (167) (equilibrated growth phase). One of the characteristic features of this phase is the maturation of the interstitium, in which primary interstitial cells begin to disappear, due to apoptosis. In the newborn rat, apoptosis causes a 20% reduction in the number of lung fibroblasts as the interstitial volume of the alveolar walls decreases (169). Overlapping this phase is the final stage of lung development, microvascular maturation. During alveolarization, the inter-air-space walls of the lung are thick and contain a capillary bilayer, but during the equilibrated growth phase, the maturation of the interstitium brings capillary bilayers closer together, so that they touch in places and focally merge their lumina. It has been hypothesized that these multiple focal fusions between adjacent capillary layers results in capillary wall restructuring followed by preferential growth of the fused areas (168,170).

The postnatal growths of other parts of the lung have not received as much attention, but there are some fundamental differences in the design of the neonatal respiratory system compared to the adult. Specifically, in the upper airway of human infants the laryngeal block is located higher, with respect to its projection on the vertebral column in the adult (171). The neonatal oropharyngeal region is therefore relatively narrower than in adults, which is fundamentally important for the generation of the negative mouth pressures required for suckling (172). In dogs, the distal airways increase approximately 10 times in length postnatally, while the proximal airways increase approximately 3 times in length (173). The number of pores of Kohn also increases in number, up to 1 year postnatally in dogs (174). Once lung maturation has occurred, the lung undergoes a natural aging process. The changes that occur as a consequence of aging are similar to, but less pronounced than, the changes that are observed in certain disease states (e.g., emphysema). These changes include: loss of lung elastic recoil, increase in closing volume, decrease in maximum expiratory flows, decreased diffusion capacity, decreased arterial oxygen tension, and changes in response to stimuli (172).

Three major postnatal lung diseases are characterized by the presence of too few alveoli: emphysema, diffuse interstitial fibrosis, and bronchopulmonary dysplasia (BPD). Alveolar destruction is the main recognized cause of alveolar insufficiency in emphysema and in interstitial fibrosis. In contrast, the hallmark of severe BPD, as it is currently seen in clinical practice, is an impairment of secondary septation, leading to a reduction in alveolar number and surface area for gas exchange (175). The cellular and molecular events regulating septation and alveolar formation in the developing and postnatal lung are not well characterized. The roles of potential suppressive signals and the responding genes that may exist to terminate the process of septation and alveolar formation are virtually unknown. The following sections delineate what is known in regards to the contribution of agents such as: hormones, nutrition, oxygen tension, transcription factors, growth factors, and physical factors in postnatal lung growth.

A. Hormones and Postnatal Lung Development

Cortisol and thyroid hormones are known to modulate the maturation of various fetal organ systems, enzymes, and biochemical pathways. Prenatally glucocorticoids stimulate lung maturation, especially the surfactant system (15). However, treatment of fetuses and preterm infants with repeated and/or high doses of corticosteroids may have considerable long-term side effects on lung growth. Morphological analysis of 60-day-old pups treated in utero with dexamethasone revealed a lower numerical density of alveoli and a larger mean alveolar radius than control pups, suggesting that antenatal administration of dexamethasone impaired normal postnatal lung growth (176). It is likely that this impairment is predominantly due to altered alveolar epithelial cell replication, as glucocorticoids inhibit proliferation. Specifically, dexamethasone has been shown to profoundly decrease the activity of cyclin E-CDK2 complexes possibly through induction of the CDK inhibitor p21[CIP1] (177), thereby blocking entry of alveolar epithelial cells into S phase. Alternatively, glucocorticoids may inhibit alveolar growth by diminishing cell–cell communication through gap junctions (178) or may also affect postnatal lung growth by decreasing thyroid-stimulating hormone secretion and reducing peripheral conversion of T(4) to T(3) (179).

In contrast to corticosteroids, thyroid hormones accelerate the formation of alveoli in newborn rats (180). In the rat, circulating thyroid hormone content (180) and lung tissue thyroid hormone receptor density (181,182) increase just prior to alveolar septation. Thyroid hormone administration accelerates DNA synthesis in newborn rats (180). It also increases the surface-to-volume ratio and surface area and, furthermore, decreases the mean chord length of the gas-exchange structures (183). All theses changes are indicative of an increase in septation. Clinically, preterm newborns have lower thyroxine serum levels compared with late-gestational fetuses (184) and in newborns the frequency and severity of respiratory distress syndrome can be correlated to lower tri-iodothyronine indices, a higher ratio of thyroxine (T4) to tri-iodothyronine (T3) and higher thyrotropin concentration when compared to infants without respiratory distress syndrome (185). These observations show that thyroid activity at birth influences lung maturation and influences the prevalence and severity of neonatal illness.

B. Nutrition and Vitamins in Postnatal Lung Growth

Malnutrition can cause functional and structural alterations of the lung parenchyma. Specifically, intermittent starvation of rat pups results in a reduced number of alveoli on postnatal day 7, and striking morphological differences on postnatal day 14, which cannot be reversed by one week of normal uninterrupted suckling (186). The effect of early protein deficiency, results in the presence of fewer and smaller cells than control lungs, along with increased surface forces, and decreased tissue elasticity (187). A deficiency in adenosine deaminase (a purine catabolic enzyme) in mice is associated with a severe enlargement of alveolar spaces due to abnormal alveogenesis (188).

Retinol deficiency (vitamin A deficiency) results in lung histopathology that is similar to bronchopulmonary dysplasia (189), which occurs frequently in human premature neonates of extremely low birth weight. Experimental evidence suggests that retinoids (vitamin A) regulate the formation of pulmonary alveoli by inducing the eruption of septa and determining the distance between septa (178). During septation, there are dramatic changes in metabolism of endogenous retinoids from storage forms (retinyl esters) to more biologically active forms, such as retinal or RA, as well as, transcriptional increases in the retinoid-binding proteins and RA receptor genes (190–192). Accordingly, when RA receptor knockout mice for RAR$\gamma^{-/-}$ and RXR$\alpha^{+/-}$ are combined the resulting double knockout mutant mice have reduced number of alveoli and less elastic fiber in their alveolar walls (193). Conversely RAR$\beta^{-/-}$ mice show early onset septation resulting in twice as many alveoli in the null mutant lungs when compared to wild-type lungs (194). This suggests that RARβ is an endogenous inhibitor of septation, while RARγ and RXRα are stimulators of septation. Together these data show the importance of retinoids in alveolar septation and suggest that not only is the amount of retinoids present important for alveolarization, but also the interplay between RA receptors.

Preterm neonates and neonates that exhibit physiological vitamin E deficiency can be at increased risk for the development of acute lung diseases. Intracellularly, vitamin E deficiency results in a reversible increase in Bax and cytosolic cytochrome C and reduces mitochondrial transmembrane potential and Hsp25 expression. All these factors have the ability to influence apoptosis, but do not initiate apoptosis themselves. However, alterations in the expression of these factors in alveolar type II cells have been shown to sensitize these cells to apoptosis when an additional insult is applied (195). Vitamin B6 deficiency may also influences postnatal lung development through its ability to affect lung elastin crosslinking (196), such that inhibition of elastin cross-linking is associated with emphysematous changes in the lung (197).

C. Oxygen and Postnatal Lung Development

Exposure of lung tissue to increased concentrations of oxygen leads to an increase in the formation of reactive oxygen species (ROS) (198). Oxidative stress has been demonstrated to be sufficient to cause a lung lesion similar to BPD, as originally described in humans (199), in baboons (200). The cytotoxicity of oxygen on the lung depends not only on concentration, but also duration of exposure. At 40% oxygen, animals exposed for three weeks show a significant reduction in lung size at day 23 (201). At 60% oxygen, there is patchy parenchymal thickening, in addition to an inhibition of secondary septation (202,203), while at higher oxygen concentrations (>85%) alveolar formation is reduced (204). Inhibition of alveolar formation by 95% oxygen can be prevented by overexpression of a ROS scavenger, extracellular superoxide dismutase (205), by prevention of neutrophil influx (206) or by treatment with RA (207). Increasing evidence suggests that ROS act as intra- and intercellular messengers (208), and their effects on modulating the growth and differentiation status of target cells have been the subject of a several comprehensive reviews (209–212). In vitro studies of premature lung cells exposed to high concentrations of O_2 have shown that they have a marked increase in prostaglandin synthesis, and cis-unsaturated fatty acids, including arachidonic acid (213,214). Exposure of pneumocytes from premature rat lung to 95% O_2 results in DNA breaks (215), which has been linked to modulation of *c-fos* expression (216). When these same cells are exposed to low concentrations of paraquat, to increase intracellular production of superoxide, there is a marked stimulation of DNA synthesis, whereas treatment with antioxidants inhibits DNA synthesis both in vitro (217) and in vivo (218). Consistent with a physiological role for ROS in early postnatal lung growth, hypoxaemia even for a very short duration perinatally, in rats, appears to inhibit lung septation (219,220). Postnatally, hypoxaemia results in a higher gas-exchange surface area per 100 g body weight (201,221).

D. Transcription Factors and Postnatal Lung Development

As aforementioned, Ttf1 is a critical regulator of embryonic lung morphogenesis (25–27). Postnatally, Ttf1 is found in adult type II cells and is likely a necessary factor for the maintenance of differentiated cellular phenotypes and influencing surfactant protein synthesis (8). This is supported by the fact that overexpression of Ttf1, causes dose-dependent alterations in postnatal lung morphology. Modest overexpression of Ttf1, using an SP-C-Ttf1 transgene, causes type II cell hyperplasia and increases the cellular content of SP-B, while higher expression levels of Ttf1 disrupts alveolar septation, causing emphysema (222). Clinically, Ttf1 has been documented in the lungs of neonates who died with bronchopulmonary dysplasia (223). These data suggest that many of the transcriptional mediators that are important in embryonic lung morphogenesis, may indeed also be critical mediators of postnatal lung development. Supporting this idea is the fact that the newborn mice with diminished Foxf1 levels exhibit abnormal formation of pulmonary alveoli and capillaries and die postnatally (224). Two additional transcriptions factors that may influence postnatal lung growth and development are Foxfa2 (46) and GATA-6 (225,226), both of which are found in the lung postnatally.

E. Growth Factors and Postnatal Lung Development

As with the lung in utero, numerous growth factors have been shown to influence postnatal lung growth and development. As described in the baboon model of BPD, chronic neonatal lung injury is associated with dysregulated lung growth, reflected in both an inhibition of alveolarization and a relative increase in epithelial cells to mesenchymal cells (227). In newborn rats, intraperitoneal injections of neutralizing antibodies to Pdgf-BB or truncated soluble PdgfRβ were found to inhibit total lung DNA synthesis, as measured by [^{3}H] thymidine incorporation (228). These results indicate that the Pdgfs are critical mediators of early postnatal lung development. Indeed, Pdgf-A deficient mice have impaired alveolar septation attributed to a lack of alveolar myofibroblast differentiation and spreading (229,230), while overexpression of PdgfA, using a SPC-PdgfA transgene, resulted in an enlarged, nonfunctional lung and perinatal lethality caused by failure to initiate ventilation (231). These results suggest that PdgfA is a potent growth factor for mesenchymal myofibroblasts in both the developing and postnatal lung. Interestingly, overexpression of PdgfB, using an SPC-PdgfB transgene, does not mimic the phenotype observed in the SPC-PdgfA over-expressing mice. In SPC-PdgfB mice, there was no excess perinatal mortality, although this may be due to the incomplete penetration of the phenotype. However, in 1-week-old neonatal SPC-PdgfB mice, morpho-metric measurements demonstrate that airspace area and septal chord length, a parameter that increases with septal thickness, were significantly increased in the transgenic mouse lungs, suggesting alterations in alveolar-ization (232). Overall, one may speculate that both Pdgf-A and Pdgf-B influence postnatal lung development, but via separate biological actions.

As mentioned, Fgfs are important regulators of prenatal lung develop-ment. Fgfs signal via Fgfs tyrosine kinase receptors of which two of them, FgfR3 and FgfR4, are expressed in postnatal pulmonary mesenchyme. While a null mutation of either FgfR3 or FgfR4 causes no obvious lung defects, silen-cing of both receptors results in a severe restriction in overall body growth and a failure of postnatal alveolar formation (71). The precise ligands mediating the Fgf signalling by these receptors are not completely known; however, Fgf7 and hepatocyte growth factor (Hgf), which has considerable homology with Fgf7 (233) have been hypothesized as potential regulators (234,235).

Proper formation of the pulmonary microvasculature is essential for normal postnatal lung development and gas exchange. When vasculariza-tion is disrupted by antiangiogenic drugs, such as, thalidomide and fumagil-lin, in newborn rats for 2 weeks, the result is a significant reduction pulmonary arterial density and a significant drop in alveolarization (236). A similar phenotype can also be produced if the actions of vascular endothelin growth factor (Vegf) are inhibited (236,237). Vegf, is a specific mitogen for endothelial cells, and is often expressed in epithelial cells in close proximity to capillary beds. In newborn rabbits, Vegf mRNA is located primarily in alveolar epithelial cells (238). While in animals models of neonatal chronic lung disease, Vegf (238,239) as well as, its receptor fms-like tyrosine kinase receptor (Flt-1) have been shown to be significantly decreased, while other angiogenic factors (i.e., angiopoietin) are not altered (239). Findings in lungs from infants dying of BPD suggest reductions in Vegf, Flt-1, as well as the Tie-2 angiogenic receptor (240). Thus, along with Pdgfs and Fgfs, Vegfs are clearly important growth factors in postnatal lung growth. Interestingly, during microvascular maturation, a surge in the antiangiogenic molecule EMAPII (166) suggests that antiangiogenic mole-cules may be important in completing the maturation process of the pulmonary vasculature.

F. Physical Factors and Postnatal Lung Development

After birth, physical forces still play an important role in regulation of lung growth, function, structure, and metabolism (167,241). In vivo experimental support for this idea comes from several sources. First, when newborn ferrets are exposed to a continuous positive airway pressure of 6 cm H_2O for two weeks their lungs demonstrate accelerated growth (242). Second, when 10–12-week-old cats and 8-week-old piglets underwent unilateral diaphragmatic paralysis by thoracic and cervical phrenectomy, respectively, there is a significant reduction in overall functional residual capacity, while growth of contralateral lungs relative to ipsilateral lungs was increased (243). This suggests that regional growth of lung parenchyma depends in part on regional distribution of respiratory muscle activity. Finally, when the left pulmonary artery was ligated in puppies 12–24 hr after birth, marked alterations in lung maturation are present by 6 months. Specifically, left lung size is decreased, oxygen consumption and static compliances are depressed and the lungs display microscopic changes typical of chronic emphysema (244).

In vitro, a variety of stretch devices have been used to mimic the changes in transpulmonary pressure produced by the cyclic expansion and relaxation of the lung muscles in the chest wall and diaphragm. These studies have demonstrated that physical forces regulate multiple activities in neonatal and adult lung cells. First, stretching of adult type II pneumocytes (even once) in vitro causes an increased mobilization of intracellular calcium (245), and this is associated with increased release of surfactant. Surfactant, which is a proteolipid complex, may be released by deformation-induced lipid trafficking. Vlahakis et al. (246) have recently demonstrated that deformation-induced lipid trafficking is a vesicular process and is associated with a large increase in cell surface area. Besides surfactant secretion, stretch also triggers the differentiation of alveolar type II to alveolar type I cells, as well as alveolar type II cell apoptosis (247,248), thereby modulating the proportion of these cells in the lung epithelium during postnatal lung growth. Interestingly, where distension favors expression of type I cell phenotype, contraction favors a type II cell phenotype (249), and thus breathing pattern may affect the state of alveolar epithelial cell differentiation.

In cultured tracheal mucosal cells, mechanical stress using a glass microprobe results in a transient increase in ciliary beat frequency (250). This effect can be transmitted to neighboring cells, potentially through gap junctions (251), and is mediated by inositol triphosphate (IP_3) (252). Mechanical stresses in airway lung epithelial can also influence liquid transport. Specifically, a 10% stretch in airway epithelial cells causes a significant increase in Na^+–K^+–ATPase activity by 30 min (253). Additionally, when cat or human airway epithelial cells are subjected to cyclic stretch prostaglandin (PG)E2, PGI2, and thromboxane A2 synthesis are downregulated in a frequency-dependent manner (254). These biological responses of airway epithelial cells to mechanical stresses could be important for control of lung mucosal, particulate and fluid removal, as well as, for regulation of airway smooth muscle tone.

Pulmonary fibroblasts located in the interstitial space of the capillary wall throughout the lung parenchyma and within the large vessels and airways are uniquely situated to sense changes in mechanical force. Under mechanical stress fibroblasts align perpendicular to the force vector (255) and show increased mRNA expression of the extracellular matrix protein alpha(1)(I) procollagen and the calcium binding protein calcyclin (255,256). Pleural mesothelial cells also sense changes in mechanical forces from distension of the lung during inflation, as well as, shear forces exerted by the fluid film between the visceral and parietal pleura. Exposure of rat visceral pleura mesothelial cells to fluid shear stress has been shown to stimulate the release of endothelin-1 (ET-1) (257) and to increase cell permeability (258). A similar ET-1 response is seen when rat visceral pleura mesothelial cells experience a cyclic stretch (20% maximum strain, 30 cycles/min), while neither stretch nor shear stress influenced Pdgf expression (257). These results suggest that cell behavior of interstitial fibroblasts and pleural mesothelial cells is regulated in part by physical forces, and together with the epithelium, these studies point to the integral part mechanical distortion plays in maintaining the overall structure and function of the postnatal lung.

V. Postnatal Lung Disease and Injury

Despite major advances in intensive care, injury-related lung disease in both preterm and full-term babies remains a major contributor to neonatal mortality and morbidity. Injury-related lung disease is also an important cause of mortality and morbidity in older patients, as emphasized in subsequent chapters. Factors that contribute to the development of postnatal lung disease in infants include adverse perinatal events, prematurity, and therapeutic medical interventions. In addition to these categories, other etiological factors that contribute to postnatal lung injury include proteases/antiprotease imbalances, oxidant production of ROS, infectious bacteria and viruses, and environmental contaminants (see Fig. 3). It is known that premature infants are more susceptible to the development of CLD than their full-term counterparts, and the incidence of CLD increases with decreasing birth weight (259). This increased vulnerability due to prematurity is associated with several airway defects, which include: poorly developed supporting structures, such as smooth muscle and cartilage,

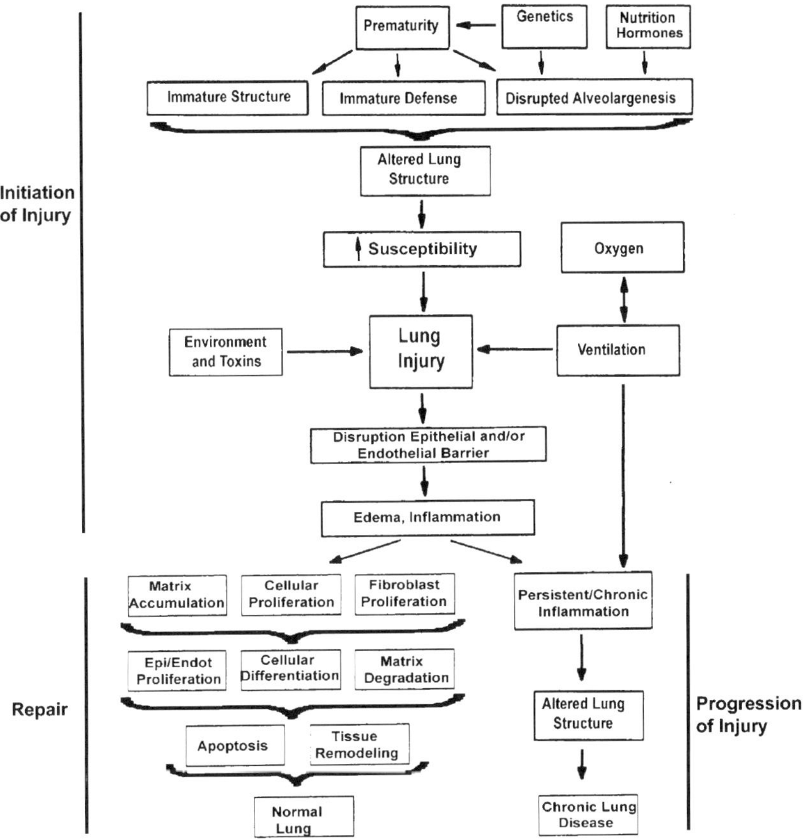

Figure 3 Mechanisms of lung injury and repair.

underdeveloped antioxidant and immune-protective responses, immature cellular mechanisms of ion transport, and incomplete development of the bronchial circulation in the airways. Parenchymal cells are not only vulnerable to injury due to immature cellular mechanisms of ion transport, and incomplete development of the pulmonary vasculature, but are also susceptible to injury due to a poorly developed gas-exchange surface, and surfactant immaturity as a result of incomplete cellular differentiation (260,261).

A. Bronchopulmonary Dysplasia

The term BPD was coined by Northway et al. (199) to reflect the involvement of all lung tissue elements in the pathology of a disorder of postnatal lung growth described in ventilated infants. The described features included airway mucosal metaplasia, airway and vascular smooth muscle hyperplasia, saccular emphysema and atelectasis. There are likely to be multiple factors, which result in the histological changes seen with the development of BPD, but the three major candidates are pulmonary oxygen toxicity, volutrauma, and cellular immaturity. Unlike injury to the adult lung, in which lung cell proliferation is superimposed on an essentially growth-arrested organ, BPD occurs in an organ that is normally in a state of active cell division. BPD is now, in the most severely affected infants, characterized by a long-term global reduction in alveolar number and surface area, consistent with an inhibition or arrest of normal maturation (262,263). This long-term failure of lung growth is also accompanied, in the early stages of injury, by reparative pneumocyte hyperplasia, proliferation of perivascular smooth muscle cells leading to pulmonary hypertension and later, in those who develop fibrosis, patchy areas of fibroblast hyperplasia. These specific cellular hyperplasias are superimposed on an overall pattern of development in which formation of new alveoli is retarded.

B. Ventilator-Induced Lung Injury

There are several mechanisms by which mechanical ventilation, a widely used intervention for treating patients with severe lung injury and respiratory disease, can itself cause pulmonary injury (see Chapter 13 for detailed discussion of ventilator-induced lung injury). Volutrauma as a result of regional overdistention of the alveoli and pulmonary airways is one mechanism thought to contribute to ventilator-induced injury (242,264–266). Ventilation with high tidal volumes can increase vascular filtration pressures, produce stress fractures of capillary endothelium, epithelium, and basement membrane and cause lung rupture (267), as well as stimulate the release of proinflammatory cytokines (268). The more premature an infant, the more susceptible their lungs are to ventilator-induced lung injury. This is due to a combination of factors including structural immaturity, the presence surfactant deficiency, fluid filled lungs, antioxidant deficiency, and a pliant chest wall (261,269). Compounding this, infection, antenatal exposure to inflammatory mediators, and malnutrition can also increase the susceptibility of the lungs to ventilator-induced lung injury.

Preventing overdistention of functional lung units during therapeutic ventilation may minimize the risk of ventilator-induced lung injury. Pohlandt et al. (270) reported that preterm infants ventilated at 60 cycles/min with a short inspiratory time (0.33 sec) had a significantly reduced incidence of extra-alveolar air leakage or death prior to air leak, when compared to infants ventilated at 30 cycles/min with a longer inspiratory time (1 sec). Meredith et al. (271) demonstrated that the use of high-frequency ventilation prevented the development of CLD in premature baboons, when compared to intermittent mandatory ventilation with positive end-expiratory pressure (271). A trial of conventional ventilation at low tidal volumes in preterm infants did not prevent the development of BPD, but did significantly reduce the duration of ventilatory support (272). While in patients <2 years of age with thermal lung injury, treatment with ventilators to employ a high-frequency progressive accumulation of subtidal volumes in a pressure-limited format decreased the incidence of pulmonary barotraumas (273). Together these studies suggest that ventilator strategies can contribute to the progression of CLD. However, a study by Bland et al. (274) has reported that sustained mechanical ventilation (3–4 weeks) of prematurely delivered lambs with high and low tidal volume strategies did not produce appreciable differences in lung pathology. The reason for this apparent difference is unclear. Therefore, although overdistension of the lung may result in CLD, changes in ventilation strategies alone, may not prevent CLD from occurring in the premature infant. The effects of various ventilation strategies on transcription factors, growth factors, and morphogens in the premature lungs, as well as later in life, are still being clarified.

C. Growth Factors in Lung Injury

Subsequent chapters detail the broad spectrum of growth factors and other mediators that are involved in lung injury, remodelling, and repair. As one relevant example, Igfs have been implicated in compensatory growth of liver (275), kidney (276), and lung (277). Igf-I has also been implicated in experimental pulmonary hypertension induced by continuous air embolization (278). Igf-I and type I-Igf receptor mRNAs and proteins are increased in the lung parenchyma of adult rats exposed to 85% O_2, with the increase in the Igf receptor occurring in the perivascular and peribronchial smooth muscle and endothelial cells (279). Exposure of newborn rats to 60% O_2 for two weeks results in an increased expression of the IgfI-R (202), while exposure of newborn rats to 80–90% O_2, for four to six weeks, results in a markedly increased expression of both Igf-I and Igf-II (280). Given that oxygen can regulate Igf gene expression in experimental models, it is very likely that Igfs will be found to play a role in BPD. In fact, a recent study suggests that changes in serum Igf-I, IgfBP-2, and IgfBP-3 reflect the nutritional status of premature infants and demonstrate that the relation between these proteins and nutritional intake differs in premature infants with and without BPD (281). Furthermore, in children with interstitial lung disease, IgfBP-2 expression is increased (282). These data emphasize that insulin-like growth factor proteins may play important roles in injury/repair processes in the lungs.

Studies with transgenic mice, in which respiratory epithelial cells overexpressed Tgfα, support a paracrine pathway for epithelial cell-derived Tgfα leading to pulmonary fibroblast hyperplasia (283). This effect appears to be dose dependent, in which high doses lead to emphysematous and fibrotic changes during postnatal alveologenesis (284). Type II pneumocytes from

O_2-exposed rabbits produce increased amounts of Tgfα (285) but, following oxidant injury, hamster lung fibroblasts also synthesize Tgfα (286). The two studies that looked at Egf/Tgfα expression in tissues from infants with BPD had conflicting results. Stahlman et al. (287) described the presence of bronchiolar Egf in infants with BPD, which was not seen in unaffected infants. Strandjord et al. (288) detected Egf and its receptor in all lung epithelium and Tgfα in airway epithelium of normal children, while children with BPD had increased Egf, Egf receptor, and Tgfα in alveolar macrophages.

Human patients with idiopathic pulmonary fibrosis have mRNA for PdgfB in both alveolar macrophages (AMs) and alveolar epithelial cells (289–291), with similar findings observed in experimental asbestosis (292). Under these conditions it seems that the major source of the peptide is the AM, to which Pdgf-BB can be localized by immunohistochemistry. PdgfB mRNA and Pdgf-BB peptide, as well as the Pdgf β-receptor mRNA and protein, have also been found by several groups (14,293,294) to be increased in adult rats subjected to hyperoxia. Under these conditions, immunoblotting suggested that the Pdgf-BB extracted from O_2-exposed lungs was not primarily of AM origin (14). Pdgf has been implicated in the obliterative bronchiolitis, sometimes seen after lung transplantation (295), and has been localized to the airways of adult rats exposed to 85% O_2. In the 60% O_2 neonatal rat model there is a marked upregulation of the Pdgf β-receptor following O_2 exposure (228). In combination, these data make it likely that Pdgf isoforms will be found to play some role in the cellular changes seen in BPD, but immunohistochemical and in situ hybridization analyses of human tissue are awaited.

A number of Fgfs play a role in normal and abnormal lung growth. Exposure to 85% O_2 for 6 days results in increased Fgf2 mRNA and protein, along with a change in Fgf2 distribution from the matrix to alveolar epithelial cells, in the adult rat (296). In common with a number of other growth factors, Fgf2 can apparently be stored in matrix, from which it can be released to exert a mitogenic effect (297). In adult rats exposed to 85% O_2 there is also a transient appearance of Fgf2 receptor (FgfR1) at a time of active pneumocyte proliferation (296). In human patients dying 10–28 days after an acute lung injury much of the observed intra-alveolar Fgf2 appears to be contributed by macrophages (298). Both Fgf1 and Fgf2 are mitogenic for type II pneumocytes (299). This property is shared by members of the Fgf family, particularly Fgf7 and hepatocyte growth factor (Hgf), which has considerable homology with Fgf7 (233). Fgf7 and FgfR2 mRNAs are constitutively expressed in lung tissue (83,234). Type II pneumocytes have the Hgf receptor (233), but Hgf mRNA in normal lung is localized to macrophages (300). An intriguing observation has been that lung endothelial cell-derived Hgf may serve an endocrine function following unilateral nephrectomy or partial hepatectomy (300).

The Tgfβs are a superfamily of multifunctional peptide growth factors that are expressed in virtually all cells, while most cells possess functional membrane-bound receptors for members of this family (301). Increased expression of Tgfβ1 expression has been reported in the lungs of animals subjected to experimental silicosis (302), bleomycin-induced pulmonary fibrosis (303), asbestosis (304), hypersensitivity pneumonitis (305), and pulmonary oxygen toxicity (306). Tgfβ has been localized to airway epithelium and to alveolar macrophages in human idiopathic pulmonary fibrosis (307). The origin of Tgfβs in the injured lung may be from a variety of cell types at differing time points following the onset of the injury process. In bleomycin-mediated injury, for example, the initial source is epithelium, followed by macrophages then interstitial cells (308). Intervention studies, using antibodies to three Tgfβ isoforms, have limited collagen deposition in experimental bleomycin-induced pulmonary fibrosis (309). Such an intervention might also be expected to limit changes in the synthesis of other collagens (310), elastin (311), and proteoglycans (312). Thus, Tgfβs may play a role in matrix remodelling in neonatal lung injury. Though the role of Tgfβs in the matrix deposition of lung injury has been confirmed by intervention studies, they may also be influencing cell proliferation. There is a temporal relationship between Tgfβ expression and cell proliferation in bleomycin-induced pulmonary fibrosis (313), however, studies have not found a significant effect of Tgfβ1 on immature lung fibroblast DNA synthesis (314). One other effect of Tgfβ that may be of relevance in BPD is a capacity, shared with Fgfs, to regulate nitric oxide synthase activity (315,316).

Exposure to 100% oxygen has been shown to impair the synthesis of Vegf by epithelial cells, which may contribute to impaired postnatal microvascular development (238). Neuroendocrine cells containing gastrin-releasing peptide increase in the airways of infants with BPD, and there is good evidence that gastrin-releasing peptide is a growth factor for airway epithelium (317). A role for 5-hydroxytryptamine as a fibroblast mitogen is suggested by studies of experimental radiation-induced pulmonary fibrosis (318). Adult cryptogenic fibrosing alveolitis is associated with an increased expression of endothelin-1 in airway and alveolar epithelial cells, particularly at sites adjacent to granulation tissue, as well as in endothelial cells (319). Endothelin-1 is a known mitogen for vascular smooth muscle cells (320), and may play a role in the pulmonary hypertension seen in BPD. Thrombin, which has also been reported to be mitogenic for smooth muscle, appears to exert this effect through Fgf2 (321).

VI. Repair in the Postnatal Lung

Repair of pulmonary tissue as an adaptation to stress or injury occurs throughout life. However, pulmonary repair processes and their efficiency are age dependent, and interact with on-going lung development and growth. Premature infants are more susceptible to CLD than their full-term counterparts (261). One reason for this vulnerability may be a fundamental difference in the ability of the premature lung to undergo an efficient and controlled repair process in the postnatal environment. Ideally, repair processes that follow lung injury should mimic ontogeny. That is, successful recovery from lung injury would utilize a cascade of events to re-establish normal lung architecture similar to those occurring during normal lung development. In situations where the inciting factor (e.g., hyperoxia) is removed, natural repair processes often work quite well. However, with a severe or prolonged insult, the repair process may lead to fibrosis, thus preventing the re-establishment of normal lung function, making the repair process part of the disease. Factors that determine whether an injury will lead to regeneration and repair, or will progress to irreversible tissue destruction and fibrosis, are now being elucidated. Hopefully, a better understanding of normal lung repair will ultimately allow effective therapeutic interventions to be developed for use when the repair process is aberrant (see Fig. 3).

The general paradigm for normal lung injury and repair can be characterized by a number of steps, with the initial insult causing a disruption of the barrier function of either the epithelium or endothelium. Vascular leakage allows the accumulation of edema fluid in the interstitium and loss of the epithelial barrier results in this interstitial fluid spilling into the alveolar space. Edema fluid is filled with cytokines, and many growth factors that may exacerbate the insult or initiate repair. The ensuing inflammatory response is a necessary component of the repair process, as it is beneficial against attacking pathogens, but if this inflammatory response is not regulated it could lead to further injury (322). The initial cellular processes involved in tissue repair include: matrix accumulation, cell migration, and proliferation of fibroblasts, while in the later phases of repair there may be transient proliferation of epithelial and endothelial cells, cellular differentiation, matrix degradation, decreased fibroblast proliferation, and finally apoptosis (323).

Apoptosis, until recently, was an underappreciated contributor to the repair process (324). It is likely to contribute to the repair of the lung in at least three ways. Firstly, excess neutrophils are cleared from the lung through apoptosis (325,326) and in a recent study, Oei et al. (327) demonstrated that preterm infants with low levels of neutrophil apoptosis are predisposed to disordered lung repair. Secondly, apoptosis is a likely mechanism for the elimination of granulation tissue such as fibroblasts. Lastly, it may rid the repairing alveolar epithelium of excess hyperplastic type II alveolar epithelial cells (328). This removal of excess type II cells would allow the remaining cells to spread and differentiate into thinner type I cells that are less of a barrier to gas diffusion.

A. Postpneumonectomy Compensatory Lung Growth: A Model for Normal Lung Repair

Children and adolescents subjected to a unilateral pneumonectomy develop a varying degree of compensatory growth in the contralateral lung (329). This phenomenon has been exploited in extensive animal studies to enhance understanding of repair processes in the neonatal lungs (330,331). With increasing age the degree of compensatory growth achieved is reduced, but if lung tissue is removed sufficiently early in life, there is an almost complete restitution of air space, capillary and tissue volumes and alveolar and capillary surface areas to normal (332,333). Physiological, pathophysiological, and morphological studies suggest that, at least in small animal species, this compensatory growth occurs within the first 2 weeks after surgery (334,335). Cellular hyperplasia is evident during compensatory lung growth (335,336), with increased mitotic indices of parenchymal cells, total DNA, and DNA synthesis as measured by incorporation of [^{3}H]thymidine having been observed in rats (335,337,338), mice (339), and rabbits (334).

Successful postpneumonectomy lung growth likely requires the coordinated expression of numerous factors, directed at the different cell types within the lung (340), and acting through autocrine, endocrine, juxtacrine, or paracrine pathways. Despite an extensive literature relating to experimental pneumonectomy, many of the mediators of compensatory growth in the residual lung tissue have not been elucidated. It has been shown that the immediate-early genes c-fos and jun-B are upregulated very rapidly (30 min) following pneumonectomy (340). It has been suggested that tumor necrosis factor (Tnf) may be one of the hormonal factors implicated in postpneumonectomy lung growth (341). The role of Igf-I compensatory lung growth is controversial, as it has been reported not to influence lung growth following pneumonectomy in rabbits (342) and rats (343), but an Igf-I has been reported stimulate lung growth following pneumonectomy in lambs (344). Serum concentrations of Hgf increase after pneumonectomy in adult humans (345) and mice (346), as did c-Met/HGF receptor expression in alveolar type II and airway epithelial cells of pneumonectomized mice (346). This suggests that Hgf may be important in lung repair. In addition, in vivo neutralization of Pdgf-BB, using a truncated soluble Pdgf β-receptor, attenuated the increased lung DNA synthesis following pneumonectomy (347), while the administration of Kgf significantly increased the lung weight index, lung volume index, and alveolar cell proliferation index at 10 and 21 days after pneumonectomy (348). Finally, eNOS may be a critical for compensatory lung growth since nitric oxide is considered an essential mediator of Vegf-induced angiogenesis, and during compensatory lung growth there is increased flow and shear stress. Supporting this idea is data showing that compensatory lung growth was severely impaired in eNOS$^{-/-}$ mice or by treating pneumonectomized mice with the nitric oxide synthase inhibitor N(G)-nitro-L-arginine methyl ester (349). In another model

of compensatory lung growth, seen after the return to air of rat pups exposed to
95% oxygen, recovery of alveolarization was prevented by treatment with a
FgfR1 soluble receptor (350). These results indicate that many factors, including eNOS, PdgfB, and Hgf, are important mediators of lung repair.

VII. Summary

This chapter has provided an overview of basic processes involved in lung
development, growth, and repair. The lungs develop prenatally as a result of
multiple interactive mechanisms, and pulmonary growth, remodelling, and
repair continue in postnatal life. Pulmonary alveolarization, essential for
effective gas exchange, proceeds through basic stages including the
embryonic development of major airways followed by a pseudoglandular
period where airways develop to terminal bronchioles, a canalicular period
involving acinar development and vascularization, a terminal sac (saccular)
period involving subdivision of saccules by secondary crests, and an alveolar period where discrete airsacs are formed. In humans, these events
result in lungs that are anatomically capable of significant gas exchange
by about two-thirds of gestation (term = 40 weeks), although the process
of alveolarization continues well into the postnatal period. Lung growth
is a basic concomitant of lung development, and both are contributed to
by processes of remodelling and repair in response to interactions with
the environment.

Detailed in this chapter have been a number of important factors and
mediators that influence how the lungs develop and grow under normal
conditions. The activity and timing of these mediators and factors, and
the consequences when they are absent or expressed abnormally, have also
been presented. Factors that influence lung development, growth, and
repair fall into several categories including transcription factors, growth
factors, nutritional factors, physical factors, and environmental factors.
These factors interact in an extremely complex web of links and associa-
tions that continued basic research is helping to unravel. Not only are these
factors crucial for normal lung development and growth, but they are also
highly relevant for pulmonary responses to injury. Ultimately, a better
understanding of the molecular basis of lung development, growth, and
repair will help in the treatment of abnormalites such as foregut malformation and pulmonary hypoplasia. Such understanding will also contribute to
the prevention and treatment of lung injury and disease in newborns, as well
as injury-related pulmonary diseases involving inflammation and aberrant
remodelling and repair in older patients. Subsequent chapters provide additional detail about the mechanistic pathophysiology of acute and chronic
lung injury, and discuss therapeutic interventions in the context of evolving
basic science perspectives.

References

1. Hopper AF, Hart NH. Foundations of Animal Development. Oxford: Oxford University Press, 1985:366–378.

2. Jeffrey PK. The development of large and small airways. Am J Respir Crit Care Med 1998; 157(5 Pt 2):S174–S180.

3. Burri PH. Fetal and postnatal development of the lung. Annu Rev Physiol 1984; 46:617–628.

4. DiFiore JW, Wilson JM. Lung development. Semin Pediatr Surg 1994; 3(4):221–232.

5. Masters JR. Epithelial–mesenchymal interaction during lung development: the effect of mesenchymal mass. Dev Biol 1976; 51(1):98–108.

6. Spooner BS, Wessells NK. Mammalian lung development: interactions in primordium formation and bronchial morphogenesis. J Exp Zool 1970; 175(4):445–454.

7. Wessells NK. Mammalian lung development: interactions in formation and morphogenesis of tracheal buds. J Exp Zool 1970; 175(4):455–466.

8. Demayo F, et al. Mesenchymal–epithelial interactions in lung development and repair: are modeling and remodeling the same process? Am J Physiol Lung Cell Mol Physiol 2002; 283(3):L510–L517.

9. Minoo P, King RJ. Epithelial–mesenchymal interactions in lung development. Annu Rev Physiol 1994; 56:13–45.

10. Kauffman SL. Cell proliferation in the mammalian lung. Int Rev Exp Pathol 1980; 22:131–191.

11. Adamson IY, King GM. Sex differences in development of fetal rat lung I Autoradiographic and biochemical studies. Lab Invest 1984; 50(4):456–460.

12. Adamson IY, Bowden DH. Derivation of type 1 epithelium from type 2 cells in the developing rat lung. Lab Invest 1975; 32(6):736–745.

13. O'Hare KH, Townes PL. Morphogenesis of albino rat lung: an autoradiographic analysis of the embryological origin of the type I and II pulmonary epithelial cells. J Morphol 1970; 132(1):69–87.

14. Buch S, et al. Ontogeny and regulation of platelet-derived growth factor gene expression in distal fetal rat lung epithelial cells. Am J Respir Cell Mol Biol 1994; 11(3):251–261.

15. Post M, Smith BT. Hormonal control of surfactant metabolism. In: Robertson B, Van Golde LMG, Batenburg JJ, eds. Pulmonary Surfactant: from Molecular Biology to Clinical Practice. New York: Elsevier, 1992:379–424.

16. Caniggia I, et al. Inhibition of fibroblast growth by epithelial cells in fetal rat lung. Am J Respir Cell Mol Biol 1995; 13(1):91–98.

17. Weinstein DC, et al. The winged-helix transcription factor HNF-3 beta is required for notochord development in the mouse embryo. Cell 1994; 78(4): 575–588.

18. Ang SL, et al. The formation and maintenance of the definitive endoderm lineage in the mouse: involvement of HNF3/forkhead proteins. Development 1993; 119(4):1301–1315.

19. Ang SL, Rossant J. HNF-3 beta is essential for node and notochord formation in mouse development. Cell 1994; 78(4):561–574.

20. Kaestner KH. The hepatocyte nuclear factor 3 (HNF3 or FOXA) family in metabolism. Trends Endocrinol Metab 2000; 11(7):281–285.

21. Dufort D, et al. The transcription factor HNF3beta is required in visceral endoderm for normal primitive streak morphogenesis. Development 1998; 125(16):3015–3025.

22. Kappen C. Hox genes in the lung. Am J Respir Cell Mol Biol 1996; 15(2): 156–162.

23. Cardoso WV. Transcription factors and pattern formation in the developing lung. Am J Physiol 1995; 269(4 Pt 1):L429–L442.

24. Motoyama J, et al. Essential function of Gli2 and Gli3 in the formation of lung, trachea and oesophagus. Nat Genet 1998; 20(1):54–57.

25. Lazzaro D, et al. The transcription factor TTF-1 is expressed at the onset of thyroid and lung morphogenesis and in restricted regions of the foetal brain. Development 1991; 113(4):1093–1104.

26. Minoo P, et al. Defects in tracheoesophageal and lung morphogenesis in Nkx2.1($-/-$) mouse embryos. Dev Biol 1999; 209(1):60–71.

27. Yuan B, et al. Inhibition of distal lung morphogenesis in Nkx2.1(–/–) embryos. Dev Dyn 2000; 217(2):180–190.

28. Chen J, et al. Mutation of the mouse hepatocyte nuclear factor/forkhead homologue 4 gene results in an absence of cilia and random left–right asymmetry. J Clin Invest 1998; 102(6):1077–1082.

29. Gage PJ, Suh H, Camper SA. Dosage requirement of Pitx2 for development of multiple organs. Development 1999; 126(20):4643–4651.

30. Lu MF, et al. Function of Rieger syndrome gene in left–right asymmetry and craniofacial development. Nature 1999; 401(6750):276–278.

31. Lin CR, et al. Pitx2 regulates lung asymmetry, cardiac positioning and pituitary and tooth morphogenesis. Nature 1999; 401(6750):279–282.

32. Keijzer R, et al. The transcription factor GATA6 is essential for branching morphogenesis and epithelial cell differentiation during fetal pulmonary development. Development 2001; 128(4):503–511.

33. Morrisey EE, et al. GATA-6: a zinc finger transcription factor that is expressed in multiple cell lineages derived from lateral mesoderm. Dev Biol 1996; 177(1):309–322.

34. Koutsourakis M, et al. Branching and differentiation defects in pulmonary epithelium with elevated Gata6 expression. Mech Dev 2001; 105(1–2):105–114.

35. Yang H, et al. GATA6 regulates differentiation of distal lung epithelium. Development 2002; 129(9):2233–2246.

36. Charron J, et al. Embryonic lethality in mice homozygous for a targeted disruption of the *N*-myc gene. Genes Dev 1992; 6(12A):2248–2257.

37. Stanton BR, et al. Loss of *N*-myc function results in embryonic lethality and failure of the epithelial component of the embryo to develop. Genes Dev 1992; 6(12A):2235–2247.

38. Moens CB, et al. A targeted mutation reveals a role for *N*-myc in branching morphogenesis in the embryonic mouse lung. Genes Dev 1992; 6(5):691–704.

39. Moens CB, et al. Defects in heart and lung development in compound heterozygotes for two different targeted mutations at the *N*-myc locus. Development 1993; 119(2):485–499.

40. Borges M, et al. An achaete-scute homologue essential for neuroendocrine differentiation in the lung. Nature 1997; 386(6627):852–855.

41. Ito T, et al. Basic helix–loop–helix transcription factors regulate the neuroendocrine differentiation of fetal mouse pulmonary epithelium. Development 2000; 127(18):3913–3921.

42. Quaggin SE, et al. The basic-helix–loop–helix protein pod1 is critically important for kidney and lung organogenesis. Development 1999; 126(24):5771–5783.

43. Bingle CD, Gitlin JD. Identification of hepatocyte nuclear factor-3 binding sites in the Clara cell secretory protein gene. Biochem J 1993; 295(Pt 1): 227–232.

44. Bingle CD, et al. Role of hepatocyte nuclear factor-3 alpha and hepatocyte nuclear factor-3 beta in Clara cell secretory protein gene expression in the bronchiolar epithelium. Biochem J 1995; 308(Pt 1):197–202.

45. Bohinski RJ, Di Lauro R, Whitsett JA. The lung-specific surfactant protein B gene promoter is a target for thyroid transcription factor 1 and hepatocyte nuclear factor 3, indicating common factors for organ-specific gene expression along the foregut axis. Mol Cell Biol 1994; 14(9):5671–5681.

46. Clevidence DE, et al. Members of the HNF-3/forkhead family of transcription factors exhibit distinct cellular expression patterns in lung and regulate the surfactant protein B promoter. Dev Biol 1994; 166(1):195–209.

47. Tichelaar JW, et al. HNF-3/forkhead homologue-4 (HFH-4) is expressed in ciliated epithelial cells in the developing mouse lung. J Histochem Cytochem 1999; 47(6):823–832.

48. Brody SL, et al. Ciliogenesis and left–right axis defects in forkhead factor HFH-4-null mice. Am J Respir Cell Mol Biol 2000; 23(1):45–51.

49. Compernolle V, et al. Loss of HIF-2alpha and inhibition of VEGF impair fetal lung maturation, whereas treatment with VEGF prevents fatal respiratory distress in premature mice. Nat Med 2002; 8(7):702–710.

50. Lawrence PA, Struhl G. Morphogens, compartments, and pattern: lessons from drosophila?. Cell 1996; 85(7):951–961.

51. Reilly KM, Melton DA. Short-range signaling by candidate morphogens of the TGF beta family and evidence for a relay mechanism of induction. Cell 1996; 86(5):743–754.

52. Wilson PA, Melton DA. Mesodermal patterning by an inducer gradient depends on secondary cell–cell communication. Curr Biol 1994; 4(8): 676–686.

53. Urase K, et al. Spatial expression of Sonic hedgehog in the lung epithelium during branching morphogenesis. Biochem Biophys Res Commun 1996; 225(1):161–166.

54. Bitgood MJ, McMahon AP. Hedgehog and Bmp genes are coexpressed at many diverse sites of cell–cell interaction in the mouse embryo. Dev Biol 1995; 172(1):126–138.

55. Litingtung Y, et al. Sonic hedgehog is essential to foregut development. Nat Genet 1998; 20(1):58–61.

56. Bellusci S, et al. Involvement of Sonic hedgehog (Shh) in mouse embryonic lung growth and morphogenesis. Development 1997; 124(1):53–63.

57. van Tuyl M, Post M. From fruitflies to mammals: mechanisms of signalling via the Sonic hedgehog pathway in lung development. Respir Res 2000; 1(1):30–35.

58. Grindley JC, et al. Evidence for the involvement of the Gli gene family in embryonic mouse lung development. Dev Biol 1997; 188(2):337–348.

59. Park HL, et al. Mouse Gli1 mutants are viable but have defects in SHH signaling in combination with a Gli2 mutation. Development 2000; 127(8): 1593–1605.

60. Ingham PW. Signalling by hedgehog family proteins in Drosophila and vertebrate development. Curr Opin Genet Dev 1995; 5(4):492–498.

61. Gavin BJ, McMahon JA, McMahon AP. Expression of multiple novel Wnt-1/int-1-related genes during fetal and adult mouse development. Genes Dev 1990; 4(12B):2319–2332.

62. Sarkar L, et al. Wnt/Shh interactions regulate ectodermal boundary formation during mammalian tooth development. Proc Natl Acad Sci USA 2000; 97(9):4520–4524.

63. Shu W, et al. Wnt7b regulates mesenchymal proliferation and vascular development in the lung. Development 2002; 129(20):4831–4842.

64. Li C, et al. Wnt5a participates in distal lung morphogenesis. Dev Biol 2002; 248(1):68–81.

65. Warburton D, et al. The molecular basis of lung morphogenesis. Mech Dev 2000; 92(1):55–81.

66. Ornitz DM, et al. Receptor specificity of the fibroblast growth factor family. J Biol Chem 1996; 271(25):15292–15297.

67. Arman E, et al. Fgfr2 is required for limb outgrowth and lung-branching morphogenesis. Proc Natl Acad Sci USA 1999; 96(21):11895–11899.

68. Peters K, et al. Targeted expression of a dominant negative FGF receptor blocks branching morphogenesis and epithelial differentiation of the mouse lung. EMBO J 1994; 13(14):3296–3301.

69. Arman E, et al. Targeted disruption of fibroblast growth factor (FGF) receptor 2 suggests a role for FGF signaling in pregastrulation mammalian development. Proc Natl Acad Sci USA 1998; 95(9):5082–5087.

70. Xu X, et al. Fibroblast growth factor receptor 2 (FGFR2)-mediated reciprocal regulation loop between FGF8 and FGF10 is essential for limb induction. Development 1998; 125(4):753–765.

71. Weinstein M, et al. FGFR-3 and FGFR-4 function cooperatively to direct alveogenesis in the murine lung. Development 1998; 125(18):3615–3623.

72. Colvin JS, et al, Lung hypoplasia and neonatal death in Fgf9-null mice identify this gene as an essential regulator of lung mesenchyme. Development 2001; 128(11):2095–2106.

73. Whitsett JA, et al. Fibroblast growth factor 18 influences proximal programming during lung morphogenesis. J Biol Chem 2002; 277(25):22743–22749.

74. Bellusci S, et al. Fibroblast growth factor 10 (FGF10) and branching morphogenesis in the embryonic mouse lung. Development 1997; 124(23): 4867–4878.

75. Min H, et al. Fgf-10 is required for both limb and lung development and exhibits striking functional similarity to *Drosophila* branchless. Genes Dev 1998; 12(20):3156–3161.

76. Sekine K, et al. Fgf10 is essential for limb and lung formation. Nat Genet 1999; 21(1):138–141.

77. Cebra-Thomas JA, et al. T-box gene products are required for mesenchymal induction of epithelial branching in the embryonic mouse lung. Dev Dyn 2003; 226(1):82–90.

78. Sakiyama J, Yamagishi A, Kuroiwa A. Tbx4-Fgf10 system controls lung bud formation during chicken embryonic development. Development 2003; 130(7):1225–1234.

79. Tichelaar JW, Lu W, Whitsett JA. Conditional expression of fibroblast growth factor-7 in the developing and mature lung. J Biol Chem 2000; 275(16): 11858–11864.

80. Simonet WS, et al. Pulmonary malformation in transgenic mice expressing human keratinocyte growth factor in the lung. Proc Natl Acad Sci USA 1995; 92(26):12461–12465.

81. Chelly N, et al. Keratinocyte growth factor enhances maturation of fetal rat lung type II cells. Am J Respir Cell Mol Biol 1999; 20(3):423–432.

82. Cardoso WV, et al. FGF-1 and FGF-7 induce distinct patterns of growth and differentiation in embryonic lung epithelium. Dev Dyn 1997; 208(3):398–405.

83. Post M, et al. Keratinocyte growth factor and its receptor are involved in regulating early lung branching. Development 1996; 122(10):3107–3115.

84. Shiratori M, et al. Keratinocyte growth factor and embryonic rat lung morphogenesis. Am J Respir Cell Mol Biol 1996; 15(3):328–338.

85. Hu MC, et al. FGF-18, a novel member of the fibroblast growth factor family, stimulates hepatic and intestinal proliferation. Mol Cell Biol 1998; 18(10):6063–6074.

86. Loewenstein WR. Cell-to-cell communication and the control of growth. Am Rev Respir Dis 1990; 142(6 Pt 2):S48–S53.

87. Munari-Silem Y, Audebet C, Rousset B. Hormonal control of cell to cell communication: regulation by thyrotropin of the gap junction-mediated dye transfer between thyroid cells. Endocrinology 1991; 128(6):3299–3309.

88. Massague J. Transforming growth factor-alpha. A model for membrane-anchored growth factors. J Biol Chem 1990; 265(35):21393–21396.

89. Raaberg L, et al. Epidermal growth factor transcription, translation, and signal transduction by rat type II pneumocytes in culture. Am J Respir Cell Mol Biol 1992; 6(1):44–49.

90. Raaberg L, et al. Fetal effects of epidermal growth factor deficiency induced in rats by autoantibodies against epidermal growth factor. Pediatr Res 1995; 37(2):175–181.

91. Kaartinen V, et al. Abnormal lung development and cleft palate in mice lacking TGF-beta 3 indicates defects of epithelial–mesenchymal interaction. Nat Genet 1995; 11(4):415–421.

92. Souza P, et al. PDGF-AA and its receptor influence early lung branching via an epithelial–mesenchymal interaction. Development 1995; 121(8): 2559–2567.

93. Weaver M, et al. Bmp signaling regulates proximal–distal differentiation of endoderm in mouse lung development. Development 1999; 126(18): 4005–4015.

94. Greenberg JM, et al. Mesenchymal expression of vascular endothelial growth factors D and A defines vascular patterning in developing lung. Dev Dyn 2002; 224(2):144–153.

95. Pichel JG, et al. Developmental cooperation of leukemia inhibitory factor and insulin-like growth factor I in mice is tissue-specific and essential for lung maturation involving the transcription factors Sp3 and TTF-1. Mech Dev 2003; 120(3):349–361.

96. Han RN, et al. Insulin-like growth factor-I receptor-mediated vasculogenesis/angiogenesis in human lung development. Am J Respir Cell Mol Biol 2003; 28(2):159–169.

97. Morris DG, et al. Loss of integrin alpha(v)beta6-mediated TGF-beta activation causes Mmp12-dependent emphysema. Nature 2003; 422(6928):169–173.

98. Li C, et al. Transforming growth factor-beta inhibits pulmonary surfactant protein B gene transcription through SMAD3 interactions with NKX2.1 and HNF-3 transcription factors. J Biol Chem 2002; 277(41):38399–38408.

99. Hyatt BA, Shangguan X, Shannon JM. BMP4 modulates fibroblast growth factor-mediated induction of proximal and distal lung differentiation in mouse embryonic tracheal epithelium in mesenchyme-free culture. Dev Dyn 2002; 225(2):153–165.

100. Farago A, Nishizuka Y. Protein kinase C in transmembrane signalling. FEBS Lett 1990; 268(2):350–354.

101. Yarden Y, Ullrich A. Growth factor receptor tyrosine kinases. Annu Rev Biochem 1988; 57:443–478.

102. Dumont JE, Jauniaux JC, Roger PP. The cyclic AMP-mediated stimulation of cell proliferation. Trends Biochem Sci 1989; 14(2):67–71.

103. Maden M. The role of retinoic acid in embryonic and post-embryonic development. Proc Nutr Soc 2000; 59(1):65–73.

104. Morriss-Kay G. Retinoic acid and development. Pathobiology 1992; 60(5):264–270.

105. Chambon P. A decade of molecular biology of retinoic acid receptors. FASEB J 1996; 10(9):940–954.

106. Krezel W, et al. RXR gamma null mice are apparently normal and compound RXR alpha +/− /RXR beta −/−/RXR gamma −/− mutant mice are viable. Proc Natl Acad Sci USA 1996; 93(17):9010–9014.

107. Mendelsohn C, et al. Retinoic acid receptor beta 2 (RAR beta 2) null mutant mice appear normal. Dev Biol 1994; 166(1):246–258.

108. Mark M, et al. A genetic dissection of the retinoid signalling pathway in the mouse. Proc Nutr Soc 1999; 58(3):609–613.

109. Lohnes D, et al. Developmental roles of the retinoic acid receptors. J Steroid Biochem Mol Biol 1995; 53(1–6):475–486.

110. Mendelsohn C, et al. Function of the retinoic acid receptors (RARs) during development (II). Multiple abnormalities at various stages of organogenesis in RAR double mutants. Development 1994; 120(10):2749–2771.

111. Kastner P, et al. Genetic evidence that the retinoid signal is transduced by heterodimeric RXR/RAR functional units during mouse development. Development 1997; 124(2):313–326.

112. Nguyen TM, et al. Evidence for a vitamin D paracrine system regulating maturation of developing rat lung epithelium. Am J Physiol 1996; 271(3 Pt 1):L392–L399.

113. Edelson JD, et al. Vitamin D stimulates DNA synthesis in alveolar type-II cells. Biochim Biophys Acta 1994; 1221(2):159–166.

114. Harding R, Hooper SB, Han VK. Abolition of fetal breathing movements by spinal cord transection leads to reductions in fetal lung liquid volume, lung growth, and IGF-II gene expression. Pediatr Res 1993; 34(2):148–153.

115. Alcorn D, et al. Morphological effects of chronic tracheal ligation and drainage in the fetal lamb lung. J Anat 1977; 123(3):649–660.

116. Griscom NT, et al. Fluid-filled lung due to airway obstruction in the newborn. Pediatrics 1969; 43(3):383–390.

117. Perlman M, Levin M. Fetal pulmonary hypoplasia, anuria, and oligohydramnios: clinicopathologic observations and review of the literature. Am J Obstet Gynecol 1974; 118(8):1119–1123.

118. Thomas IT, Smith DW. Oligohydramnios, cause of the nonrenal features of Potter's syndrome, including pulmonary hypoplasia. J Pediatr 1974; 84(6):811–815.

119. Finegold MJ, et al. Lung structure in thoracic dystrophy. Am J Dis Child 1971; 122(2):153–159.

120. George DK, et al. Hypoplasia and immaturity of the terminal lung unit (acinus) in congenital diaphragmatic hernia. Am Rev Respir Dis 1987; 136(4):947–950.

121. Harrison MR, et al. Correction of congenital diaphragmatic hernia in utero. II. Simulated correction permits fetal lung growth with survival at birth. Surgery 1980; 88(2):260–268.

122. Rcalc FR, Esterly JR. Pulmonary hypoplasia: a morphometric study of the lungs of infants with diaphragmatic hernia, anencephaly, and renal malformations. Pediatrics 1973; 51(1):91–96.

123. Liggins GC, et al. The effect of spinal cord transection on lung development in fetal sheep. J Dev Physiol 1981; 3(4):267–274.

124. Wigglesworth JS, Desai R. Effect on lung growth of cervical cord section in the rabbit fetus. Early Hum Dev 1979; 3(1):51–65.

125. Islam S, Donahoe PK, Schnitzer JJ. Tracheal ligation increases mitogen-activated protein kinase activity and attenuates surfactant protein B mRNA in fetal sheep lungs. J Surg Res 1999; 84(1):19–23.

126. Souza P, O'Brodovich H, Post M. Lung fluid restriction affects growth but not airway branching of embryonic rat lung. Int J Dev Biol 1995; 39(4):629–637.

127. Moessinger AC, et al. Oligohydramnios-induced lung hypoplasia: the influence of timing and duration in gestation. Pediatr Res 1986; 20(10):951–954.

128. Nakayama DK, et al. Experimental pulmonary hypoplasia due to oligohydramnios and its reversal by relieving thoracic compression. J Pediatr Surg 1983; 18(4):347–353.

129. Higuchi M, et al. The influence of experimentally produced oligohydramnios on lung growth and pulmonary surfactant content in fetal rabbits. J Dev Physiol 1991; 16(4):223–227.

130. Wilson JM, DiFiore JW, Peters CA. Experimental fetal tracheal ligation prevents the pulmonary hypoplasia associated with fetal nephrectomy: possible application for congenital diaphragmatic hernia. J Pediatr Surg 1993; 28(11):1433–1439; discussion 1439–1440.

131. Peters CA, et al. The role of the kidney in lung growth and maturation in the setting of obstructive uropathy and oligohydramnios. J Urol 1991; 146(2 (Pt 2)):597–600.

132. Neilson IR, et al. Congenital adenomatoid malformation of the lung: current management and prognosis. J Pediatr Surg 1991; 26(8):975–980; discussion 980–981.

133. Cooney TP, Thurlbeck WM. Lung growth and development in anencephaly and hydranencephaly. Am Rev Respir Dis 1985; 132(3):596–601.

134. DiFiore JW, et al. Experimental fetal tracheal ligation reverses the structural and physiological effects of pulmonary hypoplasia in congenital diaphragmatic hernia. J Pediatr Surg 1994; 29(2):248–256; discussion 256–257.

135. Kitano Y, et al. Fetal tracheal occlusion in the rat model of nitrofen-induced congenital diaphragmatic hernia. J Appl Physiol 1999; 87(2):769–775.

136. Wu J, et al. Pulmonary effects of in utero tracheal occlusion are dependent on gestational age in a rabbit model of diaphragmatic hernia. J Pediatr Surg 2002; 37(1):11–17.

137. O'Toole SJ, et al. Tracheal ligation does not correct the surfactant deficiency associated with congenital diaphragmatic hernia. J Pediatr Surg 1996; 31(4): 546–550.

138. Savich RD, et al. The effect of fetal breathing movements on pulmonary blood flow in fetal sheep. Pediatr Res 1994; 35(4 Pt 1):484–489.

139. Fewell JE, Lee CC, Kitterman JA. Effects of phrenic nerve section on the respiratory system of fetal lambs. J Appl Physiol 1981; 51(2):293–297.

140. Tseng BS, et al. Pulmonary hypoplasia in the myogenin null mouse embryo. Am J Respir Cell Mol Biol 2000; 22(3):304–315.

141. Liu M, Tanswell AK, Post M. Mechanical force-induced signal transduction in lung cells. Am J Physiol 1999; 277(4 Pt 1):L667–L683.

142. Liu M, Post M. Invited review: mechanochemical signal transduction in the fetal lung. J Appl Physiol 2000; 89(5):2078–2084.

143. Liu M, et al. Stretch-induced growth-promoting activities stimulate fetal rat lung epithelial cell proliferation. Exp Lung Res 1993; 19(4):505–517.

144. Xu J, Liu M, Post M. Differential regulation of extracellular matrix molecules by mechanical strain of fetal lung cells. Am J Physiol 1999; 276(5 Pt 1): L728–L735.

145. Liu M, et al. Inhibition of mechanical strain-induced fetal rat lung cell proliferation by gadolinium, a stretch-activated channel blocker. J Cell Physiol 1994; 161(3):501–507.

146. Liu M, et al. Mechanical strain-enhanced fetal lung cell proliferation is mediated by phospholipase C and D and protein kinase C. Am J Physiol 1995; 268(5 Pt 1):L729–L738.

147. Liu M, et al. Mechanical strain induces pp60src activation and translocation to cytoskeleton in fetal rat lung cells. J Biol Chem 1996; 271(12):7066–7071.

148. Skinner SJ, Somervell CE, Olson DM. The effects of mechanical stretching on fetal rat lung cell prostacyclin production. Prostaglandins 1992; 43(5): 413–433.

149. Scott JE, et al. Influence of strain on [3H]thymidine incorporation, surfactant-related phospholipid synthesis, and cAMP levels in fetal type II alveolar cells. Am J Respir Cell Mol Biol 1993; 8(3):258–265.

150. Sanchez-Esteban J, et al. Cyclic mechanical stretch inhibits cell proliferation and induces apoptosis in fetal rat lung fibroblasts. Am J Physiol Lung Cell Mol Physiol 2002; 282(3):L448–L456.

151. Roman J. Cell–cell and cell–matrix interactions in development of the lung vasculature. In: McDonald JA, ed. Lung Growth and Development. New York: Marcel Dekker, 1997:365–400.

152. deMello DE, et al. Early fetal development of lung vasculature. Am J Respir Cell Mol Biol 1997; 16(5):568–581.

153. Alameh J, et al. Alveolar capillary dysplasia: a cause of persistent pulmonary hypertension of the newborn. Eur J Pediatr 2002; 161(5):262–266.

154. Chelliah BP, et al. Alveolar capillary dysplasia—a cause of persistent pulmonary hypertension unresponsive to a second course of extracorporeal membrane oxygenation. Pediatrics 1995; 96(6):1159–1161.

155. Cullinane C, Cox PN, Silver MM. Persistent pulmonary hypertension of the newborn due to alveolar capillary dysplasia. Pediatr Pathol 1992; 12(4): 499–514.

156. Hislop A, Sanderson M, Reid L. Unilateral congenital dysplasia of lung associated with vascular anomalies. Thorax 1973; 28(4):435–441.

157. Wallen LD, Kulisz E, Maloney JE. Main pulmonary artery ligation reduces lung fluid production in fetal sheep. J Dev Physiol 1991; 16(3):173–179.

158. Wallen LD, et al. Fetal lung growth. Influence of pulmonary arterial flow and surgery in sheep. Am J Respir Crit Care Med 1994; 149(4 Pt 1):1005–1011.

159. Healy AM, et al. VEGF is deposited in the subepithelial matrix at the leading edge of branching airways and stimulates neovascularization in the murine embryonic lung. Dev Dyn 2000; 219(3):341–352.

160. Bhatt AJ, et al. Expression of vascular endothelial growth factor and Flk-1 in developing and glucocorticoid-treated mouse lung. Pediatr Res 2000; 47(5): 606–613.

161. Gebb SA, Shannon JM. Tissue interactions mediate early events in pulmonary vasculogenesis. Dev Dyn 2000; 217(2):159–169.

162. Colen KL, et al. Vascular development in the mouse embryonic pancreas and lung. J Pediatr Surg 1999; 34(5):781–785.

163. Koblizek TI, et al. Angiopoietin-1 induces sprouting angiogenesis in vitro. Curr Biol 1998; 8(9):529–532.

164. Maisonpierre PC, et al. Angiopoietin-2, a natural antagonist for Tie2 that disrupts in vivo angiogenesis. Science 1997; 277(5322):55–60.

165. Hall SM, Hislop AA, Haworth SG. Origin, differentiation, and maturation of human pulmonary veins. Am J Respir Cell Mol Biol 2002; 26(3):333–340.

166. Schwarz M, et al. EMAP II: a modulator of neovascularization in the developing lung. Am J Physiol 1999; 276(2 Pt 1):L365–L375.

167. Thurlbeck WM. Postnatal growth and development of the lung. Am Rev Respir Dis 1975; 111(6):803–844.

168. Burri PH. The postnatal growth of the rat lung. 3. Morphology. Anat Rec 1974; 180(1):77–98.

169. Bruce MC, Honaker CE, Cross RJ. Lung fibroblasts undergo apoptosis following alveolarization. Am J Respir Cell Mol Biol 1999; 20(2):228–236.

170. Caduff JH, Fischer LC, Burri PH. Scanning electron microscope study of the developing microvasculature in the postnatal rat lung. Anat Rec 1986; 216(2):154–164.

171. Bosma JF. Functional anatomy of the upper airway during development. In: Mathew OP, Sant'Ambrogio G, eds. Respiratory function of the upper airway. New York: Marcel Dekker, 1988:47–86.

172. Knudson RJ. Physiology of the aging lung. In: Crystal RG, West JB, eds. The Lung: Scientific Foundations. New York: Raven Press, 1991:1749–1759.

173. Boyden EA, Tompsett DH. The changing patterns in the developing lungs of infants. Acta Anat 1965; 61(2):164–192.

174. Martin HB. The effect of aging on the alveolar pores of Kohn in the Dog. Am Rev Respir Dis 1963; 88:773–778.

175. Bhandari A, Bhandari V. Pathogenesis, pathology and pathophysiology of pulmonary sequelae of bronchopulmonary dysplasia in premature infants. Front Biosci 2003; 8:e370–e380.

176. Okajima S, et al. Antenatal dexamethasone administration impairs normal postnatal lung growth in rats. Pediatr Res 2001; 49(6):777–781.

177. Corroyer S, Nabeyrat E, Clement A. Involvement of the cell cycle inhibitor CIPI/WAF1 in lung alveolar epithelial cell growth arrest induced by glucocorticoids. Endocrinology 1997; 138(9):3677–3685.

178. Massaro D, Massaro GD. Invited Review: pulmonary alveoli: formation, the "call for oxygen," and other regulators. Am J Physiol Lung Cell Mol Physiol 2002; 282(3):L345–L358.

179. Morishige WK, Joun NS. Influence of glucocorticoids on postnatal lung development in the rat: possible modulation by thyroid hormone. Endocrinology 1982; 111(5):1587–1594.

180. Morishige WK, Joun NS, Guernsey DL. Thyroidal influence on postnatal lung development in the rat. Endocrinology 1982; 110(2):444–451.

181. Bellabarba D, et al. Triiodothyronine nuclear receptors in liver, brain and lung of neonatal rats. Effect of hypothyroidism and thyroid replacement therapy. Biol Neonate 1984; 45(1):41–48.

182. Ruel J, Coulombe P, Dussault JH. Characterization of nuclear 3,5,3′-triiodothyronine receptors in the developing rat lung: effects of hypo- and hyperthyroidism. Pediatr Res 1982; 16(3):238–242.

183. Massaro D, Teich N, Massaro GD. Postnatal development of pulmonary alveoli: modulation in rats by thyroid hormones. Am J Physiol 1986; 250 (1 Pt 2):R51–R55.

184. Vanhole C, et al. L-Thyroxine treatment of preterm newborns: clinical and endocrine effects. Pediatr Res 1997; 42(1):87–92.

185. Cuestas RA, Lindall A, Engel RR. Low thyroid hormones and respiratory-distress syndrome of the newborn. Studies on cord blood. N Engl J Med 1976; 295(6):297–302.

186. Das RM. The effects of intermittent starvation on lung development in suckling rats. Am J Pathol 1984; 117(2):326–332.

187. Kalenga M. Henquin JC. Protein deprivation from the neonatal period impairs lung development in the rat. Pediatr Res 1987; 22(1):45–49.

188. Blackburn MR, et al. Metabolic consequences of adenosine deaminase deficiency in mice are associated with defects in alveogenesis, pulmonary inflammation, and airway obstruction. J Exp Med 2000; 192(2):159–170.

189. Zachman RD. Role of vitamin A in lung development. J Nutr 1995; 125(6 Suppl):1634S–1638S.

190. McGowan SE, Harvey CS, Jackson SK. Retinoids, retinoic acid receptors, and cytoplasmic retinoid binding proteins in perinatal rat lung fibroblasts. Am J Physiol 1995; 269(4 Pt 1):L463–L472.

191. Ong DE, Chytil F. Changes in levels of cellular retinol- and retinoic-acid-binding proteins of liver and lung during perinatal development of rat. Proc Natl Acad Sci USA 1976; 73(11):3976–3978.

192. Whitney D, et al. Gene expression of cellular retinoid-binding proteins: modulation by retinoic acid and dexamethasone in postnatal rat lung. Pediatr Res 1999; 45(1):2–7.

193. McGowan S, et al. Mice bearing deletions of retinoic acid receptors demonstrate reduced lung elastin and alveolar numbers. Am J Respir Cell Mol Biol 2000; 23(2):162–167.

194. Massaro GD, et al. Retinoic acid receptor-beta: an endogenous inhibitor of the perinatal formation of pulmonary alveoli. Physiol Genomics 2000; 4(1):51–57.

195. Sinha P, et al. Vitamin E deficiency sensitizes alveolar type II cells for apoptosis. Biochim Biophys Acta 2002; 1583(1):91–98.

196. Vitamin B6 deficiency affects lung elastin crosslinking. Nutr Rev 1986; 44(1):24–26.

197. O'Dell BL, et al. The lung of the copper-deficient rat. A model for developmental pulmonary emphysema. Am J Pathol 1978; 91(3):413–432.

198. Freeman BA, Crapo JD. Hyperoxia increases oxygen radical production in rat lungs and lung mitochondria. J Biol Chem 1981; 256(21):10986–10992.

199. Northway WH Jr, Rosan RC, Porter DY. Pulmonary disease following respirator therapy of hyaline-membrane disease. Bronchopulmonary dysplasia. N Engl J Med 1967; 276(7):357–368.

200. Chang LY, et al. A catalytic antioxidant attenuates alveolar structural remodeling in bronchopulmonary dysplasia. Am J Respir Crit Care Med 2003; 167(1):57–64.

201. Burri PH, Weibel ER. Morphometric estimation of pulmonary diffusion capacity. II. Effect of Po_2 on the growing lung, adaption of the growing rat lung to hypoxia and hyperoxia. Respir Physiol 1971; 11(2):247–264.

202. Han RN, et al. Changes in structure, mechanics, and insulin-like growth factor-related gene expression in the lungs of newborn rats exposed to air or 60% oxygen. Pediatr Res 1996; 39(6):921–929.

203. Dauger S, et al. Neonatal exposure to 65% oxygen durably impairs lung architecture and breathing pattern in adult mice. Chest 2003; 123(2):530–538.

204. Randell SH, Mercer RR, Young SL. Postnatal growth of pulmonary acini and alveoli in normal and oxygen-exposed rats studied by serial section reconstructions. Am J Anat 1989; 186(1):55–68.

205. Ahmed MN, et al. Extracellular superoxide dismutase protects lung development in hyperoxia-exposed newborn mice. Am J Respir Crit Care Med 2003; 167(3):400–405.

206. Deng H, Mason SN, Auten RL Jr. Lung inflammation in hyperoxia can be prevented by antichemokine treatment in newborn rats. Am J Respir Crit Care Med 2000; 162(6):2316–2323.

207. Veness-Meehan KA, et al. Retinoic acid attenuates O_2-induced inhibition of lung septation. Am J Physiol Lung Cell Mol Physiol 2002; 283(5):L971–L980.

208. Saran M, Bors W. Oxygen radicals acting as chemical messengers: a hypothesis. Free Radic Res Commun 1989; 7(3–6):213–220.

209. Martindale JL, Holbrook NJ. Cellular response to oxidative stress: signaling for suicide and survival. J Cell Physiol 2002; 192(1):1–15.

210. Sauer H, Wartenberg M, Hescheler J. Reactive oxygen species as intracellular messengers during cell growth and differentiation. Cell Physiol Biochem 2001; 11(4):173–186.

211. Thannickal VJ, Fanburg BL. Reactive oxygen species in cell signaling. Am J Physiol Lung Cell Mol Physiol 2000; 279(6):L1005–L1028.

212. Hensley K, et al. Reactive oxygen species, cell signaling, and cell injury. Free Radic Biol Med 2000; 28(10):1456–1462.

213. Tanswell AK, Olson DM, Freeman BA. Response of fetal rat lung fibroblasts to elevated oxygen concentrations after liposome-mediated augmentation of antioxidant enzymes. Biochim Biophys Acta 1990; 1044(2):269–274.

214. Tanswell AK, Olson DM, Freeman BA. Liposome-mediated augmentation of antioxidant defenses in fetal rat pneumocytes. Am J Physiol 1990; 258(4 Pt 1):L165–L172.

215. Christie NA, et al. A critical role for thiol, but not ATP, depletion in 95% O_2-mediated injury of preterm pneumocytes in vitro. Arch Biochem Biophys 1994; 313(1):131–138.

216. Amstad PA, Krupitza G, Cerutti PA. Mechanism of c-fos induction by active oxygen. Cancer Res 1992; 52(14):3952–3960.

217. Jankov RP, Negus A, Tanswell AK. Antioxidants as therapy in the newborn: some words of caution. Pediatr Res 2001; 50(6):681–687.

218. Luo X, et al. Effect of the 21-aminosteroid U74389G on oxygen-induced free radical production, lipid peroxidation, and inhibition of lung growth in neonatal rats. Pediatr Res 1999; 46(2):215–223.

219. Massaro GD, et al. Postnatal development of lung alveoli: suppression by 13% O_2 and a critical period. Am J Physiol 1990; 258(6 Pt 1):L321–L327.

220. Massaro D. Regulation of alveolar formation. Hosp Pract (Off Ed) 1990; 25(9):81–84, 87–88.

221. Bartlett D Jr, Remmers JE. Effects of high altitude exposure on the lungs of young rats. Respir Physiol 1971; 13(1):116–125.

222. Wert SE, et al. Increased expression of thyroid transcription factor-1 (TTF-1) in respiratory epithelial cells inhibits alveolarization and causes pulmonary inflammation. Dev Biol 2002; 242(2):75–87.

223. Stahlman MT, Gray ME, Whitsett JA. Expression of thyroid transcription factor-1(TTF-1) in fetal and neonatal human lung. J Histochem Cytochem 1996; 44(7):673–678.

224. Kalinichenko VV, et al. Wild-type levels of the mouse Forkhead Box f1 gene are essential for lung repair. Am J Physiol Lung Cell Mol Physiol 2002; 282(6):L1253–L1265.

225. Molkentin JD. The zinc finger-containing transcription factors GATA-4, -5, and -6. Ubiquitously expressed regulators of tissue-specific gene expression. J Biol Chem 2000; 275(50):38949–38952.

226. Caramori G, et al. Expression of GATA family of transcription factors in T-cells, monocytes and bronchial biopsies. Eur Respir J 2001; 18(3):466–473.

227. Maniscalco WM, et al. Increased epithelial cell proliferation in very premature baboons with chronic lung disease. Am J Physiol Lung Cell Mol Physiol 2002; 283(5):L991–L1001.

228. Buch S, et al. Changes in expression of platelet-derived growth factor and its receptors in the lungs of newborn rats exposed to air or 60% O(2). Pediatr Res 2000; 48(4):423–433.

229. Bostrom H, et al. PDGF-A signaling is a critical event in lung alveolar myofibroblast development and alveogenesis. Cell 1996; 85(6):863–873.

230. Lindahl P, et al. Alveogenesis failure in PDGF-A-deficient mice is coupled to lack of distal spreading of alveolar smooth muscle cell progenitors during lung development. Development 1997; 124(20):3943–3953.

231. Li J, Hoyle GW. Overexpression of PDGF-A in the lung epithelium of transgenic mice produces a lethal phenotype associated with hyperplasia of mesenchymal cells. Dev Biol 2001; 239(2):338–349.

232. Hoyle GW, et al. Emphysematous lesions, inflammation, and fibrosis in the lungs of transgenic mice overexpressing platelet-derived growth factor. Am J Pathol 1999; 154(6):1763–1775.

233. Mason RJ, et al. Hepatocyte growth factor is a growth factor for rat alveolar type II cells. Am J Respir Cell Mol Biol 1994; 11(5):561–567.

234. Ware LB, Matthay MA. Keratinocyte and hepatocyte growth factors in the lung: roles in lung development, inflammation, and repair. Am J Physiol Lung Cell Mol Physiol 2002; 282(5):L924–L940.

235. Mason RJ. Hepatocyte growth factor: the key to alveolar septation? Am J Respir Cell Mol Biol 2002; 26(5):517–520.

236. Jakkula M, et al. Inhibition of angiogenesis decreases alveolarization in the developing rat lung. Am J Physiol Lung Cell Mol Physiol 2000; 279(3):L600–L607.

237. Le Cras TD, et al. Treatment of newborn rats with a VEGF receptor inhibitor causes pulmonary hypertension and abnormal lung structure. Am J Physiol Lung Cell Mol Physiol 2002; 283(3):L555–L562.

238. Maniscalco WM, et al. Hyperoxic injury decreases alveolar epithelial cell expression of vascular endothelial growth factor (VEGF) in neonatal rabbit lung. Am J Respir Cell Mol Biol 1997; 16(5):557–567.

239. Maniscalco WM, et al. Angiogenic factors and alveolar vasculature: development and alterations by injury in very premature baboons. Am J Physiol Lung Cell Mol Physiol 2002; 282(4):L811–L823.

240. Bhatt AJ, et al. Disrupted pulmonary vasculature and decreased vascular endothelial growth factor, Flt-1, and TIE-2 in human infants dying with bronchopulmonary dysplasia. Am J Respir Crit Care Med 2001; 164(10 Pt 1):1971–1980.

241. Riley DJ, et al. NHLBI Workshop Summary. Effect of physical forces on lung structure, function, and metabolism. Am Rev Respir Dis 1990; 142(4): 910–914.

242. Zhang S, Garbutt V, McBride JT. Strain-induced growth of the immature lung. J Appl Physiol 1996; 81(4):1471–1476.

243. Mansell AL, et al. Diaphragmatic activity is a determinant of postnatal lung growth. J Appl Physiol 1986; 61(3):1098–1103.

244. DeVries WC, Seaber AV, Sealy WC. Unilateral pulmonary emphysema created by ligation of the left pulmonary artery in newborn puppies. Ann Thorac Surg 1979; 27(2):154–160.

245. Wirtz HR, Dobbs LG. Calcium mobilization and exocytosis after one mechanical stretch of lung epithelial cells. Science 1990; 250(4985): 1266–1269.

246. Vlahakis NE, et al. Deformation-induced lipid trafficking in alveolar epithelial cells. Am J Physiol Lung Cell Mol Physiol 2001; 280(5):L938–L946.

247. Edwards YS, et al. Cyclic stretch induces both apoptosis and secretion in rat alveolar type II cells. FEBS Lett 1999; 448(1):127–130.

248. Dobbs LG, Gutierrez JA. Mechanical forces modulate alveolar epithelial phenotypic expression. Comp Biochem Physiol A Mol Integr Physiol 2001; 129(1):261–266.

249. Wirtz HR, Dobbs LG. The effects of mechanical forces on lung functions. Respir Physiol 2000; 119(1):1–17.

250. Sanderson MJ, Dirksen ER. Mechanosensitivity of cultured ciliated cells from the mammalian respiratory tract: implications for the regulation of mucociliary transport. Proc Natl Acad Sci USA 1986; 83(19):7302–7306.

251. Isakson BE, Evans WH, Boitano S. Intercellular Ca^{2+} signaling in alveolar epithelial cells through gap junctions and by extracellular ATP. Am J Physiol Lung Cell Mol Physiol 2001; 280(2):L221–L228.

252. Boitano S, Dirksen ER, Sanderson MJ. Intercellular propagation of calcium waves mediated by inositol trisphosphate. Science 1992; 258(5080):292–295.

253. Waters CM, et al. Mechanical stretching of alveolar epithelial cells increases Na(+)–K(+)–ATPase activity. J Appl Physiol 1999; 87(2):715–721.

254. Savla U, Sporn PH, Waters CM. Cyclic stretch of airway epithelium inhibits prostanoid synthesis. Am J Physiol 1997; 273(5 Pt 1):L1013–L1019.

255. Breen EC. Mechanical strain increases type I collagen expression in pulmonary fibroblasts in vitro. J Appl Physiol 2000; 88(1):203–209.

256. Breen EC, Fu Z, Normand H. Calcyclin gene expression is increased by mechanical strain in fibroblasts and lung. Am J Respir Cell Mol Biol 1999; 21(6):746–752.

257. Waters CM, et al. Mechanical forces alter growth factor release by pleural mesothelial cells. Am J Physiol 1997; 272(3 Pt 1):L552–L557.

258. Waters CM, et al. Shear stress alters pleural mesothelial cell permeability in culture. J Appl Physiol 1996; 81(1):448–458.

259. Yoder BA, Anwar MU, Clark RH. Early prediction of neonatal chronic lung disease: a comparison of three scoring methods. Pediatr Pulmonol 1999; 27(6):388–394.

260. Bolt RJ, et al. Glucocorticoids and lung development in the fetus and preterm infant. Pediatr Pulmonol 2001; 32(1):76–91.

261. Jobe AH, Ikegami M. Mechanisms initiating lung injury in the preterm. Early Hum Dev 1998; 53(1):81–94.

262. Margraf LR, et al. Morphometric analysis of the lung in bronchopulmonary dysplasia. Am Rev Respir Dis 1991; 143(2):391–400.

263. Husain AN, Siddiqui NH, Stocker JT. Pathology of arrested acinar development in postsurfactant bronchopulmonary dysplasia. Hum Pathol 1998; 29(7):710–717.

264. Carlton DP, et al. Lung overexpansion increases pulmonary microvascular protein permeability in young lambs. J Appl Physiol 1990; 69(2):577–583.

265. Dreyfuss D, et al. High inflation pressure pulmonary edema. Respective effects of high airway pressure, high tidal volume, and positive end-expiratory pressure. Am Rev Respir Dis 1988; 137(5):1159–1164.

266. Manning HL. Peak airway pressure: why the fuss? Chest 1994; 105(1): 242–247.

267. Parker JC, Hernandez LA, Peevy KJ. Mechanisms of ventilator-induced lung injury. Crit Care Med 1993; 21(1):131–143.

268. Tremblay L, et al. Injurious ventilatory strategies increase cytokines and c-fos m-RNA expression in an isolated rat lung model. J Clin Invest 1997; 99(5):944–952.

269. Adkins WK, et al. Age effects susceptibility to pulmonary barotrauma in rabbits. Crit Care Med 1991; 19(3):390–393.

270. Pohlandt F, et al. Decreased incidence of extra-alveolar air leakage or death prior to air leakage in high versus low rate positive pressure ventilation: results of a randomised seven-centre trial in preterm infants. Eur J Pediatr 1992; 151(12):904–909.

271. Meredith KS, et al. Role of lung injury in the pathogenesis of hyaline membrane disease in premature baboons. J Appl Physiol 1989; 66(5):2150–2158.

272. Carlo WA, et al. Minimal ventilation to prevent bronchopulmonary dysplasia in extremely-low-birth-weight infants. J Pediatr 2002; 141(3):370–374.

273. Rodeberg DA, et al. Decreased pulmonary barotrauma with the use of volumetric diffusive respiration in pediatric patients with burns: the 1992 Moyer Award. J Burn Care Rehabil 1992; 13(5):506–511.

274. Bland RD, et al. Chronic lung injury in preterm lambs: abnormalities of the pulmonary circulation and lung fluid balance. Pediatr Res 2000; 48(1):64–74.

275. Scott CD, Ballesteros M, Baxter RC. Increased expression of insulin-like growth factor-II/mannose-6- phosphate receptor in regenerating rat liver. Endocrinology 1990; 127(5):2210–2216.

276. Stiles AD, et al. Relation of kidney tissue somatomedin-C/insulin-like growth factor I to postnephrectomy renal growth in the rat. Endocrinology 1985; 117(6):2397–2401.

277. Stiles AD, D'Ercole AJ. The insulin-like growth factors and the lung. Am J Respir Cell Mol Biol 1990; 3(2):93–100.

278. Perkett EA. et al. Insulin-like growth factor I and pulmonary hypertension induced by continuous air embolization in sheep. Am J Respir Cell Mol Biol 1992; 6(1):82–87.

279. Han RN, et al. Insulin-like growth factor-I and type I insulin-like growth factor receptor in 85% O_2-exposed rat lung. Am J Physiol 1996; 271(1 Pt 1): L139–L149.

280. Veness-Meehan KA, et al. Re-emergence of a fetal pattern of insulin-like growth factor expression during hyperoxic rat lung injury. Am J Respir Cell Mol Biol 1997; 16(5):538–548.

281. Price WA, et al. Relation between serum insulinlike growth factor-1, insulin-like growth factor binding protein-2, and insulinlike growth factor binding protein-3 and nutritional intake in premature infants with bronchopulmonary dysplasia. J Pediatr Gastroenterol Nutr 2001; 32(5):542–549.

282. Chadelat K, et al. Expression of insulin-like growth factors and their binding proteins by bronchoalveolar cells from children with and without interstitial lung disease. Eur Respir J 1998; 11(6):1329–1336.

283. Korfhagen TR, et al. Respiratory epithelial cell expression of human transforming growth factor-alpha induces lung fibrosis in transgenic mice. J Clin Invest 1994; 93(4):1691–1699.

284. Hardie WD, et al. Dose-dependent lung remodeling in transgenic mice expressing transforming growth factor-alpha. Am J Physiol Lung Cell Mol Physiol 2001; 281(5):L1088–L1094.

285. Waheed S, et al. Transforming growth factor alpha (TGF(alpha)) is increased during hyperoxia and fibrosis. Exp Lung Res 2002; 28(5):361–372.

286. Vivekananda J, et al. Acute inflammatory injury in the lung precipitated by oxidant stress induces fibroblasts to synthesize and release transforming growth factor-alpha. J Biol Chem 1994; 269(40):25057–25061.

287. Stahlman MT, Orth DN, Gray ME. Immunocytochemical localization of epidermal growth factor in the developing human respiratory system and in acute and chronic lung disease in the neonate. Lab Invest 1989; 60(4): 539–547.

288. Strandjord TP, et al. Immunolocalization of transforming growth factor-alpha, epidermal growth factor (EGF), and EGF-receptor in normal and injured developing human lung. Pediatr Res 1995; 38(6):851–856.

289. Antoniades HN, et al. Platelet-derived growth factor in idiopathic pulmonary fibrosis. J Clin Invest 1990; 86(4):1055–1064.

290. Marinelli WA, et al. Role of platelet-derived growth factor in pulmonary fibrosis. Am J Respir Cell Mol Biol 1991; 5(6):503–504.

291. Vignaud JM, et al. Presence of platelet-derived growth factor in normal and fibrotic lung is specifically associated with interstitial macrophages, while both interstitial macrophages and alveolar epithelial cells express the c- sis proto-oncogene. Am J Respir Cell Mol Biol 1991; 5(6):531–538.

292. Brody AR. Control of lung fibroblast proliferation by macrophage-derived platelet- derived growth factor. Ann N Y Acad Sci 1994; 725:193–199.

293. Powell PP, Wang CC, Jones R. Differential regulation of the genes encoding platelet-derived growth factor receptor and its ligand in rat lung during microvascular and alveolar wall remodeling in hyperoxia. Am J Respir Cell Mol Biol 1992; 7(3):278–285.

294. Fabisiak JP, Evans JN, Kelley J. Increased expression of PDGF-B (c-sis) mRNA in rat lung precedes DNA synthesis and tissue repair during chronic hyperoxia. Am J Respir Cell Mol Biol 1989; 1(3):181–189.

295. Hertz MI, et al. Obliterative bronchiolitis after lung transplantation: a fibroproliferative disorder associated with platelet-derived growth factor. Proc Natl Acad Sci USA 1992; 89(21):10385–10389.

296. Buch S, et al. Basic fibroblast growth factor and growth factor receptor gene expression in 85% O_2-exposed rat lung. Am J Physiol 1995; 268(3 Pt 1): L455–L464.

297. Moscatelli D, Flaumenhaft R, Saksela O. Interaction of basic fibroblast growth factor with extracellular matrix and receptors. Ann NY Acad Sci 1991; 638:177–181.

298. Henke C, et al. Macrophage production of basic fibroblast growth factor in the fibroproliferative disorder of alveolar fibrosis after lung injury. Am J Pathol 1993; 143(4):1189–1199.

299. Leslie CC, McCormick-Shannon K, Mason RJ. Heparin-binding growth factors stimulate DNA synthesis in rat alveolar type II cells. Am J Respir Cell Mol Biol 1990; 2(1):99–106.

300. Yanagita K, et al. Lung may have an endocrine function producing hepatocyte growth factor in response to injury of distal organs. Biochem Biophys Res Commun 1992; 182(2):802–809.

301. Sporn MB, Roberts AB. The transforming growth factor-betas: past, present, and future. Ann NY Acad Sci 1990; 593:1–6.

302. Williams AO, Flanders KC, Saffiotti U. Immunohistochemical localization of transforming growth factor-beta 1 in rats with experimental silicosis, alveolar type II hyperplasia, and lung cancer. Am J Pathol 1993; 142(6):1831–1840.

303. Khalil N, et al. Regulation of type II alveolar epithelial cell proliferation by TGF- beta during bleomycin-induced lung injury in rats. Am J Physiol 1994; 267(5 Pt 1):L498–L507.

304. Perdue TD, Brody AR. Distribution of transforming growth factor-beta 1, fibronectin smooth muscle actin in asbestos-induced pulmonary fibrosis in rats. J Histochem Cytochem 1994; 42(8):1061–1070.

305. Denis M, Ghadirian E. Transforming growth factor-beta is generated in the course of hypersensitivity pneumonitis: contribution to collagen synthesis. Am J Respir Cell Mol Biol 1992; 7(2):156–160.

306. Moore AM, et al. Altered expression of type I collagen, TGF-beta 1, and related genes in rat lung exposed to 85% O_2. Am J Physiol 1995; 268(1 Pt 1): L78–L84.

307. Khalil N, et al. Enhanced expression and immunohistochemical distribution of transforming growth factor-beta in idiopathic pulmonary fibrosis. Chest 1991; 99(3 suppl):65S–66S.

308. Khalil N, et al. Macrophage production of transforming growth factor beta and fibroblast collagen synthesis in chronic pulmonary inflammation. J Exp Med 1989; 170(3):727–737.

309. Giri SN, Hyde DM, Hollinger MA. Effect of antibody to transforming growth factor beta on bleomycin induced accumulation of lung collagen in mice. Thorax 1993; 48(10):959–966.

310. Grande J, et al. Transforming growth factor-beta 1 induces collagen IV gene expression in NIH-3T3 cells. Lab Invest 1993; 69(4):387–395.

311. Katchman SD, et al. Transforming growth factor-beta up-regulates human elastin promoter activity in transgenic mice. Biochem Biophys Res Commun 1994; 203(1):485–490.

312. Maniscalco WM, Campbell MH. Transforming growth factor-beta induces a chondroitin sulfate/dermatan sulfate proteoglycan in alveolar type II cells. Am J Physiol 1994; 266(6 Pt 1):L672–L680.

313. Raghow B, Irish P, Kang AH. Coordinate regulation of transforming growth factor beta gene expression and cell proliferation in hamster lungs undergoing bleomycin-induced pulmonary fibrosis. J Clin Invest 1989; 84(6):1836–1842.

314. Caniggia I, et al. Spatial and temporal differences in fibroblast behavior in fetal rat lung. Am J Physiol 1991; 261(6 Pt 1):L424–L433.

315. Perrella MA, et al. Transforming growth factor-beta 1, but not dexamethasone, down-regulates nitric-oxide synthase mRNA after its induction by interleukin-1 beta in rat smooth muscle cells. J Biol Chem 1994; 269(20): 14595–14600.

316. Goureau O, et al. Differential regulation of inducible nitric oxide synthase by fibroblast growth factors and transforming growth factor beta in bovine retinal pigmented epithelial cells: inverse correlation with cellular proliferation. Proc Natl Acad Sci USA 1993; 90(9):4276–4280.

317. Sunday ME, et al. Gastrin-releasing peptide (mammalian bombesin) gene expression in health and disease. Lab Invest 1988; 59(1):5–24.

318. Aldenborg F, et al. Mast cells and biogenic amines in radiation-induced pulmonary fibrosis. Am J Respir Cell Mol Biol 1993; 8(1):112–117.

319. Giaid A, et al. Expression of endothelin-1 in lungs of patients with cryptogenic fibrosing alveolitis. Lancet 1993; 341(8860):1550–1554.

320. Komuro I, et al. Endothelin stimulates c-fos and c-myc expression and proliferation of vascular smooth muscle cells. FEBS Lett 1988; 238(2):249–252.

321. Cucina A, et al. Autocrine production of basic fibroblast growth factor translated from novel synthesized mRNA mediates thrombin-induced mitogenesis in smooth muscle cells. Cell Biochem Funct 2002; 20(1):39–46.

322. Perkett EA. Role of growth factors in lung repair and diseases. Curr Opin Pediatr 1995; 7(3):242–249.

323. Bitterman PB, Polunovsky VA, Ingbar DH. Repair after acute lung injury. Chest 1994; 105(3 suppl):118S–121S.

324. Uhal BD. Apoptosis in lung fibrosis and repair. Chest 2002; 122(6 Suppl): 293S–298S.

325. Haslett C. Granulocyte apoptosis and its role in the resolution and control of lung inflammation. Am J Respir Crit Care Med 1999; 160(5 Pt 2):S5–S11.

326. Mecklenburgh K, et al. Role of neutrophil apoptosis in the resolution of pulmonary inflammation. Monaldi Arch Chest Dis 1999; 54(4):345–349.

327. Oei J, et al. Decreased neutrophil apoptosis in tracheal fluids of preterm infants at risk of chronic lung disease. Arch Dis Child Fetal Neonatal Ed 2003; 88(3):F245–F249.

328. Bardales RH, et al. Apoptosis is a major pathway responsible for the resolution of type II pneumocytes in acute lung injury. Am J Pathol 1996; 149(3) 845–852.

329. Laros CD, Westermann CJ. Dilatation, compensatory growth, or both after pneumonectomy during childhood and adolescence. A thirty-year follow-up study. J Thorac Cardiovasc Surg 1987; 93(4):570–576.

330. Arnup ME, et al. Dynamic lung function in dogs with compensatory lung growth. J Appl Physiol 1984; 57(5):1569–1576.

331. Cagle PT, Thurlbeck WM. Postpneumonectomy compensatory lung growth. Am Rev Respir Dis 1988; 138(5):1314–1326.

332. Burri PH, Sehovic S. The adaptive response of the rat lung after bilobectomy. Am Rev Respir Dis 1979; 119(5):769–777.

333. Holmes C, Thurlbeck WM. Normal lung growth and response after pneumonectomy in rats at various ages. Am Rev Respir Dis 1979; 120(5):1125–1136.

334. Das RM, Thurlbeck WM. The events in the contralateral lung following pneumonectomy in the rabbit. Lung 1979; 156(3):165–172.

335. Rannels DE, White DM, Watkins CA. Rapidity of compensatory lung growth following pneumonectomy in adult rats. J Appl Physiol 1979; 46(2):326–333.

336. Watkins CA. Burkhart LR, Rannels DE. Lung growth in response to unilateral pneumonectomy in rapidly growing rats. Am J Physiol 1985; 248(2 Pt 1): E162–E169.

337. Kuboi S, et al. DNA synthesis and related enzymes altered in compensatory lung growth in rats. Scand J Clin Lab Invest 1992; 52(7):707–715.

338. Thet LA, Law DJ. Changes in cell number and lung morphology during early postpneumonectomy lung growth. J Appl Physiol 1984; 56(4):975–978.

339. Brody JS, Burki R, Kaplan N. Deoxyribonucleic acid synthesis in lung cells during compensatory lung growth after pneumonectomy. Am Rev Respir Dis 1978; 117(2):307–316.

340. Gilbert KA, Rannels DE. Increased lung inflation induces gene expression after pneumonectomy. Am J Physiol 1998; 275(1 Pt 1):L21–L29.

341. Dubaybo BA, Bayasi G, Rubeiz GJ. Changes in tumor necrosis factor in postpneumonectomy lung growth. J Thorac Cardiovasc Surg 1995; 110(2): 396–404.

342. Thurlbeck WM, D-Ercole AJ, Smith BT. Serum somatomedin C concentrations following pneumonectomy. Am Rev Respir Dis 1984; 130(3):499–500.

343. Price WA, et al. Expression of the insulin-like growth factor system in postpneumonectomy lung growth. Exp Lung Res 1998; 24(2):203–217.

344. Nobuhara KK, et al. Insulin-like growth factor-I gene expression in three models of accelerated lung growth. J Pediatr Surg 1998; 33(7):1057–1060; discussion 1061.

345. Sugahara K, et al. Elevation of serum human hepatocyte growth factor (HGF) level in patients with pneumonectomy during a perioperative period. Intensive Care Med 1998; 24(5):434–437.
346. Sakamaki Y, et al. Hepatocyte growth factor stimulates proliferation of respiratory epithelial cells during postpneumonectomy compensatory lung growth in mice. Am J Respir Cell Mol Biol 2002; 26(5):525–533.
347. Yuan S, et al. A role for platelet-derived growth factor-BB in rat postpneumonectomy compensatory lung growth. Pediatr Res 2002; 52(1):25–33.
348. Kaza AK, et al. Keratinocyte growth factor enhances post-pneumonectomy lung growth by alveolar proliferation. Circulation 2002; 106(12 suppl 1): I120–I124.
349. Leuwerke SM, et al. Inhibition of compensatory lung growth in endothelial nitric oxide synthase-deficient mice. Am J Physiol Lung Cell Mol Physiol 2002; 282(6):L1272–L1278.
350. Jankov RP, et al. Fibroblast growth factor receptor-1 and neonatal compensatory lung growth after exposure to 95% oxygen. Am J Respir Crit Care Med 2003; 167(11):1554–1561.

3

Acute Lung Injury: Etiologies and Basic Features

PAUL R. KNIGHT and ALEXANDRE T. ROTTA

Departments of Anesthesiology and Microbiology, State University of New York (SUNY) at Buffalo, Buffalo, New York, U.S.A.

I. Overview

Acute lung injury is characterized by the rapid onset of a severe inflammatory response that contributes to cell and tissue injury, abnormal lung compliance, and impaired gas exchange. This chapter describes the multiple etiologies and clinical relevance of acute lung injury, with an emphasis on basic pathophysiological principles, processes, and pathways. Basic concepts of pulmonary epithelial, endothelial, and interstitial injury are presented and discussed. Pathophysiological processes such as lung edema formation, vascular abnormalities, and surfactant dysfunction in acute injury are also introduced, with more detailed discussion on these phenomena given later in Chapters 7–9. A conceptual overview of inflammatory mediators important in acute lung injury is also provided, with additional details on mediator activity and cell recruitment discussed in the following chapter. In addition to summarizing basic concepts of acute lung injury and inflammation, the present chapter defines clinical acute lung injury (ALI) and the acute respiratory distress syndrome (ARDS). These clinical syndromes are associated with severe acute respiratory failure in patients of all ages (infants to adults). Coverage here focuses primarily on the etiologies, pathological features, and clinical course of ALI/ARDS.

Therapeutic considerations for ALI/ARDS are also noted, with more detailed discussion about lung-injury therapies given later in Chapters 13–19.

II. Introduction to Acute Lung Injury

In order to promote gas exchange, the lungs minimize diffusion resistance via a very thin barrier between the external environment and the pulmonary vasculature, the so-called alveolar capillary membrane (ACM). The ACM consists of a two cell layers (endothelial and epithelial) separated by fused basal lamina. The epithelial side represents the largest surface area of the body in contact with the external environment, and the entire cardiac output passes by the endothelial surface. As a result of this anatomical organization, the lungs can be exposed both directly to environmental injurious agents via the airways, as well as bear the full brunt of systemic insults that can damage the microvascular integrity of organs. Fortunately, the pulmonary system has evolved a sophisticated system of defenses designed to effectively remove and/or limit damage caused by these insults, and effectively and rapidly institute repairs. However, significant lung injury can result when the capacity of pulmonary defense mechanisms is overwhelmed by the magnitude of the exposure to the inciting agent. Additionally, the relative capacity of the lung to maintain the integrity of the ACM by removing and/or limiting injurious insults may also be reduced by concurrent morbidities. Similarly, reparative processes may also become dysfunctional as a result of preexisting pulmonary injury or systemic disease.

Acute lung injury becomes manifest when functional impairment in respiratory ability rapidly appears. This is realized as a decrease in the efficiency of gas exchange at the ACM and is associated with an increase in the work of breathing, with or without hypoxemia and/or hypercarbia. Generalized acute lung injury should not be confused with the specific clinical syndrome of ALI bearing the same name. This clinical syndrome is characterized by a sudden, severe inflammatory response resulting in hypoxemia and loss of lung compliance in association with diverse direct (airway-delivered) and/or indirect (circulatory-delivered) etiologies. Acute lung injury, and its more severe form known as the acute respiratory distress syndrome, are functional definitions based on arterial oxygenation derangements and compatible x-ray findings. These syndromes have a high mortality (30–40%) and significant morbidity, and are frequently associated with multiorgan system failure. While the clinical designations of ALI and ARDS can be useful, they have unfortunately also been responsible for a "one-size-fits-all" approach to therapy that has been shown, on occasion, to be detrimental. This is because it is somewhat unrealistic to try to lump a widely diverse set of clinical conditions resulting from trauma, sepsis, gastric aspiration, bacterial aspiration, pulmonary viral infections such as

Hantavirus-induced ARDS (HARDS), smoke inhalation, near drowning, and a variety of other etiologies into a unified theory of pathogenesis.

In spite of the above caveat, discussion in this chapter does utilize functional definitions of clinical ALI and ARDS. However, also emphasized is an understanding of the pathogenesis of the underlying specific etiologies of ALI/ARDS, and of differences in inflammatory patterns related to these etiologies and to temporal factors that need to be taken into account in managing patients. In addition, the importance of added iatrogenic injury in patients with ALI/ARDS needs to be appreciated. Several advances in symptomatic therapy for these conditions have resulted from elimination of iatrogenic contributions to lung injury related to mechanical ventilation and other intensive care support. As a result, mortality from ALI/ARDS has decreased since the initial description of these syndromes, although it still remains unacceptably high.

Unfortunately, therapies aimed at specific aspects of the underlying inflammatory pathology of ALI/ARDS have thus far been largely unsuccessful. As detailed in later chapters, a variety of individual therapeutic strategies have been tested, including anti-inflammatory agents (e.g., steroids), inhaled nitric oxide (NO), antioxidant strategies, surfactant replacement, blockade of cytokines and the arachidonic acid cascade, antibacterial agents, and endotoxin blockade in sepsis. Recently, trials involving activated protein C show promise for reducing sepsis-associated lung injury suggesting that manipulation of the coagulation cascade may also be efficacious. However, to date none of these approaches have had a large impact on the mortality of patients with ALI/ARDS. Nonetheless, the conceptual rationale underlying many of these therapies is sound, and their relative lack of efficacy may reflect the multifactoral nature of inflammatory lung injury and the need for combined-modality interventions. Important breakthroughs in improving outcomes for patients with ALI/ARDS should be associated with continuing improvements in subgroup diagnosis to allow more specific management, as well as the use of optimal combinations of therapeutic interventions and agents directed at multiple aspects of the pathogenesis of disease (Chapters 13–19).

III. Overview of the Inflammatory Response

As stated previously, the lungs have evolved a number of sophisticated mechanisms that effectively block the access of infectious and noninfectious environmental contaminants, or remove and/or limit damage if initial barriers are breached. Structural defenses include the specific action of the glottis, the cough reflex, airway secretions, and the ascending mucociliary clearance system. The sentinel macrophages of the airways and alveoli represent the major phagocytic resident cells of the lung. In the setting of a low burden of airborne particles or micro-organisms, these cells in conjunction with the mucociliary system can rapidly remove material deposited on the surface of the respiratory tract. However, if this burden overcomes the capacity of resident cells to deal with the condition, as can occur with aspiration of gastric material or pathogenic bacteria, activation of additional nonspecific mechanisms becomes important. These mechanisms involve direct activity against injurious agents or micro-organisms, as well as promoting the recruitment of additional leukocytes. The activation and totality of these mechanisms constitutes the pulmonary inflammatory response.

In general terms, the *inflammatory response* is defined as a nonspecific defensive reaction of the body to invasion by a foreign substance or organism that involves phagocytosis by white blood cells and is often accompanied by pus (cellular liquefaction in a neutrophil-rich exudate) and an increase in local temperature. It is to be distinguished from the original definition of *inflammation*, which denoted the local tissue response to injury characterized by redness, swelling, pain, and generation of heat (1). In practice, however, the two terms are often used interchangeably. Regardless of semantics, it is important to understand that the pulmonary inflammatory response is, in principle, a protective set of mechanisms for the lungs to return to a preinjury condition or initiate and complete effective repair. There is a tendency in clinical medicine to consider the inflammatory response to be harmful to the body or, at best, as a "double edged sword" of benefit and harm. However, the primary role of this response is to maintain homeostasis under a variety of adverse environmental influences. This may account for why interference with the inflammatory response during therapy has led to long-term problems on a number of occasions.

Three distinct lung-injury patterns can directly initiate pulmonary inflammation: 1) responses to caustic physical insults; 2) responses to foreign bodies; and 3) responses involving host antimicrobial defense. Low pH gastric aspiration, inhalation of toxic fumes, and trauma are examples of physical insults that directly damage pulmonary tissue (2). In this scenario, the major goal of the inflammatory response is to limit tissue damage, repair injured tissue, and remove irreversibly damaged tissue. Responses related to the removal of foreign bodies represent a second important homeostatic function of pulmonary inflammation. The pulmonary system is constantly being barraged by environmental particulate material. Additionally, microaspiration of food particulate material is a common occurrence in several subpopulations of patients (3). While some of these inhaled particles can be directly toxic to pulmonary cells, most are not. The major goal of the pulmonary system in this scenario is to remove these foreign bodies and repair any secondary injury. Major differences between particulate (foreign body) and caustic physical injuries are that the latter are generally associated with immediate tissue damage but tend to be more transient. Caustic insults may need detoxification (e.g., buffering of low pH), but the major objective is to repair the damage after terminating direct toxicity. Conversely, particulate material often does not cause immediate tissue damage, but the offending insult can be more difficult to expel physically. Thus, removal of foreign particles is initially a higher priority of this aspect of the inflammatory response. In some cases, removal is not possible, and "walling off" the particular material via granuloma formation is the best the inflammatory response can do.

The final important aspect of the pulmonary inflammatory response relates to host antimicrobial defense. Depending on the pathogen (e.g., bacteria, virus, parasite), the innate nonadaptive antimicrobial function of the pulmonary inflammatory response plays an important role in defense of the lungs by killing and eliminating micro-organisms. This aspect of the pulmonary inflammatory response plays essential roles in initiating and interacting with adaptive immune responses (Fig. 1) (4,5). As with noninfectious particulate material, the resulting antimicrobial inflammatory response can also "wall off" injurious pathogens from unaffected regions of the lungs.

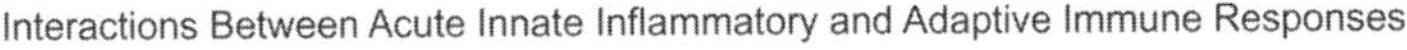
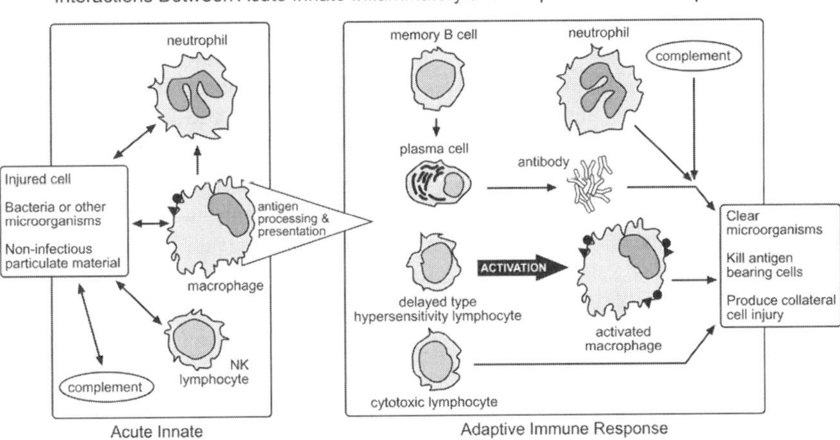

Figure 1 Interactions between the acute innate inflammatory and the adaptive immune responses. In the innate nonadaptive inflammatory response, effector cells like macrophages and neutrophils are recruited and activated directly or indirectly by signals generated as a result of cellular injury, as well as by noninfectious and infectious products. These cells phagocytize, produce toxic products, and initiate repair based on the stimuli present. Following phagocytosis, macrophages also can process antigens and present them to lymphocytes, which are part of the adaptive immune response. Antigen-specific lymphocytes can be directly cytotoxic, act indirectly via secretion of antibody, or activate macrophages and neutrophils to destroy bacteria or viral antigen bearing cells. These responses benefit the organism, but can also cause collateral damage to the lungs and other organs.

How does the totality of the remarkable pulmonary inflammatory response perform and regulate the large number of necessary tasks associated with maintaining lung homeostasis? Conceptually, the pulmonary inflammatory response can be likened to an orchestra playing a musical piece with multiple movements. The selection of the score to be played is dependent on the inciting cause. The multiple arms of the inflammatory response can be likened to the different groups of instruments present in the orchestra. Although there is a beginning and an end to any musical piece, the specific manner in which the conductor organizes and utilizes different groups of instruments varies substantially, and is analogous to the multiple varieties in which the inflammatory response can respond to a pulmonary insult. To torture the analogy further, poor orchestration, lack of timing, or a weak performance by the musicians can lead to discordant music. Similarly, dysfunction of one or more arms of the inflammatory response can lead to impairment of primary functions and, in many cases, exacerbate lung injury due to an inability of the system to maintain homeostasis.

Consistent with the above, several interacting pathways are important in the initiation and progression of pulmonary inflammatory responses. One important set of pathways involves direct local responses to tissue injury. Damaged tissue releases proteases and other peptides that activate proinflammatory mediators and lead to the hallmark responses of inflammation (6). These include increased blood flow and vascular permeability, as well as recruitment and activation of leukocytes to the site of injury. Such physiologic changes are responsible for removing irreversibly damaged tissue, and instituting the cellular signals required for repair. A second pathway involves direct activation of proinflammatory signals from resident professional cells (i.e., alveolar macrophages) or extracellular mediators (i.e., complement), whose primary functions are the recognition of foreign material and the release of mediators that activate a progressive proinflammatory cascade (7). Although these pathways are distinct, there is a high degree of interaction between them. For example, damaged cells or cellular debris that release inflammatory mediators can also be engulfed by macrophages and stimulate this arm of the initiating pathway plus activate the complement cascade. Similarly, the release of toxic leukocyte products can secondarily cause collateral tissue damage, thereby further activating that pathway. Nonetheless, pulmonary inflammatory responses can have significant qualitative and/or quantitative differences depending on their primary pathway of activation.

Host–parasite interactions that occur with pathogenic microorganisms can also impact the initiation and progression of the subsequent inflammatory response. For example, exposure to, and elimination of, nonpathogenic microbes stimulates an inflammatory pathway similar to a noninfectious inert foreign body response. In some cases, elimination may be easier for microbes since digestion can occur, which is not always the case with inert material. However, pathogenic micro-organisms have also evolved a number of mechanisms by which they can evade innate antimicrobial host defenses (8). Examples of these include virulence factors that inhibit phagocytosis and directly injure or interfere with the effector functions of leukocytes. In response, the host has evolved specific counter measures to these more aggressive infectious agents. Distinct and idiosyncratic mechanisms include specific cellular receptors to microbial antigens, preformed antibodies, direct activation of soluble mediators by bacterial products, and selective activation of multiple pathways (9). Thus, based on the infectious agent, the inflammatory response can be significantly modified by microbial-evolved virulence factors, as well as a number of host-derived counter measures.

In addition to initiating mechanisms that directly activate the inflammatory cascade, indirect pathways can also contribute to pulmonary inflammation. The most notable of these involve "spill over" from responses to systemic insults, with interactions between the cellular and humoral arms of the adaptive immune response and components of the nonadaptive inflammatory response. For example, activation of systemic inflammatory responses as occurs in sepsis may lead to infiltration of leukocytes indiscriminately into various organs including the lung (2). This occurs through direct stimulation of pulmonary vascular endothelial cells leading to increased expression of adhesion molecules required for leukocyte attachment and migration into the pulmonary interstitium and alveoli. Additionally, systemic stimulation of endothelial cells by blood-borne mediators increases leakage of proteinaceous fluids and soluble inflammatory mediators through the capillary endothelium into the lungs. This in turn activates additional proinflammatory responses in epithelial cells lining the alveolar wall and in the capillary endothelium.

Examples of how adaptive pulmonary immune responses can interact with nonadaptive inflammatory system are illustrated in Fig. 1. Activation of the Th$_1$ or cellular arm of the adaptive immune response specifically results in the elaboration of mediators that recruit and activate monocytes. Both cytotoxic lymphocytes and monocytes recruited and activated by lymphocyte-generated mediators can generate intense injury to cells and tissue, which further promote the inflammatory response. Antibodies also are intricately involved with the inflammatory response. Antibody receptors on macrophages and neutrophils specifically enhance phagocytosis and tissue destruction, and the deposition of antigen–antibody complexes in the lung can also be a potent stimulus of the proinflammatory cascade.

The acute pulmonary inflammatory response is initiated, maintained, regulated, and terminated by the actions of soluble inflammatory mediators such as those summarized in Table 1 (also see Chapters 4 and 6). The chemical classes of inflammatory mediators are diverse, and include plasma proteinases (e.g., complement, kinins, clotting factors), lipid mediators

Table 1 Soluble Mediators of Inflammation

Mediators	Major source	Activated by	Inflammatory role
Vasoactive peptides (e.g., histamine, serotonin)	Mast cells, basophils, platelets	IgE, and other physical and chemical stimuli	Vasodilatation, increased vascular permeability
Complement (e.g., C3a, C5a)	Nine soluble forms in blood primarily produced in the liver. Monocytes/macrophages and fibroblasts may produce some components	Antibodies, bacterial products, damaged tissue proteases, plasmin	Augmented phagocytosis, increased vascular permeability, chemotaxis
Kinins (e.g., bradykinin)	Soluble forms in blood	Tissue detritus, bacterial products, activated Factor XII	Vasoconstriction, increased vascular permeability, chemotaxis
Fibrinolytic peptides	Proteolytic cleavage of fibrin	Activation of the clotting cascade	Activation of complement and Factor XII
Prostaglandins	Monocytes/macrophages, neutrophils, endothelial cells, platelets	Bacterial products, antigen–antibody complexes, C3a, kinins, interleukin-1β	Increased body temperature, stimulation of nociceptors, increased vascular permeability
Leukotrienes (e.g., leukotriene B$_4$, leukotrienes C and D)	Leukocytes with metabolic conversion by other cells	Activation of leukocytes	Vasoconstriction, vascular permeability, neutrophil recruitment and activation
Platelet activating factor	Platelets, leukocytes, endothelial cells	Platelet activation	Platelet aggregation, leukocyte recruitment and activation
Cytokines (e.g., TNF-α, IL-1, IL-6, IL-8, MCP-1, IL-12, IFN-γ, IL-4, IL-10)	Resident and recruited leukocytes and structural cells of the lung	Bacteria and particulates, tissue detritus, oxidants, NO, other cytokines	Recruit and activate leukocytes, augment, modulate, and resolve the inflammatory response

(e.g., prostaglandins, leukotrienes, platelet activating factor), amines, and peptides. The latter two classes include vasoactive mediators (e.g., histamine and serotonin), neuropeptides (e.g., substance P), and proinflammatory cytokines like tumor necrosis factor-α (TNF-α), interferon-γ, and interleukins (IL) such as IL-1β, IL-6, IL-8, IL-10, IL-12. Additionally, reactive species of oxygen and NO also play important roles in modulating the inflammatory response. Mediators that are responsible for orchestrating and controlling the inflammatory response are termed chemical regulators of inflammation. These substances can directly increase capillary leakiness, initiate the recruitment and activation of leukocytes by stimulating endothelial–leukocyte interactions (e.g., increase expression of adhesion molecules), provide a chemotactic gradient to direct leukocytes to the target area, and interact with other regulators to enhance or limit their actions.

Mediators that are directly involved in enhancing phagocytosis, killing and/or digesting foreign contaminants and microbes, as well as causing collateral damage to healthy lung tissue, are termed chemical effectors of inflammation (Table 2). For example, there are ~50 toxic products released from activated neutrophils following infiltration into the lung. Most notable of these chemical effectors are reactive species of oxygen and nitrogen (Chapter 7), as well as leukocyte derived serine and matrix metallo-proteinases. Many of the inflammatory mediators have a role as both chemical regulators and effectors. For example, oxidants can cause severe damage to the functional properties of proteins, lipids, and nucleic acids. However, these agents also play a role in stimulating cellular pathways involved in the evolution of the inflammatory response, as well as terminate the action of other inflammatory mediators (i.e., leukotrienes) (10,11). This multiplicity of activites, which can have both beneficial and detrimental consequences, may be one reason why it has been difficult to find clinically effective drugs that antagonize chemical mediators of inflammation.

Cellular components of the inflammatory response can be classified analogous to the chemical inflammatory mediators (a summary of some of the important cells is given in Table 3). The role of regulator cells is to release soluble mediators that control and orchestrate the inflammatory response. Effector cells are directly engaged in eliminating foreign contaminants, microbes, as well as damaged tissue from the lung. These cells are primarily involved in phagocytosis and intracellular digestion, as well as in the release toxic products. The cellular components of the inflammatory response can be further classified as primary or "professional" inflammatory cells and accessory cells. Leukocytes, both resident and newly recruited are the professional cells as this is their major function. The accessory cells such as those of the alveoli capillary wall, as well as those lining the airways also play an important role during inflammation (7). These cells can both regulate the

Table 2 Soluble Chemical Effectors of Inflammation

Effectors	Source	Inflammatory function	Negative side effects
Oxidants	Generated by leukocytes in large amounts following stimulation (oxidative "burst"); also produced by endothelial and respiratory epithelial cells	Kill microbes and cells harboring microbes; activate cell signal pathways involved in the inflammatory response; inactivate some chemoattractants and other toxic products; induce apoptosis	Damage proteins, lipids, and nucleic acids; activate intracellular signal pathways; cause cell death; inactivate antiproteinases
Proteinases	Released from all cells following severe injury; generated by leukocytes following activation	Activate the inflammatory response; play an important role in a number of inflammatory cascades (e.g., complement); digest foreign substances; inactivate inflammatory peptides	Damage connective tissue as well as cell membranes; may inactivate antioxidants
Nitric oxide	Endothelial cells; monocytes/macrophages	Vasorelaxation; kills some microbes; activates cell signal pathways involved in the inflammatory response; scavenges superoxide	Based on conditions, may generate highly toxic reactive nitrogen compounds by combining with superoxide
Antioxidants	All cells	Terminate oxidant activity; protect healthy tissue against oxidant damage	Imbalance may cause dysfunction by altering inflammatory cascades
Antiproteinases	All cells	Terminate proteinase activity; protect healthy tissue against proteinase damage	Imbalance may cause dysfunction by altering inflammatory cascades

Table 3 Resident and Recruited Cells of the Lung Inflammatory Response

Cell type	Chemotactic and activating mediators	Regulatory role in inflammation	Role in inflammation
Neutrophils	Bacterial products, TNF-α, IL-8, GM-CSF, IFN-γ, C5a, LTB$_4$, endothelial adhesion molecules	Release mediators that augment the inflammatory response (e.g., TNF-α, IL-1β, IL-8, GM-CSF)	Phagocytosis; production of oxidants, proteinases, defensins (generate $\sim$50 toxic products)
Monocytes/ macrophages	MCP-1, MIP-1α, IFN-γ, TNF-α, IL-1β (autocrine response)	Resident macrophages are the source of proinflammatory cytokines, as well as prostaglandins and PAF. Promote the switch from acute to chronic inflammation and healing (e.g., IL-10, TGF-β, FGF), and adaptive immunity (antigen presentation)	Phagocytosis; oxidant, NO, and proteinase production; "walling off" insult (granuloma)
Lymphocytes	IL-2, IL-12, IFN-γ, IL-4, IL-10	Release cytokines that augment (IFN-γ) or down-modulate (IL-4, IL-10) the inflammatory response	Release of cytoxins that injure cells; release of preformed antibodies to foreign substance
Eosinophils	Rantes, MIP-1α, eotaxin, histamine	Poorly understood	Release of oxidants and cationic proteins; airway reactivity

(Continued)

Table 3 Resident and Recruited Cells of the Lung Inflammatory Response (*Continued*)

Cell type	Chemotactic and activating mediators	Regulatory role in inflammation	Role in inflammation
Basophils	MCP-1	Preformed TNF-α reservoir	Major source of vasoactive amines
Endothelial cells	TNF-α and IL-1β, oxidants	Express adhesion molecules for leukocyte attachment; ource of cytokines and other mediators that recruit and activate leukocytes	Generation of oxidants; increase of leakiness for leukocyte infiltration and other blood-borne mediators
Epithelial cells	TNF-α and IL-1β, oxidants	Secondary source of cytokines and other mediators that recruit and activate leukocytes	Generation of oxidants, surfactant; barrier function to protect system
Fibroblasts	TNF-α, IL-1β, FGF, TGF-β, oxidants	Secondary source of cytokines and other mediators that recruit and activate leukocytes	Generation of oxidants; "walling off" insult; initial epair to structural damage

inflammatory response and generate some of the chemical effectors. However, these functions are not their major role in the otherwise healthy lung.

Macrophages of the airways and alveoli are the principal professional phagocytes of the lung. These cells have both effector and regulator functions. Their primary role is to phagocytize foreign substances and microbes and eliminate them from the lung. As noted earlier, when the burden is small the resident macrophages can perform this function effectively and eliminate particulate contaminants, as well as kill and digest bacteria. However, when the particulate or microbial load becomes greater than the capacity of the resident macrophages to handle, or the micro-organisms are more pathogenic, or there is direct tissue damage, the recruitment of additional effector cells becomes necessary. Resident macrophages release mediators to facilitate this process. These chemical regulators in turn act by a complex set of mechanisms, which include autocrine stimulation of resident macrophages, plus recruitment and activation of other leukocytes from the circulatory system. Additionally, macrophage-derived products also stimulate other pulmonary cells such as those of the alveolar capillary wall (i.e., alveolar epithelial cells and vascular endothelial cells) to also release additional mediators important in the progression of the inflammatory response (7). Finally, if the offending insult is not eliminated, lymphocytes will release chemical regulators that can enhance (e.g., interferon-γ) or retard (e.g., IL-4, IL-10) the intensity of the inflammatory response, as well as produce chemical effectors (i.e., antibodies) that also interact with other leukocytes to enhance their effector functions.

A. Examples of the Acute Inflammatory Responses in Clinical Lung Injuries of Different Etiology

The following brief descriptions give examples of how clinical conditions involving acute lung injury from different etiologies incorporate the various arms of the inflammatory response (i.e., direct lung injury from gastric aspiration, microbial aspiration, and viral pneumonia, as well as indirect lung injury from sepsis). Each of these insults involve a somewhat different orchestration of the inflammatory response, but all cause acute injury and are risk factors for progression to severe ALI/ARDS in patients. Details about the clinical features and course of ALI/ARDS are given in the next section.

Gastric Aspiration

Gastric aspiration can elicit very different inflammatory responses based on the contents of the stomach at the time of reflux (e.g., pH, type of food, bile salts, bacterial colonization). For example, aspiration of acidic clear fluid causes a transient caustic injury in which the low pH is typically buffered within 60 sec. Experimentally, this is primarily a neutrophil mediated lung injury in which the monocytic response minimal (12,13). Proinflammatory cytokine production is limited. However, both lung and blood leukocytes are "primed" for an additional insult (14). Acutely, there is severe hypoxemia due to extravasation of fluid and serum proteins into the alveoli and surfactant dysfunction (15). Death can occur acutely from massive aspiration, but if the initial insult is tolerated and secondary complications do not arise, resolution is very rapid. Conversely, when low pH gastric contents are combined with food particles, a very severe lung injury arises with an inflammatory response that evolves through the clinical stages of a progressive inflammatory lesion (16–18). Production of both acute inflammatory and chronic inflammatory mediators are robust, as well as infiltration of neutrophils and monocytes into the lung. In this scenario, the risk of developing ALI/ARDS is dramatically increased (19,20). Interestingly, aspiration of food with a high pH does not cause such severe lung injury despite a dramatic acute proinflammatory cytokine response and a large influx of neutrophils and monocytes. If obstruction of airways does not occur, high pH food aspiration is generally well tolerated. This scenario probably occurs frequently in older debilitated patients at night. A major concern with high pH particulate aspiration is asphyxia if obstruction is caused in a major bronchus (21). There is also an increased risk of a secondary infection (22). Finally, although gastric aspiration lung injury is primarily acute, repeated aspiration events can lead to chronic inflammation and fibrotic lung injury.

Microbial Aspiration

Aspiration of extracellular bacterial pathogens elicits similar inflammatory responses as sepsis. However, these responses are primarily protective, eliminating the micro-organisms from the lung and preventing their invasion into the systemic circulation and other organs. Inhibiting acute innate inflammatory/immune responses can actually increase lung injury following bacterial infection due to proliferation of the pathogen. The proinflammatory responses that are elicited by airway inoculation of bacteria are similar to aspiration of food particles, but have several important distinctions (9). First, complement probably plays a more important role both in the magnitude of the response and in clearing the bacteria from the lung. Second, the host usually has a number of defense mechanisms directed against the bacteria that are specific to the type of bacteria involved (i.e., receptors to bacterial products, preformed antibodies). Since the bacteria are replicating, host antimicrobial defenses must not only destroy micro-organisms, but must do so faster than progeny bacteria are being produced in order to clear the pathogen from the lung. Finally, as previously noted, pathogenic bacteria can modify the host antibacterial response by structural components (e.g., capsule), as well as secreted products (i.e., necrotizing or virulence factors) (23). Progressive clinical pneumonia results when, due to the interaction of all these factors, the host cannot clear the bacteria from the lungs. The risk of such an occurrence is greater when host antibacterial mechanisms are impaired, such as secondary to additional underlying disease (e.g., gastric aspiration, viral infection, severe trauma, or sepsis). A bacterial nosocomial lung infection is often the terminal event in ARDS because of increased susceptibility of the patient due to impairment of innate inflammatory/immune pulmonary defense, exposure to very pathogenic micro-organisms in the hospital setting, or both (24–27).

Viral Pneumonia

Viral pneumonia can produce lung injury by the cellular immune (Th$_1$) response (28–30). Furthermore, viral pneumonias predispose the patient to a secondary bacterial pneumonia as a result of impairing the acute inflammatory/immune response (31–33). Not surprisingly, the leading cause of death during an influenza epidemic is secondary bacterial pneumonia (34). Experimentally, inhibiting the intensity of the Th$_1$ cellular immune response to a influenza virus respiratory tract infection decreases the lung injury without significantly impairing the clearance of the virus (29). Additionally, the propensity to develop a secondary bacterial pneumonia is decreased. Viral pneumonia probably leads to progressive lung injury as a result of an underlying disease that impairs the immune system to the extent that the virus cannot be removed or due to secondary complications associated with viral-mediated inflammatory/immune dysfunction.

Sepsis

Sepsis is a systemic disease, but often includes indirect inflammatory lung injury. Experimentally, proinflammatory mediators are increased in the blood rapidly peaking at about 4 hr following exposure to bacterial products. Cytokines including TNFα, IL-1β, IL-6, and IL-8 affect the pulmonary vascular endothelium resulting in expression of leukocyte adhesion molecules and decreases in endothelial cell to cell tight junctions (7). These changes lead to extravasation of serum proteins including albumin and proinflammatory mediators into the interstitial and alveolar spaces. Neutrophils and monocytes rapidly begin attaching to pulmonary microvascular endothelial cells via the newly expressed adhesion molecules following the appearance of bacterial products in the circulation (35). Once in the lung, these cells release toxic mediators that can damage lung tissue, thereby further promoting the inflammatory response and causing cell and tissue injury. The pathogenesis of this inflammatory lung injury progresses as long as the inciting organism(s) is present in the blood and, as detailed later, evolves through different clinical stages of acute (exudative) injury to later fibrosing alveolitis (2).

IV. Clinical ALI and ARDS
A. Functional Definitions

Understanding about clinical ALI and ARDS has increased substantially during the past three decades. The original 1967 description of ARDS by Ashbaugh et al. (36) consisted of adult patients with acute-onset respiratory distress, poor lung compliance, refractory hypoxemia, and diffuse pulmonary infiltrates on chest radiograph. The term "adult" respiratory distress syndrome, coined in their follow up publication (37), persisted for over two decades. This condition is now termed the "acute" respiratory distress syndrome owing to the fact that patients of all ages can be affected. The original definition of ARDS lacked specific criteria required to identify and study patients in a systematic manner, resulting in controversies about its incidence, natural history and mortality, as well as making it difficult to quantify the severity of disease in clinical trials. Murray et al. (38) proposed an expanded functional definition of ARDS with the intent of better characterizing the physiologic respiratory derangement through the use of a lung-injury scoring system. Commonly known as the lung-injury score, this system uses a four-point scoring grid dependent on the degree of infiltration or consolidation evident on chest radiographs, severity of hypoxemia (as a function of the ratio of the partial pressure of arterial oxygen to the fraction of inspired oxygen), respiratory system compliance, and the level of positive end-expiratory pressure (PEEP) (Table 4). A lung-injury score of 0 suggests absence of lung injury, whereas a score greater than 2.5 indicates severe lung injury (i.e., ARDS). When calculated at four to seven days after the onset of respiratory failure, lung-injury scores of 2.5 or higher are predictive of a more complicated clinical course with the need for prolonged mechanical ventilatory support (39). However, although many physicians have embraced this lung-injury scoring system to quantify the severity of acute pulmonary injury, its clinical usefulness is somewhat limited by the lack of predictive value in the first 72 hr following the onset respiratory symptoms (40).

More recently, a simplified definition by the American–European Consensus Conference Committee (41) has gained widespread clinical acceptance (Table 5). The Consensus Committee definition is applicable to patients with disease of acute onset and, unlike the lung-injury score described above, excludes patients with clinical evidence of left atrial hypertension or pulmonary-wedge pressures equal or greater than 18 mmHg. Although patients with hypoxemia and pulmonary infiltrates caused by volume overload and/or heart failure (left atrial hypertension) are excluded from these definitions of ALI and ARDS, it is conceivable that some of these patients may indeed have related injury pathology in addition to hydrostatic edema.

The simplicity of the Consensus definitions of ALI and ARDS classifies patients into two *severity-of-illness* categories that facilitate comparison and grouping of patients in clinical trials. However, the simplicity of these

Table 4 Lung Injury Score[a]

Parameter	Score
Chest roentgenogram	
No alveolar consolidation	0
Alveolar consolidation in one quadrant	1
Alveolar consolidation in two quadrants	2
Alveolar consolidation in three quadrants	3
Alveolar consolidation in four quadrants	4
Hypoxemia score	
$PaO_2/FiO_2 \geq 300$	0
PaO_2/FiO_2 225–299	1
PaO_2/FiO_2 175–224	2
PaO_2/FiO_2 100–174	3
$PaO_2/FiO_2 < 100$	4
Respiratory system compliance (when ventilated) (mL/cm H_2O)	
≥ 80	0
60–79	1
40–59	2
20–39	3
≤ 19	4
Positive end-expiratory pressure (when ventilated) (cm H_2O)	
≤ 5	0
6–8	1
9–11	2
12–14	3
≥ 15	4
Final value	
No lung injury	0
Acute lung injury	0.1–2.5
Severe lung injury (ARDS)	>2.5

[a]Obtained by dividing the aggregate sum by the number of components that were used (38).

definitions can also be a significant limitation. For example, factors such as underlying etiology, presence of multiorgan failure, or even the intensity of ventilatory support employed are not considered. Since the definitions in Table 5 disregard the level of PEEP, a patient could be classified as having ARDS while being ventilated with inappropriately low pressures, or as having ALI when higher levels of PEEP were applied, since this variable affects shunt fraction and oxygenation. Nevertheless, the use of the lung-injury score and the Consensus Committee definitions of ALI/ARDS have been widely accepted clinically, and create a standard definition of the severity of illness to serve as a framework for clinical practice and research. Finally, the application of added pertinent nonlung-injury specific scoring systems, such as the Acute Physiologic and Chronic Health Evaluations II

Table 5 The American–European Consensus Conference Criteria for ALI and ARDS

	Timing	Oxygenation	Chest radiograph	Pulmonary artery occlusion pressure
Criteria for ALI	Acute onset	$PaO_2/FiO_2 \leq 300$ mmHg (regardless of PEEP level)	Bilateral infiltrates on frontal chest radiograph	≤ 18 mmHg or no clinical evidence of left atrial hypertension
Criteria for ARDS	Acute onset	$PaO_2/FiO_2 \leq 200$ Torr (regardless of PEEP level)	Bilateral infiltrates on frontal chest radiograph	≤ 18 mmHg or no clinical evidence of left atrial hypertension

(From Ref. 41.)

(APACHE II) score (42) and the Pediatric Risk of Mortality Score (PRISM) (43), are also useful in the management of patients with ALI/ARDS and can help circumvent some of the limitations inherent to the more simplified definition.

B. Etiologies

ALI and ARDS are not specific diseases, but rather pulmonary manifestations of a broad range of clinical disorders including several already noted in the preceding section. Examples of common conditions encountered in infants, children, and adults that can lead to ALI/ARDS include aspiration of noninfectious gastric contents or bacteria colonizing the oropharynx and gastrointestinal tract, viral respiratory tract infections, near drowning, severe trauma, sepsis and the systemic inflammatory response syndrome (SIRS), and exposure to toxic gases. Etiologies of ALI and ARDS are divided into disorders causing direct lung injury (pulmonary) and those causing indirect lung injury in the setting of a systemic insult (extrapulmonary) in Table 6. This not only provides an organizational structure, but clinical evidence also suggests that these two subsets of etiologies may respond differently to therapeutic interventions (44).

Among all the individual etiologic factors noted in Table 6, sepsis carries the highest risk for ARDS, with as many as 40% of patients developing this syndrome (45). The risk of ARDS is also substantially increased when multiple predisposing disorders, such as aspiration of gastric contents, sepsis, multiple transfusions, or pulmonary contusions, are manifested in

Table 6 Clinical Disorders Associated with the Development of ALI and ARDS

Direct lung injury (pulmonary)	Indirect lung injury (extrapulmonary)
Common causes	
Aspiration of gastric contents	Sepsis, SIRS
Pneumonia	Severe trauma with shock
Less common causes	
Near drowning	Acute pancreatitis
Inhalational injuries	Transfusion of blood products
Pulmonary contusion	Drug overdose and toxins
Pulmonary embolic disorders	Anaphylaxis
Reperfusion injury (postlung transplantation, postembolectomy, postarrest)	Extracorporeal membrane oxygenation and cardiopulmonary bypass
Thoracic radiotherapy	Decompression sickness
	Heat stroke

an individual patient (20). For example, the risk of developing ARDS associated with just one factor (25%) has been reported to be compounded by the presence of two (42%) and three (85%) simultaneous factors, and this was more predictive of ARDS than the injury severity score or initial arterial oxygenation (20).

C. Pathophysiology
Alveolar Epithelial Injury

Knowledge of basic lung structure and alveolar cell types is important for understanding the pathophysiology of direct pulmonary epithelial injury caused by aspiration of gastric contents, inhalation of high-temperature gases, or other etiologies in Table 6 (46–48). The respiratory epithelium is composed of type I cells and type II cells, which cover approximately 90% and 10%, respectively, of the alveolar surface area. Type I cells provide the thin barrier between the alveolar space and the interstitium, and are often the primary target of direct alveolar epithelial injury. The epithelial barrier formed by type I cells is much less permeable than the endothelial barrier and, therefore, plays a major role in preventing fluid movement into the alveolus (49). Type II cells are cuboidal and somewhat more resistant to direct injury. Type II cells are responsible for surfactant production and play a significant role in ion transport and fluid removal from the alveolar space. These cells are also capable of differentiating into type I cells following epithelial injury, an important mechanism of alveolar epithelial repair. In addition to direct inhalational insult, the alveolar epithelium is also the target of injury from inflammation and oxidative insult from the adjacent interstitium.

Injury to type I and type II cells has a number of consequences central to the genesis of ALI/ARDS and the onset of respiratory failure (Fig. 2). The loss of epithelial integrity and disrupted junctions between type I cells allow protein-rich plasma to flood the alveolus, creating a barrier for the diffusion of gases and interfering with normal alveolar dynamics due to inactivation of surfactant (50). Surfactant function is further impaired by the action of proteolytic enzymes released by the dense inflammatory infiltrate in ARDS (51). In addition, the surfactant system can be further affected by injury or alteration of type II cells, which decrease the production and turnover of surfactant (52). A complete discussion of surfactant dysfunction and its mechanisms in acute pulmonary injury is given in Chapter 9. Injury to alveolar epithelial cells in ALI/ARDS also disrupts ion and fluid transport across the epithelium, further interfering with the removal of edema fluid accumulated in the alveolar space (53). Finally, disruption of the epithelial barrier can lead to entrance of bacteria from the alveolar space into circulation and has been implicated in the development of bacteremia and septic shock in patients with bacterial pneumonia (54).

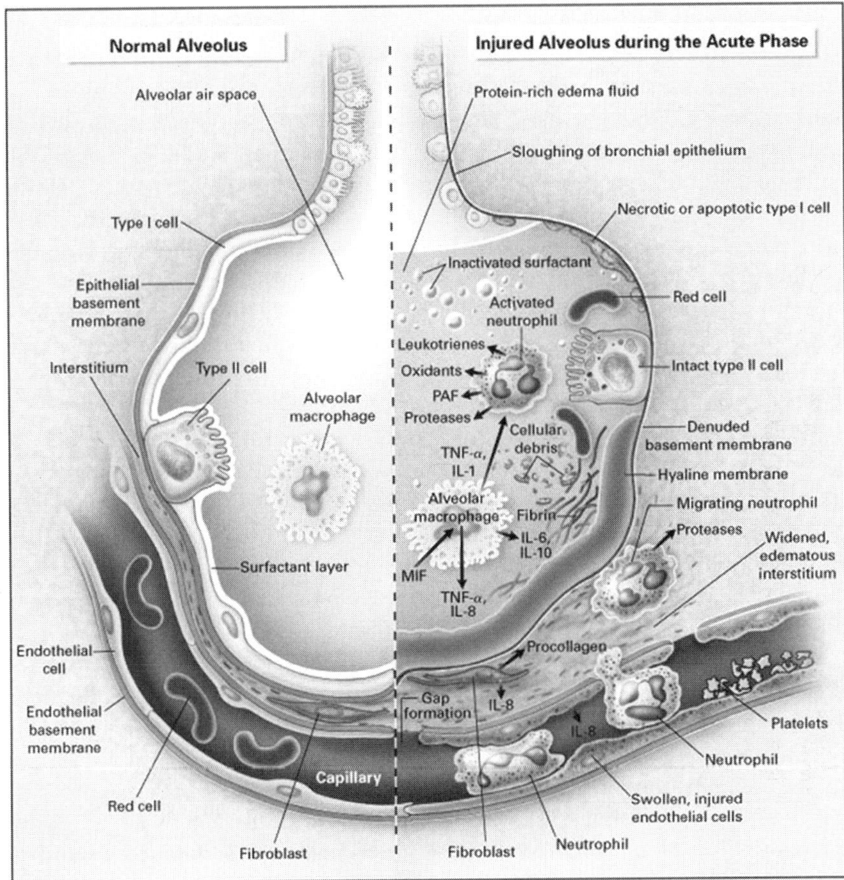

Figure 2 The normal alveolus (left-hand side) and the injured alveolus in the acute phase of ALI/ARDS (right-hand side). In the acute phase of ALI/ARDS (right-hand side), there is sloughing of bronchial and alveolar epithelial cells, with the formation of hyaline membranes on the denuded basement membrane. Neutrophils are shown adhering to the injured capillary endothelium and marginating through the interstitium into the air space, which is filled with protein-rich edema fluid. In the alveolar lumen, a macrophage is secreting proinflammatory cytokines, e.g., interleukin (IL)-1, 6, 8, and 10 and tumor necrosis factor-α (TNF-α), which act locally to stimulate chemotaxis and activate neutrophils, increase the production of extracellular matrix by fibroblasts, or promote the release of oxidants, proteases, leukotrienes, and other proinflammatory molecules like platelet-activating factor (PAF). Anti-inflammatory mediators are also present in the alveolar milieu (e.g., IL-1-receptor antagonist, soluble TNF-α receptor, autoantibodies against IL-8, and cytokines like IL-10 and 11 (not shown). The influx of protein-rich edema fluid into the alveolus has also led to the inactivation of surfactant. MIF denotes macrophage inhibitory factor. [From Ref. 2 © 2000 Massachusetts Medical Society. All rights reserved.]

Capillary Endothelial Injury and Vascular Dysfunction

Endothelial cells are often the target of injury resulting from systemic insults, such as septic shock, trauma, and pancreatitis. Regardless of the inciting event, injury causes endothelial cells to become more rounded and the intercellular junctions among them less tight, leading to increased pulmonary capillary permeability and movement of protein-rich plasma fluid to the interstitium (Fig. 2). The leakage of plasma fluid into the interstitium is accompanied by a corresponding increase in pulmonary lymphatic flow (55). When an unbalanced state is reached, characterized by a rate of capillary leak that exceed the ability of lymphatic flow to clear the interstitium, the lungs begin to accumulate edema fluid that ultimately enters the alveolus (Fig. 2). As mentioned above, the presence of proteinaceous edema fluid in alveoli contributes to respiratory failure by interfering with surfactant function and by being a diffusion barrier for gases. In addition, endothelial injury is marked by the presence of inflammatory cells, such as neutrophils, as well as the aggregation of platelets and the formation of microthrombi (56,57). The resultant impediment to regional pulmonary microcirculation, in conjunction with reflex hypoxic vasoconstriction, can lead to an increase in pulmonary vascular resistance that can further augment capillary fluid leakage and alveolar dysfunction.

Vascular function is significantly impaired early in the course of ALI/ARDS. Activation of complex interactions between the endothelium, inflammatory cells, local mediators and the coagulation system lead to platelet aggregation and formation of platelet–fibrin thrombi in the microcirculation, which in turn result in increased pulmonary vascular resistance and areas or hypoperfusion (57). This phenomenon is further exacerbated by impaired fibrinolysis that accompanies the procoagulant state (57). In addition, areas of alveolar flooding and collapse due to edema and surfactant dysfunction lead to hypoxic vasoconstriction, intrapulmonary shunting, and ventilation-perfusion mismatch. Vascular dysfunction in the pathophysiology of lung injury and ARDS is detailed in Chapter 8.

Neutrophil and Macrophage-Dependent Injury

The onset of ALI and ARDS is marked by significant accumulation of neutrophils in the lung, as evidenced by histologic analysis of tissue specimens in both humans and laboratory animals (58–60). Neutrophils are also the predominant cell type in the bronchoalveolar lavage fluid obtained from affected patients (56). The temporal relationship between the development of lung injury and the activation and infiltration of neutrophils in the lung provides circumstantial evidence of the role of these cells in the pathogenesis of ARDS. The fact that neutrophil depletion is capable of attenuating ALI in experimental models adds further support to this hypothesis (61,62). However, despite their apparent central role in initiating acute pulmonary injury and ARDS, it is unclear at this time whether the infiltration of neutrophils is a cause or consequence of the evolving lung injury. If neutrophils are indeed central initiators of injury in ALI/ARDS, current evidence suggests that they are not the sole mediators of this complex pathology. For example, patients with profound neutropenia are still capable of developing ARDS (63,64). In addition, the fact that neutropenic patients with severe pneumonia receiving granulocyte colony-stimulating factor do not develop a more severe form of lung injury (65) provides further evidence that ARDS can be neutrophil independent.

As mentioned earlier in the chapter, resident and newly recruited alveolar macrophages play a significant role in the evolution of lung injury (66). Resident macrophages release mediators that recruit and activate neutrophils and circulating monocytes, thus augmenting the response and potential injury following a noxious stimulus. Macrophages produce a complex network of cytokines and chemokines that are thought to play a major role not only locally, but also in the pathophysiology of dysfunction in other organs in patients that develop multiorgan system failure during the course of ARDS (Fig. 2). Macrophages also serve a regulatory role by releasing mediators that can further increase or retard the intensity of the inflammatory response. Cross-signaling between neutrophils and macrophages is important not only in the proinflammatory process, but also in host defense and in healing.

Ventilator-Induced Lung Injury

Considering that the vast majority of patients with ALI and ARDS require ventilatory support during the course of their illness, the concept of ventilator-induced lung injury cannot be overlooked. Once thought to be merely a necessary support modality, it is now known that mechanical ventilation can either be beneficial or injurious to patients depending on how it is used (67,68). Experimental evidence demonstrates that the use of high fractions of inspired oxygen in the acute phase following a pulmonary insult, even if for a limited period of time, can exacerbate lung injury (69). The use of large tidal volumes and very low values of PEEP is associated with progression and exacerbation of lung disease, presumably due to the overdistension of more compliant alveoli during inspiration and the cyclic opening and closing of the less compliant alveoli throughout the respiratory cycle (68). Such ventilation strategies are also associated with increases in proinflammatory cytokines (70), which may worsen local pulmonary disease as well as lead to end-organ dysfunction, a process currently termed "biotrauma" (71). Clinical trials showing that the use of protective ventilation strategies is associated with a reduced cytokine response (72) and lower mortality (73,74) underscore the importance of the interaction between specific mechanical ventilation and the course of lung disease. A complete discussion of ventilation-induced lung injury and the utility of different ventilation strategies in treating ALI/ARDS is given in Chapter 13.

D. Clinical Course

Natural History

The clinical natural history of ARDS progresses as a continuum, from the original inciting event to the development of the severe physiologic derangements that lead to death, and can be divided into four distinct clinical phases (75). Depending on the original precipitating insult these clinical phases may be well differentiated (e.g., as seen in gastric aspiration) or they may be more subtle and follow a continuum (e.g., as occurs when ARDS evolves in patients with septic shock).

Phase 1: Acute Injury

During this acute injury phase that encompasses the period immediately after the original insult, patients may have a relatively normal physical examination, often exhibiting subtle clinical signs such as hyperventilation and the resulting respiratory alkalosis. Conversely, in some cases, symptoms and signs may be more severe than definitive markers of lung injury, i.e., the chest radiograph. Patients with aspiration of gastric contents often demonstrate severe hypoxemia prior to evidence of pneumonitis on chest radiograph. Similarly, patients with septic shock frequently have a normal chest radiograph during the early phase. During this initial phase of disease, treatments such as fluid resuscitation or initiation of vasoactive drugs are often instituted in patients that come to medical attention.

Phase 2: Latent Period

Following the initial acute injury phase, patients often experience a latency period lasting between 6 and 48 hr, depending on the type and severity of the insult. This is a period of clinical stability, generally marked by minor abnormalities on chest radiograph and physical examination. Patients may continue to exhibit hyperventilation and hypocapnia, while experiencing a gradual increase in venous admixture. A latent phase is commonly observed, for example, in patients who develop ARDS following aspiration of gastric contents and those with viral respiratory tract infections, but may be absent or more subtle when septic shock is the inciting event.

Phase 3: Acute Respiratory Failure

The onset of respiratory failure is characterized by marked dyspnea, tachypnea, and the use of accessory respiratory musculature. These signs and symptoms result from the progressively worsening lung compliance and associated hypoxemia. At this stage, patients require supplemental oxygen and the initiation of mechanical ventilation in order to sustain life. From a clinician's perspective, it is often impossible to discern the type of original insult through analysis of the clinical and radiological features characterizing this phase of acute respiratory failure. This is an important diagnostic challenge that needs to be addressed in future research.

Phase 4: Severe Physiologic Derangement

Patients who do not receive medical attention, or those with the most severe forms of ALI/ARDS, progress to a phase of severe physiologic derangement. These patients exhibit significant increases in intrapulmonary shunting that lead to further severe hypoxemia, hemodynamic instability, as well as metabolic and respiratory acidosis. These severe derangements may be progressive and poorly responsive to medical therapy, particularly if it is instituted late in the clinical course. If hemodynamic compromise persists and worsens, myocardial ischemia, bradycardia, arrhythmias, and terminal asystole can follow.

Pathologic Phases

The clinical phases described above mark the evolution of a dynamic disease process over time and can be roughly correlated with different pathologic phases observed under more stringently controlled animal laboratory experiments or in clinical practice at the time of autopsy.

Exudative Phase of Pathology

This early pathologic phase occurs within hours of the initial injury and lasts approximately 1 week. During the exudative phase, the excised lungs appear erythematous, edematous, and engorged, with macroscopic characteristics resembling that of hepatic tissue ("hepatization"). The microscopic correlates for such abnormalities include vascular congestion and the extravasation of serum proteins, fluid and erythrocytes from the intravascular space into the interstitium and alveoli. An abundance of proteinaceous exudate occupies the airspaces clearly interfering with oxygenation and decreasing lung compliance. This is accompanied by infiltration of neutrophils into the lung, leading to the appearance of dense foci containing inflammatory cells. Hyaline membranes of proteinaceous material, as well as cellular debris, can be found in the alveolar spaces. During the later part of the exudative phase, an increased number of type II pneumocytes can be found in preparation for replacing irreversibly injured type I cell injury.

Fibroproliferative Phase of Pathology

The fibroproliferative phase immediately follows the exudative phase, and often persists for approximately 4 weeks. Conceptually, this phase can be considered as the beginning of an attempt to contain or isolate the still present inflammatory stimulus so as to return to a state of functional pulmonary homeostasis. This phase is marked by lungs that appear gray on macroscopic examination, while microscopic examination reveals areas of consolidation with intense fibroblast proliferation in the interstitium and alveolar spaces. The acute inflammatory cell infiltration (neutrophils and macrophages) from the earlier exudative phase gives rise to a predominantly monocytic population. Factors involved in fibroproliferative lung injury are detailed in Chapters 5 and 6.

Fibrotic Phase

The fibrotic phase of ARDS is the latest phase of lung repair, and is marked by the deposition of mature collagen, interstitial fibrosis, and healing. Patients that ultimately survive ARDS often show resolution of the increased fibroblast proliferation and collagen deposition within 4–6 months of the original insult. By that time, many of these patients exhibit little or no residual pulmonary function abnormalities.

F. Therapeutic Considerations in ALI/ARDS

Detailed discussion of therapies for lung injury is given in Chapters 13–19, but selected interventions and therapeutic considerations are illustrated here. Because ALI and ARDS exhibit significant clinical variability and are caused by a myriad of etiologies, it is not surprising that their treatment is multifaceted and should be tailored to the underlying etiology and needs of the individual patient. Commonly employed therapeutic modalities are summarized in Table 7.

Treatment of the Inciting Clinical Condition

One of the most important aspects of the management of patients with ALI and ARDS is the prompt identification and treatment of the original inciting disorder (76). Once started, the inflammatory response will continue to evolve until the underlying insult is removed. From the outset, significant efforts should be applied to search for treatable causes, such as sepsis or

Table 7 Common Therapeutic Considerations in ALI and ARDS

Treatment of the original inciting condition
Fluids, and hemodynamic management
Mechanical ventilation
Vascular-based therapies
Prone positioning therapy
Surfactant replacement therapy
Anti-inflammatory therapies
Antioxidant therapies
Alveolar edema resolution therapies
Multimodal therapies

pneumonia. Depending on the clinical history and the host's immunologic status, active surveillance and early treatment of pulmonary infections such as bacterial, atypical (*Mycoplasma pneumoniae*) and fungal pneumonia, as well as *Pneumocystis carinii* or tuberculosis should be entertained. In addition, identification of extrapulmonary sites of infection such as acute abdomen and invasive soft tissue infections should be a priority since these conditions require prompt surgical intervention and proper antibiotic therapy (77).

In a significant number of patients with ALI and ARDS, the original insult that led to the development of these conditions does not have a specific treatment. This is the case in most patients following aspiration of gastric contents or patients that develop ALI/ARDS following treatment for another condition, such as multiple blood transfusions during trauma resuscitation, reperfusion injury after lung transplantation, or cardiopulmonary bypass. These patients should be managed with therapeutic modalities that optimize the natural healing process (i.e., pulmonary toilet) and support respiratory function, optimize tissue oxygen delivery, and attenuate physiologic derangements. Additionally, during the time taken for the evolution of the natural healing process to occur, the lungs should be supported in a manner to keep further iatrogenic insults at a minimum (67–72).

Fluids and Hemodynamic Management

The clinician treating patients with ALI/ARDS must reconcile two distinct situations regarding the administration of fluids. Treatment of some conditions that lead to ALI/ARDS, such as septic shock, requires prompt and aggressive fluid resuscitation. Clinical evidence suggests that aggressive fluid resuscitation in septic shock does not increase the risk of subsequently developing ARDS and lowers the mortality from this disease (78). Conversely, experiments in animal models of ALI demonstrate that the degree of pulmonary edema and respiratory dysfunction is attenuated when left atrial pressure is reduced (79). Clinical studies demonstrating improved survival in patients with ARDS associated with reduced pulmonary artery wedge pressures lend further support to these laboratory observations (80,81). However, fluid restriction and lower left atrial pressures have not been validated as an optimal therapeutic strategy for fluid management in a large, multicentric population of patients with ALI/ARDS. Currently, the ARDS Network is conducting a large multicentric clinical trial to assess the safety and efficacy of "fluid conservative" vs. "fluid liberal" management strategies on lung function, nonpulmonary organ function, as well as mortality and the need for mechanical ventilation. While results from this study are not yet available, a reasonable strategy is to target an intravascular volume at the lowest level consistent with adequate systemic perfusion based on clinical, metabolic, and acid–base parameters.

Mechanical Ventilation

The use of mechanical ventilation is central in treating patients with acute respiratory failure in ALI/ARDS. The heterogeneity of disease distribution in affected patients (Fig. 3), as well as the desire not to cause ventilation-associated iatrogenic injury to the lungs, pose remarkable challenges to the clinician. In typical ARDS, gravitationally dependent areas of the lung are marked by dense cellular infiltrates, alveolar and interstitial edema, cellular debris, atelectasis, and consolidation, while the nondependent areas are relatively spared (Fig. 3). Unlike the healthy lung with uniform normal surface tension where the tidal volume is distributed throughout the various segments in a balanced manner, the lungs of patients with ARDS experience an abnormal distribution of tidal volumes that follow a path of least impediment. This can lead to overdistension and injury of the more compliant nondependent alveoli while failing to recruit the less compliant dependent alveoli.

Understanding of ventilation strategies for ALI/ARDS has improved significantly. As noted earlier, it is now known that high tidal volumes that cause alveolar overdistension, and low levels of PEEP that lead to cyclic opening and closing of less compliant alveoli, can cause ventilator-induced

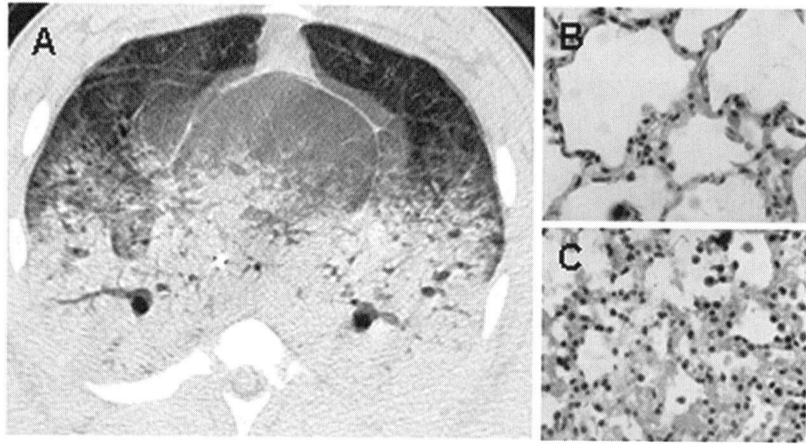

Figure 3 Computed tomographic (CT) and light microscopic findings in experimental acute lung injury in swine. Panel A: CT findings; Panel B: Light microscopy of nondependent areas of the lungs; Panel C: Light microscopy of dependent areas of the lungs. The CT image in Panel A shows the highly nonhomogeneous pattern of disease distribution in acute pulmonary injury, with severe involvement of dependent areas and relative sparing of nondependent areas. Corresponding light microscopy sections reflect the relatively preserved alveolar architecture in a nondependent area (Panel B), in contrast to edema, hyaline membrane formation, atelectasis, and inflammatory infiltrate in a dependent area (Panel C).

lung injury in an experimental setting (67,68). A recent multicentric trial conducted by the ARDS Network showed a significant reduction in hospital mortality rate when patients were ventilated with a reduced tidal volume (6 mL/kg of predicted body weight) compared to traditional tidal volume (12 mL/kg of predicted body weight) (74). Mechanical ventilation with reduced tidal volumes is now the preferred strategy for ventilating patients with ARDS (Chapter 13).

The role of PEEP to prevent cyclic alveolar collapse (or derecruitment), as employed in the so-called "open lung" strategy, has been supported by numerous animal laboratory studies (67,68,70,82). In this strategy, PEEP is used to stabilize alveoli throughout the entire respiratory cycle by maintaining alveoli above their respective closing volumes. This prevents cyclic alveolar closure upon exhalation and repeated forceful reopening at the onset of inspiration, which can lead to further lung injury in a process termed atelectrauma (Fig. 4) (83). A small single-institution trial by Amato et al. (73) showed a reduction in 28-day mortality in patients ventilated with an "open lung" strategy, consisting of low tidal volumes, pressure-controlled inverse-ratio ventilation, and a high level of PEEP set above the lower inflection point of the pressure–volume curve for each patient in attempt to prevent cyclic derecruitment during expiration (Fig. 4). The intuitive belief that higher levels of PEEP may further accentuate the benefits of a low tidal volume strategy in patients with ARDS

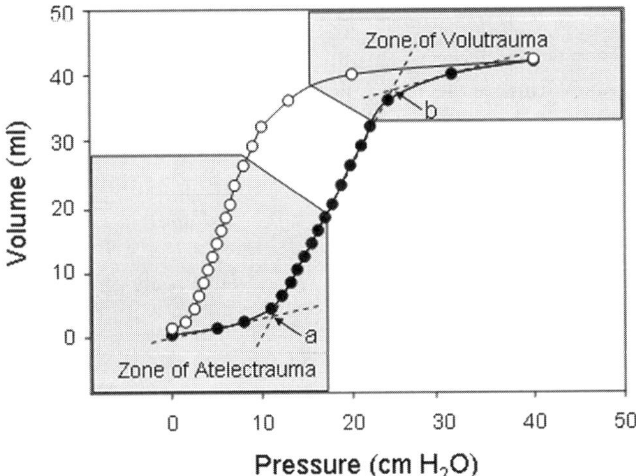

Figure 4 Static pressure–volume relationship of the total respiratory system in rabbits with acute lung injury following surfactant depletion by saline lavage. Zones of alveolar overdistension (volutrauma) and derecruitment (atelectrauma) are shown in the shaded areas. The lower (a) and upper inflection points (b) of the inspiratory curve are also designated.

awaits confirmation by larger multicentric clinical trials. Inherent to a strategy employing reduced tidal volumes and higher PEEP is the development of controlled respiratory acidosis or permissive hypercapnia. Although generally well tolerated in adults (84), permissive hypercapnia is not free of adverse effects and may be contraindicated in certain patients (increased intracranial pressure, pulmonary vascular reactivity, etc.) (85).

A promising alternative to conventional mechanical ventilation currently being accessed in clinical trials is high frequency oscillatory ventilation (HFOV). HFOV employs very small tidal volumes at supraphysiologic rates to promote optimal lung recruitment while avoiding cyclic overdistension and atelectrauma (Fig. 4). Furthermore, it does so while avoiding hypercarbia and optimizing oxygenation. HFOV attenuates lung injury in various experimental models (67,86,87). Reduced morbidity in neonatal and pediatric populations has also been observed with this ventilatory modality (88,89). HFOV is capable of maintaining acceptable ventilation and oxygenation in adult patients with severe ARDS (90). The role of HFOV in the treatment of patients with ARDS in comparison with conventional lung protective strategies still requires evaluation by large randomized controlled trials.

Vascular-Based Therapies

Nitric oxide is a potent endogenous vasodilator that can be administered via inhalation and is capable of producing relaxation of the pulmonary vasculature without significant systemic effects (91,92). Exogenously inhaled NO (iNO) can be delivered through a face mask, or more commonly, through an endotracheal tube by blending controlled amounts of this substance with the inspired gas mixture of a mechanical ventilator. Once in the alveolus, iNO readily diffuses into the adjacent vascular bed and causes direct vasodilatation prior to its rapid deactivation by binding to circulating hemoglobin. Of some concern is the interaction of iNO and oxidants to form injurious reactive nitrogen species, particularly in the presence of increased ambient oxygen concentrations. However, this issue does not appear to be of significant concern at clinically relevant low iNO concentrations. The ability of iNO to promote vasodilatation and increased perfusion to ventilated areas while not affecting poorly ventilated areas with high intrapulmonary shunt, coupled with a lack of systemic vasodilatation and hypotension, makes it an attractive therapeutic agent for patients with ALI/ARDS. Unfortunately, despite encouraging results in animal models of lung injury (93,94), clinical studies fail to show a significant benefit of using iNO in adults with ARDS (95,96). The use of iNO in this population is associated with modest improvements in oxygenation that are not sustained beyond the first 24 hr of treatment. Furthermore, iNO has not been shown to improve mortality or decrease the duration of mechanical ventilation (95,96), and it is not recommended as standard treatment in patients with ARDS. However, iNO may be useful in the acute management of subgroups of profoundly hypoxemic patients with evidence of increased pulmonary vascular resistance. The effects of other vasodilators such as intravenous prostacyclin and prostaglandin E_1 in ALI/ARDS have been disappointing due to lack of meaningful outcome improvements and the occurrence of systemic hemodynamic adverse effects. Chapter 17 provides detailed discussion about vasoactive agents available for therapeutic use in the laboratory and in clinical practice.

Prone Position Therapy

The relative simplicity and low cost of prone position therapy, and the fact that it improves oxygenation in more than 60% of patients with ARDS (97,98), have made it a popular modality in intensive care units throughout the world. Various mechanisms have been proposed to explain the improved oxygenation observed in the proned patient, including increased end-expiratory lung volumes, regional ventilation changes associated with altered chest wall mechanics, and improved ventilation-perfusion match (99–101). However, improvements in oxygenation do not necessarily translate into decreased morbidity and mortality in ARDS (74). Gattinoni et al. (102) reported the results of a multicenter-controlled trial where patients were randomized to receive conventional treatment (supine position) or prone position for 6 or more hours per day for 10 days. In this study, despite an observed improvement in oxygenation, prone position therapy was not associated with a reduction in mortality. The fact that patients were kept prone for only 30% of the time (approximately 7 hr per day) and for a maximum of 10 days may help explain the observed lack of benefit. The use of prone position therapy cannot be considered a standard therapeutic modality in patients with ARDS until it is evaluated by a clinical trial designed to maximize its impact on respiratory dysfunction. In the meantime, this simple therapy may have a role in the management of the selected patients with refractory hypoxemia.

Surfactant Replacement Therapy

As described earlier and detailed in Chapter 9, the pulmonary surfactant system is markedly abnormal in ALI/ARDS. The success of surfactant replacement therapy in newborns with hyaline membrane disease, coupled with encouraging results in a number of experimental models of ALI, has fostered optimism that this therapy may be of benefit in treating patients with ALI/ARDS (103,104). Several clinical studies have shown that surfactant replacement therapy can benefit term infants and children with clinical lung injury (Chapter 15), but current experience with surfactant therapy in adults with ALI/ARDS has been relatively unsuccessful. The largest published multicenter, randomized, placebo-controlled trial in adults with ARDS found that an aerosolized protein-free artificial surfactant (Exosurf) failed to improve oxygenation, duration of mechanical ventilation, or survival in adults with ARDS (105). Exosurf, however, is no longer widely used in surfactant therapy in infants because its activity is significantly lower than that of animal-derived surfactant preparations. More active exogenous surfactants are still under study for use in ALI and ARDS, in conjunction with more effective delivery methods (e.g., direct tracheal administration or regional instillation during bronchoscopy), as discussed in Chapter 15.

Anti-inflammatory Therapies

Since an aggressive inflammatory process has long been believed to play a major role in the pathogenesis of ALI/ARDS, anti-inflammatory drugs including glucocorticoids have been tested as potential therapeutic agents. The use of glucocorticoids, however, neither prevents the progression of ARDS in patients at risk (106) nor exerts beneficial effects when given early in the clinical course (107). Interestingly, small clinical studies suggest that glucocorticoids may be beneficial when used later in the clinical course during the resolution of the fibro-proliferate phase (108,109). Empiric use of glucocorticoids in ARDS must be weighed against the potential serious side effects, including gastrointestinal bleeding and increased risk of infection. The use of other agents with anti-inflammatory properties such as ketoconazole (110) has been largely disappointing, underscoring that the inflammatory process in ALI and ARDS plays important roles in disease resolution that must be maintained in therapy. Attempts to manipulate the pulmonary inflammatory response must be specific and precisely timed, and it is difficult to accomplish this clinically based on current understanding. Chapter 14 provides further details about the use of anti-inflammatory agents in treating lung injury.

Antioxidant Therapies

Reactive oxygen species generated during acute inflammation play a major role in the development of ALI and ARDS (111,112). In addition, exposure to high concentrations of inspired oxygen inherent to the management of ALI and ARDS further exacerbate the oxidative insult (69). Antioxidant therapy has, therefore, emerged as a logical potential therapeutic strategy. Treatment of experimental models of ALI with free radical scavengers attenuates pulmonary damage and yields better physiologic outcomes (113). However, a large randomized, placebo-controlled trial of procysteine in patients with ALI and ARDS was halted due to lack of efficacy (2). The rationale for antioxidant therapy in lung injury, and therapeutic agents of potential clinical utility, are detailed in Chapter 16.

Therapies Leading to Accelerated Resolution of Lung Injury

The resolution phase of ALI/ARDS involves the removal of accumulated alveolar edema fluid, in conjunction with restoration of the injured and denuded alveolar epithelium. Thus, therapies capable of accelerating this resolution phase have been the recent target of various investigators (114,115). Catecholamines, such as inhaled and systemic beta-agonists, markedly increase alveolar fluid clearance by influencing the active sodium transport across the alveolar epithelium (116). Recently, therapies in experimental animals employing adenoviral-mediated gene overexpression of Na,K-ATPase or β_2-adrenergic receptor function in alveolar epithelium have improved alveolar fluid clearance (117,118) (Chapter 18). Reconstitution of the disrupted alveolar epithelial surface injury with alveolar epithelial type I cells is also central in the resolution phase of ALI and ARDS. As part of the repair process, proliferation of alveolar epithelial type II cells provides a provisional epithelial barrier that restores the air–liquid interface and facilitates alveolar fluid clearance. Experimental studies support the hypothesis that keratinocyte growth factor (119,120) is capable of increasing proliferation of alveolar epithelial type II cells, raising the speculation that an epithelium growth factor could be employed to accelerate resolution of the lung injury in ARDS.

Multimodal Therapies

The recognition that ALI and ARDS involve a broad spectrum of disease caused by multiple etiologies makes it obvious that therapies cannot be employed stereotypically. Instead, clinicians must identify the needs of individual patients at a given stage of the disease process and institute the most appropriate therapy or combination of therapies. A patient with ALI secondary to shock from a penetrating gunshot wound to the abdomen may require little more than surgical intervention, broad-spectrum antibiotics, and lung protective ventilation. Conversely, a patient two weeks into the course of ARDS secondary to massive aspiration of gastric contents with refractory hypoxemia may benefit from protective ventilation in combination with prone position or NO therapy, as well as specific therapy to enhance clearance of alveolar fluid. The scope, rationale, and evaluation of specific combined-modality approaches for treating lung injury are covered in Chapter 19.

V. Summary

The lungs have sophisticated defense systems to remove and limit damage caused by direct or systemic insults. Lung injury results when the capacity of pulmonary defense mechanisms is overwhelmed by the magnitude of the inciting cause. In general terms, acute lung injury involves a rapidly evolving impairment of the alveolar capillary surface that results in inflammation, increased work of breathing, and abnormal gas exchange, with or without hypoxemia or hypercarbia. This generalized view of acute lung injury emphasizes that it encompasses a variety of processes, and is not limited to the clinical syndrome bearing the same name (i.e., ALI) or the more severe related clinical syndrome of ARDS. Regardless of its clinical presentation, acute lung injury typically incorporates a prominent inflammatory response. This inflammatory response involves a complex set of mechanisms aimed at removing or isolating noxious foreign substances or organisms and repairing the lungs to the preinjury condition. In practice, the inflammatory response accompanying pulmonary injury can have detrimental as well as beneficial aspects. In therapeutic applications, it is necessary to maintain the beneficial physiologic aspects of pulmonary inflammation while antagonizing or mitigating its detriments.

Understanding of clinical ALI and ARDS has increased significantly over the past three decades, leading to better functional definitions of these syndromes and improved treatment and support modalities. A lung-injury score (38) based on a four-point scoring grid (degree of infiltration or consolidation on chest radiograph, severity of hypoxemia, respiratory system compliance and level of PEEP) has been used to better classify clinical ALI and ARDS. More recently, a simple definition by the American–European Consensus Conference Committee involving the degree of hypoxemia, the presence of bilateral infiltrates on chest radiograph, and the absence of left atrial hypertension, has gained widespread acceptance in clinical practice.

As stated above, clinical ALI and ARDS are not specific diseases but rather syndromes that reflect a broad range of etiologies. These etiologies are generally classified as direct (pulmonary) insults like aspiration of gastric contents and pneumonias, or indirect (systemic) insults such as septic shock and pancreatitis. Regardless of specific etiology, the pathophysiology of ALI/ARDS involves injury to the alveolar epithelium and capillary endothelium, recruitment and activation of inflammatory neutrophils and macrophages, surfactant dysfunction, and abnormalities of pulmonary blood flow distribution. Injury to type I cells of the alveolar epithelium allows the influx of protein-rich edema fluid, creating a barrier to gas exchange and interfering with alveolar dynamics by inhibiting surfactant function. The surfactant system can also be further impaired by direct injury or alteration of alveolar type II cells. Capillary endothelial cell injury is also prominent in ALI/ARDS, with associated permeability edema, recruitment of activated inflammatory macrophages and neutrophils, and platelet aggregation and microthrombus formation. Resident alveolar macrophages are also crucial in ALI, serving both as effectors and regulators in this setting. These cells are professional phagocytes whose primary role is to eliminate foreign substances and micro-organisms from the lung. However, in situations where an insult overwhelms their capacity, resident macrophages also release mediators capable of autocrine stimulation as well as recruiting and activating additional effector cells. Inflammatory mediators involved in cell recruitment and activation in acute pulmonary injury are detailed further in Chapter 4, and oxidant injury, vascular dysfunction, and surfactant dysfunction are discussed in Chapters 7–9.

The natural history of clinical ARDS begins with an acute injury phase immediately after an initiating insult. This is often followed by a latent phase marked by clinical stability and minor respiratory symptoms that may last 6–48 hr. Progression of the syndrome then leads to acute respiratory failure marked by hypoxemia, abnormal lung compliance, and typical radiographic findings. The clinical phases of ARDS roughly correlate with pathologic phases observed in the experimental setting or during autopsy. Early "exudative" pulmonary pathology in ALI/ARDS is apparent within hours of injury, and may persist for more than a week. This is followed by a fibroproliferative phase of pathology that can persist for up to 4 weeks. Resolution of ARDS occurs during a late fibrotic phase, which is marked by deposition of mature collagen, interstitial fibrosis, and healing.

Considering the multiplicity of etiologies that lead to clinical ALI/ARDS, it is only natural that therapy for these syndromes should be multifaceted. One of the most important aspects of managing patients with these conditions is the identification and treatment of the original inciting disorder. The vast majority of patients with ALI/ARDS require mechanical ventilation, which is performed with the objective of supporting the patient while avoiding further insult (ventilator-induced lung injury). Administration of fluids is aimed at maintaining an intravascular volume consistent with adequate systemic perfusion while avoiding exaggerated accumulation of lung water. The use of vascular-based therapies such as iNO has been associated with transient improvements in oxygenation but no reduction in morbidity or mortality in patients with ARDS. Prone position therapy has also been shown to improve ventilation–perfusion match and oxygenation, but not to reduce mortality in clinical studies. Other therapeutic modalities currently being evaluated in patients with ARDS include exogenous surfactant therapy, anti-inflammatory and antioxidant therapies, and strategies designed to accelerate resolution of lung injury, such as enhanced alveolar fluid clearance by catecholamines or adenoviral-mediated gene overexpression of Na,K-ATPase or β_2-adrenergic receptor function in alveolar cells, and administration of keratinocyte growth factor. Therapeutic interventions for lung injury are detailed further in Chapters 13–19.

Acknowledgment

The authors gratefully acknowledge the support of NIH grants HL-48889 and AI-46534.

References

1. Parker SP. Editor for McGraw-Hill's Dictionary of Scientific and Technical Terms. 5th ed. New York, NY: McGraw-Hill, 1994.
2. Ware LB, Matthay MA. The acute respiratory distress syndrome. NEJM 2000; 342:1334–1348.
3. Marik PE. Aspiration pneumonitis and aspiration pneumonia. NEJM 2001; 344:665–671.
4. Standiford TJ, Huffnagle GB. Cytokines in host defense against pneumonia. J Inv Med 1997; 45:335–345.
5. Nelson S, Summer WR. Innate immunity, cytokines and host defense. Infect Dis Clin North Am 1998; 12:555–567.
6. Kuhns DB, DeCarlo E, Hawk DM, Gallin JI. Dynamics of the cellular and humoral components of the inflammatory response elicited in skin blisters in humans. J Clin Invest 1992; 89:1734–1740.
7. Ward PA. Role of complement, chemokines, and regulatory cytokines in acute lung injury. Ann N Y Acad Sci 1996; 796:104–112.
8. Russo TA, Davidson BA, Prior R, Carlino CB, Helinska JD, Knight PR. Capsular polysaccharide and O-specific divergently modulate pulmonary neutrophil influx in a rat *Escherichia coli* model of gram-negative pneumonitis. Immun Infect 2000; 68:2854–2862.
9. Tarmont EC, Hoover DL. General or nonspecific host defense mechanisms. In: Mandell GL, Bennett JE, Dolin R, eds. Mandell, Douglas and Bennett's Principles and Practice of Infectious Diseases. 4th ed. New York, NY: Churchill Livingstone, 1995:30–35.
10. Schreck R, Rieber P, Baeuerle PA. Reactive oxygen intermediates as apparently widely used messengers in the activation of the NF-kB transcription factor and HIV-1. EMBO J 1991; 10:2247–2258.
11. Segal BH, Kuhns DB, Ding L, Gallin JI, Holland SM. Thioglycollate peritonitis in mice lacking C5, 5-lipoxygenase, or p47(phox): complement, leukotrienes, and reactive oxidants in acute inflammation. J Leukoc Biol 2002; 71(3):410–416.
12. Knight PR, Druskovich G, Tait AR, Johnson KJ. The role of neutrophils, oxidants and proteases in the pathogenesis of acid pulmonary injury. Anesthesiology 1992; 77:772–778.
13. Goldman G, Welbourn R, Klausner JM, Kobzik L, Valeri CR, Shepro D, Hechtman HB. Leukocytes mediate acid aspiration-induced multiorgan edema. Surgery 1993; 114:13–20.
14. Nader-Djalal N, Knight PR, Thusu K, Davidson BA, Holm BA, Johnson KJ, Dandona P. Reactive oxygen species contribute to oxygen-related lung injury after acid aspiration. Anesth Analg 1998; 87:127–133.

15. Knight PR, Kurek C, Nader ND, Davidson BA, Sokolowski J, Holm BA. Acid aspiration augments sensitivity to increased ambient oxygen concentrations. Am J Physiol Lung 2000; 278:1240–1247.

16. Knight PR, Rutter T, Tait AR, Coleman EJ, Johnson KJ. Pathogenesis of gastric particulate lung injury: a comparison and interaction with acid pneumonitis. Anesth Analg 1993; 77:754–760.

17. Davidson BA, Knight PR, Helinski J, Nader DN Shanley T, Johnson KJ. The role of tumor necrosis factor alpha in the pathogenesis of aspiration pneumonitis. Anesthesiology 1999; 91:486–499.

18. Shanley T, Davidson BA, Nader ND, Bless N, Vasti N, Ward PA, Johnson KJ, Knight PR, et al. Role of macrophage inflammatory protein-2 in aspiration-induced lung injury. Crit Care Med 2000; 28:2437–2444.

19. Fowler AA, Hamman RF, Good JT, Benson KN, Baird M, Eberle DJ, Petty TL, Hyers TM. Adult respiratory distress syndrome: risk with common predispositions. Ann Intern Med 1983; 98:593–597.

20. Pepe PE, Potkin RT, Reus DH, Hudson LD, Carrico CJ. Clinical predictors of the adult respiratory distress syndrome. Am J Surg 1982; 144:124–130.

21. Mendelson CL. The aspiration of stomach contents into the lungs during obstetric anesthesia. Am J Obstet Gynecol 1946; 52:191–205.

22. Britto J, Demling RH. Aspiration lung injury. New Horiz 1993; 1:435–439.

23. Hewlett EL. Toxins and other virulence factors. In: Mandell GL, Bennett JE, Dolin R, eds. Mandell, Douglas and Bennett's Principles and Practice of Infectious Diseases. 4th ed. New York, NY: Churchill Livingstone, 1995: 2–11.

24. Seidenfeld JJ, Pohl DF, Bell RC, Harris GD, Johanson WG Jr. Incidence, site, and outcome of infections in patients with the adult respiratory distress syndrome. Am Rev Respir Dis 1986; 134:12 16.

25. Dever LL, Johanson WG Jr. Pneumonia complicating adult respiratory distress syndrome. Clin Chest Med 1995; 16:147–153.

26. Rouby JJ, Martin De Lassale E, Poete P, Nicolas MH, Bodin L, Jarlier V, Le Charpentier Y, Grosset J, Viars P. Nosocomial bronchopneumonia in the critically ill. Histologic and bacteriologic aspects. Am Rev Respir Dis 1992; 146:1059–1066.

27. Montgomery AB, Stager MA, Carrico CJ, Hudson LD. Causes of mortality in patients with the adult respiratory distress syndrome. Am Rev Respir Dis 1985; 132:485–489.

28. Monteiro JM, Harvey C, Trinchieri G. Role of interleukin-12 in primary influenza virus infection. J Virol 1998; 72:4825–4831.

29. Penna AM, Johnson KJ, Camilleri J, Knight PR. Alterations in influenza A virus specific immune injury in mice anesthetized with halothane or ketamine. Intervirology 1990; 31:188–196.

30. Oda T, Akaike T, Hamamoto T, Suzuki F, Hirano T, Maeda H. Oxygen radicals in influenza-induced pathogenesis and treatment with pyran polymer-conjugated SOD. Science 1989; 244:974–976.

31. Degre M. Interaction between viral and bacterial infections in the respiratory tract. Scand J Infect Dis 1986(suppl 49):140–145.

32. Jakab GJ. Mechanisms of bacterial superinfections in viral pneumonias. Schweiz Med Wochenschr 1985; 115:75–86.

33. Jakab GJ. Immune impairment of alveolar macrophage phagocytosis during influenza virus pneumonia. Am Rev Respir Dis 1982; 126:778–782.

34. Betts RF. Influenza virus. In: Mandell GL, Bennett JE, Dolin R, eds. Mandell, Douglas and Bennett's Principles and Practice of Infectious Diseases. 4th ed. New York, NY: Churchill Livingstone, 1995:1546–1567.

35. Goldblum SE. The role of cytokines in acute pulmonary vascular endothelial injury. In: Kimball ES, ed. Cytokines and Inflammation. Boca Raton, FL: CRC Press, 1991:191–234.

36. Ashbaugh DG, Bigelow DB, Petty TL, Levine BE. Acute respiratory distress in adults. Lancet 1967; 2:319–323.

37. Petty TL, Ashbaugh DG. The adult respiratory distress syndrome: clinical features, factors influencing prognosis and principles of management. Chest 1971; 60:233–239.

38. Murray JF, Matthay MA, Luce JM, Flick MR. An expanded definition of the adult respiratory distress syndrome. Am Rev Respir Dis 1988; 138:720–723.

39. Heffner JE, Brown LK, Barbieri CA, Harpel KS, DeLeo J. Prospective validation of an acute respiratory distress syndrome predictive score. Am J Respir Crit Care Med 1995; 152:1518–1526.

40. Doyle RL, Szaflarski N, Modin GW, Wiener-Kronish JP, Matthay MA. Identification of patients with acute lung injury: predictors of mortality. Am J Respir Crit Care Med 1995; 152:1818–1824.

41. Bernard GR, Artigas A, Brigham KL, et al. The American–European Consensus Conference on ARDS: definitions, mechanisms, relevant outcomes, and clinical trial coordination. Am J Respir Crit Care Med 1994; 149:818–824.

42. Knaus WA, Draper EA, Wagner DP, Zimmerman JE. APACHE II: a severity of disease classification system. Crit Care Med 1985; 13:818–829.

43. Pollack MM, Ruttimann UE, Getson PR. Pediatric risk of mortality (PRISM) score. Crit Care Med 1988; 16:1110–1116.

44. Goodman LR, Fumagalli R, Tagliabue P, Tagliabue M, Ferrario M, Gattinoni L, Pesenti A. Adult respiratory distress syndrome due to pulmonary and extrapulmonary causes: CT, clinical, and functional correlations. Radiology 1999; 213:545–552.

45. Hudson LD, Milberg JA, Anardi D, Maunder RJ. Clinical risks for development of the acute respiratory distress syndrome. Am J Respir Crit Care Med 1995; 151:293–301.

46. Kimmel EC, Still KR. Acute lung injury, acute respiratory distress syndrome and inhalation injury: an overview. Drug Chem Tox 1999; 22:91–128.

47. Hollingstead TC, Saffle JR, Barton RG, Craft WB, Morris SE. Etiology and consequences of respiratory failure in thermally injured patients. Am J Surg 1993; 166:592–596.

48. Laffon M, Pittet JF, Modelska K, Matthay MA, Young DM. Interleukin-8 mediates injury from smoke inhalation to both the lung endothelial and alveolar epithelial barriers in rabbits. Am J Respir Crit Care Med 1999; 160:1443–1449.

49. Wiener-Kronish JP, Albertine KH, Matthay MA. Differential responses of the endothelial and epithelial barriers of the lung in sheep to *Escherichia coli* endotoxin. J Clin Invest 1991; 88:864–875.

50. Seeger W, Grube C, Gunther A, Schmidt R. Surfactant inhibition by plasma proteins: differential sensitivity of various surfactant preparations. Eur Respir J 1993; 6:971–977.

51. Baker CS, Evans TW, Randle BJ, Haslam PL. Damage to surfactant-specific protein in acute respiratory distress syndrome. Lancet 1999; 353:1232–1237.

52. Greene KE, Wright JR, Steinberg KP, et al. Serial changes in surfactant-associated proteins in lung and serum before and after onset of ARDS. Am J Respir Crit Care Med 1999; 160:1843–1850.

53. Sznajder JI. Strategies to increase alveolar epithelial fluid removal in the injured lung. Am J Respir Crit Care Med 1999; 160:1441–1442.

54. Kurahashi K, Kajikawa O, Sawa T, et al. Pathogenesis of septic shock in *Pseudomonas aeruginosa* pneumonia. J Clin Invest 1999; 104:743–750.

55. Judges D, Sharkey P, Cheung H, et al. Pulmonary microvascular fluid flux in a large animal model of sepsis: evidence for increased pulmonary endothelial permeability accompanying surgically induced peritonitis in sheep. Surgery 1986; 99:222–234.

56. Pittet JF, MacKersie RC, Martin TR, Matthay MA. Biological markers of acute lung injury: prognostic and pathogenetic significance. Am J Respir Crit Care Med 1997; 155:1187–1205.

57. Gunther A, Mosavi P, Heinemann S, et al. Alveolar fibrin formation caused by enhanced procoagulant and depressed fibrinolytic capacities in severe pneumonia: comparison with the acute respiratory distress syndrome. Am J Respir Crit Care Med 2000; 161:454–462.

58. Rotta AT, Gunnarsson B, Hernan LJ, et al. Partial liquid ventilation influences pulmonary histopathology in an animal model of acute lung injury. J Crit Care 1999; 14:84–92.

59. Weiland JE, Davis WB, Holter JF, et al. Lung neutrophils in the adult respiratory distress syndrome. Am Rev Respir Dis 1986; 133:218–225.

60. Bachofen M, Weibel ER. Structural alterations of lung parenchyma in the adult respiratory distress syndrome. Clin Chest Med 1982; 3:35–56.

61. Heflin AC Jr, Brigham KL. Prevention by granulocyte depletion of increased vascular permeability of sheep lung following endotoxemia. J Clin Invest 1981; 68:1253–1260.

62. Kawano T, Mori S, Cybulsky M, et al. Effect of granulocyte depletion in a ventilated surfactant-depleted lung. J Appl Physiol 1987; 62:27–33.

63. Ognibene FP, Martin SE, Parker MM, et al. Adult respiratory distress syndrome in patients with severe neutropenia. N Engl J Med 1986; 315:547–551.

64. Laufe MD, Simon RH, Flint A, Keller JB. Adult respiratory distress syndrome in neutropenic patients. Am J Med 1986; 80:1022–1026.

65. Nelson S, Belknap SM, Carlson RW, et al. A randomized controlled trial of filgrastim as an adjunct to antibiotics for treatment of hospitalized patients with community-acquired pneumonia. J Infect Dis 1998; 178:1075–1080.

66. Rosseau S, Hammerl P, Maus U, et al. Phenotypic characterization of alveolar monocytes recruitment in acute respiratory distress syndrome. Am J Physiol 2000; 279:L25–L35.

67. Rotta AT, Gunnarsson B, Fuhrman BP, Hernan LJ, Steinhorn DM. Comparison of lung protective ventilation strategies in a rabbit model of acute lung injury. Crit Care Med 2001; 29:2176–2184.

68. Dreyfuss D, Saumon G. Ventilator induced lung injury: lessons from experimental studies. Am J Respir Crit Care Med 1988; 157:294–323.

69. Nader-Djalal N, Knight PR, Davidson BA, Johnson K. Hyperoxia exacerbates microvascular lung injury following acid aspiration. Chest 1997; 112:1607–1614.

70. Tremblay L, Valenza F, Ribeiro SP, et al. Injurious ventilatory strategies increase cytokines and c-fos mRNA expression in isolated rat lung model. J Clin Invest 1997; 99:944–952.

71. Slutsky AS, Tremblay LN. Multiple system organ failure: is mechanical ventilation a contributing factor? Am J Respir Crit Care Med 1998; 157: 1721–1725.

72. Ranieri VM, Suter PM, Tortorella C, et al. Effect of mechanical ventilation on inflammatory mediators in patients with acute respiratory distress syndrome: a randomized controlled trial. JAMA 1999; 282:54–61.

73. Amato MBP, Barbas CSV, Medeiros DM, et al. Effect of a protective-ventilation strategy on mortality in the acute respiratory distress syndrome. N Engl J Med 1998; 338:347–354.

74. The Acute Respiratory Distress Syndrome Network. Ventilation with lower tidal volumes as compared with traditional tidal volumes for acute lung injury and the acute respiratory distress syndrome. N Engl J Med 2000; 342: 1301–1308.

75. Brown SD. ARDS: history, definitions, and physiology. Respir Care Clin North Am 1998; 4:567–582.

76. Brower RG, Ware LB, Berthiaume Y, Matthay MA. Treatment of ARDS. Chest 2001; 120:1347–1367.

77. Anderson ID, Fearon KC, Grant IS. Laparotomy for abdominal sepsis in the critically ill. Br J Surg 1996; 83:535–539.

78. Carcillo JA, Davis AL, Zaritsky A. Role of early fluid resuscitation in pediatric septic shock. JAMA 1991; 266:1242–1245.

79. Prewitt RM, McCarthy J, Wood LDH. Treatment of acute low pressure pulmonary edema in dogs: relative effects of hydrostatic and oncotic pressure, nitroprusside, and positive end-expiratory pressure. J Clin Invest 1981; 67: 409–418.

80. Humphrey H, Hall J, Sznajder I, Silverstein M, Wood L. Improved survival in ARDS patients associated with a reduction in pulmonary capillary wedge pressure. Chest 1990; 97:1176–1180.

81. Mitchell JP, Schuller D, Calandrino FS, Schuster DP. Improved outcome based on fluid management in critically ill patients requiring pulmonary artery catheterization. Am Rev Respir Dis 1992; 145:990–998.

82. Chiumello D, Pristine G, Slutski AS. Mechanical ventilation affects local and systemic cytokines in an animal model of acute respiratory distress syndrome. Am J Respir Crit Care Med 1999; 160:109–116.

83. Slutsky AS. Lung injury caused by mechanical ventilation. Chest 1999; 116(suppl):9S–15S.

84. Carvalho CRR, Barbas CSV, Medeiros DM, et al. Temporal hemodynamic effects of permissive hypercapnia associated with ideal PEEP in ARDS. Am J Respir Crit Care Med 1997; 156:1458–1466.

85. Feihl F, Perret C. Permissive hypercapnia: how permissive should we be? Am J Respir Crit Care Med 1994; 150:1722–1737.

86. McCulloch PR, Forkert PG, Froese AB. Lung volume maintenance prevents lung injury during high frequency oscillatory ventilation in surfactant-deficient rabbits. Am Rev Respir Dis 1988; 137:1185–1192.

87. Froese AB. Role of lung volume in lung injury: HFO in the atelectasis-prone lung. Acta Anesthesiol Scand 1989; 33(suppl):126–130.

88. Gerstmann DR, Minton SD, Stoddard RA, et al. The provo multicenter early high-frequency oscillatory ventilation trial: improved pulmonary and clinical outcome in respiratory distress syndrome. Pediatrics 1996; 98: 1044–1057.

89. Arnold JH, Hanson JH, Toro-Figuero LO, et al. Prospective, randomized comparison of high-frequency oscillatory ventilation and conventional mechanical ventilation in pediatric respiratory failure. Crit Care Med 1994; 22:1530–1539.

90. Derdak S, Mehta S, Stewart TE, et al. High-frequency oscillatory ventilation for acute respiratory distress syndrome in adults: a randomized controlled trial. Am J Respir Crit Care Med 2002; 166:801–808.

91. Rossaint R, Pison U, Gerlach H, et al. Inhaled nitric oxide: its effects on pulmonary circulation and airway smooth muscle cells. Eur Heart J 1993; 14(suppl I):133–140.

92. Zapol WM, Hurford WE. Inhaled nitric oxide in the adult respiratory distress syndrome and other lung diseases. New Horiz 1993; 1:638–650.

93. Fratacci MD, Frostell CG, Chen TY, et al. Inhaled nitric oxide: a selective pulmonary vasodilator of heparin-protamine vasoconstriction in sheep. Anesthesiology 1991; 75:990–999.

94. Shah NS, Nakayama DK, Jacob TD. Efficacy of inhaled nitric oxide in a porcine model of adult respiratory distress syndrome. Arch Surg 1994; 129: 158–164.

95. Dellinger RP, Zimmerman JL, Taylor RW, et al. Inhaled Nitric Oxide in ARDS Study Group. Effects of inhaled nitric oxide in patients with acute respiratory distress syndrome: results of a randomized phase II trial. Crit Care Med 1998; 26:15–23.

96. Payen D, Vallet B, Group G. Results of the French prospective multicentric randomized double-blind placebo-controlled trial on inhaled nitric oxide in ARDS. Intensive Care Med 1999; 25:S166.

97. Pelosi P, Tubiolo D, Mascheroni D, et al. Effects of the prone position on respiratory mechanics and gas exchange during acute lung injury. Am J Respir Crit Care Med 1998; 157:387–393.

98. Nakos G, Tsangaris I, Kostanti E, et al. Effect of the prone position on patients with hydrostatic pulmonary edema compared with patients with acute respiratory distress syndrome and pulmonary fibrosis. Am J Respir Crit Care Med 2000; 161:360–368.

99. Pappert D, Rossaint R, Slama K, Gruning T, Falke KJ. Influence of positioning on ventilation-perfusion relationships in severe adult respiratory distress syndrome. Chest 1994; 106:1511–1516.

100. Douglas WW, Rehder K, Beynen FM, Sessler AD, Marsh HM. Improved oxygenation in patients with acute respiratory failure: the prone position. Am Rev Respir Dis 1977; 115:559–566.

101. Pelosi P, Tubiolo D, Mascheroni D, et al. Effects of the prone position on respiratory mechanics and gas-exchange during acute lung injury. Am J Respir Crit Care Med 1998; 157:387–393.

102. Gattinoni L, Tognoni G, Pesenti A, et al. Effect of prone positioning on the survival of patients with acute respiratory failure. N Engl J Med 2001; 345:568–573.

103. Notter RH. Lung Surfactants: Basic Science and Clinical Applications. New York: Marcel Dekker, 2000.

104. Lewis JF, Jobe AH. Surfactant and the adult respiratory distress syndrome. Am Rev Respir Dis 1993; 147:218–233.

105. Anzueto A, Baughman RP, Guntupalli KK, et al. Aerosolized surfactant in adults with sepsis-induced acute respiratory distress syndrome. N Engl J Med 1996; 334:1417–1421.

106. Luce JM, Montgomery AB, Marks JD, Turner J, Metz CA, Murray JF. Ineffectiveness of high-dose methylprednisolone in preventing parenchymal lung injury and improving mortality in patients with septic shock. Am Rev Respir Dis 1988; 136:62–68.

107. Bernard GR, Luce JM, Sprung CL, et al. High-dose corticosteroids in patients with the adult respiratory distress syndrome. N Engl J Med 1987; 317:1565–1570.

108. Meduri GU, Belenchia JM, Estes RJ, Wunderink RG, el Torky M, Leeper KV Jr. Fibroproliferative phase of ARDS: clinical findings and effects of corticosteroids. Chest 1991; 100:943–952.

109. Meduri GU, Chinn AJ, Leeper KV, et al. Corticosteroid rescue treatment of progressive fibroproliferation in late ARDS: patterns of response and predictors of outcome. Chest 1994; 105:1516–1527.

110. NIH ARDS Network. Ketoconazole does not reduce mortality in patients with the acute respiratory distress syndrome. JAMA 2000; 283:1995–2002.

111. Warshawski F, Sibbald W, Driedger A, et al. Abnormal neutrophil-pulmonary interactions in the respiratory distress syndrome. Am Rev Respir Dis 1986; 133:797–804.

112. Carey PD, Jenkin JK, Byrne K, et al. The neutrophil respiratory burst and tissue injury in septic acute lung injury: the effect of cyclo-oxygenase inhibition in swine. Surgery 1992; 112:45–55.

113. Bernard GR, Lucht WD, Niedermeyer ME, et al. Effect of *N*-acetylcysteine on the pulmonary response to endotoxin in the awake sheep and upon in vitro granulocyte function. J Clin Invest 1984; 73:1772–1784.

114. Sznajder JI. Strategies to increase alveolar epithelial fluid removal in the injured lung. Am J Respir Crit Care Med 1999; 160:1441–1442.

115. Folkesson HG, Nitenberg G, Oliver BL, Jayr C, Albertine KH, Matthay MA. Upregulation of alveolar epithelial fluid transport after subacute lung injury in rats from bleomycin. Am J Physiol 1998; 275:L478–L490.

116. Lasnier JM, Wangensteen OD, Schmitz LS, Gross CR, Ingbar DH. Terbutaline stimulates alveolar fluid resorption in hyperoxic lung injury. J Appl Physiol 1996; 81:1723–1729.

117. Azzam ZS, Dumasius V, Saldias FJ, Adir Y, Sznajder JI, Factor P. Na,K-ATPase overexpression improves alveolar fluid clearance in a rat model of elevated left atrial pressure. Circulation 2002; 105:497–501.

118. Factor P, Mendez M, Mutlu GM, Dumasius V. Acute hyperoxic lung injury does not impede adenoviral-mediated alveolar gene transfer. Am J Respir Crit Care Med 2002; 165:521–526.

119. Panos RJ, Bak PM, Simonet WS, et al. Intratracheal instillation of keratinocyte growth factor decreases hyperoxia-induced mortality in rats. J Clin Invest 1995; 96:2026–2033.

120. Yano T, Deterding RR, Simonet WS, et al. Keratinocyte growth factor reduces lung damage due to acid instillation in rats. Am J Respir Cell Mol Biol 1996; 15:433–442.

4

Mediators and Inflammatory Cell Recruitment in Acute Lung Injury

MICHAEL P. KEANE, JOHN A. BELPERIO, and ROBERT M. STRIETER

*Departments of Medicine and Pathology and Laboratory Medicine,
UCLA School of Medicine, Los Angeles, California, U.S.A.*

I. Overview

This chapter discusses mediators and leukocytic cell recruitment important in the acute pulmonary inflammatory response and related acute lung injury. The pathophysiology of acute lung injury and the acute respiratory distress syndrome (ARDS) has been described in the preceding chapter. Discussion here provides further details on mechanisms and events involved in acute pulmonary inflammation and injury, including the importance of specific cytokine mediators, cell receptors, and transcription factors in the initiation and regulation of innate host defense. The activities of early response cytokines, particularly the interleukin-1 (IL-1) and tumor necrosis factor (TNF) families, are detailed and discussed for their roles in acute pulmonary inflammation. Extensive coverage is devoted to chemotactic cytokines (chemokines) that modulate and regulate inflammatory cell recruitment during innate host defense (C, CC, CXC, and CXXXC families). Significant emphasis is placed on the roles and importance of the CXC and CC families of chemokines and their receptors in mediating leukocytic cell recruitment during acute pulmonary inflammation and injury. The importance of these chemokines in subacute and chronic inflammation and lung injury is also discussed. Subsequent chapters (Chapters 5 and 6) give further details on etiologies, mechanisms, and mediators involved in chronic lung injury and chronic respiratory disease.

II. Introduction

The lungs comprise a unique interface between the body and the environment, presenting an extensive alveolar surface area ($\sim 1\,m^2/kg$ body weight) with only a minimal barrier of 4–8 μm between the airspaces and the microvasculature. While this configuration is ideal for gas exchange, it also increases vulnerability to noxious stimuli and pathogens. Consequently, pulmonary tissue must possess the capacity to generate a brisk innate host defense characterized by acute inflammation to both inhaled and hematogenous challenges that results in prompt clearance of the offending agent without compromise of essential gas exchange function. This acute pulmonary inflammatory response typically results in local increases in vascular permeability and a predominantly early neutrophil influx followed by mononuclear cell infiltration. Once successful containment of the noxious agent has occurred, pulmonary inflammation should then resolve to allow normal repair, tissue remodeling, and a return to homeostasis. However, because of their great capacity to initiate acute inflammation of innate immunity, the lungs can be subject to tissue injury by excessive reactions generated by both local and distant mediators. In conditions such as ARDS, overexuberant tissue inflammation can result in severe irreversible lung injury mediated primarily by elicited and activated leukocytes.

Many clinical entities, including trauma, pneumonia/sepsis, ischemia–reperfusion injury, as well as ARDS, are characterized by varying degrees of acute pulmonary inflammation and impairment of normal gas exchange function (Chapter 3). The pulmonary inflammatory response is initiated, maintained, resolved and depends upon complex yet coordinated intercellular interactions between immune and nonimmune cells. For example, the host response to bacterial pneumonia is characterized by acute inflammation. The typical histopathology of bacterial pneumonia is composed of proteinaceous exudate and massive neutrophil extravasation leading to consolidation of lung tissue. Once the inciting microbe is cleared; however, the inflammatory reaction resolves and normal repair and tissue remodeling occurs. This re-establishes normal lung function without the sequela of persistent inflammation or fibroproliferation. In contrast, the acute inflammatory response associated with ARDS often culminates in severe lung injury and respiratory failure, impacting host survival. A variety of mediators and factors produced by both immune and nonimmune cells are involved in coordinating and modulating pulmonary inflammation, including reactive oxygen metabolites, carbohydrates, lipids, and protein mediators such as cytokines.

While events occurring in pulmonary inflammation often involve direct cell-to-cell adhesive interaction via specific cellular adhesion molecules, cells also signal each other through soluble mediators such as cytokines. These polypeptide molecules have pleiotropic effects on a number of biological functions including proliferation, differentiation, recognition, and leukocyte recruitment. Their actions are mediated through paracrine and autocrine signaling through receptor–ligand interactions on specific cell populations. However, under certain conditions, these molecules may behave as hormones. Cytokines display concentration-dependent effects, being expressed in low concentrations during normal homeostasis, with modest increases exerting local effects, and still greater elevations resulting in systemic effects. Individual subpopulations of immune cells possess different capacities to elaborate and secrete specific cytokines in response to particular stimuli. Nonimmune cells, including endothelial cells, fibroblasts, and epithelial cells also demonstrate particular responses to specific signals resulting in the production of other cytokines. Furthermore, cell populations vary in their expression of receptors for individual cytokines, and, as a result, differ in their capacity to respond to specific cytokine signals.

Investigations into the interactions between various cell populations have led to the concept of cytokine networking. In this process, one population of cells may respond directly to specific stimuli (i.e., exogenous and/or endogenous) leading to the elaboration of a particular cytokine to exert distinct effects upon another population of cells. The targets respond by producing cytokines, which may serve as positive and negative feedback signals to the primary cell, or alternatively, initiate a cascade of events by affecting yet another array of target cells. Inflammatory effector cells, such as neutrophils and monocytes, may be locally recruited and activated in response to specific chemotactic signals resulting in further amplification of a cytokine cascade by nonimmune resident cells (i.e., endothelial cells, fibroblasts, and epithelial cells). As many of the complexities of the innate immune cytokine cascade have been shown to mediate acute pulmonary inflammation, increasing evidence suggests that nonimmune cells play crucial roles in the generation, maintenance, and resolution of both local and systemic inflammatory responses. While a variety of factors are involved in the innate response leading to acute pulmonary inflammation, cytokines constitute the largest and most pleiotropic group of mediators that regulate this response and are the focus of this chapter. Emphasis is on recent advances in inflammation research that address mechanisms of cytokine-induced leukocyte recruitment into the lung during the pathogenesis of acute pulmonary inflammation.

III. Innate Host Defense

Cytokines that are involved in the innate immune response of the lung are not constitutively expressed, and must be called into play by specific signals that alert the host to invading micro-organisms or early triggering events. Evolution has provided the mammalian host with two major forms of host defense, the innate and adaptive immune responses (1–4). The innate defense is the gatekeeper for immediate host defense against invading micro-organisms. The adaptive immune response is naïve, delayed in development, and must be taught through somatic generation of a diverse repertoire of receptors prior to the full development of an appropriate immune response (1,3–7). This difference in behavior suggests that the innate immune response has been genetically predetermined to recognize micro-organism associated molecular patterns, and to develop strategies to directly interact with, recognize, and immediately respond to counteract the invading micro-organism. In contrast, the adaptive immune response depends on two classes of specialized lymphocytes, T- and B-cells with specific receptors that are somatically generated in response to antigen presentation by professional antigen presenting cells (i.e., dendritic cells, macrophages, and other B-cells). This process allows for antigen-dependent clonal expansion of T- and B-cells resulting in learned, and long-term humoral and cell-mediated immune memory. However, this process does not occur immediately in response to a novel antigen, and the delay in response could have devastating impact on survival of the host. Therefore, the two immune responses are coordinate in their behavior, with the innate immunity representing the most fundamental process in acute inflammation of innate host defense.

Micro-organisms are critical in initiating acute inflammation of innate host response. Micro-organism express highly conserved molecular patterns that are unique and distinguish themselves from host. The host has evolved specific pattern recognition receptors to detect these pathogen-associated molecules (2,6,7). While these receptors can be divided into secreted, endocytic, and signaling classes of receptors (2,6,7), the latter class of signaling receptors is critical in mediating the expression of a variety of cytokines that are subsequently necessary to amplify acute inflammation of innate immunity.

The mammalian Toll-like receptors (TLRs) are important signaling receptors in innate host defense, and have evolved from the Drosophila Toll gene (2–4,6–8). Although the Drosophila Toll gene was identified in mediating dorsoventral polarization during embryogenesis of the fly (9), it is a transmembrane protein with a cytoplasmic domain that is homologous to the cytoplasmic domain of the mammalian IL-1 receptor (10). This finding supports the notion that both Toll and mammalian TLRs share similar signal-transduction pathways that ultimately involve the nuclear factor-κB (NF-κB) family of transcriptional factors (10,11). Nuclear factor-κB plays an important role as a "master switch" in the transactivation of a number of cytokines that are involved in the innate immune response and development of pulmonary inflammation (11). Medzhitov et al.(12) were the first to characterize a human TLR, TLR4. The constitutively active mutant of TLR4 transfected into human cell lines induced the activation of NF-κB and the expression of proinflammatory cytokines genes for interleukin-1 (IL-1), interleukin-6 (IL-6), and interleukin-8 (IL-8/CXCL8) (12). In addition, TLR4 signal transduction and NF-κB transactivation resulted in the expression IL-12 p40 and the molecules CD80 and CD86, which are costimulatory molecules necessary to bridge the innate to the adaptive immune response and activate naïve T-cells in an antigen-dependent manner (12).

Subsequent work has identified TLR4 as the receptor for LPS signal transduction on macrophages, dendritic cells, and B-cells. In LPS resistant C3H/HeJ and C57BL/10ScCr mice, defective LPS signaling is related to mutations in TLR4 gene (13–15). However, LPS recognition and triggering of the innate host response is more complex than direct interaction with TLR4. LPS first interacts with a serum protein, lipopolysaccharide-binding protein (LBP), which transfers LPS to CD14 anchored to the cell membrane (16). While CD14 lacks a transmembrane and cytoplasmic domain for signaling coupling, it appears that the LPS/CD14 complex uses TLR4 as a coreceptor (8). Furthermore, MD-2 is a molecule that is constitutively associated with TLR4 and confers enhanced LPS responsiveness to TLR4 (17). These studies support the notion that the LPS recognition by the host is dictated by a complex of at least three components, CD14, TLR4, and MD-2 (2,6,7).

Although another Toll-like receptor, TLR2, was initially thought to also bind and signal couple LPS, studies have now shown that TLR2−/− mice are able to respond to LPS, but not to bacterial-associated molecular patterns, peptidoglycan, and lipoproteins, suggesting that TLR2 is important for detecting microbial molecular patterns other than LPS (18,19). The ability of these receptors to detect only pathogen-associated molecular patterns and result in important signal coupling supports their high degree of specificity for detecting micro-organisms and acting as sentinels in the initiation of acute inflammation of innate host response with expression of a variety of factors, including cytokines. The expression of cytokines provides further fidelity to the innate response and acute pulmonary inflammation, as not all cells that participate in the developing innate response have receptors that directly sense micro-organisms. The ability of cytokine networks to be activated after encountering a micro-organism or other triggering event leads to autocrine, paracrine, and endocrine intercellular communication between immune and nonimmune cells that ultimately amplifies the innate host defense, increases the inflammatory response, and elicits the recruitment of leukocytes that ultimately aids in the eradication of the micro-organism or triggering event.

IV. Early Response Cytokines

While the above mechanisms for pathogen recognition in the innate immune response are necessary in order to sense and to initially respond to micro-organism molecular patterns, it is increasingly clear that cytokines are necessary for the full development of the innate host defense and the promotion of acute pulmonary inflammation. Early response cytokines are cytokines that are activated initially after TLR signal coupling or in response to other triggering events; they amplify, engage, and activate additional cells; they signal the expression of more distal cytokines that are important in the recruitment of leukocytes. Two of the most important early response cytokines in innate immunity and acute pulmonary inflammation are IL-1 and TNF-α.

Although biochemically unrelated, TNF and IL-1 demonstrate similar pleiotropic and overlapping effects on a variety cellular functions (20–36). These cytokines are primarily produced by mononuclear phagocytes and, because of their role for initiating further inflammatory responses, have been termed "early response cytokines." At sites of local inflammation, modest concentrations are essential, and serve to closely regulate cellular function. These early response cytokines dictate the events leading to further initiation, maintenance, and resolution of tissue injury in a cascade of cytokine activity. In marked contrast to the controlled events of local production of TNF and IL-1, the exaggerated systemic release of these cytokines can result in a syndrome of multiorgan injury with increased host morbidity and mortality. Thus, TNF and IL-1 have a broad spectrum of biologic activity that can influence the outcome of acute pulmonary inflammatory response on both the local and the systemic levels.

A. Interleukin-1 Family of Cytokines

The IL-1 family of cytokines consists of two agonists, IL-1α and IL-1β, and one antagonist, IL-1 receptor antagonist (IL-1Ra) (24,25). The IL-1 agonists are pleiotropic cytokines that exist as two distinct genes (24,25). These two forms of IL-1 are also distinguished by whether they are found predominantly membrane associated (IL-1α) or secreted (IL-1β) (24,25).

In contrast to the two IL-1 agonists, IL-1Ra is the only known naturally occurring cytokine with specific antagonistic activity. The discovery of the IL-1Ra has led to an appreciation of a dynamic balance between IL-1 agonists and IL-1Ra in the maintenance of IL-1-dependent homeostasis and inflammation, and has necessitated investigations into the role of IL-1Ra in disease (24,25). Two structural variants of IL-1Ra have previously been described, a 17-kDa protein that is secreted by monocytes, macrophages, and neutrophils as a variably glycosylated protein (sIL-1Ra), and a second intracellular 18-kDa protein that remains in the cytoplasm of monocytes, epithelial cells, and keratinocytes (icIL-1Ra) (29). In addition, a smaller isoform of intracellular IL-1Ra has been described (37). Investigations have demonstrated that IL-1Ra acts as a pure antagonist of either IL-1α or IL-1β and, when present in sufficient quantities, can attenuate a variety of IL-1 actions in both in vitro and in vivo model systems (24,25). These studies have led to an appreciation that IL-1Ra normally modulates IL-1-dependent activity and speculation that it may play a role in the resolution of the pulmonary inflammatory cascade necessary for the lung to return to homeostasis. Interleukin-1Ra is produced in response to a variety of agents, the most potent being adherent IgG, LPS, GM-CSF, and IL-4 (29).

Interleukin-1 and IL-1Ra have been implicated in the pathogenesis of a variety of lung diseases including bronchial asthma (38), ARDS (39), pan-bronchiolitis (40), and pulmonary fibrosis (41). In ARDS, low levels of the anti-inflammatory cytokines, IL-10 and IL-1Ra, in the BAL of patients with early disease correlated with a poor prognosis (39). When LPS, IL-1 or TNF are intratracheally injected, these inflammatory mediators induce an intra-alveolar inflammatory response composed predominately of neutrophils, followed later by a mononuclear cell infiltrate (42). However, IL-1 is more potent than TNF in this response. In addition, LPS is capable of inducing both TNF and IL-1 gene expression in the lung that is important for its effect in amplifying the inflammatory response. In fact, IL-1Ra has been found to reduce the inflammatory response to LPS in the lungs (42). These findings suggest that IL-1Ra has an important immunomodulating influence on IL-1, and its production by mononuclear phagocytes and other cells in the lung may impact on the pathogenesis of the innate response.

However, genetic approaches have led to findings that are less impressive for IL-1 in the innate immune response. For example, IL-1α–/– and IL-1β–/– animals display no phenotype at birth and appear similar to their wild-type littermates (+/+) (43). To determine their response under conditions analogous to the innate host response, Horai et al.(43) generated doubly deficient knockout animals (IL-1α–/– /IL-1β–/– mice), as compared to IL-1α–/–, IL-1β–/–, and IL-1Ra –/– mice. When these mice were injected with a nonspecific inducer of inflammation (i.e., turpentine), fever was suppressed in IL-1β–/– as well as IL-1α/β–/– mice, whereas IL-1α–/– mice displayed no abnormal response. In contrast, IL-1Ra–/– mice showed an elevated febrile response (43). This response was paralleled by increased levels of circulating glucocorticoids (43). In response to LPS, IL-1β–/– mice behave very similarly to IL-1β+/+ mice in regard to generation of IL-1α, IL-6, and TNF-α, and were equally sensitive to the lethal effects of LPS (44,45). However, in response to influenza infection, IL-1β–/– mice demonstrated a higher mortality rate, as compared to IL-1β+/+ mice (46). The difference in above findings for the importance of IL-1 in mediating inflammation and participating in the innate host response may be related to the individual model systems or the development of redundancy that may have occurred during embryogenesis in the $-/-$ mice.

B. Tumor Necrosis Factor-Alpha (TNF-α)

Tumor necrosis factor is a mononuclear phagocyte and T-lymphocyte-derived cytokine, which has been increasingly recognized for its pleiotropic effects on numerous inflammatory and immunological responses. It is one of 10 known members of a family of ligands that activate a corresponding family of receptors (47). Tumor necrosis factor is produced primarily by monocytes/macrophages, and has many overlapping biologic activities with IL-1. Tumor necrosis factor was first described as a cytolytic agent that caused hemorrhagic necrosis of tumor cells in vivo, and also causes fever, cachexia, systemic shock, and the production of hepatic acute phase proteins (48,49). In solution, TNF is a homotrimer and binds to two different cell surface receptors, p55 and p75 (48). The TNF receptor family are transmembrane proteins with an extracellular domain that contains a recurring cysteine rich motif and an intracellular domain that demonstrates more variability than the extracellular domain (47). The p55 receptor and the Fas receptor contain a 60 amino acid domain known as the "death domain" which is essential for signal transduction of an apoptotic signal (47).

While low levels of TNF may be involved in the maintenance of physiologic homeostasis, elevated levels of TNF have been implicated in the pathogenesis of a number of disease states, including septic shock/sepsis syndrome (48), ARDS (50), hepatic ischemia–reperfusion injury (51), AIDS-related cachexia, (52), chronic parasitic infections (53), graft vs. host disease (54) and heart, kidney, liver, and lung allograft rejection (55). Furthermore, it has been suggested that autoimmune disorders are a result of mutations in the receptors for TNF and its related ligands, which are important in mediating apoptosis (56). The resultant defect may lead to a compensatory increase in the relevant ligand with subsequent inflammatory damage typical of complex autoimmune disorders such as rheumatoid arthritis and Crohn's disease (56). Specifically, mutations in the Fas receptor gene lead to a lymphoproliferative disorder with splenomegaly and signs of autoimmunity at an early age (57,58).

Tumor necrosis factor exhibits a variety of inflammatory effects, including: induction of neutrophil- and mononuclear cell-endothelial cell adhesion and transendothelial migration via expression of adhesion molecules and chemokines; enhancement of a procoagulant environment by upregulating the expression of tissue factor and plasminogen activator inhibitor, and suppressing the protein C pathway; and acting as an early response cytokine in the promotion of a cytokine cascade (48,59). Although TNF may be a significant mediator of proximal nonspecific inflammation, this cytokine may have a role in mediating specific immune inflammatory events in the lung. Recent studies have suggested immunoregulatory functions of TNF that include regulation of B-lymphocyte differentiation and enhanced cytolytic activity of human natural killer (NK) cells. While resting T-lymphocytes do not specifically bind TNF, Scheurich et al.(60) have identified that anti-CD3 antibody activated T-lymphocytes express specific TNF receptors in a kinetic fashion similar to the expression of IL-2 receptors. These TNF receptors have biological function, as TNF enhances the expression of MHC class II antigens, induces the expression of high-affinity IL-2 receptors, and synergizes with IL-2 to stimulate T-lymphocyte proliferation and production of gamma-interferon (IFN-γ). In addition, TNF has been shown to stimulate T-lymphocyte colony formation that may be mediated through TNF-induced production of IL-1 (61) and enhance antigen and mitogen-induced T-lymphocyte proliferation (62).

Although the pathogenesis of septic shock and the development of acute lung injury are multifactorial, the role of TNF and IL-1 in mediating septic shock and ARDS has been clearly demonstrated in a number of studies. Waage et al. (63) examined sera from patients suffering from meningococcal septicemia with acute lung injury. They found a significant correlation between serum TNF levels and mortality. In a similar study of 55 patients with a clinical diagnosis of sepsis and purpura fulminans due to meningococcemia, serum levels of both TNF and IL-1 correlated with mortality (64). In another study, patients were prospectively randomized to assess the efficacy of methylprednisolone administered in septic shock (65). Serum levels of TNF were detected in 33% of the patients with septic shock. Tumor necrosis factor levels were elevated with equal frequency in patients with shock due to either gram-positive or -negative bacteria. The magnitude of TNF measured also correlated with a higher incidence and severity of ARDS and mortality. The ratio of TNF to the anti-inflammatory cytokine IL-10 in BAL fluid has been shown to be significantly higher in ARDS patients than in at risk patients, although there was no difference in the ability of alveolar macrophages to produce IL-10 in response to endotoxin (66). In animals, systemically administered TNF has been found to induce similar pathophysiological effects to either endotoxin or infusion of live gram-negative bacteria. Administration of TNF to animals is associated with metabolic acidosis, elevated body temperature and circulating levels of catecholamines, disseminated intravascular coagulation, multiorgan dysfunction (renal, hepatic, gastrointestinal, and pulmonary), alterations in circulating leukocytes, and hypotension leading to shock (67). In addition, TNF and IL-1 have been found to be synergistic in mediating similar pathophysiological effects when administered concurrently (23).

Inhibition of endogenously produced TNF during bacteria-induced septic shock has been shown in animal models to significantly attenuate the pathogenesis of multiorgan injury and mortality. Tracey et al. (67), using a baboon model of septic shock, administered a monoclonal antihuman TNF antibody both prior to and after the injection of a LD_{100} dose of live *Escherichia coli*. Only monoclonal antibody administration prior to the lethal dose of *E. coli* decreased mortality. In contrast, Hinshaw et al. (68), employing a similar model of *E. coli*-induced lethal septicemia in a baboon model, could delay the addition of monoclonal anti-TNF antibodies for up to 30 min after *E. coli* challenge and all animals survived. The endogenous expression and regulation of TNF from murine models of endotoxemia has shown that TNF is rapidly produced after a LD_{100} infusion of endotoxin (69). Peak levels of TNF were seen at 1 hr, with a rapid decline to relatively unmeasurable levels by 8 hr. Similar findings have been seen in human volunteer subjects injected with low doses of endotoxin (70). These results suggest that TNF is under strict regulation.

While the above studies demonstrate an important role for TNF in inflammation, inhibition of TNF in humans with sepsis has been disappointing (71,72). However, a recent study has suggested that there may be subgroups of patients that may derive benefit (73). Therapy with anti-TNF antibodies is fraught with difficulty. First, anti-TNF antibodies do not prevent lymphotoxin from signaling at the TNF receptors. Second, formation of immune complexes may lead to the activation of complement with potentially harmful effects. Third, murine monoclonal antibodies, and even humanized monoclonal antibodies, are antigenic which may preclude long-term therapy. Attempts to overcome these obstacles have led to the development of chimeric inhibitor molecules. These molecules contain the extracellular domain of the TNF receptor joined to an immunoglobulin heavy chain fragment and are minimally antigenic (47). They are highly specific and neutralize all ligands for the TNF receptor including lymphotoxin-α (74). These chimeric inhibitors are being evaluated for efficacy in rheumatoid arthritis.

V. Inflammatory Cell Recruitment

The recruitment of specific leukocyte subpopulations in response to lung injury is a fundamental mechanism of acute pulmonary inflammation. The elicitation of leukocytes is dependent upon a complex series of events, including reduced leukocyte deformability, endothelial cell activation and expression of endothelial cell-derived leukocyte adhesion molecules, leukocyte–endothelial cell adhesion, leukocyte activation and expression of leukocyte-derived adhesion molecules, leukocyte transendothelial migration, and leukocyte migration beyond the endothelial barrier along established chemotactic and haptotactic gradients.

Historically, the first observations of leukocyte migration dates back to the initial observation of leukocyte adherence followed by transendothelial migration by Augustus Waller in 1846, who described extravasation of leukocytes in a frog tongue (75). This observation was followed by the first description of leukocyte migration in response to chemotactic signals, reported in the late 19th century (76). These studies demonstrated that leukocytes migrate in response to either products of other leukocytes or killed bacteria. Although these studies were descriptive in nature, they were the first to establish leukocyte extravasation in response to a chemotactic signal.

The development of a chemotactic chamber in 1962 by Boyden (77) was a historical event that allowed the quantitative analysis of leukocyte migration in vitro. While molecules may in vivo behave as leukocyte chemotaxins, the use of these chambers allowed the assessment in vitro as to whether a molecule behaves as a direct or indirect leukocyte chemotaxin. Moreover, by modifying this technique, Zigmond and Hirsch (78) could distinguish chemotaxis, a process of leukocyte migration in response to a concentration gradient, from chemokinesis, a property of random leukocyte motion. In the late 1960s, investigators identified the first chemotactic molecules (79–81). These studies demonstrated that N-formylmethionyl peptides from bacterial cell walls and the anaphylatoxin, C5a, were chemotactic for leukocytes. These findings were followed by the discovery that specific products of arachidonate metabolism were leukocyte chemotaxins. Both platelet activating factor (PAF) and leukotriene B_4 (LTB_4) were shown to have significant chemotactic activity for leukocytes at pM to nM concentrations (82,83). These findings supported the premise that leukocyte recruitment is critical to acute inflammation of innate immunity, and that a number of factors that possess potent and overlapping leukocyte chemotactic activity are necessary to assure continued leukocyte emigration at sites of inflammation.

The salient feature of acute inflammation of innate immunity and the development of acute lung injury is the extravasation of predominately neutrophils followed by mononuclear cells. These extravasating leukocytes contribute to the pathogenesis of inflammation and promote the eradication of the offending agent. In addition, the shear magnitude of increase in infiltrating cells, the activation of these cells, and the release of a variety of mediators, including additional cytokines that interact with resident nonleukocyte cellular populations leads to further amplification of acute inflammation and lung injury. The maintenance of leukocyte recruitment during inflammation requires intercellular communication between infiltrating leukocytes and the endothelium, resident stromal and parenchyma cells. These events are mediated via the recognition of the offending agent by the TLRs, the generation of early response cytokines (e.g., IL-1 and TNF), the expression of cell–surface adhesion molecules, and the production of chemotactic molecules, such as chemokines.

VI. Chemotactic Cytokines (Chemokines)
A. Chemokine Families

The salient feature of persistent inflammation is the association of leukocyte infiltration. The maintenance of leukocyte recruitment during inflammation requires intercellular communication between infiltrating leukocytes and the endothelium, resident stromal and parenchymal cells. The human CXC, CC, C, and CXXXC chemokine families of chemotactic cytokines are four closely related polypeptide families that behave, in general, as potent chemotactic factors for neutrophils, eosinophils, basophils, monocytes, mast cells, dendritic cells, NK cells, T and B-lymphocytes (Table 1). These cytokines in their monomeric form range from 7 to 10 kD and are characteristically basic heparin-binding proteins. The chemokines display highly conserved cysteine amino acid residues. The CXC chemokine family has the first two NH_2-terminal cysteines separated by one nonconserved amino acid residue, the CXC cysteine motif. The CC chemokine family has the first two NH_2-terminal cysteines in juxtaposition, the CC cysteine motif. The C chemokine has one lone NH_2-terminal cysteine amino acid, the C cysteine motif; and the CXXXC chemokine has the first two NH_2-terminal cysteines separated by three nonconserved amino acid residues. Interestingly, CXC chemokines are, in general, clustered on human chromosome 4, and exhibit between 20% and 50% homology on the amino acid level. CC chemokines are, in general, clustered on human chromosome 17, and exhibit between 28% and 45% homology on the amino acid level, the one C chemokine, lymphotactin, is located on human chromosome 1, and the one CXXXC, fractalkine, is located on human chromosome 16. There is approximately 20–40% homology between the members of the four chemokine families.

The murine homologues of the human CXC chemokines, KC/CXCL1, macrophage inflammatory protein-2 (MIP-2)/CXCL2, IP-10/CXCL10, MIG/CXCL9, and SDF-1/CXCL12 are structurally homologous to human GRO-α/CXCL1, GRO-*β*/*GRO*-*γ* (CXCL2/CXCL3), IP-10/CXCL10, MIG/CXCL9, and SDF-1/CXCL12, respectively (84,85). No murine or rat structural homologue exists for human IL-8 (84,85). The murine CC and C chemokines, in general, are known by the same names as their human counterparts (59,84–86). The CXXXC chemokine, fractalkine/CX3CL1, was initially described on nonhemopoeitic cells and it can exist as either a membrane-anchored or as a shed glycoprotein, which act as a potent adhesion molecule or chemoattractant, respectively, for T-cells and monocytes (87,88).

Chemokines have been found to be produced by an array of cells including monocytes, alveolar macrophages, neutrophils, platelets, eosinophils, mast cells, T- and B-lymphocytes, NK cells, keratinocytes, mesangial cells, epithelial cells, hepatocytes, fibroblasts, smooth muscle cells,

Table 1 The Human C, CC, CXC and CXXXC Chemokine Families of Chemotactic
Cytokines

The C chemokines	
XCL1	Lymphotactin
XCL2	SCM-1β
The CC chemokines	
CCL1	I-309
CCL2	Monocyte chemotactic protein-1 (MCP-1)
CCL3	Macrophage inflammatory protein-1 alpha (MIP-1α)
CCL4	Macrophage inflammatory protein-1 beta (MIP-1β)
CCL5	Regulated on activation normal T-cell expressed and secreted (RANTES)
CCL7	Monocyte chemotactic protein-3 (MCP-3)
CCL8	Monocyte chemotactic protein-2 (MCP-2)
CCL9	Macrophage inflammatory protein-1delta (MIP-1δ)
CCL11	Eotaxin
CCL13	Monocyte chemotactic protein-4 (MCP-4)
CCL14	HCC-1
CCL15	HCC-2
CCL16	HCC-4
CCL17	Thymus and activation-regulated chemokine (TARC)
CCL18	DC-CK-1
CCL19	Macrophage inflammatory protein-3 beta (MIP-3β)
CCL20	Macrophage inflammatory protein-3 alpha (MIP-3α)
CCL21	6Ckine
CCL22	MDC
CCL23	MPIF-1
CCL24	MPIF-2
CCL25	TECK
CCL26	Eotaxin-3
CCL27	CTACK
The CXC chemokines	
CXCL1	Growth-related oncogene alpha (GRO-α)
CXCL2	Growth-related oncogene beta (GRO-β)
CXCL3	Growth-related oncogene gamma (GRO-γ)
CXCL4	Platelet factor-4 (PF4)
CXCL5	Epithelial neutrophil activating protein-78 (ENA-78)
CXCL6	Granulocyte chemotactic protein-2 (GCP-2)
CXCL7	Neutrophil activating protein-2 (NAP-2)
CXCL8	Interleukin-8 (IL-8)
CXCL9	Monokine induced by interferon-γ (MIG)
CXCL10	Interferon-γ-inducible protein (IP-10)
CXCL11	Interferon inducible T-cell alpha chemoattractant (ITAC)
CXCL12	Stromal cell-derived factor-1 (SDF-1)
CXCL13	B-cell-attracting chemokine-1 (BCA-1)
The CXXXC chemokine	
CXC3CL1	Fractalkine

mesothelial cells, and endothelial cells. These cells can produce chemokines in response to a variety of factors, including viruses, bacterial products, IL-1, TNF, C5a, LTB$_4$, and IFNs. The production of chemokines by both immune and nonimmune cells supports the contention that these cytokines may play a pivotal role in orchestrating chronic inflammation. We will focus our discussion on the role of the CXC and CC chemokine families.

B. The CXC Chemokines

The CXC chemokines can be further divided into two groups on the basis of a structure/function domain consisting of the presence or absence of three amino acid residues (Glu-Leu-Arg; "ELR" motif) that precedes the first cysteine amino acid residue in the primary structure of these cytokines (59,84,86,89–92). The ELR$^+$ CXC chemokines are chemoattractants for neutrophils and act as potent angiogenic factors (93–95). In contrast, the ELR$^-$ CXC chemokines are chemoattractants for mononuclear cells and are potent inhibitors of angiogenesis (Table 2) (95,96).

Based on the structural/functional difference, the members of the CXC chemokine family are unique cytokines in their ability to behave in a disparate manner in the regulation of angiogenesis. The angiogenic members include interleukin-8 (IL-8)/CXCL8, epithelial neutrophil activating protein-78 (ENA-78)/CXCL5, growth related genes (GRO-α, -β, and -γ)/CXCL1, 2, and 3, granulocyte chemotactic protein-2 (GCP-2)/CXCL6, CXCL6, and NH$_2$-terminal truncated forms of platelet basic protein (PBP), which are generated by proteolytic cleavage with monocyte-derived

Table 2 The CXC Chemokines that Display Disparate Angiogenic Activity

Angiogenic CXC chemokines containing the ELR motif	
CXCL1	Growth-related oncogene alpha (GRO-α)
CXCL2	Growth-related oncogene beta (GRO-β)
CXCL3	Growth-related oncogene gamma (GRO-γ)
CXCL5	Epithelial neutrophil activating protein-78 (ENA-78)
CXCL6	Granulocyte chemotactic protein-2 (GCP-2)
CXCL7	Neutrophil activating protein-2 (NAP-2)
CXCL8	Interleukin-8 (IL-8)
Angiostatic CXC chemokines that lack the ELR motif	
CXCL4	Platelet factor-4 (PF4)
CXCL9	Monokine induced by interferon-γ (MIG)
CXCL10	Interferon-γ-inducible protein (IP-10)
CXCL11	Interferon inducible T-cell alpha chemoattractant (ITAC)
CXCL12	Stromal cell-derived factor-1 (SDF-1)

proteases and include connective tissue activating protein-III (CTAP-III), beta-thromboglobulin (β-TG), and neutrophil activating protein-2 (NAP-2). GRO-α, -β, and -γ are closely related CXC chemokines, with GRO-α/CXCL1 originally described for its melanoma growth stimulatory activity. Interleukin-8/CXCL8, ENA-78/CXCL5, and GCP-2/CXCL6 were all initially identified on the basis of neutrophil activation and chemotaxis.

The angiostatic (ELR$^-$) members of the CXC chemokine family include platelet factor 4 (PF4)/CXCL4, which was originally described for its ability to bind heparin and inactivate heparin's anticoagulation function. Other angiostatic ELR$^-$ CXC chemokines include MIG/CXCL9 and IP-10/CXCL10 (Table 2). Stromal cell-derived factor (SDF-1)/CXCL12 gained notoriety when it was shown that SDF-1/CXCL12 induces lymphocyte migration and prevents infection of T-cells by lymphotropic strains of HIV-1. Although SDF-1/CXCL12 is another ELR$^-$ CXC chemokine, it remains unclear whether it inhibits angiogenesis. SDF-1/CXCL12 was found to induce in vitro migration of human umbilical vein endothelial cells (HUVEC), whereas in another study, SDF-1/CXCL12 was found to attenuate the in vivo angiogenic activity of either ELR$^+$ CXC chemokines, bFGF, or VEGF using the rat cornea micropocket assay of neovascularization (97).

Of particular interest is the fact that IP-10/CXCL10 and MIG/CXCL9 are highly induced by interferons. IP-10/CXCL10 can be induced by all three interferons (IFN-α, -β, and -γ). MIG/CXCL9 is unique in that it is only induced by IFN-γ. In addition, IL-12 and IL-18, via the induction of IFN-γ have been found to induce the expression of IP-10/CXCL10 and MIG/CXCL9 (98). While interferons induce the production of the angiostatic CXC chemokines, IP-10/CXCL10 and MIG/CXCL9, they attenuate the expression of the angiogenic CXC chemokines IL-8/CXCL8, GRO-α/CXCL1, and ENA-78/CXCL5. This differential regulation of angiostatic vs. angiogenic CXC chemokines by interferons is likely to account for their previously documented inhibitory effect on angiogenesis.

Information on chemokine function can be obtained from transgenic animal models. Transgenic mice that overexpress IL-8/CXCL8 on a liver-specific promoter do not develop neutrophil infiltrates in their liver (99). They have high circulating IL-8/CXCL8 levels that are associated with L-selectin shedding from neutrophils and lack the ability to induce neutrophil accumulation in response to local stimuli (99). Similarly, intravenous administration of IL-8/CXCL8 in rabbits prevents local neutrophil accumulation, although L-selectin shedding was not observed (100,101). Furthermore, mice that express KC (murine homologue of GRO-α/CXCL1) on a lung CC10 promoter have demonstrated that chronic unregulated expression of KC/CXCL1 is associated with attenuated recruitment of neutrophils over time (102). Similar findings have been reported in the thymus (103). Furthermore, the neutrophil accumulation that was seen early in the lungs of KC/CXCL1 transgenic mice is not associated with tissue injury or evidence for the development of fibrosis or emphysema (102). Similarly, mice that express MCP-1/CCL2 under the control of the insulin promoter develop a monocytic insulitis without tissue damage or diabetes (104). These studies demonstrate that chemokines exert their attractant effects only when expressed locally at low levels and that chemoattraction is not always associated with leukocyte activation. Furthermore, this may explain the relative lack of neutrophils in chronic inflammatory/fibroproliferative disorders associated with significant levels of IL-8/CXCL8 or other ELR$^+$ CXC chemokines, whereas these chemokines are acting as an angiogenic factors (105–108).

C. CXC Chemokine Receptors

Chemokine activities are mediated through G-protein coupled receptors. Six CXC chemokine receptors have been identified (Table 3) (109,110). The ELR$^+$ chemokines bind to CXCR1 and CXCR2 receptors which are found on neutrophils, T-lymphocytes, monocytes, basophils, keratinocytes and mast cells and endothelial cells (111,112). The CXCR1 and CXCR2 receptor genes are found on human chromosome 2 (q34–q35), and may have arisen from duplication of a common ancestral gene. While the transmembrane and the second and third intracellular/cytoplasmic domains of these receptors are well conserved, the NH_2- and COOH-terminal ends of these receptors are variable. The intracellular COOH-terminus of these receptors is rich in serine and threonine amino acid residues that may be important in phosphorylation and signal coupling via G proteins (113–115). In general, these receptors are coupled to $G\alpha_i$ proteins that are inhibited in response to pertussis toxin (110,116–120).

Members of the herpesvirus family have been demonstrated to encode genes that mimic the chemokine receptors (121). Both herpesvirus saimiri (HVS) and Kaposi's sarcoma-associated herpesvirus (KSHV) have the genes, ECRF3 and ORF74, respectively, that encode a G-protein coupled receptor, with significant homology to CXCR2 (122,123). These receptors are functional and specific receptors for the CXC chemokines. Similarly,

Table 3 The CXC Chemokine Receptors

Receptor	Ligand
CXCR1	CXCL6, CXCL8
CXCR2	CXCL1, CXCL2, CXCL3, CXCL5, CXCL6, CXCL7, CXCL8
CXCR3	CXCL9,CXCL10, CXCL11
CXCR4	CXCL12
CXCR5	CXCL13

human CMV can encode four G-protein coupled receptors, UL33, US27, US28, and UL78 (121). US28 binds CC chemokines and has homology with CX_3CR1 and binds fractalkine (121). Human herpes virus 6 encodes a functional chemokine receptor homologue designated US12, which binds CC chemokines (121). Moreover, the expression of these receptors suggests a potential role for chemokines in mediating the pathogenesis associated with the infection of these viruses. For example, ORF74 expression on cell surface is associated with constitutive activity that can induce cellular proliferation, cell transformation, and tumorigenicity (124,125). In addition, ELR^+ CXC chemokine ligands, such as IL-8 and GRO-α, can bind to this receptor and further augment signal transduction of this receptor (126). Furthermore, the non-ELR CXC chemokine, IP-10, has been found to inhibit signaling of this receptor (126).

The receptor for IP-10 and MIG, CXCR3, is expressed on activated T-lymphocytes in the presence of IL-2; however, it is not significantly present on resting T- and B-lymphocytes, monocytes, or neutrophils (127). CXCR4 is the specific receptor for SDF-1 and is the cofactor for lymphotropic HIV-1, and SDF-1 is a potent inhibitor of HIV entry into T-lymphocytes (110,128,129). In contrast to CXCR3, CXCR4 appears to be expressed on resting T-lymphocytes (110,128,129). These findings suggest that ELR^- CXC chemokines and their receptors are important in regulating mononuclear cell function. CXCR1, CXCR2, and CXCR4 are expressed on HUVEC and the spontaneously transformed HUVEC cell line, ECV304 (130). We have found that CXCR2 is expressed on human microvascular endothelial cells (HMVEC) and that it mediates the angiogenic effects of ELR^+ chemokines (111). Recent evidence suggests that the expression of CXCR3 on HUMVEC is cell cycle dependent (131).

CXCR5 is the receptor for B-cell attracting chemokine-1 (BCA-1) (132). It was originally described on Burkitt's lymphoma cells and B-lymphocytes and was noticed to have many structural similarities to other chemokine receptors (133). BCA-1 and CXCR5 are necessary for the homing of B-lymphocytes and proper development of the B-cell-rich regions of lymphoid organs (134). CXCR6 is a receptor for the recently described CXCL16 which differs from other CXC chemokines in that its sequence predicts that it is membrane bound and suspended by a mucin stalk in a similar fashion to fractalkine/CX3C (135). CXCR6 was initially described as an orphan receptor that could serve as a coreceptor for HIV (119,136). CXCR6 is predominantly expressed on type 1 polarized T-cells suggesting it may have a role in type 1 mediated processes (137).

While the CXCRs have been demonstrated to have functional activity with ligand binding, another chemokine receptor has been identified that apparently binds chemokines without a subsequent signal coupling event. This receptor demonstrates promiscuity in that it binds both CXC and CC chemokines without apparent signal coupling (110,113–115). This receptor was originally found on human erythrocytes and felt to represent a "sink" for chemokines (115). In addition to binding of the chemokine family, this receptor has been found to be shared by the malarial parasites, *Plasmodium vivax* and *knowlesi*, and may allow their invasion into erythrocytes (115). This receptor has been cloned and found to be identical to the Duffy blood group antigen, and is now referred to as the Duffy antigen receptor for chemokines (DARC), and its structure demonstrates a seven transmembrane spanning receptor motif, similar to other chemokine receptors (110,115). Further studies are required to examine the functional nature of this receptor.

D. CXC Chemokines in Pulmonary Inflammation

CXC chemokines have also been found to play a significant role in mediating neutrophil infiltration in the lung parenchyma and pleural space in response to endotoxin and bacterial challenge. Frevert et al.(138) have passively immunized rats with neutralizing KC (homologous to human GRO-α/CXCL1) antibodies prior to intratracheal LPS, and found a 71% reduction in neutrophil accumulation within the lung. Broaddus et al. (139,140) have found that passive immunization with neutralizing IL-8/CXCL8 antibodies blocked 77% of endotoxin-induced neutrophil influx in the pleura of rabbits. However, in the context of micro-organism invasion, depletion of a CXC chemokine and reduction of infiltrating neutrophils may have a major impact on the host.

ELR$^+$ CXC chemokines have been implicated in mediating neutrophil sequestration in the lungs of patients with pneumonia. Interleukin-8/CXCL8 has been found in the bronchoalveolar lavage of patients with community acquired pneumonia and nosocomial pneumonia following trauma (141,142). In animal models of pneumonia, ELR$^+$ CXC chemokines have been found in a number of model systems of pneumonia, for example: growth related gene (GRO-α/CXCL1) has been found in *E. coli* pneumonia in rabbits (143); murine GRO-α (CXCL1) and GRO-β/γ (CXCL2/3) (KC/CXCL1 and MIP-2/CXCL2/3, respectively) have been found in murine models of *Klebsiella pneumoniae*, *Pseudomonas aeruginosa*, *Nocardia asteroides*, and *Aspergillus fumigatus* pneumonia (144–150). In a model of *A. fumigatus* pneumonia, neutralization of TNF resulted in marked attenuation of the expression of murine GRO-α (KC; CXCL1) and GRO-β/γ (MIP-2; CXCL2/3) that was paralleled by a reduction in the infiltration of neutrophils and associated with increased mortality (146,147). In addition, Laichalk et al.(151) administered a TNF agonist peptide consisting of the 11 amino acid TNF binding site (TNF70–80) to animals intratracheally inoculated with *K. pneumoniae* and found markedly elevated levels of MIP-2 (CXCL2/3) associated with increased neutrophil infiltration.

To further establish the role of ELR$^+$ CXC chemokines in mediating the innate host defense and eradication of a variety of micro-organism in the lung, Greenberger et al.(144) demonstrated that depletion of MIP-2

(CXCL2/3) during the pathogenesis of murine *K. pneumoniae* pneumonia resulted in a marked reduction in the recruitment of neutrophils to the lung that was paralleled by increased bacteremia and reduced bacterial clearance in the lung. Since ELR^+ CXC chemokine ligands in the mouse use the CXC chemokine receptor, CXCR2, and several ELR^+ CXC chemokine ligands are expressed during murine models of pneumonia, this would suggest targeting CXCR2 would delineate the importance of ELR^+ CXC chemokine ligand/CXCR2 biology during the pathogenesis of pneumonia and acute lung injury. Standiford and his associates using specific neutralizing antibodies to CXCR2 have demonstrated that blocking CXCR2 results in markedly reduced neutrophil infiltration in response to *P. aeruginosa* (148), *N. asteroides* (150), and *A. fumigatus* (147) pneumonias. The reduction in neutrophil elicitation was directly related to reduced clearance of the micro-organisms and increased mortality in these model systems. These studies have established the critical importance that ELR^+ CXC chemokine/CXCR biology plays in acute inflammation of innate immune response to a variety of micro-organisms. Moreover, with the evolving clinical presence of multidrug resistant micro-organisms, it is increasing necessary to consider alternative means to eradicate these microbial pathogens. Tsai et al.(149) have demonstrated that transgenic expression of murine GRO-α (KC; CXCL1) in the lung using a Clara cell-specific promoter in the context of *K. pneumoniae* pneumonia enhances host survival that is directly related to increased neutrophil recruitment and bacterial clearance in the lungs under these conditions. This response was not accompanied by the increased expression of other proinflammatory cytokines, such as TNF, IFN-γ, or IL-12. This study indicated that the compartmentalized overexpression of an ELR^+ CXC chemokine could represent a novel approach to the treatment of antimicrobial resistant micro-organisms. Furthermore, these studies demonstrate the importance of micro-organism recognition, early response cytokine production (i.e., TNF), and the subsequent generation of ELR^+ CXC chemokines associated with neutrophil elicitation and eradication of invading microbial pathogens.

Interestingly, Cole et al. (152) have recently demonstrated that, similar to defensins, ELR^- CXC chemokines have direct antimicrobial properties. Using a radial diffusion assay, these investigators demonstrated that the IFN inducible CXC chemokines, MIG/CXCL9, IP-10/CXCL10 and ITAC/CXCL11, had direct antimicrobial activities against *E. coli* and *L. monocytogenes*. IFN stimulated monocytes released levels of chemokines that would be microbiocidal in vivo (152). This demonstrates a role for interferon inducible chemokines in the innate host response.

Clinical studies examining elevations in pulmonary IL-8 levels and the development and mortality of the acute respiratory distress syndrome have conflicted, although most have suggested a strong correlation between the two (153–158). Of particular interest is the study of Donnelly et al. (157), which correlated early increases in IL-8/CXCL8 in bronchoalveolar lavage fluid with an increased risk of subsequent development of ARDS, and also demonstrated that alveolar macrophages were an important source of IL-8/CXCL8 prior to neutrophil influx. High concentrations of IL-8/CXCL8 CXCL8 were found in bronchoalveolar lavage fluid from trauma patients, some within 1 hr of injury and prior to any evidence of significant neutrophil influx. Patients who progressed to ARDS had significantly greater bronchoalveolar lavage fluid levels of IL-8/CXCL8 than those who failed to develop this condition. Levels of IL-8/CXCL8 in plasma, as opposed to lavage, were not found to be significantly different between patients who did or did not develop ARDS (157).

It has also been shown that anoxia/hyperoxia simulating an ischemia–reperfusion or hyperoxia environment can lead to an induction of IL-8/CXCL8 gene expression with a significant increase in IL-8/CXCL8 production by mononuclear cells and endothelial cells (159,160). Interleukin-8/CXCL8 gene induction was associated with the presence of increased binding activity in nuclear extracts from hypoxic endothelial cells for the NF-κB site (159,160). Of further clinical significance, endotoxin was found to further potentate this response (159,160). In animal studies in vivo, Sekido et al.(161) demonstrated that IL-8/CXCL8 significantly contributed to reperfusion lung injury in a rabbit model of lung ischemia–reperfusion injury. Reperfusion of the ischemic lung resulted in the production of IL-8, which correlated with maximal pulmonary neutrophil infiltration. Passive immunization of the animals with neutralizing antibodies to IL-8/CXCL8 prior to reperfusion of the ischemic lung prevented neutrophil extravasation and tissue injury, suggesting a causal role for IL-8/CXCL8 in this model. In other studies, Colletti et al.(51,162) have demonstrated that hepatic ischemia–reperfusion injury and the generation of TNF can result in pulmonary-derived ENA-78/CXCL5, showing the importance of cytokine cascades between the liver and the lung. The production of ENA-78/CXCL5 in the lung was correlated with the presence of neutrophil-dependent lung injury, and passive immunization with neutralizing ENA-78/CXCL5 antibodies resulted in significant attenuation of lung injury (51,162). These studies support the notion that CXC chemokines are important in the elicitation of neutrophils in the lung under conditions of acute inflammation. Furthermore, under conditions of micro-organism-induced pneumonia leading to acute lung injury, the expression of CXC chemokines may be beneficial to both the eradication of the organism and host survival.

E. The CC Chemokines

The CC chemokines (Table 1) are chemoattractants for monocyte, T and B-lymphocytes, NK cells, dendritic cells, basophils, mast cells, and eosinophils (84,85). The genes for CC chemokines are, in general, clustered on human chromosome 17 (q11.2–q12) (84,85). In general, the CC chemokine genes have three exons and two introns. The first and second introns of all the genes of this chemokine family are highly conserved (59,84,86). The splice junctions between the second and third exons in all CC chemokine genes occur at precisely the same position, suggesting that the CXC and CC chemokine superfamily may have diverged from a common ancestral gene (59,84,86). The CC chemokines have been found to be produced by an array of cells including monocytes, alveolar macrophages, neutrophils, platelets, eosinophils, mast cells, T-cells, B-cells, NK cells, keratinocytes, mesangial cells, epithelial cells, hepatocytes, fibroblasts, smooth muscle cells, mesothelial cells, and endothelial cells (59,84,86). These cells can produce CC chemokines in response to a variety of factors, including viruses, bacterial products, IL-1, TNF, C5a, LTB_4, and IFNs and appear to be significantly susceptible to suppression by IL-10 (59,84,86).

The primary structure of members of the CC chemokine family is similar to MCP-1/CCL2 (59,84,86,163). There is a 29–71% sequence homology on the amino acid level of the other CC chemokines with MCP-1/CCL2. The CC chemokines lack a conserved NH_2-terminal sequence analogous to the ELR motif of the CXC chemokine family (59,84,86,163). NH_2-terminal processing of CC chemokines influences their activity in the recruitment of mononuclear cells. CD26/dipeptidyl peptidase IV, a lymphocyte membrane-associated peptidase, selectively cleaves peptides with proline or alanine at the second position and cleaves dipeptides at the NH_2-terminus (164). While NH_2-terminal truncation of the CXC chemokine GCP-2 (CXCL6) by CD26 does not alter neutrophil chemotactic activity (164,165), NH_2-terminal truncation of RAN-TES/CCL5, eotaxin/CCL11, and macrophage-derived chemokine (MDC/CCL22) by CD26 has been shown to markedly impair chemotactic activity (164,165). NH_2-terminal truncation of RANTES (CCL5) by CD26 reduced activation of CCR1 and CCR3 receptors, while binding to CCR5 was preserved after proteolysis (165). Thus, proteolytic modification of RANTES (CCL5) by CD26 increased receptor selectivity and responses during innate and adaptive immune responses. In contrast, NH_2-terminal processing of LD78beta (CCL3), an isoform of macrophage inflammatory peptide-1α (MIP-1α; CCL3), by CD26 increased its chemotactic activity (166), an effect mediated by the chemokine receptors CCR1 and CCR5 (166). These studies show that extracellular processing of leukocyte chemoattractants modifies their ability to recruit leukocytes and influence inflammatory responses.

F. CC Chemokine Receptors

CC chemokine activities are mediated by seven-transmembrane-domain, G-protein coupled receptors. The CC chemokine receptors are structurally homologous. While the transmembrane and the second and third intracellular/cytoplasmic domains of these receptors are well conserved, the NH_2- and COOH-terminal ends of these receptors are highly variable. This suggests that the conserved domains are involved in G-protein signal coupling, and the variable domains are involved in specific ligand interaction and unique cellular signaling. Currently, at least 10 cellular CC chemokine receptors have been cloned, expressed, and identified to have specific ligand binding profiles (Table 4) (110,118–120,167–169).

The expression of specific CCRs may be restricted to a state of cellular activation (i.e., resting or activated) and differentiation. Mononuclear phagocytes stimulated with IL-2 express CCR2, whereas, MCP-1/CCL2 itself has no effect in regulating expression of CCR2 on these cells (170). In addition to CC chemokine ligand–receptor interaction leading to chemoattraction of mononuclear phagocytes, IL-2 induces the expression of CCR1 and CCR2 on CD45RO+ T-cells, the primary receptors for RANTES/CCL5 and MCP-1/CCL2, respectively (171). The expression of CCR1 and CCR2 was directly correlated to their migration in response to RANTES/CCL5 and MCP-1/CCL2, respectively (171). Moreover, the ability of these cells to express CCRs and respond to CC chemokine ligands was dependent on continued IL-2 exposure (171). This response was mimicked by IL-12, but not in the presence of other cytokines (171). Combined activation of TCR/CD3 complex with CD28 antigen caused rapid downregulation of CCR1 and CCR2 expression. This effect was paralleled by a decline in chemotactic response to either RANTES/CCL5 or MCP-1/CCL2, even in the presence of IL-2 (171). These findings support the notion that IL-2, by induction of specific CCRs, in conjunction with specific CC chemokine ligand production can have a significant impact on the recruitment of mononuclear cells.

Table 4 The CC Chemokine Receptors

Receptor	Ligand
CCR1	CCL3, CCL5, CCL7, CCL14, CCL15, CCL16, CCL23
CCR2	CCL2, CCL7, CCL13
CCR3	CCL5, CCL7, CCL11, CCL15, CCL26
CCR4	CCL17, CCL22
CCR5	CCL3, CCL4, CCL5
CCR6	CCL20
CCR7	CCL19
CCR8	CCL1
CCR9	CCL25
CCR10	CCL27

Type 1 T Helper cells and type 2 T Helper cells can be differentially recruited to promote different types of inflammatory reactions. It has become increasingly recognized that chemokine receptors are differentially expressed on T-cells depending on their antigenic experience and type of polarization (172). Chemokines and their receptors are essential components of type 1 and type 2 mediated responses (172). Naïve T-cells express CXCR4 and CCR7 and migrate in response to SDF-1 and MIP-3β (173). CXCR3 is present on most peripheral blood memory cells and is expressed at higher levels on type 1 cells than type 2 (172). CCR5 is mainly expressed on type 1 cells, whereas CCR3, CCR4, and CCR8 are more characteristic of type 2 cells (172,173). CXCR6 is predominantly expressed on type 1 polarized T-cells (137). Furthermore, polarized type 1/type 2 cells differentially respond to the appropriate ligand for these receptors including IP-1/CXCL10 and MIP-1β CCL4 for type 1 cells and MDC/CCL22, I309/CCL1 and eotaxin/CCL11 for type 2 cells (173). These findings demonstrate that chemokines are important in the amplification of polarization of T-cells. There is increasing evidence that pulmonary fibrosis is predominantly a type 2 mediated process.

The use of CC chemokine receptor knockout mice has provided additional insight into the biology of chemokines and their receptors in animal models of inflammation. Mice gene targeted to lack CCR2 develop normally and have no hematopoietic abnormalities, yet have profound defects in their ability to recruit mononuclear cells in response to intraperitoneal thioglycollate or to mount a DTH response in the context of granuloma formation (174–176). In addition, CCR2−/− were found to have lower levels of IFN-γ as compared to CCR+/+ mice. Furthermore, CCR2−/− mice have less tracheal obliteration with extracellular matrix and improved graft survival in a murine model of obliterative bronchiolitis (177). The beneficial effects were directly related to the absence of CCR2 expressing macrophages demonstrating the importance of a specific population of macrophages in the development of fibrosis (177). CCR1 −/− mice, as compared to littermate controls, have reduced ability to form granulomas that were associated with defects in the production of type 1 and type 2 cytokines and have improved graft survival in a cardiac transplant model (178,179). These studies support the notion that understanding the biology of CC chemokine ligands and their receptors will provide important insight into mechanisms of leukocyte trafficking during inflammation and the evolution of chronic fibrosis.

G.   CC Chemokines in Pulmonary Inflammation

The CC chemokines, RANTES/CCL5, MIP-1α/CCL3, MIP-1β/CCL4, MCP-1/CCL2), have also been implicated in mediating the innate host defense in animal models of *Influenza* A virus (180), *Paramyxovirus* pneumonia virus, *A. fumigatus*, and *Cryptococcus neoformans* pneumonias. The host response to *Influenza* A virus is characterized by an influx of mononuclear cells into the lungs that is associated with the increased expression of CC chemokine ligands (180). Dawson et al.(180) have used a genetic approach to determine the role of CC chemokines in mediating the innate response to this virus. Using a mouse adapted strain of *Influenza* A infected in CCR5−/− (note: CCR5 is the receptor for RANTES (CCL5), MIP-1α (CCL3), and MIP-1β (CCL4)) and CCR2−/− (note: CCR2 is the receptor for MCP-1 (CCL2)) mice, as compared to control+/+ mice, these investigators demonstrated that CCR5−/− mice displayed increased mortality related to severe pneumonitis, whereas CCR2−/− mice were protected from the severe pneumonitis due to defective macrophage recruitment. The delay in macrophage accumulation in CCR2−/− mice was correlated with high pulmonary viral titers (180). These studies support the potential of different roles that CC chemokine ligand/receptor biology plays in influenza infection. In addition, this study also demonstrates the importance of macrophage recruitment during the innate response is critical to the development of adaptive immunity to this microbe. Domachowske et al.(181) have examined the role of CC chemokine ligands (i.e., RANTES/CCL5 and MIP-1α/CCL3) that bind to the CC chemokine receptor CCR1 in response to *Paramyxovirus* pneumonia virus infection in mice. This infection is associated with a predominate neutrophil and eosinophil infiltration into the lung that is accompanied by expression of CCR1 ligands (181). However, in CCR1−/− mice infected with *Paramyxovirus* pneumonia virus, the inflammatory response was found to be minimal, the clearance of virus from lung tissue was reduced, and mortality was markedly increased (181). These results indicate that CC chemokine-dependent innate responses limited the rate of virus replication in vivo and played an important role in reducing mortality.

The effect of CC chemokines in mediating the recruitment of mononuclear cells during the innate host defense is not limited to viral infections. Mehrad et al.(182) have shown that MIP-1α/CCL3 and the recruitment of mononuclear cells plays an important role in the eradication of invasive pulmonary aspergillosis. They demonstrated that in both immunocompetent and neutropenic mice, MIP-1α/CCL3 is induced in the lungs in response to intratracheal inoculation of *A. fumigatus*. Depletion of endogenous MIP-1α/CCL3 by passive immunization with neutralizing antibodies to MIP-1α/CCL3 resulted in increased mortality in neutropenic mice, which was associated with a reduced mononuclear cell infiltration and markedly decreased clearance of lung fungal burden. Gao et al.(179) have confirmed this finding by assessing the importance of CCR1, the major chemokine receptor for MIP-1α (CCL3), in mice. CCR1−/− mice exposed to *A. fumigatus* had markedly increased mortality compared to wild-type CCR1+/+ control mice (179). These studies indicate that MIP-1α/CCL3 and elicitation of mononuclear cells are crucial in mediating host defense against *A. fumigatus* in the setting of neutropenia, and this understanding may be important in devising future therapeutic strategies against invasive pulmonary aspergillosis.

C. neoformans is acquired via the respiratory tract and is a significant cause of fatal mycosis in immunocompromised patients. Both the innate and adaptive immune response are necessary to clear the microbe from the lung and prevent dissemination to the meninges. Huffnagle et al.(183,184) have found that MCP-1/CCL2 and MIP-1α/CCL3 play important roles in the eradication of *C. neoformans* from the lung and prevent cryptococcal meningitis. In mice exposed to intratracheal *C. neoformans*, both MCP-1/CCL2 and MIP-1α/CCL3 expression directly correlate with the magnitude of infiltrating leukocytes. Depletion of endogenous MCP-1/CCL2 with neutralizing antibodies markedly decreased the recruitment of both macrophages and CD4+ T-cells, and inhibited cryptococcal clearance. Neutralization of MCP-1/CCL2 also resulted in decreased BAL fluid levels of TNF. Using the same model system, depletion of MIP-1α/CCL3 resulted in a significant reduction in total leukocytes and an increase in the burden of *C. neoformans* in the lungs of these animals. Interestingly, depletion of MIP-1α/CCL3 did not decrease the levels of MCP-1/CCL2, however, depletion of MCP-1/CCL2 significantly reduced MIP-1α/CCL3 levels, demonstrating that induction of MIP-1α/CCL3 was largely dependent on MCP-1/CCL2 production. Neutralization of MIP-1α/CCL3 also blocked the cellular recruitment phase of a recall response to cryptococcal antigen in the lungs of immunized mice. Thus, in both the context of active cryptococcal infection or rechallenge with cryptococcal antigen, MIP-1α/CCL3 was required for maximal leukocyte recruitment into the lungs, most notably the recruitment of phagocytic effector cells (neutrophils and macrophages). These studies support the notion that CC chemokine ligand/receptor biology plays a critical role in innate host defense and development of pulmonary inflammation that is important in eradication of micro-organisms.

VII. Summary

Inflammation, injury, and repair occur in response to a variety of insults that affect the lungs and other organs. In the absence of overexuberant pulmonary inflammation, effective remodeling and repair can occur despite significant tissue injury, leading to the return of normal function and gas exchange. However, acute lung injury can also become progressively more severe, involving on-going tissue destruction and inflammation that fail to resolve and culminate in respiratory failure or chronic fibrogenic pathology. As illustrated in this chapter, the pulmonary inflammatory response is a crucial determinant of these different outcomes, and the mechanisms and mediators involved in initiating, modulating, and regulating pulmonary inflammation are complex and interactive.

The mammalian lung exhibits complementary innate and adaptive immune responses. Innate immunity is associated with immediate host defense, and involves an acute inflammatory response that is initiated, maintained, and resolved depending on coordinated interactions between immune and nonimmune cells. Adaptive immunity depends on specialized T- and B-lymphocytes with specific receptors generated in response to antigen presentation, and involves antigen-dependent clonal expansion to generate long-term humoral and cell-mediated immune memory. The adaptive immune response is initially naïve and delayed, although it can be strengthened through repeat exposure. The innate immune response is intrinsically rapid. Cell-based receptors (e.g., TLRs) detect micro-organisms or toxins and initiate acute inflammation including the expression of factors such as cytokines. Cytokines broaden the innate host response through intercellular signaling. The activation of cytokine networks generates autocrine, paracrine, and endocrine signaling that recruits and activates leukocytes and, if properly controlled, eradicates the inciting agent or insult. Acute inflammation associated with innate pulmonary host defense has been the primary focus of coverage in this chapter.

Two of the most important families of early response cytokines are the IL-1 and TNF-α families, which are produced primarily by mononuclear phagocytes. These early response cytokines engage additional cells and promote the expression of more distal cytokines important in recruiting leukocytes. Tumor necrosis factor and IL-1 are biochemically unrelated, but have overlapping and interactive effects on many cellular functions as discussed in this chapter. When produced locally in appropriate amounts, these early response cytokines are essential in the beneficial removal of invading micro-organisms and the resolution of tissue injury. In marked contrast, the exaggerated systemic release of TNF and IL-1 can result in severe injury to the lungs and other organs, with significant host morbidity and mortality as in clinical acute lung injury and ARDS. Thus, TNF and IL-1 have a broad spectrum of biologic activities that influence the outcome of acute pulmonary inflammation on both local and systemic levels.

One crucial class of mediators in the progression of the inflammatory response are chemotactic cytokines called chemokines. The human CXC, CC, C, and CXXXC chemokine families are four closely related polypeptide families that attract neutrophils, eosinophils, basophils, monocytes, mast cells, dendritic cells, NK cells, or T- and B-lymphocytes. These chemokines have monomer molecular weights of 7–10 kD and are characteristically basic heparin-binding proteins with highly conserved cysteine amino acid residues. CXC and CC chemokines have been emphasized in discussion here. The CXC chemokine family has the first two NH_2-terminal cysteines separated by one nonconserved amino acid residue, the CXC cysteine motif. The CC chemokine family has the first two NH_2-terminal cysteines in juxtaposition, the CC cysteine motif. Human CXC chemokines are clustered primarily on chromosome 4, and exhibit between 20% and 50% homology on the amino acid level; CC chemokines are clustered primarily on chromosome 17, and exhibit between 28% and 45% amino acid homology. There are a variety of murine and other species-dependent homologues of these chemokines (e.g., KC/CXCL1, MIP-2/CXCL2, IP-10/CXCL10, MIG/CXCL9, and SDF-1/CXCL12 are murine analogs of human GRO-α/CXCL1, GRO-β/GRO-γ (CXCL2/CXCL3), IP-10/CXCL10, MIG/CXCL9, and SDF-1/CXCL12, respectively). Chemokines are produced by multiple cells including monocytes, alveolar macrophages, neutrophils, platelets, eosinophils, mast cells, T- and B-lymphocytes, epithelial cells, endothelial cells, fibroblasts, smooth muscle cells, hepatocytes, and mesothelial cells. Stimuli for chemokine production include bacteria and bacterial products, viruses, mediators such as IL-1, TNF, and many others.

Developing effective therapies for acute lung injury and ARDS depends on a firm understanding of inflammatory mediators and regulatory pathways. Numerous animal studies show that antagonizing or neutralizing individual inflammatory mediators can attenuate pulmonary or systemic injury. Experience from sepsis trials in humans, however, indicates that this is not necessarily the case in patients. Anti-inflammatory therapies for lung injury are discussed in detail in Chapter 14. Current understanding suggests that future lung injury therapy will likely include combination interventions, where monoclonal antibodies or inhibitors of several inflammatory mediators may be used along with agents or interventions targeting other aspects of lung injury. In addition, systemic or intrapulmonary gene therapy could be used to attenuate or augment the expression of specific inflammatory mediators. Regardless of how any anti-inflammatory therapy is structured and applied, it will be necessary to maintain beneficial aspects of innate host defense that protect against infection and promote normal tissue remodeling and repair, while antagonizing excessive, detrimental aspects of the inflammatory response. Therapies for acute and chronic lung injury are discussed in detail in Chapters 13–19.

Acknowledgments

This work was supported, in part, by National Institutes of Health grants P01HL67665, HL03906 (M.P.K), HL04493 (J.A.B.), P01HL67665, P50CA90388, HL66027, CA87879 (RMS). M.P.K. is the holder of a Dalsemer Scholar Award from the American Lung Association. J.A.B. holds a Research Award from the American Lung Association and the American Lung Association of California.

References

1. Delves PJ, Roitt IM. The immune system. Second of two parts. N Engl J Med 2000; 343:108–117.
2. Medzhitov R, Janeway C Jr. Innate immune recognition: mechanisms and pathways. Immunol Rev 2000; 173:89–97.
3. Brightbill HD, Libraty DH, Krutzik SR, et al. Host defense mechanisms triggered by microbial lipoproteins through toll-like receptors. Science 1999; 285:732–736.
4. Brightbill HD, Modlin RL. Toll-like receptors: molecular mechanisms of the mammalian immune response. Immunology 2000; 101:1–10.
5. Delves PJ, Roitt IM. The immune system. First of two parts. N Engl J Med 2000; 343:37–49.
6. Medzhitov R, Janeway C Jr. Innate immunity. N Engl J Med 2000; 343: 338–344.
7. Medzhitov R, Janeway CA Jr. How does the immune system distinguish self from nonself? Semin Immunol 2000; 12:185–188. Discussion 257–344.
8. Beutler B, Poltorak A. Positional cloning of Lps, and the general role of toll-like receptors in the innate immune response. Eur Cytokine Netw 2000; 11:143–152.
9. Hashimoto C, Hudson KL, Anderson KV. The Toll gene of Drosophila, required for dorsal–ventral embryonic polarity, appears to encode a transmembrane protein. Cell 1988; 52:269–279.
10. Gay NJ, Keith FJ. Drosophila Toll and IL-1 receptor [letter]. Nature 1991; 351:355–356.
11. Ghosh S, May MJ, Kopp EB. NF-kappa B and Rel proteins: evolutionarily conserved mediators of immune responses. Annu Rev Immunol 1998; 16:225–260.
12. Medzhitov R, Preston-Hurlburt P, Janeway CA Jr. A human homologue of the Drosophila Toll protein signals activation of adaptive immunity [see comments]. Nature 1997; 388:394–397.
13. Poltorak A, He X, Smirnova I, et al. Defective LPS signaling in C3H/HeJ and C57BL/10ScCr mice: mutations in Tlr4 gene. Science 1998; 282: 2085–2088.
14. Qureshi ST, Lariviere L, Leveque G, et al. Endotoxin-tolerant mice have mutations in Toll-like receptor 4 (Tlr4)[see comments] [published erratum appears in J Exp Med 1999 May 3;189(9):following 1518]. J Exp Med 1999; 189:615–625.
15. Hoshino K, Takeuchi O, Kawai T, et al. Cutting edge: Toll-like receptor 4 (TLR4)-deficient mice are hyporesponsive to lipopolysaccharide: evidence for TLR4 as the Lps gene product. J Immunol 1999; 162:3749–3752.
16. Wright SD, Tobias PS, Ulevitch RJ, Ramos RA. Lipopolysaccharide (LPS) binding protein opsonizes LPS-bearing particles for recognition by a novel receptor on macrophages. J Exp Med 1989; 170:1231–1241.
17. Shimazu R, Akashi S, Ogata H, et al. MD-2, a molecule that confers lipopolysaccharide responsiveness on Toll-like receptor 4. J Exp Med 1999; 189: 1777–1782.

18. Takeuchi O, Kaufmann A, Grote K, et al. Cutting edge: preferentially the *R*-stereoisomer of the mycoplasmal lipopeptide macrophage-activating lipopeptide-2 activates immune cells through a toll-like receptor 2- and MyD88-dependent signaling pathway. J Immunol 2000; 164:554–557.

19. Takeuchi O, Hoshino K, Kawai T, et al. Differential roles of TLR2 and TLR4 in recognition of Gram-negative and Gram-positive bacterial cell wall components. Immunity 1999;11:443–451.

20. Dinarello CA. Biology of interleukin 1. FASEB J 1988; 2:108–115.

21. Dinarello CA. An update of human interleukin 1: from molecular biology to clinical relevance. J Clin Immunol 1985; 5:287–297.

22. Dinarello CA, Cannon JG, Wolff SM, et al. Tumor necrosis factor (cachectin) is an endogenous pyrogen and induces production of interleukin 1. J Exp Med 1986; 163:1433–1450.

23. Dinarello CA. Interleukin-1 and its biologically related cytokines. Adv Immunol 1989; 44:153–205.

24. Dinarello CA. Interleukin-1 and interleukin-1 antagonism. Blood 1991; 77: 1627–1635.

25. Dinarello CA. Biologic basis for interleukin-1 in disease. Blood 1996; 87: 2095–2147.

26. Dinarello CA. Interleukin-1. Cytokine Growth Factor Rev 1997; 8:253–265.

27. Dinarello CA. Interleukin-1 beta, interleukin-18, and the interleukin-1 beta converting enzyme. Ann NY Acad Sci 1998; 856:1–11.

28. Arend WP. Interleukin-1 receptor antagonist—a new member of the interleukin-1 family. J Clin Invest 1991; 88:1445–1451.

29. Arend WP, Malyak M, Guthridge CJ, Gabay C. Interleukin-1 receptor antagonist: role in biology. Annu Rev Immunol 1998; 16:27–55.

30. Beutler B, Krochin N, Milsark IW, Luedke C, Cerami A. Control of cachectin (tumor necrosis factor) synthesis: mechanisms of endotoxin resistance. Science 1986; 232:977–979.

31. Beutler B, Cerami A. Cachectin and tumor necrosis factor as two sides of the same biological coin. Nature 1986; 320:584–588.

32. Beutler B, Cerami A. The biology of cachectin/TNF-A primary mediator of the host response. Annu Rev Immunol 1989; 7:625–650.

33. Kunkel SL, Remick DG, Strieter RM, Larrick JW. Mechanisms that regulate the production and effects of tumor necrosis factor α. Crit Rev Immunol 1989; 9:93–117.

34. Le J, Vilcek J. Tumor necrosis factor and interleukin 1: cytokines with multiple overlapping biological activities. Lab Invest 1987; 56:234–248.

35. Larrick JW, Kunkel SL. The role of tumor necrosis factor and interleukin-1 in the immunoinflammatory response. Pharmacol Res 1988; 5:129–139.

36. Cerami A. Inflammatory cytokines. Clin Immunol Immunopathol 1992; 62: S3–S10.

37. Malyak M, Guthridge JM, Hance KR, Dower SK, Freed JH, Arend WP. Characterization of a low molecular weight isoform of IL-1 receptor antagonist. J Immunol 1998; 161:1997–2003.

38. Sousa AR, Lane SJ, Nakhosteen JA, Lee TH, Poston RN. Expression of interleukin-1 beta (IL-1beta) and interleukin-1 receptor antagonist (IL-1ra)

on asthmatic bronchial epithelium. Am J Respir Crit Care Med 1996; 154: 1061–1066.

39. Donnelly SC, Strieter RM, Reid PT, et al. The association between mortality rates and decreased concentrations of interleukin-10 and interleukin-1 receptor antagonist in the lung fluids of patients with the adult respiratory distress syndrome. Ann Intern Med 1996; 125:191–196.

40. Kadota J, Matsubara Y, Ishimatsu Y, et al. Significance of IL-1beta and IL-1 receptor antagonist (IL-1Ra) in bronchoalveolar lavage fluid (BALF) in patients with diffuse panbronchiolitis (DPB). Clin Exp Immunol 1996; 103: 461–466.

41. Smith DR, Kunkel SL, Standiford TJ, et al. Increased interleukin-1 receptor antagonist in idiopathic pulmonary fibrosis. A compartmental analysis. Am J Respir Crit Care Med 1995; 151:1965–1973.

42. Ulich TR, Watson LR, Yin SM, et al. The intratracheal administration of endotoxin and cytokines. I. Characterization of LPS-induced inflammatory infiltrate. Am J Pathol 1991; 138:1485–1496.

43. Horai R, Asano M, Sudo K, et al. Production of mice deficient in genes for interleukin (IL)-1alpha, IL-1beta, IL-1alpha/beta, and IL-1 receptor antagonist shows that IL-1beta is crucial in turpentine-induced fever development and glucocorticoid secretion. J Exp Med 1998; 187:1463–1475.

44. Fantuzzi G, Dinarello CA. The inflammatory response in interleukin-1 beta-deficient mice: comparison with other cytokine-related knock-out mice. J Leukoc Biol 1996; 59:489–493.

45. Fantuzzi G, Zheng H, Faggioni R, et al. Effect of endotoxin in IL-1 beta-deficient mice. J Immunol 1996; 157:291–296.

46. Kozak W, Zheng H, Conn CA, Soszynski D, van der Ploeg LH, Kluger MJ. Thermal and behavioral effects of lipopolysaccharide and influenza in interleukin-1 beta-deficient mice. Am J Physiol 1995; 269:R969–R977.

47. Bazzoni F, Beutler B. The tumor necrosis factor ligand and receptor families. N Engl J Med 1996; 334:1717–1725.

48. Strieter RM, Kunkel SL, Bone RC. Role of tumor necrosis factor-alpha in disease states and inflammation. Crit Care Med 1993; 21:S447–S463.

49. Tomashefski JF. Pulmonary pathology of the adult respiratory distress syndrome. Clin Chest Med 1990; 11:593–619.

50. Millar AB, Foley NM, Singer M, Johnson N, Meager A, Rook GA. TNF in bronchopulmonary secretions of patients with adult respiratory distress syndrome. Lancet 1989; 2:712–714.

51. Colletti LM, Remick DG, Burtch GD, Kunkel SL, Strieter RM, Campbell DA Jr. Role of tumor necrosis factor-alpha in the pathophysiologic alterations after hepatic ischemia/reperfusion injury in the rat. J Clin Invest 1990; 85:1936–1943.

52. Lahdevirta J, Maury CPJ, Teppo AM, Reppo H. Elevated levels of circulating cachectin/tumor necrosis factor in patients with acquired immunodeficiency syndrome. Am J Med 1988; 85:289–291.

53. Scuderi P, Lam KS, Ryan KJ, et al. Raised serum levels of tumour necrosis factor in parasitic infections. Lancet 1986; 2(8520):1364–1365.

54. Piguet P-F, Grau GE, Allet B, Vassalli P. Tumor necrosis factor/cachectin is an effector of skin and gut lesions of the acute phase of graft-vs-host disease. J Exp Med 1987; 166:1280–1289.
55. DeMeester SR, Rolfe MW, Kunkel SL, et al. The bimodal expression of tumor necrosis factor-α in association with rat lung reimplantation and allograft rejection. J Immunol 1993; 150:2494–2505.
56. Beutler B, Bazzoni F. TNF, apoptosis and autoimmunity: a common thread? Blood Cells Mol Dis 1998; 24:216–230.
57. Watanabe-Fukunaga R, Brannan CI, Copeland NG, Jenkins NA, Nagata S. Lymphoproliferation disorder in mice explained by defects in Fas antigen that mediates apoptosis. Nature 1992; 356:314–317.
58. Adachi M, Watanabe-Fukunaga R, Nagata S. Aberrant transcription caused by the insertion of an early transposable element in an intron of the Fas antigen gene of lpr mice. Proc Natl Acad Sci USA 1993; 90:1756–1760.
59. Strieter RM, Lukacs NW, Standiford TJ, Kunkel SL. Cytokines and lung inflammation. Thorax 1993; 48:765–769.
60. Scheurich P, Thoma B, Ucer U, Pfizenmaier K. Immunoregulatory activity of recombinant human tumor necrosis factor (TNF)-α: induction of the TNF receptors on human T cells and TNF-α-mediated enhancement of T cell responses. J Immunol 1987; 138:1786–1790.
61. Zucali JR, Elfenbein GJ, Barth KC, Dinarello CA. Effects of human interleukin 1 and human tumor necrosis factor on human T lymphocyte colony formation. J Clin Invest 1987; 80:772–777.
62. Yokota S, Geppert TD, Lipsky PE. Enhancement of antigen- and mitogen-induced human T lymphocyte proliferation by tumor necrosis factor-α. J Immunol 1988; 140:531–536.
63. Waage A, Halstensen A, Espevik T. Association between tumor necrosis factor in serum and fatal outcome in patients with menigococcal disease. Lancet 1987; 1i:355–357.
64. Girardin E, Grau GE, Dayer JM, Roux-Lombard P, Lambert PH. Tumor necrosis factor and interleukin-1 in the serum of children with severe infectious purpura. N Engl J Med 1988; 319:397–400.
65. Marks JD, Marks CB, Luce JM, et al. Plasma tumor necrosis in patients with septic shock: mortality rate, incidence of adult respiratory distress syndrome. Am Rev Respir Dis 1990; 141:94–97.
66. Armstrong L, Millar AB. Relative production of tumour necrosis factor alpha and interleukin 10 in adult respiratory distress syndrome. Thorax 1997; 52: 442–446.
67. Tracey KJ, Beutler B, Lowry SF, et al. Shock and tissue injury induced by recombinant human cachectin. Science 1986; 234:470–474.
68. Hinshaw LB, Tekamp-Olson P, Chang ACK, et al. Survival of primates in LD$_{100}$ septic shock following therapy with antibody to tumor necrosis factor (TNF-alpha). Circ Shock 1990; 30:279–292.
69. Remick DG, Strieter RM, Lynch JPD, Nguyen D, Eskandari M, Kunkel SL. In vivo dynamics of murine tumor necrosis factor-alpha gene expression. Kinetics of dexamethasone-induced suppression. Lab Invest 1989; 60: 766–771.

70. Michie HR, Mangue KR, Spriggs DR, et al. Detection of circulating tumor necrosis factor after endotoxin administration. N Eng J Med 1988; 318: 1481–1484.

71. Wherry JC, Pennington JE, Wenzel RP. Tumor necrosis factor and the therapeutic potential of anti-tumor necrosis factor antibodies. Crit Care Med 1993; 21:S436–S440.

72. Abraham E, Wunderink R, Silverman H, et al. Efficacy and safety of monoclonal antibody to human tumor necrosis factor alpha in patients with sepsis syndrome. A randomized, controlled, double-blind, multicenter clinical trial. TNF-alpha MAb Sepsis Study Group. JAMA 1995; 273:934–941.

73. Abraham E, Glauser MP, Butler T, et al. p55 tumor necrosis factor receptor fusion protein in the treatment of patients with severe sepsis and septic shock. A randomized controlled multicenter trial. Ro 45–2081 Study Group. JAMA 1997; 277:1531–1538.

74. Peppel K, Crawford D, Beutler B. A tumor necrosis factor (TNF) receptor-IgG heavy chain chimeric protein as a bivalent antagonist of TNF activity. J Exp Med 1991; 174:1483–1489.

75. Waller A. Microscopical observations on the perforation of the capillaries by the corpuscles of the blood, and on the origin of mucous and pus-globules. Philos Mag 1846; 29:397.

76. Massart J, Bordet C. Recherches sur l'irritabilite des leucocytes et sur l'intervention de cette irritabilite dans la nutrition des cellules et dans l'inflammation. J Med Chir Pharm Brux 1890; 90:169.

77. Boyden S. The chemotactic effect of mixtures of antibody and antigens on polymorphonuclear leukocytes. J Exp Med 1962; 115:453.

78. Zigmond SH, Hirsch JG. Leukocyte locomotion and chemotaxis: new methods for evaluation and demonstration of cell-derived chemotactic factor. J Exp Med 1973; 137:387.

79. Ward PA, Newman LJ. A neutrophil chemotactic factor from human C'5. J Immunol 1969; 102:93–99.

80. Shin HS, Snyderman R, Friedman E, Mellors A, Mayer MM. Chemotactic and anaphylatoxic fragment cleaved from the fifth component of guinea pig complement. Science 1968; 162:361–363.

81. Becker EL, Ward PA. Esterases of the polymorphonuclear leukocyte capable of hydrolyzing acetyl DL-phenyl-alanine beta-naphthyl ester. Relationship to the activatable esterase of chemotaxis. J Exp Med 1969; 129:569–584.

82. Lee TC, Snyder F. Function, metabolism and regulation of platelet activating factor and related ether lipids. In: Kuo JF, ed. Phospholipids and Cellular Regulation. Boca Raton: CRC Press Inc., 1985:1–39.

83. Ford-Hutchinson AW, Bray MA, Doig MV, Shipley ME, Smith MJ. Leukotriene B, a potent chemokinetic and aggregating substance released from polymorphonuclear leukocytes. Nature 1980; 286:264–265.

84. Strieter RM, Kunkel SL. Chemokines in the lung. In: Crystal R, West J, Weibel E, Barnes P, eds.Lung: Scientific Foundations. 2nd ed. New York: Raven Press, 1997:155–186.

85. Zlotnik A, Yoshie O. Chemokines: a new classification system and their role in immunity. Immunity 2000; 12:121–127.

86. Koch AE, Strieter RM. In: Koch AE, Strieter RM, eds. Chemokines in Disease. Austin, TX: R.G. Landes, Co., Biomedical Publishers, 1996.

87. Rossi DL, Hardiman G, Copeland NG, et al. Cloning and characterization of a new type of mouse chemokine. Genomics 1998; 47:163–170.

88. Bazan JF, Bacon KB, Hardiman G, et al. A new class of membrane-bound chemokine with a CX3C motif. Nature 1997; 385:640–644.

89. Farber JM. HuMIG: a new member of the chemokine family of cytokines. Biochem Biophys Res Commun 1993; 192:223–230.

90. Taub DD, Oppenheim JJ. Chemokines, inflammation and immune system. Therapeutic Immunol 1994; 1:229–246.

91. Proost P, Wolf-Peeters CD, Conings R, Opdenakker G, Billiau A, Damme JV. Identification of a novel granulocyte chemotactic protein (GCP-1) from human tumor cells: in vitro and in vivo comparison with natural forms of GROa, IP-10, and IL-8. J Immunol 1993; 1150:1000–1010.

92. Walz A, Burgener R, Car B, Baggiolini M, Kunkel SL, Strieter RM. Structure and neutrophil-activating properties of a novel inflammatory peptide (ENA-78) with homology to interleukin-8. J Exp Med 1991; 174:1355–1362.

93. Clark-Lewis I, Dewald B, Geiser T, Moser B, Baggiolini M. Platelet factor 4 binds to interleukin 8 receptors and activates neutrophils when its N terminus is modified with Glu-Leu-Arg. Proc Natl Acad Sci USA 1993; 90: 3574–3577.

94. Hebert CA, Vitangcol RV, Baker JB. Scanning mutagenesis of interleukin-8 identifies a cluster of residues required for receptor binding. J Biol Chem 1991; 266:18989–18994.

95. Strieter RM, Polverini PJ, Kunkel SL, et al. The functional role of the 'ELR' motif in CXC chemokine-mediated angiogenesis. J Biol Chem 1995; 270:27348 27357.

96. Luster AD, Greenberg SM, Leder P. The IP-10 chemokine binds to a specific cell surface heparin sulfate shared with platelet factor 4 and inhibits endothelial cell proliferation. J Exp Med 1995; 182:219–232.

97. Arenberg DA, Polverini PJ, Kunkel SL, Shanafelt A, Strieter RM. In vitro and in vivo systems to assess role of CXC chemokines in regulation of angiogenesis. Methods Enzymol 1997; 288:190–220.

98. Coughlin CM, Salhany KE, Wysocka M, et al. Interleukin-12 and interleukin-18 synergistically induce murine tumor regression which involves inhibition of angiogenesis. J Clin Invest 1998; 101:1441–1452.

99. Simonet WS, Hughes TM, Nguyen HQ, Trebasky LD, Danilenko DM, Medlock ES. Long-term impaired neutrophil migration in mice overexpressing human interleukin-8. J Clin Invest 1994; 94:1310–1319.

100. Hechtman DH, Cybulsky MI, Fuchs HJ, Baker JB, Gimbrone MA Jr. Intravascular IL-8. Inhibitor of polymorphonuclear leukocyte accumulation at sites of acute inflammation. J Immunol 1991; 147:883–892.

101. Ley K, Baker JB, Cybulsky MI, Gimbrone MA Jr, Luscinskas FW. Intravenous interleukin-8 inhibits granulocyte emigration from rabbit mesenteric venules without altering L-selectin expression or leukocyte rolling. J Immunol 1993; 151:6347–6357.

102. Lira SA, Fuentes ME, Strieter RM, Durham SK. Transgenic methods to study chemokine function in lung and central nervous system. Methods Enzymol 1997; 287:304–318.

103. Lira SA, Zalamea P, Heinrich JN, et al. Expression of the chemokine N51/KC in the thymus and epidermis of transgenic mice results in marked infiltration of a single class of inflammatory cells. J Exp Med 1994; 180: 2039–2048.

104. Grewal IS, Rutledge BJ, Fiorillo JA, et al. Transgenic monocyte chemoattractant protein-1 (MCP-1) in pancreatic islets produces monocyte-rich insulitis without diabetes: abrogation by a second transgene expressing systemic MCP-1. J Immunol 1997; 159:401–408.

105. Keane MP, Arenberg DA, Lynch JPR, et al. The CXC chemokines, IL-8 and IP-10, regulate angiogenic activity in idiopathic pulmonary fibrosis. J Immunol 1997; 159:1437–1443.

106. Koch AE, Leibovich SJ, Polverini PJ. Stimulation of neovascularization by human rheumatoid synovial tissue macrophages. Arthritis Rheum 1989; 29:471–479.

107. Koch AE, Polverini PJ, Kunkel SL, et al. Interleukin-8 (IL-8) as a macrophage-derived mediator of angiogenesis. Science 1992; 258:1798–1801.

108. Nickoloff BJ, Mitra RS, Varani J, Dixit VM, Polverini PJ. Aberrant production of interleukin-8 and thrombospondin-1 by psoriatic keratinocytes mediates angiogenesis. Am J Pathol 1994; 144:820–828.

109. Broxmeyer HE, Kim CH. Regulation of hematopoiesis in a sea of chemokine family members with a plethora of redundant activities. Exp Hematol 1999; 27:1113–1123.

110. Premack BA, Schall TJ. Chemokine receptors: gateways to inflammation and infection. Nature Med 1996; 2:1174–1178.

111. Addison CL, Daniel TO, Burdick MD, et al. The CXC chemokine receptor 2, CXCR2, is the putative receptor for ELR(+) CXC chemokine-induced angiogenic activity [in process citation]. J Immunol 2000; 165:5269–5277.

112. Lippert U, Artuc M, Grutzkau A, et al. Expression and functional activity of the IL-8 receptor type CXCR1 and CXCR2 on human mast cells. J Immunol 1998; 161:2600–2608.

113. Ahuja SK, Gao JL, Murphy PM. Chemokine receptors and molecular mimicry. Immunol Today 1994; 15:281–287.

114. Murphy PM. The molecular biology of leukocyte chemoattractant receptors. Annu Rev Immunol 1994; 12:593–633.

115. Horuk R. Molecular properties of the chemokine receptor family. Trends Pharmacol Sci 1994; 15:159–165.

116. Rollins BJ. Chemokines. Blood 1997; 90:909–928.

117. Luster AD. Chemokines—chemotactic cytokines that mediate inflammation. N Engl J Med 1998; 338:436–445.

118. Imai T, Chantry D, Raport CJ, et al. Macrophage-derived chemokine is a functional ligand for the CC chemokine receptor 4. J Biol Chem 1998; 273: 1764–1768.

119. Liao F, Alkhatib G, Peden KW, Sharma G, Berger EA, Farber JM. STRL33, a novel chemokine receptor-like protein, functions as a fusion cofactor for

both macrophage-tropic and T cell line-tropic HIV-1. J Exp Med 1997; 185:2015–2023.

120. Liao F, Alderson R, Su J, Ullrich SJ, Kreider BL, Farber JM. STRL22 is a receptor for the CC chemokine MIP-3alpha. Biochem Biophys Res Commun 1997; 236:212–217.

121. Stine JT, Chantry D, Gray P. Virally encoded chemokines and chemokine receptors: genetic embezzlement of host DNA. In: Mantovani A, ed. Chemokines. Basel: Karger, 1999:72:161–180.

122. Ahuja SK, Murphy PM. Molecular piracy of mammalian interleukin-8 receptor type B by herpesvirus saimiri. J Biol Chem 1993; 268:20691–20694.

123. Arvanitakis L, Geras-Raaka E, Varma A, Gershengorn MC, Cesarman E. Human herpesvirus KSHV encodes a constitutively active G-protein-coupled receptor linked to cell proliferation. Nature 1997; 385:347–349.

124. Bais C, Santomasso B, Coso O, et al. G-protein-coupled receptor of Kaposi's sarcoma-associated herpesvirus is a viral oncogene and angiogenesis activator [see comments] [published erratum appears in Nature 1998; 392(6672):210]. Nature 1998; 391:86–89.

125. Geras-Raaka E, Varma A, Ho H, Clark-Lewis I, Gershengorn MC. Human interferon-gamma-inducible protein 10 (IP-10) inhibits constitutive signaling of Kaposi's sarcoma-associated herpesvirus G protein-coupled receptor. J Exp Med 1998; 188:405–408.

126. Rosenkilde MM, Kledal TN, Brauner-Osborne H, Schwartz TW. Agonists and inverse agonists for the herpesvirus 8-encoded constitutively active seven-transmembrane oncogene product, ORF-74. J Biol Chem 1999; 274: 956–961.

127. Loetscher M, Gerber B, Loetscher P, et al. Chemokine receptor specific for IP10 and mig: structure, function, and expression in activated T-lymphocytes. J Exp Med 1996; 184:963–969.

128. Oberlin E, Amara A, Bachelerie F, et al. The CXC chemokine SDF-1 is the ligand for LESTR/fusin and prevents infection by T-cell-line-adapted HIV-1. Nature 1996; 382:833–835.

129. Bleul CC, Farzan M, Choe H, et al. The lymphocyte chemoattractant SDF-1 is a ligand for LESTR/fusin and blocks HIV-1 entry. Nature 1996; 382: 829–833.

130. Murdoch C, Monk PN, Finn A. Cxc chemokine receptor expression on human endothelial cells. Cytokine 1999; 11:704–712.

131. Romagnani P, Annunziato F, Lasagni L, et al. Cell cycle-dependent expression of CXC chemokine receptor 3 by endothelial cells mediates angiostatic activity. J Clin Invest 2001; 107:53–63.

132. Legler DF, Loetscher M, Roos RS, Clark-Lewis I, Baggiolini M, Moser B. B cell-attracting chemokine 1, a human CXC chemokine expressed in lymphoid tissues, selectively attracts B lymphocytes via BLR1/CXCR5. J Exp Med 1998; 187:655–660.

133. Dobner T, Wolf I, Emrich T, Lipp M. Differentiation-specific expression of a novel G protein-coupled receptor from Burkitt's lymphoma. Eur J Immunol 1992; 22:2795–2799.

134. Forster R, Mattis AE, Kremmer E, Wolf E, Brem G, Lipp M. A putative chemokine receptor, BLR1, directs B cell migration to defined lymphoid organs and specific anatomic compartments of the spleen. Cell 1996; 87:1037–1047.

135. Wilbanks A, Zondlo SC, Murphy K, et al. Expression cloning of the STRL33/BONZO/TYMSTRligand reveals elements of CC, CXC, and CX3C chemokines. J Immunol 2001; 166:5145–5154.

136. Deng HK, Unutmaz D, KewalRamani VN, Littman DR. Expression cloning of new receptors used by simian and human immunodeficiency viruses. Nature 1997; 388:296–300.

137. Kim CH, Kunkel EJ, Boisvert J, et al. Bonzo/CXCR6 expression defines type 1-polarized T-cell subsets with extralymphoid tissue homing potential. J Clin Invest 2001; 107:595–601.

138. Frevert CW, Farone A, Danaee H, Paulauskis JD, Kobzik L. Functional characterization of rat chemokine macrophage inflammatory protein-2. Inflammation 1995; 19:133–142.

139. Boylan AM, Hebert CA, Sadick M, et al. Interleukin-8 is a major component of pleural liquid chemotactic activity in a rabbit model of endotoxin pleurisy. Am J Physiol 1994; 267:L137–L144.

140. Broaddus VC, Boylan AM, Hoeffel JM, et al. Neutralization of IL-8 inhibits neutrophil influx in a rabbit model of endotoxin-induced pleurisy. J Immunol 1994; 152:2960–2967.

141. Boutten A, Dehoux MS, Seta N, et al. Compartmentalized IL-8 and elastase release within the human lung in unilateral pneumonia. Am J Respir Crit Care Med 1996; 153:336–342.

142. Rodriguez JL, Miller CG, DeForge LE, et al. Local production of interleukin-8 is associated with nosocomial pneumonia. J Trauma 1992; 33:74–81. Discussion 81–82.

143. Johnson MC II, Kajikawa O, Goodman RB, et al. Molecular expression of the alpha-chemokine rabbit GRO in Escherichia coli and characterization of its production by lung cells in vitro and in vivo. J Biol Chem 1996; 271:10853–10858.

144. Greenberger MJ, Strieter RM, Kunkel SL, et al. Neutralization of macrophage inflammatory protein-2 attenuates neutrophil recruitment and bacterial clearance in murine Klebsiella pneumonia. J Infect Dis 1996; 173:159–165.

145. Standiford TJ, Kunkel SL, Greenberger MJ, Laichalk LL, Strieter RM. Expression and regulation of chemokines in bacterial pneumonia. J Leukoc Biol 1996; 59:24–28.

146. Mehrad B, Standiford TJ. Role of cytokines in pulmonary antimicrobial host defense. Immunol Res 1999; 20:15–27.

147. Mehrad B, Strieter RM, Moore TA, Tsai WC, Lira SA, Standiford TJ. CXC chemokine receptor-2 ligands are necessary components of neutrophil-mediated host defense in invasive pulmonary aspergillosis. J Immunol 1999; 163:6086–6094.

148. Tsai WC, Strieter RM, Mehrad B, Newstead MW, Zeng X, Standiford TJ. CXC chemokine receptor CXCR2 is essential for protective innate host response in murine *Pseudomonas aeruginosa* pneumonia. Infect Immun 2000; 68:4289–4296.

149. Tsai WC, Strieter RM, Wilkowski JM, et al. Lung-specific transgenic expression of KC enhances resistance to *Klebsiella pneumoniae* in mice. J Immunol 1998; 161:2435–2440.

150. Moore TA, Newstead MW, Strieter RM, Mehrad B, Beaman BL, Standiford TJ. Bacterial clearance and survival are dependent on CXC chemokine receptor-2 ligands in a murine model of pulmonary *Nocardia asteroides* infection. J Immunol 2000; 164:908–915.

151. Laichalk LL, Bucknell KA, Huffnagle GB, et al. Intrapulmonary delivery of tumor necrosis factor agonist peptide augments host defense in murine Gram-negative bacterial pneumonia. Infect Immun 1998; 66:2822–2826.

152. Cole AM, Ganz T, Liese AM, Burdick MD, Liu L, Strieter RM. Cutting edge: IFN-inducible ELR$^-$ CXC chemokines display defensin-like antimicrobial activity. J Immunol 2001; 167:623–627.

153. Jorens PG, Van Damme J, De Backer W, et al. Interleukin 8 (IL-8) in the bronchoalveolar lavage fluid from patients with the adult respiratory distress syndrome (ARDS) and patients at risk for ARDS. Cytokine 1992; 4:592–597.

154. Miller EJ, Cohen AB, Nagao S, et al. Elevated levels of NAP-1/interleukin-8 are present in the airspaces of patients with the adult respiratory distress syndrome and are associated with increased mortality. Am Rev Respir Dis 1992; 146:427–432.

155. Hack CE, Hart M, Strack-vanSchijndel RJM, et al. Interleukin-8 in sepsis: relation to shock and inflammatory mediators. Infect Immun 1992; 60:2835–2842.

156. Chollet-Martin S, Montravers P, Gibert C, et al. High levels of interleukin-8 in the blood and alveolar spaces of patients with pneumonia and adult respiratory distress syndrome. Infect Immun 1993; 61:4553–4559.

157. Donnelly SC, Strieter RM, Kunkel SL, et al. Interleukin-8 and development of adult respiratory distress syndrome in at-risk patient groups. Lancet 1993; 341.

158. Goodman RB, Strieter RM, Martin DP, et al. Inflammatory cytokines in patients with persistence of the acute respiratory distress syndrome. Am J Respir Crit Care Med 1996; 154:602–611.

159. Metinko AP, Kunkel SL, Standiford TJ, Strieter RM. Anoxia–hyperoxia induces monocyte derived interleukin-8. J Clin Invest 1992; 90:791–798.

160. Karakurum M, Shreeniwas R, Chen J, et al. Hypoxic induction of interleukin-8 gene expression in human endothelial cells. J Clin Invest 1994; 93:1564–1570.

161. Sekido N, Mukaida N, Harada A, Nakanishi I, Watanabe Y, Matsushima K. Prevention of lung reperfusion injury in rabbits by a monoclonal antibody against interleukin-8. Nature 1993; 365:654–657.

162. Colletti LM, Kunkel SL, Walz A, et al. Chemokine expression during hepatic ischemia/reperfusion-induced lung injury in the rat. The role of epithelial neutrophil activating protein. J Clin Invest 1995; 95:134–141.

163. Schall TJ. Biology of the RANTES/SIS cytokine family. Cytokine 1991; 3:165.

164. De Meester I, Korom S, Van Damme J, Scharpe S. CD26, let it cut or cut it down. Immunol Today 1999; 20:367–375.

165. Proost P, De Meester I, Schols D, et al. Amino-terminal truncation of chemokines by CD26/dipeptidyl-peptidase IV. Conversion of RANTES into a potent inhibitor of monocyte chemotaxis and HIV-1-infection. J Biol Chem 1998; 273:7222–7227.

166. Proost P, Menten P, Struyf S, Schutyser E, De Meester I, Van Damme J. Cleavage by CD26/dipeptidyl peptidase IV converts the chemokine LD78beta into a most efficient monocyte attractant and CCR1 agonist. Blood 2000; 96:1674–1680.

167. Nibbs RJB, Wylie SM, Pragnell IB, Graham GJ. Cloning and characterization of a novel murine beta chemokine receptor, D6. Comparison to three other related macrophage inflammatory protein-1alpha receptors, CCR-1, CCR-3, and CCR-5. J Biol Chem 1997; 272:12495–12504.

168. Nibbs RJ, Wylie SM, Yang J, Landau NR, Graham GJ. Cloning and characterization of a novel promiscuous human beta-chemokine receptor D6. J Biol Chem 1997; 272:32078–32083.

169. Rossi D, Zlotnik A. The biology of chemokines and their receptors. Annu Rev Immunol 2000; 18:217–242.

170. Sica A, Saccani A, Borsatti A, et al. Bacterial lipopolysaccharide rapidly inhibits expression of C-C chemokine receptors in human monocytes. J Exp Med 1997; 185:969–974.

171. Loetscher P, Seitz M, Baggiolini M, Moser B. Interleukin-2 regulates CC chemokine receptor expression and chemotactic responsiveness in T lymphocytes [see comments]. J Exp Med 1996; 184:569–577.

172. Sallusto F, Lanzavecchia A, Mackay CR. Chemokines and chemokine receptors in T-cell priming and Th1/Th2-mediated responses. Immunol Today 1998; 19:568–574.

173. Allavena P, Luini W, Bonecchi R, et al. Chemokines and chemokine receptors in the regulation of dendritic cell trafficking. In: Mantovani A, ed. Chemical Immunology; Chemokines. Vol. 72. Basel: Karger, 1999:69–85.

174. Boring L, Gosling J, Chensue SW, et al. Impaired monocyte migration and reduced type 1 (Th1) cytokine responses in C-C chemokine receptor 2 knockout mice. J Clin Invest 1997; 100:2552–2561.

175. Kuziel WA, Morgan SJ, Dawson TC, et al. Severe reduction in leukocyte adhesion and monocyte extravasation in mice deficient in CC chemokine receptor 2. Proc Natl Acad Sci USA 1997; 94:12053–12058.

176. Kurihara T, Warr G, Loy J, Bravo R. Defects in macrophage recruitment and host defense in mice lacking the CCR2 chemokine receptor. J Exp Med 1997; 186:1757–1762.

177. Belperio JA, Keane MP, Burdick MD, et al. Critical role for the chemokine MCP-1/CCR2 in the pathogenesis of bronchiolitis obliterans syndrome. J Clin Invest 2001; 108:547–556.

178. Gao W, Topham PS, King JA, et al. Targeting of the chemokine receptor CCR1 suppresses development of acute and chronic cardiac allograft rejection. J Clin Invest 2000; 105:35–44.

179. Gao JL, Wynn TA, Chang Y, et al. Impaired host defense, hematopoiesis, granulomatous inflammation and type 1-type 2 cytokine balance in mice lacking CC chemokine receptor 1. J Exp Med 1997; 185:1959–1968.

180. Dawson TC, Beck MA, Kuziel WA, Henderson F, Maeda N. Contrasting effects of CCR5 and CCR2 deficiency in the pulmonary inflammatory response to influenza A virus. Am J Pathol 2000; 156:1951–1959.

181. Domachowske JB, Bonville CA, Gao JL, Murphy PM, Easton AJ, Rosenberg HF. The chemokine macrophage-inflammatory protein-1 alpha and its receptor CCR1 control pulmonary inflammation and antiviral host defense in paramyxovirus infection. J Immunol 2000; 165:2677–2682.

182. Mehrad B, Moore TA, Standiford TJ. Macrophage inflammatory protein-1 alpha is a critical mediator of host defense against invasive pulmonary aspergillosis in neutropenic hosts. J Immunol 2000; 165:962–968.

183. Huffnagle GB, Strieter RM, Standiford TJ, et al. The role of monocyte chemotactic protein-1 (MCP-1) in the recruitment of monocytes and CD4+ T cells during a pulmonary *Cryptococcus neoformans* infection. J Immunol 1995; 155:4790–4797.

184. Huffnagle GB, Strieter RM, McNeil LK, et al. Macrophage inflammatory protein-1alpha (MIP-1alpha) is required for the efferent phase of pulmonary cell-mediated immunity to a *Cryptococcus neoformans* infection. J Immunol 1997; 159:318–327.

5

Chronic Lung Injury: Basic Features and Clinical Relevance

DAVID PERLMAN, PETER B. BITTERMAN, and CHRISTINE H. WENDT

Department of Medicine, University of Minnesota, School of Medicine, Minneapolis, Minnesota, U.S.A.

I. Overview

This chapter describes basic features and pathophysiological processes relevant for chronic lung injury and its clinical manifestations. Acute and chronic lung injury are not distinct and separate entities, and many of the inflammatory processes, mediators, and mechanisms discussed in the context of acute injury in preceding chapters are also relevant for pulmonary remodeling, repair, and fibrosis. This chapter describes pathophysiological pathways contributing to lung injury and its progression to chronic pathology, including generalized cellular responses to stress and pulmonary inflammatory responses and defense mechanisms. Also described are mediators and factors important in lung injury and fibroproliferation (additional discussion of mediators thought to play important roles in chronic pulmonary injury and fibroproliferative responses is provided in Chapter 6). In addition to covering the basic pathophysiology of chronic lung injury and fibroproliferation, this chapter also discusses related clinical disease. A variety of chronic obstructive pulmonary diseases contain prominent components of chronic lung injury and fibrosis. Two representative examples of such diseases (idiopathic pulmonary fibrosis and silicosis) are discussed to illustrate common clinical manifestations of chronic injury, abnormal remodeling, and fibroproliferation. Therapeutic interventions relevant for chronic lung disease and injury are detailed later in this book.

II. Introduction

The conducting airways and parenchyma of the lung can be injured by a variety of exogenous infectious, particulate, and gas phase agents. Abrupt, high intensity exposures are often associated with dramatic clinical syndromes such as the acute respiratory distress syndrome (ARDS) or severe airway obstruction with a relatively direct connection between stimulus and response. Acute injury and its associated inflammatory response can eventually resolve with beneficial remodeling and repair of damaged lung tissue. Alternatively, acute injury can progress to subacute and chronic injury with persistent inflammation and abnormal pulmonary remodeling and repair. Many aspects of the pathobiology of chronic injury and the mechanisms of pulmonary remodeling and repair remain to be elucidated. Chronic lung injury from periodic or continuous subthreshold perturbation by known or cryptic respiratory pathogens provides additional scientific and clinical challenges. Initial sections of this chapter discuss current perspectives on pulmonary inflammation, repair, and fibroproliferation. Lung injury is viewed as a continuum of events progressing from an initial insult and acute inflammation to either adaptation, repair, and resolution or chronic injury with persistent inflammation and inappropriate fibroproliferation. This continuum of events includes the concept of chronicity, since the outcome (beneficial or detrimental) of many of the processes involved depends on their timing of occurrence relative to each other. Chronic lung injury is also discussed in the context of the biology of physiological stress and the generalized responses of the organism to it. Selected examples of chronic obstructive lung disease (restrictive or interstitial lung disease) are described at the end of the chapter to illustrate common clinical manifestations.

III. Generalized Cellular Responses to Stress and Injury

The pulmonary response to injury does not involve a unique set of processes and mechanistic pathways, but rather incorporates several relevant features from other phenomena such as growth and development (Chapter 2) plus generalized responses of the organism to stress. To better understand the processes of lung injury and repair, it is useful to briefly summarize the most fundamental cellular response to injury, which is the generalized stress response. All living organisms face a continuously changing burden of physiological stress, and have evolved a repertoire of stress-inducible responses. One aspect of such responses is the family of proteins called heat shock proteins (HSP) that are involved in protein homeostasis (1–4). Stress causes the formation of non-native proteins, which aggregate and disrupt cell function. The HSP re-establish protein homeostasis by facilitating protein repair or degradation. Heat shock proteins are induced by thermal and nonthermal forms of cellular stress and are regulated transcriptionally, primarily by heat shock factor-1 (HSF1) (2,5,6). HSF1 is abundant in its inactive, cytoplasmic form sequestered by HSP. Non-native proteins associate with HSP, which disrupts the equilibrium of bound HSP to HSF1 leading to release of HSF1. Free HSF1 translocates to the nucleus, trimerizes, and binds to its cognate nucleotide sequence in the $5'$ regulatory region of HSP genes to upregulate their transcription. HSF1 serves a fundamental regulatory role in the initiation of the stress-inducible response (2,6), and the status of this system provides a valuable readout of the cellular response to stress. From an analogous perspective, lung injury and repair can be viewed as the integrated readout of stress responses in pulmonary cell populations as a result of exposure to specific insults or toxicants. The sum of these responses can either be adaptive or maladaptive for the lungs.

A. Adaptation

Once the level of imposed stress exceeds a critical threshold, cells must adapt to the new circumstances or be at risk of dysfunction. Adaptation is manifest physiologically by a change in the dose–response properties of cells exposed to further stress, and is influenced by the level and duration of the exposure. For example, reactive oxygen species (ROS) generated by particulate pollutants and many other injury-inducing substances can be toxic to cells and tissues, especially in disease states (7–10). Cells maintain homeostatic conditions using antioxidants present in the basal state. When the oxidant burden increases, key processes such as ion transport, uptake of essential nutrients, and cellular metabolism are disrupted (11). Under these conditions, genes coding for protective proteins are stably upregulated helping the cell adapt to the environmental stress. These genes include antioxidants, such as catalase and superoxide dismutase (SOD), and sodium transport proteins, such as the Na,K-ATPase and Na channel (12–14). This stable induction of genes results in a differentiated state that can persist for hours to days and allows the cell to survive in a hostile environment.

One pathway responsible for cellular adaptation is initiated by the antioxidant-responsive transcription factor, activator protein-1 (AP-1), which induces the transcription of several antioxidant genes (15,16). AP-1 is composed of homodimers and heterodimers of the proto-oncogene family fos, jun, and ATF (activating transcription factor) and upregulates genes by binding to the TPA responsive element (TRE). AP-1 is regulated by changes in cellular redox state, and activates transcription of several antioxidant genes (e.g., glutathione-*S*-transferase and NADP(H):quinone reductase) which protects cells from oxidant induced injury.

B. Ineffective Adaptation (Maladaptive Responses)

When stress exceeds the threshold for adaptation, injury occurs and innate immunity is triggered. An integral component of the innate immune response in the lung is recruitment of neutrophils and their adhesion to microvascular endothelial cells at sites of injury. Once adhesion to injured endothelium has occurred, neutrophils egress from the circulation into the lung. The early response mediators released by activated macrophages, TNFα and interleukin-1 (IL-1), initiate a cascade of reactions leading to neutrophil sequestration and chemotaxis (17,18). TNFα is also a potent inducer of endothelial cell apoptosis, impairing capillary integrity and delivery of oxygen and nutrients downstream (19,20). This response repertoire is regulated at the level of transcription. One of the most studied transcription factors in this response is NFκB (21–23). Early during physiological stress, when the ability of a cell to maintain homeostasis is in balance, NFκB remains bound to its inhibitory protein partner, IκB (24). When cellular stress is in excess, the release of NFκB and its translocation to the nucleus results in the upregulation of cytokines involved in the inflammatory response (21,25).

C. Cell Death (Apoptosis)

When stress exceeds the reparative capacity of a cell, death ensues. Some of the resultant cell death can be orchestrated by a regulated sequence of biochemical reactions into a distinct morphological pattern termed apoptosis (26). Cells detach from their neighbors and the substratum. The plasma membrane ruffles and the nucleus and cytoplasm condense. Apoptotic cells fragment and are rapidly eaten by neighboring cells or professional phagocytes. The integration of extracellular information by a cell into a decision to live or die is of fundamental importance during development, wound healing, immune responses, and tumorigenesis (27,28). The apoptotic program can be triggered through at least two distinct signaling pathways with the potential for crosstalk. One pathway, leading to activation of caspase-8, is triggered by ligation of specific cell surface death receptors, such as Fas/CD95 or TNFα receptor (29–31). The second pathway, initiated by various stressors such as cytotoxic drugs and radiation, is transduced through a series of steps into mitochondrial release of cytochrome *c*. Subsequent formation of the apoptosome, a complex containing cytochrome *c*, adapter protein Apaf-1 and procaspase-9 leads to activation of caspase-9 (32,33). When activated, caspases-8 and -9 activate effectors caspases-3, -6, and/or 7, which in turn cleave critical cellular targets resulting in death (30). Proteins in the

Bcl-2 family tightly regulate mitochondrial release of cytochrome *c.* The proapoptotic Bcl-2 proteins, such as Bid, Bax, Bad, and Bak, form pores in the outer mitochondrial membrane, while the antiapoptotic proteins, Bcl-2 and Bcl-X_L, inhibit pore formation (31). In some cells, these two pathways converge, and receptor-induced activation of caspase-8 also results in mitochondrial release of death promoters with subsequent activation of the apoptosome-dependent caspase cascade (34).

Apoptosis is generally viewed as a physiological form of death that functions to sculpt tissues into their mature shape during development, to eliminate inflammatory cells after they have served their function, or to remove excess tissue during repair of an injured organ (35,36). While apoptosis is distinguished from necrotic death, a pathological process characterized by abrupt cessation of cellular function, its role as a strictly physiological process has been partially shrouded by its occurrence during stroke, myocardial infarction and lung injury, distinctly pathological events. This paradox can be understood if apoptotic death is assumed to be the preferred mode of death. According to this formulation, during infections, tissue ischemia, or environmental stress, cells that are injured beyond their reparative capacity will in general undergo apoptosis. Necrosis is observed only in those regions where the pathological insult is sufficiently rapid and intense to cripple the generation of ATP, a requirement for the regulated biochemical reactions of apoptosis. As a consequence, the physiological process of apoptosis can be associated with a pathological clinical outcome if too many cells of an organ die. Thus, investigators studying a variety of injury models and patient samples arrive at differing conclusions regarding the frequency, distribution, and timing of apoptotic vs. necrotic cell death. This is a matter of great therapeutic import, since apoptotic death is amenable to interdiction and necrotic death probably is not. What appears to supervene in human disease associated with tissue injury is a mixture of apoptotic cells, necrotic cells, and many cells displaying features of both. This blended mode of death perhaps results when a physiological stress triggering apoptosis intensifies, aborting the process abruptly at any stage and switching it to necrosis.

IV. Lung Injury and Its Mechanisms

Following an initial insult, the lung responds in a sequential, yet often overlapping response, consisting of coagulation, inflammation, tissue formation, and tissue remodeling. This sequence of events often results in effective repair and the return of normal lung function. However, if the injury stimulus is severe, repetitive, or chronic, the stages of inflammation and tissue formation may be prolonged and exaggerated leading to fibrosis and physiological dysfunction. In some examples of lung injury, epithelial and endothelial cell damage and death may be histologically obvious within areas of inflammation and fibroproliferation. In contrast, not all fibroproliferative disorders show widespread cellular damage and cellular injury may be subtle histologically. Although the histological injury may appear inconsequential, it may trigger cellular events that will lead to fibroproliferation. Identifying the cellular responses following injury may lead to a better understanding of the patterns that are protective vs. those that will ultimately lead to fibroproliferation.

A. Lung Cellular Injury

The earliest discernible histological changes in many types of lung injury are the loss of alveolar epithelium and vascular endothelium. Damage to the airway epithelium and other cellular components of pulmonary tissue can also occur, with a timing of appearance dependent on the type of injury-inducing process or stress involved. Injury to pulmonary cells can be lethal or sublethal. Even if epithelial and endothelial cells remain viable, they may lose tight junctions and become impaired in their ability to provide a barrier to molecular transport. Type I epithelial cells cover a larger surface area than type II cells and appear to be more susceptible to many forms of injury than type II epithelial cells (37). Death of type I epithelial cells results in a large area of denuded basement membrane at the air–lung interface. Injury to capillary endothelial cells causes a loss of vascular integrity and leads to the escape of plasma and activation of the coagulation cascade. Coagulation is an important event for the development of a primordial matrix along the denuded basement membrane and subsequently, the initiation of tissue formation. Consequently, persistent cell death or lack of cell proliferation can lead to dysregulated coagulation and the continuous deposition of matrix resulting in fibrosis. Specific molecular mechanisms responsible for cell loss and fibrosis in many chronic fibroproliferative disorders, however, remain unknown. Numerous pathophysiological effectors have been proposed including oxidants and proteinases derived from resident and recruited leukocytes. However, the target stimuli inducing leukocyte recruitment and activation have not been clearly identified, nor have the pathophysiological consequences of their presence been defined.

B. Pulmonary Inflammation

In classic models of pulmonary fibrosis, injury and the associated necrotic death of epithelial and endothelial cells incite a progressive inflammatory response that eventually leads to inappropriate fibroproliferation and fibrosis. Key to the recruitment of neutrophils into the lung is their initial adhesion to endothelial cells at sites of alveolar injury. This occurs through a number of adhesion molecules found on the surface of leukocytes (e.g., members of the β_2 integrin adhesion molecule family) and on the surface of injured endothelial cells (e.g., members of the selectin family and ICAM-1).

Once adhesion to injured endothelium has occurred, neutrophils egress from the circulation into the lung. The early response mediators released by activated macrophages, TNFα and IL-1, are important in the initial inflammatory response (17,38,39). The IL-1 family of cytokines is complex and consists of agonists (IL-1α and IL-1β), receptor antagonists (IL-1ra), and two receptors (type I and II). The balance of these various compounds influences the inflammatory process and hence, fibrosis. Numerous studies have demonstrated that IL-1 recruits leukocytes through the expression of adhesion molecules and chemokines. In addition, IL-1 induces fibroblast production of procollagens, fibronectin, glycosaminogly-cans, and growth factors, such as platelet-derived growth factor (PDGF), that indirectly results in fibroblast proliferation (18).

TNF is a potent inducer of endothelial cell apoptosis. This can lead to the loss of capillary integrity as described earlier, which allows further neutrophil recruitment into the lung. Neither TNF nor IL-1 has chemotactic activity by itself. However, both can induce the expression of chemoattractants, such as IL-8, a member of the C-X-C chemokine supergene family (Chapter 4), which has both neutrophil chemoattractant and activating activity. Recruited leukocytes can produce oxidants, which in turn can induce injury and expression of cytokines, such as IL-8. In addition, TNF can induce cellular injury via the induction of nuclear factor (NF)κB, B, which can upregulate both the antiapoptotic and the proinflammatory pathways.

Additional mediators are also important in pulmonary inflammation. The CD40 receptor on fibroblasts is important in fibroblast signaling and is stimulated by CD40 ligand secreted by activated inflammatory cells, such as lymphocytes, platelets, and mast cells. This CD40 ligand, CD154, stimulates fibroblasts to synthesize several factors including interleukins (IL-6 and IL-8) and extracellular proteins such as hyaluronate. The CC chemokine family is important in the recruitment and maintenance of inflammatory cells in the chronic injury state. One chemokine, monocyte chemoattractant protein (MCP) -1, has been demonstrated to be markedly elevated in patients with idiopathic pulmonary fibrosis (IPF). In addition, reduction of MCP-1 in bleomycin induced lung injury results in an attenuation of the fibrotic response as measured by a reduction in collagen deposition. The mechanism appears to be via a reduction in inflammatory cell recruitment.

C. Reactive Oxygen/Nitrogen Species

One important effector of pulmonary injury is excessive oxidant stress, which can lead to necrotic death and inflammatory and fibrotic consequences if cellular antioxidant mechanisms are overwhelmed. However, the proinflammatory consequences of necrotic death may be avoided in instances of oxidant stress that occurs within the boundary of the epithelial cell's antioxidant capacity. Alternatively, this level of oxidants may trigger apoptosis and inhibit compensatory cellular proliferation. Whether loss of epithelial integrity in idiopathic fibroproliferative lung diseases results from necrosis, apoptosis, or failure of normal cellular proliferation is not clearly defined. In addition, it is not clear what effect the loss of cellular integrity has on the formation of fibrosis.

For some time, oxidants have been implicated in the lung injury that leads to the fibroproliferative response (40,41). In idiopathic pulmonary fibrosis (IPF), which is discussed later in the chapter, the inflammatory process is marked by an increase in macrophages and neutrophils that release significantly higher amounts of oxidants such as O_2-radicals and H_2O_2, compared to healthy subjects (42). Consequently, many of the animal models for pulmonary fibrosis can be produced by an exposure to oxidants or oxidant forming compounds such as bleomycin or FITC (43). In addition, antioxidants, such as liposome-entrapped catalase or *N*-acetylcysteine, can abrogate the effects of this injury, supporting a role for oxidant injury (43,44). Therefore, these oxidants may represent a mechanism of injury and may influence the repair process. Oxidants and antioxidants and their effects on lung injury are discussed in more detail in Chapters 7 and 16.

Oxygen is essential for all aerobic life forms, but excessive oxygen or its conversion to reactive oxidant species can be toxic to cells and tissues. In the homeopathic state, oxidant species are derived by normal respiration in the formation of cellular ATP via the four electron reduction of oxygen to form H_2O_2 within the mitochondrial electron transport system. In addition, stimulated macrophages and neutrophils generate oxidants that are helpful in host defenses against infection (45).

A number of reactive oxygen species can contribute to inflammatory lung injury. The superoxide anion radical of oxygen ($O_2^{\bullet -}$) is commonly generated by electrons leaking from the respiratory chain onto oxygen. It is a weak oxidant with a short half-life and can oxidize relatively few compounds, including ascorbate, sulfhydryl groups, and certain catecholamines. However, superoxide can exert cytotoxicity by inactivating essential cellular enzymes, such as tRNase, RNase, and glyceraldehyde-3-phosphate dehydrogenase. Although these reactions may occur, superoxide seems to exert most of its toxicity by acting as a precursor to more reactive oxidants via SOD (45).

A more potent oxidant, hydrogen peroxide (H_2O_2), is produced in mitochondria by the reduction of O_2 or the dismutation of superoxide. From the mitochondria, it readily diffuses across the cytoplasm and out of the cell. Hydrogen peroxide is a slow oxidant, however, in the presence of trace metals, it can form hydroxyl radicals such as in the iron-catalyzed Fenton reaction. This is particularly pertinent in areas of lung injury where heme and therefore iron has accumulated due to endothelial cell damage and the extravasation of erythrocytes. Although high concentrations of hydrogen peroxide are required to damage cells, low concentrations can damage cellular DNA and alter molecular events especially in the presence of trace metals. Hydrogen peroxide is converted to water by catalase or the glutathione peroxidase system (45).

One of the most potent oxidants, hydroxyl radical (OH^-), is produced from superoxide reducing hydrogen peroxide via the Haber–Weiss reaction. This reaction is accelerated by iron released from such compounds as ferritin, hemoglobin, and transferrin during inflammatory processes. Although this oxidant is short-lived, the rate of reaction is fast, approaching diffusion-limited rates, making this oxidant very reactive (45).

Reactive nitrogen compounds can also generate lung injury. Nitric oxide (NO) is a molecule with properties including signal transduction, antioxidant function, and pro-oxidant effects. For example, NO can rapidly react with superoxide anion and produce the oxidant peroxynitrite (ONOO–), which coexists with its conjugate acid peroxynitrous acid (ONOOH) at neutral pH. Various reactive metabolites of NO, such as nitrous anhydride (N_2O_3) and nitrogen dioxide (NO_2), can also be produced and react with a wide range of biological targets (46,47). The effects of reactive nitrogen species can often be detected by the presence of nitroadducts on target proteins. One nitroadduct, 3-nitrotyrosine, has been detected in many diverse lung diseases including IPF (48). Although the detection of 3-nitrotyrosine in diseased lung indicates the formation of NO-derived oxidants, the role of these oxidants and the contribution of 3-nitrotyrosine modified proteins to the lung injury and subsequent fibrosis remains unknown.

Reactive oxygen and nitrogen species can directly damage membrane lipids and cellular proteins in the lungs (49). When plasma membranes are exposed to oxidants, the membrane lipids can undergo peroxidation. This reaction is self-perpetuating and results in a decrease in membrane fluidity. In addition, oxidation can inactivate membrane proteins by the cross-linkage of aldehyde groups to lipids. Other proteins, including enzymes, can be inactivated by the oxidation of sulfhydryl groups. These changes can affect all aspects of cellular homeostasis, such as ion transport, the uptake of essential nutrients, and cellular metabolism (50). The disruption of ion and fluid transport are necessary to keep alveoli free of excess fluid and to maintain normal gas exchange.

In addition to affecting cell membrane integrity, oxidants can disrupt intracellular function. For example, oxidants can disturb cellular energy stores and damage DNA via the depression of ATP and the inhibition of ADP phosphorylation (51). In addition, cellular energy stores are affected by the inhibition of glucose uptake and glycolysis. Cellular DNA damage results from nicking by hydroxyl radicals, leading to abnormal cross-linking, mutations, and even cellular death in extreme cases (52). Oxidants can also damage extracellular proteins and lipids including components of surfactant present in the alveolar epithelial lining fluid. Surfactant proteins A and D are important as collectins in mediating the native host response to eliminate infectious agents. This is evident in the surfactant protein D knock-out mouse that demonstrates a predisposition to pulmonary fibrosis.

D. Proteinases

The turnover of extracellular matrix is essential for normal cellular growth and function. This is accomplished by proteinases in the matrix metalloproteinase (MMP) or serine proteinase families. In the lung, the alveolar macrophage is the source of several MMPs, including interstitial collagenase and stromelysin, while other cells produce gelantinases and neutrophil collagenases. These enzymes are released as zymogens, in contrast to the serine proteinases that are released as active proteins. The serine proteinases (e.g., plasminogen activators, neutrophil elastase, cathepsin G, and proteinase 3) and MMPs further enhance matrix turnover via inactivation of proteinase inhibitors.

During oxidant injury, aberrant matrix synthesis by injured cells and/or by direct oxidation of matrix proteins alters extracellular matrix composition. In addition, oxidant injury increases proteinase and plasminogen activator synthesis, which are important in the degradation and remodeling of extracellular matrix components (53,54). Collagenase activation by oxidants can result in the direct loss or fragmentation of collagen within the extracellular matrix (55). Epithelial cells are especially susceptible to aberrant matrix as they have an absolute substratum requirement to remain viable. Loss of appropriate input from cell surface receptors including integrins and possibly proteoglycans can trigger programmed death. Therefore, it is feasible that alterations of the epithelial basement membrane by inflammatory or parenchymal cell derived matrix active enzymes could create an environment no longer capable of supporting the viability of the epithelial cells. Proteolytic enzymes have been detected within the lungs of patients with idiopathic fibroproliferative disorders including collagenases, elastases, and gelatinases. What is not clear is whether these enzymes contribute to the pathogenesis of the disease, or whether they are mainly involved in tissue remodeling and disease progression.

V. Lung Defense Mechanisms

As described above, important contributors to lung injury include excessive inflammation, oxidant production, and proteinase activation from recruited leukoctyes. These factors cause cellular death and/or dysfunction, with a resultant loss of normal pulmonary architecture and function. However, in many fibroproliferative disorders, extensive cellular injury and death are not always evident. This suggests that oxidants and other injury-inducing substances can induce more subtle cellular responses that contribute to the fibroproliferative response. It also indicates that abnormalities of regulation that are less apparent than frank cell death are important in chronic injury. This is especially true during chronic or repeated exposure to injury, when loss of control of the normal reparative process occurs. Normal repair requires an orchestration of molecular and cellular events that turn on and off at appropriate times. The loss of this control may result in a maladaptive reparative process and a subsequent fibroproliferative state.

Repopulation of the denuded basement membrane is key for normal repair. Oxidants and other compounds induced by inflammation have both positive and negative effects on cellular proliferation in the lung. In animal models in vivo, cellular proliferation can be induced by acute exposures to oxidants (56). This may have a beneficial effect if it results in the proliferation of type II cells and the re-epithelialization of the denuded basement membrane. Alternatively, repeated or sustained injury results in decreased proliferation and continued loss of epithelium. Exacerbating this epithelial loss is the stimulation of fibroblasts that to invades the alveolus and results in fibrosis. During lung injury, genes are upregulated that may be protective. These include the induction of type II epithelial cell surfactant apoproteins, ion transport, and antioxidant genes (57–59). Surfactant oxidation can result in loss of host defenses and regional atelectasis subsequent organ dysfunction (59,60). The ion transport systems are important proteins for the homeostasis of the cell and ion and fluid transport in the lung. Oxidants injure cellular tight junctions and increase the amount of fluid in the alveoli. To counteract this, cells increase sodium transport via an increase in sodium channel and Na,K-ATPase expression and activity (57). Lastly, to counteract the increased oxidants present, antioxidant genes are upregulated.

A. Antioxidants

There are several antioxidant mechanisms by which the lungs protect against oxidant injury. Metals sequestered by cellular and extracellular proteins, such as ferritin and metallothionien, protect against the Fenton reaction. A variety of endogenous compounds, such as vitamins A, C and E, behave as weak antioxidants. More effective antioxidants include SOD, catalase, and glutathione (GSH). Superoxide dismutase converts superoxide anion into H_2O_2, while catalase and glutathione peroxidase break H_2O_2 down to H_2O plus oxygen. Small amounts of SOD and catalase are present in alveolar lining fluid, but these antioxidants are mainly intracellular. Glutathione is predominantly extracellular and is present in significant quantities in alveolar lining fluid (43). An initial response by several types of pulmonary cells to inhibit oxidant damage is to produce antioxidants or antioxidant enzymes.

There is increasing evidence that oxidants and/or injury modulate gene expression, including the antioxidant gene expression, in lung epithelial and endothelial cells (53,61). This includes gene expression for catalase, MnSOD and glutathione peroxidase, which are directly involved in eliminating oxidant species and protecting the epithelium and endothelium from injury (12,53,61–64). The mechanism by which these genes are upregulated has been most clearly elucidated in the glutathione-*S*-transferase and NAD(P) H quinone reductase genes in which an "antioxidant response element" has been described that upregulates gene expression in the presence of oxidants (65). Indirectly, oxidants also can modulate gene expression via signal transduction pathways, such as the activation of S6-kinase and protein kinase C by superoxide and hydrogen peroxide (61). In addition, oxidants and/or injury also induce the expression of certain acute phase reactant proteins, such as HSP, 10–40-fold (61). In contrast, other genes regulated by oxidants or injury such as certain housekeeping genes may need only a 3–5-fold increase in expression to have a significant physiological effect (53,58).

In chronic or repetitive lung injury, the persistent influx of inflammatory cells may overwhelm the endogenous antioxidant activity, tipping the balance towards continued oxidant injury. This in turn may alter the gene expression involved in the normal reparative process and contribute to an abnormal fibroproliferative response. Augmentation of antioxidant defenses may thus be a potential therapeutic intervention to mitigate the progression of fibroproliferation and facilitate normal repair. The delivery of antioxidant enzymes to lungs exposed to oxidizing agents, such as bleomycin, has an attenuating effect against lung injury and the fibroproliferative state. Detailed discussion of antioxidant therapies for lung injury are discussed in Chapter 16.

B. Cytokines

The balance of pro- and anti-inflammatory cytokines is highly important in the resolution of lung inflammation and injury. TNFα and IL-1, which trigger cytokine networks and are necessary for neutrophil chemotaxis and activation, must be down-regulated to prevent further recruitment and activation of leukocytes. Apoptosis of recruited leukocytes followed by their phagocytosis by resident macrophages is an important component (66). Apoptosis, compared to necrotic death, does not promote further cytokine release that fuels the inflammatory response. In the presence of recurrent or chronic injury, counter-regulatory processes and the orderly elimination of leukocytes are absent, and persistent inflammation with continued oxidant injury occurs. This creates a cycle of sustained cytokine production and continued injury leading to chronic disease. Basic mechanisms of pulmonary repair and how they are compromised in abnormal fibroproliferative states are not fully understood. However, research has identified a large number of inflammatory mediators and factors important in acute and chronic lung injury. Specific mediators contributing to acute inflammation and lung injury have been discussed in Chapters 3 and 4, and mediators important in chronic fibroproliferative lung injury are detailed further in Chapter 6. Ultimately, the ability of the lung to defend itself productively against injury from micro-organisms and toxic substances depends on regulating the inflammatory response to facilitate those aspects that are beneficial for the host while antagonizing those that are over-exuberant or disruptive to normal pulmonary repair.

C. Antiproteinases

To maintain a healthy substratum for lung epithelial and endothelial cells, matrix degradation by proteinases is necessary for normal matrix turnover. However, it is important to maintain a balance in proteinase activity to prevent excessive matrix degradation that leads to cellular and organ dysfunction. Proteinase activity is regulated by antiproteinases, such as alpha-1 proteinase inhibitor and the tissue inhibitors of metalloproteinases (TIMP). Injury to the lung, such as by hyperoxia, increases expression of antiproteases such as TIMP (53,67). Antiproteinases appear to play a significant role in attenuating lung injury. In addition to the inhibition of protease activity, antiproteinases have anti-inflammatory activity. These include suppression of neutrophil chemotaxis, antioxidant activity, inhibition of fibroblast proliferation, and reduced neutrophil adherence to epithelial cells. This may have a protective effect, since experimental studies have shown that bleomycin-induced fibrosis can be attenuated by the administration of antiproteinases (68).

VI. Fibroproliferation and Chronic Lung Disease

Fibroproliferation occurs in the setting of injury to the alveolus, and is part of the body's normal wound-healing response. However, in chronic lung disease, fibroproliferation becomes exaggerated and counterproductive. As detailed earlier, lung injury involves an initial exogenous insult followed by an inflammatory process that affects the alveolar epithelium, the interstitum, and the microcirculation. In regions of damaged alveolar epithelium, the airspace is repopulated by cells of mesenchymal origin termed "myofibroblasts." These cells display a motile phenotype, characterized by high levels of expression of α-smooth muscle actin (α-SMA), which allows them to migrate along the surface of the injured epithelium (69). This migration is also facilitated by changes in surface receptor expression in the epithelial cells. Transforming growth factor $\beta 1$ (TGF $\beta 1$), an important cytokine in wound healing and fibroliferation, upregulates the expression of the integrin α5β1, which has been found in increased levels in areas of fibrosis (70,71). Recent evidence has also shown that blocking the function of certain integrins (specifically αvβ3 and αvβ5) upregulates the expression of α-SMA (72) implying a role for the epithelium in modulation of myofibroblast phenotype. The fibroblasts migrate into the airspace of the injured epithelium where, in response to several signaling molecules, they undergo proliferation and collagen synthesis and deposition.

There are several signaling molecules that have been implicated in the fibrogenic process including: TGF β1, PDGF, and the family of fibroblast growth factors (73,74). The growth factors act on check points in the cell cycle, stimulating cells to emerge from a quiescent state to a proliferative state, and facilitating transit through the restriction point in the G1 phase of the cell cycle. In the case of normal healing, collagen deposition allows for re-epithelialization of the alveolar air–lung interface following injury. Once this has been accomplished the fibroblast population regresses through apoptosis, an orderly process of programmed cell death (75). In the case of chronic fibrotic disorders, there is evidence to suggest that there is interference with the apoptotic process (35). Fibroblasts recovered from patients with acute lung injury display an enhanced proliferative phenotype in vitro when compared to fibroblasts recovered from histologically normal lungs (76), and fibroblast cell lines derived from patients with pulmonary fibrosis proliferate at a much higher rate in vitro than cells derived from normal lungs (77). Fibroblasts thus continue to proliferate resulting in collagen deposition and contraction, and eventually, destruction of the alveolar airspace and loss of ventilatory function. This loss of ventilation leads to the ventilation-perfusion mismatch that is characteristic of fibrotic lung disorders. This physiology is seen in both chronic as well as acute lung injury disorders, the main difference being in the number of alveoli involved at a given time. In acute disorders, such as ARDS, histological examination reveals diffuse alveolar damage, with the fibroproliferative filling process seen throughout the lung. In chronic fibrotic diseases such as IPF, it is common to see normal lung architecture alongside organizing pneumonitis juxtaposed with completely destroyed alveoli. Pulmonary illnesses characterized by a pattern of chronic injury have been traditionally divided in a binary manner into diseases of known and unknown cause (Table 1). General concepts of chronic lung disease are illustrated here by selecting a prototypical illness from each category: IPF as a disease of unknown cause, and silicosis as a disease with a clear precipitant.

A. Idiopathic Pulmonary Fibrosis (IPF)

Idiopathic pulmonary fibrosis is a deadly disease, with an estimated incidence of 7–11 cases per 100,000, and an estimated prevalence of 27–29 per 100,000 (78). Currently, the only effective therapeutic option is lung transplantation.

Table 1 Chronic Interstitial Lung Diseases (ILDs)

	Reference
Diseases of known etiology	
Occupational/environmental	(79)
Asbestosis	(80)
Berylliosis	(81)
Coal workers pneumoconiosis	(82)
Silicosis	(80,82)
Byssinosis	(83)
Drug induced	(84,85)
Hypersensitivity pneumonitis	(86)
Collagen vascular disease associated ILD	(87)
Diseases of unknown etiology	
Sarcoidosis	(88)
Chronic eosinophilic pneumonia	(89)
Langerhans' cell histiocytosis (histocytosis X)	(90)
Lymphangioleiomyomatosis	(91)
Idiopathic interstitial pneumonias (IIP)	(92)
Idiopathic pulmonary fibrosis (IPF, usual interstitial pneumonia)	
Nonspecific interstitial pneumonia	
Cryptogenic organizing pneumonia (previously BOOP)	
Respiratory bronchiolitis—interstitial lung disease	
Desquamative interstitial pneumonia	
Lymphocytic interstitial pneumonia	
Acute interstitial pneumonia (diffuse alveolar damage)	

The chronic interstitial lung diseases can be grouped into disorders of known and unknown etiology. The diseases of known etiology consist mainly of disorders in which the cause is exposure to a known pathogen. This can be chronic exposure, as in the occupational exposures, or repeated exposures causing acute exacerbations, such as in hypersensitivity pneumonitis, or exposure to a medication with pulmonary toxicity. The diseases of unknown etiology include the IIPs which have clinically overlapping features and often have to be distinguished histologically, and chronic infiltrative/granulomatous disorders in which the causative agent or exposure is unknown. References are provided for further information.

Characteristically, fibrotic lesions are found scattered throughout the lung parenchyma at different stages of progression. Some alveolar units are inflamed, others manifest epithelial denudation with fibroblastic foci and still others are scarred shut with a mature collagenous matrix. For reasons that remain to be elucidated, fibrosis begins at the lung bases and periphery working its way towards the lung apices and hilum. Attempts to treat inflammation with the goal of interdicting fibrosis have been disappointing.

IPF evolves as if it resulted from a cryptic alveolar injury, although direct evidence to support injury as the first step in the process has not been forthcoming. Detailed morphological studies point to the subepithelial fibroblastic focus as the sentinel morphological lesion, in a pathological pattern that is designated usual interstitial pneumonitis. In diseased alveolar units, fibroblastic foci expand. There are accumulations of myofibroblasts and their connective tissue products, distorting alveolar architecture and compromising the ability to participate in normal gas exchange.

Clinically, IPF presents with the insidious onset of cough and breathlessness, typically in the sixth decade of life, a time when symptoms of breathlessness are frequently disregarded by the patient and physician as due to aging. At presentation, the disease process is frequently well established with bibasalar crackles, radiographic evidence of peripheral and basalar linear opacities with honeycombing, restrictive physiology, and a widened alveolar-arterial oxygen gradient. Clubbing of the fingers and toes are sometimes observed, and some patients have a clear family history of IPF in an autosomal dominant pattern. Therapy with traditional anti-inflammatory and immunosuppressive agents has been disappointing, with the average time from diagnosis to death estimated at 3–5 years. New therapeutics such as immune interferon that target both innate immune aberrations and the fibrotic response per se are under active investigation, however, when available transplantation remains the best option for patients.

B. Silicosis

Over the last several decades, there has been strong evidence that lung injury plays a role in some interstitial lung diseases. Epidemiological and pathological studies have demonstrated that inhalational exposure to silica crystals can result in chronic lung injury (80,82). This injury has been manifested by inflammatory cells and is a good example of an injury, namely the inhalation of crystalline silica, leading to the production of oxidative species and subsequently oxidized lipids and proteins in epithelial lining fluid. After the lung is exposed to silica, there is an immediate inflammatory reaction that involves a broad range of inflammatory cells. This includes macrophages, polymorphonuclear leukocytes, and ultimately the participation of other inflammatory cells such as lymphocytes, eosinophils, and plasma cells. The initial lesion, consisting of the silica particle, is surrounded and engulfed by macrophages and a cascade of inflammatory cells. This is followed by fibroblast proliferation and collagen deposition in an attempt to wall off and contain the inflammatory process (scar formation). Within this matrix of particles, inflammatory and fibrotic cells is evidence of oxidation. The ability of the lung to isolate the injury and keep the inflammatory and fibrotic process in check will determine the extent of affected pulmonary tissue. In certain animals models, antioxidants can abrogate chronic injury relevant for interstitial lung disease. Unfortunately, the complex cascade of events that occur in the progression of inflammatory lung injury to chronic pathology does not lend itself at present to any truly curative therapeutic intervention.

VII. Summary

The lungs are subject to physiologic stresses as a result of their constant exposure to a broad oxidizing environment containing a variety of potentially harmful substances. This physiologic stress can result in a prolonged or permanent perturbation in pulmonary homeostasis or, alternatively, lead to adaptation. In instances of repetitive or persistent stress, severe chronic injury with abnormal repair and fibroproliferation can occur. In many chronic injury states of the lung, such as those exemplified by IPF and silicosis, oxidants have been demonstrated. In an attempt to maintain homeostasis or to adapt to this increased oxidant state, the injured lung can upregulate host defenses such as antioxidant enzymes. However, in instances where the injury overwhelms host defense systems, injury may progress to an exaggerated fibroproliferative state. In many cases, this kind of pulmonary pathology is not uniform, and the progression of the physiological response may not be linear. There may be areas of lung where host defenses and adaptation are overwhelmed and fibroproliferation proceeds unabated to radically change tissue architecture. At the same time, there may be other areas of lung where homeostasis is more resonant, and tissue appears undamaged or healed.

A good deal of information has been elucidated regarding the responses and chronic adaptations of the lungs to injury as described in this chapter. Additional discussion on cellular processes and mediators involved in chronic pulmonary injury, remodeling, and repair are given in Chapter 6. At present, understanding of the mechanistic pathophysiology of chronic lung injury and chronic pulmonary disease is incomplete. Such understanding is essential for rational therapeutic development for chronic or fibrotic lung disease. In many chronic fibroproliferative states, the underlying injury largely remains occult and does not become manifest until pulmonary damage is irreversible. The scientific and clinical challenges of future research include identifying early stages of cryptic injury associated with the fibroproliferative response, and defining interventions able to modulate or regulate on-going host defense to facilitate effective pulmonary repair. Effective early modulation of innate host responses to stress can promote homeostasis and adaptation, and may allow the lung to avoid the destruction of an over-exuberant fibroproliferative response. Therapies for clinical acute and chronic lung disease and injury are discussed in detail later in this book (Chapters 13–19).

References

1. Hightower LE. Heat shock, stress proteins, chaperones, and proteotoxicity. Cell 1991; 66:191–197.
2. Morimoto RI. Cells in stress: transcriptional activation of heat shock genes. Science 1993; 259:1409–1410.

3. Sorger PK. Heat shock factor and the heat shock response. Cell 1991; 65:363–366.
4. Wong HR, Wispe JR. The stress response and the lung. Am J Physiol 1997; 273:L1–L9.
5. Nover L. HSFs and HSPs—a stressful program on transcription factors and chaperones. Stress proteins and the heat shock response, sponsored by Cold Spring Harbor Laboratory, Cold Spring Harbor, NY, USA, April 29–May 2, 1991. New Biol 1991; 3:855–859.
6. Wu C. Heat shock transcription factors: structure and regulation. Annu Rev Cell Dev Biol 1995; 11:441–469.
7. Repine JE, Bast A, Lankhorst I. Oxidative stress in chronic obstructive pulmonary disease. Oxidative Stress Study Group. Am J Respir Crit Care Med 1997; 156:341–357.
8. Carter JD, Ghio AJ, Samet JM, Devlin RB. Cytokine production by human airway epithelial cells after exposure to an air pollution particle is metal-dependent. Toxicol Appl Pharmacol 1997; 146:180–188.
9. Dreher KL, Jaskot RH, Lehmann JR, Richards JH, McGee JK, Ghio AJ, Costa DL. Soluble transition metals mediate residual oil fly ash induced acute lung injury. J Toxicol Environ Health 1997; 50:285–305.
10. Kadiiska MB, Mason RP, Dreher KL, Costa DL, Ghio AJ. In vivo evidence of free radical formation in the rat lung after exposure to an emission source air pollution particle. Chem Res Toxicol 1997; 10:1104–1108.
11. Bitterman PB, Wendt CH. Pathophysiology of pulmonary fibrosis. In: Fishman AP, ed. Pulmonary Diseases and Disorders. 3rd ed. New York: McGraw-Hill, 1998.
12. Clerch LB, Massaro D. Oxidation–reduction-sensitive binding of lung protein to rat catalase mRNA. J Biol Chem 1992; 267:2853–2855.
13. Wendt CH, Towle H, Sharma R, Duvick S, Kawakami K, Gick G, Ingbar DH. Regulation of Na-K-ATPase gene expression by hyperoxia in MDCK cells. Am J Physiol 1998; 274:C356–C364.
14. Yue G, Russell WJ, Benos DJ, Jackson RM, Olman MA, Matalon S. Increased expression and activity of sodium channels in alveolar type II cells of hyperoxic rats. Proc Natl Acad Sci USA 1995; 92:8418–8422.
15. Karin M, Liu Z, Zandi E. AP-1 function and regulation. Curr Opin Cell Biol 1997; 9:240–246.
16. Sen CK, Packer L. Antioxidant and redox regulation of gene transcription. FASEB J 1996; 10:709–720.
17. Bazzoni F, Beutler B. The tumor necrosis factor ligand and receptor families. N Engl J Med 1996; 334:1717–1725.
18. Dinarello CA, Wolff SM. The role of interleukin-1 in disease. N Engl J Med 1993; 328:106–113.
19. Polunovsky VA, Wendt CH, Ingbar DH, Peterson MS, Bitterman PB. Induction of endothelial cell apoptosis by TNF alpha: modulation by inhibitors of protein synthesis. Exp Cell Res 1994; 214:584–594.
20. Wendt CH, Polunovsky VA, Peterson MS, Bitterman PB, Ingbar DH. Alveolar epithelial cells regulate the induction of endothelial cell apoptosis. Am J Physiol 1994; 267:C893–C900.

21. Schreck R, Albermann K, Baeuerle PA. Nuclear factor kappa B: an oxidative stress-responsive transcription factor of eukaryotic cells (a review). Free Radic Res Commun 1992; 17:221–237.

22. Schreck R, Rieber P, Baeuerle PA. Reactive oxygen intermediates as apparently widely used messengers in the activation of the NF-kappa B transcription factor and HIV-1. EMBO J 1991; 10:2247–2258.

23. Devary Y, Rosette C, DiDonato JA, Karin M. NF-kappa B activation by ultraviolet light not dependent on a nuclear signal. Science 1993; 261:1442–1445.

24. Sun SC, Ganchi PA, Ballard DW, Greene WC. NF-kappa B controls expression of inhibitor I kappa B alpha: evidence for an inducible autoregulatory pathway. Science 1993; 259:1912–1915.

25. Haddad EB, Salmon M, Koto H, Barnes PJ, Adcock I, Chung KF. Ozone induction of cytokine-induced neutrophil chemoattractant (CINC) and nuclear factor-kappa b in rat lung: inhibition by corticosteroids. FEBS Lett 1996; 379:265–268.

26. Arends MJ, Wyllie AH. Apoptosis: mechanisms and roles in pathology. Int Rev Exp Pathol 1991; 32:223–254.

27. Lowe SW, Lin AW. Apoptosis in cancer. Carcinogenesis 2000; 21:485–495.

28. Thompson CB. Apoptosis in the pathogenesis and treatment of disease. Science 1995; 267:1456–1462.

29. Ashkenazi A, Pai RC, Fong S, Leung S, Lawrence DA, Marsters SA, Blackie C, Chang L, McMurtrey AE, Hebert A, DeForge L, Koumenis IL, Lewis D, Harris L, Bussiere J, Koeppen H, Shahrokh Z, Schwall RH. Safety and antitumor activity of recombinant soluble Apo2 ligand. J Clin Invest 1999; 104: 155–162.

30. Green DR. Apoptotic pathways: the roads to ruin. Cell 1998; 94:695–698.

31. Hengartner MO. The biochemistry of apoptosis. Nature 2000; 407:770–776.

32. Saleh A, Srinivasula SM, Acharya S, Fishel R, Alnemri ES. Cytochrome *c* and dATP-mediated oligomerization of Apaf-1 is a prerequisite for procaspase-9 activation. J Biol Chem 1999; 274:17941–17945.

33. Jiang X, Wang X. Cytochrome *c* promotes caspase-9 activation by inducing nucleotide binding to Apaf-1. J Biol Chem 2000; 275:31199–31203.

34. Sun XM, MacFarlane M, Zhuang J, Wolf BB, Green DR, Cohen GM. Distinct caspase cascades are initiated in receptor-mediated and chemical-induced apoptosis. J Biol Chem 1999; 274:5053–5060.

35. Polunovsky VA, Chen B, Henke C, Snover D, Wendt C, Ingbar DH, Bitterman PB. Role of mesenchymal cell death in lung remodeling after injury. J Clin Invest 1993; 92:388–397.

36. Desmouliere A, Badid C, Bochaton-Piallat ML, Gabbiani G. Apoptosis during wound healing, fibrocontractive diseases and vascular wall injury. Int J Biochem Cell Biol 1997; 29:19–30.

37. Yamaya M, Sekizawa K, Masuda T, Morikawa M, Sawai T, Sasaki H. Oxidants affect permeability and repair of the cultured human tracheal epithelium. Am J Physiol 1995; 268:L284–L293.

38. Kolb M, Margetts PJ, Anthony DC, Pitossi F, Gauldie J. Transient expression of IL-1beta induces acute lung injury and chronic repair leading to pulmonary fibrosis. J Clin Invest 2001; 107:1529–1536.

39. Dinarello CA. Interleukin-1 beta, interleukin-18, and the interleukin-1 beta converting enzyme. Ann N Y Acad Sci 1998; 856:1–11.

40. Nakashima JM, Levin JR, Hyde DM, Giri SN. Repeated exposures to enzyme-generated oxidants cause alveolitis, epithelial hyperplasia, and fibrosis in hamsters. Am J Pathol 1991; 139:1485–1499.

41. Borzi RM, Grigolo B, Meliconi R, Fasano L, Sturani C, Fabbri M, Porstmann T, Facchini A. Elevated serum superoxide dismutase levels correlate with disease severity and neutrophil degranulation in idiopathic pulmonary fibrosis. Clin Sci (Lond) 1993; 85:353–359.

42. Cantin AM, North SL, Fells GA, Hubbard RC, Crystal RG. Oxidant-mediated epithelial cell injury in idiopathic pulmonary fibrosis. J Clin Invest 1987; 79:1665–1673.

43. Ledwozyw A. Protective effect of liposome-entrapped superoxide dismutase and catalase on bleomycin-induced lung injury in rats. II. Phospholipids of the lung surfactant. Acta Physiol Hung 1991; 78:157–162.

44. Shahzeidi S, Sarnstrand B, Jeffery PK, McAnulty RJ, Laurent GJ. Oral *N*-acetylcysteine reduces bleomycin-induced collagen deposition in the lungs of mice. Eur Respir J 1991; 4:845–852.

45. Kinnula VL, Crapo JD, Raivio KO. Generation and disposal of reactive oxygen metabolites in the lung. Lab Invest 1995; 73:3–19.

46. Haddad IY, Pataki G, Hu P, Galliani C, Beckman JS, Matalon S. Quantitation of nitrotyrosine levels in lung sections of patients and animals with acute lung injury. J Clin Invest 1994; 94:2407–2413.

47. Haddad IY, Zhu S, Crow J, Barefield E, Gadilhe T, Matalon S. Inhibition of alveolar type II cell ATP and surfactant synthesis by nitric oxide. Am J Physiol 1996; 270:L898–L906.

48. van der Vliet A, Cross CE. Oxidants, nitrosants, and the lung. Am J Med 2000; 109:398–421.

49. Berger NA. Oxidant-induced cytotoxicity: a challenge for metabolic modulation. Am J Respir Cell Mol Biol 1991; 4:1–3.

50. Clerici C, Friedlander G, Amiel C. Impairment of sodium-coupled uptakes by hydrogen peroxide in alveolar type II cells: protective effect of d-alpha-tocopherol. Am J Physiol 1992; 262:L542–L548.

51. Spragg RG, Hinshaw DB, Hyslop PA, Schraufstatter IU, Cochrane CG. Alterations in adenosine triphosphate and energy charge in cultured endothelial and P388D1 cells after oxidant injury. J Clin Invest 1985; 76:1471–1476.

52. Spragg RG. DNA strand break formation following exposure of bovine pulmonary artery and aortic endothelial cells to reactive oxygen products. Am J Respir Cell Mol Biol 1991; 4:4–10.

53. Horowitz S, Dafni N, Shapiro DL, Holm BA, Notter RH, Quible DJ. Hyperoxic exposure alters gene expression in the lung. Induction of the tissue inhibitor of metalloproteinases mRNA and other mRNAs. J Biol Chem 1989; 264:7092–7095.

54. Phillips PG, Birnby L, Di Bernardo LA, Ryan TJ, Tsan MF. Hyperoxia increases plasminogen activator activity of cultured endothelial cells. Am J Physiol 1992; 262:L21–L31.

55. Kerr JF, Wyllie AH, Currie AR. Apoptosis: a basic biological phenomenon with wide-ranging implications in tissue kinetics. Br J Cancer 1972; 26:239–257.

56. Everett MM, King RJ, Jones MB, Martin HM. Lung fibroblasts from animals breathing 100% oxygen produce growth factors for alveolar type II cells. Am J Physiol 1990; 259:L247–L254.

57. Haskell JF, Yue G, Benos DJ, Matalon S. Upregulation of sodium conductive pathways in alveolar type II cells in sublethal hyperoxia. Am J Physiol 1994; 266:L30–L37.

58. Nici L, Dowin R, Gilmore-Hebert M, Jamieson JD, Ingbar DH. Upregulation of rat lung Na-K-ATPase during hyperoxic injury. Am J Physiol 1991; 261: L307–L314.

59. Minoo P, King RJ, Coalson JJ. Surfactant proteins and lipids are regulated independently during hyperoxia. Am J Physiol 1992; 263:L291–L298.

60. Engstrom PC, Holm BA, Matalon S. Surfactant replacement attenuates the increase in alveolar permeability in hyperoxia. J Appl Physiol 1989; 67: 688–693.

61. Fanburg BL, Massaro DJ, Gerutti PA, Gail DB, Berberich MA. Regulation of gene expression by O2 tension. Am J Physiol 1992; 262:L235–L241.

62. Ho YS, Dey MS, Crapo JD. Antioxidant enzyme expression in rat lungs during hyperoxia. Am J Physiol 1996; 270:L810–L818.

63. Knickelbein RG, Ingbar DH, Seres T, Snow K, Johnston RB, Jr., Fayemi O, Gumkowski F, Jamieson JD, Warshaw JB. Hyperoxia enhances expression of gamma-glutamyl transpeptidase and increases protein *S*-glutathiolation in rat lung. Am J Physiol 1996; 270:L115–L122.

64. Rahman I, Clerch LB, Massaro D. Rat lung antioxidant enzyme induction by ozone. Am J Physiol 1991; 260:L412–L418.

65. Rushmore TH, Morton MR, Pickett CB. The antioxidant responsive element. Activation by oxidative stress and identification of the DNA consensus sequence required for functional activity. J Biol Chem 1991; 266:11632–11639.

66. Dransfield I, Stocks SC, Haslett C. Regulation of cell adhesion molecule expression and function associated with neutrophil apoptosis. Blood 1995; 85:3264–3273.

67. Madtes DK, Elston AL, Kaback LA, Clark JG. Selective induction of tissue inhibitor of metalloproteinase-1 in bleomycin-induced pulmonary fibrosis. Am J Respir Cell Mol Biol 2001; 24:599–607.

68. Nagai A, Aoshiba K, Ishihara Y, Inano H, Sakamoto K, Yamaguchi E, Kagawa J, Takizawa T. Administration of alpha 1-proteinase inhibitor ameliorates bleomycin-induced pulmonary fibrosis in hamsters. Am Rev Respir Dis 1992; 145:651–656.

69. Serini G, Gabbiani G. Mechanisms of myofibroblast activity and phenotypic modulation. Exp Cell Res 1999; 250:273–283.

70. Zambruno G, Marchisio PC, Marconi A, Vaschieri C, Melchiori A, Giannetti A, De Luca M. Transforming growth factor-beta 1 modulates beta 1 and beta 5 integrin receptors and induces the de novo expression of the alpha v beta 6 heterodimer in normal human keratinocytes: implications for wound healing. J Cell Biol 1995; 129:853–865.

71. Fukuda Y, Basset F, Ferrans VJ, Yamanaka N. Significance of early intra-alveolar fibrotic lesions and integrin expression in lung biopsy specimens from patients with idiopathic pulmonary fibrosis. Hum Pathol 1995; 26:53–61.

72. Scaffidi AK, Moodley YP, Weichselbaum M, Thompson PJ, Knight DA. Regulation of human lung fibroblast phenotype and function by vitronectin and vitronectin integrins. J Cell Sci 2001; 114:3507–3516.

73. Ohta K, Mortenson RL, Clark RA, Hirose N, King TE Jr. Immunohistochemical identification and characterization of smooth muscle-like cells in idiopathic pulmonary fibrosis. Am J Respir Crit Care Med 1995; 152:1659–1665.

74. Kapanci Y, Desmouliere A, Pache JC, Redard M, Gabbiani G. Cytoskeletal protein modulation in pulmonary alveolar myofibroblasts during idiopathic pulmonary fibrosis. Possible role of transforming growth factor beta and tumor necrosis factor alpha. Am J Respir Crit Care Med 1995; 152:2163–2169.

75. Desmouliere A, Redard M, Darby I, Gabbiani G. Apoptosis mediates the decrease in cellularity during the transition between granulation tissue and scar. Am J Pathol 1995; 146:56–66.

76. Chen B, Polunovsky V, White J, Blazar B, Nakhleh R, Jessurun J, Peterson M, Bitterman P. Mesenchymal cells isolated after acute lung injury manifest an enhanced proliferative phenotype. J Clin Invest 1992; 90:1778–1785.

77. Jordana M, Schulman J, McSharry C, Irving LB, Newhouse MT, Jordana G, Gauldie J. Heterogeneous proliferative characteristics of human adult lung fibroblast lines and clonally derived fibroblasts from control and fibrotic tissue. Am Rev Respir Dis 1988; 137:579–584.

78. Crystal RG, Bitterman PB, Mossman B, Schwarz MI, Sheppard D, Almasy L, Chapman HA, Friedman SL, King TE, Jr., Leinwand LA, Liotta L, Martin GR, Schwartz DA, Schultz GS, Wagner CR, Musson RA. Future research directions in idiopathic pulmonary fibrosis: summary of a National Heart, Lung, and Blood Institute working group. Am J Respir Crit Care Med 2002; 166:236–246.

79. Schwartz DA, Peterson MW. Occupational lung disease. Adv Intern Med 1997; 42:269–312.

80. Fujimura N. Pathology and pathophysiology of pneumoconiosis. Curr Opin Pulm Med 2000; 6:140–144.

81. Saltini C, Amicosante M. Beryllium disease. Am J Med Sci 2001; 321:89–98.

82. Castranova V, Vallyathan V. Silicosis and coal workers' pneumoconiosis. Environ Health Perspect 2000; 108(Suppl 4):675–684.

83. Mc L Niven R, Pickering CA. Byssinosis: a review. Thorax 1996; 51:632–637.

84. Camus PH, Foucher P, Bonniaud PH, Ask K. Drug-induced infiltrative lung disease. Eur Respir J Suppl 2001; 32:93s–100s.

85. www.pneumotox.com. Department of Pulmonary Diseases and Intensive Care Unit. University Hospital. Dijon, France.

86. Patel AM, Ryu JH, Reed CE. Hypersensitivity pneumonitis: current concepts and future questions. J Allergy Clin Immunol 2001; 108:661–670.

87. Lamblin C, Bergoin C, Saelens T, Wallaert B. Interstitial lung diseases in collagen vascular diseases. Eur Respir J Suppl 2001; 32:69s–80s.

88. Costabel U. Sarcoidosis: clinical update. Eur Respir J Suppl 2001; 32:56s–68s.

89. Allen JN, Davis WB. Eosinophilic lung diseases. Am J Respir Crit Care Med 1994; 150:1423–1438.

90. Harari S, Comel A. Pulmonary Langerhans cell histiocytosis. Sarcoidosis Vasc Diffuse Lung Dis 2001; 18:253–262.

91. Hancock E, Osborne J. Lymphangioleiomyomatosis: a review of the literature. Respir Med 2002; 96:1–6.

92. American Thoracic Society/European Respiratory Society International Multidisciplinary Consensus Classification of the Idiopathic Interstitial Pneumonias. This joint statement of the American Thoracic Society (ATS), and the European Respiratory Society (ERS) was adopted by the ATS board of directors, June 2001 and by the ERS Executive Committee, June 2001. Am J Respir Crit Care Med 2002; 165:277–304.

6

Mediators and Mechanisms in Chronic Lung Injury and Fibrosis

JOSEPH A. LASKY, LUIS A. ORTIZ, and ARNOLD R. BRODY

*Departments of Medicine and Pathology and Laboratory Medicine,
Tulane University Health Sciences Center, New Orleans, Louisiana, U.S.A., and
Department of Environmental and Occupational Health, University of Pittsburgh,
Pittsburgh, Pennsylvania, U.S.A.*

I. Overview

This chapter discusses the roles and importance of selected mediators in chronic lung injury and fibroproliferation. A multiplicity of intracellular and extracellular mediators,factors, and signaling pathways is relevant for chronic lung injury, including many that are also involved in acute lung injury. The pathophysiology and clinical importance of chronic fibroproliferative injury to the lungs have been detailed in the preceding Chapter 5. The current chapter provides additional complementary coverage of mediators and pathways important in chronic lung injury and related clinical diseases such as idiopathic pulmonary fibrosis (IPF). Particular emphasis in the discussion here focuses on the roles and interactions of four mediators [tumor necrosis factor alpha (TNF-α), platelet-derived growth factor (PDGF), connective tissue growth factor (CTGF), and transforming growth factor beta (TGF-β)] in chronic lung injury and fibroproliferation. The importance of considering the interactions of these mediators in the pathophysiology of chronic lung injury, rather than simply viewing their individual activities in isolation, is also highlighted. Implications of mediator activity and interaction for the treatment of clinical chronic lung injury and disease are also noted in this chapter, although detailed discussion of lung injury therapies is presented later in the book (Chapters 13–19).

II. Introduction

There are a number of ways the lung can be subjected to progressive, chronic injury. Inhaled inorganic particles such as silica and asbestos, drugs like bleomycin and cyclophosphamide, or allergens and infectious organisms, all cause injury to lung cells resulting in a fibrogenic response (1,2). It appears to matter little that these very different agents cause injury by clearly different mechanisms, e.g., inorganic particles attract macrophages by a complement-dependent pathway (3), generate O_2 radicals and damage the alveolar epithelium which transports the particles to the interstitium (4–6). In comparison, certain inhaled mold spores can lead to a lymphocyte-mediated hypersensitivity (7). Although seemingly diverse, both these scenarios result in interstitial damage and fibrosis, where fibroblasts are activated to produce an increased collagenous matrix in a background of mixed inflammatory cells. Similar fibroproliferative pathology is present in many of the chronic obstructive pulmonary diseases as discussed in the preceding chapter.

There are at present no truly effective therapies other than lung transplantation for severe cases of IPF (8). A major reason for this is that many of the mediators and mechanisms involved in the fibroproliferative pathology of IPF and related chronic lung diseases are not fully understood. For example, as IPF develops, the following have been measured in abundance: (1) reactive oxygen species (ROS) such as superoxide, hydroxyl radicals, and peroxynitrate (see Ref. 4); (2) arachidonic acid metabolites such as prostaglandins and leukotrienes (see Ref. 9); (3) cytokines such as the interleukins, TGFs, PDGFs, and other potent peptides that exert multiple chemokinetic and cell-cycle controlling activities (see Ref. 10). Researchers involved in investigating the mechanisms of chronic lung injury and fibrogenesis are faced with this enormous panoply of biological mediators (e.g., Table 1). To make progress, it is essential that investigators focus on defined subsets of specific mediators and determine their interactions and roles, if any, in the molecular mechanisms of fibroproliferation. In this chapter, emphasis is placed on the roles and importance of TNF-α, PDGF isoforms, CTGF, and TGF-β in chronic fibroproliferative lung injury and the pathogenesis of IPF.

Figure 1 illustrates schematically a scenario in which injury to the alveolar epithelium results in the expression of TNF-α, PDGF isoforms, and TGF-

Table 1 Representative Mediators and Factors Relevant for Chronic Lung Injury.

Cytokines and growth factors
Cytokines (e.g., TNF-α, TGF-α, TGF-β, IL-1, IL-4, IL-6, IL-9, IL-10, IFN-γ)
Growth factors (e.g., CTGF, EGF, FGF, G-CSF, GM-CSF, KGF, PDGF, VEGF)

Chemokines
C, CC, CXC families

Other inflammatory mediators
Multiple additional inflammatory mediators (e.g., leukotrienes,
   prostaglandins, thromboxanes, heat shock proteins, complement and
   complement fragments)

Reactive oxygen/nitrogen species
Reactive oxidants and nitrating agents (e.g., hydroxyl radical, superoxide,
   nitric oxide, peroxynitrite, hydrogen peroxide, hydroperoxide)

Antioxidants and antioxidant enzymes
Multiple protein and non-protein antioxidants (e.g., GSH, GSH peroxidase,
   catalase, SODs, vitamin E)

Matrix proteins, matrix modifying enzymes and adhesion molecules
Matrix components, adhesion molecules, and related enzymes (e.g., collagen,
   elastin, fibronectin, laminin, ICAM, VCAM, β_2-integrins, L-selectins,
   metalloproteinases, TIMPs, collagenases)

A multitude of mediators and factors are relevant for chronic lung injury and fibroproliferation, many of which are also important in acute inflammatory injury (as discussed in Chapters 3 and 4). A variety of transcription factors, receptors, and transduction pathways not tabulated here are also involved in chronic lung injury processes. This complexity hampers mechanistic interpretations involving individual mediators as discussed in the text.
Abbreviations: CTGF, connective tissue growth factor; EGF, epidermal growth factor; FGF, fibroblast growth factor; G-CSF, granulocyte-colony stimulating factor; GM-CSF, granulocyte macrophage-CSF; GSH, glutathione; HSP, heat shock proteins; ICAM, intracellular adhesion molecule; IFN, interferon; IL, interleukin; KGF, keratinocyte growth factor; PDGF, platelet-derived growth factor; SODs, superoxide dismutases; TIMPs, tissue inhibitors of metalloproteinases; TGF, transforming growth factor; TNF, tumor necrosis factor; VCAM, vascular cell adhesion molecule; VEGF, vascular-endothelial growth factor.

β, leading to inflammatory cell activation and recruitment, the elaboration of ROS, and a persistent inflammatory response with increased expression of extracellular matrix constituents leading to interstitial fibroproliferation. According to the scenario in Fig. 1, the initial injury to the alveolar epithelium is from inhaled asbestos fibers, but the injurious agent could be one of a multitude of toxic particles, gases, infectious agents, or hypersensitizing allergens (2). Whatever the differences might be in the ways these agents injure the epithelium, the results are similar, i.e., release of a cytokine cascade that mediates inflammation, cell proliferation, and matrix production, culminating in fibrogenic lung disease (11).

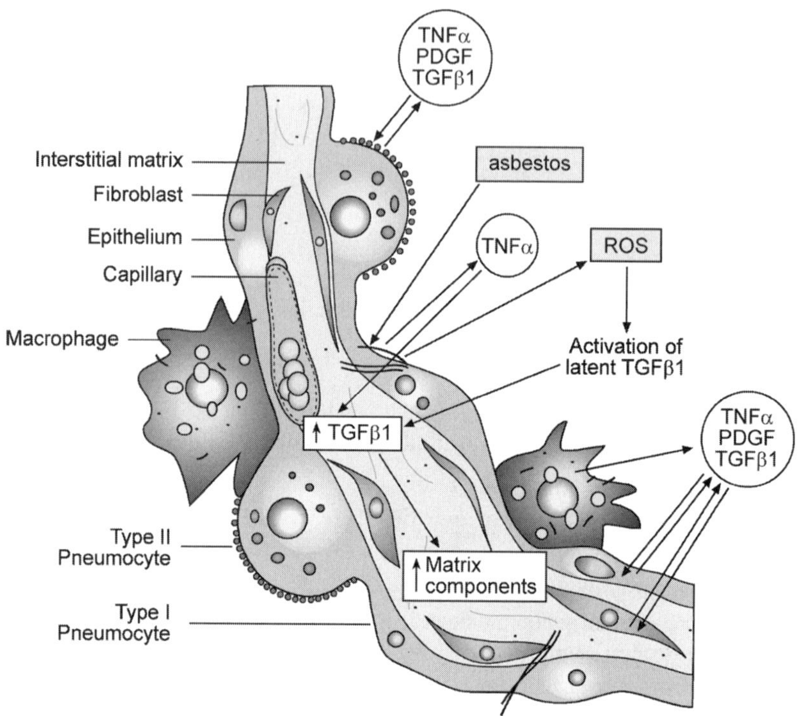

Figure 1 Simplified schematic of fibrogenic pulmonary injury. The diagram illustrates an alveolar wall injured by asbestos, a well-characterized fibrogenic agent. The evidence is that such an injury causes the rapid upregulation of growth factors such as PDGF, TGF-β, and TNF-α. It is postulated that these factors are essential components of the fibroproliferative response where PDGF controls fibroblast growth, TGF-β upregulates synthesis of extracellular matrix components, and TNF-α influences the expression of these and other growth factors. In addition, reactive oxygen species from asbestos and other sources, may play a role in activating the TGF-β protein.

Although the schematic events in Fig. 1 are highly simplified compared to actual chronic lung injury, this framework provides a focus for discussion of the activities of the mediators noted. As just described, it is necessary to analyze the activities and interactions of such subsets of mediators in order to develop a better understanding of chronic fibroproliferative lung injury. In Fig. 1, TNF-α is a "master cytokine" that plays a central role in the injury process through its known roles of activating the expression of PDGF (12) and TGF-β (13–15), attracting inflammatory cells (16), and modulating cell proliferation (14) in a pleiotropic fashion (13,14). Mouse models that have genes for TNF-α receptors knocked out provide compelling evidence for the key role of this cytokine in the pathogenesis of pulmonary fibrosis (17–20). The biology and proinflammatory activity of TNF-α is detailed in the following section.

In addition to discussing TNF-α as a presumptive "master cytokine" in persistent inflammation and chronic lung injury, attention is also focused on PDGF isoforms, two of which have been discovered only recently. Also, the activities of CTGF and TGF-β are highlighted because of their potential to work in concert and their known relevance for fibrogenesis. The influence of TGF-β isoforms on a variety of pulmonary and other cell types is well characterized.Connective tissue growth factor shares several fibrogenic characteristics with TGF-β, and its expression is dependent upon a TGF-β-response element in the CTGF promoter (21). Proliferation of the alveolar epithelial and mesenchymal cell populations consequent to lung injury is a major feature in the pathogenesis of chronic lung disease (22,23). Increased numbers of fibroblasts produce large amounts of extracellular matrix, and new epithelial cells cover this matrix and incorporate it into an expanded interstitium (5,24). Epidermal growth factor (EGF) and transforming growth factor alpha (TGF-α), which share the same receptor (25,26), are likely involved in controlling epithelial proliferation in lung injury (27,28). However, the PDGF isoforms are focused on in discussion here as the most potent mesenchymal cell mitogens yet described (29). In addition, TGF-β$_1$ also has activities relevant for fibroproliferation through its effects on the synthesis and secretion of extracellular matrix components by interstitial fibroblasts and myofibroblasts. Further details about the activities and interactions of these mediators are given in the following sections.

III. Relevance of Tumor Necrosis Factor Alpha for Pulmonary Fibrosis

A. TNF Biology

Since its discovery in the 1980s, tumor necrosis factor (TNF) has been recognized for its potent inflammatory properties (30–32). Originally identified for its ability to induce hemorrhagic necrosis of tumors, TNF was soon implicated as a major contributor to lung injury and subsequently to the pathogenesis of pulmonary fibrosis (33,34). Tumor necrosis factor is one of nine members of a ligand family with nonoverlapping functions (30–32). Virtually, every cell in the body is capable of producing TNF, but monocytes, macrophages, lymphocytes (NK, T, and B populations), brain glial, and Kupffer cells are responsible for the bulk of its production (30–32). Tumor necrosis factor production is primarily regulated by transcriptional mechanisms, and heavy methylation of the TNF gene promoter inhibits its transcription (30–32). Lipopolysaccharide (LPS) is the most powerful inductor of TNF transcription, but a number of different stimuli including activated complement, ischemia reperfusion, silica, and TNF itself stimulate TNF gene transcription (30–32). Following gene transcription, TNF protein undergoes important translational and post-translational modification (30–32). Protein synthesis is regulated by 3′ untranslated uridine- and adenine-rich elements that repress translation (30–32). Tumor necrosis factor is originally produced as a 26-kDa peptide that undergoes proteolytical cleavage to a 17-kDa molecule (30–32). Three of these molecules associate to form a biologically active homotrimer (30–32).

B. TNF Interactions with Its Receptors

Tumor necrosis factor mediates its biologic effects by binding to two different plasma membrane receptors. These receptors, designated as the 55 and 75 kDa receptors (also referred as TNFR1 and TNFR2, respectively), are two of 10 members of a receptor family with similar origins (30–32,35,36). Each member of the TNF receptor family is characterized by the presence of a repeating extracellular cysteine-rich motif (30,31). In addition to TNF, LT-α or lymphotoxin is also capable of binding to TNF receptors, while all the other ligands of the family interact with their receptors on a one-to-one basis (30,31). All of the TNF ligand family members are believed to be trimeric proteins, and exert their effects by inducing receptor multimerization at the cell surface (30–32). The TNF homotrimer is secreted, while the other members of the TNF ligand family are membrane-anchored binding a single receptor and activating the cell by direct contact (30,31). In addition to TNF and lymphotoxin-α, the other members of the family of ligands include the Fas ligand, the CD40 ligand, and the ligands for CD27, CD30, OX40, and 4-1BB receptors (30,31).

Although most cells express p55 and p75 TNF receptors, the expression of the genes encoding for the two receptors are differentially regulated (30–32,35). The expression of the gene encoding for p55 is controlled by a noninducible, housekeeping promoter, which does not respond to TNF, TGF-β, IL-1, or the interferons (32). In contrast to these observations, the gene encoding for the p75 TNF receptor demonstrates a low constitutive expression and is easily inducible (32,35,36). The p55 receptor demonstrates a low affinity ($K_d = 500\,\text{pM}$), low dissociation rate ($t_{1/2} > 3\,\text{hr}$) that allows it to bind TNF at high concentrations. In contrast, the p75 receptor demonstrates a high affinity ($K_d = 100\,\text{pM}$), high dissociation rate ($t_{1/2} = 10\,\text{min}$) that enables it to bind TNF at low concentration of the ligand (31,32,35,36). p55 mediates most TNF-induced cytotoxicity, and is responsible for the species-specific effects of TNF (30–32). p75, because of its inducibility, has been linked to the TNF-mediated proliferative effects. p75 is also cleaved and shed from the cell allowing it to bind TNF (a mechanism that can dampen or perpetuate TNF effects). These data suggest that p55 monopolizes TNF-mediated signaling while p75 plays an accessory role in enhancing p55 (32,35,36).

The function of various members of the TNF receptor and ligand families has been characterized through the identification of natural or induced mutations (knockouts) that disrupt the activity of the normal gene product. In humans, absence of the CD40 ligand leads to a form of immunodeficiency characterized by high levels of IgM and other immunoglobulin deficiency (37). In mice, mutations that involve the Fas ligand are characterized by an abnormal proliferation of CD4–/CD8– T cells, and the development of a lupus-like autoimmune disorder (38). In the past 5 years, the genes for the two TNF receptors have been deleted in mice (39–41), and genes encoding inhibitor proteins that selectively bind and neutralize homotrimeric forms of TNF have been introduced in mice (42). Deletion of the 55-kDa TNF receptor in mice is associated with an increased susceptibility to *Listeria monocytogenes* and resistance to the lethal effect of lipopolysaccharide (39,40). In contrast, the deletion of the 75-kDa receptor gene causes a minimal phenotype, in which scab formation fails to occur in response to intradermal injections of TNF, and there is moderate resistance to lethal effects of TNF (41). A combined 55- and 75-kDa receptor knockout has been developed by breeding animals with each individual mutation (43,44). These knockout animals (p55p75–/–) have been shown to be protected from the fibrogenic effects of bleomycin, silica, and asbestos, even though their genetic background is one of sensitivity to these agents (45). Confirming a central role for TNF expression on fibrogenic lung disease, these double TNF receptor deficient mice did not show increased expression of fibrogenic cytokines such as TGF-β (Fig. 2) or PDGF in their lungs (17,19).

The role of the individual TNF receptors in lung fibrosis has been studied by exposing individual TNF receptor deficient mice to fibrogenic agents such as silica (45). These animals were also developed on a silica-sensitive (C56BL/6) genetic background. As expected, wild-type mice reacted to silica with the accumulation of lymphocytes and loosely form nodules in the peribronchiolar regions of the lung (Fig. 3) (20). In contrast, p55 deficient mice did not demonstrate these nodules and reacted to silica exposure with a diffuse accumulation of proteinaceous material in the alveolar regions of the lung (Fig. 3). p75 deficient mice form silica-induced nodules, but in contrast to wild-type mice, their distribution was mostly around perivascular areas of the lung (Fig. 3). Thus, these data suggest that the p55 receptor is an important component of the granulomatous response, while p75 is relevant for processes of vascular pathology (45). Consistent with these interpretations are data demonstrating that p55 deficient mice fail to form granulomas in response to mycobacterial exposure and that p75 deficient mice are sensitive to cerebral malaria (46–48).

C. TNF and Fibrotic Lung Injury

A large body of experimental and clinical data implicate TNF as a central mediator in the pathogenesis of pulmonary fibrosis. Piguet et al. reported that the exposure of mice to bleomycin was followed by an enhanced TNF mRNA expression in the lungs of these animals (33,34). This enhanced TNF expression preceded the development of lung inflammation and the deposition of collagen

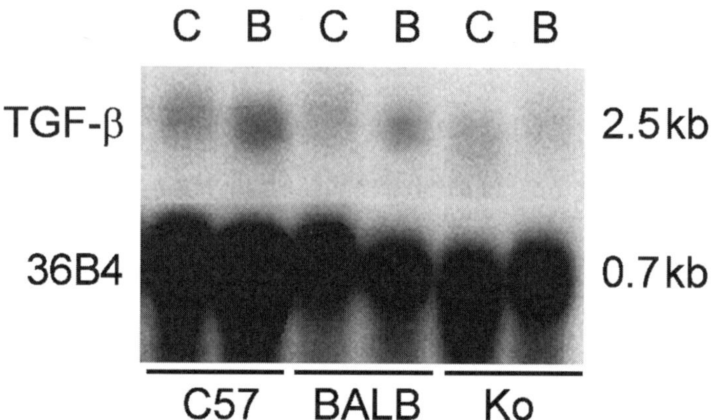

Figure 2 TGF-β mRNA expression in the lung following bleomycin exposure. Northern blot analysis of TGF-β mRNA expression in mouse lung 21 days following the intraperitoneal injection of saline as control (C) or BLM (B), 120 mg/kg, in three murine strains: C57BL/6, BALB/c, and p55−/−75−/−TNF receptor knockout (Ko). TGF-β mRNA expression is present in the lungs of control treated mice and is increased following the administration of BLM in BLM-sensitive (C57BL/6) and BLM-resistant (BALB/c), but not in TNF receptor deficient mice. (Courtesy of Taylor & Francis Group, Philadelphia, Pennsylvania) (19).

in the lungs of bleomycin-treated mice (33,34). Furthermore, these investigators were able to abrogate inflammation and bleomycin-induced lung fibrosis with the administration of anti-TNF antibodies or TNF receptors that antagonized the bioactive TNF (33,34). Subsequent reports confirmed enhanced TNF expression following the exposure of other fibrogenic agents such as dusts (silica and asbestos), toxic agents (paraquat), or hyperoxia (49–51). The use of in situ hybridization determined that the cellular source responsible for the enhanced TNF mRNA expression observed in response to these agents was predominantly the alveolar macrophages, but some hybridization for TNF mRNA was also found in lymphocytes and epithelial cells (19).

Even though this information illustrates the temporal relation between enhanced TNF expression in the lung and the development of pulmonary fibrosis, it does not constitute direct evidence that TNF is mediating the injurious response in the lung. This evidence was obtained in animal models in which mice or rats were conditioned to overexpress TNF protein in their lungs (14,52). Transgenic mice overexpressing TNF from the lung-specific SPC promoter developed alveolitis that progressed to pulmonary fibrosis (52). In addition, rats treated by endotracheal administration of an adenoviral vector coding for TNF developed pulmonary inflammation that was followed by enhanced expression of fibrogenic cytokines (such as TGF-β) and the development of pulmonary fibrosis (14). These data clearly indicate that TNF is capable of inducing lung inflammation and fibrosis. They also suggest that TNF may function as a master

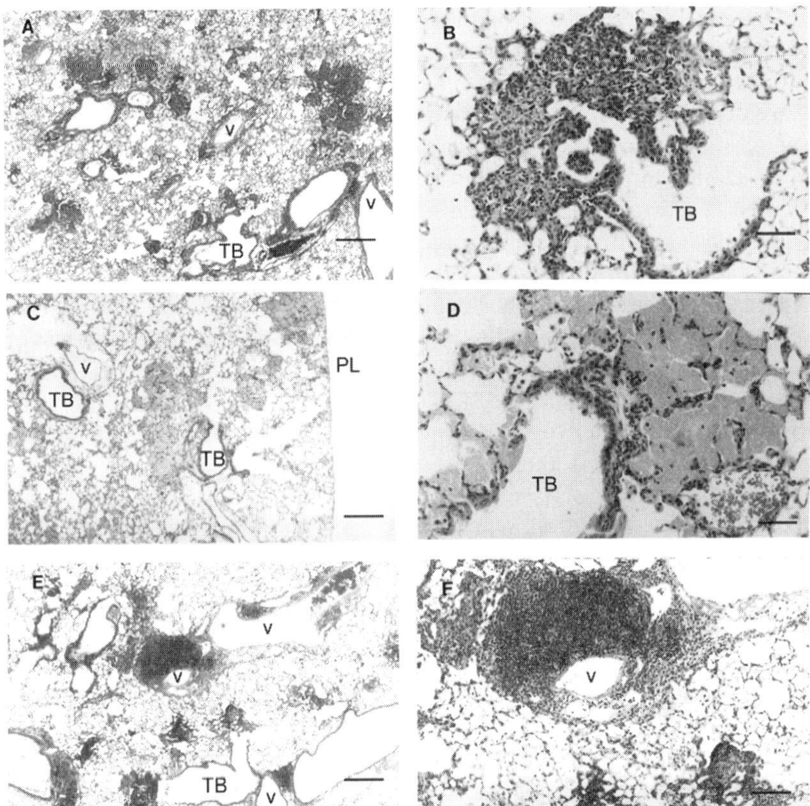

Figure 3 Silica-induced lung injury in mice. Representative low (×100) and high (×400) power magnification photomicrographs of the lung obtained from wild-type and individual (p55−/−or p75−/−) TNF receptor deficient mice 28 days following silica exposure: C57BL/6 (A and B), p55−/− (C and D), p75−/− (E and F) (*n* = 10 mice per murine strain and treatment). Silica-induced granulomatous inflammation is peribronchiolar in C57BL/6 mice and perivascular in p75−/−TNF receptor deficient mice. P55−/−mice demonstrate alveolar filling with proteinaceous material. TB, terminal bronchiole; PL, pleural surface; V, vein; bar = 20 μm. (Courtesy of American Journal of Respiratory and Critical Care Medicine, New York) (45).

switch regulating the expression of other fibrogenic (such as TGF-β) and inflammatory (CC chemokines) cytokines that participate in cytokine networks implicated in the pathogenesis of pulmonary fibrosis (53).

Enhanced TNF expression and production can also be observed in humans with fibrotic lung injuries. Alveolar macrophages retrieved from the lungs of individuals exposed to asbestos or from patients with IPF demonstrate enhanced TNF production compared to macrophages isolated from normal controls (16). Enhanced TNF expression has also been demonstrated in the alveolar epithelium of lung biopsies from patients with pulmonary fibrosis (54). Enhanced TNF expression has also been reported in the lungs of patients with rheumatoid arthritis complicated by pulmonary fibrosis (55). In patients with the diagnosis of sarcoidosis, enhanced TNF production by the alveolar macrophages has been associated with greater risk of clinical progression of lung disease (56).

To help explain the correlation between increased levels of TNF and the progression of fibrotic lung injury in some patients, it has been hypothesized that polymorphisms of the TNF gene promoter could be associated with enhanced protein synthesis and secretion (57). Several biallelic TNF polymorphisms have been described, but TNF-308 (also called TNF-A allele 2) in the promoter of the TNF gene has been mostly associated with enhanced TNF production (58). To examine this hypothesis, TNF polymorphism was studied by genotyping 88 patients with IPF compared to matched controls in England as well as 61 patients with IPF and 103 unmatched controls in Italy (59). Results showed that carriage of TNF-A allele 2 was associated with increased risk of IPF in both English (odds ratio, 1.85; 95% CI, 0.94–3.63; $p = 0.075$) and Italian (OR, 2.5; 95% CI, 1.14–5.47; $p = 0.0022$) patients (59). However, a subsequent study of 74 patients with IPF in the south of England did not show evidence of deviation in TNF genotype, allele, or haplotype frequencies when compared to the general populations (60). These mixed results indicate the necessity for continued population studies of this kind in the future.

In the case of sarcoidosis, a high frequency of the less common –857T TNF allele was demonstrated in British and Dutch patients with acute forms of Löfgren's syndrome (61). However, studies in Japanese and African-American populations of patients with sarcoidosis failed to demonstrate any significant association between TNF gene polymorphism and the development of lung injury due to sarcoidosis (62). Similarly, no enhanced TNF gene promoter polymorphism was found in populations of Black South African miners diagnosed with silicosis when compared to miners without this diagnosis (63). However, miners with severe silicosis were significantly more likely to demonstrate the –238A and –376A mutations of the TNF promoter (63). These data suggest that TNF gene polymorphisms might not be a predictor of susceptibility for a specific fibrotic lung disease in the general population, but may be a good marker for severity of disease.

D. TNFR-Related Proteins

As described above, TNF exerts its cytotoxic and regulatory activities by binding to its receptors (30–32). Binding of the TNF ligand to the receptor triggers receptor aggregation and phosphorylation activating downstream signaling pathways and promoting upregulation of transcription factors (30–32). Tumor necrosis factor-induced signal transduction pathways are initiated by activating TNFR associated proteins or by recruiting effector molecules that will interact with specific domains of the receptor (64–67). In the case of the p55 (TNFR1), an 80-amino acid region has been identified within the cytoplasmic domain (64,65). This region is required for the initiation of apoptosis and the activation of NF-κB (64,65). This region, designated the "death domain," is 28% identical to a 65-amino acid region located in the intracellular region of the Fas antigen (68–71). An understanding of the importance of the p55 signal transduction pathway has been obtained from the identification of a 34-kDa TNF receptor death domain associated protein, designated TRADD, that interacts with the intracytoplasmic domain of this receptor (64,65,68–71). TRADD interacts with the death domain of p55 and its overexpression leads to cell death and causes NF-κB activation (64,65). These data suggest that TRADD is a signal molecule downstream of TNFR1 (64,65).

Maturational studies have demonstrated that the death domain of TRADD is necessary for its known functions self-association, binding to TNFR1, induction of NF-κB activation, and induction of cell death (64). The functional portion of TRADD that contains this death domain (68-amino acids) shows a 32% homology with the death domain present in TNFR1 (64,65,68–71). The TRADD death domain allows for interaction with the TNFR1, but not the Fas death domain (64,65,68–71). Mutational analysis of TRADD, in which certain areas of the death domain have been substituted by alanines, has confirmed that the entire death domain is necessary for TRADD self-association and binding to TNFR1 (65). These studies also showed that the TRADD regions responsible for the induction of cell death and NF-κB activation overlap (65). Mutant aa296–299 demonstrated association with TNFR1, but failed to induce NF-κB activation (65). Expression of a luciferase reporter gene, under the control of a TNF sensitive NF-κB-dependent promoter, was consistently lower in cells transfected with TRADD mutant aa296–299 when stimulated with TNF compared to a control vector lacking TRADD sequences (65). In addition, the same mutation was found to eliminate TNF-induced cell cytotoxicity suggesting that the aa296–299 behaves as a dominant negative TRADD mutant (65).

The role of TRADD in the pathogenesis of fibrotic lung diseases is unknown. Recently, it has been demonstrated that exposure of mice to silica is associated with an enhanced expression of TRADD mRNA (Fig. 4) and protein (not shown) in the lungs of C57BL/6 mice (that are bleomycin- and silica sensitive), but not in BALB/c or double TNFR deficient mice (that are resistant to bleomycin and silica) (unpublished observations). In addition to these data, incubation of RAW 264.7 macrophages with silica has been shown to result in enhanced TNF production (72). Moreover, this enhanced production of TNF by silica-stimulated RAW 264.7 cells is eliminated by the transient transfection of these cells with TRADD mutant aa296–299, which inhibits NF-κB activation (Fig. 5). These data suggest

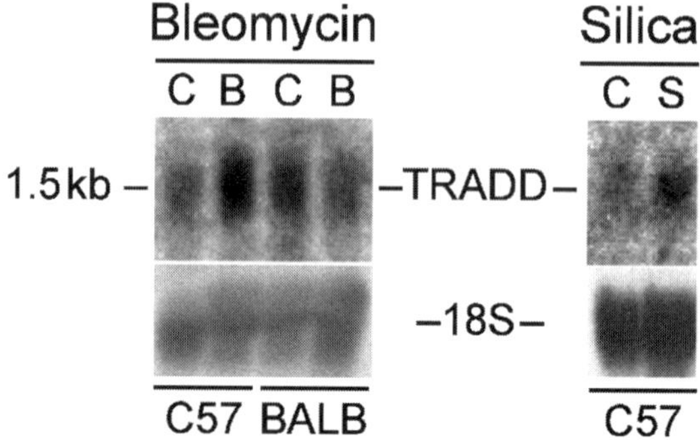

Figure 4 TRADD mRNA expression in the mouse lung following exposure to silica or bleomycin. Northern blot analysis of TRADD mRNA expression in mouse lung 28 days following the intratracheal injection of saline as control (C) or silica (S) or bleomycin (B) in C57BL/6 and BALB/c mice. TRADD mRNA expression is minimal in lungs from control treated mice and is increased in C57BL/6, but not in BALB/c mice, following the administration of silica and bleomycin. (Luis Ortiz, M.D., unpublished observations.)

that blocking TNF signaling at the level of TRADD could be of benefit in preventing the development of lung injury in mice.

The signal transduction associated with p75 (TNFR2) involves several related proteins. These proteins, designated as TNF receptor-associated factors (TRAFs), complex with the cytoplasmic domains of the receptor and induce NF-κB, and AP-1 activation (32,66,67). However, TRAF knock-out mice and mice in which dominant negative TRAF mutants have been expressed have only a slight defect in their NF-κB activation in response to TNF suggesting that TRAF may not be essential for transcription factor activation in response to TNF (68). The role of TRAF in lung fibrosis is unknown at this time.

E. TNF Receptor-Mediated Signal Transduction in Pulmonary Fibrosis

A wealth of information is available on TNF signal transduction. However, little is known about the importance of TNF signaling in the pathogenesis of fibrotic lung diseases. Research in animals in which TNF receptors have been genetically deleted has demonstrated the importance of some of these pathways in the pathogenesis of fibrotic lung injuries like silicosis (see above). Following recruitment of TNF-related proteins to the receptor, a series of phosphorylation events are triggered that eventuate in activation of NF-κB and AP-1 (73–75). This NF-κB and AP-1 activation has been shown to be of importance in mediating inflammatory and fibrogenic effects (73–78).

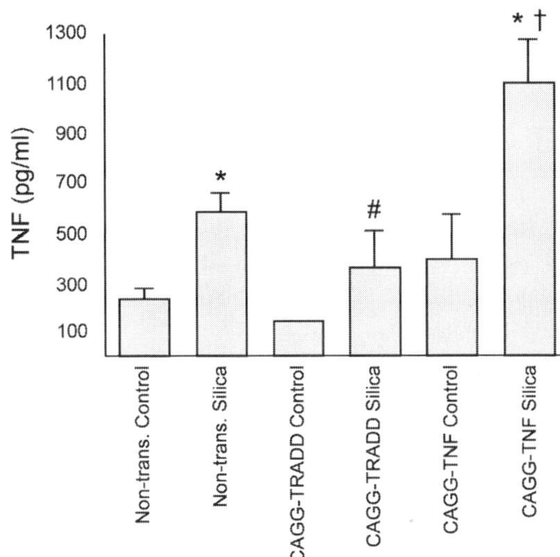

Figure 5 Silica induction of TNF production by RAW 264.7 cells following CAG-TRADD transfection. Silica enhanced TNF production in RAW 264.7 cells. A construct encoding the TRADD mutant aa296–299 was developed under the control of the CAG promoter. Because this TRADD mutant inhibits TNF-mediated NF-κB activation, the CAG-TRADD construct was used to transiently transfect silica exposed RAW 264.7 macrophages. A CAG-TNF construct was used as a positive control for the transfection efficiency. Its transfection significantly upregulates TNF production by RAW 264.7 cells. In contrast, CAG-TRADD transfection inhibits silica-induced production of TNF. * indicates significant ($p < 0.05$) difference compared to control-treated cells; †denotes significant ($p < 0.05$) difference compared to silica-treated nontransfected and CAG-TRADD transfected cells; # denotes significant ($p < 0.05$) difference compared to silica-treated nontransfected and CAG-TNF transfected cells. (Luis Ortiz, M.D., unpublished observations.)

Several NF-κB proteins have been identified (78–80). The activated form of NF-κB is a heterodimer, which usually consists of two proteins, a p65 (also called relA) and a p50 subunit (80). Other subunits, such as rel, relB, vrel, and p52, may also form part of activated NF-κB (80,81). In nonstimulated cells, the different NF-κB complexes are held in the cytoplasm by interaction with the IκB inhibitors which prevent their entrance into the nuclei (80,81). Following cell stimulation by inflammatory mediators, IκB is phosphorylated (on serines 32 and 36 residues) by the action of two kinases: IκB kinases α and β (82–84). Once phosphorylated, IκB is ubiquitinated and the NF-κB–IκB complex dissociates (81,85,86). This dissociation allows the NF-κB dimers to be translocated to the nucleus where they bind the promoter region of target genes (85–87). Exposure of murine macrophages to silica results in NF-κB activation

(76,88). The predominant product of NF-κB activation following silica is a p50/p50 homodimer (76,88).

NF-κB activation contributes to the initiation of inflammation (76,88). NF-κB activation upregulates the expression of cytokines and other mediators of inflammation (87). An example of the association between NF-κB activation and inflammation is the enhanced expression of the inducible form of nitric oxide synthase observed in asthma, ulcerative colitis, and rheumatoid arthritis (87,89–91). In these diseases, treatment with corticosteroids (that impede access of NF-κB to the nucleus) improves clinical outcomes (87,89–91).

Silica induces NF-κB activation, TNF production, and apoptosis in RAW 264.7, but not in IC-21 macrophage cell lines (72). Furthermore, treatment of RAW 264.7 with the BAY compound 2, which inhibits the TNF dependent phosphorylation of IκB, significantly reduced NF-κB activation and TNF production (92). Endotracheal injection of silica into C57BL/6 (silica sensitive), and double TNFR knockout mice is followed by early phosphorylation and disappearance of IκB in the lung of silica-sensitive mice but not in double TNFR deficient mice. This effect of silica on lung IκB expression is followed by enhanced NF-κB activation in the lungs of C57BL/6 mice.

The signal transduction pathways involved in TNF-mediated AP-1 activation in response to lung fibrosis are not completely clear. AP-1 as a transcription factor requires phosphorylation for its activation. Of particular importance to AP-1 induction is the activation of serine/threonine mitogen-activated protein kinases (MAP kinases or MAPK). Mitogen-activated protein kinases are members of a family of evolutionarily conserved enzymes involved in regulating the response of eukaryotic cells to extracellular signals (93). To date, three branches of MAPK pathways have been described (94–96). These involve the extracellular signal-regulated kinases (ERK) 1 and 2, the stress-activated protein kinase/c-Jun NH2-terminal kinase (SAP/JNK), and p38 (94–96). These kinases can be activated by a diversity of stimuli, and their role involves the transmission and amplification of extracellular signals via a double phosphorylation mechanism on a threonine and a tyrosine residue, thereby leading to transcriptionally regulated early gene induction (33,97). One of these early genes, c-Jun, is activated by SAPK/JNK phosphorylation (97), and stimulates its own transcription (98,99). In turn, SAPK/JNK is activated by phosphorylation via an MAP kinase kinase (SEK1/MKK4) (97,100). Extracellular signal-regulated kinase 1/ extracellular signal-regulated kinase 2 are activated by MAP kinase kinase (MEK), leading to the induction of another early gene, c-Fos (97). Both of these early gene products can then interact and form heterodimers of Jun and Fos proteins or homodimers of Jun proteins constituting the AP-1 binding complex (101). Of note, IκB kinases α and β can also be activated by MEKK1, MEKK2, and MKK3, the upstream kinase activating the MAP pathways

(102–104). Silicate particles, including asbestos, have been shown to cause stimulation of the MAP kinase cascade (73,74). In rat fibroblasts, silica induces phosphorylation of ERK1/2 kinases by promoting formation of ROS (74). In addition, freshly fractured silica induces p38 phosphorylation in rat lung epithelial cells (75). The effect of silica upon SAP/JNK activation is unknown.

Tumor necrosis factor has been shown to promote MAPK activation (105,106). Choi and associates report that TNF treatment of silica-sensitive macrophages (RAW 264.7) induces apoptosis and MAPK activation (106). Furthermore, inhibition of the MAPK activity with PD-098059 inhibitor protected RAW 264.7 cells from TNF-induced apoptosis (106). Therefore, these data suggest that the interaction of the TNF ligand with its receptors plays an important role in regulating MAPK activation during inflammation (106). The importance of TNFR in MAPK activation during lung injury and fibrosis has been demonstrated in TNFR deficient mice (105).

Silica exposure results in enhanced AP-1 activation in the lungs of silica-sensitive (C57BL/6), but not TNFR deficient mice (Fig. 6) (45). In addition, enhanced phosphorylation of ERK1/2, and JNK has been shown in RAW 264.7 macrophages (72). There is enhanced p38 phosphorylation in the lungs of C57BL/6 mice upon treatment with bleomycin, but this enhanced p38 phosphorylation was absent in the lungs of double TNFR deficient mice, suggesting that TNFRs are fundamental in p38 activation (data not shown). Further studies on the role of TNF receptors in regulating the activation of MAPK during silicosis and fibrogenesis in general could provide important new targets for therapeutic interventions and will provide a more complete understanding of the fundamental mechanisms of fibrogenic lung disease.

IV. Platelet-Derived Growth Factor

A second mediator discussed here as highly relevant for the pathobiology of lung fibrosis is PDGF, which plays a significant role in fibroblast proliferation. The failure of immunosuppressive agents such as corticosteroids, azathioprine, and cytoxan to retard the progression of fibrotic diseases such as IPF has led investigators to further evaluate antifibrotic mechanisms (107). There is compelling evidence that increased numbers of fibroblast foci, which are tightly packed clusters of mesenchymal cells within the airspaces of the lung, correlate with a more rapid decline in lung function in patients with IPF, whereas an overall score of inflammation does not (108). Fibroblast foci are located along the leading edge of the fibrotic parenchyma. Morphometric analysis of these foci has shown that they are comprised of tightly packed myofibroblasts along with young connective tissue matrix. Platelet-derived growth factor stands out among the many peptide factors that act as fibroblast mitogens for several reasons. Firstly, the majority of fibroblast mito-

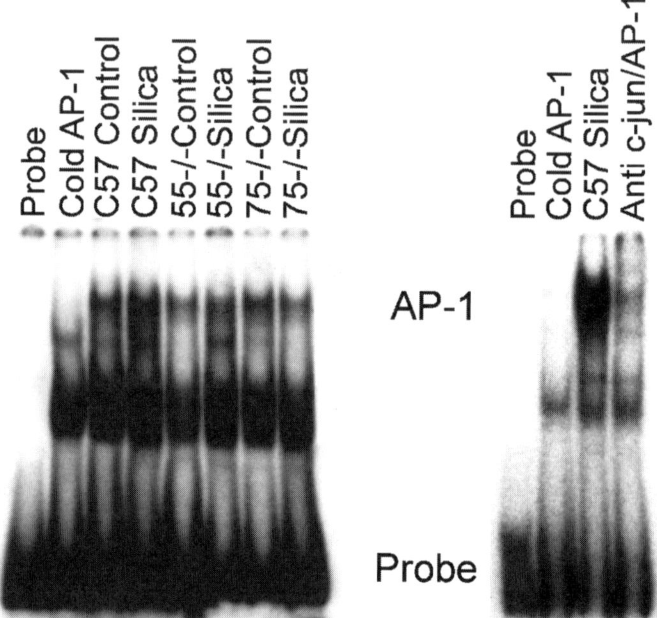

Figure 6 AP-1 activation in murine lung after silica exposure. DNA binding activity of AP-1 in crude nuclear extracts from whole lung isolated from C57BL/6, and individual TNF receptor deficient mice 28 days after silica exposure. Cold AP-1 represents AP-1 binding in lung nuclear extract of a C57BL/6 silica-treated mouse, assayed in the presence of excess unlabeled oligonucleotide as a competitor. Antibody supershifts were performed using the nuclear extract of a C57BL/6 silica-treated mouse as described (45). Densitometry analysis (not shown) of gelshifts demonstrated that decreased AP-1 activation in the lungs of TNF receptor deficient mice when compared to AP-1 activation observed in the lungs of silica-treated C57BL/6 mice. (From Ref. 45, courtesy of American Journal of Respiratory and Critical Care Medicine, New York.)

genic activity found in serum is attributable to PDGF. Secondly, many other fibroblast growth factors promote cellular growth indirectly by upregulation of PDGF and/or its receptor. Furthermore, there is considerable literature showing that PDGF expression is increased during lung fibrogenesis.

Platelet-derived growth factor was first identified in 1974 and now there are hundreds of scientific manuscripts with a focus on it and lung fibrosis. This factor is a peptide produced by multiple cell types found within the lung, including platelets, macrophages, Type II epithelial cells, endothelial cells, fibroblasts, and smooth muscle cells. It is a family of peptide isomers that shares a highly conserved cysteine knot domain, which is a region responsible for the formation of inter- and intrapeptide sulfhydryl bonds that are necessary for biologic activity (109). Monomers of PDGF are inactive since they are not able to initiate signal transduction through the paired PDGF receptor subunits designated alpha and beta. Binding of PDGF dimers results in trans-phosphorylation of receptor subunits initiating subsequent steps in signal transduction (110). Platelet-derived growth factor-A and -B chains are highly homologous peptides that dimerize as homodimers or a heterodimer. Two more recently identified PDGF isoforms (designated "C" and "D") share significant homology in the preserved cysteine knot with the PDGF-A and PDGF-B isoforms. However, unlike PDGF-A and PDGF-B isoforms, PDGF-C and PDGF-D isoforms require proteolytic cleavage before they can bind to their receptors (111). The complex binding pattern of PDGF isoforms to their receptors is shown in Fig. 7 (112).

Platelet-derived growth factor isoforms have been repeatedly shown as potent mitogens and chemoattractants for lung fibroblasts and smooth muscle cells (109). However, lung fibroblast subsets respond variably to PDGF isoforms. For example, Thy-1(−) and Thy-1(+) lung fibroblasts proliferate equally well in response to PDGF-BB, but Thy-1(+) fibroblasts, in contrast to Thy-1(−) fibroblasts, do not proliferate in response to PDGF-AA. The differences in response to the PDGF-AA isoform can be explained by the absence of PDGF-alpha receptors, that are required for the binding of the PDGF-AA isoform, in the Thy-1(+) lung fibroblast subset (113). Other investigators have also reported that cells with higher PDGF alpha-receptor expression proliferate more vigorously in response to PDGF-AA (114).

Platelet-derived growth factor also stimulates production of glycosaminoglycans and is a weak pulmonary vasoconstrictor. It induces interstitial

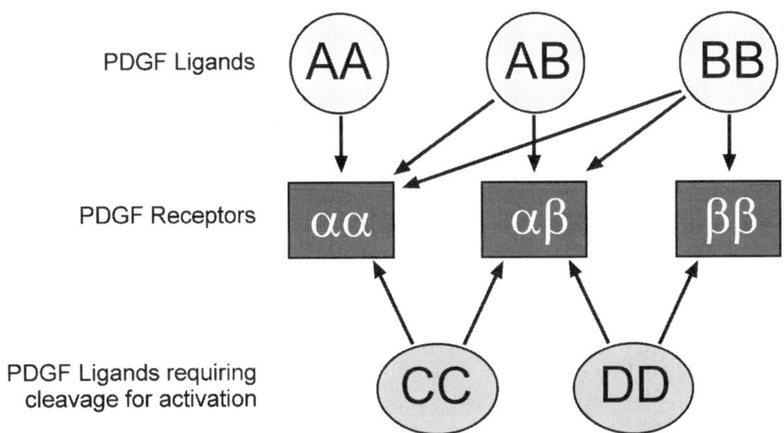

Figure 7 Diagram of the three PDGF receptor dimers and their known ligands. The PDGF-A and -B chains must dimerize to bind the receptor as indicated, and the C and D homodimers must be cleaved.

collagenase (MMP-1) production, and in combination with IL-1β and TNF-α, also induces MMP-3 and MMP-9 activity in human lung fibroblasts, as demonstrated by zymography (107). The increased production of metalloproteinases is an important process since it releases the fibroblasts to migrate and proliferate. Interestingly, investigators have reported that mast cells, which are frequently observed in fibrotic lung tissue, contain proteases and heparin that can inhibit PDGF activity (115).

Platelet-derived growth factor may also act as a vasoconstrictor in the pathogenesis of pulmonary hypertension (116). Angiotensin II (ATII) induces PDGF-A chain expression in cultured vascular smooth muscle cells (117). Platelet-derived growth factor-AB and -BB have been shown to block NOS activity and thereby reduce expression of the potent vasodilator nitric oxide (NO) (116,118,119). Conversely, eNOS has been shown to inhibit PDGF-mediated vascular smooth muscle cell proliferation (120). Notably, eNOS knockout mice have exacerbated development of hypoxic pulmonary hypertension (121). Nitric oxide, which can block the formation of pulmonary hypertension, in turn antagonizes ATII induction of PDGF-AA. It also modulates shear stress signal transduction pathways (122), which may be a mechanism for decreasing PDGF expression (123). Interestingly, one potentially therapeutic agent, Tranilast, inhibits PDGF-mediated proliferation, and restores cytokine-induced NO production and its antiproliferative effect in the presence of PDGF (118). These data suggest, but do not prove, that PDGF may be involved in the pathogenesis of pulmonary hypertension.

Inhibition of PDGF is an attractive strategy for the treatment of fibroproliferative lung disease because many other fibroblast mitogens exert their effect by increasing the expression of the PDGF ligands, PDGF receptors, or both. Upregulation of PDGF expression by other cytokines also occurs in vivo. For example, PDGF expression is increased in a murine model of lung fibrosis wherein IL-1β is overexpressed using a viral vector (124).

The role of PDGF in lung fibrosis has been most extensively studied in a murine model of asbestos-induced lung fibrosis. A single 5-hr exposure to asbestos fibers results in the formation of fibrotic lesions at sites of fiber deposition, principally the alveolar duct bifurcations (ADBs) (3,5,6,17). The fibrotic lesions at the ADB have a strikingly similar appearance to the fibroblast foci described in humans with IPF (Fig. 8). Investigations have revealed that there is upregulation of PDGF-A and PDGF-B chain (Fig. 8). as well as PDGF alpha-receptor expression within hours following the exposure at the site of the fibrotic lesion and at a time point that coincides with the fibroproliferative events (125). Moreover, there is phosphorylation of the PDGF receptors, indicative of receptor activation, in the murine model of asbestos-induced fibrosis. Both asbestos-induced PDGF receptor phosphorylation in vivo and the area of the fibrotic lesions are significantly blocked by a PDGF-selective tyrosine kinase inhibitor (126).

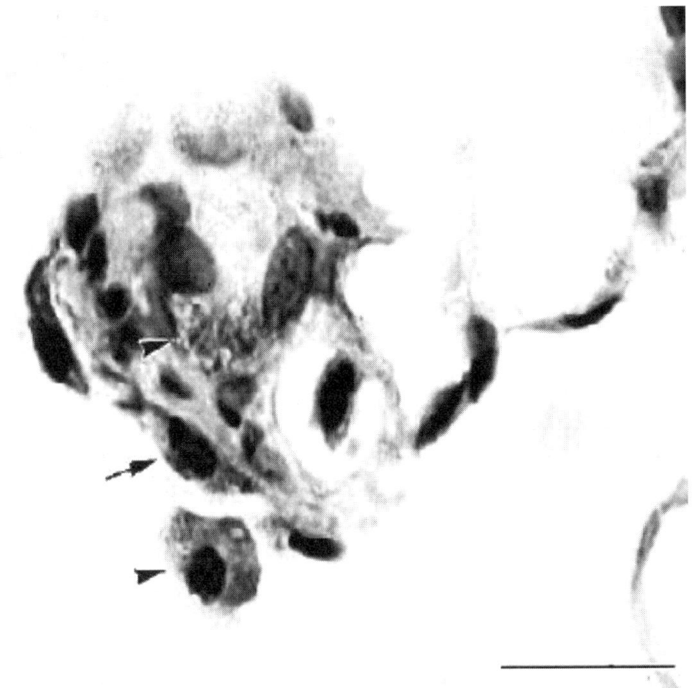

Figure 8 An alveolar duct bifurcation from a rat exposed for 5 hr to an aerosol of chrysotile asbestos fibers. Forty-eight hours postexposure, a polyclonal antibody raised against the PDGF-BB isoform strongly stains epithelial cell (arrow), macrophages (arrowhead), and interstitial cells (arrowhead in tissue). Bar equals 50 microns. (Modified from Ref. 214.)

Others have also shown that a PDGF-receptor selective tyrosine kinase inhibitor of the tyrphostin class was more than 90% effective in preventing the increase in hydroxyproline observed in vanadium pentoxide-treated rats (127). Thus, PDGF receptors are activated during lung fibrogenesis and inhibition of PDGF signal transduction reduces lung fibrosis. Accordingly, lavaged cells from bleomycin-treated hamsters have upregulated PDGF-A and PDGF-B mRNA expression when studied by RT-PCR (128). Treatment with Pirfenidone decreases the PDGF expression and reduces the lavage mitogenic activity (129).

There is no published information on PDGF-C and PDGF-D expression as of yet using asbestos or any other model of lung fibrosis. However, an abstract indicates that there is upregulation of PDGF-C mRNA expression and a decrease in PDGF-D mRNA expression, with no significant change in either PDGF-A or PDGF-B mRNA expression in the lungs of mice treated with bleomycin (130).

Knockout mice have been generated for each of the PDGF ligand chains. Mice that lack the PDGF-A chain are generally not viable, and those that are develop pulmonary emphysema, which is apparently due to a failure of alveogenesis (131,132). Furthermore, embryos with the homozygous deletion of the PDGFR die at or around day 10 in utero with a reduction in mesenchymal cell components (110,133). These findings make these animals unsuitable for lung fibrosis studies but do indicate that PDGF-A chain is involved in the generation of the proliferative mesenchymal cell phenotype observed in pulmonary fibrosis. Mice lacking either the PDGF-B chain or PDGFR-β are not viable and develop bleeding due to pericyte loss and microaneurism formation (132), and the absence of renal glomeruli (134).

Intratracheal administration of PDGF-B results in peribronchiolar fibrosis (135). Over-expression of either PDGF-A chain or PDGF-B chain through the lung specific surfactant protein-C promoter results in nonviable mice with enlarged lungs packed with mesenchymal cells or viable mice with a mixed pattern of emphysema and thickened alveolar septa, respectively (136,137). Intratracheal administration of a liposome encapsulated expression plasmid containing the extracellular portion of the PDGF-β receptor is protective in bleomycin-induced pulmonary fibrosis (138), consistent with the central role of PDGF-B in lung fibrogenesis.

Analysis of tissue sections from fibrotic human lung also demonstrates upregulation of PDGF-A and PDGF-B isoforms (139). Similar to the animal models, there are no current studies examining the expression of the PDGF-C and PDGF-D isoforms in fibrotic human lung tissue. Platelet-derived growth factor has also been implicated in the airway fibrosis that results in the syndrome of constrictive bronchiolitis postlung transplant, because PDGF peptide levels were detected in the lavage fluid of a patient who went on to develop this malady post-transplantation (140). This case report has been substantiated by a larger study showing that PDGF-B mRNA was increased in BAL samples from patients with bronchiolitis obliterens compared to unaffected recipients and controls (141). Plotting the FEV1 in percentage of vital capacity and the PDGF expression, patients with bronchiolitis obliterens revealed an increased PDGF signal preceding lung function deterioration (141).

In summary, PDGF is a potent chemoattractant and mitogen for lung fibroblasts. Animal models of lung fibrosis, and histology of fibrotic human lung sections, clearly demonstrate that PDGF is upregulated during lung fibrogenesis. Over expression of PDGF within the lungs of animals results in fibroproliferative pathology, and blocking PDGF signal transduction reduces lung fibrosis. Therefore, PDGF appears to be important in the pathogenesis of lung fibrosis and anti-PDGF trials as therapy for lung fibrosis seem promising.

V. Connective Tissue Growth Factor

Connective tissue growth factor is a peptide that shares several profibrogenic activities with TGF-β_1, namely as a promoter of collagen and fibronectin synthesis, a mitogen for mesenchymal cells under limited conditions, and an inducer of cell adhesion. Basal CTGF expression is dependent upon a novel TGF-β response element in the CTGF promoter (21), and it has been proposed that some of the profibrotic activities of TGF-β_1 may be mediated through CTGF. Despite strong evidence demonstrating the profibrotic effect of TGF-β (see the following section), a specific anti-TGF-β directed therapy for fibrotic disorders has not been forthcoming. This may reflect the fact that TGF-β has diverse biological activities in addition to its fibrogenic properties, including anti-inflammatory and immunoregulatory effects and the modulation of cell adhesion. Complete abolition of all of these TGF-β_1-mediated activities can be deleterious, as apparent in TGF-β_1 null mice that develop severe pulmonary, dermal, and bowel inflammation within weeks after birth (142). Overexuberant inflammation is counterproductive in fibrotic lung disease, since it is recognized as an early component in many models of fibrogenesis and chronic lung disease (143). There is thus significant interest in identifying factors through which TGF-β mediates collagen deposition, but not inflammation, including potential roles for CTGF.

Connective tissue growth factor, also called CCN2, is a 38-kDa cysteine-rich peptide monomer that was first isolated from human umbilical artery endothelial cells (144). It is postulated to be a member of the insulin-like growth factor binding protein superfamily (145), and thus has also been referred to as insulin-like growth factor protein-related protein 2 (146). Soluble and cell-associated forms have been characterized (147). Breakdown products of 24, 18, and 10 kDa have been described and the 10-kDa moiety has been found to possess biological activity (145,147). Subsequently, CTGF was noted to be expressed by human foreskin and dermal fibroblasts (148), smooth muscle cells, bovine aorta endothelial (BAE) cells (149), Type II epithelial cells (150), and lung fibroblasts (151). Leukocytes (152) have not been found to synthesize CTGF in vitro or in vivo. Connective tissue growth factor shares homology with several other peptides including CEF-10 (153), Cyr61 (154), and the murine homologue of CTGF, fisp-12 (155).

All three human TGF-β isoforms induce the expression of CTGF, as does thrombin and VEGF. Thrombin induces CTGF expression (156) and inhibition of thrombin signal transduction results in a modest decrease in both CTGF mRNA expression and collagen accumulation in a murine model of bleomycin-induced fibrosis. In contrast, TNF-α (149,157) and interleukin-4 (158) appear to decrease CTGF expression, which may limit the profibrotic activity of these two cytokines. Dexamethasone has been reported to increase CTGF expression in BALB/c 3T3 fibroblasts, which is a concern since corticosteroids are frequently employed in an attempt to arrest inflammation in subjects afflicted with IPF or with fibrotic lung disease associated with connective tissue disorders (157). However, dexamethasone did not increase the enhanced expression of CTGF in a model of murine wound healing (157).

There is very limited information regarding the CTGF receptor(s). Connective tissue growth factor receptors have been studied in a human chondrocytic cell line using radiolabeled CTGF (159). Scatchard analysis demonstrated two classes of CTGF receptors, but only one band at approximately 280 kDa was detected using a crosslinking study. Connective tissue growth factor binds to $\alpha V\beta 6$ integrins on fibroblasts and promotes osteocyte adhesion, and to $\alpha M\beta 2$ integrins on activated monocytes (160). The low-density lipoprotein receptor-related protein/alpha2-macroglobulin receptor also binds CTGF and may serve as a regulatory degradative pathway (161). To date, no other specific CTGF receptor has been isolated, and a CTGF receptor gene has not been cloned or sequenced.

A. CTGF Activity

In vitro studies have demonstrated that CTGF has several biologic activities that are key components of fibrogenesis. Connective tissue growth factor has been shown to be mitogenic for several types of mesenchymal cells including NIH 3T3 cells, kidney fibroblasts, and human dermal fibroblasts (144,152). Work by Hagood et al. has demonstrated that although most lung fibroblasts do not proliferate in response to CTGF, a Thy-1(−) subset will proliferate when treated with CTGF (162). This appears to be important since there is an increase in the proportion of Thy-1(−) fibroblasts in fibrotic lung in comparison to normal lung (163). Connective tissue growth factor was found to be responsible for mediating TGF-β-induced anchorage independent growth in normal rat kidney (NRK) fibroblasts (152). Further studies have shown that cAMP can inhibit TGF-β-induced anchorage independent growth, and that the block, which occurs late in the G1 phase of the cell cycle, can be overcome by the administration of CTGF (164). Other investigators have reported that CTGF alone has no mitogenic activity on human umbilical vein endothelial cells and NIH 3T3 fibroblasts, but will enhance basic fibroblast growth factor-induced DNA synthesis (165). Finally, to balance mitogenesis with cell death, CTGF was recently reported to induce apoptosis in breast cancer cell lines and in smooth muscle cell isolates (166,167). It is not known whether CTGF-induced apoptosis occurs via the same mechanism as TGF-β-mediated apoptosis.

Connective tissue growth factor is also a chemoattractant for endothelial and mesenchymal cells (168), and so may contribute to the accumulation of these cells in wounds. This is potentially important in lung fibrosis since vascular neogenesis within fibrotic lung lesions appears to correlate with reversibility of the lesion. Thus, factors that promote vascular neogenesis may lead to the development of lesions that are more susceptible to degradation. Connective tissue growth factor is expressed by BAE cells, and an antisense CTGF oligonucleotide has been employed to demonstrate that endogenous CTGF expression is involved in proliferation and migration of BAE cells in culture (168). In other cell types, such as HUVE, NIH 3T3, and mink lung epithelial cell, CTGF promotes cell adhesion in vitro (165). Thus, on one hand, CTGF appears to promote angiogenesis by acting as a chemoattractant for BAE cells, and on the other hand, CTGF may limit angiogenesis by promoting adhesion of cells. A study of three cancer cell lines showed that induction of angiogenesis correlated positively with CTGF expression and a neutralizing anti-CTGF antibody suppressed neovascularization in cancer cell implants (169). Hypoxia has been shown to induce CTGF expression in cancer cell lines, which stimulates endothelial cells to synthesize metalloproteinases that could liberate the cells from the surrounding matrix, thus initiating angiogenesis (170). Conversely, others have found that CTGF binds to VEGF and limits its activity, thereby inhibiting neovascularization (171). Thus, the net effect of CTGF on angiogenesis associated with lung fibrosis may be dependent upon coexpression of other growth factors.

Important for the discussion here is that CTGF induces collagen and fibronectin message levels. Exposure of dermal and NRK fibroblasts to CTGF in culture results in an increase in both collagen Type I and fibronectin peptide expression (172). Type I collagen synthesis has been the major focus of numerous studies of fibrotic lung disease largely because it is abundant in the normal lung and because it accounts for the greatest percentage of collagen accumulating within the lung as a consequence of lung fibrosis (173). There is a positive correlation between CTGF mRNA expression and collagen synthesis in rat lung fibroblast subsets (113). Moreover, collagen expression correlates more closely with CTGF expression than with TGF-β_1 expression in lung TGF-β_1 knockout and wild-type lung fibroblasts and in fibroblasts treated with TGF-β (Fig. 9). In view of the fact that CTGF expression can be upregulated by TGF-β_1 through an element in the CTGF promoter, the relationship between CTGF and alpha 1 Type I collagen mRNA expression has been explored in embryonic cells isolated from TGF-β_1 knockout mice (kindly provided by Dr. Doetschman, University of Cincinnati) and their wild-type littermates (Fig. 9). Increased CTGF expression is found to be present in the cells isolated from TGF-β_1 knockout mice compared with the wild-type cells. More importantly, alpha 1 Type I collagen expression correlated more closely with CTGF expression than with TGF-β_1 expression. The correlation between CTGF and collagen expression in these cell lines strongly suggests that CTGF is a factor that plays a role in developing fibrogenesis. Additional questions for further investigation include whether TGF-β_1 knockout mice that survive have

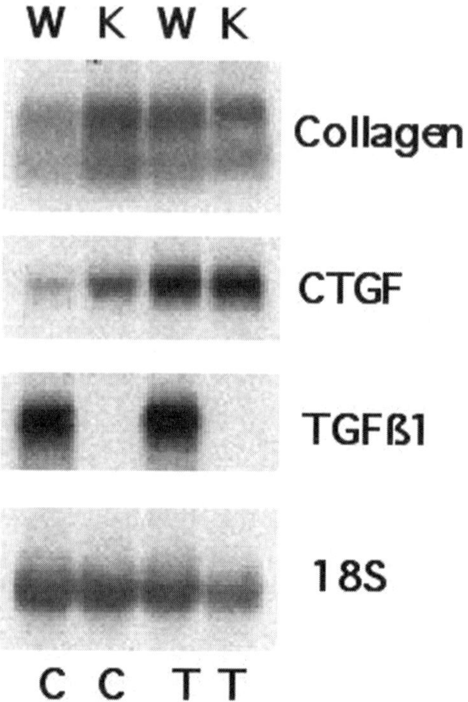

Figure 9   Expression of CTGF, TGF-β_1, alpha 1 Type I procollagen, and 18S ribosomal RNA in wild-type and TGF-β_1 knockout mice. The figure shows a composite of Northern hybridizations from a membrane probed for CTGF, and then stripped and probed for TGF-β_1, alpha 1 Type I collagen and 18S ribosomal RNA, respectively. 3T3-like cells were isolated from TGF-β_1 knockout (K) mice and their wild-type littermates (W). Cells were grown to confluence and rendered quiescent in serum-free media for 48 hr prior to the addition of 10 ng/ml of rTGF-β_1 (T) or media alone (C). In the absence of TGF-β_1 the knockout cells express more CTGF and alpha 1 Type I procollagen message than do the wild-type cells. (Joseph A. Lasky, M.D., unpublished observations.)

higher baseline CTGF expression enabling them to synthesize adequate collagen for development, and whether there are other cytokines that also upregulate CTGF expression.

In effective pulmonary repair, fibroblast proliferation and collagen accumulation should balance with matrix degradation and cell death. Apoptosis may be an important mechanism in the resolution of lung scars. Connective tissue growth factor has been shown to induce apoptosis in some epithelial cancer cell lines (166). In contrast, statins have been shown to induce apoptosis in lung fibroblasts and more recently have been shown to decrease the expression of CTGF (174). Therefore, it is conceivable that CTGF could be profibrotic by reducing fibroblast apoptosis while stimulating apoptosis in epithelial cells that are designed to contain the fibrotic response.

Mechanisms of action of CTGF, and how they relate to those of TGF-β, are still under study. Transforming growth factor beta leads to collagen accumulation by causing a decrease in collagen degradation via stimulation of metalloproteinase expression and activation. In contrast, most studies indicate that CTGF promotes expression of peptides involved in matrix degradation. Exposure of vascular smooth muscle cells to recombinant CTGF or a CTGF expression vector resulted in increased MMP-2 transcription and activity in vitro, which was blocked by neutralizing antibodies to CTGF (175). In addition, coating culture plates with CTGF leads to enhanced MMP-1 and MMP-3 mRNAs and proteins in a human lung fibroblast cell line (176). However, other investigators using a breast cancer cell line (MDA23) and human umbilical artery endothelial cells found that addition of recombinant CTGF results in increased expression of a number of metalloproteinases and a decrease in the expression of TIMP-2 (170).

B. CTGF Expression During Fibrogenesis

Fibrosis occurs through similar pathways regardless of location, and there is increasing evidence that CTGF may be involved in the pathogenesis of fibrosis in organs such as the skin. This is not unexpected since TGF-β_1 is increased in fibroproliferative dermal pathology, such as scleroderma, and because TGF-β_1, TGF-β_2, and TGF-β_3 upregulate CTGF expression in vitro. Importantly, subcutaneous injection of TGF-β_1 results in increased expression of CTGF within dermal fibroblasts and the subsequent formation of fibrotic lesions (177). In addition, a positive correlation between CTGF expression and skin sclerosis has been reported (148,178). A rat skin wound model has revealed an upregulation of CTGF mRNA expression that follows an increase in TGF-β_1 mRNA expression, suggesting that CTGF is induced by the increased expression of TGF-β_1 in vivo (148). Because dermal fibroblasts synthesize CTGF and proliferate in response to CTGF, others have proposed that CTGF may act as an autocrine mitogen induced by TGF-β_1 (177).

Connective tissue growth factor has increasingly been reported to be associated with fibrosis in other organ systems including the skin, kidney, liver, bowel, and heart. The following serve as examples:

1. In situ hybridization for CTGF revealed strong upregulation in extracapillary and severe mesangial cell proliferative lesions of crescentic glomerulonephritis, IgA nephropathy, focal and segmental glomerulosclerosis, and diabetic nephropathy in sections of human kidney. Moreover, an increase in the number of cells expressing CTGF mRNA was observed at sites of tubulointerstitial damage (179).

2. Human CTGF mRNA and protein expression are increased in atherosclerotic vessels compared with normal vessels. Connective tissue growth factor mRNA expression predominantly localizes to smooth muscle and endothelial cells in areas of fibrosis (180).
3. Serum CTGF expression, as measured by ELISA, was found to correlate with progression of biliary atresia (fibrosis of the bile ducts) (181).
4. Connective tissue growth factor is expressed in inflammatory bowel disease (157).
5. Connective tissue growth factor is expressed in cells from malignant desmoplastic melanoma and may contribute to the desmoplastic reaction (182).
6. Connective tissue growth factor mRNA is expressed within fibroblasts in desmoplastic tissue surrounding breast tumors (183).

In vivo experiments using rodent models of fibroproliferative lung disease also suggest that CTGF is involved in the pathogenesis of lung fibrosis. Connective tissue growth factor expression is upregulated in the lungs of a bleomycin-sensitive, but not a bleomycin-resistant, mouse strain following the intratracheal administration of this chemotherapeutic drug known to cause lung fibrosis (151). Furthermore, intratracheal administration of an adenovirus expressing an active TGF-β_1 construct results in upregulation of CTGF mRNA expression and lung fibrosis in mice (125), whereas administration of the viral vector lacking the TGF-β_1 construct does not cause an increase in CTGF expression or fibrosis. The increased CTGF expression in these animal models of lung fibrosis are consistent with recent reports of elevated CTGF expression in lavage specimens derived from fibrotic human lung (146). Others have confirmed that CTGF mRNA expression is upregulated in fibrotic lung tissue compared with controls and that expression is localized by in situ hybridization to proliferating Type II epithelial cells and activated fibroblasts (150). Moreover, CTGF mRNA expression is diminished in a cohort of patients with IPF who showed an improvement in lung physiologic parameters following treatment with interferon-gamma (184). Thus, CTGF appears at the site of fibrotic reactions and has the biological potential to induce fibrosis.

Even though CTGF expression is increased in many fibrotic diseases and has profibrotic activity in vitro, no one has yet answered the question as to whether or not overexpression of CTGF mediates fibrosis in any organ system. Transgenic mice that overexpress CTGF on the surfactant protein-C promoter display a normal lung phenotype (185) even though they express abundant CTGF in lavage fluid and homogenized lung. Lung hydroxyproline content as a measure of lung collagen content is the same between CTGF transgenic mice and their wild-type littermates, as is their expression of alpha-1 Type I collagen mRNA (185). The lack of fibrosis in CTGF transgenic mice should not be interpreted as lack of involvement of CTGF in lung collagen homeostasis, since CTGF is constitutively expressed in the lung (151) and could be involved in dynamic collagen turnover in unperturbed lungs (186). Moreover, there are new data showing that inhibition of CTGF reduces the production of collagen and fibronectin in vitro (187). Antisense CTGF oligodeoxynucleotides decrease fibronectin and collagen mRNA expression, as well as the synthesis of collagen in rat mesangial cells (188). A CTGF neutralizing antibody was shown to limit the induction of fibronectin mRNA in human dermal fibroblasts exposed to advanced glycosylation end products (189). Further experiments that block CTGF expression and signaling are necessary to better define the role of CTGF in lung fibrogenesis.

VI. Transforming Growth Factor Beta

As described earlier in the chapter, TGF-β influences cell proliferation and migration and is a potent stimulator of extracellular matrix deposition (190). The most abundant member of the three TGF-β isoforms, which have similar but nonoverlapping activities, is TGF-β_1 (190). A large percentage of the experiments on TGF-β have emphasized the β_1 isoform, and the following discussion is concentrated largely upon this specific peptide.

A. Activation of TGF-β_1

Transforming growth factor beta 1 is synthesized and secreted in a latent form as a high molecular weight complex that can be converted to the biologically active molecule which binds to membrane-bound receptor complexes (190,191). The latent form is comprised of the TGF-β_1 molecule covalently bound to the latent associated peptide (LAP) (192). Understanding the mechanism(s) through which the LAP is cleaved is essential for establishing how TGF-β plays a role in lung fibrogenesis. Current evidence supports at least four separate biologically relevant mechanisms for releasing active TGF-β: (1) binding to thrombospondin (193), (2) proteolysis involving plasmin (194), (3) $\alpha V\beta 6$ and the integrin receptor (195), and (4) ROS (196,197).

Although the removal of LAP appears to be a critical step in the control of TGF-β_1 activity, the mechanisms involved remain poorly understood. In vitro, physicochemical means such as chaotropes, detergents, heat, and pH extremes (198) are capable of activating TGF-β. Research also suggests that TGF-β is redox sensitive. Immunohistochemistry data show activation after irradiation in breast tissue (197). Redox activation of TGF-β has also been demonstrated in vitro in the presence of iron-induced free radicals

(196). Glycosidases have been demonstrated to remove carbohydrate groups which bind to the LAP, destabilizing the LAP:TGF-β complex leading to activation (198). Proteolysis of LAP by serine proteases, plasmin, and cathepsin D has been shown to cleave the N-terminal of LAP leading to release of active TGF-β_1 (194). Matrix metalloproteinases (MMP9 and MMP2) have also been implicated in the proteolytic activation of TGF-β at the cell surface (199). Nonenzymatic activation of TGF-β can also occur through binding and conformational changes. Thrombospondin-1 (TSP-1), for example, is capable of forming complexes with TGF-β_1, allowing the cytokine to become active (193). In an elegant study by Munger et al. (195), it was demonstrated that LAP:TGF-β is able to bind to αVβ6 integrin on the cell surface, causing a conformational change in the LAP:TGF-β complex, and exposing the active TGF-β. This allows TGF-β to bind to its receptors, thus inducing signaling.

B. Receptor Binding and Biological Activity

Upon activation of TGF-β, binding to the receptors can proceed. In this process, Type I and Type II transmembrane receptors apparently operate in concert, with the Type II domains binding TGF-β with high affinity and consequently recruiting the Type I receptors leading to its phosphorylation of TGF-β on a cluster of glycine and serine residues (190). Upon receptor binding, signal transduction molecules known as SMADs are essential for activating expression of the genes influenced by TGF-β (191). It is at this point that the astounding array of biological effects controlled by TGF-β can be observed. For example, active TGF-β_1 inhibits proliferation of lung epithelial cells, both in vivo (200) and in vitro (201). On the other hand, TGF-β_1 has been shown to have both a positive (202) and negative (203) influence on mesenchymal cell growth. It has also been shown that PDGF-induced mitogenesis of primary rat lung fibroblasts can be blocked in vitro by active TGF-β_1 (203,204).

Studies of lung development and transgenic mouse models indicate essential roles for TGF-β in immune regulation and lung morphogenesis. As examples, genetically altered mice lacking the TGF-β_1 genes die with chronic multifocal inflammation (142). Transforming growth factor beta 1 also inhibits branching morphogenesis of the embryonic mouse lung (200), while lack of the TGF-β_1 isoform causes mice to die shortly after birth with abnormally developed lungs. As mentioned above, there is a strong association between high levels of TGF-β expression and deposition of extracellular matrix components, including several collagen types and fibronectin (142,205,206). Given this clear relation between TGF-β expression and chronic fibroproliferative lung disease, this peptide has been proposed as one of the major factors in inducing, maintaining, and perhaps, ameliorating chronic fibrogenesis. Several of the models used to test this postulate are described below.

C. Exposure to an Aerosol of Asbestos Fibers

Inhalation of asbestos fibers has long been known to cause interstitial fibrogenesis in humans (1) and a variety of animal models (5). Asbestos-exposed rats (5,22) and mice (17,207) have been used for many years in attempts to understand the mechanisms of the fibrogenic process. Understanding has progressed from the very first look at where inhaled fibers are initially deposited on alveolar duct bifurcations (208) to a description of the complement-mediated mechanisms of macrophage accumulation at the sites of fiber deposition (209). As the inhaled fibers are transported across cell membranes (210) and anatomic compartments (6), the epithelial (211), mesenchymal (211,212), and endothelial (212) cell populations are induced to proliferate while the extracellular matrix is deposited in the alveolar interstitium (205). Once this pathogenetic sequence of events had been established, mechanisms controlling this disease process could be sought, and the role of other peptide growth factors (as discussed above) elucidated. Tumor necrosis factor alpha (33,213), PDGF isoforms (214–216), and TGF-β all appear to have key roles in the disease process. While TNF-α and PDGF are detailed above, and TGF-β is emphasized here, it appears that the pathobiological influences that each factor exhibits are interconnected.

Within the first 24 hr after asbestos exposure, TNF-α, PDGF (Fig. 8), and TGF-β_1 can be readily detected by immunohistochemistry (IHC), in situ hybridization (ISH), and Northern analysis (214,217,218). Transforming growth factor beta 1 is detected primarily in macrophages and the alveolar and airway epithelial cell populations, with faint staining in the interstitium in both rats and mice (219). Interestingly, in mice with both the Type I and II TNF-α receptors knocked out, asbestos-induced fibroproliferative lung disease fails to develop (17) (Fig. 10), and there is little expression of TGF-β_1. Similar findings were reported in the 129J mouse strain, which exhibits a genetic resistance to developing asbestos-induced disease in a proportion of the exposed animals (220). In these mice, histopathology revealed reduced levels of interstitial disease and ISH showed little expression of TGF-β_1 (220).

It was clear from studies with the 129J mouse strain that, even though these animals are inbred, there are significant differences among individual responses to asbestos exposure (220). Thus, an F1 generation was produced by crossing 129J mice (some fibrogenic resistant) with C57BL/6 mice (uniformly susceptible). When the F1 mice were exposed to asbestos, there was a broad range of responses from severe disease to no response (221). F1 mice then were backcrossed to either the 129J or C57 founders and the offspring exposed to asbestos. The C57 backcross produced essentially all susceptible individuals. In contrast, the backcross with the 129J mice produced offspring, 26% of which exhibited no fibrogenic response to asbestos (221). These individual mice exhibited reduced immunohistochemical staining for

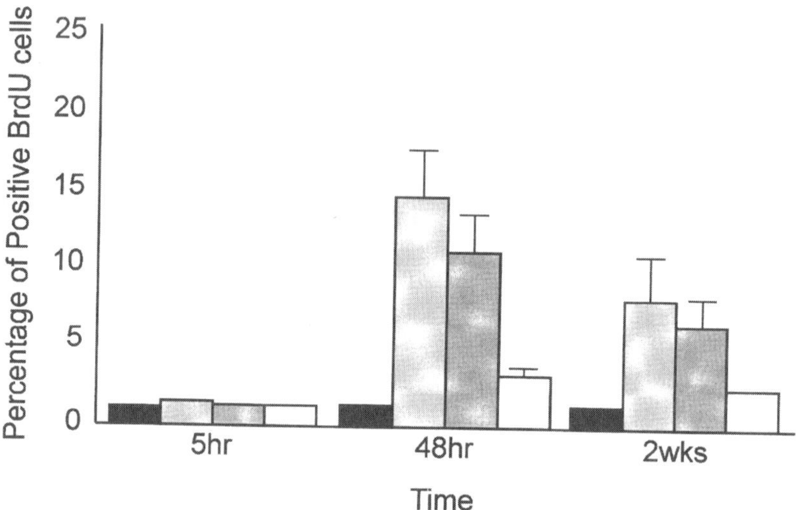

Figure 10 Tumor necrosis factor α receptor knockout mice are protected from the fibrogenic effects of asbestos. This figure demonstrates protection from fibrosis in TNF receptor knockout mice at both 48 hr and 2 weeks postexposure by quantifying incorporation of bromodoxyuridine (BrdU) into epithelial and interstitial cells following asbestos exposure. Both cell types in the knockout mice exhibited significantly reduced BrdU uptake, indicating less lung injury, inflammation, and consequent cell proliferation, thus indicating a prominent role for TNF-α in the disease process. (From Ref. 17.)

TGF-β_1 and will be invaluable in ongoing studies where the gene or gene cluster which imparts resistance in these mice is sought.

D. Isolation of Primary Mouse Alveolar Epithelial Cells and Fibroblasts

Another way to understand the biological activity of TGF-β_1 is by isolating target and secretory cell populations to determine whether or not there is gene expression, subsequent protein production, and the expected biological responses. These sorts of studies have been performed in a number of laboratories and form the basis for drawing conclusions on the multiple functions of TGF-β in controlling cell growth (15).

A reliable system for isolating primary bronchiolar–alveolar epithelial cells from mice (15,222,223) has been developed. If these cells are a source of TGF-β that could bind to appropriate receptors on mesenchymal cells in the lung interstitium, the mRNA transcript that codes for TGF-β_1 as well as the protein should be readily identified in vitro. This turns out to be the case, and most interesting were the findings that treatment of the cell cultures with TNF-α upregulated TGF-β_1 expression (15). Transforming growth factor beta 1 is expressed constitutively in primary epithelial and mesenchymal cells (15). Whether or not TGF-β is constitutively expressed in vivo is not entirely clear because studies using in situ hybridization have failed to demonstrate TGF-β_1 expression at the alveolar level in normal rats or mice, although some macrophages were always positive (219). Certainly, removal of any cell population from its normal anatomic position in the lung could stimulate gene expression, and this is what probably occurs with TGF-β_1 expression. As noted above, brief exposure to asbestos quickly upregulates TGF-β_1 expression in mice in vivo unless the animals are resistant to developing fibrogenesis (219) (Fig. 11). Studies in fibrotic human lungs have demonstrated strong expression of TGF-β_1 by immunohistochemistry (224).

Isolated cell studies have also examined primary fibroblasts from the lungs of fibrogenic-resistant 129J mice (225). These cells were found to be less responsive to PDGF, TGF-β, and TNF-α in their ability to proliferate and produce the extracellular matrix protein, α1-procollagen compared to fibroblasts from normal mice (225). These findings support the concept that the 129 mice exhibit an inherent reduction in response to asbestos (220) and to

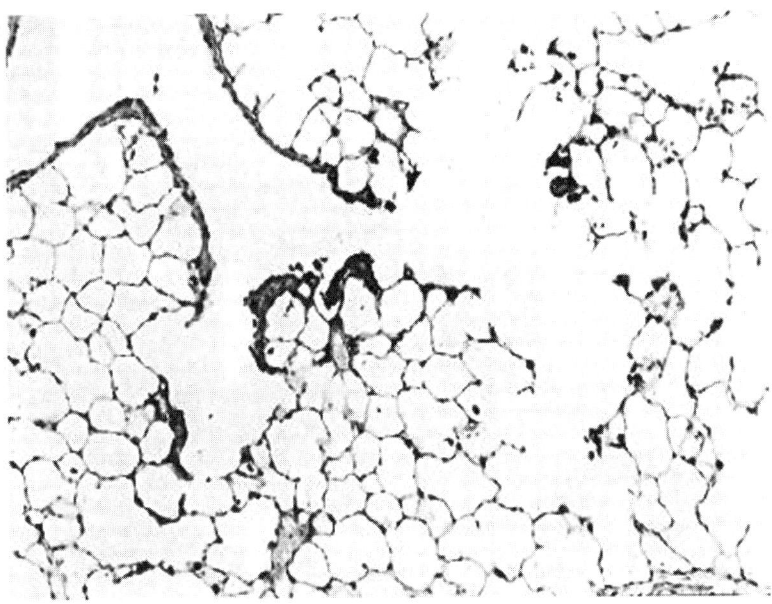

Figure 11 Gene expression of TGF-β_1 following asbestos exposure in rodents. Numerous cells along the bronchiolar–alveolar duct regions express the gene coding for TGF-β_1 within 48 hr after asbestos exposure in rats and mice. The alveolar epithelium and macrophages are clearly stained by nonradioactive in situ hybridization. (From Ref. 219.)

TGF-β overexpression (see below) because of key factors in the interstitial mesenchymal cells.

E. An Adenovirus Vector Transduces Overexpression of TGF-β₁ at the Alveolar Level

A nonreplicating adenovirus has been used for years as a vector to transduce the expression of a variety of genes in the lungs and other organs (226). This adenovirus vector (AdV) was used in 1998 to overexpress active TGF-β₁ in the lungs of rats (227). A high concentration of virus was used (10^9 pfu), and the resulting disease was a severe diffuse interstitial fibrosis (227). When the gene construct that codes for latent TGF-β was used, only slight focal inflammation was produced (227). These studies were central in demonstrating that TGF-β₁ alone can induce IPF. However, as discussed earlier, it is also clear that TGF-β₁ modulates the production and expression of a number of chemotactic factors, interleukins, latent TGF-β₁, and other mediators. Just what role(s) each of these plays in the development of fibroproliferative lung injury has yet to be established, and the use of genetically defined mouse models will be instrumental in such determinations.

When the AdV–TGF-β₁ construct was used in C57BL/6 mice (228), the response was the same as reported in rats (227). However, it was possible to titrate the viral dose and find a no-effect level of TGF-β₁ expression at 10^6 pfu (228). Also, 10^7 and 5×10^7 pfu were minimal-effect viral doses that allowed studies of histopathology, cell division rates and levels of TGF-β produced at the alveolar level, both active and latent (228). Establishing appropriate dose levels of viral vector is important in allowing investigators to further examine how TGF-β influences cell growth and inflammation, as is currently being done in several laboratories. For example, the AdV–TGF-β₁ construct has been used in the 129J mouse strain to ask if these animals are resistant to the fibrogenic effects of TGF-β₁ expression. Interestingly, the answer is yes or no, depending upon the dose and time after treatment (221). At doses of 10^8 and 10^9 pfu, C57BL/6 and 129 mice had essentially the same levels of severe IPF. At 10^7 and 5×10^7 pfu, the 129 strain had significantly fewer animals with disease, and this finding remained significantly different through 1 week post-treatment. By 2 weeks post-treatment, all the animals in both strains of mice exhibited severe disease which began to ameliorate 1 month later (221). Since there was considerable variability within the 129 strain regarding the degree of disease development, a question of genetically dependent susceptibility was raised. This has been answered in part in the studies reported above using the asbestos inhalation model with C57 × 129J crosses (221). Here, using the AdV–TGF-β₁, some of the 129J mice studied were found to exhibit a clear delay in the response to TGF-β₁. Perhaps the same gene or gene cluster that protected this subset of mice from the fibrogenic effects of asbestos is delaying the response to TGF-β_1 overexpression. Determining if this is the case will require identification of the gene and its function. The search for such susceptibility factors is an important cooncept that is being pursued by several research groups (57).

Transforming growth factor beta 1, as described earlier, is a potent inhibitor of epithelial cell proliferation (15). If this important biological activity were operating during the development of TGF-β_1-induced IPF, it should be possible to measure this effect on bronchiolar–alveolar epithelial lining cells. These cells are among the first to be damaged upon exposure to toxic agents (229,230), and a number of investigators have quantified significantly increased mitogenic responses in these cells consequent to lung injury (211,229). In the IPF induced by TGF-β_1 overexpression, the bronchiolar–alveolar epithelium remains remarkably quiescent (18,228). Even though the interstitial cell populations exhibit significantly increased rates of BrdU incorporation, and there is a robust inflammatory cell infiltrate, the epithelial cells are only slightly above normal levels, suggesting that the high levels of TGF-β_1 are influencing epithelial proliferation (18,228). If this is true, it will be important to understand if this is a beneficial effect that limits the degree and duration of disease. One way to test this postulate will be to increase the activation of latent TGF-β_1 at the alveolar level and monitor the consequent effects on epithelial cell populations and disease development.

Finally, a provocative question was addressed when the TNF-α receptor knockout (TNF-αRKO) mice were treated with the AdV–TGF-β_1 construct (18). Recall that these mice are resistant to the fibrogenic effects of asbestos (17), silica, and bleomycin (19,20). Since active TGF-β_1 is such a potent fibrogenic factor, the question was whether AdV–TGF-β_1 treatment would induce interstitial fibrogenesis in these mice? If the answer were "No," it would be possible to conclude that signaling through TNF-α receptors was necessary for a fibrogenic response to ensue. If the answer were "Yes," then it would be clear that TGF-β_1 alone, and the factors consequent to its expression, were sufficient without TNF-α to induce disease. The answer was "Yes" (18) (Fig. 12), suggesting that the TGF-β_1 cascade is particularly important for investigation. In normal mice exposed to fibrogenic agents in vivo, TNF-α kicks off a series of events that includes upregulation of TGF-β_1 and multiple other cytokines and factors (16,33). However, based on the finding above, a fibrogenic cascade can also begin with TGF-β_1. The extent to which fibroproliferative lung diseases mediated by TNF-α or by TGF-β_1 are similar or different is an essential concept to address in continuing research.

VII. Summary

This chapter has addressed a number of important mediators and pathophysiological pathways involved in lung injury and its progression to fibro-

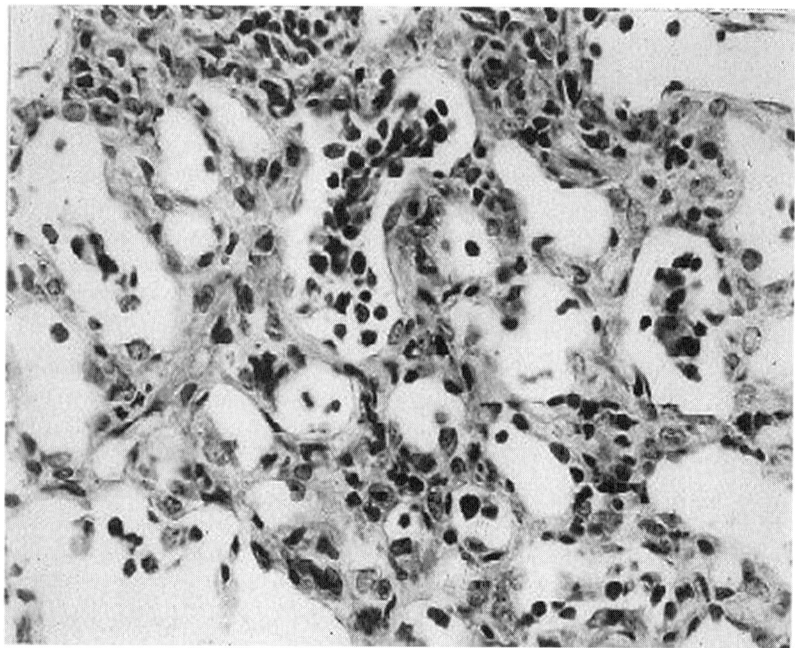

Figure 12   Inflammation and fibrosis in the lung of a TNF-α receptor knockout mouse treated with an adenovirus vector transducing expression of TGF-β_1. This diffuse interstitial inflammation and fibrosis is from the lung of a TNF-α receptor knockout mouse that is resistant to the fibrogenic effects of asbestos, silica, and bleomycin (17). This is a trichrome stain that marks interstitial fibrosis at the alveolar level, demonstrating that TGF-β_1 is sufficient to mediate the disease process. (From Ref. 18.)

proliferation and chronic lung disease. A multiplicity of inflammatory mediators is relevant for chronic fibroproliferative lung injury, including many that have been discussed in earlier chapters as important in acute inflammation and injury (e.g., Table 1). Although a large number of relevant mediators exist, much of the discussion in this chapter has focused on four specific peptide growth factors: TNF-α, PDGF, CTGF, and TGF-β. Focusing attention on these mediators allows more specific assessments of their interactions and importance in the development of chronic pulmonary fibroproliferative responses. At the same time, it should also be emphasized that these four mediators are only a few of many that warrant study in terms of their activities and interactions in lung injury.

Although inflammatory mediators have individual activities, it is becoming more and more clear that disease develops consequent to interactions among these factors. The biological effects of cytokines, growth factors, and other mediators do not occur in isolation, but instead are part of an orchestrated set of pulmonary responses. If appropriately regulated, the complex interplay of mediator expression and activity leads to the resolution of lung injury and effective pulmonary remodeling and repair. Conversely, if inflammation is unregulated, overexuberant, or persistent, repair and remodeling are compromised and fibroproliferative chronic lung injury can occur. The complex pathophysiology of inflammatory lung injury cannot be elucidated by considering mediators as distinct and noninteracting. For example, when it is found that increases in TNF-α are associated with increases in fibrogenesis, it is necessary to understand how and to what extent TNF-α upregulates the expression of growth factors like TGF-β which is the most potent known inducer of extracellular matrix component synthesis. Although much information exists about TNF-α and its activities as described in this chapter, intracellular signaling pathways from the TNF-α membrane receptors, through TGF-β, to promotion sequences in the CTGF and the α1 procollagen gene have yet to be elucidated. Although intuition suggests that CTGF should be central to the fibrogenic process by virtue of its biological activity, mouse models have thus far failed to reveal a significant role for this growth factor in fibroproliferation and this remains the subject of on-going research.

Stimulated by the prevalence and importance of chronic fibroproliferative lung injury and related clinical diseases including IPF and others, there is significant interest in elucidating the basic molecular mechanisms that control pulmonary fibrogenesis. The consensus of current research strengthens the hypothesis that a group of potent peptide growth factors interacts at multiple levels in mediating fibroproliferative chronic lung injury and disease. Just how large this group of essential factors may ultimately prove to be, and the precise molecular mechanisms through which these factors control the development of disease, are still being revealed. Basic research is progressing to the point where relevant pathophysiological targets can be identified, and new therapeutic approaches can be designed. Specific therapies for clinical lung injury are detailed later in Chapters 13–19. Prior to the discussion of therapies, intervening chapters examine the mechanistic pathophysiology of specific aspects of lung injury (oxidant injury, vascular dysfunction, and surfactant dysfunction) as well as introduce experimental models (animal and cell, transgenic, and inhalation) used in studying mechanisms and evaluating potential therapeutic agents.

Acknowledgments

This work was supported by NIH Grants ES-60766 (A.B.), HL-60532 (A.B.), ES-10046 (J.L.), and ES-10859 (L.O.) as well as by an award from the State of Louisiana's Health Excellence Fund, HEF (2001-06)-05. The authors are also grateful to Ms. Odette Marquez for assistance in preparation of the manuscript.

References

1. Crouch E. Pathobiology of pulmonary fibrosis. Am J Physiol 1990; 259: L159–L184.
2. Morris GF, Brody AR. Molecular mechanisms of particle-induced lung disease. In: Rom WR, ed. Environmental and Occupational Medicine. Philadelphia, PA: Lippincott–Raven Publishers, 1998:305–334.
3. Warheit DB, Overby LH, Brody AR. Pulmonary macrophages are attracted to inhaled particles through complement activation. Exp Lung Res 1988; 14: 51–66.
4. Quinlan TR, Marsh JP, Janssen YMW, Borm PA, Mossman BT. Oxygen radicals and asbestos-mediated disease. Environ Health Perspect 1994; 102:107–110.
5. Brody AR. Asbestos exposure as a model of inflammation inducing interstitial pulmonary fibrosis. In: Gallin JI, Goldstein IM, Snyderman R, eds. Inflammation: Basic Principles and Clinical Correlates. New York: Raven Press, Ltd., 1992:1033–1049.
6. Coin PG, Roggli VL, Brody AR. Persistence of long thin chrysotile asbestos fibers in the lungs of rats. Environ Health Perspect 1994; 102:195–200.
7. Ostro MG, Bloch KJ. Hypersensitivity pneumonitis in humans and experimental animals. In: Kradin RL, Robinson BWS, eds. Immunopathology of Lung Disease. Boston, MA: Butterworth-Heinemann, 1996:133–146.
8. American Thoracic Society. Idiopathic pulmonary fibrosis: diagnosis and treatment. International consensus statement. American Thoracic Society (ATS), and the European Respiratory Society (ERS). Am J Respir Crit Care Med 2000; 161:646–664.
9. Fine A, Matsui R, Zhan X, Poliks C, Smith B, Goldstein R. Discordant regulation of human type I collagen genes by prostaglandin E2. Biochim Biophys Acta 1992; 1135: 67–72.
10. Sporn MB, Roberts AR. Peptide Growth Factors and their Receptors. Heidelberg: Springer-Verlag, 1991.
11. Driscoll KE, Maurer JK, Higgins J, Poynter J. Alveolar macrophage cytokine and growth factor production in a rat model of crocidolite-induced pulmonary inflammation and fibrosis. J Toxicol Environ Health 1995; 46:155–169.
12. Paulsson Y, Austgulen R, Hofsli E, Heldin CH, Westermark B, Nissen-Meyer J. Tumor necrosis factor-induced expression of platelet-derived growth factor A-chain messenger RNA in fibroblasts. Exp Cell Res 1989; 180:490–496.
13. Phan SH, Gharaee-Kermani M, McGarry B, Kunkel SL, Wolber FW. Regulation of rat pulmonary artery endothelial cell transforming growth factor-β production by IL-1β and tumor necrosis factor-α1. J Immunol 1992; 149:103–106.
14. Sime PJ, Marr RA, Gauldie D, Xing Z, Helwett BR, Graham FL, Gauldie J. Transfer of tumor necrosis factor-α to rat lung induces severe pulmonary inflammation and patchy interstitial fibrogenesis with induction of transforming growth factor-β1 and myofibroblasts. Am J Pathol 1998; 153:825–832.
15. Warshamana GS, Corti M, Brody AR. TNF-α, PDGF and TGF-β_1 expression by primary mouse bronchiolar–alveolar epithelial and mesenchymal cells: TNF-α induces TGF-β_1. Exp Mol Pathol 2001; 71:13–33.

16. Zhang Y, Lee TC, Guillemin B, Yu M, Rom W. Enhanced IL-1 beta and tumor necrosis factor-alpha release and messenger RNA expression in macrophages from idiopathic pulmonary fibrosis or after asbestos exposure. J Immunol 1993; 150:4188–4196.

17. Liu J-Y, Brass DM, Hoyle GW, Brody AR. TNF-α receptor knock out mice are protected from the fibroproliferative effects of inhaled asbestos fibers. Am J Pathol 1998; 153:1839–1847.

18. Liu J-Y, Sime PJ, Wu T, Warshamana GS, Pociask D, Tsai S-Y, Brody AR. Transforming growth factor β_1 overexpression in tumor necrosis factor-α receptor knockout mice induces fibroproliferative lung disease. Am J Respir Cell Mol Biol 2001; 25:3–7.

19. Ortiz LA, Lasky JA, Hamilton RF, Holian A, Hoyle GW, Banks W, Peschon JJ, Brody AR, Lungarella G, Friedman M. Expression of TNF and the necessity of TNF receptors in bleomycin-induced lung injury in mice. Exp Lung Res 1998; 24:721–743.

20. Ortiz LA, Lasky J, Lungarella G, Cavarra E, Martorana P, Banks WA, Peschon JJ, Schmidts H-L, Brody AR, Friedman M. Upregulation of the p75 but not the p55 TNF-α receptor mRNA after silica and bleomycin exposure and protection from lung injury in double receptor knockout mice. Am J Respir Cell Mol Biol 1999; 20:825–833.

21. Grotendorst GR, Okochi H, Hayashi N. A novel transforming growth factor beta response element controls the expression of the connective tissue growth factor gene. Cell Growth Differ 1996; 7:469–480.

22. Chang LY, Overby LH, Brody AR, Crapo JD. Progressive lung cell reactions and extracellular matrix production after a brief exposure to asbestos. Am J Pathol 1988; 131:156–170.

23. Brody AR, Overby LH. Incorporation of tritiated thymidine by epithelial and interstitial cells in bronchiolar-alveolar regions of asbestos-exposed rats. Am J Pathol 1989; 134:133–144.

24. Finkelstein JN, Kramer C. Alveolar epithelial proliferation and production of growth factors and cytokines in pulmonary fibrosis. Am Rev Respir Dis 1993; 147:A153.

25. Schreiber AB, Winkler ME, Derynck R. Transforming growth factor-α: a more potent angiogenic mediator than epidermal growth factor. Science 1986; 232:250–253.

26. Strandjord TP, Clark CJ, Madtes DK. Expression of TGF-α, EGF, and EGF receptor in fetal rat lung. Am J Physiol 1994; 267:L384-L389.

27. Liu J-Y, Morris GF, Lei W-H, Corti M, Brody AR. Up-regulated expression of transforming growth factor-α in the bronchiolar-alveolar duct regions of asbestos-exposed rats. Am J Pathol 1996; 149:205–217.

28. Korfhagen TR, Swantz RJ, Wert SE, McCarty JM, Kerlakian CB, Glasser SW, Whitsett JA. Respiratory epithelial cell expression of human transforming growth factor-α induces lung fibrosis in transgenic mice. J Clin Invest 1994; 93: 1691–1699.

29. Battegay E, Raines E, Colbert T, Ross R. TNF-alpha stimulation of fibroblast proliferation. Dependence on platelet-derived growth factor (PDGF) secretion and alteration of PDGF receptor expression. J Immunol 1995; 154:6040–6047.

30. Beutler B, Van Huffel C. Unreveling function in the TNF ligand and receptor families. Science 1994; 265:667–668.

31. Bazzoni F, Beutler B. The tumor necrosis factor ligand and receptor families. N Engl J Med 1996; 334:1717–1725.

32. Vandenabeele P, Declerq W, Beyaert R, Fiers W. Two tumor necrosis factor receptors: structure and function. Trends Cell Biol 1995; 5:392–399.

33. Piguet PF, Collart MA, Grau GE, Sappino A-P, Vassalli P. Requirement of tumour necrosis factor for development of silica-induced pulmonary fibrosis. Nature 1990; 344:245–247.

34. Piguet PF, Vesin C. Treatment by human recombinant soluble TNF receptor of pulmonary fibrosis induced by bleomycin or silica in mice. Eur Respir J 1994; 7:515–518.

35. Goodwin RG, Anderson D, Jerzy R, Davis T, Brannan CI, Copeland NG, Jenkins NA, Smith C. Molecular cloning and expression of the type 1 and type 2 murine receptor for tumor necrosis factor. Mol Cell Biol 1991; 11:3020–3026.

36. Lewis M, Tartaglia LA, Lee A, Bennett GL, Rice GC, Wong GHW, Chen EY, Goeddel D. Cloning and expression of cDNAs for two distinct murine tumor necrosis factor receptors demonstrate one receptor is species specific. Proc Natl Acad Sci USA 1991; 88.

37. Allen RC, Armitage RJ, Conley ME, Rosenblatt H, Jenkins NA, Copeland NG, Bedell MA, Edelhoff S, Disteche CM, Simoneaux DK, Fanslow WC, Belmont J, Spriggs MK. CD40 ligand gene defects responsible for X-linked hyper-IgM syndrome. Science 1993; 259:990–993.

38. Matsuzawa A, Moriyama T, Kneko T, Tanaka M, Kimura M, Ikeda H, Katagiri T. A new allele of the lpr locus, lprgc, that complements the gld gene in induction of lymphadenopathy in the mouse. J Exp Med 1990; 171:519–531.

39. Rothe J, Lessiauer W, Lotscher H, Lang Y, Koebel P, Kontgen F, Althage A, Zinkernagel R, Steinmetz M, Bluethmann H. Mice lacking the tumour necrosis factor receptor 1 are resistant to TNF-mediated toxicity but highly susceptible to infection by Listeria monocytogenes. Nature 1993; 364:798–802.

40. Pfeffer K, Matsuyama T, Kundig TM, Wakeham A, Kishihara K, Shahinian A, Wiegmann K, Ohashi PS, Kronke M, Mak TW. Mice deficient for the 55 kD tumor necrosis factor receptor are resistant to endotoxic shock, yet succumb to L. monocytogenes infection. Cell 1993; 73:457–467.

41. Erickson SL, DeSauvage FJ, Kildy K, Carver-Moore K, Pitts-Meek S, Gillette N, Sheehan KCF, Schreiver RD, Goeddel DV, Moore MW. Decreased sensitivity to tumor necrosis factor but normal T cell development in TNF receptor-2-deficient mice. Nature 1994; 372:560–563.

42. Kolls J, Peppel K, Silva M, Beutler B. Prolonged and effective blockade of tumor necrosis factor activity through adenovirus-mediated gene transfer. Proc Natl Acad Sci USA 1994; 91:215–219.

43. Peschon JJ, Torrance DS, Stocking KL, Glaccum MB, Otten C, Willis CR, Charrier K, Morrissey PJ, Ware CB, Mohler KM. TNF receptor-deficient mice reveal divergent roles for p55 and p75 in several models of inflammation. J Immunol 1998; 160(2):943–952.

44. Zheng L, Fisher G, Miller RE, Peschon J, Lynch D, Lenardo MJ. Induciton of apoptosis in mature T cells by tumor necrosis factor. Nature 1995; 377: 348–351.

45. Ortiz LA, Lasky JA, Gozal E, Lungarella G, Cavarra E, Martorana P, Ruiz V, Pardo A, Brody AR, Friedman M, Selman M. Tumor necrosis factor receptor deficiency alters metalloproteinase 13/tissue inhibitor of metalloproteinase 1 expression in murine silicosis. Am J Respir Crit Care Med 2001; 163: 244–252.

46. Senaldi G, Yin S, Shaklee CL, Piguet PF, Mak TW, Ulich TR. Corynebacter-iujm parvum- and Mycobacterium bovis bacillus Calmette-Guerin-induced granuloma formation is inhi-bited in TNF receptor 1 (TNF-R1) knockout mice and by treatment with soluble TNF-R1. J Immunol 1996; 157: 5022–5026.

47. Lucas R, Juillard P, Decoster E, Redard M, Burger D, Donati Y, Giroud C, Monso-Hinard C, De Kesel T, Buurman WA, Moore MW, Dayer JM, Fiers W, Bluethmann H, Grau GE. Crucial role of tumor necrosis factor (TNF) receptor 2 and membrane-bound TNF in experimental cerebral malaria. Eur J Immunol 1997; 27:1719–1725.

48. Lucas R, Lou J, Morel DR, Ricou B, Suiter PM, Grau GE. TNF receptors in the microvascular pathology of acute respiratory distress syndrome and cere-bral malaria. J Leukoc Biol 1997; 61:551–558.

49. Erroi A, Bianchi M, Ghezzi P. The pneumotoxicant paraquat potentiates IL-1 and TNF production by human mononuclear cells. Agents Actions 1992; 36: 66–69.

50. Horinouchi H, Wang CC, Shepherd KE, Jones R. TNF alpha gene and pro-tein expression in alveolar macrophages in acute and chronic hyperoxia-induced lung injury. Am J Respir Cell Mol Biol 1996; 14(6):548–555.

51. Barazzone C, Tacchini-Cottier F, Vesin C, Rochat AF, Piguet PF. Hyperoxia induces platelet activation and lung sequestration: an event dependent on tumor necrosis factor-alpha and CD11. Am J Respir Cell Mol Biol 1996; 15: 107–114.

52. Miyazaki Y, Araki K, Vesin C, Garcia I, Kapanci Y, Whitsett JA, Piguet PF, Vassalli P. Expression of a tumor necrosis factor-alpha transgene in murine lung causes lymphocytic and fibrosing alveolitis: a mouse model of progres-sive pulmonary fibrosis. J Clin Invest 1995; 96:250–259.

53. Smith RE, Strieter RM, Phan SH, Kunkel SL. C–C chemokines: novel mediators of pro-fibrotic inflammatory response to bleomycin challenge. Am J Respir Cell Mol Biol 1996; 15:693–702.

54. Piguet PF, Ribaux C, Karpuz V, Grau GE, Kapanci Y. Expression and loca-lization of tumor necrosis factor α and its mRNA in idiopathic pulmonary fibrosis. Am J Pathol 1993; 143:651–655.

55. Gosset P, Perez T, Lassalle P, Duquesnoy B, Farre JM, Tonnel AB, Capron A. Increased TNF-α secretions by alveolar macrophages from patients with rheumatoid arthritis. Am Rev Respir Dis 1991; 143:593–597.

56. Ziegenhagen MW, Benner UK, Zissel GT, Zabel P, Schlaak M, Müller-Quernheim J. Sarcoidosis: TNF-release from alveolar macrophages and

serum level of sIL-2R are prognostic markers. Am Respir Crit Care Med 1997; 156:1586–1592.

57. DuBois RM. The genetic predisposition to interstitial lung disease: functional relevance. Chest 2002; 121:14S–20S.

58. Wilson AG, di Giovane FS, Blakemore AI, Duff GW. Single base polymorphism in the human tumor necrosis factor α (TNFα) gene detectable b NcoI restriction of PCR product. Hum Mol Genet 1992; 1:353.

59. Whyte M, Hubbard R, Meliconi R, Whidborne M, Eaton V, Bingle C, Timms J, Duff G, Facchini A, Pacilli A, Fabbri M, Hall I, Britton J, Johnston I, Di Giovine F. Increased risk of fibrosing alveolitis associated with interleukin-1 receptor antagonist and tumor necrosis factor-alpha gene polymorphisms. Am J Respir Crit Care Med 2000; 162(2 Pt 1):755–758.

60. Pantelidis P, Fanning GC, Wells AU, Welsh KI, Du Bois RM. Analysis of tumor necrosis factor-alpha, lymphotoxin-alpha, tumor necrosis factor receptor II, and interleukin-6 polymorphisms in patients with idiopathic pulmonary fibrosis. Am J Respir Crit Care Med 2001; 163:1432–1436.

61. Grutters JC, Sato H, Pantelidis P, Lagan AL, McGrath DS, Lammers JW, van den Bosch JM, Wells AU, du Bois RM, Welsh KI. Increased frequency of the uncommon tumor necrosis factor-857T allele in British and Dutch patients with sarcoidosis. Am J Respir Crit Care Med 2002; 165:1119–1124.

62. Pandey JP, Frederick M, Group AR. TNF-α, IL1, and immunoglobulin (GM and KM) gene polymorphisms in sarcoidosis. Hum Immunol 2002; 63: 485–491.

63. Corbett EL, Mozzato-Chamay N, Butterworth AE, De Cock KM, Williams BG, Churchyard GJ, Conway DJ. Polymorphisms in the tumor necrosis factor-alpha gene promoter may predispose to severe silicosis in black South African miners. Am J Respir Crit Care Med 2002; 165:690–693.

64. Hsu H, Xiong J, Goeddel DV. The TNF receptor 1-associated protein TRADD signals cell death and NF-κB activation. Cell 1995; 81:495–504.

65. Park A, Baichwal VJ. Systematic mutational analysis of the death domain of the tumor necrosis factor receptor 1-associated protein TRADD. J Biol Chem 1996; 16:9858–9862.

66. Rothe M, Wong SC, Henzel WJ, Goeddel DV. A novel family of putative signal transducers associated with the cytoplasmic domain of the 75kDa tumor necrosis factor receptor. Cell 1994; 78:681–692.

67. Rothe M, Sarma V, Dixit VM, Goeddel DV. TRAF-2 mediated activation of NF-κB by TNF receptor 2 and CD40. Science 1995; 269:1424–1427.

68. Ashkenazi A, Dixit M. Death receptors: signaling and modulation. Science 1998; 281:1305–1308.

69. Cleveland JL, Ihle J. Contenders in Fas/TNF death signaling. Cell 1995; 81:479–482.

70. Nagata S. Apoptosis by death factor. Cell 1997; 88:355–365.

71. Baker SJ, Redy P. Transducers of life and death: TNF receptor superfamily associated proteins. Oncogenes 1996; 12:1–9.

72. Gozal E, Ortiz LA, Zou X, Burow M, Lasky JA, Friedman M. Silica-induced apoptosis in murine macrophage: involvement of TNF-α and NF-κB activation. Am J Respir Cell Mol Biol 2002; 27(1):91–98.

73. Zanella CL, Posada J, Tritton TR, Mossman BT. Asbestos causes stimulation of the extracellular signal-regulated kinase 1 mitogen-activated protein kinase cascade after phosphorylation of the epidermal growth factor receptor. Cancer Res 1996; 56:5334–5338.

74. Cho YJ, Seo MS, Kim JK, Lim Y, Chae G, Ha KS, Lee KH. Silica-induced generation of reactive oxygen species in Rat2 fibroblast: role in activation of mitogen-activated protein kinase. Biochem Biophys Res Commun 1999; 7:708–712.

75. Ding M, Shi X, Dong Z, Chen F, Lu Y, Castranova V, Vallyanthan V. Freshly fractured crystalline silica induces activator protein-1 activation through ERKs and p38 MAPK. J Biol Chem 1999; 22:30611–30616.

76. Claudio E, Segade F, Wrobel K, Ramos S, Bravo R, Lazo P. Molecular mechanisms of TNF-α cytotoxicity: activation of NF-κB and nuclear translocation. Exp Cell Res 1996; 224:63–71.

77. Rojanasakul Y, Ye J, Chen F, Wang L, Cheng N, Castranova V, Vallyathan V, Shi X. Dependence of NF-kappaB activation and free radical generation on silica-induced TNF-alpha production in macrophages. Mol Cell Biochem 1999; 200:119–125.

78. Baeuerle PA, Henkel T. Function and activation of NF-κB in the immune system. Ann Rev Immunol 1994; 12:141–179.

79. Sen R, Baltimore D. Multiple nuclear factors interact with the immunoglobulin enhancer sequences. Cell 1986; 46:705–712.

80. Baeuerle PA, Baltimore D. NF-κB: ten years after. Cell 1996; 87:13–20.

81. Liou H-C, Baltimore D. Regulation of the NF-κB/rel transcription factor and the IκB inhibitor system. Curr Opin Cell Biol 1993; 5:477–487.

82. Ling L, Cao Z, Goeddel DV. NF-κB-inducing kinase activates IKK-α by phosphorylation of Scr-176. Proc Natl Acad Sci USA 1998; 95:3792–3797.

83. Mercurio F, Zhu H, Murray BW, Shevchenko A, Bennett BL, Li JW, Young DB, Barbosa M, Mann M. IKK-1 and IKK-2: cytokine-activated IκB kinases essential for NF-κB activation. Science 1997; 278:860–866.

84. Woronicz JD, Gao X, Cao Z, Rothe M, Goeddel DV. IκB kinase-β: NF-κB activation and complex formation with IκB kinase-α and NIK. Science 1997; 278:866–869.

85. Ghosh S, Baltimore D. Activation in vitro of NF-κB by phosphorylation of its inhibitor IκB. Nature 1990; 344:678–682.

86. Chen ZJ, Parent L, Maniatis T. Site-specific phosphorylation of IκB by a novel ubiquitination-dependent protein kinase activity. Cell 1996; 84:853–862.

87. Barnes PJ, Karin M. Nuclear Factor-κB a pivotal transcription factor in chronic inflammatory diseases. N Engl J Med 1997; 336:1066–1071.

88. Chen F, Sun SC, Kuh DC, Gaydos LJ, Demers LM. Essential role for NF-κB activation in silica-induced inflammatory mediator production in macrophages. Biochem Biophys Res Commun 1995; 214:985–992.

89. Hamid Q, Springall DR, Riveros-Moreno V, Chanez P, Howarth P, Redington A, Bousquet J, Godard P, Holgate S, Polak JM. Induction of nitric oxide synthase in asthma. Lancet 1993; 342:1510–1523.

90. Rachmilewitz D, Stamler JS, Bachwich D, Karmeli F, Ackerman Z, Podolsky DK. Enhanced colonic nitric oxide generation and nitric oxide synthase activity in ulcerative colitis and crohn's disease. Gut 1995; 36:718–723.

91. Evans CH, Stefanovic-Racic R, Lancaster J. Nitric oxide and its role in orthopeadic disease. Clin Orthop 1995; 312:275–294.

92. Pierce JW, Schoenleber R, Jasmoke G, Best J, Moore SA, Collins T, Geritsen ME. Novel inhibitors of cytokine-induced IκBa phosphorylation and endothelial cell adhesion molecule expression show anti-inflammatory effects in vivo. J Biol Chem 1997; 272:21096–21103.

93. Boulton TG, Yancoupolous GD, Gregory JS, Slaughter C, Moomaw C, Hsu J, Cobb MH. An insulin-stimulated protein kinase similar to yeast kinases involved in cell cycle control. Science 1990; 249:64–67.

94. Seger R, Krebs EG. The MAPK signaling cascade. FASEB J 1995; 9: 726–735.

95. Woodgett JR, Avruch J, Kyriakis J. The stress activated protein kinase pathway. Cancer Surv 1996; 27:127–138.

96. Xia Z, Dickens M, Raingeaud J, Davis RJ, Greenberg ME. Opposing effects of ERK and JNK-p38 MAP kinases on apoptosis. Science 1995; 270:1326–1331.

97. Karin M, Hunter T. Transcriptional control by protein phosphorylation: signal transmission from the cell surface to the nucleus. Curr Biol 1995; 5: 747–757.

98. Angel P, Allegretto EA, Okino ST, Hattory K, Boyle W, Hunter T, Karin M. Oncogene jun encodes a sequence-specific trans-activator similar to AP-1. Nature 1988; 332:166–171.

99. Angel P, Hattori K, Smeal T, Karin M. The jun proto-oncogene is positively autoregulated by its product Jun/ AP-1. Cell 1988; 55:875–885.

100. Derijard B, Raingeaud J, Barrett T, Wu I-H, Han J, Ulevitch RJ, Davis RJ. Independent human MAP kinase signal transduction pathways defined by MEK and MKK isoforms. Science 1995; 267:682–685.

101. Rahmsdorf HJ. Jun: transcription factor and oncoprotein. J Mol Med 1996; 74:725–747.

102. Nakano H, Shindo M, Sakon S, Nishinaka S, Mihara M, Yagita H, Okomura K. Differential regulation of IκB kinase α and β by two upstream kinases, NF-κβ-inducing kinase and mitogen-activated protein kinase/ERK kinase kinase-1. Proc Natl Acad Sci USA 1998; 95:3537–3542.

103. Karin M, Delhase M. JNK or IKK, AP-1 or NF-κB, which are the targets for MEK kinase1 action? Proc Natl Acad Sci USA 1998; 95:9067–9069.

104. Zhao Q, Lee FS. Mitogen-activated protein kinase/ERK kinase kinases 2 and 3 activate nuclear factor-κB through IκB kinase-α and IκB kinase α. J Biol Chem 1999; 26:8355–8358.

105. Chin BY, Choi ME, Burick MD, Strieter RM, Risby TH, Choi AMK. Transduction of apoptosis by particulate matter: role of TNF-α and MAPK. Am J Physiol: Lung Cell Mol Physiol 1998; 275:L942–L949.

106. Kalb A, Bluethmann H, Moore MW, Lesslauer W. Tumor necrosis factor receptor (TNF) in mouse fibroblast deficient in TNFR1 or TNFR2 are signal-

ing competent and activate the mitogen-activated protein kinase pathway with differential kinetics. J Biol Chem 1996; 271:28097–28104.

107. Raghu G. Idiopathic pulmonary fibrosis: a need for treatment with drugs other than corticosteroids—a role for antifibrotic agents? Mayo Clin Proc 1997; 72:285–287.

108. King TE Jr, Schwarz MI, Brown K, Tooze JA, Colby TV, Waldron JA Jr, Flint A, Thurlbeck W, Cherniack RM. Idiopathic pulmonary fibrosis: relationship between histopathologic features and mortality. Am J Respir Crit Care Med 2001; 164:1025–1032.

109. Raines EA. PDGF. In: Sporn MB, Roberts AR, eds. Peptide Growth Factors and their Receptors. New York: Springer-Verlag, 1991.

110. Betscholtz C, Raines EW. Platelet-derived growth factor: a key regulator of connective tissue cells in embryogenesis and pathogenesis. Kidney Int 1997; 51:1361–1368.

111. Li X, Ponten A, Aase K, Karlsson L, Abramsson A, Uutela M, Backstrom G, Hellstrom M, Bostrom H, Li H, Soriano P, Betsholtz C, Heldin CH, Alitalo K, Ostman A, Eriksson U. PDGF-C is a new protease-activated ligand for the PDGF alpha-receptor. Nat Cell Biol 2000; 2:302–309.

112. LaRochelle WJ, Jeffers M, McDonald WF, Chillakuru RA, Giese NA, Lokker NA, Sullivan C, Boldog FL, Yang M, Vernet C, Burgess CE, Fernandes E, Deegler LL, Rittman B, Shimkets J, Shimkets RA, Rothberg JM, Lichenstein HS. PDGF-D, a new protease-activated growth factor. Nat Cell Biol 2001; 3:517–521.

113. Hagood JS, Miller PJ, Lasky JA, Tousson A, Guo B, Fuller GM, McIntosh JC. Differential expression of platelet-derived growth factor-alpha receptor by Thy-1(−) and Thy-1(+) lung fibroblasts. Am J Physiol 1999; 277: L218–L224.

114. Bonner JC, Goodell AL, Coin PG, Brody AR. Chrysotile asbestos upregulates gene expression and production of alpha-receptors for platelet-derived growth factor (PDGF-AA) on rat lung fibroblasts. J Clin Invest 1993; 92:425–430.

115. Sasaki M, Kashima M, Ito T, Watanabe A, Sano M, Kagaya M, Shioya T, Miura M. Effect of heparin and related glycosaminoglycan on PDGF-induced lung fibroblast proliferation, chemotactic response and matrix metalloproteinases activity. Mediators Inflamm 2000; 9:85–91.

116. Yamawaki H, Sato K, Hori M, Ozaki H, Nakamura S, Nakayama H, Doi K, Karaki H. Impairment of EDR by a long-term PDGF treatment in organ-cultured rabbit mesenteric artery. Am J Physiol 1999; 277:H318–H323.

117. Day FL, Rafty LA, Chesterman CN, Khachigian LM. Angiotensin II (ATII)-inducible platelet-derived growth factor A-chain gene expression is p42/44 extracellular signal-regulated kinase-1/2 and Egr-1-dependent and mediated via the ATII type 1 but not type 2 receptor. Induction by ATII antagonized by nitric oxide. J Biol Chem 1999; 274:23726–23733.

118. Hishikawa K, Nakaki T, Hirahashi J, Marumo T, Saruta T. Tranilast restores cytokine-induced nitric oxide production against platelet-derived growth factor in vascular smooth muscle cells. J Cardiovasc Pharmacol 1996; 28: 200–207.

119. Schini VB, Durante W, Elizondo E, Scott-Burden T, Junquero DC, Schafer AI, Vanhoutte PM. The induction of nitric oxide synthase activity is inhibited by TGF-beta 1, PDGFAB and PDGFBB in vascular smooth muscle cells. Eur J Pharmacol 1992; 216:379–383.
120. Sharma RV, Tan E, Fang S, Gurjar MV, Bhalla RC. NOS gene transfer inhibits expression of cell cycle regulatory molecules in vascular smooth muscle cells. Am J Physiol 1999; 276:H1450–H1459.
121. Fagan KA, Fouty BW, Tyler RC, Morris KG Jr, Hepler LK, Sato K, LeCras TD, Abman SH, Weinberger HD, Huang PL, McMurtry IF, Rodman DM. The pulmonary circulation of homozygous or heterozygous eNOS-null mice is hyperresponsive to mild hypoxia. J Clin Invest 1999; 103:291–299.
122. Chiu JJ, Wung BS, Hsieh HJ, Lo LW, Wang DL. Nitric oxide regulates shear stress-induced early growth response-1. Expression via the extracellular signal-regulated kinase pathway in endothelial cells. Circ Res 1999; 85:238–246.
123. Kourembanas S, McQuillan LP, Leung GK, Faller DV. Nitric oxide regulates the expression of vasoconstrictors and growth factors by vascular endothelium under both normoxia and hypoxia. J Clin Invest 1993; 92:99–104.
124. Kolb M, Margetts PJ, Anthony DC, Pitossi F, Gauldie J. Transient expression of IL-1beta induces acute lung injury and chronic repair leading to pulmonary fibrosis. J Clin Invest 2001; 107:1529–1536.
125. Lasky JA, Brody AR. Interstitial fibrosis and growth factors. Environ Health Perspect 2000; 108(suppl 4):751–762.
126. Lasky JA, Goza E, Brass D, Lu H, Frieidman M, Brody A. A PDGF-selective tyrosine kinase inhibitor significantly blocks asbestos-induced lung fibroblast proliferation. Am J Respir Crit Care Med 1999; 159:A72.
127. Rice AB, Moomaw CR, Morgan DL, Bonner JC. Specific inhibitors of platelet-derived growth factor or epidermal growth factor receptor tyrosine kinase reduce pulmonary fibrosis in rats. Am J Pathol 1999; 155:213–221.
128. Gurujeyalakshmi G, Hollinger MA, Giri SN. Pirfenidone inhibits PDGF isoforms in bleomycin hamster model of lung fibrosis at the translational level. Am J Physiol 1999; 276(2 Pt 1):L311–L318.
129. Song M, He B, Qiu Z. Expressions of TNF alpha, PDGF in alveolar type II epithelial cells of rats with bleomycin-induced pulmonary. Chin J Tuber Respir Dis 1998; 21(4):221–223.
130. Zhuo Y, Pham D, Ortiz L, Zhang J, Hoyle G, Lasky J. PDGF-C and -D expression is differentially regulated during bleomycin-induced lung fibrosis. Am J Respir Crit Care Med 2002; 165:A169.
131. Bostrom H, Gritli-Linde A, Betsholtz C. PDGF-A/PDGF alpha-receptor signaling is required for lung growth and the formation of alveoli but not for early lung branching morphogenesis. Dev Dyn 2002; 223:155–162.
132. Lindahl P, Johansson BR, Leveen P, Betsholtz C. Pericyte loss and microaneurysm formation in PDGF-B-deficient mice. Science 1997; 277:242–245.
133. Soriano P. The PDGF alpha receptor is required for neural crest cell development and for normal patterning of the somites. Development 1997; 124:2691–2700.

134. Leveen P, Pekny M, Gebre-Medhin S, Swolin B, Larsson E, Betsholtz C. Mice deficient for PDGF B show renal, cardiovascular, and hematological abnormalities. Genes Dev 1994; 8:1875–1887.

135. Yoshida M, Sakuma J, Hayashi S, Abe K, Saito I, Harada S, Sakatani M, Yamamoto S, Matsumoto N, Kaneda Y, et al. A histologically distinctive interstitial pneumonia induced by overexpression of the interleukin 6, transforming growth factor beta 1, or platelet-derived growth factor B gene. Proc Natl Acad Sci USA 1995; 92:9570–9574.

136. Li J, Hoyle GW. Overexpression of PDGF-A in the lung epithelium of transgenic mice produces a lethal phenotype associated with hyperplasia of mesenchymal cells. Dev Biol 2001; 239:338–349.

137. Hoyle GW, Li J, Finkelstein JB, Eisenberg T, Liu JY, Lasky JA, Athas G, Morris GF, Brody AR. Emphysematous lesions, inflammation, and fibrosis in the lungs of transgenic mice overexpressing platelet-derived growth factor. Am J Pathol 1999; 154:1763–1775.

138. Yoshida M, Sakuma-Mochizuki J, Abe K, Arai T, Mori M, Goya S, Matsuoka H, Hayashi S, Kaneda Y, Kishimoto T. In vivo gene transfer of an extracellular domain of platelet-derived growth factor beta receptor by the HVJ-liposome method ameliorates bleomycin-induced pulmonary fibrosis. Biochem Biophys Res Commun 1999; 265:503–508.

139. Antoniades HN, Bravo MA, Avila RE, Galanopoulos T, Neville-Golden J, Maxwell M, Selman M. Platelet-derived growth factor in idiopathic pulmonary fibrosis. J Clin Invest 1990; 86:1055–1064.

140. Hertz MI, Henke CA, Nakhleh RE, Harmon KR, Marinelli WA, Fox JM, Kubo SH, Shumway SJ, Bolman RM III, Bitterman PB. Obliterative bronchiolitis after lung transplantation: a fibroproliferative disorder associated with platelet-derived growth factor. Proc Natl Acad Sci USA 1992; 89: 10385–10389.

141. Bergmann M, Tiroke A, Schafer H, Barth J, Haverich A. Gene expression of profibrotic mediators in bronchiolitis obliterans syndrome after lung transplantation. Scand Cardiovasc J 1998; 32:97–103.

142. Shull MM, Ormsby I, Kier AB, Pawlowski S, Diebold RJ, Yin M, Allen R, Sidman C, Proetzel G, Calvin D, et al. Targeted disruption of the mouse transforming growth factor-beta 1 gene results in multifocal inflammatory disease. Nature 1992; 359:693–699..

143. Crystal RG, Wolff G. . The Lung Scientific Foundations. Philadelphia, PA: Lippincott-Raven Publishers, 1997.

144. Bradham DM, Igarashi A, Potter RL, Grotendorst GR. Connective tissue growth factor: a cysteine-rich mitogen secreted by human vascular endothelial cells is related to the SRC-induced immediate early gene product CEF-10. J Cell Biol 1991; 114:1285–1294.

145. Yang DH, Kim HS, Wilson EM, Rosenfeld RG, Oh Y. Identification of glycosylated 38-kDa connective tissue growth factor (IGFBP-related protein 2) and proteolytic fragments in human biological fluids, and up-regulation of IGFBP-rP2 expression by TGF-beta in Hs578T human breast cancer cells. J Clin Endocrinol Metab 1998; 83:2593–2596.

146. Allen JT, Knight RA, Bloor CA, Spiteri MA. Enhanced insulin-like growth factor binding protein-related protein 2 (connective tissue growth factor) expression in patients with idiopathic pulmonary fibrosis and pulmonary sarcoidosis. Am J Respir Cell Mol Biol 1999; 21:693–700.

147. Steffen CL, Ball-Mirth DK, Harding PA, Bhattacharyya N, Pillai S, Brigstock DR. Characterization of cell-associated and soluble forms of connective tissue growth factor (CTGF) produced by fibroblast cells in vitro. Growth Factors 1998; 15:199–213.

148. Igarashi A, Okochi H, Bradham DM, Grotendorst GR. Regulation of connective tissue growth factor gene expression in human skin fibroblasts and during wound repair. Mol Biol Cell 1993; 4:637–645.

149. Lin J, Liliensiek B, Kanitz M, Schimanski U, Bohrer H, Waldherr R, Martin E, Kauffmann G, Ziegler R, Nawroth PP. Molecular cloning of genes differentially regulated by TNF-alpha in bovine aortic endothelial cells, fibroblasts and smooth muscle cells. Cardiovasc Res 1998; 38:802–813.

150. Pan LH, Yamauchi K, Uzuki M, Nakanishi T, Takigawa M, Inoue H, Sawai T. Type II alveolar epithelial cells and interstitial fibroblasts express connective tissue growth factor in IPF. Eur Respir J 2001; 17:1220–1227.

151. Lasky JA, Ortiz LA, Tonthat B, Hoyle GW, Corti M, Athas G, Lungarella G, Brody A, Friedman M. Connective tissue growth factor mRNA expression is upregulated in bleomycin-induced lung fibrosis. Am J Physiol 1998; 275:L365–L371.

152. Kothapalli D, Frazier KS, Welply A, Segarini PR, Grotendorst GR. Transforming growth factor beta induces anchorage-independent growth of NRK fibroblasts via a connective tissue growth factor-dependent signaling pathway. Cell Growth Differ 1997; 8:61–68.

153. Simmons DL, Levy DB, Yannoni Y, Erikson RL. Identification of a phorbol ester-repressible v-src-inducible gene. Proc Natl Acad Sci USA 1989; 86:1178–1182.

154. O'Brien TP, Yang GP, Sanders L, Lau LF. Expression of cyr61, a growth factor-inducible immediate-early gene. Mol Cell Biol 1990; 10:3569–3577.

155. Ryseck RP, Macdonald-Bravo H, Mattei MG, Bravo R. Structure, mapping, and expression of fisp-12, a growth factor-inducible gene encoding a secreted cysteine-rich protein. Cell Growth Differ 1991; 2:225–233.

156. Howell DC, Goldsack NR, Marshall RP, McAnulty RJ, Starke R, Purdy G, Laurent GJ, Chambers RC. Direct thrombin inhibition reduces lung collagen, accumulation, and connective tissue growth factor mRNA levels in bleomycin-induced pulmonary fibrosis. Am J Pathol 2001; 159:1383–1395.

157. Dammeier J, Brauchle M, Falk W, Grotendorst GR, Werner S. Connective tissue growth factor: a novel regulator of mucosal repair and fibrosis in inflammatory bowel disease? Int J Biochem Cell Biol 1998; 30:909–922.

158. Rishikof DC, Ricupero DA, Kuang PP, Liu H, Goldstein RH. Interleukin-4 regulates connective tissue growth factor expression in human lung fibroblasts. J Cell Biochem 2002; 85:496–504.

159. Nishida T, Nakanishi T, Shimo T, Asano M, Hattori T, Tamatani T, Tezuka K, Takigawa M. Demonstration of receptors specific for connective tissue

growth factor on a human chondrocytic cell line (HCS-2/8). Biochem Biophys Res Commun 1998; 247:905–909.

160. Schober JM, Chen N, Grzeszkiewicz TM, Jovanovic I, Emeson EE, Ugarova TP, Ye RD, Lau LF, Lam SC. Identification of integrin alpha(M)beta(2) as an adhesion receptor on peripheral blood monocytes for Cyr61 (CCN1) and connective tissue growth factor (CCN2): immediate-early gene products expressed in atherosclerotic lesions. Blood 2002; 99:4457–4465.

161. Segarini PR, Nesbitt JE, Li D, Hays LG, Yates JR III, Carmichael DF. The low density lipoprotein receptor-related protein/alpha2-macroglobulin receptor is a receptor for connective tissue growth factor. J Biol Chem 2001; 276:40659–40667.

162. Hagood JS, Lasky JA, Nesbitt JE, Segarini P. Differential expression, surface binding, and response to connective tissue growth factor in lung fibroblast subpopulations. Chest 2001; 120:64S–66S.

163. McIntosh JC, Hagood JS, Richardson TL, Simecka JW. Thy1 (+) and (−) lung fibrosis subpopulations in LEW and F344 rats. Eur Respir J 1994; 7:2131–2138.

164. Kothapalli D, Hayashi N, Grotendorst GR. Inhibition of TGF-beta--stimulated CTGF gene expression and anchorage-independent growth by cAMP identifies a CTGF-dependent restriction point in the cell cycle. FASEB J 1998; 12:1151–1161.

165. Kireeva ML, Latinkic BV, Kolesnikova TV, Chen CC, Yang GP, Abler AS, Lau LF. Cyr61 and Fisp12 are both ECM-associated signaling molecules: activities, metabolism, and localization during development. Exp Cell Res 1997; 233:63–77.

166. Hishikawa K, Oemar BS, Tanner FC, Nakaki T, Luscher TF, Fujii T. Connective tissue growth factor induces apoptosis in human breast cancer cell line MCF-7. J Biol Chem 1999; 274:37461–374616.

167. Hishikawa K, Nakaki T, Fujii T. Connective tissue growth factor induces apoptosis via caspase 3 in cultured human aortic smooth muscle cells. Eur J Pharmacol 2000; 392:19–22.

168. Shimo T, Nakanishi T, Kimura Y, Nishida T, Ishizeki K, Matsumura T, Takigawa M. Inhibition of endogenous expression of connective tissue growth factor by its antisense oligonucleotide and antisense RNA suppresses proliferation and migration of vascular endothelial cells. J Biochem (Tokyo) 1998; 124:130–140.

169. Shimo T, Nakanishi T, Nishida T, Asano M, Sasaki A, Kanyama M, Kuboki T, Matsumura T, Takigawa M. Involvement of CTGF, a hypertrophic chondrocyte-specific gene product, in tumor angiogenesis. Oncology 2001; 61: 315–322.

170. Kondo S, Kubota S, Shimo T, Nishida T, Yosimichi G, Eguchi T, Sugahara T, Takigawa M. Connective tissue growth factor increased by hypoxia may initiate angiogenesis in collaboration with matrix metalloproteinases. Carcinogenesis 2002; 23:769–776.

171. Inoki I, Shiomi T, Hashimoto G, Enomoto H, Nakamura H, Makino K, Ikeda E, Takata S, Kobayashi K, Okada Y. Connective tissue growth factor

binds vascular endothelial growth factor (VEGF) and inhibits VEGF-induced angiogenesis. FASEB J 2002; 16:219–221.

172. Frazier K, Williams S, Kothapalli D, Klapper H, Grotendorst GR. Stimulation of fibroblast cell growth, matrix production, and granulation tissue formation by connective tissue growth factor. J Invest Dermatol 1996; 107(3): 404–411.

173. Rennard SI, Crystal RG. Collagen in health and disease. In: Weiss JB, Jayson MIV, eds. Lung. London: Churchill Livingstone, 1982:424–444.

174. Eberlein M, Heusinger-Ribeiro J, Goppelt-Struebe M. Rho-dependent inhibition of the induction of connective tissue growth factor (CTGF) by HMG CoA reductase inhibitors (statins). Br J Pharmacol 2001; 133:1172–1180.

175. Fan WH, Karnovsky MJ. Increased MMP-2 expression in connective tissue growth factor over-expression vascular smooth muscle cells. J Biol Chem 2002; 277:9800–9805.

176. Chen CC, Chen N, Lau LF. The angiogenic factors Cyr61 and connective tissue growth factor induce adhesive signaling in primary human skin fibroblasts. J Biol Chem 2001; 276:10443–10452.

177. Shinozaki M, Kawara S, Hayashi N, Kakinuma T, Igarashi A, Takehara K. Induction of subcutaneous tissue fibrosis in newborn mice by transforming growth factor beta-simultaneous application with basic fibroblast growth factor causes persistent fibrosis. Biochem Biophys Res Commun 1997; 237: 292–296.

178. Igarashi A, Nashiro K, Kikuchi K, Sato S, Ihn H, Grotendorst GR, Takehara K. Significant correlation between connective tissue growth factor gene expression and skin sclerosis in tissue sections from patients with systemic sclerosis. J Invest Dermatol 1995; 105:280–284.

179. Ito Y, Aten J, Bende RJ, Oemar BS, Rabelink TJ, Weening JJ, Goldschmeding R. Expression of connective tissue growth factor in human renal fibrosis. Kidney Int 1998; 53:853–861.

180. Oemar BS, Luscher TF. Connective tissue growth factor. Friend or foe? Arterioscler Thromb Vasc Biol 1997; 17:1483–1489.

181. Tamatani T, Kobayashi H, Tezuka K, Sakamoto S, Suzuki K, Nakanishi T, Takigawa M, Miyano T. Establishment of the enzyme-linked immunosorbent assay for connective tissue growth factor (CTGF) and its detection in the sera of biliary atresia. Biochem Biophys Res Commun 1998; 251:748–752.

182. Kubo M, Kikuchi K, Nashiro K, Kakinuma T, Hayashi N, Nanko H, Tamaki K. Expression of fibrogenic cytokines in desmoplastic malignant melanoma. Br J Dermatol 1998; 139:192–197.

183. Frazier KS, Grotendorst GR. Expression of connective tissue growth factor mRNA in the fibrous stroma of mammary tumors. Int J Biochem Cell Biol 1997; 29:153–161.

184. Ziesche R, Hofbauer E, Wittmann K, Petkov V, Block LH. A preliminary study of long-term treatment with interferon gamma-1b and low-dose prednisolone in patients with idiopathic pulmonary fibrosis. N Engl J Med 1999; 341:1264–1269.

185. Lasky JA, Friedman M, Warshamana S, Liu H, Zhuo Y, Brody AR, Hoyle GW. Normal lung development in transgenic mice overexpressing connective tissue growth factor. Am J Respir Crit Care Med 1998; 161:A480.

186. Laurent GJ, McAnulty RJ. Protein metabolism during bleomycin-induced pulmonary fibrosis in rabbits. In vivo evidence for collagen accumulation because of increased synthesis and decreased degradation of the newly synthesized collagen. Am Rev Respir Dis 1983; 128:82–88.

187. McAnulty RJ, Laurent GJ. Collagen synthesis and degradation in vivo. Evidence for rapid rates of collagen turnover with extensive degradation of newly synthesized collagen in tissues of the adult rat. Coll Relat Res 1987; 7:93–104.

188. Yokoi H, Mukoyama M, Sugawara A, Mori K, Nagae T, Makino H, Suganami T, Yahata K, Fujinaga Y, Tanaka I, Nakao K. Role of connective tissue growth factor in fibronectin expression and tubulointerstitial fibrosis. Am J Physiol Renal Physiol 2002; 282:F933–F942.

189. Twigg SM, Joly AH, Chen MM, Tsubaki J, Kim HS, Hwa V, Oh Y, Rosenfeld RG. Connective tissue growth factor/IGF-binding protein-related protein-2 is a mediator in the induction of fibronectin by advanced glycosylation end-products in human dermal fibroblasts. Endocrinology 2002; 143: 1260–1269.

190. Massague J. TGF-beta signaling: receptors, transducers, and Mad proteins. Cell 1996; 85:947–950.

191. Attisano L, Wrana J. Signal transduction by the TGF-beta superfamily. Science 2002; 296:1646–1647.

192. Harpel JG, Metz CN, Kojima S, Rifkin DB. Control of TGF-β activity: latency vs activation. Prog Growth Factor Res 1992; 4:321–335.

193. Sasaki A, Naganuma H, Satoh E, Kawataki T, Amagasaki K, Nukui H. Participation of thrombospondin-1 in the activation of latent transforming growth factor-beta in malignant glioma cells. Neurol Med Chir (Tokyo) 2001; 41:253–258; discussion 258–259.

194. Lyons R, Gentry L, Purchio A, Moses H. Mechanism of activation of latent recombinant transforming growth factor beta 1 by plasmin. J Cell Biol 1990; 110:1361–1367.

195. Munger J, Huang X, Kawakatsu H, Griffiths M, Dalton S, Wu J, Pittet J, Kaminski N, Garat C, Matthay M, Rifkin D, Sheppard D. The integrin alpha v beta 6 binds and activates latent TGF beta 1: a mechanism for regulating pulmonary inflammation and fibrosis. Cell 1999; 96:319–328.

196. Barcellos-Hoff M, Dix T. Redox-mediated activation of latent transforming growth factor-beta 1. Mol Endocrinol 1996; 10:1077–1083.

197. Ehrhart E, Segarini P, Tsang M, Carroll A, Barcellos-Hoff M. Latent transforming growth factor beta1 activation in situ: quantitative and functional evidence after low-dose gamma-irradiation. FASEB J 1997; 11:1191–1202.

198. Miyazono K, Heldin C. Role for carbohydrate structures in TGF-beta 1 latency. Nature 1989; 338:158–160.

199. Yu Q, Stamenkovic I. Cell surface-localized matrix metalloproteinase-9 proteolytically activates TGF-beta and promotes tumor invasion and angiogenesis. Genes Dev 2000; 14:163–176.

200. Zhou L, Dey CR, Wert SE, Whitsett JA. Arrested lung morphogenesis in transgenic mice bearing an SP-C-TGF-beta 1 chimeric gene. Dev Biol 1996; 175:227–238.

201. Borset M, Waage A, Sundan A. Hepatocyte growth factor reverses the TGF-beta-induced growth inhibition of CCL-64 cells. A novel bioassay for HGF and implications for the TGF-beta bioassay. J Immunol Methods 1996; 189:59–64.

202. Dkhissi F, Jullien RS, Lawrence DA. Growth stimulation of murine fibroblasts by TGF-beta1 depends on the expression of a functional p53 protein. Oncogene 1999; 18:703–711.

203. Bonner JC, Badgett A, Lindroos PM, Osornio-Varga AR. Transforming growth factor-beta-1 (TGF-beta-1) down-regulates the platelet-derived growth factor (PDGF) alpha-receptor subtype on human lung fibroblasts in vitro. Am J Respir Cell Mol Biol 1995; 13:496.

204. Kalter VG, Brody AR. Receptors for transforming growth factor-β on rat lung fibroblasts have higher affinity for TGF-β_1 than for TGF-β_2. Am J Respir Cell Mol Biol 1991; 4:397.

205. Perdue TD, Brody AR. Distribution of transforming growth factor-β1, fibronectin, and smooth muscle actin in asbestos-induced pulmonary fibrosis in rats. J Histochem Cytochem 1994; 42:1061–1070.

206. Keski-Oja J, Raghow R, Sawdey M, Loskutoff DJ, Postlethwaite AE, Kang AH, Moses HL. Regulation of mRNAs for type-1 plasminogen activator inhibitor, fibronectin, and type I procollagen by transforming growth factor-β. Divergent responses in lung fibroblasts and carcinoma cells. J Biol Chem 1988; 263:3111–3115.

207. Bozelka BE, Sestini P, Gaumer R, Hammad Y, Heather C, Salvaggio J. A murine model of asbestosis. Am J Pathol 1983; 112:326.

208. Brody AR, Roe MW. Deposition pattern of inorganic particles at the alveolar level in the lungs of rats and mice. Am Rev Respir Dis 1983; 128:724–729.

209. Warheit DB, George G, Hill LH, Snyderman R, Brody AR. Inhaled asbestos activates a complement-dependent chemotactic factor for macrophages. Lab Invest 1985; 52:505–514.

210. Cole RW, Ault JC, Hayden JH, Rieder CL. Crocidolite asbestos fibers undergo size-dependent microtubule-mediated transport after endocytosis in vertebrate lung epithelial cells. Cancer Res 1991; 51:4942–4947.

211. Gardner SY, Brody AR. Incorporation of bromodeoxyuridine as a method to quantify cell proliferation in bronchiolar–alveolar duct regions of asbestos-exposed mice. Inhal Toxicol 1995; 7:215–224.

212. McGavran PD, Moore LM, Brody AR. Inhalation of chrysotile asbestos induces rapid cellular proliferation in small pulmonary vessels of mice and rats. Am J Pathol 1990; 136:695–705.

213. Gossart S, Cambon C, Orfila C, Seguelas MH, Lepert JC, Rami J, Carre P, Pipy B. Reactive oxygen intermediates as regulators of TNF-alpha production in rat lung inflammation induced by silica. J Immunol 1996; 156:1540–1548.

214. Liu J-Y, Morris G, Lei W-H, Hart C, Lasky J, Brody AR. Rapid activation of PDGF-A and -B expression at sites of lung injury in asbestos-exposed rats. Am J Respir Cell Mol Biol 1997; 17:129–140.

215. Lasky JA, Coin PG, Lindroos PM, Ostrowski LE, Brody AR, Bonner JC. Chrysotile asbestos stimulates gene expression and secretion of PDGF-AA by rat fibroblasts in vitro: evidence for an autocrine loop. Am J Respir Cell Mol Biol 1995; 12:162–170.

216. Bonner JC, Brody AR. Asbestos-induced alveolar injury: evidence for macrophage-derived PDGF as a mediator of the fibrogenic response. Chest 1991; 99(3):54s–55s.

217. Lasky JA, Tonthat B, Liu J-Y, Friedman M, Brody AR. Up-regulation of the PDGF-alpha-receptor precedes asbestos-induced lung fibrosis in rats. Am J Respir Crit Care Med 1997; 1998:1652–1657.

218. Brody AR, Liu J-Y, Brass D, Corti M. Analyzing the genes and peptide growth factors expressed in the lung consequent to asbestos exposure, Proceedings of the International Conference on Toxicology of Natural and Man Made Particles. Environ Health Perspect 1997; 105.

219. Liu J-Y, Brody AR. Increased TGF-β_1 in the lungs of asbestos-exposed rats and mice: reduced expression in TNF-α receptor knockout mice. J Environ Pathol Toxicol Oncol 2001; 20:77–87.

220. Brass DM, Hoyle GW, Poovey HG, Liu J-Y, Brody AR. Reduced TNF-α and TGF-β1 expression in the lungs of inbred mice that fail to develop fibroproliferative lesions consequent to asbestos exposure. Am J Pathol 1999; 154:853–862.

221. Warshamana GS, Pociask DA, Sime PJ, Schwartz DA, Brody AR. Susceptibility to asbestos-induced and TGF-β1-induced fibroproliferative lung disease in two strains of mice. Am J Respir Cell Mol Biol 2002; 27:705–713.

222. Corti M, Brody AR, Harrison JH. Isolation and primary culture of murine alveolar type II cells. Am J Respir Cell Mol Biol 1996; 14:309–315.

223. Corti M, Brody AR. The influences of sera and substrate on transepithelial resistances and morphology of cultured mouse ATII cells. Am J Respir Crit Care Med 1996; 153(4):A510.

224. Khalil N, O'Connor RN, Flanders KC, Unruh H. TGF-β_1, but not TGF-β_2 or TGF-β_3, is differentially present in epithelial cells of advanced pulmonary fibrosis: an immunohistochemical study. Am J Respir Crit Care Med 1996; 14:131–138.

225. Brass DM, Tsai S-Y, Brody AR. Primary lung fibroblasts from the 129 mouse strain exhibit reduced growth factor responsiveness "in vitro". Exp Lung Res 2001; 27:639–653.

226. Brody S, Crystal R. Adenovirus-mediated in vivo gene transfer. Ann N Y Acad Sci 1994; 716:90–101.

227. Sime PJ, Xing Z, Graham FL, Csaky KG, Gauldie J. Adenovector-mediated gene transfer of active transforming growth factor-β1 induces prolonged severe fibrosis in rat lung. J Clin Invest 1997; 100:768–776.

228. Warshamana GS, Pociask DA, Fisher KJ, Liu J-Y, Sime PJ, Brody AR. Titration of non-replicating adenovirus as a vector for transducing active TGF-β_1 gene expression causing inflammation and fibrogenesis in the lungs of C57BL/6 mice. Int J Exp Pathol 2002; 83:1–19.

229. McGavran PD, Brody AR. Chrysotile asbestos inhalation induces tritiated thymidine incorporation by epithelial cells of distal bronchioles. Am J Respir Cell Mol Biol 1989; 1:231–235.

230. Mossman BT, Marsh JP, Shatos MA. Alteration of superoxide dismutase activity in tracheal epithelial cells by asbestos and inhibition of cytotoxicity by antioxidants. Lab Invest 1986; 54:204–212.

7

Roles of Reactive Oxygen and Nitrogen Species in Lung Injury

IAN C. DAVIS, JOHN D. LANG, and SADIS MATALON

Departments of Anesthesiology, and Physiology and Biophysics, University of Alabama at Birmingham, Birmingham, Alabama, U.S.A.

I. Overview

This chapter covers reactive oxygen and nitrogen species and their importance in inflammatory lung injury. As described in prior chapters, the pathophysiology of lung injury is multifaceted, and includes the elaboration of reactive oxygen and nitrogen species by inflammatory cells. Reactive oxygen and nitrogen species are of considerable importance in innate immunity and cellular regulation, but their release also results in collateral damage to lung tissue that can ultimately compromise both gas exchange and host defense. For example, reactive nitrogen species (RNS) produced by macrophages in the presence of physiologic CO_2 tensions can induce nitration of surfactant protein A (SP-A) and compromise its ability to act as a collectin during host defense. Endogenous reactive oxygen and nitrogen species can also cause cell and tissue injury by a variety of other mechanisms. In addition, exogenous reactive oxygen and nitrogen species can also be involved in generating lung injury (e.g., from environmental exposure to hyperoxia, ozone, nitric oxide, or related gases). This chapter reviews the fundamental chemistry of reactive oxygen and nitrogen species, as well as their positive and negative biological effects. Emphasis is on the roles of reactive species in acute injury and pulmonary disease based on basic science and clinical perspectives. Pulmonary antioxidant defenses against reactive oxygen and nitrogen species are also discussed. Therapeutic applications targeting oxidant-related pathophysiology are noted, with further details on antioxidant therapies for lung injury given later in Chapter 16.

II. Introduction

The primary function of the lungs is to promote gas exchange between inspired air and the blood. Two kinds of epithelial cells are present in the alveolar air-sacs to promote respiratory function. The pulmonary gas exchange surface is mainly composed of a single thin layer of epithelial cells, the alveolar type I cells. Interspersed among these are larger cuboidal alveolar type II cells, which produce the alveolar lining fluid and synthesize, secrete, and recycle pulmonary surfactant. The cytoplasm of alveolar type I cells and the adjacent fluid layer are by necessity small in thickness to permit efficient gas exchange across a broad surface area into capillary blood. Despite its small thickness, the alveolar epithelium has low permeability to electrolytes and plasma proteins. It actively transports sodium ions away from the lumenal surface, and contains tight junctions between cells to provide a high-resistance barrier to fluid movement from the interstitium into the alveolar space (1). Pulmonary surfactant secreted by type II cells into the alveolar liquid lining layer adsorbs to the air–water interface and lowers surface tension, reduces respiratory work, and promotes alveolar stability and inflation uniformity (2). The activity of pulmonary surfactant and its dysfunction during lung injury are detailed in Chapter 9. Free ranging phagocytic alveolar macrophages (AMs) are a third cell type found in varying numbers in the extracellular lining fluid on the alveolar surface. These cells patrol the interior of the alveoli and ingest inspired particulates and invading pathogens (3).

The alveolar epithelium is continuously exposed to reactive oxygen and nitrogen species from both endogenous and exogenous sources. Prolonged exposure to these reactive species results in damage to the pulmonary surfactant system and alveolar epithelium, causing protein leakage into the alveolar space, pulmonary atelectasis, and hypoxemia. Reactive oxygen species (ROS) are generated as intermediates in mitochondrial electron transport systems and during microsomal metabolism of endogenous cytoplasmic compounds and xenobiotics, such as drugs and environmental pollutants (4). In addition, during the innate inflammatory response to injury, neutrophils, AMs, and other inflammatory cells can generate and release ROS by an NADPH-oxidase-dependent mechanism (5,6). In addition, nitric oxide ($^\bullet$NO) also contributes to the alveolar epithelium's oxidant burden and induces the formation of other reactive oxygen–nitrogen intermediates (7,8). Lung tissues may be exposed to increased concentrations of

•NO in inhaled polluted air (9,10), or as a consequence of its overproduction by AMs, or pulmonary epithelial, interstitial, and endothelial cells (see below). Overproduction of •NO and other RNS has been implicated in a variety of inflammatory diseases, including clinical acute lung injury (ALI) and the acute respiratory distress syndrome (ARDS).

III. Chemistry and Biochemistry of Reactive Oxygen and Nitrogen Species

A. Reactive Oxygen Species

At normal oxygen tensions in humans, approximately 98% of oxygen undergoes a four-electron catalytic reduction by mitochondrial cytochrome *c* oxidase to form water (11). The remaining 2% of oxygen, however, may undergo sequential incomplete reduction by the mitochondrial electron transport chain to form the superoxide anion radical ($O_2^{\bullet-}$) (12). H_2O_2 also can be formed by spontaneous, or superoxide dismutase (SOD)-catalyzed dismutation of $O_2^{\bullet-}$ (13). The latter may occur when SOD expression is induced without concomitant upregulation of catalase activity. Neutrophil myeloperoxidase (MPO) can also convert H_2O_2 to hypochlorous acid (HOCl) (14). HOCl is a highly reactive oxidant, capable of oxidizing thiols, thioethers, heme groups, and iron–sulfur centers, as well chlorinating amines (15).

$O_2^{\bullet-}$ and H_2O_2 are relatively long-lived compounds in biologic systems, and both can enter cells (H_2O_2 directly crosses cell membranes by simple diffusion, while $O_2^{\bullet}$ enters via anion channels) (4). H_2O_2 is less reactive than $O_2^{\bullet-}$, but it can exert toxic effects more distally. However, the limited reactivity of $O_2^{\bullet-}$ and H_2O_2 with many biological molecules and their low intracellular concentrations (10 pM and 1–100 nM, respectively) has raised questions about their toxicity in vivo. Likewise, the degree to which the MPO/HOCl system contributes to host antimicrobial defenses is still unclear, although microbicidal activity of MPO against *Mycobacterium tuberculosis* has been demonstrated (16). Moreover, studies with gene "knock-out" mice lacking MPO have demonstrated increased susceptibility to pneumonia induced by intratracheal administration of *Candida albicans* (17).

A more potent reactive metabolite of $O_2^{\bullet-}$ that is generated in a variety of biologic systems is the hydroxyl radical (•OH) (18). In the Haber–Weiss reaction, $O_2^{\bullet-}$ directly reduces H_2O_2 to produce •OH, together with molecular O_2 and hydroxide ion (OH^-). Alternatively, in the modified Haber–Weiss reaction (the Fenton reaction), $O_2^{\bullet-}$ can reduce trace metal ions (usually Fe^{3+}, sometimes Cu^{2+}) to form molecular O_2 (19). The reduced form of the metal ion can then react with H_2O_2 to regenerate an oxidized metal ion, with concomitant production of OH^- and •OH. While there are no known enzymatic scavenging systems for •OH radical in vivo, its reactivity is so high and nonspecific that the site of its reaction with target molecules is confined to within a few molecular radii of the site of its generation. Moreover, because generation of $^\bullet$OH by the Fenton reaction requires the interaction of two different reactive species ($O_2^{\bullet-}$ and H_2O_2) in the presence of iron, at relatively slow reaction rates, it is unlikely to occur in the normal lung where most of the iron in the epithelial lining fluid is chelated in an inactive form by transferrin and ceruloplasmin (20). In addition, ascorbate, which is present in the epithelial lining fluid in higher concentrations than $O_2^{\bullet-}$, also reduces Fe^{3+}, and so can compete with $O_2^{\bullet-}$. Nevertheless, formation of $^\bullet$OH via the Fenton reaction may still occur in vivo, especially in situations where the intracellular load of free iron is increased (21), or when antioxidant defenses are perturbed (22). Moreover, Beckman et al. have described a second pathway for the generation of potential oxidants with the reactivity of $^\bullet$OH in the absence of metal catalysis (23).

The normal lung is protected from the buildup of ROS to toxic concentrations by several antioxidant systems. Lung cells contain three forms of SOD: CuZnSOD, found mainly in cell cytoplasm but also in peroxisomes; and MnSOD, localized in mitochondria. An extracellular form of SOD (EC-SOD) also has been identified in the lung matrix and is thought to play a major role in the scavenging of extracellular $O_2^{\bullet-}$ (24). Peroxisomes also contain catalase, which will degrade H_2O_2. In addition, lung tissues contain high concentrations of a number of nonenzymatic antioxidants, including vitamin E and reduced glutathione and ascorbate (25).

Several factors may exacerbate production of ROS in acute and chronic lung diseases. First, treatment with increased concentrations of oxygen is commonly used to alleviate hypoxemia in patients with lung disease. Exposure of lung cells, subcellular organelles, and tissues to hyperoxia (100% O_2) results in a 10- to 15-fold increase in mitochondrial H_2O_2 production (26). Second, proinflammatory chemokines and cytokines released by damaged lung cells during inflammatory responses trigger migration of neutrophils into the lungs. These proinflammatory stimuli also trigger receptor-mediated activation signals, transduced through protein kinase C and phospholipase C, that lead to translocation of cytosolic components of the NADPH-oxidase complex (gp40^{phox}, gp47^{phox}, gp67^{phox}, and the Rho-family GTPase, Rac2) to a membrane-bound complex (gp91^{phox}/gp22^{phox}/Rap1a) that carries cytochrome *c*. Once activated, the membrane-bound NADPH-oxidase complex generates large quantities of $O_2^{\bullet-}$ (27). Transgenic mice that lack specific components of the NADPH-oxidase complex show increased susceptibility to pulmonary infection with *M. tuberculosis* (28,29) or *Aspergillus fumigatus* (30). However, the extent to which AMs use this system to generate ROS is not clear. Third, under conditions of ischemia, decreased perfusion, low oxygen tension, or trauma, xanthine dehydrogenase, an innocuous enzyme, acquires oxidase activity and uses xanthine and molecular oxygen to produce partially reduced oxygen species. Indeed, results of several studies suggest that xanthine oxidase may be released from intestine or liver into the circulation and bind to pulmonary endothelium, where it can serve as a locus for the intense production of ROS (31).

B. Reactive Nitrogen Species

•NO, one of the smallest and most unique biological mediators, is generated by nitric oxide synthase (NOS). •NO synthesis involves the five-electron oxidation of the guanidino nitrogen of L-arginine (32). In this reaction, molecular O_2 and NADPH act as cosubstrates, while tetrahydrobiopterin (H_4B) (33), flavin nucleotides (FMN and FAD), and thiols serve as enzyme cofactors (34). N^G-hydroxy-L-arginine is formed as a short-lived intermediate and L-citrulline is the by-product (35). •NO is an important mediator of normal physiological effects in a variety of different cell types, including neurons, smooth and skeletal muscle cells, hepatocytes, neutrophils, macrophages, and epithelial cells.

Endogenous nitric oxide synthases can be broadly classified into three types, based on their source, substrate dependency, and molecular biology: neuronal (nNOS, isoform I), endothelial (eNOS, isoform III), and inducible (iNOS, isoform II) (36). All NOS isoforms are homodimeric heme proteins, with oxygenase and reductase domains in the amino- and carboxy-termini, respectively (37). These domains are separated by a calcium/calmodulin-binding region. Formation of an active, dimeric enzyme complex also is dependent on H_4B. The reductase domain is homologous to NADPH-cytochrome P450 (38), and includes binding sites for NADPH, FMN, and FAD. During •NO synthesis, electrons donated by NADPH are transferred via the flavins and calmodulin to the catalytic heme (39). The constitutive forms have different phosphorylation sites, and eNOS has a unique amino-terminal myristylation site (40). Although the three human *Nos* genes are located on different chromosomes, considerable homology exists between them, suggesting common ancestry, with subsequent gene duplication and transposition.

nNOS and eNOS are constitutively expressed in cells as monomers, but their activity is regulated by the availability of calcium/calmodulin within the cell cytoplasm. When intracellular calcium concentrations increase in response to stimulation, binding of calmodulin allows dimerization and enzymatic activity (38). These isoforms generate •NO in small quantities for brief periods of time.

In contrast to nNOS and eNOS, iNOS protein generally is not constitutively expressed. Rather, transcription of *Nos2* in AMs, and possibly neutrophils, is triggered by proinflammatory stimuli, including endorphin-mediated stress (41), oxidative injury (42), depletion of nonferritin-bound iron (Fe^{2+}) (43), reduced oxygen tension (44), low environmental pH (45), bacterial endotoxin (46) or exotoxins (47), cross-linking of cell-surface CD23 (Fcγ receptor IIb) (48) or CD69 receptors (49), and cytokines (particularly IFN-α/β, IFN-γ, TNF-α, and IL-1β) (reviewed in Ref. 50). IFN-γ also stabilizes *Nos2* mRNA. Many anti-inflammatory agents, including glucocorticoids, cytokines (IL-4, IL-8, and IL-10), and growth factors (TGF-β) inhibit *Nos2* expression or decrease stability of *Nos2* mRNA (51). A number of signal transduction pathways have been implicated in regulation of *Nos2* gene transcription, including the Janus kinases, mitogen-activated protein kinases, protein kinase C, phosphatidylinositol-3 kinase, and protein phosphatases (52). Induction of IRF-1 and NF-κB transcription factor activity seems to be central to activation of *Nos2* transcription. It is important to note that, although iNOS and the NADPH-oxidase system are differentially regulated, they are both induced by similar proinflammatory stimuli, and so are likely to be simultaneously active and generating reactive species during an inflammatory response.

Once synthesized, iNOS localizes to the cytoplasm and intracellular vesicles (53). iNOS-like activity also has been identified in rat mitochondria (54). Because iNOS tightly binds calcium, its activity is calcium- and calmodulin-independent, permitting sustained catalysis (55). Provided substrate and cofactors are available, iNOS can generate large amounts of $^\bullet$NO for an extended period of time (56,57). Interestingly, in the absence of available L-arginine, iNOS can generate $O_2^{\bullet-}$ (58,59). iNOS does not appear to play a significant role in homeostasis in the normal animal. iNOS gene "knock-out" ($Nos2^{-/-}$) mice are born with a normal Mendelian frequency, show no deficits in growth and development, no evidence of pathology related to deletion of the gene, and reproduce normally (60). However, *Nos2* gene deletion does appear to result in upregulated pulmonary capillary endothelial transcytosis (61), although it is unclear whether this effect is related to some deficiency of $^\bullet$NO production, or is merely an epigenetic effect associated with deletion of the *Nos2* gene. Moreover, it appears that the lack of phenotype of $Nos2^{-/-}$ mice may be partly a result of redundancy of function between the iNOS and the NADPH-oxidase systems, because transgenic "double knock-out" mice lacking both functional systems ($Nos2^{-/-}/$ gp91phox$^{-/-}$) have significant defects in normal immunity to enteric commensal microbes (62).

Potential sources of $^\bullet$NO in the lungs include activated rat and human AMs (7,63), neutrophils (64), alveolar type II cells (65), endothelial cells (66), and airway cells (57). Both nNOS and eNOS have been identified in human lungs. nNOS is localized to nerve terminals that likely contribute to nonadrenergic/noncholinergic airway innervation, and is present in human and rat airway epithelial cells (66). eNOS is localized to pulmonary endothelium and bronchial epithelium (67). Studies have suggested that iNOS is constitutively expressed in human upper airway epithelium (68) and occasional AMs (66), but this may be a result of chronic exposure of these cells to inhaled pollutants and microbes (69). Expression of iNOS in other regions of the normal lung is believed to be minimal. However, iNOS has been immunolocalized to airway cells or human lung tissue obtained from patients with ARDS (70), bacterial pneumonia (71), hantavirus cardiopulmonary syndrome (72), lung cancer (73), pulmonary sarcoidosis (74), idiopathic pulmonary fibrosis (75), and asthma (62). Alveolar macrophages isolated from lungs of patients with tuberculosis (76) or ARDS following sepsis (77) have been shown to express iNOS. These findings raise the possibility that increased amounts of $^{\bullet}$NO may be released during lung inflammation into the epithelial lining fluid, where it may have both beneficial (antimicrobial) and detrimental (tissue-damaging) effects.

IV. Biological Effects of Reactive Oxygen and Nitrogen Species

A. The Dark Side of $^{\bullet}$NO

$^{\bullet}$NO is inactivated upon entering the blood stream because of its rapid and irreversible reaction with *oxy*-hemoglobin or *oxy*-myoglobin (78), resulting in formation of nitrate (NO_3^-) and methemoglobin (79):

$$Hb-Fe^{2+}-O_2 + {^{\bullet}NO} \longrightarrow Hb-Fe^{2+}-ONOO + NO_3^-$$

Therefore, inhaled $^{\bullet}$NO has been proposed to be of therapeutic value as a selective pulmonary vasodilator in treatment of bronchopulmonary dysplasia and ARDS (80). However, $^{\bullet}$NO is a free radical, and therefore can react with other free radicals, either to detoxify them or to create more toxic reactive species (81). Because cytotoxic effects of $^{\bullet}$NO are nonspecific, they are not limited to invading microbes but also can damage the cells and tissues that produce it (82). Moreover, $^{\bullet}$NO may contribute to the systemic morbidity of pathologic processes through its proposed activity as a peripheral arteriodilator (83), and because it can act as a myocardial depressant. Clinical use of $^{\bullet}$NO may therefore prove to be a double-edged sword.

There is now substantial experimental evidence that RNS may be involved in pulmonary epithelial injury in a variety of pathological situations. Induction of immune complex alveolitis in rat lungs results in increased alveolar epithelial permeability, which is associated with the presence of elevated concentrations of $^{\bullet}$NO decomposition products in bronchoalveolar lavage (BAL) fluid (84). Alveolar instillation of the NOS inhibitor L-NMMA ameliorates $^{\bullet}$NO production and alveolar epithelial injury. Similarly, paraquat-induced (85) and ischemia–reperfusion-induced (86) lung injury are both associated with stimulation of $^{\bullet}$NO synthesis, and are abrogated by NOS inhibitors. Tracheal epithelial cytopathology induced by *Bordetella pertussis* is associated with induction of $^{\bullet}$NO synthesis, and is remarkably attenuated by inhibition of NOS (82). Likewise, influenza virus-induced lung pathology in mice results from increased expression of iNOS and increased generation of $^{\bullet}$NO (87). Administration of NOS inhibitors significantly improves survival of influenza-infected mice. Additional evidence that RNS play a role in pulmonary inflammation is derived from studies utilizing transgenic $Nos2^{-/-}$ mice. Lung damage induced by either injection of LPS (88), influenza virus infection (89), or hemorrhage and resuscitation (90), is markedly reduced in these mutant mice. Similarly, in an experimental murine model of allergic airway disease, deletion of the $Nos2$ gene results in a significant decrease in eosinophil infiltration into the lungs (91).

Since $^{\bullet}$NO has an unpaired electron, it can readily react with other free radicals. At high (nonphysiologic) concentrations, $^{\bullet}$NO molecules can react with molecular oxygen to form the highly toxic agent nitrogen dioxide (NO_2). However, when $^{\bullet}$NO is present at physiologic and even pathologic concentrations, the low probability of two $^{\bullet}$NO molecules interacting makes formation of NO_2 unlikely (81). In pathologic states, most of the toxic effects of $^{\bullet}$NO have been attributed instead to its reaction with $O_2^{\bullet-}$ to form peroxynitrite ($ONOO^-$), which is a potent oxidizing and nitrating agent. When both $^{\bullet}$NO and $O_2^{\bullet-}$ are present, this reaction occurs extremely rapidly, at a near diffusion-limited rate (k_m is approximately $6.7 \times 10^9\ M^{-1}\ sec^{-1}$) (92,93). By trans-isomerization, peroxynitrous acid ($ONOOH$), the protonated form of $ONOO^-$, also can form nitrogen dioxide ($^{\bullet}NO_2$) and an intermediate with reactivity equivalent to the $^{\bullet}$OH radical (23):

$$O_2^{\bullet-} + {^{\bullet}NO} \longrightarrow ONOO^- + H^+ \longrightarrow ONOOH \longrightarrow [{^{\bullet}OH} \cdots {^{\bullet}NO_2}]$$

Under physiological conditions, a minimum of 25% of $ONOO^-$ will decompose to form [$^{\bullet}$OH $^{\bullet}NO_2$], the remainder recombining to form NO_3^-. In addition, metal ions, such as Fe^{3+} and Cu^{3+} (in the active site of SOD) can catalyze heterolysis of $ONOO^-$ to form a nitronium-ion-like species (NO_2^+) (94,95). While being highly reactive, its slow rate of decomposition under physiological conditions allows $ONOO^-$ to diffuse for up to several cell diameters (probably as peroxynitrous acid, $ONOOH$) before becoming inactive (96). Moreover, because of its neutrality and low Stokes' radius, smooth muscle- and endothelium-derived $^{\bullet}$NO can easily diffuse across membranes into the alveolar space (97), where it can combine with epithelial cell- or AM-derived $O_2^{\bullet-}$ to form $ONOO^-$ in the epithelial lining fluid. Interactions between reactive oxygen and nitrogen species that may be of biologic importance are summarized in Fig.1.

It can be argued that alveolar cells and the epithelial lining fluid contain a number of antioxidant substances, such as SODs, catalase, reduced glutathione, and urate, which will limit the steady-state concentrations of reactive oxygen and nitrogen species in vivo. Indeed, under normal conditions, intracellular $O_2^{\bullet-}$ concentrations are kept low ($< 10\,pM$), and forma-

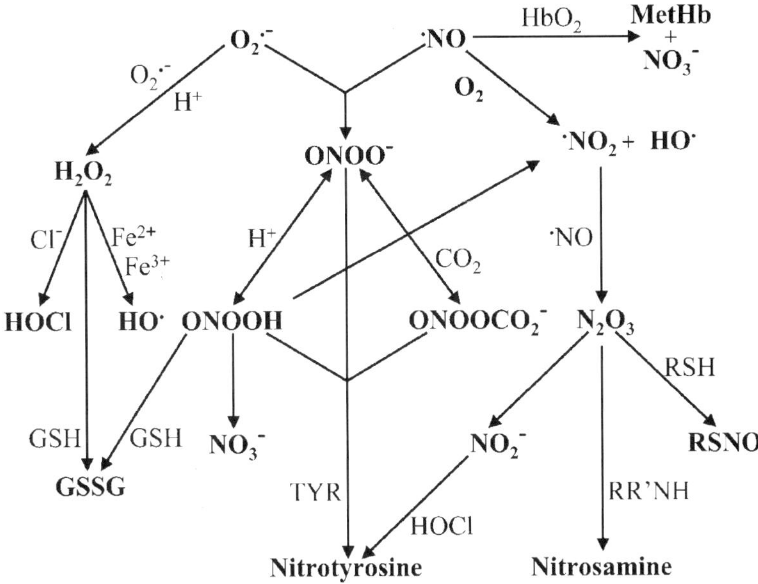

Figure 1 Interactions between reactive oxygen and nitrogen species that may be of biologic importance. Superoxide ($O_2^{\bullet-}$) generated by the mitochondrial electron transport chain or the NADPH-oxidase complex can dismutate to H_2O_2 (spontaneously, or in the presence of SOD). H_2O_2 can oxidize glutathione (GSH). Alternatively, in the presence of neutrophil myeloperoxidase and chloride ions (Cl^-), H_2O_2 is converted to the potent oxidizing agent hypochlorous acid (HOCl). In the presence of free iron (Fe^{2+} or Fe^{3+}), H_2O_2 is reduced to the highly reactive hydroxyl radical ($^{\bullet}OH$). Nitric oxide ($^{\bullet}NO$), generated by nitric oxide synthase, is rapidly inactivated by interaction with *oxy*-hemoglobin (HbO_2), generating *met*-hemoglobin (MetHb) and nitrate (NO_3^-). However, when $O_2^{\bullet-}$ is present, it rapidly reacts with $^{\bullet}NO$ to form the potent oxidizing and nitrating agents peroxynitrite ($ONOO^-$) and peroxynitrous acid (ONOOH), which can nitrate thiols (RSH), GSH, or tyrosine residues (TYR). In the presence of CO_2, $ONOO^-$ forms the nitrosoperoxycarbonate anion ($ONOOCO_2^-$), which may also be a potent nitrating agent. Alternatively, ONOOH can isomerize to form nitrogen dioxide ($^{\bullet}NO_2$) and an intermediate with reactivity equivalent to $^{\bullet}OH$. In turn, $^{\bullet}NO_2$ can react with $^{\bullet}NO$ to form dinitrogen trioxide (N_2O_3), which is capable of nitrating RSH and amines (RR'NH), and which degrades to nitrite (NO_2^-). In the presence of HOCl, NO_2^- may also nitrate TYR.

tion of $ONOO^-$ prevented, because eukaryotic cells contain large amounts of SOD (4–10 μM). However, when synthesis of $O_2^{\bullet-}$ and $^{\bullet}NO$ increase during an inflammatory response, micromolar quantities of $^{\bullet}NO$ can effectively compete with SOD for $O_2^{\bullet-}$, and $ONOO^-$ is generated. Moreover, because of its high reactivity, $ONOO^-$ can attack biologic targets even in the presence of antioxidant substances (98). Production of $ONOO^-$ by human neutrophils

(99), rat AMs (7), and bovine aortic endothelial cells (66), has been demonstrated using a luminol-dependent chemiluminescence assay.

One of the major cytotoxic effects of RNS is that they can inhibit eukaryotic gene expression by several mechanisms. Firstly, $^{\bullet}$NO and $ONOO^-$ can induce nucleotide deamination, resulting in abasic sites and DNA strand breaks (100). These trigger activation of the nuclear enzyme poly-ADP-ribosyl transferase (PART) (101). Activated PART catalyzes the attachment of ADP-ribose units to nuclear proteins, resulting in depletion of energy stores and reduced protein synthesis (102,103). Secondly, stimulated macrophages can produce enough $^{\bullet}$NO to inhibit activity of the iron–sulfur center of ribonucleotide reductase, the enzyme that converts ribonucleotides to the deoxyribonucleotides necessary for DNA synthesis (104). $ONOO^-$ and high concentrations of $^{\bullet}$NO can inactivate critical mitochondrial enzymes, such as aconitase, cytochrome *c* oxidase, and NADH:ubiquinone oxidoreductase, by interacting with the nonheme iron of iron–sulfur centers (105–108). Inhibition of mitochondrial respiration results in dissipation of mitochondrial transmembrane electrochemical proton-motive force, reduced ATP generation, and decreased protein synthesis (109). In addition, $^{\bullet}$NO can modulate the activity of redox-sensitive transcription factors including nuclear factor-kappa B (NF-κB) and AP-1 components (110). For example, $^{\bullet}$NO decreases cytokine-induced endothelial cell activation by altering expression of I-κBα (the α isoform of the inhibitor of NF-κB) to prevent nuclear translocation of NF-κB. This may block transcription of both vascular cell adhesion molecule (111) and iNOS itself (112). In contrast, in other studies, $^{\bullet}$NO has been shown to directly enhance gene activity by eliciting nuclear translocation of NF-κB (113) and AP-1 subunits *c-fos*, and *jun*B (110). Finally, $ONOO^-$ can initiate iron-independent peroxidation of lipids, resulting in damage to cellular membranes (114).

Protein thiols are important cellular targets of RNS. Although $^{\bullet}$NO can directly react with thiol groups, this reaction is kinetically unfavorable and requires the nearby presence of a strong electron acceptor such as Fe^{3+}. In contrast, $ONOO^-$ (and other species such as N_2O_3 and NO^+) can oxidize thiols to form *S*-nitrosothiols (RS-NO) at high rates. Many transcription factors contain thiol residues in motifs critical for DNA binding (e.g., zinc-finger proteins). These thiols can be modified by $ONOO^-$, and this may inhibit DNA binding and gene transcription (115). Normal function of other biologically important proteins may also be modified by *S*-nitrosylation. For example, *S*-nitrosylation of glyceraldehyde-3-phosphate dehydrogenase inhibits its enzymatic activity (101). Similarly, nitrosylation of the neuronal *N*-methyl D-aspartate (NMDA) receptor results in decreased calcium transport and neuroprotection (116). Alternatively, formation of RS-NO adducts may serve to stabilize $^{\bullet}$NO, decreasing its cytotoxic potential while maintaining its bioactive properties. Micromolar concentrations of *S*-nitrosoglutathione (GS-NO) have been detected in normal human BAL fluid ex vivo and levels are significantly increased in the lungs of patients with pneumonia or during inhalation of 80 ppm $^\bullet$NO (117).

It has been proposed that a low level of constitutive iNOS expression in cells of the human respiratory tract may result in formation of RS-NO in the alveolar lining fluid, and that this pool of stored $^\bullet$NO has important physiologic functions in the lung (61). Besides having some degree of microbistatic effect at the level of the respiratory mucosa (see below), RS-NO may regulate pulmonary endothelial and/or epithelial fluid transport, and have important effects on peripheral blood flow. It recently has been demonstrated that when hemoglobin passes through the lung, cysteine 93 of the β chain becomes charged with a nitroso group, possibly derived from alveolar RS-NO (83). Discharge of this group as $^\bullet$NO in peripheral arterioles, in response to changing arterial O_2 tension, may regulate their diameter and resistance to flow. However, other studies have shown that nitrosylation of *oxy*-hemoglobin increases its affinity for O_2. This implies that $^\bullet$NO transfer from deoxygenated SNO-hemoglobin in vivo would be limited to regions of extremely low O_2 tension. Furthermore, the kinetics of the transnitrosation reactions between GSH and SNO-hemoglobin are relatively slow, making transfer of $^\bullet$NO from SNO-hemoglobin to GSH less likely as a mechanism to elicit vessel relaxation under conditions of low oxygen tension and over the circulatory lifetime of a given red blood cell. Moreover, the physiological relevance of $^\bullet$NO release in precapillary arterioles is unclear, since it is unlikely that $^\bullet$NO released at this site can diffuse far enough into the relatively thick vessel wall to alter its tone.

Another potential role for RS-NO is in the regulation of apoptotic cell death. Activation of caspase enzymes, which is central to the execution of the apoptotic program, requires proteolytic removal of an N-terminal prodomain, can be triggered autocatalytically by proenzyme dimerization or by other active caspase molecules (reviewed in Ref. 118). Recently, it has been shown that *S*-nitrosylation of procaspase-3 also prevents its activation, and that *S*-nitrosylated procaspase-3 is present in T- and B-cell lines (119). However, there are clear differences in pathways of caspase activation in primary lymphocytes and lymphocyte cell-lines (120,121), and it is unclear whether procaspase activation is regulated by *S*-nitrosylation in primary lymphocytes, or if this phenomenon merely contributes to the capacity of leukemic cell lines to grow in an immortalized fashion.

Both $ONOO^-$ and NO_2^+ can nitrate phenolic compounds, including proteins containing tyrosine and tryptophan amino acid residues. Due to the relatively higher concentration of CO_2 in plasma (1.2 mM), the majority of $ONOO^-$ generated in biological fluids, such as the epithelial lining fluid, will react with CO_2 to form the nitrosoperoxycarbonate anion ($O{=}N{-}OOCO_2^-$) (122,123). This reaction can enhance the nitrating activity of $ONOO^-$ while at the same time, bicarbonate prevents ascorbate and urate from inhibiting $ONOO^-$-induced nitration (122–125). However, it is not clear that this reaction is biologically relevant. Berlett et al. have reported that in the absence of CO_2, $ONOO^-$ is an oxidizing but not a nitrating agent (126), while Pfeiffer and Mayer (127) have shown that $ONOO^-$ does not nitrate free tyrosine in either the presence or absence of CO_2. Alternatively, physiological levels of CO_2 may enhance nitration by increasing the activity of iNOS, by an as-yet uncharacterized mechanism (128).

Another possible mechanism for tyrosine nitration involves the interaction of HOCl, the product of neutrophil MPO, with H_2O_2, NO_2^-, and $ONOO^-$. iNOS is colocalized with MPO within neutrophils (129), suggesting that alternate substrates for MPO are present simultaneously. van der Vliet et al. have demonstrated that heme peroxidases can catalyze the nitration of phenolic compounds (including tyrosine) by oxidation products of NO_2^- in the presence of H_2O_2 (130). In addition, Eiserich et al. found that NO_2^- can act as a substrate for MPO, resulting in the nitration, chlorination, and oxidation of tyrosine residues in proteins (131). The physiological relevance of these nitration reactions was first demonstrated using neutrophils or monocytes as the source of MPO and H_2O_2 (132,133). Subsequent studies have determined in more detail the extent to which these species can nitrate, chlorinate, oxidize specific target proteins, and inhibit their function in vivo during lung inflammation. MacPherson et al. (134) have identified eosinophils and eosinophil peroxidase (EPO) as a major source of oxidants during asthma. Similarly, Hickman-Davis et al. (135) have demonstrated that neutrophils are absolutely required for formation of nitrated protein adducts in the lungs of *Mycoplasma pulmonis*-infected mice. In addition, Gaut et al. (136) have shown that both chlorotyrosine and nitrotyrosine are concomitantly produced in inflammatory foci. Finally, elegant studies by Brennan et al. (137) show that the extent to which EPO- and MPO-catalyzed reactions contribute to tyrosine nitration in vivo is very much dependent on the underlying cause of the inflammatory response, and that nitrogen dioxide ($^\bullet NO_2$), which is the one-electron oxidation product of NO_2^-, may be involved in these nitration reactions. However, the specific proteins modified by these reactions, and the functional consequences of such modification remain undefined.

The classical mechanism of oxygen atom transfer between HOCl and NO_2^- ($NO_2^- + HOCl \rightarrow HCl + NO_3^-$) cannot account for tyrosine nitration and chlorination by these reactive species. Instead, a reaction involving Cl^+ transfer from HOCl to NO_2^- has been proposed, which would yield the strong nitrating and chlorinating species $Cl-NO_2$ (131). The Cl^+ character of $Cl-NO_2$ in aqueous solution makes it possible to react directly with tyrosine via electron transfer to yield an intermediate radical pair (tyrosyl radical–$Cl^\bullet-NO_2^-$). Radical collapse of this complex will lead to the formation of chlorotyrosine and NO_2^-. Alternatively, dissociation of the radical pair complex and the subsequent oxidation of NO_2^- by $Cl^\bullet$ will result in the formation of tyrosyl radicals and $^\bullet NO_2$. Tyrosyl radicals in proteins, which are more long-lived than free tyrosyl radicals, are targets for nitration by $^\bullet NO_2$ via rapid radical–radical reaction ($k = 3 \times 10^9 \, M^{-1} \, sec^{-1}$) (138) and two tyrosyl radicals can combine to form dityrosine. However, it should be noted that the reactive intermediate $Cl\text{-}NO_2$ has a short half-life, and is rapidly hydrolyzed to NO_3^- and Cl^- ($Cl\text{-}NO_2 + H_2O \rightarrow NO_3^- + Cl^- + 2H^+$) when there are no other targets such as tyrosine or proteins in the solution.

Because the formation of $ONOO^-$ requires only the spontaneous and diffusion-limited reaction of $^\bullet NO$ and $O_2^{\bullet -}$, it is likely that $ONOO^-$ would be the first strong oxidant generated during an inflammatory response. Any $^\bullet NO$ that avoids collision with $O_2^{\bullet -}$ might then be slowly oxidized to NO_2^-, which would then serve as a substrate for MPO-catalyzed reactions. Alternatively, NO_2^- from other tissues could leak into the alveolar space and act as a MPO substrate. Consequently, in the presence of H_2O_2, both direct NO_2^- oxidation or oxidation through HOCl and $Cl\text{-}NO_2$ generation by MPO may be significant sources of NT during inflammation. It should be noted that these reactions can be catalyzed by neutrophils in the absence of macrophages, and that these reactions may have more pathologic significance for tyrosine nitration of extracellular proteins, such as SP-A, than for nitration of intracellular proteins, such as actin (137).

Irrespective of mechanism, several studies have provided evidence that nitration reactions occur in vivo during inflammatory processes. 3-nitrotyrosine residues, products of the addition of a nitro group (NO_2) to the ortho position of the hydroxyl group of tyrosine, are stable end-products of RNS-mediated reactions (139). They therefore serve as footprints of RNS action, which are readily detectable by immunohistochemistry and ELISA (140). Nitrotyrosine residue formation has been detected in the lungs of infants who died with respiratory failure or ARDS (141), adults with ARDS (141) or idiopathic pulmonary fibrosis (75), and adults who died of hantavirus cardiopulmonary syndrome (72). Nitrated ceruloplasmin, transferrin, α_1-protease inhibitor, α_1-antichymotrypsin, and β-chain fibrinogen have also been detected in the plasma of patients with ARDS (142). Experimentally, nitrotyrosine can be found in the lungs of rats exposed to endotoxin (143) or hyperoxia (141), and in the lungs of mice infected with *M. pulmonis* (57). Such findings indicate that in vivo injury to the alveolar epithelium and pulmonary surfactant system during pulmonary inflammation, which has previously been attributed to ROS, may be caused instead by RONS such as $ONOO^-$ (144,145).

Several reports have indicated that protein nitration may lead to loss of function. Nitration of tyrosine residues in human IgG, but not rabbit IgG, abrogated C_{1q}-binding activity (146). This is consistent with the presence of a tyrosine residue at the C_{1q} receptor-binding site in human but not rabbit IgG. The inactivation of *Escherichia coli* dUTPase by nitration and the occurrence of a tyrosine residue in a strictly conserved sequence motif suggests the critical importance of this residue for the function of the enzyme (147). Nitration of tyrosine residues in the α_1-protease inhibitor resulted in selective loss of elastase inhibitory activity but not chymotrypsin or trypsin inhibitory activity (148). Tyrosine nitration also inhibits protein phosphorylation by tyrosine kinases in vitro (149), although the in vivo relevance of this finding has not been demonstrated. Likewise, exposure of SP-A to tetranitromethane or ONOO$^-$ led to nitration of a single tyrosine residue in its carbohydrate recognition domain and reduced the ability of SP-A to aggregate lipids and bind to mannose in vitro (145,150,151). Nitrated SP-A also failed to enhance opsonophagocytosis of *Pneumocystis carinii* by rat AMs, a necessary event in the killing of *P. carinii* (152). This finding may be of in vivo relevance since human AMs have recently been shown to nitrate SP-A (128). Similarly, in vitro exposure to nitrating agents did not alter the activity of α_1-antichymotrypsin, but reduced the ferroxidase activity of ceruloplasmin and the elastase-inhibiting activity of α_1-protease inhibitor, and enhanced the rate of interaction of fibrinogen with thrombin (142). However, it is not yet clear that levels of protein nitration and chlorination detected in vivo are sufficient to result in significant loss of function.

Despite such caveats, there is some experimental evidence to suggest that $^\bullet$NO may damage pulmonary surfactant by nitration in vivo. Exposure of newborn piglets to 100 ppm $^\bullet$NO in 95% O$_2$ for 48 hr resulted in significant injury to the surfactant system (153). Similarly, pulmonary surfactant samples from neonatal lambs exposed to $^\bullet$NO gas (200 ppm) for 6 hr exhibited abnormal surfactant properties and reduced ability to aggregate lipids in vitro (154). Together, these studies indicate that prolonged inhalation of therapeutic $^\bullet$NO by ARDS patients may lead to subacute lung injury, exacerbating pulmonary dysfunction. However, it should be noted that these effects were seen with high concentrations of inhaled $^\bullet$NO, and it is not yet clear that similar effects occur when therapeutic doses of $^\bullet$NO are used.

B. The Good Side of $^\bullet$NO

Although formation of ONOO$^-$ can result in tissue damage, $^\bullet$NO can ameliorate tissue injury by several mechanisms. $^\bullet$NO binds the heme group of soluble guanylate cyclase, increasing synthesis of cyclic guanosine-3′-5′-monophosphate (cGMP) (155). Effects of cGMP are mediated through cGMP-associated protein kinases (PKGs), which act to lower intracellular calcium (156). Activation of guanylate cyclase by $^\bullet$NO can result in inhibition of platelet and neutrophil adhesion to endothelium, and thereby reduce cell-mediated inflammatory damage (157). It can also result in increased ciliary motility (158) and increased mucin production (159). $^\bullet$NO may directly inhibit activity of the NADPH-oxidase complex (160), while reaction of $^\bullet$NO with any O$_2$$^{\bullet-}$ that is generated may protect $O_2^{\bullet-}$-sensitive target molecules. The reaction with $^{\bullet}NO$ outcompetes SOD kinetically, and forces $O_2^{\bullet-}$ through $ONOO^-$ oxidation and decomposition pathways. As well as reducing steady-state levels of $O_2^{\bullet-}$, this reaction limits H_2O_2 buildup, which may be especially important under conditions favoring $O_2^{\bullet-}$-dependent $^{\bullet}OH$ formation (161). Additionally, $^{\bullet}NO$ can bind to the free coordination sites of heme-bound iron (162), and thereby indirectly acts as an iron chelator (163). $^{\bullet}NO$ has also been shown to induce synthesis of the antioxidant glutathione (GSH) (164), and to react rapidly with tyrosyl radicals (k_m is $1 \pm 0.3 \times 10^9\,M^{-1}\,sec^{-1}$) to limit the extent of nitrotyrosine formation (165). Finally, by annihilating lipid radical species, such as alkoxyl ($LO^{\bullet}$) and peroxyl ($LOO^{\bullet}$) radicals, $^{\bullet}NO$ can inhibit oxidant-induced membrane and lipoprotein oxidation and terminate chain radical propagation reactions (114). These reactions may be of particular importance, since $^{\bullet}NO$ significantly concentrates in lipophilic cellular compartments (166). However, species resulting from the reaction of $^{\bullet}NO$ with lipid peroxides may themselves be toxic.

Several observations have suggested that $^{\bullet}NO$ can protect the lungs from oxidant stress. In buffer-perfused isolated rabbit lungs, inhaled $^{\bullet}NO$ (24 ppm) ameliorated the increase in pulmonary vascular permeability produced by intravascular generation of H_2O_2, while inhibition of endogenous $^{\bullet}NO$ exacerbated an oxidant-mediated increase in capillary filtration (167). Moreover, treatment of rats with the NOS inhibitor aminoguanidine exacerbated hyperoxia-induced lung injury (168). However, effects of NOS inhibitors may be nonspecific, and results of such studies must be interpreted with caution.

Many studies have provided evidence that RNS may have antimicrobial roles in host defense, during both the innate and adaptive phases of the immune response. Reactive nitrogen species have been most strongly implicated in host defense against intracellular pathogens. However, not all pulmonary pathogens are equally susceptible to the activity of RNS. For example, $Nos2^{-/-}$ mice are extremely susceptible to death from *Chlamydia pneumoniae* (169) or *M. tuberculosis* (170) infection, but have normal resistance to infection of *Legionella pneumophila* (171). However, the reasons for these differences in pathogen susceptibility to RNS remain poorly defined.

The role of RNS in protecting the murine lung from infection with *M. pulmonis* has been examined in several studies (e.g., Refs. 172–175). Infection of mice with this pathogen provides an animal model that reproduces the essential features of human respiratory mycoplasmosis (caused by *M. pneumoniae*), which is responsible for 20–30% of all pneumonias in the general population of the United States. Mouse strains differ markedly in their resistance to *M. pulmonis*, with C57BL/6 being highly resistant to respiratory infection with this pathogen (172). During the first 72 hr postinfection, the number of mycoplasma decreases by more than 83% in the lungs of C57BL/6 mice, with maximal mycoplasmacidal activity occurring in the first 8 hr postinfection. Demonstration of specific antibody in serum, as well as an increase in the number of macrophages, neutrophils, or lymphocytes in the lungs, does not occur until at least 72 hr postinfection (173,174). Thus, nonspecific intrapulmonary killing of *M. pulmonis* is apparently involved, most likely mediated by rapidly activated resident AMs. The collectin SP-A binds to mycoplasma in a concentration- and partially Ca^{2+}-dependent manner, and significantly enhances the killing of these organisms in vitro (57). SP-A probably serves to modulate AM function, rather than acting as a nonspecific opsonin of mycoplasma. Addition of the iNOS inhibitor, N^G-monomethyl-l-arginine (L-NMMA), to AM cultures abrogates SP-A-mediated mycoplasmacidal activity. Concentrations of nitrate and nitrite (NO_2^-) (the decomposition products of $^\bullet NO$) were significantly increased in cultures containing SP-A and decreased in cultures containing l-NMMA (57). Moreover, when resistant C57BL/6 and strain-matched transgenic C57BL $Nos2^{-/-}$ were infected with *M. pulmonis*, the gene knockout mice had significantly greater mycoplasmal growth in the lungs and significantly more severe lung pathology after infection than did control C57BL $Nos2^{+/+}$ mice (175) (Fig. 2).

While $^\bullet NO$ is a well-recognized product of microbicidal macrophages, the mechanism(s) by which $^\bullet NO$ facilitates host defense remain undefined. $^\bullet NO$ may have direct microbicidal effects by reacting with iron or thiol groups on proteins to form iron-nitrosyl complexes and thereby inactivate enzymes important in DNA replication or mitochondrial respiration (see above). In circumstances in which $ONOO^-$ has no apparent effect, $^\bullet NO$ is directly microbicidal for some pathogens, including *Staphylococcus aureus* (176), *Leishmania major* (177), and *Giardia lamblia* (178). In contrast, other pathogens, such as *Salmonella typhimurium* (179), *E. coli* (180,181) and *Rhodococcus equi* (182), are killed by $ONOO^-$, but not by $^\bullet NO$ alone. Indeed, IFN-γ-activated murine AMs have been shown to produce $^\bullet NO$ ($1.1\,\mu M/hr/10^5$ AMs) in the presence of SP-A and mycoplasmas and to cause a significant decrease in mycoplasmal numbers (57). However, in the absence of AMs, even the significant amounts of $^\bullet NO$ (4–6 μM) produced by PAPANONOate had no effect on mycoplasmal survival, while the combination of $^\bullet NO$ and $O_2^{\bullet -}$ (generated by SIN-1) was toxic (175). $ONOO^-$ generation by 1 mM SIN-1 at 37°C was $\sim 1\,\mu M/min$ and caused a significant decrease in mycoplasma CFUs by 20 min, with complete killing by 90 min. Mycoplasmal killing was concentration dependent, with significant reduction of CFUs occurring only after exposure to $\sim 20\,\mu M$ of $ONOO^-$: 500 μM SIN-1 caused significant mycoplasmal killing by 45 min (22 μM $ONOO^-$) and 200 μM SIN-1 caused significant killing by 90 min (18 μM $ONOO^-$) (Fig. 3). The addition of bovine copper–zinc SOD (Cu,Zn-SOD) attenuated SP-A-mediated mycoplasmal killing by activated AMs (Fig. 4). Similarly, in the absence of AMs, inhibition of $>90\%$ of $ONOO^-$ production by bovine Cu,ZnSOD was protective against the mycoplasmaci-

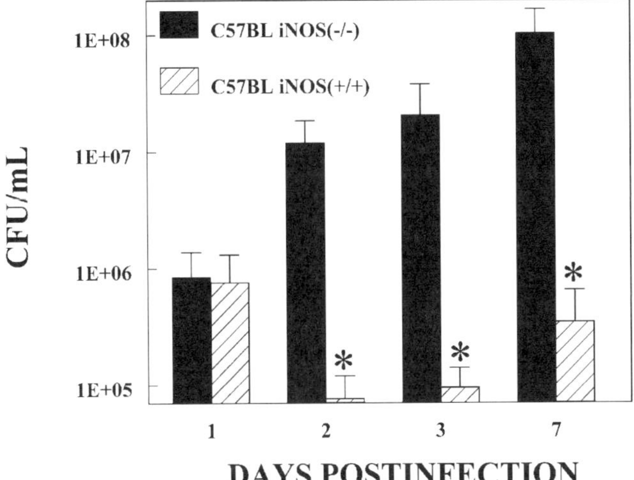

DAYS POSTINFECTION

Figure 2   Effect of iNOS deficiency on resistance to *M. pulmonis* infection in vivo. C57BL $Nos2^{-/-}$ and control C57BL $Nos2^{+/+}$ mice were infected intranasally with 1.5×10^7 CFU/mL *M. pulmonis*. All mice were euthanized at 1, 2, 3 or 7 days p.i., and the mean numbers of CFU (total recoverable mycoplasmas) were determined on whole lung homogenates. *Significant difference between control and experimental groups at each time point, $p < 0.05$. Results of quantitative cultures are means $\pm$ SE; $n = 18$. (Adapted from Ref. 175.)

dal effects of SIN-1. Catalase, however, had no effect on mycoplasma growth, indicating that H_2O_2 was not important in killing. Likewise, the generation of H_2O_2 or ${}^{\bullet}OH$ by xanthine oxidase (in the presence of xanthine and Fe^{3+}) had only a minimal effect on mycoplasmal. These data indicate that $O_2^{\bullet-}$ as well as ${}^{\bullet}NO$ is necessary for mycoplasma killing and further implicate $ONOO^-$ as the primary bactericidal reactive oxygen–nitrogen metabolite growth (57,175).

A number of pathogenic bacteria appear to have developed resistance to killing by ROS and RNS (reviewed in Ref. 183). For instance,*M. tuberculosis* contains two gene products (NoxR1 and NoxR3) thatprotect against both ROS and RNS by an undefined mechanism; these gene products are absent from nonpathogenic or opportunistic mycobacteria (184,185).

C. Other Effects of ${}^{\bullet}NO$

RNS have important immunomodulatory functions that may impact on pulmonary host defense and modulate pulmonary inflammation. Clearly, dependent on the circumstance and the effect, immunomodulation by RNS may have both beneficial and detrimental effects on the host. Besides inhibiting lymphocyte proliferation, RNS have been shown to modulate activity of a wide range of signal transduction pathways in leukocytes,

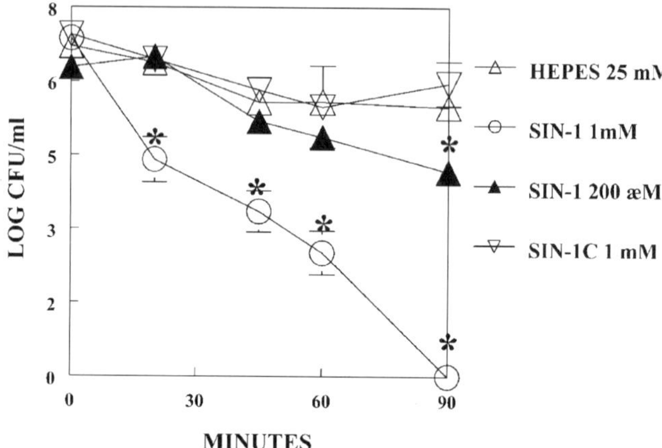

Figure 3 Effect of reactive oxygen and nitrogen species on mycoplasmal killing in the absence of AMs. *Mycoplasma pulmonis* was grown to late log phase, washed to remove serum and resuspended in 10 mL of 25 mM HEPES buffer, pH 7.4. All experiments were performed in sterile 130 mL centrifuge tubes and agitated constantly in a shaking water bath at 37°C. Aliquots were taken at 0, 20, 45, 60, and 90 min for determination of CFU. (A) HEPES 25 mM: mycoplasmas alone; SIN-1 1 mM: mycoplasmas + 1 mM SIN-1; SIN-1 200 µM: mycoplasmas + 200 µM SIN-1; SIN-1C: mycoplasmas + 1 mM SIN-1C. (B) HEPES 25 mM: mycoplasmas alone; PAPA 100 µM: mycoplasmas + 100 µM PAPANONOate; Cu,ZnSOD 3000 U/mL: mycoplasmas + 1 mM SIN-1 + 3000 U/mL Cu,ZnSOD; Cu,ZnSOD 500 U/mL: mycoplasmas + 1 mM SIN-1 + 500 U/mL Cu,ZnSOD. *Significant difference between control and experimental groups at each time point, $p < 0.05$. (Adapted from Ref. 175.)

including ion channels, G proteins, protein kinases, protein phosphatases, and caspases, by mechanisms as diverse as *S*-nitrosylation, *S*-glutathionylation, disruption of zinc fingers, or formation of iron-nitrosyl complexes (reviewed in Ref. 50). Reactive nitrogen species also influence production of both pro- and anti-inflammatory cytokines in host leukocytes. Of particular importance, native $^{\bullet}$NO, GS-NO, and ONOO^{-}, have variously been shown to either induce or prevent apoptosis of leukocytes. For example, high concentrations of exogenous $^{\bullet}$NO are proapoptotic for T cells and macrophages, partly because $^{\bullet}$NO inhibits degradation of polyubiquitinated p53 by the proteasome (186), but also because $^{\bullet}$NO can induce increased expression of Fas ligand (CD95L) on these cells (187). In contrast, low-level endogenous generation of $^{\bullet}$NO appears to be antiapoptotic in macrophages (188,189) and lymphocyte cell lines (119), possibly because *S*-nitrosylation of procaspase-3 prevents its activation (see above). However, the relevance of these effects to normal function of pulmonary immune cells has not been investigated.

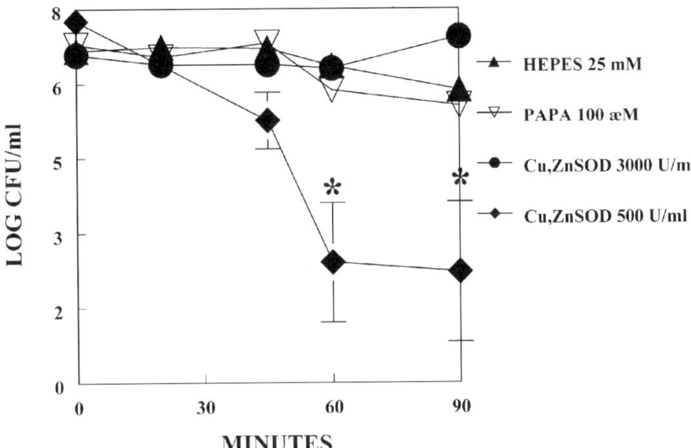

Figure 4 Effect of Cu,ZnSOD on SP-A-mediated killing of *M. pulmonis* by C57BL AMs. AMs were cultured for 18 hr with 100 U/mL of IFN-γ, washed and incubated with 1000 U/mL of Cu,ZnSOD at 37°C for 30 min. AMs were treated with SP-A (25 μg/mL) or HEPES (5 mM), infected with 10^{10} CFU of *M. pulmonis* and incubated at 37°C for 0 and 6 hr. Positive control AM cultures lacking Cu,ZnSOD were processed at the same time. Results of quantitative cultures are means ± SE from a total of three experiments with 12–15 data points per group. *Significant difference between control and experimental groups at each time point, $p < 0.05$. (Adapted from Ref. 175.)

V. Reactive Species in ALI and ARDS

The clinical syndrome of ALI/ARDS represents a common response of the lung to insults including sepsis, endotoxemia, trauma, aspiration, and pneumonia (190) (Chapter 3). Pulmonary edema is a major component of clinical ALI/ARDS, and results primarily from increased permeability of the alveolar capillary barrier (191). Many studies have provided evidence that RNS are involved in the development and progression of experimental ALI/ARDS (1,141,192–199).

A. Evidence from In Vitro and Ex Vivo Experiments

Exposure of mouse or rat AMs in vivo or in vitro to diverse proinflammatory stimuli, such as cytokines (IL-1, TNF-α, IFN-γ), lipopolysaccharide (LPS), various pathogens, respirable dusts, or oxidant gases, induces upregulated activity of both iNOS (183) and membrane-bound NADPH oxidase (200), and results in increased elaboration of both •NO and $O_2^{•-}$. Although, mitogen-activated human AMs can generate $ONOO^-$ in vitro (7), it has been unclear whether activated AMs, which are present in large numbers in the alveolar lining fluid in inflammatory conditions, but which lack MPO, contribute to the nitration and oxidation of proteins detected in the edema fluid (EF) of patients with ALI (201). Zhu et al. (128) addressed this question by assessing whether RONS generated by AMs could nitrate and oxidize human SP-A in vitro. Exposure of SP-A to LPS-activated rat AMs in the presence of physiological concentrations of CO_2 (1.2 mM) resulted in enhanced SP-A nitration (Fig. 5), and nitration on three tyrosine residues (128). Interestingly, in the presence of CO_2, AM iNOS activity was increased, as measured both by higher levels of NO_2^- and NO_3^- in the medium (Fig. 6) and enhanced conversion of L-[U-^{14}C] arginine to L-[U-^{14}C] citrulline (128). These findings indicate that physiological quantities of $ONOO^-$, which are likely to be similar to those encountered in vivo during an inflammatory response, can nitrate proteins such as SP-A and that CO_2 increases nitration both by enhancing NOS activity and by allowing formation of more efficient nitrating intermediates such as $ONO_2CO_2^-$. Enhanced NOS activity may result partly from formation of the short-lived ONO_2CO^- adduct itself, which may mitigate the oxidative inactivation of NOS by longer-lived $ONOO^-$ molecules.

B. Evidence from Clinical Studies

Clinical ALI and ARDS are characterized by severe diffuse inflammation in the lung parenchyma. Unfortunately, it is technically difficult to find direct evidence to implicate RONS as pathologic mediators of lung damage in ARDS. Attempts to directly measure RONS generation in situ are nearly always unsuccessful because the biological half-life of these molecules is in the range of nanoseconds to milliseconds in length. Moreover, concentra-

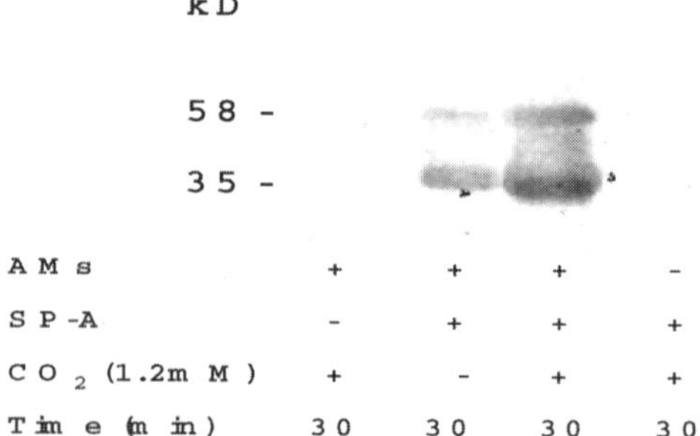

Figure 5 CO_2 enhanced nitration of SP-A by LPS-activated AMs. SP-A was added to AMs activated with LPS (100 ng/ml) for 6 hr and coincubated for an additional 30 or 60 min in the absence (–) or presence (+) of 1.2 mM CO_2. SP-A was immunoprecipitated with a polyclonal rabbit antihuman SP-A antibody, and protein nitration was detected by Western blotting with a polyclonal antinitrotyrosine antibody. (Adapted from Ref. 128.)

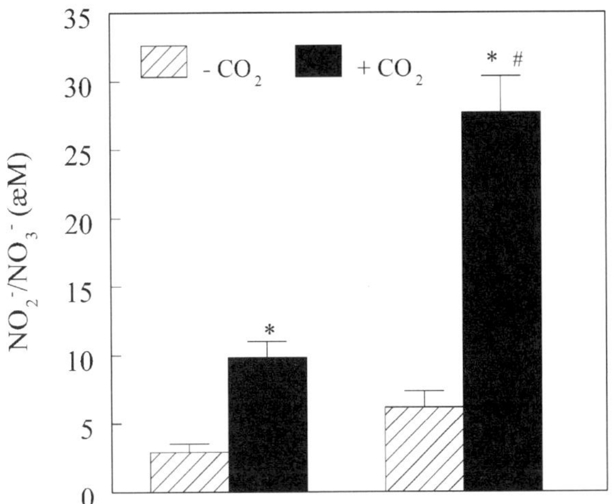

Figure 6 Enhancement of AM NO_2^- plus NO_3^- production by LPS and CO_2. AM activation and CO_2 exposure were performed as in Fig. 5. NO_2^- plus NO_3^- was measured in medium at that time using the Griess reagent. Values are means $\pm$ SE; $n = 6$ experiments. $^*p < 0.01$ compared with AMs cultured in the absence of 1.2 mM CO_2. $^\#p < 0.01$ compared with AMs cultured in the presence of 1.2 mM CO_2 but in absence of LPS. (Adapted from Ref. 128.)

tions of RONS may vary dramatically within the timecourse of disease. Nevertheless, Sittipunt et al.(70) found that NO_2^- and NO_3^- (NO_x) concentrations were significantly higher than normal in the BAL fluid from patients at risk for developing ARDS, as well as those with ARDS, and remained elevated throughout the course of the disease. In all cases, the majority of the products detected were in the form of NO_3^- ($> 90\%$ NO_3^-, and $< 10\%$ NO_2^-). NO_x was barely above background in BAL fluid from normal subjects (range 2.5–4.3 µM, median 2.5 µM). In patients at risk for ARDS, NO_x concentrations in BAL fluid from days 1 and 3 after onset of ARDS risk factors (such as multiple trauma, sepsis or multiple transfusions) have been shown to be significantly higher than in normal subjects. Levels of tyrosine nitration and chlorination (a marker of neutrophil activation) in BALF were also increased after inhaled $^\bullet$NO therapy for ARDS (202) (Fig. 7).

Levels of NO_x in the epithelial lining fluid of patients cannot be easily estimated since they are diluted considerably (as much as 50-fold) by BAL fluid. To address this issue, Zhu et al. (201) measured NO_x levels in pulmonary edema fluid and plasma samples from patients with ALI/ARDS and for comparison, in samples from patients with hydrostatic pulmonary edema. All patients studied were admitted to intensive care units at the University of California at San Francisco (UCSF) or San Francisco General Hospital

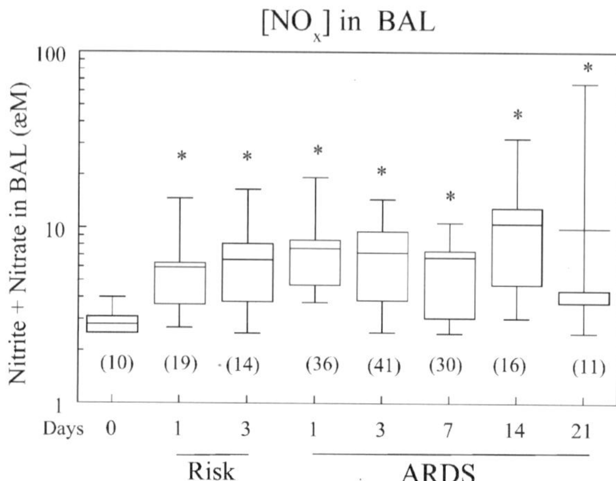

Figure 7 NO$_2^-$ and NO$_3^-$ concentration (NO$_x$) in BAL from normal volunteers (NL), patients at risk for ARDS (RISK), and patients with established ARDS (ARDS) studied at sequential times. The horizontal axis shows the patient group and the day on which the BAL was performed. (*n*) is the number of subjects in each group. The data are presented as box plots showing the 10th, 25th, 75th, and 90th percentiles and the median. $^*p \leq 0.005$ vs. normal subjects. (Reprinted with permission from Ref. 70.)

between 1985 and 1998. Pulmonary EF was collected from each patient within 30 min after endotracheal intubation by passing a standard 14 Fr tracheal suction catheter through the endotracheal tube into a wedged position in a distal airway. Pulmonary EF from patients with ALI had significantly higher levels of NO$_x$ compared to pulmonary EF from patients with hydrostatic pulmonary edema (108 ± 13 μM vs. 66 ± 9 μM; Mean $\pm$ SEM; $P < 0.05$). In addition, patients with shock had higher plasma NO$_x$ levels than those without shock (79 ± 11 μM vs. 53 ± 12 μM, $p < 0.05$). The ratios of NO$_2^-$ to NO$_3^-$ in 11 edema and 9 plasma samples were 0.01 ± 0.005 vs. 0.008 ± 0.004, indicating that more than 90% of NO$_x$ were present as nitrate, in agreement with BAL data (see above) (201).

Acidemia and increased anion gap, markers of systemic hypoperfusion, have also been associated with twofold higher plasma NO$_x$ levels. RONS in clinical ALI/ARDS are most likely produced primarily by activated pulmonary inflammatory cells. Hickman-Davis et al. (63) have recently shown that AMs isolated from the BALF of patients with lung transplants produce very large amounts of •NO when coincubated with either SP-A or with pathogens. In contrast, AMs from normal volunteers could not be stimulated to produce •NO (63).

There is significant evidence for the existence of nitrated and oxidized proteins in the plasma and alveolar spaces of patients with inflammatory diseases. For example, Gole et al. (142) reported the presence of nitrated ceruloplasmin, transferrin, α_1-protease inhibitor (α_1-PI), α_1-antichymotrypsin, and β-chain fibrinogen in the plasma of patients with ALI/ARDS. Interestingly, Cochrane et al. (203) also showed that α_1-PI was inactivated in BALF samples from patients with ARDS. In contrast, α_1-PI in plasma samples from the same patients retained $> 90\%$ activity, implicating the lung as the source of α_1-PI oxidation. Shortly, thereafter, Sznajder et al. (204) measured expired fractions of H_2O_2, a more stable membrane-permeable and volatile oxidant, in patients with normal lungs undergoing elective surgery and in critically ill patients suffering from acute hypoxemic respiratory failure (AHRF). Expired breath condensates of H_2O_2 were significantly elevated in patients suffering from AHRF with focal pulmonary infiltrates compared to those without pulmonary infiltrates (2.34 ± 1.15 vs. $0.99 \pm 0.72\,\mu\text{mol}/\text{L}$). H_2O_2 concentrations were greatest in patients with head injury and sepsis whether pulmonary infiltrates were present or not, suggesting the added participation of oxidants in septic injury to other vital organs such as the brain (204). The importance of oxidant-induced pathology in clinical lung injury is also supported by the findings of Quinlan et al. (205) that plasma concentrations of hypoxanthine, a key cofactor for the production of O_2^- and H_2O_2, were significantly elevated in patients with ARDS and were highest in those who did not survive ($37.48 \pm 3.1\,\mu\text{M}$ in nonsurvivors, $15.24 \pm 2.09\,\mu\text{M}$ in survivors, $p < 0.001$).

Significant levels of protein-associated nitrotyrosine ($\sim$400–500 pmol/mg protein) have been reported in EF from patients with ALI/ARDS ARDS and with hydrostatic pulmonary edema (201), as well as in BAL from patients with ARDS (70). These levels of nitrotyrosine are at least one order of magnitude higher than those found in proteins in normal human BAL fluid (28 pmol/mg protein) (206) or normal rat lung tissue ($\sim$30 pmol/mg protein) (207). Lamb et al. (208) also measured nitrotyrosine content in the BAL fluid of patients with severe ARDS and healthy volunteers using HPLC, although their reported values were considerably higher than those of Sittipunt et al. (70) and Zhu et al. (201). In the latter study of Zhu et al. (201), nitrated pulmonary SP-A was also detected in the EF, but not the plasma, of patients with ALI, after immunoprecipitation with specific antibody. This was the first direct evidence of injury-induced nitration of a specific protein in the human alveoli in vivo, although it had previously been demonstrated that SP-A could be nitrated and oxidized in vitro using LPS-stimulated rat AMs as the source of reactive species (128). In vitro studies also indicate that nitrated SP-A loses its ability to enhance the adherence of *P. carinii* to rat AMs (152), and is less effective in promoting the killing of *M. pulmonis* by mouse AMs (Hickman-Davis et al., unpublished observations). Nitration of human SP-A by $ONOO^-$ or tetranitromethane has also been found to inhibit its lipid aggregation and mannose binding activities in vitro (151). SP-A isolated from the lungs of lambs exposed to high concentrations of inhaled nitric oxide also has a decreased ability to aggregate lipids (209). Nitration of SP-A may be one of the factors responsible for increased susceptibility of patients with ARDS to nosocomial infections. Additional discussion of the effects of nitration on the biophysical and biological activity of this important lung surfactant protein is given in Chapter 9.

While the direct measurement of RONS in vivo poses problems, antioxidant concentrations and/or oxidant–antioxidant balance in patients are more readily assessed. For instance, plasma levels of ascorbate (a major plasma antioxidant) have been shown to be significantly decreased in patients with ARDS compared to control patients, although it is unclear whether this decrease results from reduced synthesis following organ damage, or increased consumption by oxidants (210,211). Levels of ubiquinol, a key lipid-soluble antioxidant in mitochondrial membranes, were also significantly decreased in the same patient group, while plasma levels of the antioxidant α-tocopherol were unchanged. In a separate study, incubation of plasma from a healthy donor with activated PMNs resulted in rapid oxidation of ascorbate, a slow decline in ubiquinol levels, and very little effect on α-tocopherol (210).

GSH, the most abundant nonprotein thiol, is a potent antioxidant that is particularly effective at reducing H_2O_2 and HOCl. BAL fluid and EF GSH content have been shown to be reduced in 10 patients with ARDS when compared to normal individuals (212). In subsequent studies, administration of the GSH agonist *N*-acetylcysteine to patients with ARDS did not elicit significant improvements in oxygenation, pulmonary mechanics, or total plasma GSH concentrations (213,214). Indeed, levels of catalase, a scavenger of H_2O_2, were actually found to increase in patients with sepsis with and without evolution to ARDS (215). GSH peroxidase activity was unchanged in all groups. Endothelial injury (as measured by ^{51}Cr release) was greatest in the control group and least in patients with sepsis and ARDS. Additional studies have confirmed that antioxidant responses are significantly elevated in the pro-oxidant pulmonary milieu observed in sepsis and ALI (216).

Nutritional supplementation might serve as a means to counter the undesirable chemical and cellular effects of RONS in ALI/ARDS and sepsis. While a paucity of data exists, the impact of nutritional supplementation has been evaluated in eight patients suffering from ARDS receiving "standardized" total parenteral nutrition (TPN) (211). Measurements of plasma antioxidants and antioxidant enzyme systems obtained at baseline and at days 3 and 6 after initiation of TPN were compared to controls fed a standard diet without vitamin or trace element supplementation. In addition, concentrations of the lipid peroxidation product malondiadehyde (MDA), $O_2^{\bullet-}$, and H_2O_2 were measured at the same time points. Despite TPN, plasma levels of α-tocopherol, ascorbate, β-carotene, and selenium were reduced in the ARDS patients compared to controls. MDA was significantly increased compared to controls and increased significantly over the 6-day interval studied (211). These results suggest that "standardized" TPN is not sufficient to provide the increased systemic requirement for antioxidants in patients with ARDS whose antioxidant system is severely compromised. In contrast, beneficial anti-inflammatory effects have been reported in patients with ARDS who received a specialized enteral formulation containing eicosapentaenoic acid (fish oil), γ-linolenic acid (borage seed oil), and supplementation with antioxidants (vitamin A, α-tocopherol, ascorbate, and β-carotene), compared to patients who received an isonitrogenous, isocaloric, standard diet (217). These effects translated into a reduction in days of mechanical ventilation, a decreased length of stay in the ICU and reduction in new organ failure (217). The enteral formulation also significantly increased the PaO_2/FiO_2 ratio, and decreased BALF total leukocyte and neutrophil counts over a 4–7-day interval. While RONS generation was not directly measured, it was inferred that pulmonary inflammatory responses were reduced as a consequence of a decrease in neutrophil adhesion and RONS production (217). Antioxidant therapies and supplementation strategies for patients with lung injury are discussed further in Chapter 16.

VI. Summary

Reactive oxygen and nitrogen molecules, ions, and radicals are generated by a variety of endogenous metabolic and injury processes, as well as by exposure to drugs and external toxicants. Neutrophils, macrophages, and resident pulmonary cells generate and release these substances during acute and chronic inflammation and in host defense. Reactive oxygen species of physiologic relevance include superoxide anion radical ($O_2^{\bullet-}$), hydrogen peroxide (H_2O_2), hypochlorous acid (HOCl), and the hydroxyl radical ($^{\bullet}OH$). In the Haber–Weiss reaction, $O_2^{\bullet-}$ reduces H_2O_2 to produce $^{\bullet}OH$, molecular O_2, and hydroxide ion (OH^-). In the modified Haber–Weiss reaction (the Fenton reaction), $O_2^{\bullet-}$ reduces trace metal ions such as Fe^{3+}, which then react with H_2O_2 to regenerate an oxidized metal ion plus OH^- and $^{\bullet}OH$. These reactive oxygen species have benefical activities such as in killing micro-organisms during innate host defense, but they also have the potential to cause lung injury.

Reactive nitrogen species are also important in the pathophysiology of lung injury. Nitric oxide is an important mediator of normal physiological effects in many cell types including neutrophils, macrophages, epithelial cells, neurons, muscle cells, and hepatocytes. Nitric oxide is produced by NOSs of three primary types: neuronal (nNOS, isoform I), endothelial (eNOS, isoform III), and inducible (iNOS, isoform II). All NOS isoforms are homodimeric heme proteins with oxygenase and reductase domains in the N- and C-terminal regions, respectively. All three forms of NOS exist in the lungs, but the expression of nNOS and eNOS is largely constitutive while iNOS expression is normally low in lung tissue. The production of iNOS (mediated by the *Nos2* gene) is triggered by a variety of proinflammatory stimuli including endorphin-mediated stress, oxidative injury, reduced oxygen tension, low pH, bacterial toxins, and inflammatory cytokines such as IFN-α/β, IFN-γ, TNF-α, and IL-1β. iNOS has been immunolocalized to pulmonary cells or tissue from patients with ARDS, bacterial pneumonia, idiopathic pulmonary fibrosis, hantavirus cardiopulmonary syndrome, lung cancer, sarcoidosis, tuberculosis, asthma, or sepsis. These findings raise the possibility that iNOS-induced increases in $^\bullet$NO may have both beneficial (antimicrobial) and detrimental (tissue-damaging) effects in lung injury. Other inflammation-associated RNS include peroxynitrite ($ONOO^-$), peroxynitrous acid ($ONOOH$), nitrogen dioxide ($^\bullet NO_2$), and nitronium ion (NO_2^+). Many of these species, particularly the highly reactive peroxynitrite ion, have both oxidizing and nitrating activities as described in this chapter.

While there is no doubt that endogenous reactive oxygen and nitrogen species are of considerable importance in innate pulmonary defense, their excessive release results in tissue damage and the compromise of lung function. In addition, exposure to increased concentrations of oxygen or nitric oxide during clinical therapy for hypoxemia can result in a substantial increase in the pulmonary oxidant burden (e.g., exposure of lung tissue to 100% O_2 can increase mitochondrial H_2O_2 production by an order of magnitude or more depending on duration). Overproduction of RONS has been implicated in the pathophysiology of inflammatory lung injury in multiple animal models and in human patients with clinical ALI/ARDS. The normal lungs are protected from the buildup of RONS by a variety of antioxidants. Lung cells contain three forms of SOD: CuZnSOD, found mainly in cell cytoplasm but also in peroxisomes; MnSOD, localized in mitochondria; and extracellular SOD (EC-SOD) identified in the lung matrix. All these SODs convert superoxide anion to hydrogen peroxide, which is degraded to water by catalase. The reduced glutathione–glutathione peroxidase system also contributes important antioxidant activity in the lungs. In addition, lung tissue contains high concentrations of other nonenzymatic antioxidants, including vitamin E and ascorbate. If these antioxidant defenses are inadequate or overwhelmed, injury to lung cells, interstitial matrix, and alveolar surfactant occurs. Future research needs to address specific molecular mechanisms involved in lung injury from RONS, as well as to identify more precisely the cell and tissue protein targets of these substances, and the functional consequences of reactive species-induced damage (damage to complement components or other host defense proteins, damage to channel proteins such as epithelial sodium channels, or damage to adhesion or extracellular matrix proteins, etc.). Research also needs to take into account aspects of normal pulmonary environment such as pH, CO_2 tension, and other variables that can affect the generation or activity of reactive species. Therapeutic interventions to protect lung cells and tissue against oxidant-induced lung injury are discussed in detail in Chapter 16.

Acknowledgments

This work was supported by NIH grants HL31197 (S.M.), HL51173 (S.M.), and a grant from the Office of Naval Research (N00014-97-1-0309; S.M.). I.C.D. is a Parker B. Francis Families Fellow in Pulmonary Research.

References

1. Matalon S, Egan EA. Effects of 100% O_2 breathing on permeability of alveolar epithelium to solute. J Appl Physiol 1981; 50:859–863.
2. Holm BA, Matalon S. Role of pulmonary surfactant in the development and treatment of adult respiratory distress syndrome. Anesth Analg 1989; 69: 805–818.
3. Nicod LP. Pulmonary defence mechanisms. Respiration 1999; 66:2–11.
4. Fridovich I. Fundamental aspects of reactive oxygen species, or what's the matter with oxygen? Ann N Y Acad Sci 1999; 893:13–18.
5. Nauseef WM. The NADPH-dependent oxidase of phagocytes. Proc Assoc Am Phys 1999; 111:373–382.
6. Kobayashi T, Seguchi H. Novel insight into current models of NADPH oxidase regulation, assembly and localization in human polymorphonuclear leukocytes. Histol Histopathol 1999; 14:1295–1308.
7. Ischiropoulos H, Zhu L, Beckman JS. Peroxynitrite formation from macrophage-derived nitric oxide. Arch Biochem Biophys 1992; 298:446–451.
8. Punjabi CJ, Laskin JD, Pendino KJ, Goller NL, Durham SK, Laskin DL. Production of nitric oxide by rat type II pneumocytes: increased expression of inducible nitric oxide synthase following inhalation of a pulmonary irritant. Am J Respir Cell Mol Biol 1994; 11:165–172.
9. Barnes PJ. Air pollution and asthma: molecular mechanisms. Mol Med Today 1995; 1:149–155.
10. Martin LD, Krunkosky TM, Dye JA, Fischer BM, Jiang NF, Rochelle LG, Akley NJ, Dreher KL, Adler KB. The role of reactive oxygen and nitrogen species in the response of airway epithelium to particulates. Environ Health Perspect 1997; 105(suppl 5):1301–1307.
11. Imlay JA, Fridovich I. Assay of metabolic superoxide production in *Escherichia coli*. J Biol Chem 1991; 266:6957–6965.
12. Aust SD, Roerig DL, Pederson TC. Evidence for superoxide generation by NADPH-cytochrome c reductase of rat liver microsomes. Biochem Biophys Res Commun 1972; 47:1133–1137.
13. Boveris A. Mitochondrial generation of superoxide and hydrogen peroxide. Adv Exp Med Biol 1977; 78:67–82.

14. Winterbourn CC, Vissers MC, Kettle AJ. Myeloperoxidase. Curr Opin Hematol 2000; 7:53–58.

15. Albrich JM, McCarthy CA, Hurst JK. Biological reactivity of hypochlorous acid: implications for microbicidal mechanisms of leukocyte myeloperoxidase. Proc Natl Acad Sci USA 1981; 78:210–214.

16. Borelli V, Banfi E, Perrotta MG, Zabucchi G. Myeloperoxidase exerts microbicidal activity against *Mycobacterium tuberculosis*. Infect Immun 1999; 67:4149–4152.

17. Aratani Y, Koyama H, Nyui S, Suzuki K, Kura F, Maeda N. Severe impairment in early host defense against Candida albicans in mice deficient in myeloperoxidase. Infect Immun 1999; 67:1828–1836.

18. Nohl H, Jordan W, Hegner D. Identification of free hydroxyl radicals in respiring rat heart mitochondria by spin trapping with the nitrone DMPO. FEBS Lett 1981; 123:241–244.

19. Winterbourn CC. Hydroxyl radical production in body fluids. Roles of metal ions, ascorbate and superoxide. Biochem J 1981; 198:125–131.

20. Coonrod JD. Role of leukocytes in lung defenses. Respiration 1989; 55(suppl 1):9–13.

21. Shah M, Bry K, Hallman M. Protective effect of exogenous transferrin against hyperoxia: a study on premature rabbits. Pediatr Pulmonol 1997; 24:429–437.

22. Chao CC, Park SH, Aust AE. Participation of nitric oxide and iron in the oxidation of DNA in asbestos-treated human lung epithelial cells. Arch Biochem Biophys 1996; 326:152–157.

23. Beckman JS, Beckman TW, Chen J, Marshall PA, Freeman BA. Apparent hydroxyl radical production by peroxynitrite: implications for endothelial injury from nitric oxide and superoxide. Proc Natl Acad Sci USA 1990; 87:1620–1624.

24. Oury TD, Chang LY, Marklund SL, Day BJ, Crapo JD. Immunocytochemical localization of extracellular superoxide dismutase in human lung. Lab Invest 1994; 70:889–898.

25. Cantin AM, North SL, Hubbard RC, Crystal RG. Normal alveolar epithelial lining fluid contains high levels of glutathione. J Appl Physiol 1987; 63: 152–157.

26. Turrens JF, Freeman BA, Crapo JD. Hyperoxia increases H_2O_2 release by lung mitochondria and microsomes. Arch Biochem Biophys 1982; 217: 411–421.

27. Babior BM. Activation of the respiratory burst oxidase. Environ Health Perspect 1994; 102(suppl 10):53–56.

28. Adams LB, Dinauer MC, Morgenstern DE, Krahenbuhl JL. Comparison of the roles of reactive oxygen and nitrogen intermediates in the host response to *Mycobacterium tuberculosis* using transgenic mice. Tuber Lung Dis 1997; 78:237–246.

29. Cooper AM, Segal BH, Frank AA, Holland SM, Orme IM. Transient loss of resistance to pulmonary tuberculosis in p47(phox–/–) mice. Infect Immun 2000; 68:1231–1234.

30. Morgenstern DE, Gifford MA, Li LL, Doerschuk CM, Dinauer MC. Absence of respiratory burst in X-linked chronic granulomatous disease mice leads to abnormalities in both host defense and inflammatory response to Aspergillus fumigatus. J Exp Med 1997; 185:207–218.

31. Weinbroum A, Nielsen VG, Tan S, Gelman S, Matalon S, Skinner KA, Bradley E Jr, Parks DA. Liver ischemia–reperfusion increases pulmonary permeability in rat: role of circulating xanthine oxidase. Am J Physiol 1995; 268:G988–G996.

32. Moncada S, Palmer RM, Higgs EA. Biosynthesis of nitric oxide from L-arginine. A pathway for the regulation of cell function and communication. Biochem Pharmacol 1989; 38:1709–1715.

33. Tayeh MA, Marletta MA. Oxidation of *l*-arginine to nitric oxide, nitrite, and nitrate: tetrahydrobiopterin is required as a cofactor. J Biol Chem 1989; 264:19654–19658.

34. Stuehr DJ, Kwon NS, Nathan CF. FAD and GSH participate in macrophage synthesis of nitric oxide. Biochem Biophys Res Commun 1990; 168:558–565.

35. Kwon NS, Nathan CF, Gilker C, Griffith OW, Matthews D, Stuehr DJ. L-Citrulline production from L-arginine by macrophage nitric oxide synthase: the ureido oxygen derives from dioxygen. J Biol Chem 1990; 265: 13442–13445.

36. Garvey EP, Furfine ES, Sherman PA. Purification and inhibitor screening of human nitric oxide synthase isozymes. Methods Enzymol 1996; 268: 339–349.

37. Masters BSS, McMillan K, Sheta EA, Nishimura JS, Roman LJ, Martasek P. Neuronal nitric oxide synthase, a modular enzyme formed by convergent evolution: structure studies of a cysteine thiolate-liganded heme protein that hydroxylatcs L-argininc to produce NO as a cellular signal. FASEB J 1996; 10:552–558.

38. Bredt DS, Hwang PM, Glatt CE, Lowenstein C, Reed RR, Snyder SH. Cloned and expressed nitric oxide synthase structurally resembles cytochrome P-450 reductase. Nature 1991; 351:714–718.

39. Abu-Soud HM, Stuehr DJ. Nitric oxide synthases reveal a role for calmodulin in controlling electron transfer. Proc Natl Acad Sci USA 1993; 90: 10769–10772.

40. Shaul PW, Smart EJ, Robinson LJ, German Z, Yuhanna IS, Ying Y, Anderson RGW, Michel T. Acylation targets endothelial nitric-oxide synthase to plasmalemmal caveolae. Proc Natl Acad Sci USA 1996; 271:6518–6522.

41. Aymerich MS, Bengoechea-Alonso MT, Lopez-Zabalza MJ, Santiago E, Lopez-Moratalla N. Inducible nitric oxide synthase (iNOS) expression in human monocytes triggered by beta-endorphin through an increase in cAMP. Biochem Biophys Res Commun 1998; 245:717–721.

42. Adcock IM, Brown CR, Kwon O, Barnes PJ. Oxidative stress induces NF kappa B DNA binding and inducible NOS mRNA in human epithelial cells. Biochem Biophys Res Commun 1994; 199:1518–1524.

43. Weiss G, Bogdan C, Hentze MW. Pathways for the regulation of macrophage iron metabolism by the anti-inflammatory cytokines IL-4 and IL-13. J Immunol 1997; 158:420–425.

44. Melillo G, Taylor LS, Brooks A, Musso T, Cox GW, Varesio L. Functional requirement of the hypoxia-responsive element in the activation of the inducible nitric oxide synthase promoter by the iron chelator desferrioxamine. J Biol Chem 1997; 272:12236–12243.

45. Bellocq A, Suberville S, Philippe C, Bertrand F, Perez J, Fouqueray B, Cherqui G, Baud L. Low environmental pH is responsible for the induction of nitric oxide synthase in macrophages. J Biol Chem 1998; 273:5086–5092.

46. Gao JJ, Filla MB, Fultz MJ, Vogel SN, Russell SW, Murphy WJ. Autocrine/paracrine IFN-α/β mediates the lipopolysaccharide-induced activation of transcription factor Stat-1α in mouse macrophages: pivotal role of Stat-1α in induction of the inducible nitric oxide synthase gene. J Immunol 1998; 161:4803–4810.

47. Braun JS, Novak R, Gao G, Murray PJ, Shenep JL. Pneumolysin, a protein toxin of *Streptococcus pneumoniael*, induces nitric oxide production from macrophages. Infect Immun 1999; 67:3750–3756.

48. Vouldoukis I, Riveros-Moreno V, Dugas B, Ouaaz F, Becherel P, Debre P, Moncada S, Mossalayi MD. The killing of *Leishmania major* by human macrophages is mediated by nitric oxide induced after ligation of the Fc epsilon RII/CD23 surface antigen. Proc Natl Acad Sci USA 1995; 92:7804–7808.

49. DeMaria R, Cifone MG, Trotta R, Rippo MR, Festuccia C, Santoni A, Testi R. Triggering of human monocyte activation through CD69, a member of the natural killer cell gene complex family of signal transducing receptors. J Exp Med 1994; 180:1999–2004.

50. Bogdan C, Rollinghoff M, Diefenbach A. Reactive oxygen and reactive nitrogen intermediates in innate and specific immunity. Curr Opin Immunol 2000; 12:64–76.

51. MacMicking J, Xie QW, Nathan C. Nitric oxide and macrophage function. Annu Rev Immunol 1997; 15:323–350.

52. Hecker M, Cattaruzza M, Wagner AH. Regulation of inducible nitric oxide synthase gene expression in vascular smooth muscle cells. Gen Pharmacol 1999; 32:9–16.

53. Vodovotz Y, Russell D, Xie QW, Bogdan C, Nathan C. Vesicle membrane association of nitric oxide synthase in primary mouse macrophages. J Immunol 1995; 154:2914–2925.

54. Tatoyan A, Giulivi C. Purification and characterization of a nitric oxide synthase from rat liver mitochondria. J Biol Chem 1998; 273:11044–11048.

55. Cho HJ, Xie QW, Calaycay J, Mumford RA, Swiderek KM, Lee TD, Nathan C. Calmodulin is a subunit of nitric oxide synthase from macrophages. J Exp Med 1992; 176:599–604.

56. Vodovotz Y, Kwon NS, Pospischil M, Manning J, Paik J, Nathan C. Inactivation of nitric oxide synthase after prolonged incubation of mouse macrophages with IFN-gamma and bacterial lipopolysaccharide. J Immunol 1994; 152:4110–4118.

57. Hickman-Davis JM, Lindsey JR, Zhu S, Matalon S. Surfactant protein A mediates mycoplasmacidal activity of alveolar macrophages. Am J Physiol 1998; 274:L270–L277.

58. Xia Y, Roman LJ, Masters BS, Zweier JL. Inducible nitric-oxide synthase generates superoxide from the reductase domain. J Biol Chem 1998; 273:22635–22639.

59. Xia Y, Tsai AL, Berka V, Zweier JL. Superoxide generation from endothelial nitric-oxide synthase. A Ca^{2+}/calmodulin-dependent and tetrahydrobiopterin regulatory process. J Biol Chem 1998; 273:25804–25808.

60. MacMicking JD, Nathan C, Hom G, Chartrain N, Fletcher DS, Trumbauer M, Stevens K, Xie QW, Sokol K, Hutchinson N. Altered responses to bacterial infection and endotoxic shock in mice lacking inducible nitric oxide synthase. Cell 1995; 81:641–650.

61. Nathan C. Inducible nitric oxide synthase: what difference does it make? J Clin Invest 1997; 100:2417–2423.

62. Shiloh MU, MacMicking JD, Nicholson S, Brause JE, Potter S, Marino M, Fang F, Dinauer M, Nathan C. Phenotype of mice and macrophages deficient in both phagocyte oxidase and inducible nitric oxide synthase. Immunity 1999; 10:29–38.

63. Hickman-Davis JM, O'Reilly P, Davis IC, Peti-Peterdi J, Davis G, Young KR, Devlin RB, Matalon S. Killing of *Klebsiella pneumoniae* by human alveolar macrophages. Am J Physiol Lung Cell Mol Physiol 2002; 282:L944–L956.

64. Fierro IM, Nascimento-DaSilva V, Arruda MA, Freitas MS, Plotkowski MC, Cunha FQ, Barja-Fidalgo C. Induction of NOS in rat blood PMN in vivo and in vitro: modulation by tyrosine kinase and involvement in bactericidal activity. J Leukoc Biol 1999; 65:508–514.

65. Kooy NW, Royall JA. Agonist-induced peroxynitrite production from endothelial cells. Arch Biochem Biophys 1994; 310:352–359.

66. Kobzik L, Bredt DS, Lowenstein CJ, Drazen J, Gaston B, Sugarbaker D, Stamler JS. Nitric oxide synthase in human and rat lung: immunocytochemical and histochemical localization. Am J Respir Cell Mol Biol 1993; 9: 371–377.

67. Asano K, Chee CB, Gaston B, Lilly CM, Gerard C, Drazen JM, Stamler JS. Constitutive and inducible nitric oxide synthase gene expression, regulation, and activity in human lung epithelial cells. Proc Natl Acad Sci USA 1994; 91:10089–10093.

68. Guo FH, De Raeve HR, Rice TW, Stuehr DJ, Thunnissen FB, Erzurum SC. Continuous nitric oxide synthesis by inducible nitric oxide synthase in normal human airway epithelium in vivo. Proc Natl Acad Sci USA 1995; 92: 7809–7813.

69. Pendino KJ, Laskin JD, Shuler RL, Punjabi CJ, Laskin DL. Enhanced production of nitric oxide by rat alveolar macrophages after inhalation of a pulmonary irritant is associated with increased expression of nitric oxide synthase. J Immunol 1993; 151:7196–7205.

70. Sittipunt C, Steinberg KP, Ruzinski JT, Myles C, Zhu S, Goodman RB, Hudson LD, Matalon S, Martin TR. Nitric oxide and nitrotyrosine in the lungs of patients with acute respiratory distress syndrome. Am J Respir Crit Care Med 2001; 163:503–510.

71. Tracey WR, Xue C, Klinghofer V, Barlow J, Pollock JS, Förstermann U, Johns RA. Immunochemical detection of inducible NO synthase in human lung. Am J Physiol Lung Cell Mol Physiol 1994; 266:L722–L727.

72. Davis IC, Zajac AJ, Nolte KB, Botten J, Hjelle B, Matalon S. Elevated generation of reactive oxygen/nitrogen species in hantavirus cardiopulmonary syndrome. J Virol 2002; 76:8347–8359.

73. Liu CY, Wang CH, Chen TC, Lin HC, Yu CT, Kuo HP. Increased level of exhaled nitric oxide and up-regulation of inducible nitric oxide synthase in patients with primary lung cancer. Br J Cancer 1998; 78:534–541.

74. Moodley YP, Chetty R, Lalloo UG. Nitric oxide levels in exhaled air and inducible nitric oxide synthase immunolocalization in pulmonary sarcoidosis. Eur Respir J 1999; 14:822–827.

75. Saleh D, Barnes PJ, Giaid A. Increased production of the potent oxidant peroxynitrite in the lungs of patients with idiopathic pulmonary fibrosis. Am J Respir Crit Care Med 1997; 155:1763–1769.

76. Nicholson S, Bonecini-Almeida MdG, Lapa eSJ, Nathan C, Xie QW, Mumford R, Weidner JR, Calaycay J, Geng J, Boechat N. Inducible nitric oxide synthase in pulmonary alveolar macrophages from patients with tuberculosis. J Exp Med 1996; 183:2293–2302.

77. Kobayashi A, Hashimoto S, Kooguchi K, Kitamura Y, Onodera H, Urata Y, Ashihara T. Expression of inducible nitric oxide synthase and inflammatory cytokines in alveolar macrophages of ARDS following sepsis. Chest 1998; 113:1632–1639.

78. Moncada S, Palmer RM, Higgs EA. Nitric oxide: physiology, pathophysiology, and pharmacology. Pharmacol Rev 1991; 43:109–142.

79. Doyle MP, Hoekstra JW. Oxidation of nitrogen oxides by bound dioxygen in hemoproteins. J Inorg Biochem 1981; 14:351–358.

80. Rossaint R, Falke KJ, Lopez F, Slama K, Pison U, Zapol WM. Inhaled nitric oxide for the adult respiratory distress syndrome. N Engl J Med 1993; 328:399–405.

81. Beckman JS, Koppenol WH. Nitric oxide, superoxide, and peroxynitrite: the good, the bad, and ugly. Am J Physiol 1996; 271:C1424–C1437.

82. Heiss LN, Lancaster JR Jr, Corbett JA, Goldman WE. Epithelial autotoxicity of nitric oxide: role in the respiratory cytopathology of pertussis. Proc Natl Acad Sci USA 1994; 91:267–270.

83. Jia L, Bonaventura J, Stamler JS. *S*-nitrosohaemoglobin: a dynamic activity of blood involved in vascular control. Nature 1996; 380:221–226.

84. Mulligan MS, Hevel JM, Marletta MA, Ward PA. Tissue injury caused by deposition of immune complexes is L-arginine dependent. Proc Natl Acad Sci USA 1991; 88:6338–6342.

85. Berisha HI, Pakbaz H, Absood A, Said SI. Nitric oxide as a mediator of oxidant lung injury due to paraquat. Proc Natl Acad Sci USA 1994; 91:7445–7449.

86. Ischiropoulos H, al-Mehdi AB, Fisher AB. Reactive species in ischemic rat lung injury: contribution of peroxynitrite. Am J Physiol 1995; 269: L158–L164.

87. Akaike T, Noguchi Y, Ijiri S, Setoguchi K, Suga M, Zheng YM, Dietzschold B, Maeda H. Pathogenesis of influenza virus-induced pneumonia: involvement of both nitric oxide and oxygen radicals. Proc Natl Acad Sci USA 1996; 93:2448–2453.

88. Kristof AS, Goldberg P, Laubach V, Hussain SN. Role of inducible nitric oxide synthase in endotoxin-induced acute lung injury. Am J Respir Crit Care Med 1998; 158:1883–1889.

89. Karupiah G, Chen JH, Mahalingam S, Nathan CF, MacMicking JD. Rapid interferon gamma-dependent clearance of influenza A virus and protection from consolidating pneumonitis in nitric oxide synthase 2-deficient mice. J Exp Med 1998; 188:1541–1546.

90. Szabo C, Billiar TR. Novel roles of nitric oxide in hemorrhagic shock. Shock 1999; 12:1–9.

91. Xiong Y, Karupiah G, Hogan SP, Foster PS, Ramsay AJ. Inhibition of allergic airway inflammation in mice lacking nitric oxide synthase 2. J Immunol 1999; 162:445–452.

92. Huie RE, Padmaja S. The reaction of NO with superoxide. Free Radic Res Commun 1993; 18:195–199.

93. Goldstein S, Czapski G. The reaction of $NO^\bullet$ with $O_2^{\bullet-}$ and $HO_2^\bullet$: a pulse radiolysis study. Free Radic Biol Med 1995; 19:505–510.

94. Ischiropoulos H, Zhu L, Chen J, Tsai M, Martin JC, Smith CD, Beckman JS. Peroxynitrite-mediated tyrosine nitration catalyzed by superoxide dismutase. Arch Biochem Biophys 1992; 298:431–437.

95. Sampson JB, Rosen H, Beckman JS. Peroxynitrite-dependent tyrosine nitration catalyzed by superoxide dismutase, myeloperoxidase, and horseradish peroxidase. Methods Enzymol 1996; 269:210–218.

96. Tsai J-HM, Hamilton TP, Harrison JG, Jablowski M, van der Woerd M, Martin JC, Beckman JS. Role of peroxynitrite: conformation with its stability and toxicity. J Am Chem Soc 1994; 116:4115–4116.

97. Lancaster JR Jr. Simulation of the diffusion and reaction of endogenously produced nitric oxide. Proc Natl Acad Sci USA 1994; 91:8134–8141.

98. van der Vliet A, Smith D, O'Neill CA, Kaur H, Darley-Usmar V, Cross CE, Halliwell B. Interactions of peroxynitrite with human plasma and its constituents: oxidative damage and antioxidant depletion. Biochem J 1994; 303:295–301.

99. Carreras MC, Pargament GA, Catz SD, Poderoso JJ, Boveris A. Kinetics of nitric oxide and hydrogen peroxide production and formation of peroxynitrite during the respiratory burst of human neutrophils. FEBS Lett 1994; 341:65–68.

100. Wink DA, Kasprzak KS, Maragos CM, Elespuru RK, Misra M, Dunams TM, Cebula TA, Koch WH, Andrews AW, Allen JS. DNA deaminating ability and genotoxicity of nitric oxide and its progenitors. Science 1991; 254:1001–1003.

101. Molina yVL, McDonald B, Reep B, Brune B, Di Silvio M, Billiar TR, Lapetina EG. Nitric oxide-induced *S*-nitrosylation of glyceraldehyde-3-phosphate dehydrogenase inhibits enzymatic activity and increases endogenous ADP-ribosylation [published erratum appears in J Biol Chem 1993 Feb 5; 268(4):3016]. J Biol Chem 1992; 267:24929–24932.

102. Curran RD, Ferrari FK, Kispert PH, Stadler J, Stuehr DJ, Simmons RL, Billiar TR. Nitric oxide and nitric oxide-generating compounds inhibit hepatocyte protein synthesis. FASEB J 1991; 5:2085–2092.

103. Delaney CA, Green MH, Lowe JE, Green IC. Endogenous nitric oxide induced by interleukin-1 beta in rat islets of Langerhans and HIT-T15 cells causes significant DNA damage as measured by the 'comet' assay. FEBS Lett 1993; 333:291–295.

104. Kwon NS, Stuehr DJ, Nathan CF. Inhibition of tumor cell ribonucleotide reductase by macrophage-derived nitric oxide. J Exp Med 1991; 174: 761–767.

105. Hausladen A, Fridovich I. Superoxide and peroxynitrite inactivate aconitases, but nitric oxide does not. J Biol Chem 1994; 269:29405–29408.

106. Castro L, Rodriguez M, Radi R. Aconitase is readily inactivated by peroxynitrite, but not by its precursor, nitric oxide. J Biol Chem 1994; 269:29409–29415.

107. Torres J, Davies N, Darley-Usmar VM, Wilson MT. The inhibition of cytochrome *c* oxidase by nitric oxide using *S*-nitrosoglutathione. J Inorg Biochem 1997; 66:207–212.

108. Cassina AM, Hodara R, Souza JM, Thomson L, Castro L, Ischiropoulos H, Freeman BA, Radi R. Cytochrome *c* nitration by peroxynitrite. J Biol Chem 2000; 275:21409–21415.

109. Stuehr DJ, Nathan CF. Nitric oxide. A macrophage product responsible for cytostasis and respiratory inhibition in tumor target cells. J Exp Med 1989; 169:1543–1555.

110. Pilz RB, Suhasini M, Idriss S, Meinkoth JL, Boss GR. Nitric oxide and *c*GMP analogs activate transcription from AP-1-responsive promoters in mammalian cells. FASEB J 1995; 9:552–558.

111. De Caterina R, Libby P, Peng HB, Thannickal VJ, Rajavashisth TB, Gimbrone MA Jr, Shin WS, Liao JK. Nitric oxide decreases cytokine-induced endothelial activation. Nitric oxide selectively reduces endothelial expression of adhesion molecules and proinflammatory cytokines. J Clin Invest 1995; 96:60–68.

112. Colasanti M, Persichini T, Menegazzi M, Mariotto S, Giordano E, Caldarera CM, Sogos V, Lauro GM, Suzuki H. Induction of nitric oxide synthase mRNA expression. Suppression by exogenous nitric oxide. J Biol Chem 1995; 270:26731–26733.

113. Lander HM, Sehajpal P, Levine DM, Novogrodsky A. Activation of human peripheral blood mononuclear cells by nitric oxide-generating compounds. J Immunol 1993; 150:1509–1516.

114. Rubbo H, Radi R, Trujillo M, Telleri R, Kalyanaraman B, Barnes S, Kirk M, Freeman BA. Nitric oxide regulation of superoxide and peroxynitrite-dependent lipid peroxidation. Formation of novel nitrogen-containing oxidized lipid derivatives. J Biol Chem 1994; 269:26066–26075.

115. Crow JP, Beckman JS, McCord JM. Sensitivity of the essential zinc-thiolate moiety of yeast alcohol dehydrogenase to hypochlorite and peroxynitrite. Biochemistry 1995; 34:3544–3552.

116. Lipton SA, Choi YB, Pan ZH, Lei SZ, Chen HS, Sucher NJ, Loscalzo J, Singel DJ, Stamler JS. A redox-based mechanism for the neuroprotective and neurodestructive effects of nitric oxide and related nitroso-compounds. Nature 1993; 364:626–632.

117. Gaston B, Reilly J, Drazen JM, Fackler J, Ramdev P, Arnelle D, Mullins ME, Sugarbaker DJ, Chee C, Singel DJ. Endogenous nitrogen oxides and bronchodilator *S*-nitrosothiols in human airways. Proc Natl Acad Sci USA 1993; 90:10957–10961.

118. Rathmell JC, Thompson CB. The central effectors of cell death in the immune system. Annu Rev Immunol 1999; 17:781–828.

119. Mannick JB, Hausladen A, Liu L, Hess DT, Zeng M, Miao QX, Kane LS, Gow AJ, Stamler JS. Fas-induced caspase denitrosylation. Science 1999; 284:651–654.

120. Scaffidi C, Fulda S, Srinivasan A, Friesen C, Li F, Tomaselli KJ, Debatin KM, Krammer PH, Peter ME. Two CD95 (APO-1/Fas) signaling pathways. EMBO J 1998; 17:1675–1687.

121. Scaffidi C, Schmitz I, Zha J, Korsmeyer SJ, Krammer PH, Peter ME. Differential modulation of apoptosis sensitivity in CD95 type I and type II cells. J Biol Chem 1999; 274:22532–22538.

122. Denicola A, Freeman BA, Trujillo M, Radi R. Peroxynitrite reaction with carbon dioxide/bicarbonate: kinetics and influence on peroxynitrite-mediated oxidation. Arch Biochem Biophys 1996; 333:49–58.

123. Gow A, Duran D, Thom SR, Ischiropoulos H. Carbon dioxide enhancement of peroxynitrite-mediated protein tyrosine nitration. Arch Biochem Biophys 1996; 333:42–48.

124. Lymar SV, Hurst JK. Carbon dioxide: physiological catalyst for peroxynitrite-mediated cellular damage or cellular protectant? Chem Res Toxicol 1996; 9:845–850

125. Lymar SV, Jiang Q, Hurst JK. Mechanism of carbon dioxide-catalyzed oxidation of tyrosine by peroxynitrite. Biochemistry 1996; 35:7855–7861.

126. Berlett BS, Levine RL, Stadtman ER. Carbon dioxide stimulates peroxynitrite-mediated nitration of tyrosine residues and inhibits oxidation of methionine residues of glutamine synthetase: both modifications mimic effects of adenylylation. Proc Natl Acad Sci USA 1998; 95:2784–2789.

127. Pfeiffer S, Mayer B. Lack of tyrosine nitration by peroxynitrite generated at physiological pH. J Biol Chem 1998; 273:27280–27285.

128. Zhu S, Basiouny KF, Crow JP, Matalon S. Carbon dioxide enhances nitration of surfactant protein A by activated alveolar macrophages. Am J Physiol Lung Cell Mol Physiol 2000; 278:L1025–L1031.

129. Evans TJ, Buttery LD, Carpenter A, Springall DR, Polak JM, Cohen J. Cytokine-treated human neutrophils contain inducible nitric oxide synthase that produces nitration of ingested bacteria. Proc Natl Acad Sci USA 1996; 93:9553–9558.

130. van der Vliet A, Eiserich JP, Halliwell B, Cross CE. Formation of reactive nitrogen species during peroxidase-catalyzed oxidation of nitrite. A potential additional mechanism of nitric oxide-dependent toxicity. J Biol Chem 1997; 272:7617–7625.

131. Eiserich JP, Cross CE, Jones AD, Halliwell B, van der Vliet A. Formation of nitrating and chlorinating species by reaction of nitrite with hypochlorous acid. A novel mechanism for nitric oxide-mediated protein modification. J Biol Chem 1996; 271:19199–19208.

132. Eiserich JP, Hristova M, Cross CE, Jones AD, Freeman BA, Halliwell B, van der Vliet A. Formation of nitric oxide-derived inflammatory oxidants by myeloperoxidase in neutrophils. Nature 1998; 391:393–397.

133. Hazen SL, Zhang R, Shen Z, Wu W, Podrez EA, MacPherson JC, Schmitt D, Mitra SN, Mukhopadhyay C, Chen Y, et al. Formation of nitric oxide-derived oxidants by myeloperoxidase in monocytes: pathways for monocyte-mediated protein nitration and lipid peroxidation in vivo. Circ Res 1999; 85: 950–958.

134. MacPherson JC, Comhair SA, Erzurum SC, Klein DF, Lipscomb MF, Kavuru MS, Samoszuk MK, Hazen SL. Eosinophils are a major source of nitric oxide-derived oxidants in severe asthma: characterization of pathways available to eosinophils for generating reactive nitrogen species. J Immunol 2001; 166:5763–5772.

135. Hickman-Davis JM, Lindsey JR, Matalon S. Cyclophosphamide decreases nitrotyrosine formation and inhibits nitric oxide production by alveolar macrophages in mycoplasmosis. Infect Immun 2001; 69:6401–6410.

136. Gaut JP, Byun J, Tran HD, Lauber WM, Carroll JA, Hotchkiss RS, Belaaouaj A, Heinecke JW. Myeloperoxidase produces nitrating oxidants in vivo. J Clin Invest 2002; 109:1311–1319.

137. Brennan ML, Wu W, Fu X, Shen Z, Song W, Frost H, Vadseth C, Narine L, Lenkiewicz E, Borchers MT, et al. A tale of two controversies: i) Defining the role of peroxidases in nitrotyrosine formation in vivo using eosinophil peroxidase and myeloperoxidase deficient mice; and ii) Defining the nature of peroxidase-generated reactive nitrogen species. J Biol Chem 2002; 277:17415–17427.

138. Prutz WA, Monig H, Butler J, Land EJ. Reactions of nitrogen dioxide in aqueous model systems: oxidation of tyrosine units in peptides and proteins. Arch Biochem Biophys 1985; 243:125–134.

139. Beckman JS, Ischiropoulos H, Zhu L, van der WM, Smith C, Chen J, Harrison J, Martin JC, Tsai M. Kinetics of superoxide dismutase- and iron-catalyzed nitration of phenolics by peroxynitrite. Arch Biochem Biophys 1992; 298:438–445.

140. Beckman JS, Ye YZ, Anderson PG, Chen J, Accavitti MA, Tarpey MM, White CR. Extensive nitration of protein tyrosines in human atherosclerosis detected by immunohistochemistry. Biol Chem Hoppe Seyler 1994; 375: 81–88.

141. Haddad IY, Pataki G, Hu P, Galliani C, Beckman JS, Matalon S. Quantitation of nitrotyrosine levels in lung sections of patients and animals with acute lung injury. J Clin Invest 1994; 94:2407–2413.

142. Gole MD, Souza JM, Choi I, Hertkorn C, Malcolm S, Foust RF III, Finkel B, Lanken PN, Ischiropoulos H. Plasma proteins modified by tyrosine nitration in acute respiratory distress syndrome. Am J Physiol Lung Cell Mol Physiol 2000; 278:L961–L967.

143. Wizemann TM, Gardner CR, Laskin JD, Quinones S, Durham SK, Goller NL, Ohnishi ST, Laskin DL. Production of nitric oxide and peroxynitrite in the lung during acute endotoxemia. J Leukoc Biol 1994; 56:759–768.

144. Haddad IY, Ischiropoulos H, Holm BA, Beckman JS, Baker JR, Matalon S. Mechanisms of peroxynitrite-induced injury to pulmonary surfactants. Am J Physiol 1993; 265:L555–L564.

145. Haddad IY, Zhu S, Ischiropoulos H, Matalon S. Nitration of surfactant protein A results in decreased ability to aggregate lipids. Am J Physiol 1996; 270:L281–L288.

146. McCall MN, Easterbrook-Smith SB. Comparison of the role of tyrosine residues in human IgG and rabbit IgG in binding of complement subcomponent C1q. Biochem J 1989; 257:845–851.

147. Vertessy BG, Zalud P, Nyman OP, Zeppezauer M. Identification of tyrosine as a functional residue in the active site of *Escherichia coli* dUTPase. Biochim Biophys Acta 1994; 1205:146–150.

148. Feste A, Gan JC. Selective loss of elastase inhibitory activity of α_1-proteinase inhibitor upon chemical modification of its tyrosyl residues. J Biol Chem 1981; 256:6374–6380.

149. Kong SK, Yim MB, Stadtman ER, Chock PB. Peroxynitrite disables the tyrosine phosphorylation regulatory mechanism: lymphocyte-specific tyrosine kinase fails to phosphorylate nitrated cdc2(6-20)NH2 peptide. Proc Natl Acad Sci USA 1996; 93:3377–3382.

150. Greis KD, Zhu S, Matalon S. Identification of nitration sites on surfactant protein A by tandem electrospray mass spectrometry. Arch Biochem Biophys 1996; 335:396–402.

151. Zhu S, Haddad IY, Matalon S. Nitration of surfactant protein A (SP-A) tyrosine residues results in decreased mannose binding ability. Arch Biochem Biophys 1996; 333:282–290.

152. Zhu S, Kachel DL, Martin WJ, Matalon S. Nitrated SP-A does not enhance adherence of *Pneumocystis carinii* to alveolar macrophages. Am J Physiol 1998; 275:L1031–L1039.

153. Robbins CG, Davis JM, Merritt TA, Amirkhanian JD, Sahgal N, Morin FC3, Horowitz S. Combined effects of nitric oxide and hyperoxia on surfactant function and pulmonary inflammation. Am J Physiol 1995; 269:L545–L550.

154. Matalon S, DeMarco V, Haddad IY, Myles C, Skimming JW, Schurch S, Cheng S, Cassin S. Inhaled nitric oxide injures the pulmonary surfactant system of lambs in vivo. Am J Physiol 1996; 270:L273–L280.

155. Ignarro LJ. Haem-dependent activation of cytosolic guanylate cyclase by nitric oxide: a widespread signal transduction mechanism. Biochem Soc Trans 1992; 20:465–469.

156. Lincoln TM, Cornwell TL. Intracellular cyclic GMP receptor proteins. FASEB J 1993; 7:328–338.

157. Kubes P, Suzuki M, Granger DN. Nitric oxide: an endogenous modulator of leukocyte adhesion. Proc Natl Acad Sci USA 1991; 88:4651–4655.

158. Jain B, Rubinstein I, Robbins RA, Sisson JH. TNF-alpha and IL-1 beta upregulate nitric oxide-dependent ciliary motility in bovine airway epithelium. Am J Physiol 1995; 268:L911–L917.

159. Adler KB, Fischer BM, Li H, Choe NH, Wright DT. Hypersecretion of mucin in response to inflammatory mediators by guinea pig tracheal epithelial cells in vitro is blocked by inhibition of nitric oxide synthase. Am J Respir Cell Mol Biol 1995; 13:526–530.

160. Andonegui G, Trevani AS, Gamberale R, Carreras MC, Poderoso JJ, Giordano M, Geffner JR. Effect of nitric oxide donors on oxygen-dependent cytotoxic responses mediated by neutrophils. J Immunol 1999; 162:2922–2930.

161. Wink DA, Hanbauer I, Laval F, Cook JA, Krishna MC, Mitchell JB. Nitric oxide protects against the cytotoxic effects of reactive oxygen species. Ann N Y Acad Sci 1994; 738:265–278.

162. Sharma VS, Traylor TG, Gardiner R, Mizukami H. Reaction of nitric oxide with heme proteins and model compounds of hemoglobin. Biochemistry 1987; 26:3837–3843.

163. Kanner J, Harel S, Granit R. Nitric oxide as an antioxidant. Arch Biochem Biophys 1991; 289:130–136.

164. White AC, Maloney EK, Boustani MR, Hassoun PM, Fanburg BL. Nitric oxide increases cellular glutathione levels in rat lung fibroblasts. Am J Respir Cell Mol Biol 1995; 13:442–448.

165. Eiserich JP, Butler J, van der Vliet A, Cross CE, Halliwell B. Nitric oxide rapidly scavenges tyrosine and tryptophan radicals. Biochem J 1995; 310:745–749.

166. Liu X, Miller MS, Joshi MS, Thomas DD, Lancaster JRJ. Accelerated reaction of nitric oxide with O_2 within the hydrophobic interior of biological membranes. Proc Natl Acad Sci USA 1998; 95:2175–2179.

167. Poss WB, Timmons OD, Farrukh IS, Hoidal JR, Michael JR. Inhaled nitric oxide prevents the increase in pulmonary vascular permeability caused by hydrogen peroxide. J Appl Physiol 1995; 79:886–891.

168. McElroy MC, Wiener-Kronish JP, Miyazaki H, Sawa T, Modelska K, Dobbs LG, Pittet JF. Nitric oxide attenuates lung endothelial injury caused by sublethal hyperoxia in rats. Am J Physiol 1997; 272:L631–L638.

169. Rottenberg ME, Gigliotti Rothfuchs AC, Gigliotti D, Svanholm C, Bandholtz L, Wigzell H. Role of innate and adaptive immunity in the outcome of primary infection with *Chlamydia pneumoniae,* as analyzed in genetically modified mice. J Immunol 1999; 162:2829–2836.

170. MacMicking JD, North RJ, LaCourse R, Mudgett JS, Shah SK, Nathan CF. Identification of nitric oxide synthase as a protective locus against tuberculosis. Proc Natl Acad Sci USA 1997; 94:5243–5248.

171. Heath L, Chrisp C, Huffnagle G, LeGendre M, Osawa Y, Hurley M, Engleberg C, Fantone J, Brieland J. Effector mechanisms responsible for gamma interferon-mediated host resistance to *Legionella pneumophila* lung infection: the role of endogenous nitric oxide differs in susceptible and resistant murine hosts. Infect Immun 1996; 64:5151–5160.

172. Cartner SC, Simecka JW, Briles DE, Cassell GH, Lindsey JR. Resistance to mycoplasmal lung disease in mice is a complex genetic trait. Infect Immun 1996; 64:5326–5331.

173. Davis JK, Parker RF, White H, Dziedzic D, Taylor G, Davidson MK, Cox NR, Cassell GH. Strain differences in susceptibility to murine respiratory mycoplasmosis in C57BL/6 and C3H/HeN mice. Infect Immun 1985; 50:647–654.

174. Parker RF, Davis JK, Blalock DK, Thorp RB, Simecka JW, Cassell GH. Pulmonary clearance of *Mycoplasma pulmonis* in C57BL/6N and C3H/HeN HeNmice.InfectImmun1987; 55 : 2631–2635.

175. Hickman-Davis J, Gibbs-Erwin J, Lindsey JR, Matalon S. Surfactant protein A mediates mycoplasmacidal activity of alveolar macrophages by production of peroxynitrite. Proc Natl Acad Sci USA 1999; 96:4953–4958.

176. Kaplan SS, Lancaster JR Jr, Basford RE, Simmons RL. Effect of nitric oxide on staphylococcal killing and interactive effect with superoxide. Infect Immun 1996; 64:69–76.

177. Assreuy J, Cunha FQ, Epperlein M, Noronha-Dutra A, O'Donnell CA, Liew FY, Moncada S. Production of nitric oxide and superoxide by activated macrophages and killing of *Leishmania major.* Eur J Immunol 1994; 24:672–676.

178. Fernandes PD, Assreuy J. Role of nitric oxide and superoxide in *Giardia lamblia* killing. Braz J Med Biol Res 1997; 30:93–99.

179. De Groote MA, Granger D, Xu Y, Campbell G, Prince R, Fang FC. Genetic and redox determinants of nitric oxide cytotoxicity in a *Salmonella typhimurium* model. Proc Natl Acad Sci USA 1995; 92:6399–6403.

180. Brunelli L, Crow JP, Beckman JS. The comparative toxicity of nitric oxide and peroxynitrite to *Escherichia coli.* Arch Biochem Biophys 1995; 316: 327–334.

181. Pacelli R, Wink DA, Cook JA, Krishna MC, DeGraff W, Friedman N, Tsokos M, Samuni A, Mitchell JB. Nitric oxide potentiates hydrogen peroxide-induced killing of *Escherichia coli.* J Exp Med 1995; 182:1469–1479.

182. Darrah PA, Hondalus MK, Chen Q, Ischiropoulos H, Mosser DM. Cooperation between reactive oxygen and nitrogen intermediates in killing of *Rhodococcus equi* by activated macrophages. Infect Immun 2000; 68:3587–3593.

183. Fang FC. Perspectives series: host/pathogen interactions. Mechanisms of nitric oxide-related antimicrobial activity. J Clin Invest 1997; 99:2818–2825.

184. Ehrt S, Shiloh MU, Ruan J, Choi M, Gunzburg S, Nathan C, Xie Q, Riley LW. A novel antioxidant gene from *Mycobacterium tuberculosis.* J Exp Med 1997; 186:1885–1896.

185. Ruan J, St John G, Ehrt S, Riley L, Nathan C. noxR3 a novel gene from Mycobacterium tuberculosis, protects *Salmonella typhimurium* from nitrosative oxidative stress. Infect Immun 1999; 67:3276–3283.

186. Glockzin S, von Knethen A, Scheffner M, Brune B. Activation of the cell death program by nitric oxide involves inhibition of the proteasome. J Biol Chem 1999; 274:19581–19586.

187. Williams MS, Noguchi S, Henkart PA, Osawa Y. Nitric oxide synthase plays a signaling role in TCR-triggered apoptotic death. J Immunol 1998; 161: 6526–6531.

188. von Knethen A, Callsen D, Brune B. Superoxide attenuates macrophage apoptosis by NF-kappa B and AP-1 activation that promotes cyclooxygenase-2 expression. J Immunol 1999; 163:2858–2866.

189. von Knethen A, Callsen D, Brune B. NF-kappaB and AP-1 activation by nitric oxide attenuated apoptotic cell death in RAW 264.7 macrophages. Mol Biol Cell 1999; 10:361–372.

190. Ware LB, Matthay MA. The acute respiratory distress syndrome. N Engl J Med 2000; 342:1334–1349.

191. Matthay MA, Folkesson HG, Campagna A, Kheradmand F. Alveolar epithelial barrier and acute lung injury. New Horiz 1993; 1:613–622.

192. Barnard ML, Baker RR, Matalon S. Mitigation of oxidant injury to lung microvasculature by intratracheal instillation of antioxidant enzymes. Am J Physiol 1993; 265:L340–L345.

193. Robbins CG, Horowitz S, Merritt TA, Kheiter A, Tierney J, Narula P, Davis JM. Recombinant human superoxide dismutase reduces lung injury caused by inhaled nitric oxide and hyperoxia. Am J Physiol 1997; 272:L903–L907.

194. Flick MR, Hoeffel JM, Staub NC. Superoxide dismutase with heparin prevents increased lung vascular permeability during air emboli in sheep. J Appl Physiol 1983; 55:1284–1291.

195. Bernard GR, Lucht WD, Niedermeyer ME, Snapper JR, Ogletree ML, Brigham KL. Effect of *N*-acetylcysteine on the pulmonary response to endotoxin in the awake sheep and upon in vitro granulocyte function. J Clin Invest 1984; 73:1772–1784.

196. Gonzalez PK, Zhuang J, Doctrow SR, Malfroy B, Benson PF, Menconi MJ, Fink MP. EUK-8, a synthetic superoxide dismutase and catalase mimetic, ameliorates acute lung injury in endotoxemic swine. J Pharmacol Exp Ther 1995; 275:798–806.

197. Al-Mehdi A, Shuman H, Fisher AB. Fluorescence microtopography of oxidative stress in lung ischemia–reperfusion. Lab Invest 1994; 70:579–587.

198. Matalon S, Haddad IY. Natural surfactant and hyperoxic lung injury in primates. J Appl Physiol 1994; 76:989–990.

199. Matthay MA, Wiener-Kronish JP. Intact epithelial barrier function is critical for the resolution of alveolar edema in humans. Am Rev Respir Dis 1990; 142:1250–1257.

200. Warner RL, Paine R3, Christensen PJ, Marletta MA, Richards MK, Wilcoxen SE, Ward PA. Lung sources and cytokine requirements for in vivo expression of inducible nitric oxide synthase. Am J Respir Cell Mol Biol 1995; 12:649–661.

201. Zhu S, Ware LB, Geiser T, Matthay MA, Matalon S. Increased levels of nitrate and surfactant protein a nitration in the pulmonary edema fluid of patients with acute lung injury. Am J Respir Crit Care Med 2001; 163: 166–172.

202. Lamb NJ, Quinlan GJ, Westerman ST, Gutteridge JM, Evans TW. Nitration of proteins in bronchoalveolar lavage fluid from patients with acute respiratory distress syndrome receiving inhaled nitric oxide. Am J Respir Crit Care Med 1999; 160:1031–1034.

203. Cochrane CG, Spragg R, Revak SD. Pathogenesis of the adult respiratory distress syndrome. Evidence of oxidant activity in bronchoalveolar lavage fluid. J Clin Invest 1983; 71:754–761.

204. Sznajder JI, Fraiman A, Hall JB, Sanders W, Schmidt G, Crawford G, Nahum A, Factor P, Wood LD. Increased hydrogen peroxide in the expired breath of patients with acute hypoxemic respiratory failure. Chest 1989; 96: 606–612.

205. Quinlan GJ, Lamb NJ, Tilley R, Evans TW, Gutteridge JM. Plasma hypoxanthine levels in ARDS: implications for oxidative stress, morbidity, and mortality. Am J Respir Crit Care Med 1997; 155:479–484.

206. de Andrade JA, Crow JP, Viera L, Bruce AC, Randall YK, McGiffin DC, Zorn GL, Zhu S, Matalon S, Jackson RM. Protein nitration, metabolites of reactive nitrogen species, and inflammation in lung allografts. Am J Respir Crit Care Med 2000; 161:2035–2042.

207. Tanaka S, Choe N, Hemenway DR, Zhu S, Matalon S, Kagan E. Asbestos inhalation induces reactive nitrogen species and nitrotyrosine formation in the lungs and pleura of the rat. J Clin Invest 1998; 102:445–454.

208. Lamb NJ, Gutteridge JM, Baker C, Evans TW, Quinlan GJ. Oxidative damage to proteins of bronchoalveolar lavage fluid in patients with acute respiratory distress syndrome: evidence for neutrophil-mediated hydroxylation, nitration, and chlorination. Crit Care Med 1999; 27:1738–1744.

209. Matalon S, DeMarco V, Haddad IY, Myles C, Skimming JW, Schurch S, Cheng S, Cassin S. Inhaled nitric oxide injures the pulmonary surfactant system of lambs in vivo. Am J Physiol 1996; 270:L273–L280.

210. Cross CE, Forte T, Stocker R, Louie S, Yamamoto Y, Ames BN, Frei B. Oxidative stress and abnormal cholesterol metabolism in patients with adult respiratory distress syndrome. J Lab Clin Med 1990; 115:396–404.

211. Metnitz PG, Bartens C, Fischer M, Fridrich P, Steltzer H, Druml W. Antioxidant status in patients with acute respiratory distress syndrome. Intensive Care Med 1999; 25:180–185.

212. Pacht ER, Timerman AP, Lykens MG, Merola AJ. Deficiency of alveolar fluid glutathione in patients with sepsis and the adult respiratory distress syndrome. Chest 1991; 100:1397–1403.

213. Bernard GR, Wheeler AP, Arons MM, Morris PE, Paz HL, Russell JA, Wright PE, The Antioxidant in ARDS Study Group. A trial of antioxidants *N*-acetylcysteine and procysteine in ARDS. Chest 1997; 112:164–172.

214. Molnar Z, Shearer E, Lowe D. *N*-acetylcysteine treatment to prevent the progression of multisystem organ failure: a prospective randomized placebo-controlled study. Crit Care Med 1999; 27:1100–1104.

215. Leff JA, Parsons PE, Day CE, Moore EE, Moore FA, Oppegard MA, Repine JE. Increased serum catalase activity in septic patients with the adult respiratory distress syndrome. Am Rev Respir Dis 1992; 146:985–989.

216. Leff JA, Parsons PE, Day CE, Taniguchi N, Jochum M, Fritz H, Moore FA, Moore EE, McCord JM, Repine JE. Serum antioxidants as predictors of adult respiratory distress syndrome in patients with sepsis. Lancet 1993; 341:777–780.
217. Gadek JE, DeMichele SJ, Karlstad MD, Pacht ER, Donahoe M, Albertson TE, Van Hoozen C, Wennberg AK, Nelson JL, Noursalehi M, Enteral Nutrition in ARDS Study Group. Effect of enteral feeding with eicosapentaenoic acid, gamma-linolenic acid, and antioxidants in patients with acute respiratory distress syndrome. Crit Care Med 1999; 27:1409–1420.

8

Vascular Dysfunction in Lung Injury

STEPHEN WEDGEWOOD, JEFFREY R. FINEMAN, and STEPHEN M. BLACK

*Department of Pediatrics, Northwestern University Medical School, Chicago,
Illinois, U.S.A., Department of Pediatrics and Cardiovascular Research Institute
University of California, San Francisco, California, U.S.A., and
Department of Biomedical and Pharmaceutical Sciences,
The University of Montana, Missoula, Montana, U.S.A.*

I. Overview

Abnormalities in the pulmonary vasculature are associated with many
forms of lung injury. This chapter reviews current understanding of normal
pulmonary vascular development and function, and the potential mechanisms that result in clinical manifestations of lung injury. The growth of
the pulmonary vascular bed, and the mechanisms that regulate vascular
tone are also discussed (additional details on lung growth and development
are in Chapter 2). Relevant examples of pulmonary vascular diseases are
presented, concentrating primarily on fetal and neonatal disorders. Pulmonary hypertension secondary to congenital heart disease is associated with
vascular remodeling. Abnormal structural development of the pulmonary
vasculature has also been implicated in persistent pulmonary hypertension
of the newborn (PPHN), a condition that accounts for 1% of all admissions to newborn intensive care units. Irregular vascular reactivity and
morphology have also been well characterized in adult patients with primary and secondary pulmonary hypertensive disorders. Vascular dysfunction is thought to play a significant role in the pathophysiology of both

acute lung injury (ALI) and chronic lung injury in children and adults. Relevant animal models of lung injury and vascular dysfunction, and the insights they provide in identifying underlying mechanisms are discussed in this chapter. Potential therapeutic strategies resulting from this knowledge are also described, with further details about vascular-based therapies for clinical lung injury given in Chapter 17.

II. Normal Growth and Development of the Pulmonary Vascular Bed

In the human fetus, the main pulmonary artery arises from the truncus arteriosus and the branch pulmonary (pre- and intra-acinar) arteries arise from the sixth branchial arch. The peripheral pulmonary arteries arise from the lung buds and develop at the same time as the airways (1,2). By 16 weeks gestation, all preacinar pulmonary artery branches are present. With advancing gestation, these arteries increase in diameter and length; the intra-acinar arteries develop later, along with the respiratory bronchiole, primitive alveolar ducts, and alveoli (3). After birth, the peripheral pulmonary arteries increase in diameter and length. These pulmonary arteries dilate in response to the increase in pulmonary blood flow that occurs with ventilation and oxygenation at birth. Furthermore, they increase in number as the alveoli proliferate. In the newborn, there is an artery for every 20 alveoli; in the 2-year-old, an artery for every 12 alveoli; in the adult an artery for every 8 alveoli (1–5). This increases the cross-sectional area of the pulmonary vascular bed and allows pulmonary blood flow to increase without changes in pulmonary arterial pressure or vascular resistance (4–8).

In the fetus, the structure of the pulmonary artery varies with the size of the vessel. The pulmonary arteries from the hilum to 1500 µm in diameter are elastic; from 1500 to 200 µm in diameter are fully muscular; from 200 to 100 µm in diameter are partially muscular; and less than 100 µm (intra-acinar) in diameter are nonmuscular (4–8). After birth, there is a gradual extension of muscle into more peripheral pulmonary arteries; in the adult, muscular arteries are found associated with the alveolar wall (<100 µm). Extension of muscle results from the differentiation of precursor cells, the pericyte, and intermediate cells into mature vascular smooth muscle cells (4–8).

III. Regulation of Neonatal Vascular Tone

After birth, with initiation of ventilation, pulmonary vascular resistance (PVR) decreases and pulmonary blood flow increases 8 to 10-fold to match systemic blood flow (9–12). This process is regulated by a complex and incompletely understood interplay between mechanical and metabolic factors (13). These include mechanical vascular distention and replacement of a fluid interface with air, and prostaglandin production that is associated with lung distention. Recent evidence suggests that normal pulmonary vascular tone is regulated by a complex interaction of vasoactive substances produced by the vascular endothelium (Fig. 1) (13–16). These substances include nitric oxide (NO) and endothelin-1 (ET-1). Nitric oxide is an endothelium-derived relaxing factor synthesized by the oxidation of L-arginine after activation of endothelial NO synthase (eNOS) (17). Once released from endothelial cells (EC), NO diffuses into vascular smooth muscle cells (SMC) and activates soluble guanylate cyclase (sGC), which catalyzes the production of cGMP from GTP. cGMP induces vascular SMC relaxation through activation of a cGMP-dependent protein kinase (PKG) (18). Although the exact mechanism is unclear, PKG-mediated relaxation in response to NO and cGMP has been shown to influence interactions between proteins within the smooth muscle contractile apparatus (19). Basal NO production rises 2-fold from late gestation to 1 week of life and another 1.6-fold from 1 to 4 weeks of life in intrapulmonary arteries (20). Coinciding with these data, eNOS mRNA and protein increase in late gestation then decrease postnatally in rat and sheep lung parenchyma (21–23). In addition, sGC mRNA levels are 7-fold higher in late-gestation fetal and neonatal rats than those in adult rats (24). In addition, L-arginine and inhaled NO increases pulmonary blood flow in fetal and newborn lambs, while inhibition of NO synthesis increases pulmonary vascular

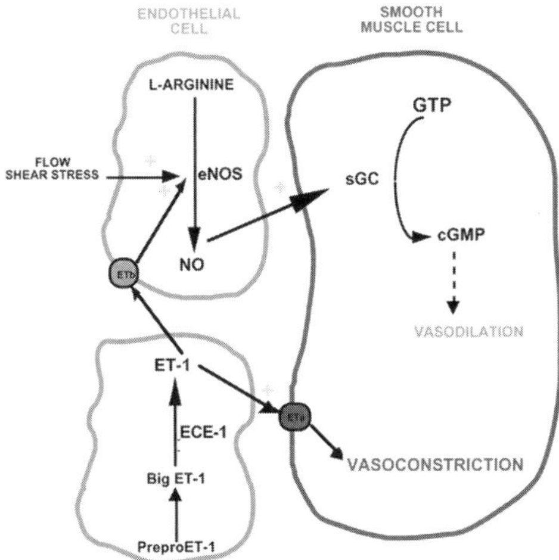

Figure 1 Schematic diagram depicting the regulation of eNOS and ET-1 gene expression and the regulation of vascular tone in the normal pulmonary circulation.

resistance in fetal and newborns (25–27). Taken together, these data strongly suggest that NO activity mediates, in part, the fall in pulmonary vascular resistance during the fetal to newborn transition, as well as basal fetal and postnatal pulmonary vascular tone.

ET-1, a 21-amino acid polypeptide produced by vascular EC, has potent vasoactive properties and is mitogenic for vascular SMC (16,28). ET-1 is produced by the cleavage of a 203-amino acid precursor (pre-proET-1) to form proET-1 (Big ET-1). Big ET-1 is then cleaved by endothelin-converting enzyme-1 (ECE-1) into its functional form (29). The complex pulmonary vasoactive effects of ET-1, which may include either vasoconstriction and/or vasodilation, are mediated by at least two different receptors: ET_A and ET_B. ET_A receptors, located predominantly on vascular SMC, mediate vasoconstriction, whereas ET_B receptors, located on vascular EC, mediate vasodilation (30–32). Increasing data suggest that NO and ET-1 regulate each other through an autocrine feedback loop (33). For example, ET-1 stimulates eNOS activity via ET_B receptor activation, whereas NO-cGMP production increases ET_A receptors in vascular SMC and inhibits ET-1 secretion and gene expression in vascular EC (34,35). Animal studies suggest that basal ET-1 production has minimal effects on normal fetal, transitional, and postnatal pulmonary vascular tone. However, both animal and human studies suggest that ET-1 plays a significant role in pulmonary vascular pathophysiology.

IV. Clinical Pulmunary Vascular Dysfunction

A. Pulmonary Hypertension Secondary to Congenital Heart Disease

Survival for children with congenital heart defects has improved significantly, although substantial morbidity and mortality still occurs even after corrective surgery. In subsets of children, this is due, in part, to an abnormal structural development of the pulmonary circulation. For example, after birth as pulmonary vascular resistance decreases, the presence of a systemic arterial to pulmonary arterial communication results in increasing pulmonary blood flow (1,2,36). This abnormal postnatal hemodynamic state may result in progressive functional and structural abnormalities of the pulmonary vascular bed (37,38). Pulmonary morphometric analysis of the lungs of children with congenital heart defects shows altered pulmonary vascular growth and remodeling correlating with the child's hemodynamic state (38). These changes are characterized by abnormal extension of muscle into small peripheral arteries and a mild medial hypertrophy of normally muscular arteries, more severe medial hypertrophy of normally muscular arteries, and reduced arterial number and concentration. Uncorrected, these vascular changes result in obliteration of the pulmonary vascular bed and death secondary to severe cyanosis and myocardial failure. After surgical correction, early vascular changes are usually reversible (38,39). However, more severe changes are irreversible and progressive. Conversely, in newborns with pulmonary atresia and decreased pulmonary blood flow, the pulmonary arteries are small, fewer in number, and less muscular (40,41). Therefore, the status of the pulmonary vasculature is often the principal determinant of the clinical course and feasibility of surgical treatment.

Several studies have demonstrated increased ET-1 plasma concentrations and impaired endothelium-dependent pulmonary vasodilation in children with congenital heart disease associated with increased pulmonary blood flow and pulmonary hypertension (42–45). Overall, several mechanisms affecting growth factor production and endothelial reactivity are likely to contribute to the vascular remodeling and vasoconstriction characteristic of pulmonary hypertension secondary to increased blood flow. Animal models and mechanisms of vascular dysfunction in pulmonary hypertension and the other pulmonary diseases described in this section are covered in detail later (Secs. V and VI).

B. Persistent Pulmonary Hypertension of the Newborn

With the initiation of ventilation and oxygenation at birth, pulmonary vascular resistance decreases and pulmonary blood flow increases. However, in a number of clinical conditions, there is a failure of the pulmonary circulation to undergo the normal transition to postnatal life, resulting in PPHN (46–49). In PPHN, pulmonary vascular resistance does not decrease normally at birth, resulting in pulmonary hypertension, right-to-left shunting, and hypoxemia (50). Newborns who die of PPHN exhibit an increase both in the thickness of the smooth muscle layer within small pulmonary arteries and an extension of this muscle to nonmuscular arteries (51). Often, microvascular thrombi occlude these arteries, and there is also proliferation of adventitial tissues (52). These structural changes indicate that in utero events have altered the pulmonary circulation. These abnormalities are associated with an increase in the expression of genes that induce vasoconstriction and a reduction in those that induce vasodilation. In particular, there is an inability to regulate properly the production of NO and ET-1 such that NO levels are suppressed and ET-1 levels are increased (Fig. 2) (47). However, it is not understood how this apparent co-ordinated regulation occurs, nor is it clear how proliferation of the smooth muscle cells in the pulmonary vasculature is stimulated to produce the observed, abnormal muscularization. Animal models of PPHN, and the roles played by NO and ET-1 in the vascular remodeling manifested in clinical condition are discussed in later sections.

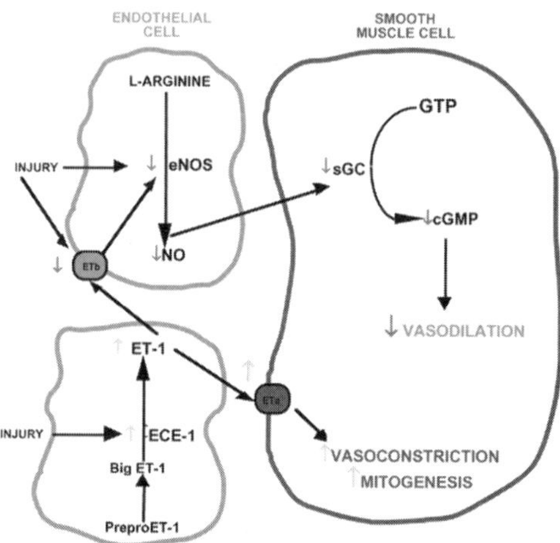

Figure 2   Schematic diagram depicting the abnormal regulation of eNOS and ET-1 gene expression and vascular tone in the hypertensive pulmonary circulation.

C. Adult Pulmonary Hypertension

Primary pulmonary hypertension (PPH) is characterized by vascular cell proliferation and obliteration of small pulmonary arteries, which leads to severe pulmonary hypertension (PH) and right ventricular failure. Adults with advanced pulmonary hypertension have impaired endothelium-dependent pulmonary vasodilation and decreased eNOS gene expression within pulmonary vascular EC (53,54). In addition, there is a correlation between the levels of circulating ET-1 and the severity of PPH (55). This suggests that aberrations in the NO-cGMP and ET-1 cascades play a significant role in the development of PPH as discussed later.

D. Hypoxia-Induced Pulmonary Hypertension

Hypoxia plays a significant role in the pulmonary hypertension associated with chronic obstructive airway disease (46). Alveolar hypoxia leads to pulmonary hypertension and subsequent vascular remodeling, particularly within the distal pulmonary arterioles (56). Studies have shown that the NO-cGMP cascade plays an important role in hypoxia-induced vascular remodeling, although the detailed mechanisms involved are unclear (57–64).

E. Vascular Dysfunction in Clinical ALI
     and ARDS

Acute lung injury and acute respiratory distress syndrome (ARDS) arise from a variety of causes with the common clinical manifestations being hypoxemia and bilateral pulmonary infiltrates (see Chapter 3) (65). A mild to moderate degree of pulmonary hypertension is common in these patients. This may worsen pulmonary edema, and impair right ventricular performance. The initial increase in pulmonary arterial pressure is not an indicator of mortality, although pulmonary arterial pressure continues to increase in patients with increased mortality. Since hypoxic pulmonary vasoconstriction is adaptive in minimizing ventilation–perfusion mismatch, the use of nonselective intravenous vasodilators may reduce pulmonary arterial pressures, but is commonly associated with worsening arterial hypoxemia secondary to impaired ventilation–perfusion matching. Inhalational vasodilators, such as NO, may selectively improve blood flow to well-ventilated lung regions and thereby improve oxygenation. A major feature of ALI/ARDS is impaired function of the pulmonary endothelium, secondary to the activation and adhesion of platelets, neutrophils, and monocytes (66,67). This may result in a decrease in vasodilators including NO. This contributes to the widespread pulmonary vasoconstriction seen in ALI/ARDS, resulting in pulmonary hypertension and hypoxemia. Mechanisms of inflammation-induced loss of endothelium function in ALI/ARDS are discussed in more detail later.

V. Animal Models
A. Animal Model of Congenital Heart Disease

A model which mimics a congenital heart defect with increased pulmonary blood flow was established in the lamb with in utero placement of an aorta-to-pulmonary artery vascular graft (68). This model is associated with increased pulmonary blood flow and pressure. At 4 weeks of age, these "shunt" lambs have clinical and pathologic sequelae similar to children with congenital heart defects associated with increased pulmonary blood flow and pulmonary hypertension. Pulmonary morphometric analysis shows pulmonary arterial medial muscular hypertrophy with abnormal extension of muscle to generally nonmuscularized small peripheral arteries. There is an increase in the number of arteries per alveoli, representing angiogenesis. Similarly, in children with congenital heart defects associated with increased pulmonary blood flow and normal pulmonary arterial pressure, wedge pulmonary arteriograms performed during cardiac catheterization show a dense capillary blush suggesting an increase in the number of peripheral pulmonary arteries (69). Therefore, this increase in pulmonary artery number likely represents an early adaptation to increased pulmonary blood flow.

B. Animal Models of PPHN

In fetal lambs, ligation, mechanical compression, or pharmacological constriction of the ductus arteriosus produces fetal and neonatal pulmonary hypertension (46–49). This model is associated with decreased pulmonary blood flow with increased pressure. Similar to newborns who die of PPHN, these lambs have an increase in the thickness of smooth muscle within the small pulmonary arteries, complete muscularization of normally partially muscularized pulmonary arteries, and extension of muscle to non-muscularized arteries. Like newborns who die of PPHN, ET-1 gene expression is increased in this ductal ligation model of fetal pulmonary hypertension (47).

C. Animal Models of Primary Pulmonary Hypertension

The compound monocrotaline has been used to induce pulmonary hypertension in several animal models. This form of hypertension is associated with pulmonary vascular remodeling, including a significantly higher pulmonary arterial medial wall thickness (70). Monocrotaline-treated animals exhibit decreased eNOS expression (71) and increased ET-1 expression (72). Several studies have demonstrated the efficacy of ET receptor antagonists in the attenuation of monocrotaline-induced pulmonary hypertension (73–75). The use of ET receptor antagonists in treating pulmonary hypertension is discussed further in Sec. VII. Monocrotaline-induced pulmonary hypertension was reversed in rats treated with serine elastase inhibitors (76). Pulmonary arterial pressure and muscularization were reduced due to myocyte apoptosis and loss of extracellular matrix, with pulmonary arterial pressure and structure returning to normal after 2 weeks.

D. Animal Models of Hypoxia and of ALI/ARDS

In chronic hypoxia-treated rats, there is an increase in eNOS and sGC expression, with an accompanying increase in sGC activity and elevated cGMP levels (77). ET-1 is also increased in the plasma and lungs of rats exposed to hypoxia (78,79). Treatment with either ET_A or combined ET_A and ET_B receptor antagonists has been shown to attenuate the development of hypoxic pulmonary hypertension (80,81). The use of ET receptor antagonists in the treatment of pulmonary hypertension is discussed in more detail later. Data relating to vascular dysfunction have also been obtained in several animal models of ALI and ARDS (see Chapter 10 for details on animal models of ALI/ARDS). Examples of relevant animal models of ALI/ARDS include intravenous injection of rabbits with bacterial endotoxin (82), and acid aspiration in rats (83). Experimental acute lung injury of these and other types results in increased levels of ET-1 in circulating blood, bronchoalveolar lavage, and lung tissue (84) (Table 1).

Table 1 Changes in gene expression in animal models of pulmonary hypertension

Model	ET-1	ECE-1	ETA-R	ETB-R	eNOS	sGC	PDE5
Shunt	↑ (98)	↑ (99)	↑ (99)	↓ (99)	↑ (101)[a]	↑ (104)	↑ (104)
Ductal ligation	↑ (118)	→ (118)		↓ (47)	↓ (47)	↓ (47)	↑ (47)
Monocrotaline	↑ (72)				↓ (71)		
Hyperoxia	↑ (78,79)				↑ (57–64)	↑ (77)	
ARDS	↑ (84)				↓[b]		

[a]eNOS expression is increased in this model. However, additional data suggests that enzyme activity is decreased (100).
[b]loss of endothelial integrity results in reduced NO bioavailability

VI. Mechanisms of Vascular Dysfunction

A common characteristic of the diseases and animal models presented in preceding sections is the loss of endothelial function, in particular NO production. This section discusses current understanding of the mechanisms that regulate normal endothelial activity, and the potential reasons for abnormal regulation in states of lung injury and in certain pulmonary diseases. Additional mechanisms that contribute to pulmonary vascular pathology in specific diseases are also detailed.

A. Regulation of eNOS Gene Expression by Shear Stress

Endothelial NO synthase gene expression is influenced by several stimuli, with laminar shear stress making an important contribution. NOS activity, NO production, and eNOS mRNA and protein levels are increased in ECs exposed to shear stress (85–92), although the mechanisms involved are unclear. In fetal pulmonary arterial endothelial cells (FPAEC) exposed to shear, NO production is biphasic with an increased concentration up to 1 hr, a plateau phase until 4 hr, and then a second release between 4 and 8 hr (93). The initial release may be due to the activation of preformed enzyme. In contrast, the second NO release coincides with an increase in eNOS mRNA and protein and may be stimulated by factors that regulate eNOS gene transcription. Interestingly, the eNOS promoter contains a cis-acting regulatory element identical to the previously identified shear stress-responsive element (94), raising the possibility that shear stress-induced factors regulate eNOS transcription via this sequence. Increasing evidence has shown that the PKC system is also stimulated by shear stress (87,89–91,95). PKC inhibition reduced the amount of NO released and prevented increases in eNOS mRNA and protein levels in sheared FPAECs (93). Furthermore, stimulation of PKC activity with phorbol ester increased eNOS gene expression without increasing NO release in FPAECs (93). These data suggest a role for PKC in shear stress regulation of eNOS gene expression in these cells. Endothelial NO synthase enzyme activity is regulated by several proteins, and the positive regulation by calmodulin and HSP90 is enhanced by shear stress (reviewed by Fulton et al. (96)). Shear stress also increases eNOS activation via Akt-mediated phosphorylation (96), and recent evidence suggests that shear stress increases eNOS mRNA half-life via c-Src activation (97). Overall, shear stress regulates NO release at the level of eNOS transcription, mRNA stability, and enzyme activity.

B. Abnormal Regulation of NO and ET-1 Cascades in Congenital Heart Disease

Several studies have demonstrated increased ET-1 plasma concentrations in children with congenital heart disease associated with increased pulmonary blood flow and pulmonary hypertension (42–44). In the shunt animal model of pulmonary hypertension, plasma ET-1 concentrations were higher (98), and levels of ECE-1 mRNA and protein were elevated in lung tissue prepared from 4-week-old lambs relative to age-matched controls (99). Furthermore, ET_A receptor mRNA and protein levels were increased, while ET_B receptor mRNA and protein levels were decreased, in lung tissue from the shunts relative to controls (99). The predicted result of these gene alterations is increased production of ET-1, increased ET-1-mediated pulmonary vasoconstriction, and decreased ET-1-mediated vasodilation. Shunt lambs also exhibit physiologic alterations in the NO-cGMP cascade, including a selective impairment of endothelium-dependent pulmonary vasodilation. This is suggestive of decreased NO activity since the endothelium-dependent pulmonary vasodilating effects of acetylcholine and ATP were attenuated compared to control lambs (68). Using isolated pulmonary arteries, it was found that removal of superoxide enhanced endothelium-dependent relaxation in shunt vessels (100). Thus, the endothelial dysfunction associated with pulmonary hypertension may be due, in part, to excessive superoxide production. Although endothelial activity is decreased in the shunt model, expression of eNOS and sGC is elevated (101). Shear stress-induced eNOS transcription, arising from increased pulmonary blood flow, may be involved. However, excessive levels of superoxide present in this model are predicted to inhibit NOS activity (102) and NO bioactivity (103). The NO-cGMP cascade is also influenced by the activity of cyclic nucleotide phosphodiesterases (PDEs), which regulate intracellular levels of cGMP by catalyzing its conversion to GMP. Recently, expression and activity of PDE type 5 (PDE5), the predominant cGMP-metabolizing PDE in pulmonary tissues, were shown to be increased in shunted lambs relative to controls (104). It is possible that the increased PDE5 activity present in lungs from shunted lambs may be sufficient to limit cGMP accumulation, thereby reducing SMC relaxation These potential interactions in the normal and hypertensive are shown in Figures 1 and 2.

C. Role of Increased Pulmonary Blood Flow and Growth Factors

In vivo, blood vessels are exposed to a variety of physiologic stimuli, including alterations in shear stress, stretch, pressure, and oxygenation. These stimuli can modify the structure and function of endothelial and vascular smooth muscle cells, and alter gene expression (105). Shear stress may be altered in the pulmonary circulation of children with congenital heart defects because: (1) increased or decreased pulmonary blood flow alters blood flow velocity, (2) blood hematocrit, related to viscosity, is increased, and (3) there may be under- or over-development of the pulmonary circulation. Shear stress induces gene expression of several endothelial cell-specific genes including basic fibroblast growth factor (bFGF) (106). Basic fibroblast growth factor stimulates the migration of, and is mitogenic for, endothelial and vascular smooth muscle cells, and fibroblasts (107). Stretch is the mechanical deformation of the blood vessel wall produced by a pulse wave. Stretch may be altered in the pulmonary circulation of children with congenital heart defects because of increased or decreased pulmonary arterial blood flow, velocity, or pressure. Mechanical stretch has been shown to increase vascular smooth muscle and endothelial cell proliferation and regulate the expression of several genes (108–111). The increased pulmonary blood flow in patients with congenital heart disease may stimulate the production of growth factors such as bFGF, thereby giving rise to vascular remodeling.

D. ET-1-Mediated Vascular SMC Proliferation in PPHN

Due to conflicting reports, the role of ET-1 in vascular SMC proliferation remains controversial (112–115). However, it has been shown that ET-1 has a direct mitogenic effect on pulmonary arterial SMC isolated from fetal lambs (116). This effect was mediated via an ET_A receptor-induced increase in superoxide production, and was prevented by ET_A receptor blockade or by antioxidant treatment. The pathway is likely to involve protein G_i, phosphotidylinositol 3-kinase, and NADPH oxidase since pharmacologic inhibitors of these proteins prevented ET-1-induced SMC proliferation. In a previous study, ET_A receptor antagonism attenuated fetal pulmonary hypertension and inhibited the SMC hypertrophy normally associated with ductal ligation (117). Thus, the vascular remodeling characteristic of PPHN may be mediated, in part, by ET-1-induced superoxide production.

E.   Abnormal Regulation of NO and ET-1 Cascades in PPHN

The effects of ET-1-induced vascular remodeling are likely to be compounded by increased pulmonary vasoconstriction in PPHN. Ligation of the ductus arteriosus in fetal lambs has been associated with a decrease in eNOS and sGC expression, and with an increase in PDE5 expression (118). In addition, an increase in the expression of preproET-1 and a decrease in the expression of ET_B receptor are also found (118). These results suggest a decrease in NO and cGMP concentrations, thereby decreasing pulmonary vasodilator activity. Furthermore, increased ET-1 concentration and limited ET_B receptor activation would increase pulmonary vasoconstrictor activity. Constriction of the ductus arteriosus in fetal lambs is associated with a 106% increase in plasma ET-1 levels and a 43% decrease in total NO synthase activity (118). ET_A receptor antagonism completely blocked the vasoconstriction and preserved NOS activity in this animal model (118). It has also been shown that peroxynitrite, formed in the reaction between superoxide, NO, and nitrates, irreversibly inhibits eNOS (119). This nitration is found to be significantly reduced by ET_A receptor blockade (119). Overall, ET_A receptor-mediated increases in superoxide production resulting in SMC proliferation and NOS inhibition, coupled with ET_A receptor-mediated vasoconstriction, are likely to play a significant role in PPHN.

F.   NO-ET-1 Interactions in PPH

The down-regulation of eNOS expression and up-regulation of ET-1 expression in PPH is likely to play a significant role in the increased vasoconstriction and vascular remodeling via the same mechanisms prevalent in PPHN discussed above.

G.   Mechanisms of Vascular Dysfunction in Hypoxia

Hypoxia is associated with an increase in muscularization of the pulmonary arteries. The up-regulation of ET-1 in chronic hypoxia has been implicated in this vascular remodeling through its mitogenic effects on vascular smooth muscle cells. However, unlike the vascular remodeling seen in patients with congenital heart disease, PPHN, and PPH, there is also an increase in eNOS expression (57–64). Therefore, the mechanisms involved are less clear and remain controversial. Increased eNOS expression during hypoxia does not automatically correlate with increased NO production. Studies have demonstrated a decrease in L-arginine uptake (120) and HSP90 expression (121) during hypoxia, both predicted to reduce eNOS activity. Furthermore, no significant increase in NO metabolites is found following hypoxia (122). These results suggest that hypoxia-induced expression of mitogens such as ET-1 may play a predominant role in vascular remodeling independent of eNOS expression.

H. Mechanisms of Vascular Dysfunction in ALI/ARDS

A major feature of ALI/ARDS is damage to the pulmonary vascular endothelium, secondary to the activation and adhesion of platelets, neutrophils, and monocytes (66,67). This is associated with an increased pulmonary vascular resistance that may reflect, in part, a loss of endothelium-derived vasodilators such as NO. In addition to its intrinsic vasodilatory activity, NO also inhibits the release of cytokines and prevents the expression of adhesion molecules in EC, smooth muscle cells, leukocytes, and platelets (123). Reduced endothelium-derived NO production in ALI/ARDS may therefore promote adhesion of platelets and leukocytes, leading to increased inflammation. Acute tissue injury in ALI/ARDS is associated with an over-exuberant inflammatory response involving a variety of mediators produced by pulmonary and leukocytic cells (see Chapters 3 and 4). Elevated levels of ET-1 may contribute to inflammatory lung injury by inducing the expression of cytokines including tumor necrosis factor and IL-6 and IL-8 (124). In addition, the increased respiratory burst, a surge of superoxide released from leucocytes and neutrophils to destroy bacteria, directly damages EC (125,126). As gaps appear in the endothelial layer, activated neutrophils come into contact with vascular SMC and continue the cascade of inflammation and injury.

VII. Therapies for Vascular Dysfunction

This section briefly reviews selected therapies and agents currently used to treat the pulmonary vascular diseases presented above. Further details about vascular-based therapies are given later in Chapter 17, and additional therapeutic modalities for lung injury are described in Chapters 13–16 and 18–19.

A. Inhaled NO Therapy

Exogenously administered inhaled NO is currently utilized as an adjuvant therapy for a number of pulmonary hypertensive disorders. In both animal and human studies, inhaled NO (5–80 ppm) induces rapid and selective pulmonary vasodilation (127–129). When administered into the airways in gaseous form, NO diffuses into pulmonary vascular smooth muscle cells where it increases cGMP levels, causing potent pulmonary vasodilation. No systemic vasodilation occurs because NO is rapidly inactivated by binding with hemoglobin when it reaches the intravascular space (130). Nonrandomized studies demonstrate that inhaled NO selectively decreases pulmonary arterial pressure and pulmonary vascular resistance in patients with congenital heart disease. In addition, NO decreases pulmonary vascular resistance and improves oxygenation in adults and children with acute lung injury, although randomized trials suggest that the effect is transient and does not change long-term outcome (127,129,131). However, multicentered randomized trials have demonstrated that inhaled NO improves oxygenation and reduces the need for extracorporeal life support in newborns with persistent pulmonary hypertension (128). Although these data are encouraging, several concerns regarding the safety of inhaled NO remain. One of the most important issues is the safety of acute NO withdrawal. Several studies have noted a potentially life-threatening increase in pulmonary vascular resistance on acute withdrawal of inhaled NO. This "rebound pulmonary hypertension" is manifested by an increase in pulmonary vascular resistance, compromised cardiac output, and/or severe hypoxemia (132)(133–135). Exogenous NO exposure inhibits endogenous eNOS activity (136), suggesting that a transient decrease in endogenous eNOS activity during inhaled NO therapy may be a potential mechanism for rebound pulmonary hypertension.

B. ET Receptor Antagonists

Both combined ET_A and ET_B receptor and selective ET_A receptor antagonists have recently been developed for potential clinical use. In adults with advanced pulmonary vascular disease, bosentan, a combined ET receptor antagonist, decreases pulmonary vascular resistance and improves exercise tolerance (137). Randomized trials are currently ongoing. Other potential therapeutic uses for ET receptor antagonists include PPHN and pulmonary hypertension associated with congenital heart disease. For example, ET_A receptor blockade prevents ET-1-induced fetal pulmonary arterial SMC proliferation (116), and has been shown to attenuate the vascular remodeling normally associated with ductal ligation in lambs (117). In addition, ET receptor antagonists induce potent pulmonary vasodilation in a lamb model of congenital heart disease with increased pulmonary blood flow. Human data are currently lacking. In an animal study looking at the causes of rebound pulmonary hypertension, plasma ET-1 levels were increased by 119.5% in lambs receiving inhaled NO for 24 hr (138). Upon acute withdrawal of NO, pulmonary vascular resistance increased by 77.8%. In contrast, there was no significant increase in pulmonary vascular resistance in lambs infused with PD156707, an ET_A receptor antagonist (138). ET-1 induces superoxide production in pulmonary arterial SMC, which, in the presence of NO, forms peroxynitrite (119). Peroxynitrite can then diffuse into the adjacent EC where it nitrates and inhibits eNOS protein. Nitrated eNOS protein was detected in lung tissue of lambs that received inhaled NO, but was reduced in animals treated with PD156707 (119). These results suggest that ET_A receptor antagonism may be beneficial in preventing rebound pulmonary hypertension upon acute NO withdrawal.

C. Antioxidant Therapy

Ascorbic acid, an antioxidant, has been shown to prevent ET-1 stimulated fetal pulmonary arterial SMC proliferation resulting from an induction of reactive oxygen species (116). Results were dependent on the levels of ascorbic acid used, with higher concentrations of ascorbic acid inducing apoptosis in these cells (116). Similarly, antioxidant treatment (139) or over-expression of catalase (140) has been shown to reduce viability and induce apoptosis in other vascular SMC. Antioxidant treatment at the appropriate levels may prove useful in the prevention or reversal of ET-1-induced vascular remodeling seen in PPHN. However, the effects of anti-oxidants on other cell types, especially fetal pulmonary arterial EC, have yet to be determined.

D. PDE5 Inhibitors

Cyclic nucleotide phosphodiesterases (PDEs) regulate intracellular levels of cGMP by catalyzing the conversion of cGMP to GMP (141). PDE type 5 is the predominant PDE in pulmonary tissues (142), and was elevated in a shunt lamb model of pulmonary hypertension secondary to increased pulmonary blood flow (104). This elevation of PDE5 may be partly responsible for impaired endothelium-dependent pulmonary vasodilation and resulting hypertension in these animals. Indeed, studies demonstrate that PDE inhibitors produce potent pulmonary vasodilation in animals and children with pulmonary hypertension (143–145). In addition, a PDE5 inhibitor has been shown to attenuate hypoxia-induced pulmonary hypertension in humans and mice (146). Additional discussion of agents to antagonize various aspects of vascular dysfunction in lung injury and related pulmonary diseases is given in Chapter 17.

VIII. Summary

Several clinical manifestations of lung injury arise from abnormalities within the pulmonary vasculature. Growth and development of the pulmonary vascular bed are complex processes that occur throughout fetal and postnatal life. Irregular control of these processes contributes to several congenital and neonatal pulmonary diseases, as well as to the pathophysiology of lung injury and disease in older individuals. Pulmonary vascular tone is also regulated by a series of complex mechanisms. Nitric oxide, a vasodilator, and ET-1, a vasoconstrictor, are just two of many factors involved in the regulatory process. Nitric oxide, synthesized in the endothelium by eNOS, stimulates relaxation of the adjacent smooth muscle layer via the activation of sGC. ET-1, also synthesized by the endothelium, stimulates vasoconstriction via ET_A receptors on smooth muscle cells. Data suggest that NO and ET-1 levels are closely controlled. Furthermore, eNOS, sGC, and ET-1 expression are developmentally regulated. Although the mechanisms involved are incompletely understood, biomechanical forces within blood vessels are likely to exert considerable influence on vascular development, growth, and tone. For example, shear stress increases eNOS gene expression via the activation of PKC isoforms, with regulation occurring at the level of eNOS transcription, mRNA stability, and enzyme activity.

Studies have demonstrated abnormal regulation of the NO and ET-1 cascades in several clinical pulmonary disorders. In children with pulmonary hypertension secondary to congenital heart defects, abnormal development of the pulmonary circulation is associated with increased pulmonary blood flow. Elevated levels of plasma ET-1 have been detected in these children. In PPHN, there is a failure of the pulmonary circulation to undergo a normal transition to postnatal life, resulting in neonatal pulmonary hypertension. Newborns who die of PPHN exhibit pulmonary vascular remodeling associated with decreased NO production and elevated ET-1 levels. Similarly, in adults with advanced pulmonary hypertension, there is impaired eNOS gene expression and increased circulating ET-1. The NO cascade is also thought to contribute to pulmonary hypertension arising from hypoxia and ALI/ARDS.

Animal models provide invaluable insights into the processes involved in vascular abnormalities in lung disease and injury. For example, a lamb model of pulmonary hypertension secondary to congenital heart disease has been generated by placement of an aorta-to-pulmonary artery vascular graft. These "shunt" animals exhibit increased pulmonary blood flow and vascular remodeling analogous to that seen in children with congenital heart disease. Ligation of the ductus arteriosus generates a lamb model that exhibits the vascular remodeling and pulmonary hypertension seen in subsets of neonates with PPHN. A number of additional animal models of PPH, hypoxia-induced pulmonary hypertension, and ALI/ARDS have also been developed as discussed in this chapter.

From research in animal and cell models, potential mechanisms of lung disease have been hypothesized. In the shunt model, abnormal regulation of several components of the NO and ET-1 cascades have been identified. Impaired NO production and decreased cGMP are likely to contribute to vasoconstriction. This is exacerbated by elevated ET-1-induced vasoconstriction arising from increases in ET-1, ECE-1, and ET_A receptor expression. Furthermore, increased pulmonary blood flow is likely to raise the expression of various growth factors, thus stimulating vascular remodeling. In the ductal ligation model of PPHN, vascular remodeling and pulmonary hypertension are associated with decreased NO production and increased

ET-1 levels. In addition to ET_A receptor-mediated vasoconstriction, ET-1 is also likely to stimulate vascular remodeling by exerting a direct mitogenic effect on smooth muscle cells.

Several potential therapies have been developed from current mechanistic understanding about vascular dysfunction in lung disease and injury. Inhaled NO therapy has been used to decrease pulmonary vascular resistance in patients with congenital heart disease and with PPHN. ET_A receptor antagonism has proved successful in attenuating the vascular remodeling seen in PPHN, probably by preventing ET_A receptor-induced SMC proliferation. Furthermore, a similar approach has been demonstrated to preserve NOS activity in patients receiving inhaled NO therapy, thereby preventing rebound pulmonary hypertension. Additional potential interventions to improve vascular dysfunction have also been developed. For example, antioxidant therapy may be useful in preventing vascular remodeling stimulated by reactive oxygen species, while PDE5 inhibition may induce pulmonary vasodilation by raising cGMP levels.

By adopting a multifaceted approach that integrates basic science and clinical perspectives in studying vascular dysfunction in lung injury, it can be hoped that understanding about the mechanisms involved will continue to improve. Data obtained from patients with pulmonary vascular diseases identify relevant abnormalities at the physiological and tissue level. These vascular abnormalities can then be studied in more detail in animal models to help identify the regulatory and pathophysiological mechanisms involved. Additional complementary cellular research can further probe the mechanistic basis of vascular abnormalities, as well as determine the specific efficacy of potential therapeutic agents in normalizing intracellular responses. Information on agent activity at the cellular and subcellular level can in turn be taken back to animal models, and ultimately extended to patients to define improved treatment strategies for injury-related pulmonary vascular dysfunction and respiratory disease.

References

1. Burrows FA, Rabinovitch M. The pulmonary circulation in children with congenital heart disease: morphologic and morphometric considerations. Can Anaesth Soc J 1985; 32:364–373.
2. Rabinovitch M. Morphology of the developing pulmonary bed: pharmacologic implications. Pediatr Pharmacol 1985; 5:31–48.
3. Hislop A, Reid L. Intra-pulmonary arterial development during fetal life: branching pattern and structure. J Anat 1972; 113:35–48.
4. Hislop A, Reid L. Pulmonary arterial development during childhood: branching pattern and structure. Thorax 1973; 28:129–135.
5. Rendas A, Branthwaite M, Reid L. Growth of pulmonary circulation in normal pig: structural analysis and cardiopulmonary function. J Appl Physiol 1978; 45:806–817.

6. Reid L. The pulmonary circulation: remodeling in growth and disease. Am Rev Resp Dis 1979; 119:531–546.

7. Haworth SG, Hislop AA. Adaptation of the pulmonary circulation to extra-uterine life in the pig and its relevance to the human infant. Cardiovasc Res 1981; 15:108–119.

8. Rabinovitch M. Structure and function of the pulmonary vascular bed: an update. Cardiol Clin 1989; 7:227–238.

9. Cassin S, Dawes GS, Mott JC, Ross BB, Strang LB. The vascular resistance of the foetal and newly ventilated lung of the lamb. J Physiol 1964; 171: 61–79.

10. Dawes GS, Mott JC, Widdicombe JG, Wyatt DG. Changes in the lungs of the newborn lamb. J Physiol 1953; 121:141–162.

11. Iwamoto HS, Teitel D, Rudolph AM. Effects of birth-related events on blood flow distribution. Pediatr Res 1987; 22:634–640.

12. Rudolph AM. Fetal and neonatal pulmonary circulation. Annu Rev Physiol 1979; 41:383–395.

13. Fineman JR, Soifer SJ, Heymann MA. Regulation of pulmonary vascular tone in the perinatal period. Annu Rev Physiol 1995; 57:115–134.

14. Furchgott RF, Vanhoutte PM. Endothelium-derived relaxing and contracting factors. FASEB J 1989; 3:2007–2018.

15. Wiklund N, Persson M, Gustafsson L, Moncada S, Hedqvist P. Modulatory role of endogenous nitric oxide in pulmonary circulation in vivo. Eur J Pharmacol 1990; 185:123–124.

16. Hassoun P, Thappa V, Landman M, Fanburg B. Endothelin 1: mitogenic activity on pulmonary artery smooth muscle cells and release from hypoxic endothelial cells. Proc Exp Biol Med 1992; 199:165–170.

17. Palmer RMJ, Ashton DS, Moncada S. Vascular endothelial cells synthesize nitric oxide from L-arginine. Nature 1988; 333:664–666.

18. Carvajal JA, Germain AM, Huidobro-Toro JP, Weiner CP. Molecular mechanism of cGMP-mediated smooth muscle relaxation. J Cell Physiol 2000; 184:409–420.

19. Surks HK, Mochizuki N, Kasai Y, Georgescu SP, Tang KM, Ito M, Lincoln TM, Mendelsohn ME. Regulation of myosin phosphatase by a specific interaction with cGMP-dependent protein kinase Ialpha. Science 1999; 286: 1583–1587.

20. Shaul PW, Farrar MA, Magness RR. Pulmonary endothelial nitric oxide production is developmentally regulated in the fetus and newborn. Am J Physiol 1993; 265:H1056–H1063.

21. Halbower AC, Tuder RM, Franklin WA, Pollock JS, Forstermann U, Abman SH. Maturation-related changes in endothelial nitric oxide synthase immunolocalization in developing ovine lung. Am J Physiol 1994; 267:L585–L591.

22. Kawai N, Bloch DB, Filippov G, Rabkina D, Suen HC, Losty PD, Janssens SP, Zapol WM, de la Monte S, Bloch KD. Constitutive endothelial nitric oxide synthase gene expression is regulated during lung development. Am J Physiol 1995; 268:L589–L595.

23. North AJ, Star RA, Brannon TS, Ujiie K, Wells LB, Lowenstein CJ, Snyder SH, Shaul PW. Nitric oxide synthase type I and type III gene expression are developmentally regulated in rat lung. Am J Physiol 1994; 266: L635–L641.

24. Bloch KD, Filippov G, Sanchez LS, Nakane M. Pulmonary soluble guanylate cyclase, a nitric oxide receptor, is increased during the perinatal period. Am J Physiol 1997; 272:L400–L406.

25. Abman SH, Chatfield BA, Hall SL, McMurtry IF. Role of endothelium-derived relaxing factor during transition of pulmonary circulation at birth. Am J Physiol 1990; 259:H1921–H1927.

26. Fineman JR, Chang R, Soifer SJ. L-Arginine, a precursor of EDRF in vitro, produces pulmonary vasodilation in lambs. Am J physiol 1991; 261: H1563–H1569.

27. Cornfield DN, Chatfield BA, McQueston JA, McMurtry IF, Abman SH. Effects of birth-related stimuli on L-arginine-dependent pulmonary vasodilation in ovine fetus. Am J Physiol 1992; 262:H1474–H1481.

28. Yanagisawa M, Kurihara H, Kimura S, Tomobe Y, Kobayashi M, Mitsui Y, Yazaki Y, Goto K, Masaki T. A novel potent vasoconstrictor peptide produced by vascular endothelial cells. Nature 1988; 332:411–415.

29. Turner AJ, Murphy LJ. Molecular pharmacology of endothelin converting enzymes. Biochem Pharmacol 1996; 51:91–102.

30. Arai H, Hori S, Aramori I, Ohkubo H, Nakanishi S. Cloning and expression of a cDNA encoding an endothelin receptor. Nature 1990; 348:730–732.

31. Sakurai T, Yanagisawa M, Takuwa Y, Miyazaki H, Kimura S, Goto K, Masaki T. Cloning of a cDNA encoding a non-isopeptide-selective subtype of the endothelin receptor. Nature 1990; 348:732–735.

32. Shetty SS, Okada T, Webb RL, DelGrande D, Lappe RW. Functionally distinct endothelin B receptors in vascular endothelium and smooth muscle. Biochem Biophys Res Commun 1993; 191:459–464.

33. Luscher TF, Yang Z, Tschudi M, von Segesser L, Stulz P, Boulanger C, Siebenmann R, Turina M, Buhler FR. Interaction between endothelin-1 and endothelium-derived relaxing factor in human arteries and veins. Circ Res 1990; 66:1088–1094.

34. Boulanger C, Luscher TF. Release of endothelin from the porcine aorta. Inhibition by endothelium-derived nitric oxide. J Clin Invest 1990; 85:587–590.

35. Redmond EM, Cahill PA, Hodges R, Zhang S, Sitzmann JV. Regulation of endothelin receptors by nitric oxide in cultured rat vascular smooth muscle cells. J Cell Physiol 1996; 166:469–479.

36. Burrows FA, Klinck JR, Rabinovitch M, Bohn DJ. Pulmonary hypertension in children: perioperative management. Can Anaesth Soc J 1986; 33:606–628.

37. Heath D, Edwards JE. The pathology of hypertensive pulmonary vascular disease: a description of six grades of structural changes in the pulmonary arteries with special reference to congenital cardiac septal defects. Circulation 1958; 18:533–547.

38. Rabinovitch M, Keane JF, Norwood WI, Castaneda AR, Reid L. Vascular structure in lung tissue obtained at biopsy correlated with pulmonary hemo-

dynamic findings after repair of congenital heart defects. Circulation 1984; 69:655–667.

39. Hall SM, Haworth SG. Onset and evolution of pulmonary vascular disease in young children: abnormal postnatal remodelling studied in lung biopsies. J Pathol 1992; 166:183–193.

40. Haworth SG, Reid L. Quantitative structural study of pulmonary circulation in the newborn with pulmonary atresia. Thorax 1977; 32:129–133.

41. Rabinovitch M, Reid LM. Quantitative structural analysis of the pulmonary vascular bed in congenital heart defects. Cardiovasc Clin North Am 1977; 11:149–169.

42. Vincent JA, Ross RD, Kassab J, Hsu JM, Pinsky WW. Relation of elevated plasma endothelin in congenital heart disease to increased pulmonary blood flow. Am J Cardiol 1993; 71:1204–1207.

43. Yamamoto K, Ikeda U, Mito H, Fujikawa H, Sekiguchi H, Shimada K. Endothelin production in pulmonary circulation of patients with mitral stenosis. Circulation 1994; 89:2093–2098.

44. Yoshibayashi M, Nishioka K, Nakao K, Saito Y, Matsumura M, Ueda T, Temma S, Shirakami G, Imura H, Mikawa H. Plasma endothelin concentrations in pati-ents with pulmonary hypertension associated with conge-nital heart defects. Evidence for increased production of endothelin in pulmonary circulation. Circulation 1991; 84:2280–2285.

45. Celermajer DS, Cullen S, Deanfield JE. Impairment of endothelium-dependent pulmonary artery relaxation in children with congenital heart disease and abnormal pulmonary hemodynamics. Circulation 1993; 87:440–446.

46. Abman SH, Shanley PF, Accurso FJ. Failure of postnatal adaptation of the pulmonary circulation after chronic intrauterine pulmonary hypertension in fetal lambs. J Clin Invest 1989; 83:1849–1858.

47. Black S, Johengen M, Soifer S. Coordinated regulation of genes of the nitric oxide and endothelin pathways during the development of pulmonary hypertension in fetal lambs. Pediatr Res 1998; 44:821–830.

48. Morin FC III. Ligating the ductus arteriosus before birth causes persistent pulmonary hypertension in the newborn lamb. Pediatr Res 1989; 25:245–250.

49. Wild LM, Nickerson PA, Morin FC III. Ligating the ductus arteriosus before birth remodels the pulmonary vasculature of the lamb. Pediatr Res 1989; 25:251–257.

50. Steinhorn R, Millard S, Morin F III. Persistent pulmonary hypertension of the newborn: role of nitric oxide and endothelin in pathophysiology and treatmnet. Clin Perinatol 1995; 22:405–428.

51. Haworth S, Reid L. Persistent fetal circulation: newly recognized structural features. J Pediatr 1976; 88:614–620.

52. Mecham R, Whitehouse L, Wren D, Parks W, Griffin G, Senior R, Crouch E, Vœlkel N, Stenmark K. Smooth muscle-mediated connective tissue remodeling in pulmonary hypertension. Science 1987; 237:423–426.

53. Dinh Xuan AT, Higenbottam TW, Clelland C, Pepke-Zaba J, Cremona G, Wallwork J. Impairment of pulmonary endothelium-dependent relaxation in patients with Eisenmenger's syndrome. Br J Pharmacol 1990; 99:9–10.

54. Giaid A, Saleh D. Reduced expression of endothelial nitric oxide synthase in the lungs of patients with pulmonary hypertension. N Engl J Med 1995; 333:214–221.

55. Rubens C, Ewert R, Halank M, Wensel R, Orzechowski HD, Schultheiss HP, Hoeffken G. Big endothelin-1 and endothelin-1 plasma levels are correlated with the severity of primary pulmonary hypertension. Chest 2001; 120: 1562–1569.

56. Rabinovitch M, Gamble W, Nadas AS, Miettinen OS, Reid L. Rat pulmonary circulation after chronic hypoxia: hemodynamic and structural features. Am J Physiol 1979; 236:H818–H827.

57. Fagan JM, Rex SE, Hayes-Licitra SA, Waxman L. L-Arginine reduces right heart hypertrophy in hypoxia-induced pulmonary hypertension. Biochem Biophys Res Commun 1999; 254:100–103.

58. Fagan KA, Fouty BW, Tyler RC, Morris KG Jr, Hepler LK, Sato K, LeCras TD, Abman SH, Weinberger HD, Huang PL, McMurtry IF, Rodman DM. The pulmonary circu-lation of homozygous or heterozygous eNOS-null mice is hyperresponsive to mild hypoxia. J Clin Invest 1999; 103:291–299.

59. Le Cras TD, Xue C, Rengasamy A, Johns RA. Chronic hypoxia upregulates endothelial and inducible NO synthase gene and protein expression in rat lung. Am J Physiol 1996; 270:L164–L170.

60. Shaul PW, North AJ, Brannon TS, Ujiie K, Wells LB, Nisen PA, Lowenstein CJ, Snyder SH, Star RA. Prolonged in vivo hypoxia enhances nitric oxide synthase type I and type III gene expression in adult rat lung. Am J Respir Cell Mol Biol 1995; 13:167–174.

61. Xue C, Johns RA. Upregulation of nitric oxide synthase correlates temporally with onset of pulmonary vascular remodeling in the hypoxic rat. Hypertension 1996; 28:743–753.

62. Steudel W, Ichinose F, Huang PL, Hurford WE, Jones RC, Bevan JA, Fishman MC, Zapol WM. Pulmonary vasoconstriction and hypertension in mice with targeted disruption of the endothelial nitric oxide synthase (NOS 3) gene. Circ Res 1997; 81:34–41.

63. Steudel W, Scherrer-Crosbie M, Bloch KD, Weimann J, Huang PL, Jones RC, Picard MH, Zapol WM. Sustained pulmonary hypertension and right ventri-cular hypertrophy after chronic hypoxia in mice with congenital deficiency of nitric oxide synthase 3. J Clin Invest 1998; 101:2468–2477.

64. Quinlan TR, Li D, Laubach VE, Shesely EG, Zhou N, Johns RA. eNOS-deficient mice show reduced pulmonary vascular proliferation, remodeling to chronic hypoxia. Am J Physiol 2000; 279:L641–L650.

65. Singh S, Evans TW. The pulmonary circulation in acute lung injury. In: Marini JJ, Evans TW, eds. Update in Intensive Care and Emergency Medi-cine. 30: Acute Lung Injury. Berlin: Springer-Verlag 1999 :129–146.

66. Hickey MJ, Kubes P. Role of nitric oxide in regulation of leucocyte-endothelial cell interactions. Exp Physiol 1997; 82:339–348.

67. Kubes P, Suzuki M, Granger DN. Nitric oxide: an endogenous modulator of leukocyte adhesion. Proc Natl Acad Sci USA 1991; 88:4651–4655.

68. Reddy VM, Meyrick B, Wong J, Khoor A, Liddicoat JR, Hanley FL, Fineman JR. In utero placement of aortopulmonary shunts. A model of postnatal

pulmonary hypertension with increased pulmonary blood flow in lambs. Circulation 1995; 92:606–613.

69. Nihill MR, McNamara DG. Magnification pulmonary wedge angiography in the evaluation of children with congenital heart disease and pulmonary hypertension. Circulation 1978; 58:1094–1106.

70. Gust R, Schuster DP. Vascular remodeling in experimentally induced subacute canine pulmonary hypertension. Exp Lung Res 2001; 27:1–12.

71. Kanno S, Wu YJ, Lee PC, Billiar TR, Ho C. Angiotensin-converting enzyme inhibitor preserves p21 and endothelial nitric oxide synthase expression in monocrotaline-induced pulmonary arterial hypertension in rats. Circulation 2001; 104:945–950.

72. Frasch HF, Marshall C, Marshall BE. Endothelin-1 is elevated in monocrotaline pulmonary hypertension. Am J Physiology 1999; 276:L304–L310.

73. Ueno M, Miyauchi T, Sakai S, Yamauchi-Kohno R, Goto K, Yamaguchi I. A combination of oral endothelin-A receptor antagonist and oral prostacyclin analogue is superior to each drug alone in ameliorating pulmonary hypertension in rats. J Am Coll Cardiol 2002; 40:175–181.

74. Tilton RG, Munsch CL, Sherwood SJ, Chen SJ, Chen YF, Wu C, Block N, Dixon RA, Brock TA. Attenuation of pulmonary vascular hypertension and cardiac hypertrophy with sitaxsentan sodium, an orally active ET(A) receptor antagonist. Pulm Pharmacol Ther 2000; 13:87–97.

75. Jasmin JF, Lucas M, Cernacek P, Dupuis J. Effectiveness of a nonselective ET(A/B) and a selective ET(A) antagonist in rats with monocrotaline-induced pulmonary hypertension. Circulation 2001; 103:314–318.

76. Cowan KN, Heilbut A, Humpl T, Lam C, Ito S, Rabinovitch M. Complete reversal of fatal pulmonary hypertension in rats by a serine elastase inhibitor. Nat Med 2000; 6:698–702.

77. Li D, Laubach VE, Johns RA. Upregulation of lung soluble guanylate cyclase during chronic hypoxia is prevented by deletion of eNOS. Am J Physiol 2001; 281:L369–L376.

78. Li H, Chen SJ, Chen YF, Meng QC, Durand J, Oparil S, Elton TS. Enhanced endothelin-1 and endothelin receptor gene expression in chronic hypoxia. J Appl Physiol 1994; 77:1451–1459.

79. Nakanishi K, Tajima F, Nakata Y, Osada H, Tachibana S, Kawai T, Torikata C, Suga T, Takishima K, Aurues T, Ikeda T. Expression of endothelin-1 in rats developing hypobaric hypoxia-induced pulmonary hypertension. Lab Invest 1999; 79:1347–1357.

80. DiCarlo VS, Chen SJ, Meng QC, Durand J, Yano M, Chen YF, Oparil S. ETA-receptor antagonist prevents and reverses chronic hypoxia-induced pulmonary hypertension in rat. Am J Physiol 1995; 269:L690–L697.

81. Bonvallet ST, Zamora MR, Hasunuma K, Sato K, Hanasato N, Anderson D, Stelzner TJ. BQ123, an ETA-receptor antagonist, attenuates hypoxic pulmonary hypertension in rats. Am J Physiol 1994; 266:H1327–H1331.

82. Rotta AT, Gunnarsson B, Hernan LJ, Fuhrman BP, Steinhorn DM. Partial liquid ventilation with perflubron attenuates in vivo oxidative damage to proteins and lipids. Crit Care Med 2000; 28:202–208.

83. Nader ND, Knight PR, Davidson BA, Safaee SS, Steinhorn DM. Systemic perfluorocarbons suppress the acute lung inflammation after gastric acid aspiration in rats. Anesth Analg 2000; 90:356–361.

84. Michael JR, Markewitz BA. Endothelins and the lung. Am J Respir Crit Care Med 1996; 154:555–581.

85. Korenaga R, Ando J, Tsuboi H, Yang W, Sakuma I, Toyo-oka T, Kamiya. A. Laminar flow stimulates ATP- and shear stress-dependent nitric oxide production in cultured bovine endothelial cells. Biochem Biophys Res Comm 1994; 198:213–219.

86. Kuchan MJ, Frangos JA. Role of calcium and calmodulin in flow-induced nitric oxide production in endothelial cells. Am J Physiol 1994; 266:C628–C636.

87. Kuchan MJ, Jo H, Frangos JA. Role of G proteins in shear stress-mediated nitric oxide production by endothelial cells. Am J Physiol 1994; 267:C753–C758.

88. Nishida K, Harrison DG, Navas JP, Fisher AA, Dockery SP, Uematsu M, Nerem RM, Alexander RW, Murphy TJ. Molecular cloning and characterization of the constitutive bovine aortic endothelial cell nitric oxide synthase. J Clin Invest 1992; 90:2092–2096.

89. Noris M, Morigi M, Donadelli R, Aiello S, Foppolo M, Todeschini M, Orisio S, Remuzzi G, Remuzzi A. Nitric oxide synthesis by cultured endothelial cells is modulated by flow conditions. Circ Res 1995; 76:536–543.

90. Ranjan V, Xiao Z, Diamond SL. Constitutive NOS expression in cultured endothelial cells is elevated by fluid shear stress. Am J Physiol 1995; 269:H550–H555.

91. Uematsu M, Ohara Y, Navas JP, Nishida K, Murphy TJ, Alexander RW, Nerem RM, Harrison DG. Regulation of endothelial cell nitric oxide synthase mRNA expression by shear stress. Am J Physiol 1995; 269:C1371–C1378.

92. Vane JR, Anggard EE, Botting RM. Regulatory functions of the vascular endothelium. N Engl J Med 1990; 323:27–36.

93. Wedgwood S, Bekker JM, Black SM. Shear stress regulation of endothelial NOS in fetal pulmonary arterial endothelial cells involves PKC. Am J Physiol 2001; 281:L490–L498.

94. Resnick N, Collins T, Atkinson W, Bonthron DT, Dewey CF Jr, Gimbrone MA Jr. Platelet-derived growth factor B chain promoter contains a cis-acting fluid shear-stress-responsive element. Proc Natl Acad Sci USA 1993; 90:4591–4595.

95. Kuchan MJ, Frangos JA. Shear stress regulates endothelin-1 release via protein kinase C and cGMP in cultured endothelial cells. Am J Physiol 1993; 264:H150–H156.

96. Fulton D, Gratton JP, Sessa WC. Post-translational control of endothelial nitric oxide synthase: why isn't calcium/calmodulin enough? J Pharmacol Exp Ther 2001; 299:818–824.

97. Davis ME, Cai H, Drummond GR, Harrison DG. Shear stress regulates endothelial nitric oxide synthase expression through c-Src by divergent signaling pathways. Circ Res 2001; 89:1073–1080.

98. Wong J, Reddy VM, Hendricks-Munoz K, Liddicoat JR, Gerrets R, Fineman JR. Endothelin-1 vasoactive responses in lambs with pulmonary hypertension and increased pulmonary blood flow. Am J Physiol 1995; 269:H1965–H1972.

99. Black SM, Bekker JM, Johengen MJ, Parry AJ, Soifer SJ, Fineman JR. Altered regulation of the ET-1 cascade in lambs with increased pulmonary blood flow and pulmonary hypertension. Pediatr Res 2000; 47:97–106.

100. Steinhorn R, Russell J, Lakshminrusimha S, Gugino S, Black S, Fineman J. Altered endothelium-dependent relaxations in lambs with high pulmonary blood flow and pulmonary hypertension. Am J Physiol Heart Circ Physiol 2001; 280:H311–H317.

101. Black SM, Fineman JR, Steinhorn RH, Bristow J, Soifer SJ. Increased endothelial NOS in lambs with increased pulmonary blood flow and pulmonary hypertension. Am J Physiol 1998; 275:H1643–H1651.

102. Sheehy AM, Burson MA, Black SM. Nitric oxide exposure inhibits endothelial NOS activity but not gene expression: a role for superoxide. Am J Physiol 1998; 274:L833–L841.

103. Solzbach U, Hornig B, Jeserich M, Just H. Vitamin C improves endothelial dysfunction of epicardial coronary arteries in hypertensive patients. Circulation 1997; 96:1513–1519.

104. Black SM, Sanchez LS, Mata-Greenwood E, Bekker JM, Steinhorn RH, Fineman JR. sGC, PDE5 are elevated in lambs with increased pulmonary blood flow, pulmonary hypertension. Am J Physiol 2001; 281:L1051–L1057.

105. Resnick N, Gimbrone MA Jr. Hemodynamic forces are complex regulators of endothelial gene expression. FASEB J 1995; 9:874–882.

106. Sterpetti AV, Cucina A, Fragale A, Lepidi S, Cavallaro A, Santoro-D'Angelo L. Shear stress influences the release of platelet derived growth factor and basic fibroblast growth factor by arterial smooth muscle cells. Eur J Vasc Surg 1994; 8:138–142.

107. Schott RJ, Morrow LA. Growth factors and angiogenesis. Cardiovasc Res 1993; 27:1155–1161.

108. Birukov KG, Shirinsky VP, Stepanova OV, Tkachuk VA, Hahn AW, Resink TJ, Smirnov VN. Stretch affects phenotype and proliferation of vascular smooth muscle cells. Mol Cell Biochem 1995; 144:131–139.

109. Osol G. Mechanotransduction by vascular smooth muscle. J Vasc Res 1995; 32:275–292.

110. Iba T, Maitz S, Furbert T, Rosales O, Widmann MD, Spillane B, Shin T, Sonoda T, Sumpio BE. Effect of cyclic stretch on endothelial cells from different vascular beds. Circ Shock 1991; 35:193–198.

111. Iba T, Shin T, Sonoda T, Rosales O, Sumpio BE. Stimulation of endothelial secretion of tissue-type plasminogen activator by repetitive stretch. J Surg Res 1991; 50:457–460.

112. Hirata Y, Takagi Y, Fukuda Y, Marumo F. Endothelin is a potent mitogen for rat vascular smooth muscle cells. Atherosclerosis 1989; 78:225–228.

113. Komuro I, Kurihara H, Sugiyama T, Yoshizumi M, Takaku F, Yazaki Y. Endothelin stimulates c-fos and c-myc expression and proliferation of vascular smooth muscle cells. FEBS Lett 1988; 238:249–252.

114. Jahan H, Kobayashi S, Nishimura J, Kanaide H. Endothelin-1 and angiotensin II act as progression but not competence growth factors in vascular smooth muscle cells. Eur J Pharmacol 1996; 295:261–269.

115. Scott-Burden T, Resink TJ, Hahn AW, Vanhoutte PM. Induction of endothelin secretion by angiotensin II: effects on growth and synthetic activity of vascular smooth muscle cells. J Cardiovasc Pharmacol 1991; 17(suppl 7): S96–S100.

116. Wedgwood S, Dettman RW, Black SM. ET-1 stimulates pulmonary arterial smooth muscle cell proliferation via induction of reactive oxygen species. Am J Physiol 2001; 281:L1058–L1067.

117. Ivy DD, Parker TA, Ziegler JW, Galan HL, Kinsella JP, Tuder RM, Abman SH. Prolonged endothelin A receptor blockade attenuates chronic pulmonary hypertension in the ovine fetus. J Clin Invest 1997; 99:1179–1186.

118. Ovadia B, Bekker JM, Fitzgerald RK, Kon A, Thelitz S, Johengen MJ, Hendricks-Munoz K, Gerrets R, Black SM, Fineman JR. Nitric oxide-endothelin-1 interactions after acute ductal constriction in fetal lambs. Am J Physiol 2002; 282:H862–H871.

119. Wedgwood S, McMullan DM, Bekker JM, Fineman JR, Black SM. Role for endothelin-1-induced superoxide and peroxynitrite production in rebound pulmonary hypertension associated with inhaled nitric oxide therapy. Circ Res 2001; 89:357–364.

120. Fike CD, Kaplowitz MR, Rehorst-Paea LA, Nelin LD. L-Arginine increases nitric oxide production in isolated lungs of chronically hypoxic newborn pigs. J Appl Physiol 2000; 88:1797–1803.

121. Su Y, Block ER. Role of calpain in hypoxic inhibition of nitric oxide synthase activity in pulmonary endothelial cells. Am J Physiol 2000; 278: L1204–L1212.

122. Fagan KA, Morrissey B, Fouty BW, Sato K, Harral JW, Morris KG Jr, Hoedt-Miller M, Vidmar S, McMurtry IF, Rodman DM. Upregulation of nitric oxide synthase in mice with severe hypoxia-induced pulmonary hypertension. Respir Res 2001; 2:306–313.

123. De Caterina R, Libby P, Peng HB, Thannickal VJ, Rajavashisth TB, fsGimbrone MA Jr, Shin WS, Liao JK. Nitric oxide decreases cytokine-induced endothelial activation. Nitric oxide selectively reduces endothelial expression of adhesion molecules and proinflammatory cytokines. J Clin Invest 1995; 96:60–68.

124. McMillen MA, Sumpio BE. Endothelins: polyfunctional cytokines. J Am Coll Surg 1995; 180:621–637.

125. Harlan JM. Leukocyte-endothelial interactions. Blood 1985; 65:513–525.

126. Smedly LA, Tonnesen MG, Sandhaus RA, Haslett C, Guthrie LA, Johnston RB Jr, Henson PM, Worthen GS. Neutrophil-mediated injury to endothelial cells. Enhancement by endotoxin and essential role of neutrophil elastase. J Clin Invest 1986; 77:1233–1243.

127. Atz AM, Wessel DL. Inhaled nitric oxide in the neonate with cardiac disease. Semin Perinatol 1997; 21:441–455.

128. Roberts JD Jr, Fineman JR, Morin FC III, Shaul PW, Rimar S, Schreiber MD, Polin RA, Zwass MS, Zayek MM, Gross I, Heymann MA, Zapol

WM. Inhaled nitric oxide and persistent pulmonary hypertension of the newborn. The Inhaled Nitric Oxide Study Group. N Engl J Med 1997; 336: 605–610.

129. Rossaint R, Falke KJ, Lopez F, Slama K, Pison U, Zapol WM. Inhaled nitric oxide for the adult respiratory distress syndrome. N Engl J Med 1993; 328:399–405.

130. Iwamoto J, Morin FC III. Nitric oxide inhibition varies with hemoglobin saturation. J Appl Physiol 1993; 75:2332–2336.

131. Markewitz BA, Michael JR. Inhaled nitric oxide in adults with the acute respiratory distress syndrome. Respir Med 2000; 94:1023–1028.

132. Atz A, Adatia I, Wessel D. Rebound pulmonary hypertension after inhalation of nitric oxide. Ann Thorac Surg 1996; 62:1759–1764.

133. Cueto E, Lopez-Herce J, Sanchez A, Carrillo A. Life-threatening effects of discontinuing inhaled nitric oxide in children. Acta Paediatr 1997; 86: 1337–1339.

134. Lavoie A, Hall JB, Olson DM, Wylam ME. Life-threatening effects of discontinuing inhaled nitric oxide in severe respiratory failure. Am J Respir Crit Care Med 1996; 153:1985–1987.

135. Miller OI, Tang SF, Keech A, Celermajer DS. Rebound pulmonary hypertension on withdrawal from inhaled nitric oxide. Lancet 1995; 346:51–52.

136. Black SM, Heidersbach RS, McMullan DM, Bekker JM, Johengen MJ, Fineman JR. Inhaled nitric oxide inhibits NOS activity in lambs: potential mechanism for rebound pulmonary hypertension. Am J Physiol 1999; 277:H1849–H1856.

137. Rubin LJ, Badesch DB, Barst RJ, Galie N, Black CM, Keogh A, Pulido T, Frost A, Roux S, Leconte I, Landzberg M, Simonneau G. Bosentan therapy for pulmonary arterial hypertension. N Engl J Med 2002; 346:896–903.

138. McMullan DM, Bekker JM, Johengen MJ, Hendricks-Munoz K, Gerrets R, Black SM, Fineman JR. Inhaled nitric oxide-induced rebound pulmonary hypertension: role for endothelin-1. Am J Physiol 2001; 280:H777–H785.

139. Tsai J, Jain M, Hsieh C, Lee W, Yoshizumi M, Patterson C, Perralla M, Cook C, Wang H, Haber E, Schlegal R, Lee M. Induction of apoptosis by pyrrolidinedithiocarbamate and *N*-acetylcysteine in vascular smooth muscle cells. J Biol Chem 1996; 271:3667–3670.

140. Brown M, Miller F, Li W, Ellingson A, Mozena J, Chatterjee P, Engelhardt J, Zwacka R, Oberley L, Fang X, Spector A, Weintraub N. Overexpression of human catalase inhibits proliferation and promotes apoptosis in vascular smooth muscle cells. Circ Res 1999; 85:524–533.

141. Beavo JA. Cyclic nucleotide phosphodiesterases: functional implications of multiple isoforms. Physiol Rev 1995; 75:725–748.

142. Sanchez LS, de la Monte SM, Filippov G, Jones RC, Zapol WM, Bloch KD. Cyclic-GMP-binding, cyclic-GMP-specific phosphodiesterase (PDE5) gene expression is regulated during rat pulmonary development. Pediatr Res 1998; 43:163–168.

143. Atz AM, Wessel DL. Sildenafil ameliorates effects of inhaled nitric oxide withdrawal. Anesthesiology 1999; 91:307–310.

144. Dukarm RC, Russell JA, Morin III FC, Perry BJ, Steinhorn RH. The cGMP-specific phosphodiesterase inhibitor E4021 dilates the pulmonary circulation. Am J Respir Crit Care Med 1999; 160:858–865.
145. Ziegler JW, Ivy DD, Wiggins JW, Kinsella JP, Clarke WR, Abman SH. Effects of dipyridamole and inhaled nitric oxide in pediatric patients with pulmonary hypertension. Am J Respir Crit Care Med 1998; 158:1388–1395.
146. Zhao L, Mason NA, Morrell NW, Kojonazarov B, Sadykov A, Maripov A, Mirrakhimov MM, Aldashev A, Wilkins MR. Sildenafil inhibits hypoxia-induced pulmonary hypertension. Circulation 2001; 104:424–428.

9

Surfactant Activity and Dysfunction in Lung Injury

ZHENGDONG WANG, BRUCE A. HOLM, SADIS MATALON, and
ROBERT H. NOTTER

*Departments of Pediatrics and Environmental Medicine,
University of Rochester, Rochester, New York, U.S.A.,
Departments of Pediatrics and Obstetrics and Gynecology,
State University of New York (SUNY) at Buffalo, Buffalo, New York, U.S.A., and
Departments of Anesthesiology and Physiology and Biophysics,
University of Alabama at Birmingham, Birmingham, Alabama, U.S.A.*

I. Overview

This chapter details the composition and activity of pulmonary surfactant,
and the mechanisms by which it becomes dysfunctional during lung injury.
Pulmonary surfactant has physiologically essential actions in decreasing
the work of breathing, stabilizing alveolar inflation-deflation, and reducing
the hydrostatic driving force for edema formation. These actions depend
on the ability of lung surfactant to lower and vary surface tension effectively within the alveolar network. Surfactant dysfunction occurs when
surface activity is disrupted by chemical or physical processes during
injury, leading to deficits in pressure–volume mechanics and gas exchange.
Surfactant metabolism can also be compromised during lung injury by

alterations in type II pneumocytes, and the host defense activities of surfactant proteins (SP)-A and SP-D can be impaired. Surfactant dysfunction is an important contributor to the pathophysiology of clinical acute lung injury (ALI) and the acute respiratory distress syndrome (ARDS). This chapter discusses mechanisms and characteristics of surfactant dysfunction from biophysical interactions with plasma proteins, cell membrane lipids, and other inhibitors in edema. Activity detriments from chemical interactions between lung surfactant components and inflammatory phospholipases, proteases, and reactive oxidants are also detailed, along with decreased surface activity from depletion or alteration of large surfactant aggregates. Mechanistic understanding of the biophysics and physiology of lung surfactant activity and dysfunction is crucial for developing effective surfactant-based therapies for clinical ALI/ARDS and related pulmonary diseases as discussed in Chapter 15.

II. Endogenous Surfactant and Its Activity

Before addressing lung surfactant dysfunction in inflammatory injury, it is necessary first to understand the normal functioning of this essential material. Active pulmonary surfactant has an extraordinary ability to lower surface tension. Although surface tension is not a major force in many macroscopic systems, it is highly important in the lungs. Much of the extensive alveolar surface ($\sim 1 m^2$/kg body weight) is covered by a thin aqueous layer or "alveolar hypophase." This hypophase is contacted by inspired air, resulting in a large air–liquid interfacial area with associated surface tension forces. The significant contribution of surface tension forces to the mechanics of breathing was demonstrated by von Neergaard in 1929 (1), who showed that much higher pressures were needed to inflate animal lungs or maintain them at fixed volume during air-filling compared to liquid-filling. This difference is due to surface tension forces, which are present along with tissue forces in air-filled lungs but not in liquid-filled lungs. Although von Neergaard's early experiments documented the importance of pulmonary surface tension forces, it was not immediately recognized that normal respiration depended on surface active agents (surfactants) to moderate these forces during breathing. The existence of lung surfactant (2,3) and the linkage between surfactant-deficiency and the respiratory distress syndrome (RDS or Hyaline Membrane Disease) in premature infants were demonstrated in the 1950s (4–7).

The biochemical components that make up pulmonary surfactant are synthesized, packaged, stored, secreted, and recycled by alveolar type II epithelial cells (for review, see Refs. 8–18).[a] Secreted surfactant in the alveolar hypophase exists as a heterogeneous population of phospholipid-rich aggregates with incorporated apoproteins. These aggregates vary in size from tens of nanometers to several microns, with larger forms generally having the greatest surface activity and apoprotein content (22–31). Surfactant in the hypophase adsorbs at the air–water interface to form a highly active film that lowers and varies alveolar surface tension during breathing. By lowering surface tension, lung surfactant reduces the nonflow component of the work of breathing (increases quasistatic lung compliance). In addition, by equalizing the ratio of surface tension to radius in different sized alveoli, surfactant reduces atelectasis and promotes more uniform inflation based on the Laplace equation $\Delta P = 2\sigma/R$, where ΔP is the pressure drop across the alveolar air–liquid interface, σ is surface tension, and R is alveolar radius.[b]Alveolar stability in vivo is further enhanced by specialized connective tissue support fibers plus an interconnected network structure that allows airsacs sharing common septa to help each other resist collapse. However, biophysically active surfactant is crucial for alveolar stability and normal lung function (Fig. 1). The consequences of surfactant deficiency are strikingly apparent in premature infants with RDS, who exhibit alveolar collapse and overdistension, decreased lung volumes and compliance, intrapulmonary shunting with reduced arterial oxygenation, and diffuse pulmonary edema (33–35). Surfactant dysfunction is also associated with acute respiratory failure in patients of all ages with ALI/ARDS.

The biophysical and physiological activity of lung surfactant is directly linked to its composition. Lung surfactant is a complex mixture of lipids and specific proteins (e.g., see Refs. 9, 36–38). Phospholipids make up about 85–90% by weight of lung surfactant material (Table 1). Phosphatidylcholine (PC) is by far the major phospholipid class, comprising about 80% of total surfactant phospholipid. Dipalmitoyl phosphatidylcholine (DPPC) is the most prevalent single compound, accounting for 40–50% of

---

[a] All the components of whole, biophysically active surfactant are synthesized in alveolar type II cells. Some surfactant components are additionally expressed or synthesized in airway cells (e.g., nonciliated bronchiolar epithelial cells or Clara cells). In addition to producing lung surfactant, type II cells are stem cells for the alveolar epithelium, and proliferate and dedifferentiate following injury to type I cells (8,10,11,19–21). Type II cells also elaborate and respond to multiple mediators during growth, development, inflammatory injury, and repair as discussed in other chapters.

[b] The Laplace equation holds for a spherical interface of radius R. A similar stability argument can be made for an alveolar interface of arbitrary curvature from the more comprehensive Young and Laplace equation, which incorporates the two principal radii of curvature R_1 and R_2 that define an interface of general shape: $\Delta P = \sigma(1/R_1 + 1/R_2)$ (32).

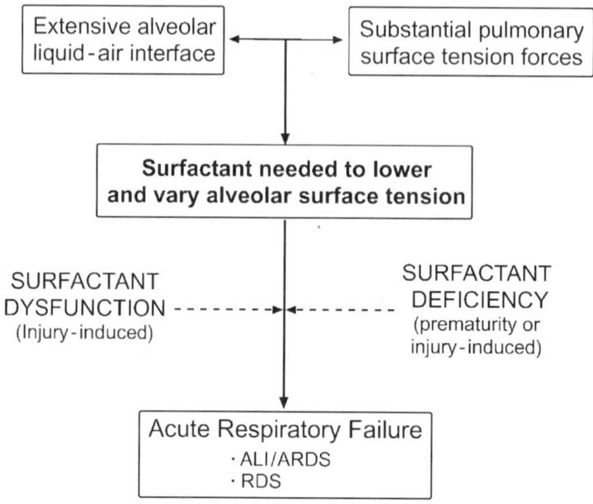

Figure 1 Necessity for lung surfactant in respiration. Surface tension forces at the extensive air–water interface in the alveolar network significantly impact pulmonary mechanics and function. By lowering and varying surface tension during breathing, lung surfactant plays essential physiological roles in reducing the work of breathing, normalizing alveolar inflation/deflation behavior, and facilitating gas exchange. Surfactant deficiency causes the respiratory distress syndrome (RDS) in premature infants, and surfactant dysfunction is an important contributor to the pathophysiology of clinical acute lung injury (ALI) and the acute respiratory distress syndrome (ARDS) in patients of all ages. ALI and ARDS can also have a component of surfactant deficiency. Lung surfactant activity and mechanisms underlying its dysfunction during injury are detailed in this chapter.

the PC fraction. Other disaturated PC compounds in lung surfactant include isomers of C14:0, C16:0 PC plus smaller amounts of C14:0, C14:0 PC and C16:0, C18:0 PC (39,40). Multiple unsaturated PC compounds including C16:0, C16:1 PC and C16:0, C18:1 PC are also present (39,40). Other phospholipid classes in lung surfactant similarly contain a mix of disaturated and unsaturated compounds (PG, PI, PS, PE, Sph, Table 1). The protein content of lung surfactant is much smaller than the lipid content. Surfactant contains approximately 7–10% protein by weight, including three biophysically active surfactant proteins (SP) -A, SP-B, and SP-C. SP-D, a fourth protein not implicated in biophysical function but important in host defense, is also present. Molecular characteristics of the four surfactant proteins are summarized in Table 2. Lung surfactant also contains about 4–7% neutral lipids, primarily cholesterol plus small amounts of cholesterol esters, diglycerides, and triglycerides (Table 1).

The physiological actions of lung surfactant depend on its ability to generate specific surface behaviors (Table 3). Since surfactant is initially

Table 1 Biochemical Composition of Endogenous Pulmonary Surfactant

---

85–90% Phospholipids
  80% Phosphatidylcholine (PC)
    40–50% DPPC
    15–20% other disaturated PCs
    35–45% unsaturated PCs
  15% Anionic phospholipids (PG, PI, PS)
  5% Other phospholipid classes (PE, Sph)

7–10% Apoproteins
  SP-A
  SP-B
  SP-C
  SP-D (not involved in biophysical function)

4–7% Neutral lipids
  Cholesterol
  Cholesterol esters, glycerides

Tabulated values are representative averages or ranges in weight percent for surfactant lavaged from animals of different species and ages. *Abbreviations*: PC, phosphatidylcholine; PG, phosphatidylglycerol; PI, phosphatidylinositol; PS, phosphatidylserine; PE, phosphatidylethanolamine; Sph, sphingomyelin; SP, surfactant protein. Lung surfactant composition and component biophysics are discussed in detail in the text by Notter (9) and in reviews such as Refs. 16, 36–38, 43, 44, 263, 264.

secreted into the alveolar hypophase, it must be able to adsorb to form a film at the air–water interface. This film must then reduce surface tension to low values during dynamic compression, and it must also vary surface tension as a function of interfacial area during cycling. Theory does not predict a unique level of surface tension lowering required for "active" lung surfactant. However, multiple studies have shown that films and dispersions of lavaged lung surfactant and related organic solvent extracts can lower surface tension to $< 1\,\text{mN/m}$ under rapid physiologic rates of compression at 37°C (e.g., see Refs. 9,36 for review). Lung surfactant films must also have the ability to respread effectively at the air–water interface during cycling, i.e., molecules lost from the surface film during compression must reintegrate with remaining film material during expansion. Rapid respreading from film-associated structures in the interfacial region, along with on-going adsorption from the hypophase, ensure that sufficient surfactant is available in the film to lower surface tension effectively during repetitive breathing cycles (9,36).

The lipid and protein components of lung surfactant interact at the molecular level to achieve the overall set of surface behaviors in Table 3. A summary of the biophysical contributions of lung surfactant components to surface activity is as follows (for further review and discussion, see Refs.

Table 2 Molecular Characteristics of Lung Surfactant Proteins

Surfactant protein (SP)	Selected molecular characteristics and functional activities
SP-A	MW 26-38 kD (monomer), 228 AA in length in humans Most abundant surfactant protein; acidic glycoprotein with multiple post-translational isoforms; C-type lectin; member of the collectin family of host defense proteins; forms an active octadecamer (six triplet monomers); aggregates and orders phospholipids (Ca^{++}-dependent); required for tubular myelin formation (with SP-B, Ca^{++}); increases the ability of surfactant to resist biophysical inhibition; important in surfactant metabolism (e.g., helps regulate reuptake and recycling).
SP-B	MW 8.5-9 kD (monomer), 79 AA in humans (active peptide); Hydrophobic structure contains 2-3 amphipathic helices plus β-sheet regions; forms dimers and other oligomers of probable functional significance; human form has 10 positive Arg/Lys and 2 negative Glu/Asp residues at neutral pH; interacts biophysically with both phospholipid headgroups and chains; necessary for tubular myelin formation (with SP-A, Ca^{++}); disrupts and fuses lipid bilayers, and promotes lipid insertion/mixing into surface films; enhances the adsorption, film spreading, and dynamic surface activity of lipids; most active surfactant apoprotein in increasing overall dynamic surface activity.
SP-C	MW 4.2 kD (monomer), 35 AA in humans (active peptide); Very hydrophobic, with only 2 charged Arg/Lys residues; forms dimers and other oligomers of possible biophysical significance; in humans has 2 palmitoylated cysteine residues; primarily α-helical in structure, with a length that spans a lipid bilayer; interacts biophysically primarily with hydrophobic phospholipid chains; disrupts and fuses lipid bilayers; enhances the adsorption, film spreading, and dynamic surface activity of lipids.
SP-D	MW 39-46 kD (monomer), 355 AA in length in humans Has significant structural similarity to SP-A; oligomerizes to a dodecamer (four triplet monomers); C-type lectin and member of the collectin family of host defense proteins; not implicated in lung surfactant biophysics; may participate in surfactant metabolism in addition to host defense.

(Adapted from Ref. 9.)

Table 3 Physiological Actions and Required Surface Properties of Functional Lung Surfactant Material

Physiological actions of functional lung surfactant
  Reduces the work of breathing (increases lung compliance)
  Increases alveolar stability against collapse during expiration
  Improves alveolar inflation uniformity
  Reduces the hydrostatic driving force for edema formation

Biophysical (surface) properties of functional lung surfactant
  Adsorbs rapidly to the air–water interface
  Reaches very low minimum surface tensions during dynamic film
    compression
  Varies surface tension with area during dynamic cycling
  Respreads from collapse phases or other film-associated structures
    during cycling

See text for discussion.
(Adapted from Ref. 9.)

9, 16, 36–38, 41–44). Disaturated phospholipids like DPPC form tightly packed, rigid films capable of extreme degrees of surface tension lowering during dynamic compression (45–53). The presence of DPPC and related disaturated phospholipids in lung surfactant films not only facilitates surface tension lowering, but also helps to vary surface tension with area during cycling. However, rigid disaturated phospholipids like DPPC do not adsorb readily to the air–water interface or respread effectively in cycled films. Fluid liquid–crystal phospholipids in lung surfactant have a major impact in improving film respreading (54), and also help increase adsorption relative to DPPC (55–57). Neutral lipids like cholesterol also facilitate adsorption and respreading, but can be detrimental to dynamic surface tension lowering if present in excess amounts (54,57).

Lung surfactant proteins make major contributors to surface activity and the ability to resist inhibition. SP-A, SP-B, and SP-C all have extensive molecular interactions with phospholipids (Table 2), and are essential in facilitating lung surfactant adsorption. Surfactant proteins (particularly SP-B and SP-C) also enhance film respreading, and aid in refining the surface film during compression to optimize dynamic surface tension lowering. SP-A functions biophysically as a large octadecamer containing six triplet monomers. Hydrophobic SP-B and SP-C also form oligomers including dimers, although the relative activities of oligomeric vs. monomeric forms of these proteins are not fully defined. SP-A in the presence of calcium acts to increase phospholipid aggregation and order, including the formation of tubular myelin, a distinctive three-dimensional network of intersecting phospholipid bilayers with incorporated apoproteins found in the aqueous phase microstructure of lung surfactant dispersions. SP-B is also required for tubular myelin formation. Tubular myelin and other large aggregate forms of lung surfactant are highly active in adsorbing to the air–water interface (23,25,26,30,58). SP-B and SP-C have been shown to disrupt and fuse phospholipid bilayers consistent with an important role in surfactant adsorption (59–61), and SP-B directly promotes the insertion and mixing of phospholipids into surface films (59). The amphipathic structure of SP-B allows it to interact with both the headgroups and chains of phospholipids in films and bilayers, while the extreme hydrophobicity of SP-C limits its interactions largely to the hydrophobic fatty chain region. Multiple studies have shown that SP-B is more active than SP-C in enhancing adsorption and overall dynamic surface tension lowering in natural and synthetic lung surfactants (59–69). SP-B is also more active than SP-C in increasing the ability of phospholipid mixtures to resist inhibition by plasma proteins and related compounds (63,65). The functional lipid and protein constituents of endogenous lung surfactant and their specific effects on surface activity are summarized in Fig. 2.

DPPC and related long-chain disaturated phospholipids
Give low minimum surface tension on dynamic compression
Vary surface tension with area during cycling

Surfactant proteins SP-A, SP-B and SP-C
Greatly increase phospholipid adsorption to the air-water interface
Improve film respreading on successive cycles
Participate in refining the surface film during dynamic compression

Fluid phospholipids (and neutral lipids)
Greatly increase film respreading during cycling
Increase adsorption relative to DPPC

Figure 2 Functional biophysical roles of lung surfactant components. Lung surfactant contains a mixture of phospholipids, apoproteins, and neutral lipids. These components interact biophysically to generate the surface active behavior exhibited by the surfactant system as a whole. The molecular biophysical roles of different chemical constituents in lung surfactant are detailed in the text. (Adapted from Refs. 9, 36.)

III. Deficiency and Dysfunction of Lung Surfactant

Surfactant deficiency refers to a decreased total amount of surfactant material in the alveoli, while surfactant dysfunction (also called inhibition or inactivation) implies a decrease in surface activity. Surfactant deficiency and dysfunction are not independent, since surface activity is reduced if total surfactant concentration is decreased. Nonetheless, understanding the relative degree of surfactant dysfunction vs. surfactant deficiency in injured lungs can be very helpful in mechanistic and pathophysiologic understanding. Surfactant deficiency is most often associated with deficits in type II cell function, either because these cells are not fully developed as in premature infants or because they are altered during injury. Surfactant dysfunction, on the other hand, frequently arises from biophysical or chemical interactions of alveolar surfactant and its essential components with injury-induced inhibitors, inflammatory enzymes, or reactive species. Alterations in type II cells or alveolar processing that deplete specific large surfactant aggregate subtypes or reduce their activity can also contribute to surfactant dysfunction. Figure 3 illustrates some of the pathways by which surfactant dysfunction can occur during acute pulmonary injury. Mechanisms and features of lung surfactant dysfunction are detailed further in subsequent sections.

Abnormalities in surfactant activity, content, or composition have been documented in a number of important respiratory diseases (9,70–83). The major disease of surfactant-deficiency worldwide is RDS or Hyaline Membrane Disease in premature infants. The incidence of RDS increases as gestational age and birth weight decrease (33–35,84–86). In the absence of prophylactic surfactant therapy, the incidence of RDS is > 50% in premature infants less than 29-week gestation, 10–20% in premature infants of 32–34-week gestation, and <5% in infants ≥35-week gestation. The incidence of RDS is increased by maternal diabetes, male sex, Caucasian race, and perinatal factors such as caesarian section (33–35). As many as 50,000 premature infants are at risk for RDS in the United States each year. Although RDS is initiated by surfactant deficiency in premature infants, acute and chronic lung injury and surfactant dysfunction can enter its clinical course as a result of mechanical ventilation, hyperoxia, and diverse complications of prematurity. However, lung surfactant dysfunction is most common in the clinical syndromes of ALI and ARDS.

In contrast to RDS in premature infants, ALI and ARDS can occur in patients of all ages. ARDS was initially described primarily in adults (87,88), and was often termed the "adult" respiratory distress syndrome. The now standard nomenclature of the "acute" respiratory distress syndrome reflects the pathophysiology of this condition as a severe rapid-onset lung injury in infants, children, and adults. The diagnosis of ARDS in early

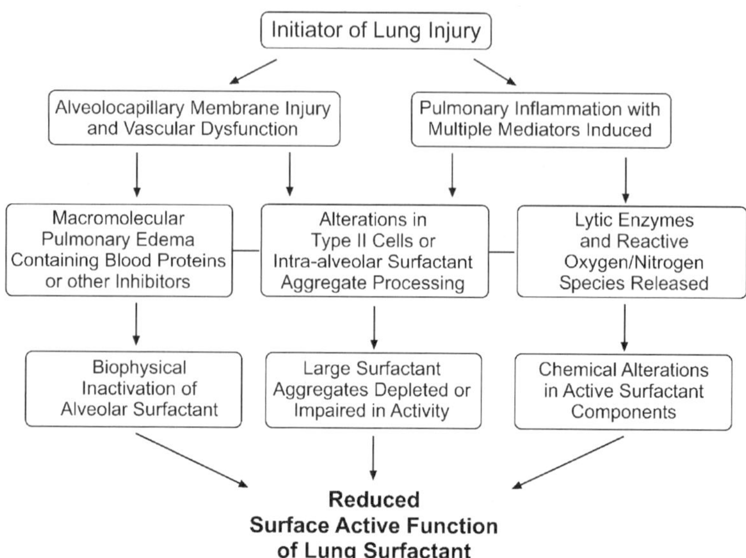

Figure 3 Surfactant-related abnormalities during acute pulmonary injury. Surfactant dysfunction (reduced surface activity) can occur by multiple pathways during lung injury. Surfactant can be inactivated by biophysical interactions with inhibitor compounds in edema or the inflammatory response, and specific active surfactant components can be chemically altered by lytic enzymes or reactive oxygen/nitrogen nitrogen species. Injury-induced changes in type II cells or the alveolar hypophase that decrease the surface activity or content of large surfactant aggregates can also cause surfactant dysfunction. The total amount of available surfactant material may also be decreased as a result of type II cell alterations during lung injury, but surfactant deficiency is typically less prominent than surfactant dysfunction. (Modified from Ref. 9.)

studies was based on the qualitative presence of bilateral edema, decreased lung volumes and compliance, and intrapulmonary shunting apparent as arterial hypoxemia resistant to high levels of inspired oxygen in the absence of left heart failure (88,89). The American-European Consensus Committee in 1994 defined clinical ARDS more specifically as requiring an acute onset, bilateral infiltrates on frontal chest radiograph, a PaO_2/FiO_2 ratio ≤ 200 mmHg, and a pulmonary capillary wedge pressure ≤ 18 mmHg (if measured) or no evidence of left atrial hypertension (90). The Consensus Committee defined ALI identically to ARDS except for a PaO_2/FiO_2 ratio ≤ 300 mmHg (90). Depending on its definition, ALI/ARDS affects 50,000–150,000 patients in the United States each year and has substantial mortality rates of 30–50% despite sophisticated intensive care (90–95). A recent analysis by Goss et al. (96) has estimated that the incidence of clinical ALI in adults in the United States is 22–64 cases per 100,000 persons per year. Surfactant abnormalities in bronchoalveolar lavage from patients with ALI/ARDS are well documented (70–77). A major focus of discussion in this chapter is on surfactant dysfunction and the mechanisms by which it occurs in ALI/ARDS.

IV. Methods for Measuring Lung Surfactant Surface Activity and Dysfunction

In order to study surfactant activity and dysfunction, it is necessary to measure the functional surface properties given earlier in Table 3 (adsorption, dynamic surface tension lowering, film respreading). Two instruments that are widely used to assess the overall surface activity and inhibition of lung surfactant materials during dynamic cycling are the pulsating bubble surfactometer and the captive bubble surfactometer. In addition, the Wilhelmy surface balance is used to measure the properties of cycled interfacial films, and adsorption behavior is isolated and measured in a dish with a stirred subphase to minimize diffusion resistance. Adsorption can also be assessed in the pulsating and captive bubble surfactometers in the absence of pulsation. A brief overview of these methods is given below.

The pulsating bubble surfactometer developed by Enhorning (97) is an important tool for assessing lung surfactant activity and dysfunction. Measurements with this instrument reflect a physiologically relevant combination of adsorption, dynamic surface tension lowering, and film respreading during rapid cycling at body temperature and high humidity. Surface tension is calculated from the Laplace equation based on measured pressure differences across the interface of a tiny air bubble, communicating with ambient air, formed and pulsated in a surfactant dispersion (97,98). The bubble is typically pulsated at 20 cycles/min between radii of 0.55 and 0.40 mm (a 50% area compression). Data are generally reported as the surface tension at minimum bubble radius (minimum surface tension) as a function of total time of pulsation in the presence or absence of inhibitors. The captive bubble apparatus developed by Schurch (99) can also be used to evaluate lung surfactant activity and inhibition. This instrument assesses surface tension in an ellipsoidal bubble formed in a surfactant dispersion and "captured" against an agar layer. The bubble is compressed/expanded by an external piston, and surface tension is calculated from its thermodynamic relationship to pressure, volume, area, and other dimensional parameters in the captive bubble. The captive bubble surfactometer is free from artifacts involving surfactant film migration that can potentially affect data during initial pulsations in the pulsating bubble surfactometer (100). However, this instrument requires more complex data analysis based on computer solutions to the equations of interfacial phenomena in conjunction with bubble dimensional parameters measured from recorded video images during cycling (100,101).

The Langmuir–Wilhelmy surface balance is used to study molecular behavior directly in surfactant films at the air–water interface. The typical apparatus consists of a hydrophobic trough (e.g., Teflon®) with a movable dam or ribbon barrier to confine the surface film, plus a Wilhelmy slide and force transducer to measure surface tension. The film is generally spread in a volatile solvent directly at the surface of a liquid subphase in the balance trough, although films can also be formed by adsorption from the subphase or by layering surfactant dispersed in saline at the interface. Data are reported as surface pressure or tension as a function of surface area or concentration during cycling at fixed temperature (surface pressure is the amount by which the surfactant film lowers surface tension below that of the pure subphase). Surface pressure–area isotherms from the Wilhelmy balance are invaluable in defining molecular behavior in well-defined surfactant films, although this instrument is less widely used to study lung surfactant dysfunction. Finally, surfactant adsorption in the presence or absence of inhibitor compounds is often measured in a Teflon® dish containing a subphase that is continuously stirred with a coated magnetic bar to minimize diffusion (102–104). Surfactant dispersed in saline is typically added to the stirred subphase at time zero, and surface tension (or pressure) is measured as a function of time from the force on a hanging Wilhelmy slide. Further details on interfacial and molecular biophysical methods used in studying lung surfactant films and bilayers are given in the research text by Notter (9).

V. Overview of Inhibitors and Mechanisms

The most common cause of injury-induced lung surfactant dysfunction is through physicochemical interactions with endogenous compounds present in edema or the inflammatory response (Fig. 3). A variety of compounds are capable of reducing the surface activity of alveolar surfactant (Table 4). Probably the most widely recognized biophysical inhibitors of surfactant activity are plasma proteins like albumin, fibrinogen, and fibrin monomer (102–114). Hemoglobin, which can be present in the lungs through lysis of red blood cells in hemorrhagic injury, is a related protein inhibitor (104,105,110,115). Lung surfactant can also be inactivated biophysically by interactions with cell membrane lipids and lysophospholipids (103,111,115–117), cholesterol (47,118), glycolipids (119), and sphingolipids (120). Lysophospholipids not only inhibit surface activity through direct biophysical interactions, but also can damage the pulmonary endothelial–epithelial barrier and increase the concentration of plasma-derived inhibitors (121). Fluid free fatty acids like oleic acid also cause both biophysical detriments to lung surfactant surface activity (118,122–124) and capil-

Table 4 Examples of Endogenous Compounds that Inhibit Lung Surfactant Activity Through Physical or Chemical Interactions

---

Biophysical inhibitors
  Plasma and blood proteins (e.g., albumin, hemoglobin, fibrinogen, fibrin monomer)
  Cell membrane lipids
  Lysophospholipids
  Fluid free fatty acids
  Glycolipids and sphingolipids
  Meconium
Chemically acting inhibitors
  Lytic enzymes (proteases, phospholipases)
  Reactive oxygen and nitrogen species (ROS, RNS)
  Antibodies to surfactant proteins

Tabulated inhibitors are examples only. See text for literature citations and discussion

lary permeability injury (125–130). Another relevant inhibitor of lung surfactant activity is meconium, a complex fetal product containing cell membrane lipids, proteins and fatty acids that cause severe acute inflammatory injury and respiratory failure if aspirated by infants during delivery (131–133). Examples of inflammation-related inhibitors that can degrade functional surfactant lipids or proteins are proteases (134), phospholipases (118,135–137), and reactive oxidants (122,138–142). Antibodies to surfactant apoproteins can also bind to these essential surfactant components and impair their activity (143–145).

Lung surfactant inhibitors act by several physicochemical mechanisms detailed in subsequent sections (Table 5). Plasma and blood proteins act primarily by competitive adsorption to reduce the entry of active lung surfactant components into the air–water interface (9,103,104). In contrast, fluid free fatty acids and membrane lipids can mix into the interfacial film itself and compromise its ability to lower surface tension during dynamic compression (9,103,123). Phospholipases, proteases, or reactive oxidants act chemically to degrade or alter essential surfactant components, and also produce reaction products able to cause further biophysical inhibition (e.g., phospholipase activity produces inhibitory lysophospholipids and fluid free fatty acids). Finally, selective depletion and/or alteration of active large surfactant aggregate subtypes has been documented in several forms of acute pulmonary injury (28,146–150). Changes in large surfactant aggregates can result from direct interactions with inhibitory substances or secondary to impaired intra-alveolar processing or injury to type II cells. Surfactant dysfunction from any of these mechanisms can severely impair mechanics and gas exchange in injured lungs, but in many cases surfactant dysfunction is reversible. Biophysical

Table 5 Examples of Mechanisms of Lung Surfactant Dysfunction

Competitive adsorption by inhibitor substances that hinder the entry of active lung
   surfactant components into the air–water interface
Mixing of fluid inhibitors directly into the interfacial film to impair surface tension
   lowering during dynamic compression
Chemical degradation of functional surfactant lipids or proteins that generate
   inhibitory byproducts and reduce the content of active surfactant components
Binding or association of inhibitors with active surfactant components that impair
   functional molecular interactions (e.g., antibodies to surfactant apoproteins)
Depletion or reduced activity of large surfactant aggregate subtypes from physical or
   chemical interactions with inhibitors or from injury-related alterations in
   surfactant metabolism and processing

See text for literature citations and examples illustrating the tabulated mechanisms.
(Adapted from Ref. 9.)

studies show that many forms of surfactant dysfunction are more severe at
low surfactant concentration, and become mitigated or abolished at high
surfactant concentration despite the continued presence of inhibitory
substances (9,36). This gives a rationale for the use of exogenous surfactant therapy to increase alveolar surfactant concentrations and reverse
dysfunction in ALI/ARDS (Chapter 15).

VI. Surfactant Inactivation by Blood Proteins

A variety of studies have shown that whole serum, albumin, hemoglobin,
fibrinogen, and other blood proteins reduce lung surfactant activity in a
concentration-dependent manner (102–115). The ability of albumin to
impair the adsorption of lavaged endogenous surfactant is illustrated in
Table 6 (102). Albumin is seen to decrease both the rate and magnitude
of adsorption at a low surfactant phospholipid concentration of 0.063
mg/mL. Inhibition becomes less severe when surfactant concentration is
increased to 0.125 mg/mL even in the presence of a higher albumin concentration (Table 6). If lung surfactant concentration is raised sufficiently, inhibitory effects on adsorption from albumin or other plasma proteins can be
completely abolished (data not shown) (102). A similar pattern of concentration-dependent lung surfactant inhibition from blood proteins is also
found to exist for dynamic surface activity (102,115). At surfactant
phospholipid concentrations of 0.5 μmol/mL, albumin (10 mg/mL) and
hemoglobin (25 mg/mL) prevent endogenous surfactant from reaching
surface tensions below 26–29 mN/m after 10 min of rapid cycling on a pulsating bubble surfactometer (Table 7). However, when surfactant phospho-

Table 6 Inhibitory Effects of Albumin on the Adsorption of Endogenous Lung Surfactant

Mixtures	Surfactant phospholipid concentration (mg/mL)	Albumin concentration (mg/mL)	Adsorption surface tension (mN/m) at time (min)		
			0	5	10
Albumin	—	0.2–1.9	56	53	51
Lung surfactant (LS)	0.063	—	55	24	23
LS + albumin	0.063	1.1	52	48	45
LS + albumin	0.063	1.9	52	49	47
LS	0.125	—	25	23	23
LS + albumin	0.125	2.5	51	29	25

Time 0 is within 15 sec following addition of surfactant or surfactant/albumin mixtures to a stirred subphase containing 0.15 M NaCl + 1.4 mM $CaCl_2$ at 37 °C. Endogenous lung surfactant (LS) was isolated by centrifugation at 12,000 × g from cell-free bronchoalveolar lavage of calf lungs.
(Data from Ref. 102.)

lipid concentration is doubled to 1 μmol/mL, minimum surface tensions < 1 mN/m are found even in the presence of larger concentrations of inhibitory proteins. Protein-induced surfactant dysfunction similar to that in Tables 6 and 7 also occurs for clinical exogenous surfactants used in replacement therapy (see Chapter 15 for coverage of the activity and inhibition of clinical exogenous surfactants). The ability of clinical exogenous surfactants to resist inhibitor-induced dysfunction is particularly important for their efficacy in ALI/ARDS.

The primary mechanism by which plasma and blood proteins inhibit lung surfactant activity is by competitive adsorption and interfacial shielding (103,104). These large protein molecules contain polar and nonpolar amino acids and have a degree of surface activity. When they adsorb at the interface, they hinder and limit the entry of lung surfactant constituents. Since the surface tension lowering ability of plasma proteins is not nearly as great as lung surfactant, this competitive adsorption reduces overall surface activity. The role of competitive adsorption in plasma protein inhibition of lung surfactant activity can be demonstrated experimentally (Table 8). Albumin alone adsorbs to a high equilibrium surface tension of 49 ± 2 mN/m, while calf lung surfactant extract (CLSE) adsorbs to a much lower equilibrium surface tension of 23 ± 1 mN/m (similar to whole surfactant) (Table 8). When albumin at 1.25 mg/mL is allowed to adsorb simultaneously with a low concentration of CLSE (0.063 mg phospholipid/mL), the mixture reaches a final equilibrium surface tension equivalent

Table 7 Inhibitory Effects of Plasma Proteins on the Dynamic Surface Activity of Endogenous Lung Surfactant

Mixtures	Surfactant phospholipid concentration (μmol/mL)	Plasma protein concentration (mg/mL)	Minimum surface tension (mN/m) at time (min)		
			0	5	10
Albumin	—	2–200	45	45	45
Hemoglobin	—	2–200	36	35	35
Lung surfactant (LS)	0.5	—	20	6	<1
LS + albumin	0.5	10	45	44	29
LS + hemoglobin	0.5	25	34	29	26
LS	1.0	—	19	3	<1
LS + albumin	1.0	100	44	3	<1
LS + hemoglobin	1.0	25–100	36	25	<1

Large aggregate lung surfactant (LS) was pelleted at 12,000 × *g* from cell-free bronchoalveolar lavage of intact calf lungs. Minimum surface tension was measured on a pulsating bubble apparatus (20 cycles/min, 50% area compression, 37 °C) at the tabulated surfactant/inhibitor concentrations in 0.15 M NaCl and 1.4 mM CaCl2. Time 0 was <15 sec from the start of bubble pulsation. (Data from Refs. 102,115.)

to that of albumin alone. This is consistent with albumin occupying a significant fraction of the interface at low surfactant concentration. However, if CLSE at the same low concentration of 0.063 mg/mL is first allowed to adsorb and form a surface film, albumin subsequently added

Table 8 Competitive Adsorption in Albumin-Induced Surfactant Dysfunction

Lung surfactant and/or inhibitor	Concentration (mg/mL)	Experimental condition	Equilibrium surface tension (mN/m)
CLSE	0.063 or 0.25	Adsorbing alone	23 ± 1
Albumin	1.25 or 2.5	Adsorbing alone	49 ± 2
CLSE + albumin	0.063 + 1.25	Simultaneous addition	49 ± 2
CLSE + albumin	0.063 + 2.5	CLSE added first	23 ± 1
CLSE + albumin	0.25 + 1.25	Simultaneous addition	23 ± 1
CLSE + albumin	0.25 + 1.25	Albumin added first	49 ± 2

CLSE (calf lung surfactant extract) is a chloroform:methanol extract of lavaged surfactant from calves. Equilibrium surface tensions (mean ± SEM) are final plateau values measured at 37 °C in a teflon dish with a 0.15 M NaCl subphase stirred with a magnetic bar to minimize diffusion resistance. When one substance was added first, it was allowed to reach its equilibrium value prior to addition of the second substance and determination of the final tabulated surface tension. [Data from Ref. 104 as adapted by Notter (9). See text for discussion.]

at 2.5 mg/mL beneath this film is unable to penetrate to the surface and raise equilibrium surface tension (Table 8). In the converse experiment, CLSE at a higher concentration of 0.25 mg/mL out-competes albumin (1.25 mg/mL) for the interface when the two are adsorbing simultaneously. However, if albumin at 1.25 mg/mL is allowed to adsorb first at the air–water interface, CLSE at a concentration of 0.25 mg/mL is not able to penetrate the preformed inhibitory albumin film (Table 8).

VII. Surfactant Inactivation by Cell Membrane Lipids, Fluid Free Fatty Acids, and Lysophospholipids

In addition to large blood proteins, smaller molecules can also interact biophysically with lung surfactant to reduce its surface activity. This is particularly true for compounds that are miscible with surfactant phospholipids and can penetrate into the surface film more readily than plasma proteins. Examples of inhibitor substances of this type are cell membrane lipids, lysophospholipids, and fluid free fatty acids (47,103,111,115–118,122–124). Lung surfactant inhibition by oleic acid is illustrated in Fig. 4. At a low surfactant phospholipid concentration of 0.5 mM, oleic acid at a molar ratio of 0.5 relative to phospholipid raises minimum surface tension to ~20 mN/m (Fig. 4A). Inhibition by oleic acid persists even at a very high surfactant concentration of 12 mM phospholipid (9 mg/mL) when the molar ratio of this fatty acid relative to surfactant phospholipid is 0.67 or more (Fig. 4B). Inhibition by oleic acid can be overcome by raising surfactant concentration, but the concentration increase must be sufficient to reduce the molar ratio of free fatty acid to surfactant phospholipid to 0.5 or below in the example shown. A conceptually similar pattern of concentration-dependent behavior also is found for lung surfactant inhibition by lysophosphatidylcholine (LPC) and red blood cell membrane lipids (103,115). Dynamic surface activity detriments induced by LPC in mixtures with CLSE are shown in Fig. 5. Minimum surface tension values after 5 min of cycling on the pulsating bubble are shown to be ≥15 mN/m when the ratio of LPC relative to surfactant phospholipid is 25% by weight or greater even at relatively high surfactant concentrations of 3 and 6 mg phospholipid/mL (Fig. 5).

The ability of LPC, fluid free fatty acids, and cell membrane lipids to penetrate and impair the activity of lung surfactant and phospholipid surface films has been directly demonstrated by Hall et al. (123) and Holm et al. (103). Experiments with spread binary films of DPPC plus oleic acid or C16:0 LPC show that these compounds are at least partially miscible and interact molecularly within the surface film (103,123). Fluid oleic acid and LPC (which has detergent-like properties) adsorb to relatively high equilibrium surface pressures, but do not reduce surface tension substan-

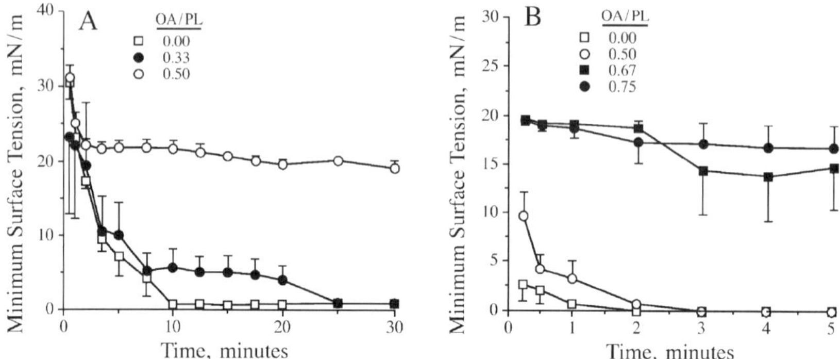

Figure 4 Inhibition of lung surfactant activity by oleic acid. Panel A: surfactant concentration 0.5 mM phospholipid; panel B: surfactant concentration 12 mM phospholipid. Mixtures of oleic acid (OA) and lavaged calf lung surfactant were studied at different molar ratios in a pulsating bubble surfactometer (20 cycles/min, 50% area change, 37 °C). OA inhibited dynamic surface tension lowering even at a high surfactant concentration of 12 mM when present at molar ratios of 0.67 and 0.75 relative to surfactant phospholipid. A lower OA molar ratio of 0.5 relative to phospholipid was inhibitory at low surfactant concentration (0.5 mM phospholipid), but inhibition was significantly reduced at high surfactant concentration (12 mM phospholipid). (From Ref. 123.)

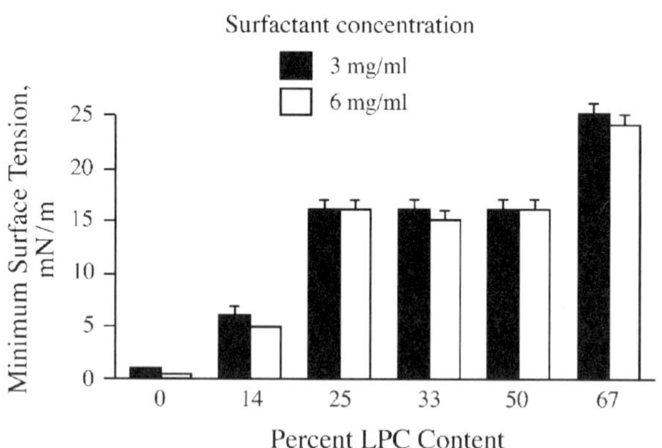

Figure 5 Inhibition of lung surfactant by lysophosphatidylcholine (LPC). Minimum surface tension after 5 min of cycling on a pulsating bubble surfactometer is shown for mixtures of LPC with a chloroform:methanol extract of lavaged calf lung surfactant (CLSE). LPC above a threshold level inhibited surface activity even at a high surfactant phospholipid concentration of 6 mg/mL (8 mM). Cycling rate 20 cycles/min, 50% area compression, 37 °C. LPC content is percent by weight in the total mixture with CLSE. (From Ref. 103.)

tially below equilibrium values under dynamic compression in films. When oleic acid or LPC are present in mixed films with lung surfactant, they fluidize the film and compromise its ability to achieve low surface tensions during dynamic compression. The ability of LPC to penetrate and reduce the activity of lung surfactant films is shown in Fig. 6 (103). An aqueous dispersion of CLSE was allowed to adsorb and form a film having a minimum surface tension <1 mN/m in a bubble apparatus with a specialized hypophase exchange system (pre-exchange, Fig. 6). This film was then isolated on a buffered saline hypophase, with its ability to reach minimum surface tensions <1 mN/m during cycling maintained (first exchange, Fig. 6). The surfactant film was then exposed to a second hypophase containing C16:0 LPC and minimum surface tension was measured after 5 min of additional cycling. The observed rise in minimum surface tension to values of ~9 mN/m indicates that LPC penetrated the film and impaired its dynamic surface tension lowering (second exchange, Fig. 6). Parallel experiments with albumin demonstrated that this protein could not penetrate a preformed surfactant film and raise minimum surface tension consistent with the results shown earlier in Table 8 (103). The differing mechanisms of action of albumin and LPC result in different patterns of concentration-dependent surfactant inhibition. Surface activity detriments from albumin are less directly related to inhibitor/surfactant concentration ratios than is the case for LPC (103). Inhibition from plasma proteins can typically be overcome

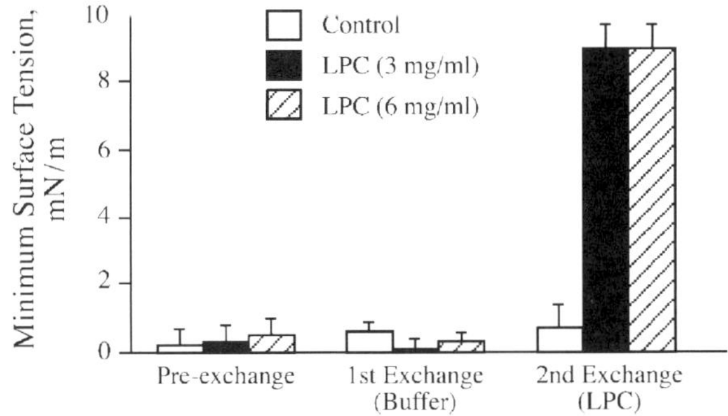

Figure 6 Mechanism of surfactant inhibition by LPC. Extracted calf lung surfactant (CLSE) was allowed to adsorb and form a film with a stable minimum surface tension <1 mN/m in a pulsating bubble surfactometer. The surfactant film was then isolated on a buffered saline subphase by hypophase exchange (first exchange), followed by exposure to a subphase containing 0, 3, or 6 mg/mL of LPC (second exchange). LPC penetrated the film and raised minimum surface tension to ~9 mN/m after 5 min of cycling (37 °C, 20 cycles/min, 50% area compression). Other compounds like fluid free fatty acids and membrane lipids are also thought to inhibit surfactant activity by penetrating and fluidizing the surface film to impair dynamic surface tension lowering. See text for details. (From Ref. 103.)

more easily by raising surfactant concentration than is true for inhibition by LPC, free fatty acids and cell membrane lipids. However, even activity detriments from these latter substances can be mitigated or abolished if surfactant concentration is raised sufficiently to reduce the percentage levels of inhibitors below threshold values (103,111,123).

VIII. Surfactant Dysfunction from Interactions with Reactive Oxygen or Nitrogen Species

Reactive oxygen and nitrogen species are important contributors to the innate pulmonary inflammatory response and to lung injury. As part of host defense, activated inflammatory cells like alveolar macrophages (AM) kill pathogens by producing a variety of reactive oxygen and nitrogen species. For example, exposure of mouse or rat AM in vivo or in vitro to inflammatory cytokines, lipopolysaccharide (LPS), pathogens, respirable dusts, or oxidant gases results in the production of nitric oxide ($^{\bullet}$NO) via upregulation of Nos2 or iNOS (the Ca^{2+}-independent form of nitric oxide synthase) (151–153), and in the production of superoxide anion ($O_2^{\bullet-}$) via the membrane-bound NADPH oxidase (154). Human alveolar macrophages from inflamed lungs also produce significant levels of reactive oxygen and nitrogen species when incubated in vitro with pathogens (155). Superoxide and $^{\bullet}$NO combine with each other, or react with thiols, molecular oxygen and other biological molecules, to form hydrogen peroxide (H_2O_2), hydroxyl radical ($^{\bullet}$OH), or additional reactive species like peroxynitrite ($ONOO^-$), nitrogen dioxide (NO_2), dinitrogen trioxide (N_2O_3), and *S*-nitrosothiols (RSNO) (156–158) (see Chapter 7 for further discussion of the chemistry of reactive nitrogen and oxygen species).

At high concentrations, $^{\bullet}$NO can inactivate critical enzymes by interacting with their iron-sulfur centers (159), cause DNA strand breaks resulting in the activation of nuclear poly-ADP-ribosyl transferase (159), and inhibit DNA and protein synthesis (160,161). At physiological concentrations, the reactivity of $^{\bullet}$NO is mild and most of its toxicity has been attributed to $ONOO^-$ or higher oxides of nitrogen. Peroxynitrite is a potent oxidizing and nitrating agent that oxidizes thiols at rates at least 1000-fold greater than H_2O_2 at pH 7 (162), causes iron-independent peroxidation of lipids and low density lipoproteins (163,164), nitrates phenol-containing amino acids including tyrosine (165,166), and oxidizes proteins (167). Because of this diverse reactivity, $ONOO^-$ can damage a spectrum of biological targets including DNA (168), the mitochondrial electron transport chain (169), lung ion channels (170–172), and the pulmonary surfactant system (140,173). Peroxynitrite can attack biological targets even in the presence of antioxidant substances (174). Physiological concentrations of carbon dioxide and bicarbonate enhance the reactivity of $ONOO^-$ and increase the extent of nitration through the formation of the nitrosoperoxycarbonate anion (175,176). Bicarbonate can also reverse the mitigating effects of ascorbate and urate on ONOO$^-$-induced nitration (175). Significant levels of nitrite and nitrate, the stable byproducts of nitric oxide metabolism, have been found in bronchoalveolar lavage (BAL) from patients at risk for or having ARDS (177,178). The production of reactive oxygen–nitrogen species in the alveoli in inflammatory injury is also indicated by the presence of nitrotyrosine in lung tissue sections and BAL from patients who have died from ARDS (178,179).

Among the many targets of reactive nitrogen and oxygen species in lung injury are surfactant proteins such as SP-A (178,180). Interactions of SP-A with reactive oxygen and nitrogen species can impair both its biophysical and biological activities. As noted earlier in this chapter, SP-A has multiple functions in vivo (Table 2). It acts biophysically to promote lipid aggregation and tubular myelin formation in lung surfactant, and enhances adsorption and film behavior (31,181–185) SP-A also has been shown to improve the ability of hydrophobic lung surfactant extracts to resist inhibition by plasma proteins (105,117,186). The potential use of recombinant SP-A or synthetic regional SP-A peptides to enhance inhibition resistance in clinical exogenous surfactants is discussed in Chapter 15. SP-A also has important biological roles other than its biophysical activity in lung surfactant. SP-A binds to type II cell receptors, regulates surfactant reuptake and recycling, and participates in host defense by enhancing macrophage function and bacterial clearance (9,180,187–189). SP-A deficient (–/–) transgenic mice maintain a high level of surfactant biophysical activity due to the continued presence of the hydrophobic surfactant proteins, but these mice have a decreased ability to clear Group B Streptococci and *Pneumocystis aeruiginosa* and mycoplasmas (190–192). SP-D also has significant roles in host defense in vivo that could potentially be disrupted by interactions with reactive nitrogen and oxygen species (11,188). In addition, these reactive species can chemically alter the hydrophobic components of lung surfactant (i.e., lipids and SP-B/C) and compromise their crucial contributions to surface active function.

A. Examples of the Nitration of SP-A and Other Proteins During Inflammatory Lung Injury

Nitration of proteins through interactions with reactive nitrogen species almost certainly occurs in vivo during inflammatory lung injury (discussion of the nitration of SP-A and other proteins in lung injury is also given in Chapter 7). 3-Nitrotyrosine residues, products of the addition of NO_2 to the *ortho* position of the hydroxyl group of tyrosine, are stable end-products of nitration reactions that can be detected by immunohistochemistry, ELISA, or high-pressure liquid chromatography (HPLC) (177,179,193,194).

Significant levels of protein-associated nitrotyrosine (400–500 pmol/mg protein) have been demonstrated by ELISA and HPLC in extracellular fluid or BAL from patients with ALI/ARDS and hydrostatic edema (177,178). These levels of protein-associated nitrotyrosine are an order of magnitude higher than reported in normal human BAL (28 pmol/mg protein) (195), normal rat lung tissue (∼30 pmol/mg protein) (196), or normal human serum albumin (∼30 pmol/mg protein) (197). Nitrated SP-A has been specifically detected in edema-derived fluid but not in plasma from patients with ALI/ARDS (178) (Fig. 7). Despite being present at high concentrations in the epithelial lining fluid of these patients, albumin was nitrated to a much lesser degree than SP-A (data not shown) (178). A variety of in vitro studies have also shown that reactive nitrogen and oxygen species produced by activated macrophages or neutrophils can interact with SP-A or other biologically important proteins such as α_1-proteinase inhibitor (140,142,173,176,198–202). An example quantitating the presence of

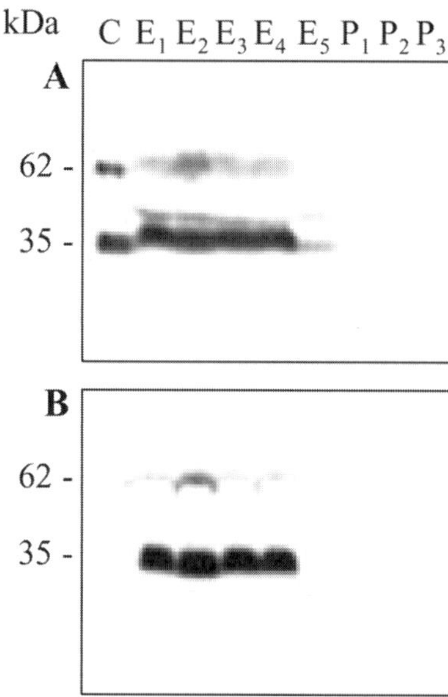

Figure 7   Nitration of surfactant protein A (SP-A) in pulmonary edema fluid samples from ALI/ARDS patients. SP-A was assessed by specific immuno-precipitation and Western blotting (panel A) and by detection of nitrotyrosine (panel B) in pulmonary edema fluid and plasma. SP-A was present as a prominent band near 35 kDa in the pulmonary edema fluid of four out of five patients with ALI/ARDS (E₁–E₄, panel A). SP-A in edema from these patients was nitrated as shown by the presence of nitrotyrosine (E₁–E₄, panel B). SP-A was present but not nitrated in edema fluid from a control patient (C) with alveolar proteinosis. SP-A was not present in plasma from any patient studied (P₁–P₃, panels A, B). (From Ref. 178.)

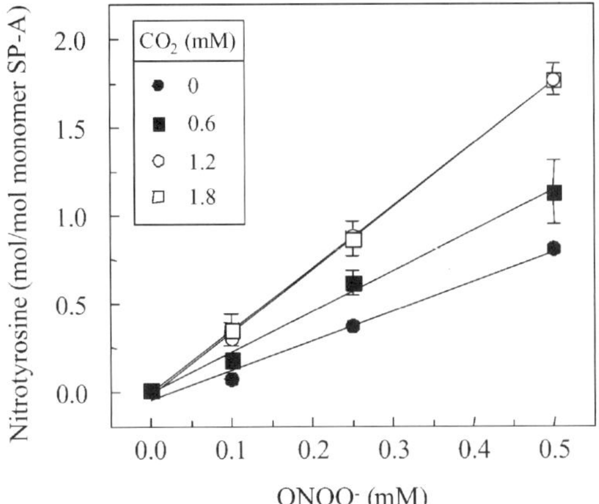

Figure 8 Peroxynitrite-induced nitration of SP-A and its enhancement by CO_2. SP-A (0.1 mg/mL in 15 mM HEPES buffer, pH 7.4) was exposed to varying concentrations of peroxynitrite ($ONOO^-$) in the absence (0 mM) or presence of CO_2 (0.6, 1.2, and 1.8 mM). Corresponding mean partial pressure values of CO_2 in the media as measured by a blood-gas analyzer were 0, 20, 40, and 59 torr. Nitrotyrosine was quantified by ELISA with nitrated bovine serum albumin as a standard. Values are means ± SEM for $n \geq 4$. Peroxynitrite is shown to induce nitration of SP-A, and this effect increases in the presence of CO_2. (From Ref. 176.)

nitrotyrosine residues in SP-A as a result of exposure to peroxynitrite is shown in Fig. 8. The added presence of CO_2 is seen to increase peroxynitrite-induced nitration of SP-A (Fig. 8).

B. Examples of Nitration-Related Functional Impairments in SP-A

Exposure of SP-A to nitrating agents, reactive nitrogen species, or compounds that generate reactive nitrogen species can alter protein activity. For example, nitration of SP-A with a concomitant reduction in its ability to bind mannose and aggregate lipids occurs following exposure to 3-morpholinosydnonimine (SIN-1), which generates $^\bullet NO$ and $O_2^\bullet$ and forms $ONOO^-$ (Fig. 9) (201). SP-A nitration and an associated loss of function have also been observed after exposure to tetranitromethane (TNM, a specific nitrating agent at pH 7.4 and 8 but not at pH 6–6.5), $ONOO^-$, or spermine NONOate and xanthine oxidase plus lumazine (140,142,173,200,201). SP-A nitration in these studies, as assessed by amino acid analysis, semi-quantitative ELISA, and Western blotting, correlated directly with a decreased ability to aggregate lipids and bind mannose in the presence of Ca^{2+}. Exposure of SP-A to $^\bullet NO$ alone (SIN-1 + SOD), xanthine and xanthine oxidase, or TNM at pH 6, did not cause SP-A nitration and did

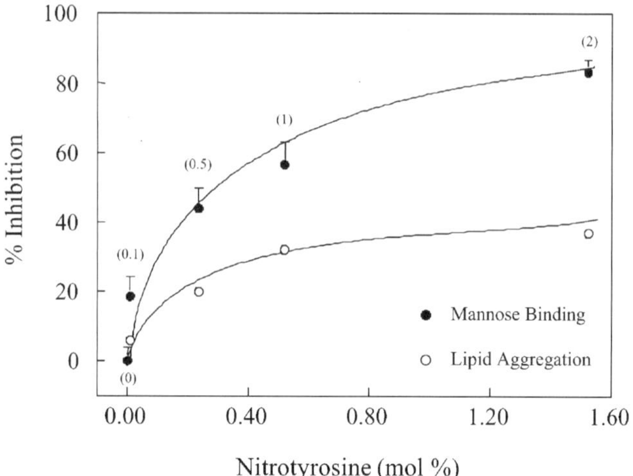

Figure 9 Correlation between nitrotyrosine formation and inhibition of SP-A mannose-binding and lipid aggregation by SIN-1. Nitrotyrosine induced by SIN-1 (3-morpholinosydnonimine) was measured by ELISA using a polyclonal anti-nitrotyrosine as the primary antibody, and is expressed as mol% (moles of nitrotyrosine per 100 amino acids). Mannose-binding (•) was assayed with immobilized d-mannose–agarose chromatography, and lipid aggregation (○) by measuring the light absorbance of a lipid liposome (PC/PG)/SP-A complex at 400 nm. Numbers in parentheses are SIN-1 concentrations in mM. Results are means ± SEM for $n \geq 4$. Some error bars are smaller than the symbols. (Data from Ref. 201.)

not inhibit its ability to aggregate lipids or bind mannose (166,173,201). Mannitol, which scavenges hydroxyl radicals, did not prevent SIN-1-induced SP-A nitration or decrease mannose binding. In contrast, cysteine or urate, which scavenge $ONOO^-$, prevented SIN-1-induced nitration and loss of function (166,173,201).

Each monomer of SP-A contains eight tyrosine residues in the C-terminal carbohydrate recognition domain responsible for carbohydrate binding and lipid aggregation (203,204). Evidence suggests that nitration of a single tyrosine in this domain of monomeric SP-A can decrease its ability to aggregate lipids and bind mannose. HPLC amino acid analysis of TNM-treated SP-A at pH 8 by Haddad et al. (173) showed a linear dose-dependent increase in nitrotyrosine and a decrease in tyrosine levels. Treatment with TNM (0.5 mM; pH 8) resulted in 0.33 ± 0.052 mole% nitrotyrosine, indicative of $11 \pm 2\%$ of tryosine residues being nitrated. These findings are consistent with the nitration of an average single tyrosine residue for each SP-A monomer (173). Mass spectroscopy has shown that the major nitrated peptide on both TNM-exposed and $ONOO^-$-exposed SP-A is the tryptic fragment $Tyr^{161}–Arg^{179}$ (YNTYAYVGL-

TEGPSPGDFR) located in the carbohydrate recognition domain (166). Sequencing of this peptide demonstrated that nitration was equally distributed on Tyr^{164} and Tyr^{166} (either tyrosine could be nitrated but not both simultaneously) (166), and no other nitrated or oxidized amino acids were detected in agreement with HPLC results (173). An additional nitration site on SP-A (Tyr^{161}) has been identified when SP-A is exposed to $ONOO^-$ in the presence of HCO_3^- (176).

Nitration of human SP-A has also been found to alter its binding to mannose-containing saccharides on *P. carinii* and its ability to help mediate adherence to AM (199) (Fig. 10). Calcium-dependent binding of SP-A to *P. carinii* was significantly reduced following nitration by $ONOO^-$ (K_d was increased from 7.8×10^{-9} to 1.6×10^{-8} M without a significant alteration in number of binding sites) (Fig. 10A). Nitration of SP-A by TNM was similarly found to reduce its ability to adhere to *P. carinii* (199). Nitration of SP-A by $ONOO^-$ also removed the ability of the apoprotein to mediate the adherence and phagocytosis of *P. carinii* by rat AM (Fig. 10B). However, the binding of SP-A itself to rat AM was not altered by nitration. These findings suggest that nitration may interfere with the ability of SP-A to serve

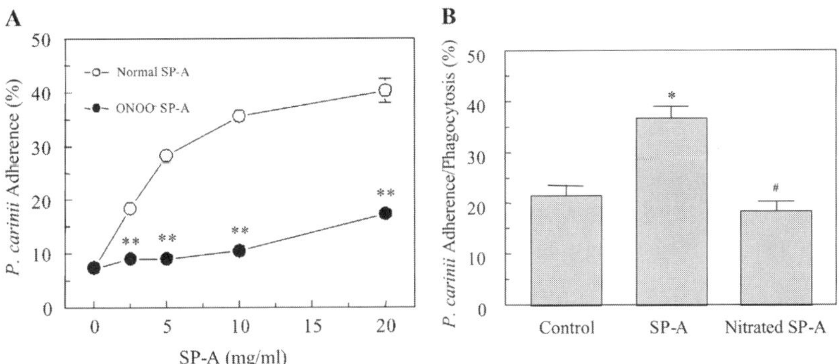

Figure 10 Role of normal and nitrated SP-A in *P. carinii* adherence or adherence/phagocytosis to alveolar macrophages. (Panel A) ^{51}Cr-labeled *P. carinii* were incubated with rat alveolar macrophages (AM) cultured in DMEM containing 0.1% BSA at 4°C for 4 hr in the absence and presence of normal or peroxynitrite ($ONOO^-$)-treated SP-A (0–20 µg/mL). *P. carinii* adherence to AM was significantly lower in the presence of $ONOO^-$-treated SP-A compared to normal SP-A at all concentrations. Results are means ± SEM for two experiments performed in duplicate. $^{**}P < 0.01$ compared with the same concentrations of normal SP-A. (Panel B) ^{51}Cr-labeled *P. carinii* were incubated with rat AM in DMEM containing 0.1% BSA at 37°C for 2 hr in the absence (*control*) and presence of normal or $ONOO^-$-treated SP-A (10 µg/mL). Normal SP-A significantly enhanced adherence/phagocytosis of *P. carinii* by AM whereas $ONOO^-$-treated SP-A lost its ability to mediate an interaction between *P. carinii* and AM. $^*P < 0.05$ compared with control; $^#P < 0.05$ compared with 10 µg/mL normal SP-A. (Data from Ref. 199.)

as a ligand for *P. carinii* adherence to AM at the site of interaction between the surfactant protein and surface protein PR30 on *P. carinii* (199).

Several lines of evidence indicate that nitration is more important than oxidation in causing activity reductions in SP-A. SP-A from the epithelial lining fluid of patients with ARDS is oxidized as well as nitrated (178). However, exposure of SP-A to TNM at pH 6–6.5 where it acts as an oxidizing agent does not decrease the ability of the apoprotein to aggregate lipids or bind mannose (173). In contrast, exposure to TNM at pH 7.5 where it functions as a nitrating agent leads to a decrease in SP-A activity (173). Carbon dioxide, which augments peroxynitrite-induced SP-A nitration but decreases oxidation in a dose-dependent fashion, exacerbates the effects of peroxynitrite in impairing the ability of SP-A to aggregate lipids (176) (Fig. 8). Finally, exposure of SP-A to generators of reactive oxygen intermediates (such as xanthine and xanthine oxidase) does not result in decreased function (142).

C. Examples of Surface Activity Detriments from Reactive Oxygen/Nitrogen Species

Exposure of animals or lung surfactant to peroxynitrite or high levels of $^{\bullet}$NO can directly impair surface active function (138,140,173,205–209). For example, surfactant lavaged from newborn lambs breathing 21% or 60% oxygen plus high levels of 80 or 200 ppm $^{\bullet}$NO has been shown to have lower surface activity than surfactant from lambs breathing 0 or 20 ppm $^{\bullet}$NO (205). Abnormal surface properties were observed in 36% and 60% of lavaged surfactant samples from lambs that breathed 80 or 200 ppm $^{\bullet}$NO, respectively. SP-A from the lambs breathing 200 ppm $^{\bullet}$NO had decreased ability to aggregate lipids in vitro (205), consistent with $^{\bullet}$NO-induced chemical changes. Reactive nitrogen and oxygen species can also directly interact with surfactant lipids and hydrophobic apoproteins. For example, exposure to peroxynitrite reduces the surface activity of calf lung surfactant extract containing all of the hydrophobic components of alveolar surfactant (140). The presence of peroxynitrite (1 mM) plus 100 μM Fe^{3+} EDTA kept CLSE from reaching minimum surface tension values below 10 mN/m during dynamic compression in pulsating bubble experiments (140). Peroxynitrite and its byproducts reacted with unsaturated lipids in CLSE, as evidenced by the appearance of conjugated dienes and thiobarbituric acid products, and also damaged the hydrophobic surfactant proteins. A mixture of hydrophobic SP-B/C exposed to peroxynitrite had greatly reduced surface activity when combined and studied with phospholipids (140). The above results demonstrate that reactive nitrogen/oxygen species like peroxynitrite have the potential to inhibit the surface activity of lung surfactant by lipid peroxidation and by damage to any or all of the surfactant proteins.

IX. Surfactant Dysfunction Involving Large Aggregates

Another mechanism that can lead to surfactant dysfunction during lung injury is the depletion or alteration of active large surfactant aggregate subtypes. As noted earlier, surfactant in the alveolar hypophase exists as a size-distributed population of phospholipid-rich aggregates, the larger of which normally have the greatest surface activity and the highest content of surfactant apoproteins (22–31). The percentage of large surfactant aggregates and their content of SP-A and SP-B have been shown to be reduced in bronchoalveolar lavage from patients with ARDS (75–77). Research in animal models of acute pulmonary injury has similarly shown that active large surfactant aggregates can be depleted in amount or reduced in activity by physicochemical interactions with inhibitors or by injury-induced changes in alveolar processing and surfactant metabolism (28,146–150,210). In addition, the rate of conversion of large to small surfactant aggregates during in vitro cycling has been shown to be increased by direct exposure to pathogenic *Escherichia coli* (211). Figure 11 illustrates the depletion and alteration of active large surfactant aggregates in rabbits with ALI following

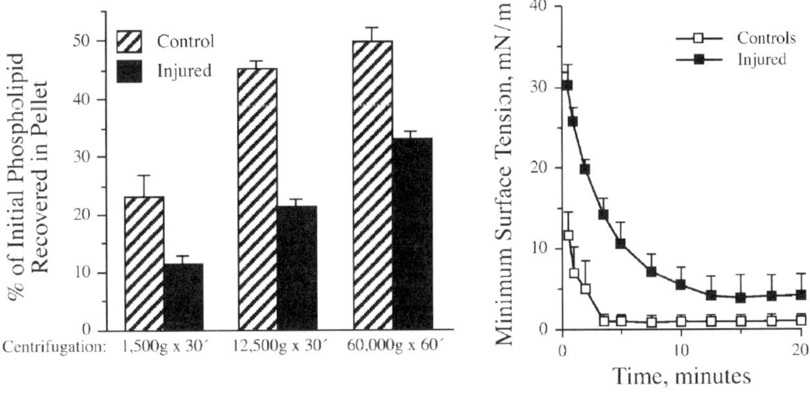

Figure 11 Depletion and alteration of large surfactant aggregates in oleic acid lung injury. Bronchoalveolar lavage from rabbits given intravenous oleic acid (OA) and from control rabbits was centrifuged at $150 \times g$ to remove cells, and surfactant aggregates pelleted under various centrifugation conditions were then examined. Panel A: Percent of total phospholipid in cell-free lavage pelleting at either $1500 \times g$, $12,500 \times g$, or $60,000 \times g$. Aggregate content is reduced in OA-injured vs. control rabbits in all cases. Panel B: Minimum surface tension of large aggregates pelleted at $12,500 \times g$ for 30 min from cell-free lavage on a pulsating bubble surfactometer (20 cycles/min, 37 °C, 50% area compression, 2 mM surfactant phospholipid concentration). The surface activity of large surfactant aggregates from OA rabbits is reduced compared to controls. See text for details. (From Ref. 28.)

intravenous infusion of oleic acid (28). The percentages of total phospholipid pelleted from BAL by centrifugation at either $1500 \times g$, $12{,}500 \times g$, or $60{,}000 \times g$ are shown to be reduced in injured animals compared to controls (Fig. 11A). Additional experiments applying these three centrifugation conditions successively to individual lavage samples demonstrated that the primary process occurring was a loss of large aggregates sedimenting at $1500 \times g$ (28). Injured animals also had a decrease in large aggregates sedimenting between 1500 and $12{,}500 \times g$, as well as an increase in small aggregates left in the supernatant after centrifugation at $60{,}000 \times g$ (28). Large surfactant aggregates in injured animals were not only depleted in amount, but also had impaired surface tension lowering ability compared to control large aggregates in pulsating bubble studies (Fig. 11B).

X. Additivity of Lung Surfactant Inhibitors

Multiple blood-derived and tissue-derived inhibitors of surfactant activity can be present simultaneously in injured lungs as a result of alveolocapillary membrane damage, edema, and inflammation. It is thus important to understand the extent to which mixtures of inhibitors can generate additive detriments to surface activity over and above their individual effects at the same concentration. Several combinations of protein and nonprotein inhibitors have been found to exhibit some degree of additivity in reducing the surface activity of lung surfactant. For example, albumin or hemoglobin mixed with LPC or red blood cell membrane lipids (RBCML) generate additive detriments to lung surfactant surface activity at selected concentrations (111). Mixtures of hemoglobin with fluid free fatty acids also can cause additive inhibition, while mixtures of albumin plus free fatty acids do not because of albumin binding of free fatty acid (111). Examples of inhibitor additivity in reducing lung surfactant activity are shown in Table 9. At lung surfactant phospholipid concentrations of 0.5 mg/mL, surface activity is impaired more severely by mixtures of hemoglobin plus arachadonic acid or RBCML, and albumin plus RBCML, than by the same concentrations of the individual inhibitors alone. However, the magnitudes of the added surface activity detriments over and above the effects of the most severe individual inhibitor present are not large for any of the mixtures shown. Moreover, the effects of the mixed inhibitors are still mitigated when surfactant phospholipid concentration is raised to 1 mg/mL (Table 9). Additivity in the inhibitory effects of blood proteins, fatty acids, and membrane lipids has also been shown to be reduced as their concentration rises and their detrimental effects as individuals become greater (111). In principle, additivity among lung surfactant inhibitors will be most pronounced for substances that function by "complementary" mechanisms. For example, an inhibitor that acts biophysically to reduce surface activity may be

Table 9 Additivity of Selected Protein and Nonprotein Inhibitors of Lung Surfactant Surface Activity

Mixtures	Inhibitor concentrations[a]	Minimum surface tension (mN/m) after bubble pulsation for (min)				
		1	5	10	15	20
LS (0.5 mg/mL)		17.7 ± 1.4	< 1			
+Hb	2.5	25.3 ± 0.8	17.7 ± 0.7	7.6 ± 1.7	2.9 ± 1.5	< 1 (16)[b]
+BSA	2.5	23.5 ± 1.3	14.0 ± 2.5	2.2 ± 1.8	< 1 (11)	
+RBCML	0.10	18.5 ± 0.5	15.2 ± 0.7	12.3 ± 1.5	6.4 ± 1.4	< 1
+AA	0.15	18.9 ± 0.4	14.3 ± 1.0	10.1 ± 2.0	3.1 ± 1.3	< 1
+Hb/RBCML	2.5/0.10	22.2 ± 0.8	16.2 ± 0.8	15.3 ± 1.4	11.3 ± 1.5	5.7 ± 1.0
+Hb/AA	2.5/0.15	21.6 ± 0.8	16.3 ± 1.4	14.9 ± 0.8	8.7 ± 1.5	3.8 ± 0.6
+BSA/RBCML	2.5/0.10	20.4 ± 0.6	17.0 ± 0.8	16.4 ± 0.8	10.5 ± 1.8	5.3 ± 1.0
+BSA/AA	2.5/0.15	19.5 ± 0.4	10.5 ± 2.3	< 1		
LS (1.0 mg/mL)						
+Hb/AA	2.5/0.15	18.0 ± 0.4	2.4 ± 1.3	< 1 (6)		
+Hb/RBCML	2.5/0.10	17.3 ± 0.8	3.5 ± 1.1	< 1 (7)		
+BSA/RBCML	2.5/0.10	17.0 ± 0.8	3.6 ± 0.4	< 1 (7)		

Lavaged calf lung surfactant (LS) was pelleted by centrifugation at $12,000 \times g$ and resuspended in 0.15 M NaCl and 2 mM CaCl2. Minimum surface tension was measured on a pulsating bubble surfactometer (20 cycles/min, 37°C).

[a]Inhibitor concentrations are in mg/mL for hemoglobin (Hb) and bovine serum albumin (BSA), and in mM for arachidonic acid (AA) and red blood cell membrane lipids (RBCML).

[b]Numbers in () are time in minutes when surface tension < 1 mN/m was reached if prior to that in the heading. Data are mean $\pm$ SEM for $n = 4$–6 from Ref. 111.

additive with a chemically acting inhibitor that degrades surfactant and reduces its effective functional concentration. Similarly, biophysical inhibitors of lung surfactant activity may be additive with substances or processes that deplete active large surfactant aggregates. Despite possible inhibitor additivity, however, current findings indicate that the resultant activity decreases can be reversed or mitigated by raising lung surfactant concentration, as noted above (e.g., Table 9).

XI. Physiological Correlates of Lung Surfactant Dysfunction and Replacement in Animals

Decades of research have shown the importance of correlating data on lung surfactant composition and biophysics with physiological effects in intact lungs or living animals. Complementary compositional, biophysical and animal research was essential in laying the basis for successful clinical surfactant replacement therapy in premature infants. Integrated biophysical and physiological research on surfactant dysfunction is similarly essential for effectively extending surfactant therapy to ALI/ARDS. Lung surfactant dysfunction has been shown to be present in multiple animal models of acute pulmonary injury, many of which are found to respond favorably to supplementation with active exogenous surfactants (see Chapter 15 plus Refs. 9, 36, 212–215 for additional review). The consensus of current animal research indicates that exogenous surfactants having the greatest surface activity and ability to resist inhibition have the highest physiological activity in reversing surfactant dysfunction and deficiency. Several examples of physiological correlates of surfactant dysfunction and replacement in lung injury are given below.

A. Example of Inhibitor-Induced Changes in Pulmonary Pressure–Volume (P–V) Mechanics in Excised Rat Lungs

Direct physiological correlates of surfactant dysfunction can be obtained by instilling plasma proteins or other inhibitors into normal lungs and measuring the effects on quasistatic P–V mechanics. Changes in P–V deflation mechanics indicating decreased compliance are found when albumin, hemoglobin, or red blood cell membrane lipids are instilled into normal or partially lavaged excised rat lungs (Fig. 12) (115). Consistent with biophysical studies with these inhibitors, mechanical detriments are more pronounced when endogenous surfactant concentration is reduced by a single lavage prior to inhibitor instillation (Fig. 12B vs. A). Also consistent with biophysical findings is that P–V mechanics can be restored almost to normal in the continued presence of inhibitors by instillation of exogenous

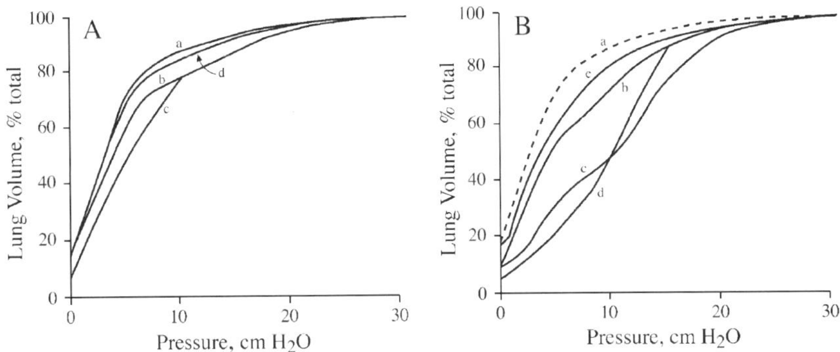

Figure 12 Alteration of pulmonary mechanics by instillation of lung surfactant inhibitors. Albumin, hemoglobin, or extracted red blood cell membrane lipids were instilled in 2.5 mL of 0.15 M NaCl into excised rat lungs (freshly excised or after a single lavage to partially deplete endogenous surfactant). Changes shown in P–V deflation mechanics are consistent with reductions in surface activity that were greater at low surfactant concentrations. Instilled CLSE (25 mg in 2.5 mL saline) restored mechanics toward normal, consistent with reversal of inhibition by increased surfactant concentration. (Panel A) (a) Normal lung, no inhibitors; (b) 4.5 mg red blood cell membrane lipids instilled; (c) 400 mg albumin or hemoglobin instilled; (d) 400 mg albumin/hemoglobin or 4.5 mg cell membrane lipids instilled, followed by 25 mg CLSE. (Panel B) (a) Normal lung; (b) partially surfactant-deficient lung (one lavage); (c) partially deficient lung instilled with 400 mg albumin or hemoglobin; (d) partially deficient lung instilled with 4.5 mg cell membrane lipids; (e) partially deficient lung instilled with 400 mg albumin/hemoglobin or 4.5 mg cell membrane lipids, followed by 25 mg CLSE. (Redrawn from Ref. 115.)

CLSE to raise surfactant concentration. Mechanical detriments analogous to those in Fig. 12 have also been demonstrated when oleic acid is instilled into excised rat lungs, and these detriments can similarly be reversed by instilled CLSE (123). These findings again agree with biophysical data showing that oleic acid reduces lung surfactant activity, and that inhibition can be overcome by increasing the concentration of active surfactant (Fig. 4). Physiological studies have also shown the additional correlate that exogenous surfactants that are easily compromised in surface activity by plasma proteins lack the ability to improve P–V mechanics in lungs containing these inhibitory substances (109).

B. Example Showing an Association Between Inflammation and Surfactant Dysfunction in Animals with *P. carinii*-Induced Lung Injury

P. carinii is an opportunistic micro-organism that is widely disseminated in the general population (216–219). Although normally benign, it can cause life-threatening pneumonia in an immunocompromised host. *P. carinii* pneumonia (PcP) has been the major presenting complaint in over 50% of HIV-positive patients with the acquired immune deficiency syndrome (216–219). In addition, *P. carinii* is estimated to account for 10–40% of pneumonia cases in HIV-negative patients who are immunosuppressed during treatment for organ transplantation, malignancies, or auto-immune connective tissue diseases. Mortality rates for PcP in immunodeficient or immunosuppressed patients in intensive care units range from 10% to 50% (216–219). Reductions in surfactant activity have been documented in several animal models of PcP, including steroid-treated rats (220), severe combined immunodeficient (SCID) mice (210), and CD4$^+$-depleted wild-type mice (221). Improvements in pulmonary function from surfactant replacement therapy have also been reported in rats (222) and human infants (223) with PcP, providing further evidence for the presence of surfactant dysfunction in this condition.

Studies by Wright et al. (221) have found a direct association between surfactant dysfunction and pulmonary inflammation in PcP. Lung injury in murine PcP includes a significant inflammatory response with elevated mRNAs for multiple cytokines and chemokines including interleukin (IL) -1α, IL-1β, IL-3, IL-6, MIP-1, MIP-2, RANTES, interferon-γ (IFNγ), and tumor necrosis factor (TNF)α and β (224–226). In association with inflammation, P–V compliance is decreased and protein/phospholipid ratios in lavage are increased in CD4$^+$ T cell-depleted mice with PcP compared to Pc-infected wild-type mice that do not develop PcP (Table 10). In addition, the surface activity of bronchoalveolar lavage from CD4$^+$-depleted mice with PcP is significantly decreased (Fig. 13) (221). Surfactant dysfunction and abnormalities in compliance and lavage protein/phospho-phospholipid are much less severe in mice with PcP that do not mount a CD8$^+$-mediated inflammatory/immune response (CD4$^+$/CD8$^+$-depleted mice, Table 10, Fig. 13) (221). A similar association of inflammation with surfactant dysfunction in PcP was also shown by Wright et al. (221) in studies with SCID mice vs. immune-reconstituted SCID mice. Nine weeks after exposure to *P. carinii* by housing in an infected colony, SCID mice with PcP had no reduction in compliance or lavage surface activity (reduced compliance and lavage surface activity were apparent at later times of 12- and 15-week postexposure). In contrast, at 9-week postexposure to *P. carinii*, SCID mice reconstituted with normal murine spleen cells 12 days prior to sacrifice had severe detriments in compliance and lavage surface activity (221).

Lung injury associated with PcP involves altered surfactant composition and metabolism in addition to reduced surface activity. Surfactant phospholipids are decreased in lavage from rats (227) and humans (228–230) with PcP, while SP-A levels are increased (231–233). The expression of SP-A and SP-D also increases in murine PcP (210,234). The expression of hydrophobic SP-B has been reported either to be decreased

Table 10 Alterations in Compliance and Lavage Phospholipid/Protein Ratios in Mice with Pneumonia and Lung Injury from *P. carinii* Infection

Experimental mouse group	Days after inoculation	Protein/phospholipid ratio (%) in BAL	P–V compliance (% control)
C57BL/6 (uninfected control)	0	70 ± 5	—
C57BL/6 (infected)	34	64 ± 5	100 ± 3
CD4$^+$/CD8$^+$T cell-depleted (infected)	34	63 ± 6	86 ± 6
CD4$^+$ T cell-depleted (infected)	34	126 ± 20 *	49 ± 4 *

Immunocompetent C57BL/6 mice (uninfected or infected with *P. carinii* organisms) do not develop PcP, in contrast to C57BL/6 mice depleted in CD4$^+$ or CD4$^+$/CD8$^+$ T-cells by specific antibody treatment followed by infection with *P. carinii*. Infection was on day 0 by intratracheal inoculation with homogenized lung tissue from mice in an infected colony. *Protein/phospholipid ratio and compliance are significantly worse in CD4$^+$ -depleted mice with PcP compared to all the other groups studied (p < 0.05 or less). Surface activity data in cell-free lavage are given in Fig. 13. See text for discussion. (Data from Ref. 221.)

(210,234,235) or unaltered (221) in murine PcP depending upon the timing and nature of injury. *P. carinii* and at least one of its cell wall components gpA (MSG, gp120) have been shown to bind surfactant apoproteins SP-A and SP-D (236–238). gpA is a mannosylated glycoprotein that interacts with SP-A (236,237) and SP-D (238) because of their lectin-like activity and homology with mannose-binding proteins. *P. carinii* organisms and/or gpA may also interfere with the synthesis/secretion of surfactant components (210,235,239,240).

C. Example of Surfactant Dysfunction and Replacement in Endotoxin-Induced Acute Lung Injury

Because of the importance of sepsis as a cause of ALI/ARDS, a number of studies have investigated surfactant dysfunction and replacement in animals with acute pulmonary injury from bacteria or bacterial toxins. As an example, Tashiro et al. (241) studied adult rats given *E. coli* endotoxin by tracheal instillation (53 ± 19 mg/kg). A second dose of instilled endotoxin was used in some animals in order to meet prospectively defined levels of oxygenation consistent with clinical ARDS ($PaO_2 < 200$ mmHg despite ventilation with 100% oxygen at a peak inspiratory pressure of 25 cm H_2O and a PEEP of

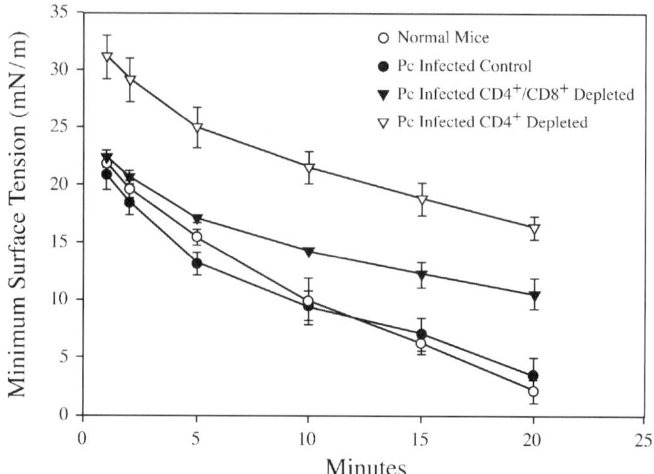

Figure 13   Inhibition of lung surfactant activity in association with inflammatory *P. carinii* pneumonia (PcP) in mice. Mice were lavaged 34 days after intratracheal inoculation with homogenized lung from mice in a *P. carinii*-infected colony. Cells were removed by centrifugation at $150 \times g$ for 10 min, and surface activity was measured as a function of time of pulsation on a bubble surfactometer (37 °C, 20 cycles/min, 50% area compression) at a uniform concentration of 2.5 mg phospholipid/mL. Surface activity is shown to be severely compromised in lavage from CD4$^+$-depleted C57BL/6 mice with PcP, but is less affected in CD4$^+$/CD8$^+$-depleted C57BL/6 mice with PcP. Control groups are immunocompetent C57BL/6 mice that do not develop PcP even if infected with *P. carinii* organisms. Data on lung compliance and lavage protein/phospholipid ratios are given in Table 10. See text for details. (Redrawn from Ref. 221.)

7.5 cm H$_2$O). After meeting criteria for ARDS, injured animals were randomly assigned to receive a porcine lung surfactant extract instilled at a dose of 100 mg/kg in 2 mL/kg saline or either air or saline as a placebo. Following assignment and treatment, mechanical ventilation with 100% oxygen was continued for 3 hr (or until death) while pulmonary function was monitored. Chest x-rays were obtained during the initial baseline period and just before treatment, as well as at the end of study prior to measurements of quasistatic P–V deflation mechanics. Rats instilled with exogenous surfactant had significant improvements in arterial oxygenation and P–V compliance compared to rats given air or saline (Fig. 14). PaO$_2$ increased to 390 ± 116 mmHg within 15 min of surfactant treatment, and stayed at a high level throughout the study period. Placebo-treated rats continued to be severely hypoxemic with PaO$_2$ values in the range of 100 mmHg and decreased static compliance compared to uninjured controls (Fig. 14). Dynamic lung-thorax compliance was improved less substantially

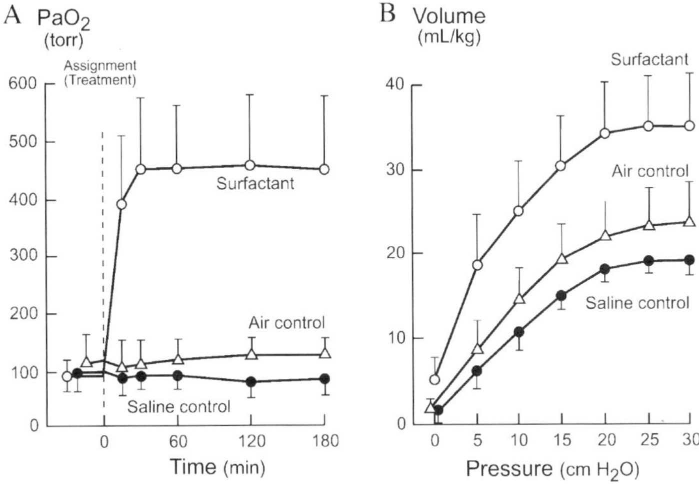

Figure 14 Effects of surfactant supplementation on pulmonary mechanics and function in endotoxin-injured rats. Panel A: partial pressure of arterial oxygen; Panel B: quasistatic P–V deflation mechanics at end-experiment. Rats with acute pulmonary injury from intratracheal instillation of *E. coli* endotoxin were randomized to receive a porcine lung surfactant extract (100 mg/kg in 2 mL/kg saline) by intratracheal instillation or placebo (saline or air). All animals were mechanically ventilated with 100% oxygen. Surfactant treatment significantly improved oxygenation and P–V mechanics, consistent with the existence of surfactant dysfunction in injured animals and its reversal by exogenous surfactant supplementation. See text for details. (Redrawn from Ref. 241.)

by surfactant treatment (data not shown) (241). Surfactant-treated rats also had reduced pulmonary edema on chest radiographs compared to placebo-treated animals, and better alveolar aeration in histological lung sections (241). These findings are consistent with surfactant dysfunction in endotoxin-injured animals that was mitigated by exogenous surfactant therapy. They also indicate the potential clinical utility of exogenous surfactant supplementation in ARDS, although benefits reported for surfactant therapy in animals injured by intravenous rather than instilled endotoxin have been less impressive (242–244). Exogenous surfactant therapy to mitigate surfactant dysfunction in clinical ALI/ARDS is detailed in Chapter 15.

D. Example of Surfactant Dysfunction in Animals with Acute Lung Injury from Acid Aspiration Plus Hyperoxia

Aspiration of gastric contents occurs in one of every 2000–3000 anesthetized patients (245,246), leading to lung injuries ranging from mild acute pneumonitis to severe, progressive inflammatory pathology consistent with ALI/ARDS (247). Oxygen is also a well-known inducer of acute and chronic lung injury despite its therapeutic benefits in patients with respiratory failure (see Refs. 9, 248–250 for review). The character of hyperoxic lung injury varies with the severity and duration of exposure, animal species, and age. Adult animals typically have a greater sensitivity to pulmonary oxygen toxicity than newborn animals, in contrast to retinal oxygen toxicity which is more severe in newborns. Severe acute pulmonary injury from prolonged exposure to high levels of oxygen (95–100%) includes inflammation, edema, increased alveolocapillary membrane permeability, type II cell dysfunction, and surfactant dysfunction (e.g., see Refs. 251– 257). Lower levels of hyperoxia of 40–80% can cause adaptive responses, but may also lead to chronic fibrogenic injury (248–250). Several studies have shown that pulmonary aspiration of acid can sensitize animals to subsequent hyperoxic lung injury (258–260) or to nitric oxide-induced injury (261).

Knight et al. (259) examined specific effects on pulmonary function, surfactant activity, and type II cell choline incorporation when adult rabbits were exposed to 50% oxygen or air for 24 hr following intratracheal instillation of 2.4 mL/kg of saline-HCl (pH 1.25) to simulate acid aspiration. This low level of oxygen exposure would normally not be expected to cause significant pulmonary toxicity. Exposure of normal adult rabbits to 60% oxygen for up to three weeks has been found to increase lung surfactant synthesis without significant acute respiratory distress (262). However, rabbits receiving 50% oxygen for 24 hr following instilled saline-HCl (pH 1.25) were found to have impaired gas exchange, decreased surfactant activity, and reduced choline incorporation in type II cells compared to rabbits receiving saline-HCl alone (259).

As shown in Fig. 15, rabbits receiving acid plus hyperoxia had a significantly decreased ratio of arterial partial pressure of oxygen to inspired oxygen fraction (PaO_2/FiO_2 ratio) measured after a 15-min period of breathing 100% oxygen at end-experiment (259). Rabbits injured with acid plus hyperoxia also had increased pulmonary edema based on lung wet to dry weight ratios compared to animals receiving acid alone (13 ± 2.5 g/kg body weight vs. 7.5 ± 1.5 g/kg body weight, $P < 0.01$). Quasistatic P–V curves in acid/hyperoxia animals indicated decreased lung compliance between 25% and 75% of the maximum volume normalized to animal body weight ($dV/dP_{25-75\%}$) (Fig. 16). Values for $dV/dP_{25-75\%}$ decreased from means of 1.4–1.5 mL/kg/cm H_2O in control animals and those receiving acid or hyperoxia alone to 0.564 ± 0.054 mL/kg/cm H_2O in animals receiving acid/hyperoxia. Consistent with decreased P–V compliance, surfactant activity was reduced in acid/hyperoxia animals. Minimum surface tension values in cell-free BAL on a pulsating bubble apparatus (20 cycles/min, 50% area compression, 37 °C, 1 μmol phospholipid/mL) were 2 ± 1 mN/m

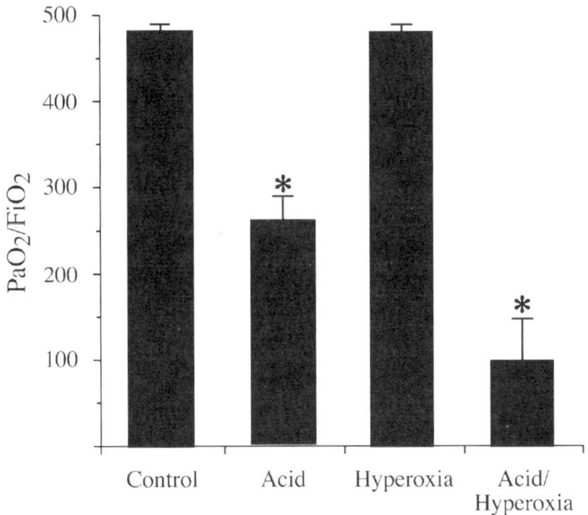

Figure 15 Arterial oxygenation in rabbits exposed to acid aspiration, hyperoxia, or both. The ratio of arterial oxygen partial pressure to inspired fraction of oxygen is shown for different groups of adult rabbits that breathed 100% oxygen for 15 min prior to sampling. Animal groups are uninjured controls ($n=5$), animals instilled with 2.4 mL/kg of normal saline-HCl (pH 1.25) (acid, $n=5$), animals exposed to 50% oxygen for 24 hr (hyperoxia, $n=5$), and animals receiving acid followed by 50% oxygen for 24 hr (acid/hyperoxia, $n=5$). Values are all mean $\pm$ SEM. (From Ref. 259.)

(uninjured controls), 2 ± 2 mN/m (hyperoxia alone), 4 ± 2 mN/m (acid alone), and 28 ± 2 mN/m (acid/hyperoxia). Surfactant metabolic abnormalities were also present in the acid/hyperoxia group based on decreased ^{3}H-choline incorporation in isolated type II cells (259). In a related study, Knight et al. (258) showed that microvascular injury was exacerbated in rabbits with acid aspiration plus short-term hyperoxic exposure. These findings suggest that acid aspiration in rabbits significantly alters the set point for oxygen toxicity, possibly by activating or priming inflammatory cells and cytokine pathways that exacerbate edema formation, surfactant dysfunction, and abnormalities in compliance and gas exchange. Underlying initial lung injury in patients with ALI/ARDS may similarly sensitize these individuals to detrimental effects from hyperoxia and/or mechanical ventilation during intensive care.

XII. Summary

Pulmonary surfactant is a highly active mixture of lipids and proteins produced by type II cells in the alveolar epithelial lining of air-breathing animals. Active lung surfactant is essential for normal respiration. Surfactant

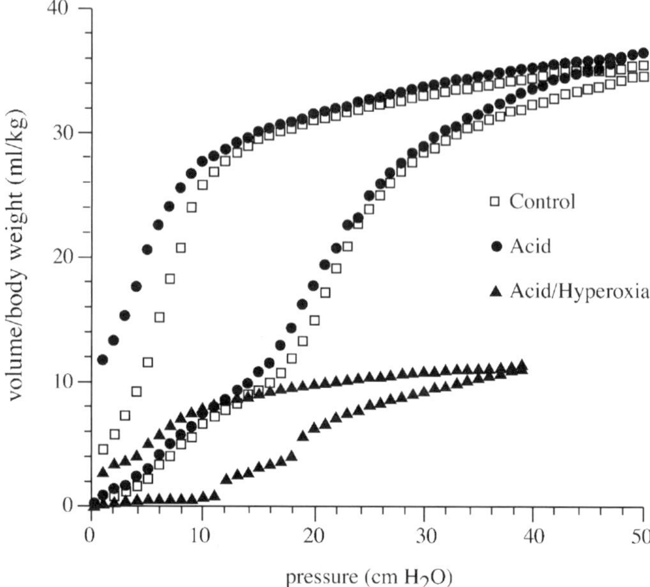

Figure 16 Representative quasistatic P–V curves at end-experiment in rabbits with acid aspiration, hyperoxia, or both. Representative P–V curves are plotted for uninjured control rabbits and for rabbits receiving intratracheal acid alone or acid/hyperoxia as in Fig. 15. Lung volumes and compliance ($dV/dP_{25-75\%}$) were significantly reduced in rabbits receiving acid plus hyperoxia. Rabbits receiving hyperoxia alone (50% oxygen for 24 hr) had P–V curves equivalent to uninjured controls (not shown). See text for details. (From Ref. 259.)

lowers the work of breathing, stabilizes alveoli against collapse and overdistension, and reduces the hydrostatic driving force for edema fluid to move from the microvasculature into the pulmonary interstitium and alveoli. Lung surfactant generates these physiological actions through surface active properties that arise from molecular biophysical interactions among its multiple components. Functional surface properties include the ability to adsorb rapidly to the air–water interface, to reduce surface tension to extremely low values < 1 mN/m during dynamic compression, to vary surface tension with surface area during dynamic cycling, and to respread rapidly and effectively at the interface during successive cycles of compression and expansion. Biophysically important components of endogenous surfactant include DPPC and related rigid disaturated phospholipids, a mix of fluid unsaturated phospholipids, and three active apoproteins SP-A, SP-B, and SP-C. SP-D, a fourth surfactant protein, does not participate in surfactant biophysical function but is important in host defense along with SP-A and possibly other surfactant components.

Significant respiratory deficits arise when lung surfactant is dysfunctional or deficient. Surfactant dysfunction (inhibition, inactivation) is an important contributor to the pathophysiology of acute inflammatory lung injury and clinical ALI/ARDS. Surfactant dysfunction can occur during lung injury by a variety of pathways. Multiple endogenous substances in edema or present in the lungs as a result of inflammation have the capacity to interact biophysically with pulmonary surfactant to reduce its surface activity. Such substances include plasma and blood proteins and lipids, cell membrane lipids, cholesterol, lysophospholipids, and fluid free fatty acids. Meconium, a complex mixture of protein and nonprotein substances in the fetus, is another powerful inhibitor of surfactant activity. Several biophysical mechanisms involved in inhibitor-induced surfactant dysfunction have been elucidated. Plasma and blood proteins, for example, adsorb to the air–water interface and reduce the entry of more active lung surfactant components into the surface. Lysophospholipids, free fatty acids, and cell membrane lipids inhibit lung surfactant activity at least in part by mixing into the surface film itself, compromising its ability to lower surface tension effectively during dynamic compression.

Additional substances present in injured, inflamed lungs act to decrease the surface tension lowering ability of lung surfactant by chemically degrading or altering its active components. Chemically acting inhibitors of this kind include phospholipases, proteases, and reactive oxygen and nitrogen species. Phospholipases A_1, A_2, C, and D degrade both saturated and unsaturated surfactant phospholipids. In addition to depleting specific active phospholipids, phospholipases generate reaction products (free fatty acids and lysophospholipids) that are capable of further inhibiting surface activity. Surfactant lipids can also be oxidized or peroxidized during lung injury by reactive nitrogen and oxygen species including peroxynitrite, nitric oxide, superoxide anion, and many others. Detriments to lung surfactant activity also result if functionally important apoproteins are degraded, nitrated, or oxidized in injured lungs by reactive oxygen/nitrogen species or by proteases like neutrophil elastase. Chemical degradation or alteration of surfactant proteins not only impairs interfacial biophysical activity, but also can compromise their metabolic and immunomodulatory activities (e.g., SP-A, SP-D).

Another form of surfactant dysfunction described in this chapter is depletion or alteration in active large surfactant aggregate subtypes. Endogenous lung surfactant and related exogenous surfactants exist in the aqueous phase as complex size-distributed aggregates containing phospholipids and proteins. In alveolar surfactant, the largest aggregates are generally the most active and contain the highest levels of surfactant apoproteins. Reductions in the content or activity of large aggregates cause decreased overall surface activity even if the total amount of alveolar surfactant material remains unchanged. Decreases in surfactant activity associated with depletion or alteration of active large aggregates have been demonstrated in several forms of acute pulmonary injury. Aggregate-related surfactant dysfunction can result from injury-induced changes in intra-alveolar processing or surfactant metabolism in type II pneumocytes, or from physicochemical interactions of inhibitory or reactive substances with surface active material in the alveoli.

Lung surfactant dysfunction has been extensively documented not only in biophysical studies in vitro, but also in multiple animal models of acute pulmonary injury. Physiological studies of surfactant dysfunction in intact lungs are consistent with in vitro biophysical studies in several important ways. Instilled inhibitors have been shown directly to induce P–V mechanical changes in excised animal lungs indicative of reduced surfactant activity. Similarly, the severity of surfactant dysfunction in bronchoalveolar lavage from animals with acute pulmonary injury in vivo in general correlates with the presence of substances known to cause surfactant dysfunction in biophysical research in vitro (e.g., plasma proteins, membrane lipids, phospholipases, etc.). Decreased surface activity in lavage is also found in association with deficits in respiratory mechanics and function consistent with decreased surfactant activity in vivo. Moreover, lung function and/or mechanics in animals with acute pulmonary injury can be improved by the delivery of active exogenous surfactants, in conceptual agreement with biophysical data showing that surfactant dysfunction can be mitigated or abolished by raising surfactant concentration. These consistent biophysical and physiological findings suggest that surfactant dysfunction in lung-injured patients should, in principle, respond to exogenous surfactant therapy assuming that active preparations able to resist inactivation are delivered effectively to the alveoli. Surfactant therapy to mitigate clinical ALI and ARDS is detailed further in Chapter 15.

Acknowledgment

The authors gratefully acknowledge the support of grants HL-56176, HL-69763, and PO1-HL-71659 from the National Institutes of Health.

References

1. von Neergaard K. Neue auffassungen uber einen grundbegriff der atemme-chanik. Dieretraktionskraft der lunge, abhangig von der oberflachenspannung in den alveolen. Z Ges Exp Med 1929; 66:373–394.
2. Pattle RE. Properties, function, and origin of the alveolar lining layer. Nature 1955; 175:1125–1126.
3. Clements JA. Surface tension of lung extracts. Proc Soc Exp Biol Med 1957; 95:170–172.

4. Pattle RE. Properties, function and origin of the alveolar lining layer. Proc R Soc (Lond) Ser B 1958; 148:217–240.
5. Gruenwald P. The mechanism of abnormal expansion of the lungs of mature and premature newborn infants. Bull Margaret Hague Maternity Hosp 1955; 8:100–106.
6. Gruenwald P. The significance of pulmonary hyaline membranes in newborn infants. J Am Med Assoc 1958; 166:621–623.
7. Avery ME, Mead J. Surface properties in relation to atelectasis and hyaline membrane disease. Am J Dis Child 1959; 97:517–523.
8. Fehrenbach H. Alveolar epithelial type II cell: defender of the alveolus revisited. Respir Res 2001; 2:33–46.
9. Notter RH. Lung Surfactants: Basic Science and Clinical Applications. New York: Marcel Dekker, 2000.
10. Dobbs LG. Isolation and culture of alveolar type II cells. Am J Physiol 1990; 258:L134–L147.
11. Mason RJ, Williams MC. Alveolar type II cells. In: Crystal R, West JB, Weibel ER, Barnes PJ, eds. The Lung: Scientific Foundations. 2d ed. Philadelphia: Lipincott-Raven, 1997:235–246.
12. Batenburg JJ. Surfactant phospholipids: synthesis and storage. Am J Physiol 1992; 262:L367–L385.
13. Haagsman HP, van Golde LMG. Synthesis and assembly of lung surfactant. Ann Rev Physiol 1991; 53:441–464.
14. Hawgood S. Pulmonary surfactant apoproteins—a review of protein and genomic structure. Am J Physiol 1989; 257:L13–L22.
15. Jobe AH, Ikegami M. Surfactant metabolism. Clin Perinatol 1993; 20:683–696.
16. Johansson J, Curstedt T, Robertson B. The proteins of the surfactant system. Eur Respir J 1994; 7:372–391.
17. Rooney SA, Young SL, Mendelson CR. Molecular and cellular processing of lung surfactant. FASEB J 1994; 8:957–967.
18. Wright JR. Clearance and recycling of pulmonary surfactant. Am J Physiol 1990; 259:L1–L12.
19. Finkelstein JN. Physiologic and toxicologic response of alveolar type II cells. Toxicology 1990; 60:41–52.
20. Witschi H. Responses of the lung to toxic injury. Environ Health Perspect 1990; 85:5–13.
21. Dormans JA, Vanbree L. Function and response of type II cells to inhaled toxicants. Inhal Tox 1995; 7:319–342.
22. Benson BJ, Williams MC, Sueishi K, Goerke J, Sargeant T. Role of calcium ions on the structure and function of pulmonary surfactant. Biochim Biophys Acta 1984; 793:18–27.
23. Gross NJ, Narine KR. Surfactant subtypes in mice: characterization and quantitation. J Appl Physiol 1989; 66:342–349.
24. Gross NJ. Extracellular metabolism of pulmonary surfactant: the role of a new serine protease. Ann Rev Physiol 1995; 57:135–150.
25. Putman E, Creuwels LAJM, Van Golde LMG, Haagsman HP. Surface properties, morphology and protein composition of pulmonary surfactant subtypes. Biochem J 1996; 320:599–605.

26. Magoon MW, Wright JR, Baritussio A, Williams MC, Goerke J, Benson BJ, Hamilton RL, Clements JA. Subfractionation of lung surfactant: implications for metabolism and surface activity. Biochim Biophys Acta 1983; 750:18–31.

27. Wright JR, Benson BJ, Williams MC, Goerke J, Clements JA. Protein composition of rabbit alveolar surfactant subfractions. Biochim Biophys Acta 1984; 791:320–332.

28. Hall SB, Hyde RW, Notter RH. Changes in subphase surfactant aggregates in rabbits injured by free fatty acid. Am J Respir Crit Care Med 1994; 149: 1099–1106.

29. Hawgood S, Benson BJ, Hamilton RJ. Effects of a surfactant-associated protein and calcium ions on the structure and surface activity of lung surfactant lipids. Biochemistry 1985; 24:184–190.

30. Putz G, Goerke J, Clements JA. Surface activity of rabbit pulmonary surfactant subfractions at different concentrations in a captive bubble. J Appl Physiol 1994; 77:597–605.

31. Veldhuizen RAW, Hearn SA, Lewis JF, Possmayer F. Surface-area cycling of different surfactant preparations: SP-A and SP-B are essential for large aggregate integrity. Biochem J 1994; 300:519–524.

32. Adamson AW, Gast AP. Physical Chemistry of Surfaces. 6th ed. New York: Wiley-Interscience, 1997.

33. Taeusch HW, Ballard RA. Avery's Diseases of the Newborn. 7th ed. Philadelphia: WB Saunders, 1998.

34. Cotran RS, Kumar V, Collins T. Robbins Pathologic Basis of Disease. 6th ed. Philadelphia: W.B. Saunders, 1999.

35. Taussig LM, Landau LI, Le Souef PN, Morgan WJ, Martinez FD, Sly PDE. Pediatric Respiratory Medicine. St. Louis: Mosby, 1999.

36. Notter RH, Wang Z. Pulmonary surfactant: physical chemistry, physiology and replacement. Rev Chem Eng 1997; 13:1–118.

37. Hawgood S. Surfactant: composition, structure, and metabolism. In: Crystal RG, West JB, Weibel ER, Barnes PJ, eds. The Lung: Scientific Foundations. 2nd ed. Philadelphia: Lippincott-Raven, 1997:557–571.

38. Creuwels LAJM, van Golde LMG, Haagsman HP. The pulmonary surfactant system: biochemical and clinical aspects. Lung 1997; 175:1–39.

39. Kahn MC, Anderson GJ, Anyan WR, Hall SB. Phosphatidylcholine molecular species of calf lung surfactant. Am J Physiol 1995; 13:L567–L573.

40. Hunt AN, Kelly FJ, Postle AD. Developmental variation in whole human lung phosphatidylcholine molecular species: a comparison with guinea pig and rat. Early Hum Devel 1991; 25:157–171.

41. Notter RH. Physical chemistry and physiological activity of pulmonary surfactant. In: Shapiro DL, Notter RH, eds. Surfactant Replacement Therapy. New York: AR Liss, 1989:19–70.

42. Keough KMW. Physical chemistry of pulmonary surfactant in the terminal air spaces. In: Robertson B, van Golde LMG, Batenburg JJ, eds. Pulmonary Surfactant: From Molecular Biology to Clinical Practice. Amsterdam: Elsevier, 1992:109–164.

43. Kuroki Y, Voelker DR. Pulmonary surfactant proteins. J Biol Chem 1994; 269:25943–25946.

44. Whitsett JA, Baatz JE. Hydrophobic surfactant proteins SP-B and SP-C: molecular biology, structure and function. In: Robertson B, van Golde LMG, Batenburg JJ, eds. Pulmonary Surfactant: From Molecular Biology to Clinical Practice. Amsterdam: Elsevier Science Publishers, 1992:55–75.

45. Notter RH. Surface chemistry of pulmonary surfactant: the role of individual components. In: Roberson B, van Golde LMG, Batenburg JJ, eds. Pulmonary Surfactant. Amsterdam: Elsevier Science Publishers, 1984:17–53.

46. Notter RH, Finkelstein JN. Pulmonary surfactant: an interdisciplinary approach. J Appl Physiol 1984; 57:1613–1624.

47. Notter RH, Tabak SA, Mavis RD. Surface properties of binary mixtures of some pulmonary surfactant components. J Lipid Res 1980; 21:10–22.

48. Tabak SA, Notter RH. A modified technique for dynamic surface pressure and relaxation measurements at the air-water interface. Rev Sci Instrum 1977; 48:1196–1201.

49. Tabak SA, Notter RH. Effect of plasma proteins on the dynamic π-A characteristics of saturated phospholipid films. J Colloid Interface Sci 1977; 59: 293–300.

50. Tabak SA, Notter RH, Ultman JS, Dinh S. Relaxation effects in the surface pressure behavior of dipalmitoyl lecithin. J Colloid Interface Sci 1977; 60:117–125.

51. Keough KMW. Physical chemical properties of some mixtures of lipids and their potential for use in exogenous surfactants. Prog Respir Res 1984; 18:257–262.

52. Hawco MW, Coolbear KP, Davis PJ, Keough KMW. Exclusion of fluid during compression of monolayers of mixtures of dipalmitoylphosphatidylcholine with some other phosphati-dylcholines. Biochim Biophys Acta 1981; 646:185–187.

53. Hawco MW, Davis PJ, Keough KMW. Lipid fluidity in lung surfactant: monolayers of saturated and unsaturated lecithins. J Appl Physiol 1981; 51: 509–515.

54. Wang Z, Hall SB, Notter RH. Dynamic surface activity of films of lung surfactant phospholipids, hydrophobic proteins, and neutral lipids. J Lipid Res 1995; 36:1283–1293.

55. Notter R, Taubold R, Finkelstein J. Comparative adsorption of natural lung surfactant, extracted phospholipids, and synthetic phospholipid mixtures. Chem Phys Lipids 1983; 33:67–80.

56. Notter RH, Smith S, Taubold RD, Finkelstein JN. Path dependence of adsorption behavior of mixtures containing dipalmitoyl phosphatidylcholine. Pediatr Res 1982; 16:515–519.

57. Wang Z, Hall SB, Notter RH. Roles of different hydrophobic constituents in the adsorption of pulmonary surfactant. J Lipid Res 1996; 37:790–798.

58. Notter RH, Penney DP, Finkelstein JN, Shapiro DL. Adsorption of natural lung surfactant and phospholipid extracts related to tubular myelin formation. Pediatr Res 1986; 20:97–101.

59. Oosterlaken-Dijksterhuis MA, van Eijk M, van Golde LMG, Haagsman HP. Lipid mixing is mediated by the hydrophobic surfactant protein SP-B but not by SP-C. Biochim Biophys Acta 1992; 1110:45–50.

60. Oosterlaken-Dijksterhuis MA, Haagsman HP, van Golde LM, Demel RA. Characterization of lipid insertion into monomolecular layers mediated by lung surfactant proteins SP-B and SP-C. Biochemistry 1991; 30:10965–10971.
61. Oosterlaken-Dijksterhuis MA, Haagsman HP, van Golde LM, Demel RA. Interaction of lipid vesicles with monomolecular layers containing lung surfactant proteins SP-B or SP-C. Biochemistry 1991; 30:8276–8281.
62. Curstedt T, Jornvall H, Robertson B, Bergman T, Berggren P. Two hydrophobic low-molecular-mass protein fractions of pulmonary surfactant: characterization and biophysical activity. Eur J Biochem 1987; 168:255–262.
63. Wang Z, Gurel O, Baatz JE, Notter RH. Differential activity and lack of synergy of lung surfactant proteins SP-B and SP-C in surface-active interactions with phospholipids. J Lipid Res 1996; 37:1749–1760.
64. Yu SH, Possmayer F. Comparative studies on the biophysical activities of the low-molecular-weight hydrophobic proteins purified from bovine pulmonary surfactant. Biochim Biophys Acta 1988; 961:337–350.
65. Seeger W, Günther A, Thede C. Differential sensitivity to fibrinogen inhibition of SP-C- vs. SP-B-based surfactants. Am J Physiol 1992; 261:L286–L291.
66. Sarin VK, Gupta S, Leung TK, Taylor VE, Ohning BL, Whitsett JA, Fox JL. Biophysical and biological activity of a synthetic 8.7 kDa hydrophobic pulmonary surfactant protein SP-B. Proc Natl Acad Sci USA 1990; 87: 2633–2637.
67. Johansson J, Gustafsson M, Zaltash S, Robertson B, Curstedt T. Synthetic surfactant protein analogs. Biol Neonate 1998; 74(suppl):9–14.
68. Revak SD, Merritt TA, Degryse E, Stefani L, Courtney M, Hallman M, Cochrane CG. The use of human low molecular weight (LMW) apoproteins in the reconstitution of surfactant biological activity. J Clin Invest 1988; 81: 826–833.
69. Notter RH, Wang Z, Egan EA, Holm BA. Component-specific surface and physiological activity in bovine-derived lung surfactants. Chem Phys Lipids 2002; 114:21–34.
70. Petty T, Reiss O, Paul G, Silvers G, Elkins N. Characteristics of pulmonary surfactant in adult respiratory distress syndrome associated with trauma and shock. Am Rev Respir Dis 1977; 115:531–536.
71. Hallman M, Spragg R, Harrell JH, Moser KM, Gluck L. Evidence of lung surfactant abnormality in respiratory failure. J Clin Invest 1982; 70:673–683.
72. Seeger W, Pison U, Buchhorn R, Obestacke U, Joka T. Surfactant abnormalities and adult respiratory failure. Lung 1990; 168(suppl):891–902.
73. Pison U, Seeger W, Buchhorn R, Joka T, Brand M, Obertacke U, Neuhof H, Schmit-Neuerberg K. Surfactant abnormalities in patients with respiratory failure after multiple trauma. Am Rev Respir Dis 1989; 140:1033–1039.
74. Gregory TJ, Longmore WJ, Moxley MA, Whitsett JA, Reed CR, Fowler AA, Hudson LD, Maunder RJ, Crim C, Hyers TM. Surfactant chemical composition and biophysical activity in acute respiratory distress syndrome. J Clin Invest 1991; 88:1976–1981.
75. Günther A, Siebert C, Schmidt R, Ziegle S, Grimminger F, Yabut M, Temmesfeld B, Walmrath D, Morr H, Seeger W. Surfactant alterations in

severe pneumonia, acute respiratory distress syndrome, and cardiogenic lung edema. Am J Respir Crit Care Med 1996; 153:176–184.

76. Veldhuizen R, McCaig L, Akino T, Lewis J. Pulmonary surfactant subfractions in patients with the acute respiratory distress syndrome. Am J Respir Crit Care Med 1995; 152:1867–1871.

77. Griese M. Pulmonary surfactant in health and human lung diseases: state of the art. Eur Respir J 1999; 13:1455–1476.

78. Mander A, Langton-Hewer S, Bernhard W, Warner JO, Postle AD. Altered phospholipid composition and aggregate structure of lung surfactant is associated with impaired lung function in young children with respiratory infections. Am J Respir Cell Mol Biol 2002; 27:714–721.

79. Schmidt R, Meier U, Markart P, Grimminger F, Velcovsky HG, Morr H, Seeger W, Gunther A. Altered fatty acid composition of lung surfactant phospholipids in interstitial lung disease. Am J Physiol 2002; 283:L1079–L1085.

80. Skelton R, Holland P, Darowski M, Chetcuti P, Morgan L, Harwood J. Abnormal surfactant composition and activity in severe bronchiolitis. Acta Paediatr 1999; 88:942–946.

81. LeVine AM, Lotze A, Stanley S, Stroud C, O'Donnell R, Whitsett J, Pollack MM. Surfactant content in children with inflammatory lung disease. Crit Care Med 1996; 24:1062–1067.

82. Dargaville PA, South M, McDougall PN. Surfactant abnormalities in infants with severe viral bronchiolitis. Arch Dis Child 1996; 75:133–136.

83. Whitsett JA, Weaver TJ. Mechanisms of disease: hydrophobic surfactant proteins in lung function and disease. N Engl J Med 2002; 347:2141–2148.

84. Hack M, Horbar JD, Malloy MH, Tyson JE, Wright E, Wright L. Very low birth weight outcomes of the National Insititute of Child Health and Human Development neonatal network. Pediatrics 1991; 87:587 597.

85. National Center for Health Statistics, MacDorman MF, Rosenberg HM. Trends in infant mortality by cause of death and other characteristics, 1960–1988. Vital and health statistics. DHHS Publication PHS 1993; 93–1857:1–51.

86. Hulsey TC, Alexander GR, Robillard PY, Annibale DJ, Kennan A. Hyaline membrane disease: the role of ethnicity and maternal risk characteristics. Am J Obstet Gynecol 1993; 168:572–576.

87. Ashbaugh DG, Bigelow DB, Petty TL, Levine BE. Acute respiratory distress in adults. Lancet 1967; 2:319–323.

88. Petty TL, Ashbaugh DG. The adult respiratory distress syndrome. Clinical features, factors influencing prognosis and principles of management. Chest 1971; 60:233–239.

89. Hopewell PC, Murray J. The adult respiratory distress syndrome. In: Shibel EM, Moser KM, eds. Respiratory Emergencies. St Louis: CV Mosby, 1977: 101–128.

90. Bernard GR, Artigas A, Brigham KL, Carlet J, Falke K, Hudson L, Lamy M, Legall JR, Morris A, Spragg R. The American-European Consensus Conference on ARDS: definitions, mechanisms, relevant outcomes, and clinical trial coordination. Am J Respir Crit Care Med 1994; 149:818–824.

91. Hudson LD, Milberg JA, Anardi D, Maunder RJ. Clinical risks for development of the acute respiratory distress syndrome. Am J Respir Crit Care Med 1995; 151:293–301.

92. Hyers TM. Prediction of survival and mortality in patients with the adult respiratory distress syndrome. New Horizons 1993; 1:466–470.

93. Doyle RL, Szaflarski N, Modin GW, Wiener-Kronish JP, Matthay MA. Identification of patients with acute lung injury: predictors of mortality. Am J Respir Crit Care Med 1995; 152:1818–1824.

94. Milberg JA, Davis DR, Steinberg KP, Hudson LD. Improved survival of patients with acute respiratory distress syndrome. JAMA 1995; 273:306–309.

95. Krafft P, Fridrich P, Pernerstorfer T, Fitzgerald RD, Koc D, Schneider B, Hammerle AF, Steltzer H. The acute respiratory distress syndrome: definitions, severity, and clinical outcome. An analysis of 101 clinical investigations. Intensive Care Med 1996; 22:519–529.

96. Goss CH, Brower RG, Hudson LD, Rubenfeld GD. ARDS Network. Incidence of acute lung injury in the United States. Crit Care Med 2003; 31: 1607–1611.

97. Enhorning G. Pulsating bubble technique for evaluation of pulmonary surfactant. J Appl Physiol 1977; 43:198–203.

98. Hall SB, Bermel MS, Ko YT, Palmer HJ, Enhorning GA, Notter RH. Approximations in the measurement of surface tension with the oscillating bubble surfactometer. J Appl Physiol 1993; 75:468–477.

99. Schurch S, Bachofen H, Goerke J, Possmayer F. A captive bubble method reproduces the in situ behavior of lung surfactant monolayers. J Appl Physiol 1989; 67:2389–2396.

100. Putz G, Goerke J, Taeusch HW, Clements JA. Comparison of captive and pulsating bubble surfactometers with use of lung surfactants. J Appl Physiol 1994; 76:1425–1431.

101. Putz G, Goerke J, Schurch S, Clements JA. Evaluation of pressure-driven captive bubble surfactometer. J Appl Physiol 1994; 76:1417–1424.

102. Holm BA, Notter RH, Finkelstein JH. Surface property changes from interactions of albumin with natural lung surfactant and extracted lung lipids. Chem Phys Lipids 1985; 38:287–298.

103. Holm BA, Wang Z, Notter RH. Multiple mechanisms of lung surfactant inhibition. Pediatr Res 1999; 46:85–93.

104. Holm BA, Enhorning G, Notter RH. A biophysical mechanism by which plasma proteins inhibit lung surfactant activity. Chem Phys Lipids 1988; 49:49–55.

105. Venkitaraman A, Hall S, Whitsett J, Notter R. Enhancement of biophysical activity of lung surfactant extracts and phospholipid-apoprotein admixtures by surfactant protein A. Chem Phys Lipids 1990; 56:185–194.

106. Ikegami M, Jobe A, Jacobs H, Lam R. A protein from airways of premature lambs that inhibits surfactant function. J Appl Physiol 1984; 57:1134–1142.

107. Seeger W, Stohr G, Wolf HRD, Neuhof H. Alteration of surfactant function due to protein leakage: special interaction with fibrin monomer. J Appl Physiol 1985; 58:326–338.

108. Fuchimukai T, Fujiwara T, Takahashi A, Enhorning G. Artificial pulmonary surfactant inhibited by proteins. J Appl Physiol 1987; 62:429–437.

109. Holm BA, Venkitaraman AR, Enhorning G, Notter RH. Biophysical inhibition of synthetic lung surfactants. Chem Phys Lipids 1990; 52:243–250.

110. Venkitaraman AR, Baatz JE, Whitsett JA, Hall SB, Notter RH. Biophysical inhibition of synthetic phospholipid-surfactant protein admixtures by plasma proteins. Chem Phys Lipids 1991; 57:49–57.

111. Wang Z, Notter RH. Additivity of protein and non-protein inhibitors of lung surfactant activity. Am J Respir Crit Care Med 1998; 158:28–35.

112. Keough KWM, Parsons CS, Tweeddale MG. Interactions between plasma proteins and pulmonary surfactant: pulsating bubble studies. Can J Physiol Pharmacol 1989; 67:663–668.

113. Kobayashi Y, Nitta K, Ganzuka M, Inui S, Grossman G, Robertson B. Inactivation of exogenous surfactant by pulmonary edema fluid. Pediatr Res 1991; 29:353–356.

114. Nitta K, Kobayashi T. Impairment of surfactant activity and ventilation by proteins in lung edema fluid. Respir Physiol 1994; 95:43–51.

115. Holm BA, Notter RH. Effects of hemoglobin and cell membrane lipids on pulmonary surfactant activity. J Appl Physiol 1987; 63:1434–1442.

116. Cockshutt A, Possmayer F. Lysophosphatidylcholine sensitizes lipid extracts of pulmonary surfactant to inhibition by plasma proteins. Biochim Biophys Acta 1991; 1086:63–71.

117. Cockshutt AM, Weitz J, Possmayer F. Pulmonary surfactant-associated protein A enhances the surface activity of lipid extract surfactant and reverses inhibition by blood proteins in vitro. Biochemistry 1990; 19:8424–8429.

118. Tierney DF, Johnson RP. Altered surface tension of lung extracts and lung mechanics. J Appl Physiol 1965; 20:1253–1260.

119. Rauvala H, Hallman M. Glycolipid accumulation in bronchoalveolar space in adult respiratory distress syndrome. J Lipid Res 1984; 25:1257–1262.

120. Ryan AJ, McCoy DM, McGowan SE, Salome RG, Mallampalli RK. Alveolar sphingolipids generated in response to TNF-α modifies surfactant biophysical activity. J Appl Physiol 2003; 94:253–258.

121. Niewoehner D, Rice K, Sinha A, Wangensteen D. Injurious effects of lysophosphatidylcholine on barrier properties of alveolar epithelium. J Appl Physiol 1987; 63:1979–1986.

122. Seeger W, Lepper H, Hellmut RD, Neuhof H. Alteration of alveolar surfactant function after exposure to oxidant stress and to oxygenated and native arachadonic acid in vitro. Biochim Biophys Acta 1985; 835:58–67.

123. Hall SB, Lu ZR, Venkitaraman AR, Hyde RW, Notter RH. Inhibition of pulmonary surfactant by oleic acid: mechanisms and characteristics. J Appl Physiol 1992; 72:1708–1716.

124. Hall SB, Notter RH, Smith RJ, Hyde RW. Altered function of pulmonary surfactant in fatty acid lung injury. J Appl Physiol 1990; 69:1143–1149.

125. Zelter M, Escudier BJ, Hoeffel JM, Murray JF. Effects of aerosolized artificial surfactant on repeated oleic acid injury in sheep. Am Rev Respir Dis 1990; 141:1014–1019.

126. Uchida T, Nakazawa K, Yokoyama K, Makita K, Amaha K. The combination of partial liquid ventilation and inhaled nitric oxide in the severe oleic acid lung injury model. Chest 1998; 113:1658–1666.

127. Shuster D. ARDS: clinical lessons from the oleic acid model of acute lung injury. Am J Respir Crit Care Med 1994; 149:245–260.

128. Malik AB. Pulmonary edema after pancreatitis: role of humoral factors. Circ Shock 1983; 10:71–80.

129. Shah NS, Nakayama DK, Jacob TD, Nishio I, Imai T, Billiar TR, Exler R, Yousem SA, Motoyama EK, Peitzman AB. Efficacy of inhaled nitric oxide in oleic acid-induced acute lung injury. Crit Care Med 1997; 25:153–158.

130. Zhu GF, Sun B, Niu S, Cai YY, Lin K, Lindwall R, Robertson B. Combined surfactant therapy and inhaled nitric oxide in rabbits with oleic acid-induced acute respiratory distress syndrome. Am J Respir Crit Care Med 1998; 158:437–443.

131. Moses D, Holm BA, Spitale P, Liu M, Enhorning G. Inhibition of pulmonary surfactant function by meconium. Am J Obstet Gynecol 1991; 164:477–481.

132. Teraska D, Clark D, Singh B, Rokahr J. Free fatty acids in meconium. Biol Neonate 1986; 50:16–20.

133. Clark DA, Nieman GF, Thompson JE, Paskanik AM, Rokhar JE, Bredenberg CE. Surfactant displacement by meconium free fatty acids: an alternative explanation for atelectasis in meconium aspiration syndrome. J Pediatr 1987; 110:765–770.

134. Pison U, Tam EK, Caughey GH, Hawgood S. Proteolytic inactivation of dog lung surfactant-associated proteins by neutrophil elastase. Biochim Biophys Acta 1989; 992:251–257.

135. Holm BA, Keicher L, Liu M, Sokolowski J, Enhorning G. Inhibition of pulmonary surfactant function by phospholipases. J Appl Physiol 1991; 71:1–5.

136. Enhorning G, Shumel B, Keicher L, Sokolowski J, Holm BA. Phospholipases introduced into the hypophase affect the surfactant film outlining a bubble. J Appl Physiol 1992; 73:941–945.

137. Vadas P, Pruzanski W. Biology of disease: role of secretory phospholipases A_2 in the pathobiology of disease. Lab Invest 1986; 55:391–404.

138. Robbins CG, Davis JM, Merritt TA, Amirkhanian JD, Sahgal N, Morin FC, Horowitz S. Combined effects of nitric oxide and hyperoxia on surfactant function and pulmonary inflammation. Am J Physiol 1995; 269:L545–L550.

139. Amirkhanian JD, Merritt TA. Inhibitory effects of oxyradicals on surfactant function: utilizing in vitro Fenton reaction. Lung 1998; 176:63–72.

140. Haddad IY, Ischiropoulos H, Holm BA, Beckman JS, Baker JR, Matalon S. Mechanisms of peroxynitrite-induced injury to pulmonary surfactants. Am J Physiol 1993; 265:L555–L564.

141. Gilliard N, Heldt GP, Loredo J, Gasser H, Redl H, Merritt TA, Spragg RG. Exposure of the hydrophobic components of porcine lung surfactant to oxidant stress alters surface tension properties. J Clin Invest 1994; 93: 2608–2615.

142. Haddad IY, Crow JP, Hu P, Ye Y, Beckman J, Matalon S. Concurrent generation of nitric oxide and superoxide damages surfactant protein A. Am J Physiol 1994; 267:L242–L249.

143. Strayer D, Herting E, Sun B, Robertson B. Antibody to surfactant protein A increases sensitivity of pulmonary surfactant to inactivation by fibrinogen. Am J Respir Crit Care Med 1996; 153:1116–1122.

144. Kobayashi T, Nitta K, Takahashi K, Kurashima B, Robertson B, Suzuki Y. Activity of pulmonary surfactant after blocking the associated protein SP-A and SP-B. J Appl Physiol 1991; 71:530–536.

145. Robertson B, Kobayashi T, Ganzuka M, Grossmann G, Li WZ, Suzuki Y. Experimental neonatal respiratory failure induced by a monoclonal antibody to the hydrophobic surfactant-associated protein SP-B. Pediatr Res 1991; 30: 239–243.

146. Lewis JF, Ikegami M, Jobe AH. Altered surfactant function and metabolism in rabbits with acute lung injury. J Appl Physiol 1990; 69:2303–2310.

147. Gross NJ. Inhibition of surfactant subtype convertase in radiation model of adult respiratory distress syndrome. Am J Physiol 1991; 4:L311–L317.

148. Gross NJ. Surfactant subtypes in experimental lung damage: radiation pneumonitis. Am J Physiol 1991; 4:L302–L310.

149. Belai Y, Hernandez-Juviel JM, Bruni R, Waring AJ, Walther FJ. Addition of α1-antitrypsin to surfactant improves oxygenation in surfactant-deficient rats. Am J Respir Crit Care Med 1999; 159:917–923.

150. Putman E, Boere AJ, van Bree L, van Golde LMG, Haagsman HP. Pulmonary surfactant subtype metabolism is altered after short-term ozone exposure. Toxicol Appl Pharmacol 1995; 134:132–138.

151. Assreuy JF, Cunha Q, Epperlein M, Noronha-Dutra A, O'Donnell CA, Liew FY, Moncada S. Production of nitric oxide and superoxide by activated macrophages and killing of Leishmania major. Eur J Immunol 1994; 24: 672–676.

152. Pendino KJ, Laskin JD, Shuler RL, Punjabi CJ, Laskin DL. Enhanced production of nitric oxide by rat alveolar macrophages after inhalation of a pulmonary irritant is associated with increased expression of nitric oxide synthase. J Immunol 1993; 151:7196–7205.

153. Fang FC. Perspectives series: host/pathogen interactions. Mechanisms of nitric oxide-related antimicrobial activity. J Clin Invest 1997; 99:2818–2825.

154. Babior BM. Activation of the respiratory burst oxidase. Environ Health Perspect 1994; 102(suppl 10):53–56.

155. Hickman-Davis JM, O'Reilly P, Davis IC, Peti-Peterdi J, Davis G, Young KR, Devlin RB, Matalon S. Killing of *Klebsiella pneumoniae* by human alveolar macrophages. Am J Physiol 2002; 282:L944–L956.

156. Beckman JS, Beckman TW, Chen J, Marshall PA, Freeman BA. Apparent hydroxyl radical production by peroxynitrite: implications for endothelial injury from nitric oxide and superoxide. Proc Natl Acad Sci USA 1990; 87: 1620–1624.

157. Beckman JS, Koppenol WH. Nitric oxide, superoxide, and peroxynitrite: the good, the bad, and the ugly. Am J Physiol 1996; 271:C1424–C1437.

158. Stamler JS. Redox signaling: nitrosylation and related target interactions of nitric oxide. Cell 1994; 78:931–936.

159. Molina YV, McDonald LB, Reep B, Brune B, Di Silvio M, Billiar TR, Lapetina EG. Nitric oxide-induced *S*-nitrosylation of glyceraldehyde-3-phos-

phate dehydrogenase inhibits enzymatic activity and increases endogenous ADP-ribosylation [published erratum appears in J Biol Chem 1993; 268:3016]. J Biol Chem 1992; 267:24929–24932.

160. Curran RD, Ferrari FK, Kispert PH, Stadler J, Stuehr DJ, Simmons RL, Billiar TR. Nitric oxide and nitric oxide-generating compounds inhibit hepatocyte protein synthesis. FASEB J 1991; 5:2085–2092.

161. Delaney CA, Green MH, Lowe JE, Green IC. Endogenous nitric oxide induced by interleukin-1β in rat islets of Langerhans and HIT-T15 cells causes significant DNA damage as measured by the 'comet' assay. FEBS Lett 1993; 333:291–295.

162. Radi R, Beckman JS, Bush KM, Freeman BA. Peroxynitrite oxidation of sulfhydryls. The cytotoxic potential of superoxide and nitric oxide. J Biol Chem 1991; 266:4244–4250.

163. Radi R, Beckman JS, Bush KM, Freeman BA. Peroxynitrite-induced membrane lipid peroxidation: the cytotoxic potential of superoxide and nitric oxide. Arch Biochem Biophys 1991; 288:481–487.

164. Graham A, Hogg N, Kalyanaraman B, O'Leary V, Darley-Usmar V, Moncada S. Peroxynitrite modification of low-density lipoprotein leads to recognition by the macrophage scavenger receptor. FEBS Lett 1993; 330:181–185.

165. Haddad IY, Pitt BR, Matalon S. Nitric oxide and lung injury. In: Fishman AP, ed. Pulmonary Diseases and Disorders. 3 New York: McGraw-Hill, 1996: 337–346.

166. Greis KD, Zhu S, Matalon S. Identification of nitration sites on surfactant protein A by tandem electrospray mass spectrometry. Arch Biochem Biophys 1996; 335:396–402.

167. Pryor WA, Jin X, Squadrito GL. One- and two-electron oxidation of methionine by peroxynitrite. Proc Natl Acad Sci USA 1994; 91:11173–11177.

168. Inoue S, Kawanishi S. Oxidative DNA damage induced by simultaneous generation of nitric oxide and superoxide. FEBS Lett 1995; 371:86–88.

169. Radi R, Rodriguez M, Castro L, Telleri R. Inhibition of mitochondrial electron transport by peroxynitrite. Arch Biochem Biophys 1994; 308:89–95.

170. Hu P, Ischiropoulos H, Beckman JS, Matalon S. Peroxynitrite inhibition of oxygen consumption and sodium transport in alveolar type II cells. Am J Physiol 1994; 266:L628–L634.

171. Devall MD, Zhu S, Fuller CM, Matalon S. Peroxynitrite inhibits amiloride-sensitive Na^+ currents in *Xenopus* oocytes expressing α,β,γ-rENaC. Am J Physiol 1998; 274:C1417–C1423.

172. Guo Y, Devall MD, Crow JP, Matalon S. Nitric oxide inhibits Na^+ absorption across cultured alveolar type II monolayers. Am J Physiol 1998; 274: L369–L377.

173. Haddad IY, Zhu S, Ischiropoulos H, Matalon S. Nitration of surfactant protein A results in decreased ability to aggregate lipids. Am J Physiol 1996; 270:L281–L288.

174. van der Vliet A, Hu ML, O'Neill CA, Cross CE, Halliwell B. Interactions of human blood plasma with hydrogen peroxide and hypochlorous acid. J Lab Clin Med 1994; 124:701–707.

175. Denicola A, Freeman BA, Trujillo M, Radi R. Peroxynitrite reaction with carbon dioxide/bicarbonate: kinetics and influence on peroxynitrite-mediated oxidation. Arch Biochem Biophys 1996; 333:49–58.
176. Zhu S, Basiouny KF, Crow JP, Matalon S. Carbon dioxide enhances nitration of surfactant protein A by activated alveolar macrophages. Am J Physiol 2000; 278:L1025–L1031.
177. Sittipunt, C, Steinberg KP, Ruzinski JT, Myles C, Zhu S, Goodman RB, Hudson LD, Matalon S, Martin TR. Nitric oxide and nitrotyrosine in the lungs of patients with acute respiratory distress syndrome. Am J Respir Crit Care Med 2001; 163:503–510.
178. Zhu S, Ware LB, Geiser T, Matthay MA, Matalon S. Increased levels of nitrate and surfactant protein A nitration in the pulmonary edema fluid of patients with acute lung injury. Am J Respir Crit Care Med 2001; 163: 166–172.
179. Haddad IY, Pataki G, Hu P, Galliani C, Beckman JS, Matalon S. Quantitation of nitrotyrosine levels in lung sections of patients and animals with acute lung injury. J Clin Invest 1994; 94(6):2407–2413.
180. Hickman-Davis JM, Fang FC, Nathan C, Shepherd VL, Voelker DR, Wright JR. Lung surfactant and reactive oxygen-nitrogen species: antimicrobial activity and host–pathogen interactions. Am J Physiol 2001; 281:L517–L523.
181. Ross GF, Notter RH, Meuth J, Whitsett JA. Phospholipid binding and biophysical activity of pulmonary surfactant-associated protein SAP-35 and its non-collagenous C-terminal domains. J Biol Chem 1985; 261:14283–14291.
182. Yu SH, Possmayer F. Adsorption, compression, and stability of surface films of natural, lipid extract, and reconstituted pulmonary surfactants. Biochim Biophys Acta 1993; 1167:264–271.
183. Schurch S, Possmayer F, Cheng S, Cockshutt AM. Pulmonary SP-A enhances adsorption and appears to induce surface sorting of lipid extract surfactant. Am J Physiol 1992; 263:L210–L218.
184. Taneva S, McEachren T, Stewart J, Keough KM. Pulmonary surfactant protein SP-A with phospholipids in spread monolayers at the air–water interface. Biochemistry 1995; 34:10279–10289.
185. Hawgood S, Benson BJ, Schilling J, Damm D, Clements JA, White RT. Nucleotide and amino acid sequences of pulmonary surfactant protein SP 18 and evidence for cooperation between SP 18 and SP 28–36 in surfactant lipid adsorption. Proc Natl Acad Sci USA 1987; 84:66–70.
186. Yukitake K, Brown CL, Schlueter MA, Clements JA, Hawgood S. Surfactant apoprotein A modifies the inhibitory effect of plasma proteins on surfactant activity in vivo. Pediatr Res 1995; 37:21–25.
187. Haagsman HP, Hawgood S, Sargeant T, Buckley D, White RT, Drickamer K, Benson BJ. The major lung surfactant protein, SP 28–36, is a calcium-dependent, carbohydrate-binding protein. J Biol Chem 1987; 262:13877–13800.
188. Wright JR. Immunomodulatory functions of surfactant. Physiol Rev 1997; 77:931–962.
189. Mason RJ, Greene K, Voelker DR. Surfactant protein A and surfactant protein D in health and disease. Am J Physiol 1998; 275:L1–L13.

190. Korfhagen TR, Bruno MD, Ross GF, Huelsman KM, Ikegami M, Jobe AH, Wert SB, Stripp BR, Morris RE, Glasser SW, Bachurski CJ, Iwamoto HS, Whitsett JA. Altered surfactant function and structure in SP-A gene targeted mice. Proc Natl Acad Sci USA 1996; 93:9594–9599.

191. Hickman-Davis JM, Lindsey JR, Zhu S, Matalon S. Surfactant protein A mediates mycoplasmacidal activity of alveolar macrophages. Am J Physiol 1998; 274:L270–L277.

192. Ikegami M, Korfhagen TR, Bruno MD, Whitsett JA, Jobe AH. Surfactant metabolism in surfactant protein A-deficient mice. Am J Physiol 1997; 272:L479–L485.

193. Beckman JS, Ye YZ, Anderson PG, Chen J, Accavitti MA, Tarpey MM, White CR. Extensive nitration of protein tyrosines in human artherosclerosis detected by immunohistochemistry. Biol Chem Hoppe Seyler 1994; 375:81–88.

194. Gole MD, Souza JM, Choi I, Hertkorn C, Malcolm S, Foust RF, Finkel B, Lanken PN, Ischiropoulos H. Plasma proteins modified by tyrosine nitration in acute respiratory distress syndrome. Am J Physiol 2000; 278:L961–L967.

195. de Andrade JA, Crow JP, Viera L, Bruce AC, Randall YK, McGiffin DC, Zorn GL, Zhu S, Matalon S, Jackson RM. Protein nitration, matobolites of reactive nitrogen species, and inflammation in lung allografts. Am J Respir Crit Care Med 2000; 161:2035–2042.

196. Tanaka S, Choe N, Hemenway DR, Zhu S, Matalon S, Kagan E. Asbestos inhalation induces reactive nitrogen species and nitrotyrosine formation in the lungs and pleura of the rat. J Clin Invest 1998; 102:445–454.

197. Kahn J, Brennand DM, Bradley N, Gao B, Bruckdorfer R, Jacobs M, Brennan DM. 3-Nitrotyrosine in the proteins of human plasma determined by an ELISA method. Biochem J 1998; 330:795–801.

198. Moreno JJ, Pryor WA. Inactivation of alpha 1 protease inhibitor by peroxynitrite. Chem Res Toxicol 1992; 5:425–431.

199. Zhu S, Kachel DL, Martin WJ, Matalon S. Nitrated SP-A does not enhance adherence of *Pneumocystis carinii* to alveolar macrophages. Am J Physiol 1998; 275:L1031–L1039.

200. Haddad IY, Beckman JS, Garver RI, Matalon S. Structural and functional alterations of surfactant protein A by peroxynitrite. Chest 1994; 105:84S.

201. Zhu S, Haddad IY, Matalon S. Modification of SP-A mannose-binding properties by reactive oxygen and nitrogen species. Arch Biochem Biophys 1996; 333:282–290.

202. van der Vliet A, Eiserich JB, Halliwell B, Cross CE. Formation of reactive nitrogen species during peroxidase-catalyzed oxidation of nitrate. A potential additional mechanism of nitric oxide-dependent toxicity. J Biol Chem 1997; 272:7617–7625.

203. Floros J, Steinbrink R, Jacobs K, Phelps D, Kriz R, Rency M, Sultzman L, Jones S, Taeusch HW, Frank HA, Fritsch EF. Isolation and characterization of cDNA clones for the 35 kDa pulmonary surfactant associated protein. J Biol Chem 1986; 261:9029–9033.

204. McCormack F, Calvert XHM, Watson PA, Smith DL, Mason RJ, Voelker DR. The structure and function of surfactant protein A. Hydroxyproline-

and carbohydrate-deficient mutant proteins. J Biol Chem 1994; 269: 5833–5841.

205. Matalon S, DeMarco V, Haddad IY, Myles C, Skimming JW, Schurch S, Cheng S, Cassin S. Inhaled nitric oxide injures the pulmonary surfactant system of lambs in vivo. Am J Physiol 1996; 270:L273–L280.

206. Hallman M. Molecular interactions between nitric oxide and lung surfactant. Biol Neonate 1997; 71(suppl 1):44–48.

207. Hallman M, Bry K. Nitric oxide and lung surfactant. Semin Perinatol 1996; 20:173–185.

208. Hallman M, Bry K, Lappalainen U. A mechanism of nitric oxide-induced surfactant dysfunction. J Appl Physiol 1996; 80:2035–2043.

209. Hallman M, Waffarn F, Bry K, Turbow R, Kleinman MT, Mautz WJ, Rasmussen RE, Bhalla DK, Phalen RF. Surfactant dysfunction after inhalation of nitric oxide. J Appl Physiol 1996; 80:2026–2034.

210. Atochina E, Beers NMF, Scanlon ST, Preston AM, Beck JM. *P. carinii* induces selective alterations in component expression biophysical activity of lung surfactant. Am J Physiol 2000; 278:L599–L609.

211. Russo T, Bartholomew ALA, Davidson BA, Helinski JD, Carlino UB, Knight PR, Beers M, Atochina EN, Notter RH, Holm BA. Total extracellular surfactant is increased but abnormal in a rat model of Gram-negative bacterial pneumonitis. Am J Physiol 2002; 283:L655–L663.

212. Lachmann B, van Daal GJ. Adult respiratory distress syndrome: animal models. In: Robertson B, van Golde LMG, Batenburg JJ, eds. Pulmonary Surfactant: From Molecular Biology to Clinical Practice. Amsterdam: Elsevier Science Publishers, 1992:635–663.

213. Notter R, Apostolakos HM, Holm BA, Willson D, Wang B, Finkelstein JN, Hyde RW. Surfactant therapy and its potential use with other agents in term infants, children and adults with acute lung injury. Perspect Neonatol 2000; 1(4):4–20.

214. Windsor ACJ. Acute lung injury: what have we learned from animal models? Am J Med Sci 1993; 306:111–116

215. Lewis J, Brackenbury FA. Role of exogenous surfactant in acute lung injury. Crit Care Med 2003; 31(suppl):S324–S328.

216. Mandell G, Bennett LJE, Dolin R. Mandell, Douglas, and Bennett's Principles and Practice of Infectious Diseases. 5th ed. New York: Churchill Livingstone, 2000.

217. Merigan TC, Bartlett JG, Bolognesi D, eds. Textbook of AIDS Medicine. 2nd ed. Baltimore: Williams and Wilkins, 1999.

218. Dei-Cas, E. Pneumocystis infections: the tip of the iceberg? Med Mycol 2000; 38(suppl 1):23–32

219. Su TH, Martin WJ. Pathogenesis and host response in *Pneumocystis carinii* pneumonia. Ann Rev Med 1994; 45:261–272.

220. Su TH, Natarajan V, Kachel DL, Moxley MA, Longmore WJ, Martin WJ. Functional impairment of bronchoalveolar lavage phospholipids in early *P. carinii* pneumonia in rats. J Lab Clin Med 1996; 127:263–271.

221. Wright TW, Notter RH, Wang Z, Harmsen AG, Gigliotti F. Pulmonary inflammation disrupts surfactant function during *P. carinii* pneumonia. Infect Immun 2001; 69:758–764.

222. Eijking EP, van Daal EJ, Tenbrinck R, Luyenduijk A, Sluiters JF, Hannappel E, Lachmann B. Effect of surfactant replacement on *Pneumocystis carinii* pneumonia in rats. Intensive Care Med 1990; 17:475–478.

223. Creery W, Hashmi DA, Hutchison JS, Singh RN. Surfactant therapy improves pulmonary function in infants with *Pneumocystis carinii* pneumonitis and acquired immunodeficiency syndrome. Pediatr Pulm 1997; 24:370–373.

224. Wright TW, Johnston CJ, Harmsen AG, Finkelstein JN. Analysis of cytokine gene expression in the lungs of *Pneumocystis carinii*-infected mice. Am J Respir Cell Mol Biol 1997; 17:491–500.

225. Wright TW, Gigliotti F, Finkelstein JN, McBride JT, An CL, Harmsen AG. Immune-mediated inflammation directly impairs pulmonary function, contributing to the pathogenesis of *Pneumocystis carinii* pneumonia. J Clin Invest 1999; 104:1307–1317.

226. Wright TW, Johnston CJ, Harmsen AG, Finkelstein JN. Chemokine gene expression during *Pneumocystis carinii*-driven pulmonary inflammation. Infect Immun 1999; 67:34452–3460.

227. Sheehan PM, Stokes DC, Yeh Y, Hughes WT. Surfactant phospholipids and lavage phospholipase A_2 in experimental *Pneumocystis carinii* pneumonia. Am Rev Respir Dis 1986; 134:526–531.

228. Hoffman AG, Lawrence MG, Ognibene FP, Suffredini AF, Lipschik AY, Kovacs JA, Masur H, Shelhamer JH. Reduction of pulmonary surfactant in patients with human immunodeficiency virus infection and *P. carinii* pneumonia. Chest 1992; 102:1730–1736.

229. Escamilla R, Prevost MC, Hermant C, Caratero A, Cariven C, Krempf M. Surfactant analysis during *P. carinii* pneumonia in HIV-infected patients. Chest 1992; 101:1558–1562.

230. Rose RM, Catalano PJ, Koziel H, Furlong ST. Abnormal lipid composition of bronchoalveolar fluid obtained from individuals with AIDS-related lung disease. Am J Respir Crit Care Med 1994; 149:332–338.

231. Sternberg RI, Whitsett JA, Hull WM, Baughman RP. *P. carinii* alters surfactant protein A concentration in bronchoalveolar lavage fluid. J Lab Clin Med 1995; 125:462–469.

232. Phelps DS, Rose RM. Increased recovery of surfactant protein A in AIDS-related pneumonia. Am Rev Respir Dis 1991; 143:1072–1075.

233. Phelps DS, Unstead TM, Rose RM, Fishman JA. Surfactant protein-A levels increase during *P. carinii* pneumonia in the rat. Eur Respir J 1996; 9:565–570.

234. Atochina EN, Beck JM, Scanlon ST, Preston AM, Beers M. *P. carinii* pneumonia alters expression distribution of lung collectins SP-A and SP-D. J Lab Clin Med 2001; 137:429–439.

235. Beers MF, Atochina EN, Preston AM, Beck JM. Inhibition of lung surfactant protein B expression during *Pneumocystis carinii* pneumonia in mice. J Lab Clin Med 1999; 133:423–433.

236. Zimmerman PE, Voelker DR, McCormack FX, Paulsrud JR, Martin WJ. 120-kD surface glycoprotein of *P. carinii* is a ligand for surfactant protein A. J Clin Invest 1992; 89:143–149.

237. McCormack FX, Festa AL, Andrews RP, Linke MJ, Walzer PD. The carbohydrate recognition domain of surfactant protein A mediates binding to the major surface glycoprotein of *P. carinii*. Biochemistry 1997; 36:8092–8099.

238. O'Riordan DM, Standing JE, Kwon KY, Chang D, Crouch EC, Limper AH. Surfactant protein D interacts with *P. carinii* and mediates organism adherence to alveolar macrophages. J Clin Invest 1995; 95:2699–2710.

239. Rice WR, Singleton FM, Linke MJ, Walzer PD. Regulation of surfactant phosphatidylcholine secretion from alveolar type II cells during *P. carinii* pneumonia in the rat. J Clin Invest 1993; 92:2778–2782.

240. Lipschik GY, Treml JF, Moore SD, Beers MF. *P. carinii* glycoprotein A inhibits surfactant phospholipid secretion by rat alveolar type II cells. J Infect Dis 1998; 177:182–187.

241. Tashiro K, Li W-Z, Yamada K, Matsumoto Y, Kobayashi T. Surfactant replacement reverses respiratory failure induced by intratracheal endotoxin in rats. Crit Care Med 1995; 23:149–156.

242. Lutz C, Carney D, Finck C, Picone A, Gatto L, Paskanik A, Langenbeck E, Nieman G. Aerosolized surfactant improves pulmonary function in endotoxin-induced lung injury. Am J Respir Crit Care Med 1998; 158:840–845.

243. Lutz CJ, Picone A, Gatto LA, Paskanik A, Landas S, Nieman G. Exogenous surfactant and positive end-expiratory pressure in the treatment of endotoxin-induced lung injury. Crit Care Med 1998; 26:1379–1389.

244. Nieman G, Gatto L, Paskanik A, Yang B, Fluck R, Picone A. Surfactant replacement in the treatment of sepsis-induced adult respiratory distress syndrome in pigs. Crit Care Med 1996; 24:1025 1033.

245. Warner MA, Warner ME, Weber JG. Clinical significance of pulmonary aspiration during the perioperative period. Anesthesiology 1993; 78:56–62.

246. Olsson GL, Hallen B, Hambraeus-Jonzon K. Aspiration during anaesthesia: a computer-aided study of 185,358 anaesthetics. Acta Anaesthesiol Scand 1986; 30:84–92.

247. Marik PE. Aspiration pneumonitis and aspiration pneumonia. N Engl J Med 2001; 344:665–671.

248. Deneke SM, Fanburg BL. Normobaric oxygen toxicity of the lung. N Engl J Med 1980; 303:76–86.

249. Clark JM, Lambertsen CJ. Pulmonary oxygen toxicity: a review. Pharmacol Rev 1971; 23:37–133.

250. D'Angio CT, Finkelstein JN. Oxygen regulation in gene expression: a study in opposites (review). Molec Gen Metab 2000; 71:371–380.

251. Holm BA, Notter RH. Pulmonary surfactant effects in sublethal hyperoxic lung injury. In: Taylor AE, Matalon S, eds. Physiology of Oxygen Radicals. Bethesda, MD: American Physiological Society Press, 1986:71–86.

252. Holm BA, Matalon S, Finkelstein JN, Notter RH. Type II pneumocyte changes during hyperoxic lung injury and recovery. J Appl Physiol 1988; 65:2672–2678.

253. Holm BA, Notter RH, Siegle J, Matalon S. Pulmonary physiological and surfactant changes during injury and recovery from hyperoxia. J Appl Physiol 1985; 59:1402–1409.

254. Matalon S, Holm BA, Loewen GM, Baker RR, Notter RH. Sublethal hyperoxic injury to the alveolar epithelium and the pulmonary surfactant system. Exp Lung Res 1988; 14:1021–1033.

255. Matalon S, Holm BA, Notter RH. Mitigation of pulmonary hyperoxic injury by administration of exogenous surfactant. J Appl Physiol 1987; 62:756–761.

256. Matalon S, Egan EA. Effects of 100% O_2 breathing on permeability of alveolar epithelium to solute. J Appl Physiol 1981; 50:859–863.

257. Matalon S, Egan EA. Interstitial fluid volumes and albumin spaces in pulmonary oxygen toxicity. J Appl Physiol 1984; 57:1767–1722.

258. Nadar-Djalal N, Knight PR, Davidson BA, Johnson K. Hyperoxia exacerbates microvascular injury following acid aspiration. Chest 1997; 112: 1607–1614.

259. Knight PR, Kurek C, Davidson BA, Nader ND, Patel A, Sokolowski J, Notter RH, Holm BA. Acid aspiration increases sensitivity to increased ambient oxygen concentrations. Am J Physiol 2000; 278:L1240–L1247.

260. Nadar-Djalal N, Knight NR, Thusu K, Davidson BA, Holm BA, Johnson KJ, Dandona P. Reactive oxygen species contribute to oxygen-related lung injury after acid aspiration. Anesth Analg 1998; 87:127–133.

261. Nadar ND, Knight PR, Bobela I, Davidson BA, Johnson KJ, Morin F. High-dose nitric oxide inhalation increases lung injury after gastric aspiration. Anesthesiology 1999; 91:741–749.

262. Holm BA, Notter RH, Leary JF, Matalon S. Alveolar epithelial changes in rabbits following a 21 day exposure to 60% O_2. J Appl Physiol 1987; 62: 2230–2236.

263. Haagsman HP. Surfactant protein A and D. Biochem Soc Trans 1994; 22: 100–106.

264. Cockshutt AM, Possmayer F. Metabolism of surfactant lipids and proteins in the developing lung. In: Robertson B, van Golde, LMG, Batenburg JJ, eds. Pulmonary Surfactant: From Molecular Biology to Clinical Practice. Amsterdam: Elsevier, 1992:339–378.

10

Cell and Animal Models of Lung Injury

JACOB N. FINKELSTEIN, MICHAEL A. O'REILLY, BRUCE A. HOLM, PATRICIA R. CHESS, and ROBERT H. NOTTER

Departments of Pediatrics and Environmental Medicine,
University of Rochester, Rochester, New York, U.S.A., and
Departments of Pediatrics and Obstetrics and Gynecology,
State University of New York (SUNY) at Buffalo, Buffalo, New York, U.S.A.

I. Overview

This chapter describes cell and animal models used in studying the mechanisms, pathophysiology, and therapy of lung injury. The complex phenomenology of lung injury requires complementary investigations in whole animals in vivo, lung tissue in situ, and cells in vitro. A variety of specific models and assessments within these general categories are used in research applications. In vitro research on lung injury examines cultured cell lines as well as isolated native pulmonary or leukocytic cells in suspension or culture. In vitro research also includes studies on cultured lung tissue explants exposed to injury stimuli. The responses of specific cells in lung tissue are also often examined in situ during acute and chronic injury. Cell-based research is particularly important in mechanistic assessments of injury-related signal transduction pathways, transcriptional events, and other biochemical and regulatory processes. Such research is complemented by animal studies in vivo that elucidate responses to injury at the level of the whole organism. Multiple animal models of acute and chronic lung injury are summarized in this chapter. Examples are also presented to illustrate specific experimental assessments relating to antioxidant activity, DNA damage, cell proliferation and death, and pulmonary surfactant alterations in hyperoxia/oxidant-induced injury. Further coverage of experimental models used in lung injury research is given in Chapter 11 (genetically modified mouse models of lung injury and repair) and Chapter 12 (models and considerations relevant for inhalation toxicology).

II. General Concepts of Cell Models

A major strength of in vitro models is that they allow direct assessments of cell-specific processes under controlled conditions. Although the behavior of cells can be examined biochemically and histologically in animals, in vitro experiments assess behavior without many of the complications inherent in studies with the whole organism. In choosing in vitro models, it is important to consider whether the objective is to replicate pulmonary responses to a given injury stimulus or to examine specific mechanistic questions at the cellular level. In many cases, in vitro models are better suited for the latter than the former. The complex multicellular nature of lung tissue and the importance of cell–cell and tissue–cell interactions during injury are substantial impediments to whole organ modeling in vitro. Several multicellular in vitro systems have been devised (1–4), but it is not currently feasible to isolate the full mix of relevant pulmonary cells and use them to rebuild or "model" a meaningful three-dimensional lung ex vivo. Thus, a major focus of in vitro research on lung injury involves the use of isolated and/or cultured pulmonary cells, or cultured tumor cell lines, to examine cell-specific mechanistic responses to injury-inducing stimuli. An additional approach that has received less attention is the study of explant tissue cultures, where cubic blocks ($\sim$1 mm^3 in volume) of lung tissue are prepared and maintained in incubated dishes and intermittently exposed to air and media on a rocker platform.

In vitro research in isolated/cultured cells or tissue is subject to several limitations. Individual cells in suspension or culture can vary significantly in their degree of viability and properties relative to the lung in vivo (5). Also, as noted above, in vitro models do not maintain the range of intercellular and tissue communications (paracrine or endocrine) that are present in vivo. In general, explant tissue cultures maintain more of these interactions than suspended or cultured cells. However, tissue explants are more subject to viability concerns, and still do not account for many in vivo interactions such as those mediated by recruited inflammatory leukocytes during lung injury. Moreover, tissue explants are subject to the selective overgrowth of specific cell types such as fibroblasts. For these and other reasons, greater emphasis in lung injury research has been placed on in vitro studies in isolated/cultured pulmonary cells or tumor cell lines. Methods exist for isolating several important types of pulmonary cells, although maintaining their differentiated state in culture can in some cases be difficult. Continuous tumor cell lines or viral-transformed cells are convenient because they provide an unlimited supply of material and are not subject to isolation-related artifacts that potentially affect native pulmonary cells harvested from animals. On the negative side, tumor cell lines frequently contain mutations in genes critical for growth and survival, necessitating caution in studying regulatory pathways involving cell proliferation and death. Despite the limitations of in vitro studies of pulmonary cells or tumor cell lines, cell-based research of this kind has provided important insights into how specific cells respond during lung injury. When information from in vitro cell studies is combined and integrated with complementary biological assessments in whole animals in vivo, it provides a powerful framework for understanding mechanisms of lung injury and repair and developing optimal treatments for related pulmonary diseases.

III. Examples of Pulmonary Cells Studied in Vitro

A number of different kinds of resident pulmonary cells can be isolated, cultured, and studied in vitro in injury-related research (e.g., Table 1). Examples discussed below include: pulmonary (alveolar) macrophages, alveolar type II epithelial cells, tracheobronchial cells, and pulmonary vascular endothelial cells.

A. Pulmonary Macrophages

Macrophages are the most abundant nonparenchymal cells in the normal lung. These cells are mononuclear phagocytes derived from bone marrow precursors. They secrete multiple inflammatory cytokines, and are thought to play crucial roles in lower respiratory tract responses to injury stimuli such as inhalation exposure to toxicants or pollutants. Macrophages are mobile cells that are free to migrate. Depending on their specific morphology and localization, pulmonary macrophages are classified as alveolar macrophages (AMs), interstitial macrophages/monocytes, dendritic cells, or plural macrophages (6–9). AMs are the first cells of the innate host defense system to interact with foreign substances, and are highly important in modulating the ensuing inflammatory response. As a result of their biological importance and accessibility, the behavior and responses of AMs in culture have been examined in a variety of injury-related studies (e.g., Refs. 6,10–16). AMs are easily collected by bronchoalveolar lavage with a balanced salt solution like Hanks solution (12,16–18), followed by further

Table 1 Examples of Pulmonary Cell Types and Isolation Procedures Used in Lung Injury Research

Pulmonary cell type	Isolation method	Specialized characteristics	Selected limitations
Alveolar macrophage	Bronchoalveolar lavage	Cells are quiescent in culture	Adherence can lead to activation of cultured cells
Tracheobronchial epithelium	Microdissection and protease digestion	Cells are cultured at the air–liquid interface; mucus secretion can be observed	Maintenance of differentiated function/proliferation
Alveolar epithelium (Type II cells)	Intratracheally instilled proteases	Surfactant metabolism can be studied; cultures display tight junctions for studies on ion transport	Subject to culture instability with loss of differentiated function(s)
Vascular endothelium	Protease perfusion plus subculture	Cells are proliferative in culture; good preservation of function	Subpopulations of microvascular and arterial/venous endothelial cells may be present
Pulmonary interstitium (e.g., fibroblasts)	Explant and/or protease digestion clonal expansion	Spindle shape/collagen production	Subpopulations of cells may be present

Details on several of the cell models in Table 1 are discussed in the text.

purification by centrifugation. AMs obtained in this way can be studied in suspension for short-term experiments, or placed in serum-containing media for incubation and culture. Cultures of rodent AMs prepared with this kind of methodology have been reported to contain $>95\%$ viable AMs (12,16–18). Human AMs have also been obtained by bronchoscopic instillation of saline into the airways, followed by filtration of recovered fluid through surgical gauze and purification by centrifugation (11,15,19). The purity of AMs obtained from healthy control subjects by this technique has been reported to be 95%, with cell viability $>90\%$ (15).

B. Alveolar Epithelial Cells

The alveolar epithelium is characterized by the presence of two major cell types: the membranous pneumocytes (type I cells) and the granular pneumocytes (type II cells). Type I cells account for only about 5–10% of pulmonary parenchymal cells, but cover $>95\%$ of the alveolar surface. These large thin cells have an extensive cytoplasm, and comprise the major epithelial component of structure for the alveolar wall. Type II cells, on the other hand, account for nearly 15% of lung parenchymal cells but only cover 4–5% of the alveolar surface. Type II pneumocytes have primary importance in the synthesis, secretion, reuptake, and recycling of pulmonary surface-active material. In addition, as progenitors of type I alveolar epithelial cells, type II pneumocytes are crucial in regenerating a continuous alveolar epithelium after injury. These cells also elicit and respond to a variety of mediators during innate pulmonary host defense and inflammatory injury. Because of the multifaceted biological importance of alveolar type II cells, significant effort has been devoted to techniques for their isolation, purification, and characterization in vitro.

Methods have been described to isolate alveolar type II cells from a variety of different animal species including rabbits, rats, mice, and humans (20–24). The majority of these methods depend on the use of proteolytic enzymes such as trypsin and/or elastase to dissociate the pulmonary epithelium, followed by lung mincing and tissue filtration to generate a crude cell mix that is subsequently enriched in type II pneumocytes by density gradient centrifugation methods. The details of isolation protocols used to obtain type II cells vary significantly, however, and specific methodologic selection generally takes into account requirements such as the need to avoid certain enzymes, the necessity to achieve defined cell yields, or the need to characterize particular cellular characteristics relating to the physiological state of the animals. Regardless of the isolation method used, it is wise to monitor the yield and purity of each cell preparation, which may vary considerably from day-to-day or from animal-to-animal. Common problems that affect the yield or purity of isolated type II cells include subclinical infections in laboratory animals that generate large increases in contaminating AMs and granulocytes, as well as lot-to-lot variations in the activity of proteolytic enzymes used to dissociate the pulmonary parenchyma. A number of histochemical methods are available to assess the yield and purity of isolated type II cells (20,25,26). The typical purity of alveolar type II pneumocyte isolates prepared by enzymatic dissociation and density gradient centrifugation in rabbits and rats is >90%, with approximately 95% cell viability by trypan blue exclusion (20,22,23,25,27,28).

While reasonably pure populations of type II cells have been prepared from rabbits and rats by enzymatic dissociation and density gradient centri-fugation, isolates obtained by these methods from mice generally have lower purity because of contaminating Clara cells and macrophages (25,29,30). Because of the research importance of genetically modified mouse models, alternative methods to isolate murine type II cells have been developed, albeit with varied success. One method involves labeling isolated lung cells with lipid soluble phosphine dye, followed by sorting by laser flow cytome-try (31). Labeling macrophages with anti-CD32 has been reported to allow separation from contaminating macrophages, resulting in increased type II cell purity (80–90%) at a yield of 10^6 cells/mouse. Unfortunately, this isolation method can damage the cells. Type II cells have also been obtained in relatively high purity from mouse lungs instilled with dispase followed by low-melt agarose to prevent dissociation of airway cells (32,33). Cell isolates are subsequently incubated with biotin-labeled anti-CD32 and anti-CD45, and type II cells purified using streptavidin-coated magnetic beads resulting in >90% purity and yields of 5×10^6 cells/mouse (32,33). A new technique that may facilitate isolation of type II pneumo-cytes from transgenic mice involves the use of green fluorescent protein (GFP) and mutated enhanced GFP (EGFP) to provide intrinsic green fluor-escence in these cells in vivo (34). Type II pneumocytes have been reported to be obtained by flow cytometry in high purity (>95%) from transgenic mice in which EGFP was targeted to these cells in the alveolar epithelium (34). However, while purity was extremely high, yields were only ~10^5 cells per mouse because a significant number of type II cells did not express EGFP in the mouse strain used (34). Nonetheless, these results show that mouse type II cells can be isualized in real-time and isolated based upon endogenous green fluorescence.

C. Tracheobronchial (Airway) Epithelial Cells

The tracheobronchial mucosa consists of a stratified, mucociliary epithelium from which it is possible to isolate specific cells or tissue for in vitro assess-ments. Starting material for tracheobronchial epithelial cell cultures comes from both isolated cells and explants. Initiation of tracheobronchial cultures with isolated cells is the method of choice, and primary cell cultures can be established with uniform seeding density in multiple vessels. When limited amounts of airway surface are involved (e.g., small bronchi), explant techniques can be useful in establishing cell cultures, although they must be passaged to achieve uniformity (35). A number of enzymes and methods are available to dissociate and isolate tracheobronchial cells and place them in primary culture (22,35–44). After initial dissociation to obtain dispersed cells in small clumps, for example, a brief exposure to a trypsinizing solution releases single cells that can then be placed in culture. Tracheobronchial surface epithelial cells have been isolated and cultured from a variety of animal species including rats (41), hamsters (44), guinea pigs (42,43), and rabbits (22,44), among others. In a number of cases, long-term propagation of cultured airway epithelial cells has proven feasible (36,40,45,46). Human tracheobronchial epithelial cells have also been isolated by enzymatic dissociation/disaggregation from bronchial brushings, surgical resections, or lungs removed for organ transplantation (45,47–50). Cultured tracheobronchial epithelial cells are generally able to grow to confluency, and cell proliferation, differentiation, and intracellular complexity is enhanced when the apical surface of the cultured cells is exposed to air at the liquid interface (e.g., Refs. 51,52).

Nonciliated bronchiolar epithelial cells (Clara cells) are an important specific example of tracheobronchial cells that have been studied in culture. These cells are crucial components of the mature bronchiolar epithelium (53,54). During development and following injury, they also serve as progenitor cells for the distal airway epithelium (53–55). Nonciliated bronchiolar cells were first isolated from rabbit lung by Devereux and Fouts (56) using enzymatic digestion, elutriation, and density gradient centrifugation. Later, similar methods also proved efficient for isolating rat nonciliated bronchiolar epithelial cells (28,57). In addition, Oreffo et al (58) developed a related but simplified technique for isolating mouse nonciliated bronchiolar cells that did not require elutriation. A different approach using fluorescent cell-sorting methodology has also been developed to isolate rat nonciliated bronchiolar cells in high purity (59), but cells obtained by this latter technique have not yet been studied in culture.

D. Pulmonary Vascular Endothelial Cells

Understanding about the mechanisms that lead to dysfunction in the pulmonary circulation during injury has been advanced by studies in isolated cultured vascular endothelial cells. Bovine pulmonary artery epithelial cells for culture were first obtained by Ryan (60), using a technique that involved luminal instillation of collagenase. Pulmonary microvascular endothelial cells and pulmonary endothelial cells have now been isolated from the lungs by a number of techniques (e.g., Refs. 61–67). This includes methods for mechanically isolating pulmonary endothelial cells on polyacrylamide beads that avoid exposure to enzymes during isolation (67). Nonhuman vascular endothelial cells are generally cultured in modifications of medium 199 or Dulbecco's Modified Eagle's Medium supplemented with fetal bovine and/or bovine serum (65,68–70). Gorfien et al (71,72) have introduced a serum-free medium that supports the growth of nonhuman vascular endothelium from a number of species. Subculture techniques for pulmonary endothelial cells have also been developed to allow propagation of cultures with preserved cell enzymes, receptors, and transport molecules in vitro. Primary cultures on microcarrier beads are easily propagated simply by transferring beads. Subculturing of cells grown in flasks requires mechanical scraping and dispersion by repetitive pipetting prior to transfer to another culture vessel. Bovine pulmonary artery cultures that can undergo multiple passages without loss of characteristics are available through the American Type Culture Collection (ATCC) (Rockville, MD). Human lung microvascular endothelial cells have been isolated and placed in subculture from mixed lung cell cultures using fluorescence-activated cell sorting (62).

IV. Examples of Cultured Cell Lines

Multiple cell lines have proved to be extremely helpful surrogates to isolated pulmonary cells in investigating injury-associated responses (Table 2). Cell lines such as those in Table 2 all share the characteristic of being maintained by continuous passage in culture and are thus defined as immortalized. Cell lines of human origin are typically derived from primary tumors. In addition, a number of cell lines have now been immortalized by the overexpression of a viral oncogene such as simian virus (SV)-40 large tumor antigen. Viral-transformed cells have the advantage of being somewhat better characterized than tumor cell lines in terms of their cell-specific origin and growth control characteristics. Several cell lines related to alveolar type II epithelial cells are discussed below as representative examples of immortalized in vitro models used in research on the pulmonary system and its responses to injury.

Until relatively recently, alveolar type II cells were difficult to study in culture, necessitating the use of immortalized cell lines. One of the most widely used type II cell models has been the A549 pulmonary epithelial cell line derived from a patient with alveolar cell carcinoma (73–75). These cells can be obtained for study from the ATCC (Rockville, MD). A549 cells examined by electron microscopy at both early and late passage levels contain multilamellar cytoplasmic inclusion bodies typical of those found in type II alveolar epithelial cells. Initial studies with these cells appeared to indicate that they were capable of producing and secreting components of the pulmonary surfactant system (disaturated phosphatidylcholine)

Table 2 Selected Cell Lines Used in Studying Injury-Induced Cellular Responses

Type of cell line	Derivation	Selected qualities	Considerations
Epithelial			
A549	Human lung	Type II-like	Lack of SP genes
MvlLu	Mink lung	Responsive to TGF-β	p53 pathway is defective
MLE15	Mouse lung	Type II-like	Immortalized with SV40
C10	Mouse lung	Type II-like	Spontaneous transformed
SV40-T2	Rat lung	Derived from type II epithelia cells	Immortalized with SV40
RLE-6TN	Rat lung	Type II-like	Spontaneous transformation
HCT116	Human colon	Clones lacking p53/p21 exist	Not related to lung cells
Tracheobronchial			
BEAS-2B	Human lung	Squamous differentiation	Immortalized with SV40
16HBE14o-	Human lung	Express CFTR solute transport	Immortalized with SV40
Endothelial	Human lung	Venous	Immortalized with SV40
HMEC			
Monocyte/macrophage			
RAW 264.7	Mouse leukemia	Macrophage/monocyte	Derived from peritoneal cavity
MHS-C	Mouse	Macrophage	SV40 immortalized alveolar macrophage
NR8383	Rat macrophage	Alveolar macrophage	Spontaneous transformation
U937	Human	Monocyte/macrophage	Nonalveolar undifferentiated
THP-1	Human	Monocyte/macrophage	Nonalveolar undifferentiated

A number of general cell lines including HeLa cells or CHO cells are also used in studying oxidant and other injuries relevant for the lungs. In vitro research on cellular responses in lung injury also includes assessments in leukocytes and pulmonary epithelial, endothelial, and interstitial cells isolated from the lungs of injured animals. See text for details. SV40, simian virus 40.

(73–75). However, when compared to freshly isolated rat type II cells and fibroblasts the cellular lipid composition in A549 cells resembles fibroblasts more closely (76). Also, A549 cells do not express surfactant proteins in culture regardless of conditions (77). Despite these differences, A549 cells continue to find extensive use as an in vitro model. While inappropriate to study the details of surfactant metabolism, these cells are useful to examine other properties of epithelial cells. Studies of cytokine production (78–81) or inflammatory cell–epithelial interactions (82–84) have all used A549 cells effectively. The A549 cell line has also proven to be useful in studying responses to oxidative stress and hyperoxia as described later.

Among the more recent cell models of the alveolar type II epithelial cell is the MLE15 cell line developed by Wikenheiser et al. (85). This cell line was produced from lung tumors generated in transgenic mice harboring the viral oncogene SV40 large tumor antigen under the transcriptional control of a promoter region from the human surfactant protein C (SP-C) gene. In culture, the MLE15 cell line exhibits several features similar to type II cells, including epithelial cell microvilli and multilamellar inclusion bodies. In contrast to A549 cells, MLE15 cells have an ability to express surfactant proteins and mRNAs. These cells also secrete phospholipids. A number of recent studies have used MLE15 cells to study cytokine expression and other injury-related phenomena (86–89). Several other rodent type II cell lines also exist. Dwyer-Nield et al. (90) and Nicks et al. (91) have produced a murine type II cell line designated as C10 by cloning cell lines arising from explanted mouse lung. The C10 cell line has been found to be nontumorigenic and to exhibit many properties of normal type II cells (reviewed in Ref. 92). A similar approach was used by Driscoll et al. (27) in rats to create a type II-like cell line designated as RLE-6TN. In addition, a related line, RLE-6T, expresses SV-40 large T-antigen, which is not found in the 6TN line (27). Likewise, the SV40T2 line was created by over-expression of SV-40 large T-antigen in neonatal rat type II cells (355).

V. Exposures of Cells to Injury Stimuli

Cellular studies investigating responses to toxicants or other injurious stimuli require effective, reproducible, quantitative exposure systems. Exposure of cells to injurious agents can be accomplished by several approaches. One approach is to expose animals to inhaled pollutants, toxic gases, or airway-instilled soluble chemical agents in vivo, followed by rapid isolation and study of specific cell populations in vitro. A second potentially more controlled approach is the direct in vitro exposure of cells in suspension or in culture. In the case of soluble chemicals, this is typically accomplished by direct addition into the media containing the cells. Cell suspensions or cultures in media can also be exposed to gases or insoluble aerosol particles in vitro, although effective concentrations in the liquid phase must then be determined. Studies involving the responses of cells to liquid, solid, or gaseous substances in vitro have several advantages. The independent responses of particular cell types to direct exposures in vitro can typically be examined under more controlled and reproducible conditions compared to whole animals in vivo (18,93–96). Moreover, in the case of human cells, such studies can address the effects of toxic agents that cannot be examined in living subjects.

Several requirements need to be met by optimal in vitro exposure systems. One primary requirement is that agents be delivered in accurate and precisely determined concentrations. In the case of agents delivered by inhalation, the test atmosphere should contact the cells as closely as possible while soluble chemicals should be distributed to achieve a uniform exposure concentration for individual cells. Cells directly exposed to ambient atmospheres can rapidly be affected by drying, and methods that maintain a humid atmosphere or keep the cells moistened in some other way are required for extended exposure studies. In addition, in vitro exposure systems must allow cells to be easily recovered or sampled to permit desired testing during and after exposure. Moreover, sterile conditions must be able to be maintained during exposure and sampling so that cells can be continued in culture.

Cell cultures in vitro are normally immersed in a liquid medium in a flask or dish on a supporting microporous membrane. The dose of active substances then relates to the concentration of these substances in the medium (97–99). Roller bottles, rotating platforms, and/or rocking platforms have been used to help meet the requirements of close exposure defined above (96). In such systems, the culture medium is periodically placed over the apical surface and exposed directly to pollutants or toxicants, thus acting as a possible sink and a variable diffusion barrier (100,101). Additional in vitro set-ups are available to expose cells at the air–liquid interface (5,102–104). One such system involves exposing cells grown on a membrane filter at an air–liquid interface in a biphasic culture (103,104). Another in vitro exposure model has used cells plated onto a collagen–gel substratum on top of a nitrocellulose membrane to study the effects of pollutants on bronchial epithelial cells (41–43). The upper surface of the growing cells is not exposed to medium, but instead is exposed to air as occurs in vivo (41–43).

VI. Animal Models of Lung Injury

Studies in animal models of acute and chronic pulmonary injury provide crucial information to supplement and complement findings in cell models in vitro. Animal models allow for proof of concept that is a key element in the development of diagnostic markers and new therapeutic agents and interventions. They also incorporate the full range of cell–cell and tissue–cell interactions present in the functioning lung in vivo, although extrapolation of experimental findings to human lungs is still required. Pulmonary function and mechanics, edema, inflammatory mediator responses, vascular and blood flow alterations, surfactant abnormalities, fibroproliferative changes, and a variety of other lung injury-associated phenomena have been examined through studies in animal models (see Refs. 105–114 for review). A number of animal models used in research on acute and chronic lung injury are listed in Table 3. Animal models that involve a prominent component of acute inflammatory pulmonary pathology are often studied in the context of applications relating to clinical acute lung injury (ALI) and the acute respiratory distress syndrome (ARDS). Animal models involving persistent inflammation and fibroproliferative pathology are generally examined in applications relating to interstitial lung disease or other forms of chronic pulmonary disease (including the later fibroproliferative phase of ARDS). Selected animal models of lung injury are summarized below.

Table 3 Examples of Animal Models Used in Studying Acute and Chronic Lung Injury

---

I. Animal models of acute pulmonary injury[a]
  Antibody-induced lung injury
  Aspiration lung injury (e.g., acid, gastric particulates, meconium)
  Airway-instilled microorganisms (e.g., bacteria, fungi)
  Bacterial sepsis or endotoxin-induced lung injury
  Viral-induced lung injury (e.g., influenza A, respiratory syncytial virus)
  Fatty acid lung injury (e.g., oleic acid lung injury)
  Oxidant-induced lung injury (e.g., severe acute exposure to oxygen, ozone)
  In vivo lung lavage (with or without mechanical ventilation)
  Neurogenic edema (e.g., vagotomy-induced lung injury)
  NNNMU-induced lung injury

II. Animal models of chronic pulmonary injury
  Oxidant-induced lung injury (e.g., prolonged lower level exposure to oxygen, ozone)
  Radiation lung injury
  Drug-induced fibroproliferative lung injury (e.g., BCNU, Cytoxan, bleomycin, and methotrexate)
  Toxicant-induced lung injury (e.g., paraquat, phorbol myristate acetate, butylated hydroxytoluene)
  Particulate/fiber-induced lung injury (e.g., silica, asbestos)

---

[a]The acute vs. chronic classification of animal models in the table is to some extent arbitrary. Models listed under acute injury can display elements of pathology relevant for chronic injury, and models listed under chronic injury can also be studied for acute pathology. NNNMU, *N*-nitroso-*N*-methylurethane. BCNU, bischlorethylnitrosourea; Cytoxan, cyclophosphamide.

A. Antibody-Induced Lung Injury

Antibodies against pulmonary tissue are known to be present in the lungs under pathological conditions and to contribute to respiratory disease (115). In addition, immune complexes or antibodies directed against lung tissue or components in lung surfactant can be infused or instilled in animals to cause acute pulmonary injury (116–120). Among other applications, animal models of this kind have been used to study surfactant dysfunction and replacement in ALI/ARDS. For example, antilung antibodies injure the alveolocapillary membrane and cause severe acute inflammatory injury with edema and surfactant dysfunction if infused into guinea pigs (116). Acute pulmonary injury with surfactant dysfunction can also be induced in animals by intraperitoneal injection of hybridoma cells that produce antibodies to surfactant protein SP-B (117,118).

B. Aspiration Lung Injury

Aspiration lung injury can involve inactive or reactive aspirants alone or in combination. Acute pulmonary injury can be induced, for example, by aspiration of hydrochloric acid (121–123), hydrochloride/pepsin (124), nonacidified gastric particles with or without added acid (125–128), or meconium (129–134). Animal models of this kind have significant clinical relevance. Aspiration of gastric contents (acid or particulates) is an important cause of ALI/ARDS in humans (135), and meconium aspiration by term infants at birth results in severe lung injury and potentially lethal respiratory failure (136,137). Animal models of aspiration lung injury generally have a multifaceted pathology including inflammation, edema, tissue injury, surfactant dysfunction, and impaired gas exchange with intrapulmonary shunting. Inflammatory mediators and cells have been extensively examined in animals with pneumonitis from aspirated acid, particulates, or combined acid-particulates (125–128,138–143). Animal models of aspiration exhibit progressive injury over several days, and thus permit assessments of pulmonary responses and putative therapies for ALI/ARDS over a clinically relevant timescale. For example, one focus of research in animal studies of meconium aspiration has been on using exogenous surfactant to improve pulmonary mechanics and gas exchange when instilled intratracheally as a bolus or as a therapeutic lavage (129–132,134). Animal studies showing that surfactant replacement therapy can be beneficial in meconium aspiration lung injury are consistent with clinical investigations documenting the efficacy of this therapy in human infants (144–147) (Chapter 15).

C. Bacterial (Microorganism) or Endotoxin-Induced Lung Injury

Bacterial infection, including both sepsis and pulmonary infection (pneumonia), is a prevalent cause of acute respiratory failure and clinical

ALI/ARDS in adult and pediatric patients (136,137,148–150). The administration of lipopolysaccharide (LPS or endotoxin) or *Escherichia coli* bacteria has been widely used to induce acute inflammatory lung injury in animal models (e.g., Refs. 110, 151–163). *Pseudomonas aeruginosa* (164,165) and group B *Streptococcus* (166,167), among other bacteria, have also been used to generate acute pulmonary injury in animals. In addition, severe lung injury in immunocompromised or immunodeficient animals can be induced by exposure to fungal-like microorganisms such as *Pneumocystis carinii* (168–174). As is true in many animal models of ALI/ARDS, administration of microorganisms or bacterial toxins causes multifaceted pulmonary pathology with prominent inflammation, permeability injury and edema, intrapulmonary shunting, surfactant dysfunction, decreased compliance and lung volumes, and impaired gas exchange. Animal models of microorganism-induced or endotoxin-induced lung injury generally permit studies to be carried out over sufficient times to allow the testing of interventions targeting inflammation, surfactant dysfunction, or other aspects of pathophysiology. Such models can also be modified to include concurrent exposure to aspiration, hyperoxia, or mechanical ventilation to examine "multihit" lung injury scenarios. Studies of this kind are highly relevant for clinical ALI/ARDS, since affected patients are often exposed to multiple inducers of lung injury during the course of disease and medical intensive care. Moreover, microorganism clearance and other host defense responses may undergo significant set point changes when multiple injury inducers are present concomitantly.

D. Viral-Induced Lung Injury

Viruses, like bacteria and other microorganisms, can also cause acute inflammatory pulmonary injury pathology relevant for ALI/ARDS. Examples of viruses that have been utilized in animal models of acute inflammatory lung injury include influenza A (175), respiratory syncytial virus (176), and Sendai virus (177,178). These animal models of viral-induced lung injury typically exhibit prominent inflammation and other abnormalities at the level of the airways and pulmonary interstitium. In addition, they also include damage to the alveolocapillary membrane that generates edema and surfactant dysfunction.

E. Fatty Acid Lung Injury

Acute fatty acid lung injury in animals is directly relevant for clinical ALI/ARDS in association with pancreatitis (179) or fat emboli from long-bone fractures. Intravenous infusion of fluid free fatty acids such as oleic acid in animals severely damages the capillary endothelium and alveolar epithelium leading to rapid and extensive permeability edema (110) (180–186). Related injury to the alveolar membrane in animals can also be induced by tracheal instillation of lyso-phosphatidylcholine, which disrupts endothelial and epithelial integrity similarly to fatty acids (187). The widely studied animal model of oleic acid lung injury includes substantial inflammation, microvascular and epithelial permeability damage, and venti-lation–perfusion mismatching. Animals injured with intravenous oleic acid also have severe surfactant dysfunction from biophysical interactions with inhibitors and from the depletion of active large surfactant aggregate sub-types (180,181,188). One complicating factor in animal studies of oleic acid injury is that the pulmonary pathology induced by fatty acid infusion can be relatively nonhomogeneous in distribution. In addition, the rapid and fulmi-nant nature of the resultant respiratory failure makes it difficult to assess the details and progression of inflammatory injury over an extended period.

F. Hyperoxic Lung Injury

The significant pulmonary toxicity of oxygen has been known for decades (for review see Refs. 189–194). Acute exposure to high levels of oxygen has been widely used to induce pulmonary injury in animal models of ALI/ARDS. In addition, longer-term exposures to moderate levels of hyperoxia can be used to generate animal models of fibrogenic chronic lung injury. Depending on the severity and duration of exposure, and on animal species and age, hyperoxia can induce pulmonary responses ranging from adaptive to lethal. Adult animals exposed to high levels of 95–100% oxygen for several days (e.g., 64 hr for rabbits, 96 hr for rats) exhibit a severe acute pulmonary injury with inflammation, edema, increased alveolocapillary membrane permeability, type II cell dysfunction, and surfactant dysfunc-tion (12,194–215). More prolonged exposures to lower levels of hyperoxia (50–85%) can be used to generate progressive chronic pathology with ele-ments of fibroproliferation and fibrosis (189,196,216–221). At a fixed level of oxygen exposure, normal newborn animals generally have a significantly higher resistance to pulmonary oxygen toxicity than adult animals (192,215,216,222–226). Animal models of hyperoxic lung injury also exhibit significant species-related variability in the details of pathology, as is the case for many animal models of pulmonary injury. Representative examples of research in animal models of hyperoxic lung injury are described in more detail later.

G. In Vivo Lung Lavage

A relatively specialized model of acute pulmonary injury involves mechani-cally ventilated small adult animals such as rats, guinea pigs, or rabbits that have been depleted in exogenous surfactant by in vivo lavage. The lavage procedure is typically done with normal saline until arterial oxygenation is reduced below a predefined level while the animals are supported by mechanical ventilation. The in vivo lavage model has been used most com-monly to investigate surfactant replacement interventions for ALI/ARDS

(227–242). However, the model inherently involves a more prominent degree of surfactant deficiency as opposed to surfactant dysfunction than is typically found in clinical ALI/ARDS. The severity of lung injury and inflammation in this model can also be quite variable, and depends on the extent of surfactant depletion, the conditions of mechanical ventilation, and the level of supplemental oxygen (if present).

H. Neurogenic Edema and Bilateral Vagotomy

Increased alveolocapillary membrane permeability and pulmonary edema can be caused neurogenically in animals by cranial injury or ligation of appropriate nerves (243–247). In animals subjected to bilateral cervical vagotomy, inflammatory lung injury has been shown to include a prominent component of surfactant dysfunction from interactions with plasma proteins or related inhibitory substances in edema (243,244). Consistent with surfactant dysfunction, the lungs of animals injured with bilateral cervical vagotomy exhibit decreased compliance, atelectasis, and hyaline membrane formation. Exogenous surfactant therapy has been shown to improve pulmonary function and compliance in this animal model of ALI/ARDS (244).

I. *N*-Nitroso-*N*-Methylurethane (NNNMU) Injury

Subcutaneous injection of the nitrogenated urethane compound NNNMU gives rise to a progressive lung injury over several days that has a number of features relevant for ALI/ARDS (248–253). Animals with NNNMU injury have pulmonary edema along with increased levels of plasma proteins and decreased levels of phospholipid in bronchoalveolar lavage. Arterial hypoxemia is also present in NNNMU-injured animals, and lung pressure–volume compliance is decreased. Surfactant activity in bronchoalveolar lavage is reduced not only by interactions with plasma proteins and other inhibitors in edema, but also from depletion of active large surfactant aggregates (248,252). NNNMU is also known to have toxic effects on pulmonary cells including alveolar type II pneumocytes (254). NNNMU-induced lung injury has been found to respond favorably to exogenous surfactant supplementation in several studies (249–252).

J. Radiation-Induced Lung Injury

Ionizing radiation to the thorax of animals or human patients can generate a severe lung injury that includes prominent features of fibroproliferation and fibrosis. The nature and severity of the early radiation-induced inflammatory pneumonitis and later organizing alveolitis/fibrosis are dependent on total dose, number of doses (fraction size), interval between doses, and the lung volume irradiated (255–260). Fibrosis typically occurs at total thoracic ionizing radiation doses of 12–17 Gy, although significantly higher total doses have also been used. Radiation can be delivered in a single dose, or with fractionation schedules such as once per day or once per week. The histopathological features of radiation-induced lung injury have been well documented (e.g., Refs. 261–263), although the mechanisms underlying the pathogenesis of fibrosis are still uncertain. In humans, fibrotic lesions in irradiated lung typically occur after a latent period of approximately 6–24 months. In C57BL/6J mice, the onset of fibrotic lesions generally occurs about 100–120 days after thoracic irradiation (256,262–265). In animal models of thoracic irradiation, chronic inflammation appears to be important in stimulating the development of fibrosis through the release of cytokines and growth factors (266–269). Mouse models using thoracic irradiation have consistently demonstrated a temporal correlation between increases in extracellular matrix, mRNA alterations of the profibrotic cytokine transforming growth factor-β (TGFβ), and the development of fibrosis (263,266,269–271). In addition, the proinflammatory cytokines tumor necrosis factor-α (TNFα), interleukin (IL)-lα, and IL-1β are induced in the early latent phase of radiation injury and persist until the development of pneumonitis and/or fibrosis (272–281). It was once thought that radiation-induced injury was confined to cells and tissue within the irradiated field. However, it is now recognized that numerous inflammatory cells are recruited into the irradiated field subsequent to injury. A prominent feature of radiation-induced lung injury is the development of a significant lymphocytic alveolitis (282–284), indicating a role for these leukocytic cells in the eventual fibrosis (270,271,282,285). Mediators produced by recruited out-of-field macrophages, monocytes, and neutrophils also likely contribute to fibroproliferative pathology in radiation lung injury (262,263,267,286–288).

K. Drug-Induced Fibroproliferative Lung Injury

Lung injury with elements of fibroproliferation and fibrosis is a well-recognized consequence of treatment with pharmaceutical agents such as those used in cancer chemotherapy. Drugs like bischlorethylnitrosourea (BCNU), cyclophosphamide (Cytoxan), bleomycin and methotrexate all generate recognized pathologies of this kind, and all have been used as models of lung injury (see Ref. 289 for review). Among these drugs, bleomycin has been most widely studied as an experimental model for fibroproliferative lung injury and fibrosis. The initial pathologic lesions in bleomycin lung injury are focal areas of diffuse alveolar damage (290), with elements of edema, intra-alveolar fibrin deposition, and hemorrhage, followed by type II pneumocyte hyperplasia and bronchial epithelial squamous metaplasia. These initial lesions at least partially resolve into self-limited foci of intra-alveolar and alveolar wall collagen deposition in association with diffuse interstitial fibrosis with microcyst formation. Myofibroblasts are also present in the interstitium at least transiently (291). Bleomycin-induced fibrosis is typically more limited and less progressive than can occur in diseases like idiopathic pulmonary fibrosis (IPF). However, the bleomycin model at the microscopic level does appear to mimic several aspects of developing fibroproliferative pathology relevant for such conditions (292–294). The potential also exists in the future to develop modified bleomycin models in genetically modified mice that display progressive rather than self-limited fibrosis and serve as even closer analogs to human fibrotic lung diseases.

VII. Examples of Cell and Animal Assessments Involving Hyperoxia and Oxidative Stress

A variety of phenomena are studied in lung injury research in cell and animal models (e.g., Table 4). Assessments of pulmonary injury in whole animals in vivo and in cells in vitro are, in principle, complementary in nature. Research that directly integrates data and mechanistic interpretations from compatible cell and animal studies is very powerful, but accomplishing this in practice is not always possible. Although many useful cell and animal models of lung injury are available as described in preceding sections, optimal experimental systems for many aspects of acute and chronic lung injury and disease have not yet been defined. The phenomenological and anatomical complexity of the lungs impede mechanistic assessments in vivo, while cell-based studies in vitro often lack important paracrine and autocrine interactions with adjacent cells and substratum. Nonetheless, examining responses to a common injury inducer in both intact lungs and cells offers an opportunity to improve understanding about a range of relevant physiological and molecular events. Discussion below focuses on examples of research findings in cell and animal models of hyperoxia-induced and oxidant-induced lung injury.

Because of the extensive alveolar surface and pulmonary microvascular network, the lungs are uniquely challenged by oxidative stress from aerobic respiration and from circulating or inhaled toxicants. Reactive oxygen species (ROS) released by resident pulmonary cells or recruited leukocytes during the innate inflammatory response also contribute to oxidant lung injury. The ability of the lungs to maintain adequate host defense while resisting, limiting, and repairing oxidant injury is critical for the physiological function of this essential organ system. Effective tissue remodeling, in which stem cells proliferate and differentiate to replace dead cells, is also required in order to recover from pulmonary oxidant injury. Significant research emphasis has thus been placed on investigating how lung cells detoxify oxidants, repair oxidant damage, die when severely injured by oxidants, and participate in the repair or remodeling of oxidant-injured tissue.

Table 4 Examples of Different Kinds of Assessments Made in Cell and Animal Models of Lung Injury

---

Cell and tissue-related injury assessments
  DNA damage
  Altered gene expression or regulation
  Cell proliferation
  Cell death (apoptotic, necrotic)
  Altered metabolism of intracellular organelles or biochemical pathways
  Changes in cell membrane potential and cell redox status
  Cellular production of (and responses to) specific inflammatory mediators
  Cellular production of specific products (e.g., surfactant, extracellular matrix
    components)
  Signal transduction pathways and related regulatory pathways

Injury assessments in whole lung
  Histopathological alterations (e.g., morphology, immunohistochemistry,
    markers of injury)
  Microvascular permeability (protein leakage)
  Vascular function (e.g., vasoconstriction/dilation, shunting, pulmonary
    blood flow)
  Edema (e.g., determined by histology or wet-to-dry weight ratio)
  Pulmonary function and gas exchange (e.g., arterial blood gases)
  Pulmonary mechanics (e.g., lung volumes, pressure–volume
    inflation/deflation relations)
  Phospholipid composition, protein composition, and surface activity of
    bronchoalveolar lavage
  Inflammatory mediator concentrations in bronchoalveolar lavage and in blood

---

The table lists some of the many different assessments made in cell-based and whole-animal research on the mechanistic pathophysiology of lung injury. Examples of several of the tabulated assessments in hyperoxic and oxidant-induced lung injury are described in Sec. VII in the text.

Multiple reactive oxidants including superoxide anion (O_2^-), hydrogen peroxide (H_2O_2), and hydroxyl radical ($\cdot OH$) are formed during normal aerobic respiration (295). These substances are thought to contribute to a variety of processes such as cancer and aging. Indeed, exposing cells or animals to high levels of oxygen (hyperoxia) has itself been argued to be a model of aging (296). Hyperoxia can also be considered a clinically induced pollutant because it is used therapeutically to reduce tissue hypoxia in patients with respiratory distress. Whether ROS are derived during respiration or by extrinsic sources, cells have developed several mechanisms to combat their damaging effects. ROS can be reduced to less toxic species by enzymatic and nonenzymatic antioxidant defenses (Chapter 7). These antioxidant defenses usually afford protection against the damaging effects of normal aerobic respiration, but may be challenged when levels of oxidative stress increase (297). Damage to macromolecules occurs when endogenous antioxidant capacity is overwhelmed. One of the important targets affected by ROS is DNA. All biological macromolecules can in principle be oxidized, but irreversible damage to DNA is often limiting for cell survival since it is the template by which damaged enzymes and structural proteins are replaced. When damage to cellular function is sufficiently severe, cells die by apoptosis or necrosis (298). Apoptosis is thought to be a beneficial form of death for maintaining tissue architecture and function because the orderly degradation and absorption of cell remnants by remaining normal cells avert inflammation. Necrosis, on the other hand, tends to occur when damage is so severe that apoptotic pathways cannot function, and is more likely to promote inflammation and compromise tissue remodeling. Examples showing how research in cells and in animal models has been used to improve understanding about antioxidant function, DNA damage (genotoxicity), cell proliferation, cell death, and other aspects of hyperoxia-induced or oxidant-induced lung injury are given below.

A. Examples of Cell and Animal Studies on Antioxidant Defenses

The predominant antioxidant enzymes in the lungs are the superoxide dismutases (SODs), catalase, and glutathione peroxidase. Although all of these enzymes have important antioxidant activity, the dismutases play major roles in protecting the lungs from hyperoxic injury. Transgenic mice that overexpress copper–zinc SOD or manganese SOD have been shown to be markedly more resistant to hyperoxia-induced injury and death compared to wildtype controls (299). Conversely, mice lacking one or more alleles of manganese-SOD are more sensitive to oxidant injury than normal control mice (300). Other antioxidant enzymes also participate in protecting cells from hyperoxia. The expression of thioredoxin reductase, a protein disulfide oxidoreductase that detoxifies H_2O_2, increases in newborn primate lungs exposed to hyperoxia (301). Peroxiredoxin, which obtains reducing equivalents from thioredoxin, similarly increases when newborn primates are exposed to hyperoxia (302). In addition, over-expression of heme oxygenase-1 (HO-1) by viral gene transfer in adult rats has been shown to protect against hyperoxic lung injury (303).

Antioxidants in cultured cells have not been investigated as intensely as in whole animals. Carnosine has been shown to protect cultured CHO cells against the clastogenic (chromosome fragmentation) effects of hyperoxia (304). However, other antioxidants such as ascorbic acid, α-tocopherol, imidazole-4-acetic acid, glutathione monoethylester, *N*-acetylcystenine, and ethoxyguin have been found to be either ineffective or to potentiate genotoxicity in this system (296). A549 cells and small airway epithelial cells treated with the antioxidant vitamins C and E have been reported to be protected against hyperoxia-induced killing (305). In analogy with results found in animal models (303), over-expression of HO-1 in A549 cells enhances survival during hyperoxia (306). Increased cell survival was associated with a marked reduction in proliferation, which is discussed later as a process that may be linked to enhanced DNA repair. Additional research is needed to clarify the mechanistic basis of the protective effects of HO-1 against hyperoxia in cell and animal studies. HO-1 degrades heme to bilirubin, and its reaction products have a variety of anti-inflammatory, antiapoptotic and antioxidant properties (307). Antioxidants like PEG-catalase have also been shown to protect cultured pulmonary cells (alveolar type II cells) from oxidant injury. Type II cells in primary culture incubated with PEG-catalase exhibit a nine-fold increase in cellular catalase levels (308). Subsequent exposure of these augmented cells to mixed oxidants (superoxide anion, hydrogen peroxide, hydroxyl radical) results in minimal damage, while control type II cells exhibit substantial losses in metabolic function and increased cell death (308).

B. Examples of Cell and Animal Studies on Genotoxicity in Hyperoxic/Oxidant Injury

Genotoxicity from oxidative stress is likely to be indirect because oxygen does not affect the integrity of pure DNA during direct exposure (309). One common hypothesis argues that damage to DNA or other cellular constituents during hyperoxia results from the intracellular production of ROS such as O_2^-, H_2O_2, ·OH, or singlet oxygen ($^1O_2$) in amounts that overwhelm cellular defenses (310). However, as discussed by Joenje (311), the precise damaging species contributing to hyperoxic/oxidant injury are often difficult to identify. Electron paramagnetic spin resonance indicates that hyperoxia increases levels of O_2^- and ·OH in pulmonary endothelial cells (312). Nonetheless, H_2O_2 has more frequently been used to model the toxicity of hyperoxia in vitro because it is easy to apply experimentally and is a physiologically relevant intermediate found in vivo after hyperoxic exposure and other inflammatory injuries.

Although H_2O_2 is often used to model hyperoxia in vitro, the two do not have identical effects on cells. For example, human peripheral lymphocytes exposed to H_2O_2 exhibit DNA single strand breaks rather than double strand breaks necessary for clastogenicity (chromosomal fragmentation) (313). Also, ATP depletion is observed in CHO cells exposed directly to hyperoxia, while only NAD(H) levels are reduced when these cells are exposed to H_2O_2 (314). Similarly, oxygen-resistant HeLa-80 cells do not exhibit equivalent resistance when challenged with a dose of H_2O_2 that produces the same degree of toxicity as hyperoxia in parental HeLa cells (315). Other studies suggest that there is some degree of mechanistic similarity between cell injury from hyperoxia and H_2O_2 exposure. For example, primary cultures of alveolar type II epithelial cells exposed to sublethal levels of H_2O_2 show a sequential loss of both NAD(H) and ATP, ultimately leading to a reduction in metabolic processes within the cell including decreased production of pulmonary surfactant (316,317). This same phenomenon is observed in type II cells freshly isolated from rabbits exposed to hyperoxia in vivo (200). In addition, alterations in type II pneumocytes in hyperoxic animals and in cell cultures exposed to H_2O_2 can be mitigated by treatment with poly ADP-ribose polymerase inhibitors (316). However, additional mechanisms beyond direct damage from oxidants such as H_2O_2 are almost certainly involved in alveolar epithelial alterations in hyperoxic lung injury in vivo.

DNA damage from oxygen-free radicals is associated with depurination, depyrimidiation, and phosphodiester single and double strand breaks as well as the production of oxidized nucleotides and sugars (318). In addition, ROS can indirectly attack DNA through oxidized lipid intermediates (319). The ability of hyperoxia to induce DNA strand breaks has been known for over 50 years, beginning with the observation that exposure to >80% oxygen induced chromosome breaks in gametocytes of the flagellate Trichonympha (320). Using dried Tradescantia pollen grains, increasing DNA strand breaks have been observed over an oxygen concentration range of 50–100% (321). The number of DNA breaks after 1 hr of hyperoxia can be extrapolated as being equivalent to the effects of 1200 rads of ionizing radiation. These findings and others demonstrate that hyperoxia is highly clastogenic, i.e., that it induces sufficient DNA strand breakage to cause observable chromosome aberrations (for review of the early literature see Ref. 311). However, although hyperoxia is clastogenic, it is not considered to be highly mutagenic as is the case with ionizing radiation (322). Thus, the types of oxidative damage to DNA caused by hyperoxia, H_2O_2, and ionizing radiation appear to be distinct in some of their features.

CHO cells and HeLa cells were once the favored cell lines for investigating how oxidative stress and hyperoxia damage DNA. The ability of hyperoxia to cause single strand breaks in DNA was first demonstrated in CHO cells using an alkaline-elution assay (315). By eluting DNA under alkaline conditions over a sizing column, the number of single strand breaks was measured as quickly eluted fragments (314). In addition, hyperoxia was shown to promote chromatid gaps and breaks, with only a few chromatid exchanges (323). Increasing chromosome aberrations have also been observed as HeLa cells become resistant to 80% oxygen by sequential selection at increasing exposure levels (315). Studies utilizing a DNA unwinding assay have shown that hyperoxia promotes DNA strand breaks in mouse hybridoma cells (324). More recently, the comet assay has been used to demonstrate that hyperoxia induces DNA fragmentation in the mink lung adenocarcinoma line MvlLu (325). The comet assay is a highly sensitive indicator of DNA damage, since it can assess single or double strand breaks within a single cell (326). In contrast, growth-arrested MvlLu cells exhibited significantly less DNA damage during hyperoxia (325). Hyperoxia has also been shown to induce DNA strand breaks in human lung adenocarcinoma A549 cells (327), even though these and MvlLu cells fail to exhibit TUNEL staining (328,329).

In animal models, hyperoxia induces damage to DNA, causes cessation of cell growth, and decreases survival. DNA strand breaks, as assessed by TUNEL staining, have been reported in adult and newborn rodents exposed to >90% oxygen (34,328,330–336). TUNEL staining is often assumed to reflect apoptosis, but it also can be used as an identifier of damaged DNA (34,337,338). Airway epithelial cells and type II epithelial cells in hyperoxic animal lungs exhibit TUNEL staining even though death of these cells is not widely observed (34,332,335). Hyperoxia induces TUNEL staining in adult mice, but not in cultured A549 cells (328). The presence of TUNEL staining in hyperoxic whole lung as opposed to cultured A549 cells may indicate the presence of different types of DNA strand breaks in vivo as a result of paracrine or other interactions (328). Evidence to support this possibility comes from a study showing attenuated TUNEL staining when neutrophil recruitment in vivo is blocked with chemokine neutralizing antisera (336). Additional studies are needed to clarify mechanisms of hyperoxia-induced DNA damage in the whole lung in vivo and in cells in vitro.

C. Examples of Studies on Cell Proliferation in Hyperoxic/Oxidant Injury

In addition to damaging DNA, hyperoxia also inhibits cell proliferation. The overall mitotic index of adult rodent lungs is quite low (< 2%), with dividing cells being distributed approximately as 50% leukocytes, 30% endothelial cells, 10% type II epithelial cells, and 10% interstitial cells (339). Proliferation of all of these cell types is inhibited by hyperoxia (340). A significant portion of this reduced proliferation appears to result from the direct effects of hyperoxia, since it occurs before inflammatory cell recruitment and increased cytokine production is detected (225). The inhibitory actions of hyperoxia on cell proliferation can be observed even more readily in premature lungs where the mitotic index is much higher. Hyperoxia and mechanical ventilation have long been considered to be important injury inducers contributing to classic bronchopulmonary dysplasia (BPD) in premature infants (341). In addition, a newer form of chronic lung disease has emerged in extremely low birth weight premature infants that is characterized by reduced vascular and alveolar development consistent with arrested cell proliferation (342). Oxygen-exposed rats, mice, rabbits, lambs, and primates have been used to model BPD and related neonatal chronic lung disease. Perhaps the best model of human BPD is one in which premature baboons are delivered at 125 or 140 days gestation (term = 185 days), and receive exogenous surfactant and positive pressure ventilation with supplemental oxygen as in clinical practice (343,344). These animals exhibit type II pneumocyte hyperplasia and disrupted vascular development reminiscent of impaired alveolarization in humans (345,346). In newborn rodents, alveolarization occurs during the first few weeks of life (347,348), and hyperoxia has been shown to inhibit lung cell proliferation based on reduced BrdU uptake over the first 72 hr of exposure (349).

Recent studies have led to an appreciation that growth arrest is mediated by cell cycle checkpoints activated in response to damaged DNA. Checkpoints do not permanently arrest cell growth, but rather delay proliferation in the Gl or G2 phases for several hours to days. DNA repair is thought to occur during these delays. DNA damage leads to stabilization of the tumor suppressor protein p53, which inhibits proliferation in the Gl phase of the cell cycle by transcriptionally increasing expression of the cyclin-dependent kinase inhibitor p21 Cipl/WAFl/Sdil (350). As expected when DNA is damaged, hyperoxia increases p53 and p21 in adult and newborn mice (330,332,351,352). Hyperoxia does not inhibit DNA replication in adult p21-deficient mice, which are significantly more sensitive to hyperoxic injury (353). This latter finding suggests that hyperoxia-induced inhibition of cell proliferation through checkpoint activation may be a protective response that allows additional time for repair to occur. Effects on cell proliferation mediated by p21 may also be important during normal postnatal lung development (352).

A study using HeLa cells was one of the first to show that > 40% oxygen directly inhibited cell proliferation in vitro (354). Since histone and thymidine kinases are inhibited in hyperoxic SV40-transformed rat type II epithelial cells (SV40-T2), reduced proliferation is thought to occur at least in part through overt cytotoxicity (355). Other studies with SV40-T2 cells have shown that hyperoxia also increases expression of p21 and inhibits Gl cyclin E-dependent kinases (356). The SV40 large T-antigen also blocks p53 activity and disrupts Gl cyclin kinase complexes during hyperoxia (357). Because p53 is a major factor in regulating p21, it is difficult to separate the roles of the two proteins in mechanistic assessments. It has been argued that p21 may be induced in SV40-T2 cells by TGF-β, a cytokine that is increased in mouse lungs exposed to hyperoxia (358). Other studies using the epithelial mink lung MvlLu cell line and clonal variants lacking TGF-β receptors indicate that hyperoxia inhibits proliferation independent of TGF-β signaling (329). Expression of p21 is not increased during hyperoxia in MvlLu cells, which arrest in S and in G2 (359). In contrast, p53 and p21 are induced in A549 cells that arrest predominantly in Gl. Perhaps the most convincing evidence linking hyperoxia-induced growth arrest in Gl with p53-dependent expression of p21 comes from a study using colon carcinoma HCT116 cells (360). In addition to the parental tumor line that expresses p53 and p21, clonal variants were created in which p53 or p21 was deleted using homologous recombination. Cells deficient in p21 were found to growth arrest in S and G2 when exposed to hyperoxia (77). Among the challenges for future research will be to determine what pulmonary cells in vivo express p21 during hyperoxia, and whether additional checkpoint processes observed in cell lines also occur in the intact lung.

D. Examples of Cell and Animal Studies on Cell Death in Hyperoxic/Oxidant Injury

A common theme in both in vitro and in vivo studies of hyperoxia is that high oxygen concentrations have direct toxicity in killing cells by either apoptosis or necrosis. In fact, the direct vs. indirect effects of hyperoxia and ROS in causing cell death during lung injury are uncertain. In addition to increased TUNEL staining, hyperoxia increases the expression of proteins involved in apoptosis, including p53, Bax, Fas, mitogen-activated protein kinases (MAPKs), and nuclear factor (NF)-κB (330,334,361,362). However, the roles of these proteins in cell killing by hyperoxia remain unclear. In contrast, evidence exists that apoptotic proteins are important in hyperoxic killing. For example, antiapoptotic Bcl-2 levels are elevated in transgenic mice that overexpress IL-6 and are more tolerant to hyperoxia, suggesting that this factor may be cytoprotective (363). The antiapoptotic serine–threonine kinase Akt has also been shown to protect mice from hyperoxia (335). There is also evidence that extracellular signal regulated kinases (ERK) 1 and 2, also known as p42/44 MAPK, may protect rat type II cells recovering from hyperoxia (364). A variety of nonapoptotic mediators and factors are also likely to influence cell death in hyperoxic lung injury in vivo.

The intact lung contains nearly 40 different cell types that may be differentially affected by hyperoxia, and only a fraction of these can currently be isolated in high purity and/or placed in culture. In vitro research has not yet been successful in clarifying several important issues relating to mechanisms of hyperoxia-induced and oxidant-induced cell death. Hyperoxia-induced apoptosis or DNA damage as defined by TUNEL staining or DNA laddering is detected in the RAW 264.7 mouse macrophage cell line (365), but not in many epithelial cell lines. In contrast, failure to exclude vital dyes (an indicator of necrosis) has been reported in A549, MvlLu, HCTl 16, and MLE15 cells exposed to hyperoxia for several days (87,328,359,360). The fact that some cell lines exhibit hyperoxia-induced necrosis, while others exhibit hyperoxia-induced apoptosis, is consistent with the observation that both processes occur in the lungs during hyperoxic injury in vivo (e.g.,(330,334)). Factors contributing to specific pathways of cell death in vitro are still under investigation. Over-expression of Bcl-X$_L$ in Ratla fibrosarcoma cells has been reported to reduce hyperoxia-induced cell death (366). However, another study has reported that

Bcl-X$_L$ does not protect A549 cells against hyperoxic injury (367). Since necrosis may occur when apoptosis cannot be executed properly (298), early expression of antiapoptotic proteins may be involved in hyperoxia-induced cell death in epithelial cell lines in vitro. In addition, cells may become more sensitive to hyperoxia as a result of substratum damage. For example, hyperoxia enhances plasminogen activator activity in pulmonary calf endothelial cells, which could enhance their sensitivity to oxidative stress (368). Further research, including refinements of existing in vitro and in vivo models, will be required in order to better define the mechanisms contributing to hyperoxia-induced cell death.

E. Cellular and Animal Studies on Hyperoxic Lung Injury and Pulmonary Surfactant

Hyperoxic lung injury has been examined extensively for surfactant-related abnormalities and for its response to surfactant replacement therapy. One widely studied animal model of severe acute hyperoxic lung injury is adult rabbits exposed to 100% oxygen (195,197,201,202,369,370). Alveolocapillary permeability in adult rabbits begins to increase after 48 hr in 100% oxygen and reaches a plateau at 64 hr of exposure (195,201,202,370). Rabbits removed to room air at this time exhibit a progressive lung injury that peaks at about 24 hr postexposure. Arterial oxygenation in injured animals is decreased, and bronchoalveolar lavage is found to have increased levels of protein, decreased levels of phospholipid, and elevated minimum surface tension (195,369–371). Consistent with severe surfactant dysfunction in injured animals, pulmonary volumes and compliance are decreased compared to uninjured controls, while lung tissue forces are unchanged based on saline P-V measurements (195). Surfactant metabolism in type II pneumocytes is also altered by this kind of hyperoxic injury. Type II epithelial cells isolated from rabbits exposed to 64 hr of 95–100% oxygen demonstrate loss of NAD(H), ATP, and surfactant metabolic capability (200). In addition, these isolated cells display a cell cycle arrest by the end of the direct hyperoxic exposure (200), providing a direct in vivo correlate with in vitro cell cycling studies. Studies on isolated type II pneumocytes are particularly important in this context, since primary cultures of these cells exposed to hyperoxia in vitro can be affected by culture-associated losses of phenotype.

The direct importance of surfactant dysfunction in the pathophysiology of hyperoxic lung injury has been further demonstrated by surfactant replacement studies in animals (197,198,212,369,370). Intratracheal instillation of calf lung surfactant extract (CLSE, 75 mg/kg) to adult rabbits at the end of a 64 hr exposure to 95–100% oxygen, and again following an additional 12 hr in room air, significantly mitigated the severity of lung injury (369,370). At 24 hr postexposure to hyperoxia, surfactant-treated rabbits had minimum surface tensions of $< 1\,\mathrm{mN/m}$ in lavage compared to values of $26 \pm 2\,\mathrm{mN/m}$ for rabbits receiving saline-placebo. Pulmonary edema was also decreased in surfactant-treated vs. saline-treated rabbits based on lower lavage protein levels (36 ± 3 vs. 60 ± 2 mg/kg) and lower lung wet-to-dry weight ratios (5.6 ± 0.1 vs. 6.3 ± 0.3) (369,370). Total lung capacity and deflation volumes were almost doubled in CLSE-treated rabbits compared to saline-treated rabbits at 24 hr postexposure. Arterial oxygenation was also significantly better in CLSE-treated vs. saline-treated rabbits breathing 100% oxygen during a 20 min measurement period, consistent with a reduced right-to-left shunt from pulmonary atelectasis after surfactant therapy (369,370). Prophylactic administration of CLSE to adult rabbits prior to exposure to 100% oxygen has additionally been found to improve arterial oxygenation and survival time, while decreasing histological evidence of lung injury and atelectasis (197). The ability of exogenous surfactant therapy to mitigate the effects of severe hyperoxia in animals is consistent with a significant mechanistic contribution from surfactant dysfunction in the injury process. Moreover, these findings suggest that exogenous surfactant therapy has the potential to benefit patients with ALI/ARDS (Chapter 15 gives details on clinical surfactant therapy for lung injury).

VIII. Summary

This chapter has provided an overview of cell and animal models used in studying lung injury. Because of the complex pathophysiology of lung injury, and the broad range of cellular and physiological responses that contribute to it, a hierarchy of complementary cell and animal models is required in research investigations. All cell and animal models of lung injury have individual limitations, and different classes of models (e.g., cultured cell lines, cells isolated from lung tissue, whole animal studies) are also subject to constraints in data analysis and interpretation. In addition, results obtained in cell and animal models require extrapolation when applications to human disease are involved. Nonetheless, research in animal and cell models is fundamentally important for defining the mechanistic pathophysiology of acute and chronic lung injury, as well as for identifying interventions able to modulate pulmonary inflammation, antagonize oxidant damage, mitigate surfactant and vascular dysfunction, and facilitate effective tissue remodeling and repair.

Conceptually, several different kinds of in vitro cell models are used in lung injury research, including cultured tumor cell lines, pulmonary cells, and leukocytes. In addition, the behavior of freshly isolated (uncultured) pulmonary cells or leukocytes is also frequently examined in research applications, and cell-specific assessments can also be done in sectioned pulmonary tissue in situ. Examples of cell lines used in lung injury research include epithelial cell lines (e.g., A549 cells, MvlLu cells, MLE15 cells, and HCT116 cells), tracheobronchial cell lines (e.g., BEAS-2B, 16HBE14o- cells), endothelial cell lines (e.g., HMEC cells), and leukocytic cell lines (e.g., RAW 264.7, U937, THP-1 cells). Examples of pulmonary cell populations that can be isolated and studied in suspension or in culture include type II alveolar epithelial cells, pulmonary vascular endothelial cells, airway cells such as Clara cells, and interstitial cells such as fibroblasts.

Although cell-based research can be highly mechanistic, research in animal models of lung injury provides crucial information on responses occurring in the whole organism. Research in animal models also allows investigations on the effects of agents and interventions in mitigating or repairing lung injury, providing a crucial link between laboratory studies and the development of clinical therapies for injury-related pulmonary diseases. A variety of animal models are used in research on lung injury and its therapy. Examples of animal models of ALI/ARDS include: antibody-induced lung injury, aspiration lung injury (e.g., acid, gastric participates, meconium), bacterial-, viral-, or fungal-induced lung injury, fatty acid lung injury, hyperoxic or oxidant-induced lung injury, and several others. Animal models of chronic pulmonary injury or fibrosis include radiation lung injury, drug-induced lung injury (e.g., bleomycin), particulate/fiber-induced lung injury (e.g., silica, asbestos), hyperoxic lung injury (prolonged lower levels of exposure compared to acute injury), and injury from toxicants such as paraquat, phorbol myristate acetate, or butylated hydroxytoluene.

In addition to general descriptions of cell and animal models used in lung injury research, this chapter has also presented a number of examples illustrating specific research assessments from cell and animal studies on hyperoxia-induced and oxidant-induced injury. In particular, examples of in vitro and in vivo assessments are discussed relating to antioxidant defenses, DNA damage (genotoxicity), cell proliferation, cell death, and the function and metabolism of pulmonary surfactant during hyperoxic/oxidant injury. Experience from such research supports the perspective that understanding is enhanced by an integrated approach that examines the consistency of data and interpretations across cell and animal model systems to take advantage of the strengths of each. The utility of this kind of integrative approach is also inherent in much of the research on acute and chronic lung injury detailed in other chapters throughout this book. Further discussion of animal models used in investigating the pathophysiology and therapy of lung injury is given in Chapter 11, which covers the important topic of genetically modified mouse models of pulmonary injury and repair. In addition, Chapter 12 includes coverage on animal and cell models utilized in the broad area of inhalation toxicology research.

Acknowledgment

We gratefully acknowledge the support of grants P30 ES-01247 (J.N.F.), HL-71659 (J.N.F., R.H.N.), HL-56176 (R.H.N., B.A.H., P.R.C.), HL-58774 (M.O.), HL-67392 (M.O.), and HL-03910 (P.C.) from the National Institutes of Health, as well as EPA Airborne Particulate Matter Center grant R827354 (J.N.F.).

References

1. Tao F, Kobzik L. Lung macrophage–epithelial cell interactions amplify particle-mediated cytokine release. Am J Respir Cell Mol Biol 2002; 26(4): 499–505.
2. Hjort MR, Brenyo AJ, Finkelstein JN, Frampton MW, LoMonaco MB, Stewart JC, Johnston CJ, D'Angio CT. Alveolar epithelial cell–macrophage interactions affect oxygen-stimulated interleukin-8 release. Inflammation 2003; 27(3):137–145.
3. Hirano S. Interaction of rat alveolar macrophages with pulmonary epithelial cells following exposure to lipopolysaccharide. Arch Toxicol 1996; 70(3–4): 230–236.
4. Mogel M, Kruger E, Krug HF, Seidel A. A new coculture-system of bronchial epithelial and endothelial cells as a model for studying ozone effects on airway tissue. Toxicol Lett 1998; 96–97:25–32.
5. Aufderheide M, Knebel JW, Ritter D. Novel approaches for studying pulmonary toxicity in vitro. Toxicol Lett 2003; 140–141:205–211.
6. Dethloff LA, Lehnert BE. Pulmonary interstitial macrophages: isolation and flow cytometric comparisons with alveolar macrophages and blood monocytes. J Leukoc Biol 1988; 43(1):80–90.
7. Franke-Ullmann G, Pfortner C, Walter P, Steinmuller C, Lohniann-Matthes ML, Kobzik L. Characterization of murine lung interstitial macrophages in comparison with alveolar macrophages in vitro. J Immunol 1996; 157(7):3097–3104.
8. Gordon S, Crocker PR, Morris L, Lee SH, Perry VH, Hume DA. Localization and function of tissue macrophages. Ciba Found Symp 1986; 118:54–67.
9. Miyamoto K, Schultz E, Heath T, Mitchell MD, Albertine KH, Staub NC. Pulmonary intravascular macrophages and hemodynamic effects of liposomes in sheep. J Appl Physiol 1988; 64(3):1143–1152.
10. Bennett B. Isolation and cultivation in vitro of macrophages from various sources in the mouse. Am J Pathol 1966; 48(1):165–181.
11. Blaschke E, Eklund A, Skog S, Danielsson B. Isolation of human alveolar macrophages and lymphocytes from bronchoalveolar lavage fluid by centrifugal elutriation. Scand J Clin Lab Invest 1985; 45(8):691–696.
12. Brandes ME, Finkelstein JN. Stimulated rabbit alveolar macrophages secrete a growth factor for type II pneumocytes. Am J Respir Cell Mol Biol 1989; 1(2):101–109.
13. Cohn ZA. The isolation and cultivation of mononuclear phagocytes. Methods Enzymol 1974; 32(PartB):758–765.

14. Fox ML. The bovine alveolar macrophage. 1. Isolation, in vitro cultivation, ultrastructure, and phagocytosis. Can J Microbiol 1973; 19(10):1207–1210.

15. Holian A, Scheule RK. Alveolarmacrophage biology. Hosp Pract (Off Ed) 1990; 25(12):53–62.

16. Lavnikova N, Prokhorova S, Helyar L, Laskin DL. Isolation and partial characterization of subpopulations of alveolar macrophages, granulocytes, and highly enriched interstitial macrophages from rat lung. Am J Respir Cell Mol Biol 1993; 8(4):384–392.

17. Myrvik QN. The role of the alveolar macrophage. J Occup Med 1973; 15(3):190–193.

18. Wallaert B, Voisin C. In vitro study of gas effects on alveolar macrophages. Cell Biol Toxicol 1992; 8(3):151–156.

19. Davis GS, Moehring JM, Absher PM, Brody AR, Kelley J, Low RB, Green GM. Isolation and characterization of fibroblasts obtained by pulmonary lavage of human subjects. In Vitro 1979; 15(8):612–623.

20. Kikkawa Y, Yoneda K. The type II epithelial cell of the lung. I. Method of isolation. Lab Invest 1974; 30(l):76–84.

21. Dobbs LG, Mason RJ. Pulmonary alveolar type II cells isolated from rats. Release of phosphatidylcholine in response to beta-adrenergic stimulation. J Clin Invest 1979; 63(3):378–387.

22. Finkelstein JN, Shapiro DL. Isolation of type II alveolar epithelial cells using low protease concentrations. Lung 1982; 160(2):85–98.

23. Finkelstein JN, Maniscalco WM, Shapiro DL. Properties of freshly isolated type II alveolar epithelial cells. Biochim Biophys Acta 1983; 762(3): 398–404.

24. Lafranconi WM, Spall RD, Sipes IG, Duhamel RC, Meezan E, Brendel K. Rapid isolation of type II pneumocytes with magne-tic removal of macrophages. Exp Lung Res 1983; 4(3):191–204.

25. Dobbs LG. Isolation and culture of alveolar type II cells. Am J Physiol 1994; 258(4 Pt 1):L134–147.

26. Shapiro DL, Finkelstein JN, Van Diver T. Isolation of alveolar epithelial cells from lung tissue obtained at autopsy. In Vitro Cell Dev Biol 1989; 25(11):1051–1054.

27. Driscoll KE, Carter JM, Iype PT, Kumari HL, Crosby LL, Aardema MJ, Isfort RJ, Cody D, Chestnut MH, Bums JL, et al. Establishment of immortalized alveolar type II epithelial cell lines from adult rats. In Vitro Cell Dev Biol Anim 1995; 31(7):516–527.

28. Devereux TR. Alveolar type II and Clara cells: isolation and xenobiotic metabolism. Environ Health Perspect 1984; 56:95–101.

29. Kumar V, Cotran RS, Robbins SL. Basic Pathology. 6th ed. Philadelphia: WB Saunders, 1997.

30. Rahman L, Li XY, Donaldson K, Harrison DJ, MacNee W. Glutathione homeostasis in alveolar epithelial cells in vitro and lung in vivo under oxidative stress. Am J Physiol 1995; 269(3 Pt 1):L285–L292.

31. Harrison JH Jr, Porretta CP, Leming K. Purification of murine pulmonary type II cells for flow cytometric cell cycle analysis. Exp Lung Res 1995; 21(3):407–421.

32. Corti M, Brody AR, Harrison JH. Isolation and primary culture of murine alveolar type II cells. Am J Respir Cell Mol Biol 1996; 14(4):309–315.

33. Rice WR, Conkright JJ, Na CL, Bcegami M, Shannon JM, Weaver TE. Maintenance of the mouse type II cell phenotype in vitro. Am J Physiol Lung Cell Mol Physiol 2002; 283(2):L256–L264.

34. Roper JM, Staversky RJ, Finkelstein JN, Keng PC, O'Reilly MA. Identification and isolation of mouse type II cells on the basis of intrinsic expression of enhanced green fluorescent protein. Am J Physiol Lung Cell Mol Physiol 2003; 285(3):L691–L700.

35. Gruenert DC, Finkbeiner WE, Widdicombe JH. Culture and transformation of human airway epithelial cells. Am J Physiol 1995; 268(3 Pt l): L347–L360.

36. Koyama S, Rennard SI, Shoji S, Romberger D, Linder J, Ertl R, Robbins RA. Bronchial epithelial cells release chemoattractant activity for monocytes. Am J Physiol 1989; 257(2 Pt l):L130–L136.

37. Takizawa H. Airway epithelial cells as regulators of airway inflammation [Rev]. Int J Mol Med 1998; l(2):367–378.

38. Rosenfeld MA, Chu CS, Seth P, Danel C, Banks T, Yoneyama K, Yoshimura K, Crystal RG. Gene transfer to freshly isolated human respiratory epithelial cells in vitro using a replication-deficient adenovirus containing the human cystic fibrosis transmembrane conductance regulator cDNA. Hum Gene Ther 1994; 5(3):331–342.

39. Zhang S, Smartt H, Holgate ST, Roche WR. Growth factors secreted by bronchial epithelial cells control myofibroblast proliferation: an in vitro co-culture model of airway remodeling in asthma. Lab Invest 1999; 79(4): 395–405.

40. Lang DS, Jorres RA, Muckc M, Sicgfricd W, Magnussen H. Interactions between human broncho epithelial cells and lung fibroblasts after ozone exposure in vitro. Toxicol Lett 1998; 96–97:13–24.

41. Kaartinen L, Nettesheim P, Adler KB, Randell SH. Rat tracheal epithelial cell differentiation in vitro. In Vitro Cell Dev Biol Anim 1993; 29A(6):481–492.

42. Adler KB, Holden-Stauffer WJ, Repine JE. Oxygen metabolites stimulate release of high-molecular-weight glycoconjugates by cell and organ cultures of rodent respiratory epithelium via an arachidonic acid-dependent mechanism. J Clin Invest 1990; 85(l):75–85.

43. Cohn LA, Adler KB. In vitro studies of mechanisms of lung injury in the rodent. Toxicol Pathol 1991; 19(4 Pt l):419–427.

44. Wu R, Nolan E, Turner C. Expression of tracheal differentiated functions inserum-free hormone-supplemented medium. J Cell Physiol 1985; 125(2): 167–181.

45. Forbes II. Human airway epithelial cell lines for in vitro drug transport and metabolism studies Pharm Sci Technol Today 2000; 3(1):18–27.

46. Reiss TF, Gruenert DC, Nadel JA, Jacoby DB. Infection of cultured human airway epithelial cells by influenza A virus. Life Sci 1991; 49(16):1173–1181.

47. Alcorn JL, Smith ME, Smith JF, Margraf LR, Mendelson CR. Primary cell culture of human type II pneumocytes—maintenance of a differentiated

phenotype and transfection with recombinant adenoviruses. Amer J Respir Cell Mol Biol 1997; 17:672–682.

48. Lechner JF, Haugen A, Autrup H, McClendon IA, Trump BF, Harris CC. Clonal growth of epithelial cells from normal adult human bronchus. Cancer Res 1981; 41(6):2294–2304.

49. Lechner JF, Haugen A, McClendon IA, Pettis EW. Clonal growth of normal adult human bronchial epithelial cells in a serum-free medium. In Vitro 1982; 18(7):633–642.

50. Kelsen SG, Mardini IA, Zhou S, Benovic JL, Higgins NC. A technique to harvest viable tracheobronchial epithelial cells from living human donors. Am J Respir Cell Mol Biol 1992; 7(l):66–72.

51. Martin LD, Norford D, Voynow J, Adler KB. Response of human airway epithelium in vitro to inflammatory mediators: dependence on the state of cellular differentiation. Chest 2000; 117(5 suppl 1):267S.

52. Kinnula VL, Adler KB, Ackley NJ, Crapo JD. Release of reactive oxygen species by guinea pig tracheal epithelial cells in vitro. Am J Physiol 1992; 262(6 Pt l):L708–L712.

53. Widdicombe JG, Pack RJ. The Clara cell. Eur J Respir Dis 1982; 63(3): 202–220.

54. Massaro GD, Singh G, Mason R, Plopper CG, Malkinson AM, Gail DB. Biology of the Clara cell. Am J Physiol 1994; 266(1 Pt l):L101–L106.

55. Plopper CG, Nisbio SJ, Alley JL, Kass P, Hyde DM. The role of the nonciliated bronchiolar epithelial (Clara) cell as the progenitor cell during bronchiolar epithelial differentiation in the perinatal rabbit lung. Am J Respir Cell Mol Biol 1992; 7(6):606–613.

56. Devereux TR, Fouts JR. Isolation and identification of Clara cells from rabbit lung. In Vitro 1980; 16(11):958–968.

57. Boyd MR, Reznik-Schuller HM. Metabolic basis for the pulmonary Clara cell as a target for pulmonary carcinogenesis. Toxicol Pathol 1984; 12(1):56–61.

58. Oreffo VI, Morgan A, Richards RI. Isolation of Clara cells from the mouse lung. Environ Health Perspect 1990; 85:51–64.

59. Martin J, Dinsdale D, White IN. Characterization of Clara and type II cells isolated from rat lung by fluorescence-activated flow cytometry. Biochem J 1983; 295(Pt l):73–80.

60. Ryan US. Isolation and culture of pulmonary endothelial cells. Environ Health Perspect 1984; 56:103–114.

61. Lombard Y, Bartholeyns J, Chokri M, Ulinger D, Hartmann D, Dumont S, Kaufmann SH, Landmann R, Loor F, Poindron P. Establishment and characterization of long-term cultured cell lines of murine resident macrophages. J Leukoc Biol 1988; 44(5):391–401.

62. Carley WW, Tanoue L, Merker M, Gillis CN. Isolation of rabbit pulmonary microvascular endothelial cells and characterization of their angiotensin converting enzyme activity. Pulm Pharmacol 1990; 3(l):35–40.

63. Magee JC, Stone AE, Oldham KT, Guice KS. Isolation, culture, and characterization of rat lung microvascular endothelial cells. Am J Physiol 1994; 267(4 Pt 1):L433–L441.

64. Gerritsen ME, Shen CP, McHugb MC, Atkinson WJ, Kiely JM, Milstone DS, Luscinskas FW, Gimbrone MA Jr. Activation-dependent isolation and culture of murine pulmonary microvascular endothelium. Microcirculation 1995; 2(2):151–163.

65. Muanza K, Gay F, Behr C, Scherf A. Primary culture of human lung microvessel endothelial cells: a useful in vitro model for studying *Plasmodium falciparum*-infected erythrocyte cytoadherence. Res Immunol 1996; 147(3): 149–163.

66. Kawanami O. The endothelium of the pulmonary micro vessels. Nippon Ika Daigaku Zasshi 1997; 64(6):495–511.

67. Ryan US, White LA, Lopez M, Ryan JW. Use of microcarriers to isolate and culture pulmonary microvascular endothelium. Tissue Cell 1982; 14(3): 597–606.

68. Dong QG, Bemasconi S, Lostaglio S, De Calmanovici RW, Martin-Padura I, Breviario F, Garlanda C, Ramponi S, Mantovani A, Vecchi A. A general strategy for isolation of endothelial cells from murine tissues. Characterization of two endothelial cell lines from the murine lung and subcutaneous sponge implants. Arterioscler Thromb Vase Biol 1997; 17(8):1599–1604.

69. Ryan US, Clements E, Habliston D, Ryan JW. Isolation and culture of pulmonary artery endothelial cells. Tissue Cell 1978; 10(3):535–554.

70. Habliston DL, Wbitaker C, Hart MA, Ryan US, Ryan JW. Isolation and culture of endothelial cells from the lungs of small animals. Am Rev Respir Dis 1979; 119(6):853–868.

71. Gorfien SF, Kitazawa K, Brodkin MA, Noble B, Andres GA, Brentjens JR. Studies on cell proliferation and tracer localization in the kidneys of guinea pigs with experimental autoimmune anti-tubular basement membrane nephritis. J Pathol 1988; 155(2):171–180.

72. Gorfien S, Spector A, DeLuca D, Weiss S. Growth and physiological functions of vascular endothelial cells in a new serum-free medium (SFM). Exp Cell Res 1993; 206(2):291–301.

73. Lieber M, Smith B, Szakal A, Nelson-Rees W, Todaro G. A continuous tumor-cell line from a human lung carcinoma with properties of type II alveolar epithelial cells. Int J Cancer 1976; 17(l):62–70.

74. Smith BT. Cell line A549: a model system for the study of alveolar type II cell function. Am Rev Respir Dis 1977; 115(2):285–293.

75. Nardone LL, Andrews SB. Cell line A549 as a model of the type II pneumocyte. Phospholipid biosynthesis from native and organometallic precursors. Biochim Biophys Acta 1979; 573(2):276–295.

76. Mason RJ, Williams MC. Phospholipid composition and ultrastructure of A549 cells and other cultured pulmonary epithelial cells of presumed type II cell origin. Biochim Biophys Acta 1980; 617(l):36–50.

77. Balis JU, Bumgarner SD, Paciga JE, Paterson JF, Shelley SA. Synthesis of lung surfactant-associated glycoproteins by A549 cells: description of an in vitro model for human type II cell dysfunction. Exp Lung Res 1984; 6(3–4):197–213.

78. DeForge LE, Preston AM, Takeuchi E, Kenney J, Boxer LA, Remick DG. Regulation of interleukin 8 gene expression by oxidant stress. J Biol Chem 1993; 268(34):25568–25576.

79. Crestani B, Comillet P, Dehoux M, Rolland C, Guenounou M, Aubier M. Alveolar type II epithelial cells produce interleukin-6 in vitro and in vivo. Regulation by alveolar macrophage secretory products. J Clin Invest 1994; 94(2):731–740.

80. Smart SJ, Casale TB. Pulmonary epithelial cells facilitate TNF-alpha-induced neutrophil chemotaxis. A role for cytokine networking. J Immunol 1994; 152(8):4087–4094.

81. Standiford TJ, Kunkel SL, Basha MA, Chensue SW, Lynch JP III, Toews GB, Westwick J, Strieter RM. Interleukin-8 gene expression by a pulmonary epithelial cell line. A model for cytokine networks in the lung. J Clin Invest 1990; 86(6):1945–1953.

82. Paine R III, Chavis A, Gaposchkin D, Christensen P, Mody CH, Turka LA, Toews GB. A factor secreted by a human pulmonary alveolar epithelial-like cell line blocks T-cell proliferation between Gl and S phase. Am J Respir Cell Mol Biol 1992; 6(6):658–666.

83. Brown KA, Vora A, Biggerstaff J, Edgell CJ, Oikle S, Mazure G, Taub N, Meager A, Hill T, Watson C, et al. Application of an immortalized human endothelial cell line to the leucocyte:endothelial adherence assay. J Immunol Methods 1993; 163(l):13–22.

84. Koyama S, Sato E, Nomura H, Kubo K, Miura M, Yamashita T, Nagai S, Izumi T. Monocyte chemotactic factors released from type II pneumocyte-like cells in response to TNF-alpha and EL-1 alpha. Eur Respir J 1999; 13(4): 820–828.

85. Wikenheiser KA, Vorbroker DK, Rice WR, Clark JC, Bachurski CJ, Oie HK, Whitsett JA. Production of immortalized distal respiratory epithelial cell lines from surfactant protein C/simian virus 40 large tumor antigen transgenic mice. Proc Natl Acad Sci USA 1993; 90(23):11029–11033.

86. Barrett EG, Johnston C, Oberdorster G, Finkelstein JN. Silica-induced chemokine expression in alveolar type II cells is mediated by TNF-alpha. Am J Physiol 1998; 275(6 Pt 1):L1110–L1119.

87. O'Reilly MA, Staversky RJ, Finkelstein JN, Keng PC. Activation of the G2 cell cycle checkpoint enhances survival of epithelial cells exposed to hyperoxia. Am J Physiol Lung Cell Mol Physiol 2003; 284(2):L368–L375.

88. Salinas D, Sparkman L, Berhane K, Boggaram V. Nitric oxide inhibits surfactant protein B gene expression in lung epithelial cells. Am J Physiol Lung Cell Mol Physiol 2003; 285(5):L1153–1165.

89. Waters CM, Ridge KM, Sunio G, Venetsanou K, Sznajder JI. Mechanical stretching of alveolar epithelial cells increases Na(+)-K(+)-ATPase activity. J Appl Physiol 1999; 87(2):715–721.

90. Dwyer-Nield LD, Miller AC, Neighbors BW, Dinsdale D, Malkinson AM. Cytoskeletal architecture in mouse lung epithelial cells is regulated by protein-kinase C-alpha and calpain II. Am J Physiol 1996; 270(4 Pt l): L526–L534.

91. Nicks KM, Droms KA, Fossli T, Smith GJ, Malkinson AM. Altered function of protein kinase C and cyclic adenosine monophosphate-dependent protein kinase in a cell line derived from a mouse lung papillary tumor. Cancer Res 1989; 49(18):5191–5198.

92. Malkinson AM, Dwyer-Nield LD, Rice PL, Dinsdale D. Mouse lung epithelial cell lines — tools for the study of differentiation and the neoplastic phenotype. Toxicology 1997; 123(1–2):53–100.

93. Driscoll KE, Simpson L, Carter J, Hassenbein D, Leikauf GD. Ozone inhalation stimulates expression of a neutrophil chemotactic protein, macrophage inflammatory protein 2. Toxicol Appl Pharmacol 1993; 119(2):306–309.

94. Leikauf GD, Simpson LG, Santrock J, Zhao Q, Abbinante-Nissen J, Zhou S, Driscoll KE. Airway epithelial cell responses to ozone injury. Environ Health Perspect 1995; 103(suppl 2):91–95.

95. Wallaert B, Gosset P, Boitelle A, Tonnel AB. In vitro assessment of environmental toxicology using alveolar cells as target. Cell Biol Toxicol 1996; 12(4–6):251–256.

96. Wallaert B, Fahy O, Tsicopoulos A, Gosset P, Tonnel AB. Experimental systems for mechanistic studies of toxicant-induced lung inflammation. Toxicol Lett 2000; 112–113:157–163.

97. Garrett NE, Campbell JA, Stack HF, Jackson MA, Lewtas J. Cellular toxicity in Chinese hamster ovary cell cultures. II. A statistical appraisal of sensitivity with the rabbit alveolar macrophage, Syrian hamster embryo, BALB 3T3 mouse, and human neonatal fibroblast cell systems. Environ Res 1983; 32(2):466–473.

98. Samet JM, Reed W, Ghio AJ, Devlin RB, Carter JD, Dailey LA, Bromberg PA, Madden MC. Induction of prostaglandin H synthase 2 in human airway epithelial cells exposed to residual oil fly ash. Toxicol Appl Pharmacol 1996; 141(1):159–168.

99. Becker S, Soukup JM, Gilmour MI, Devlin RB. Stimulation of human and rat alveolar macrophages by urban air particulates: effects on oxidant radical generation and cytokine production. Toxicol Appl Pharmacol 1996; 141(2): 637–648.

100. Valentine R. An in vitro system for exposure of lung cells to gases: effects of ozone on rat macrophages. J Toxicol Environ Health 1985; 16(1):115–126.

101. Fisher GL, Placke ME. In vitro models of lung toxicity. Toxicology 1987; 47(1–2):71–93.

102. Aufderheide M, Mohr U. CULTEX — an alternative technique for cultivation and exposure of cells of the respiratory tract to airborne pollutants at the air/liquid interface. Exp Toxicol Pathol 2000; 52(3):265–270.

103. Voisin C, Aerts C, TomeL AB, Petitprez A, Plancke Y. The human alveolar macrophage. Methods of extraction and study of cellular behavior in in vitro survival. Ann Inst Pasteur Lille 1971; 22:283–292.

104. Voisin C, Aerts C, Tonnel AB, Houdret JL, Ramon P. Survival in gaseous phase and reconstitution "in vitro" of the natural microenvironment of alveolar macrophages. Pathol Biol (Paris) 1975; 23(6):453–459.

105. Holm BA, Notter RH. Surfactant therapy in adult respiratory distress syndrome and lung injury. In: Shapiro DL, Notter RH, eds. Surfactant Replacement Therapy. New York: Alan R Liss, 1989:273–304.

106. Lewis JF, Jobe AH. Surfactant and the adult respiratory distress syndrome. Am Rev Respir Dis 1993; 147:218–233.

107. Seeger W, Giinther A, Walmrath HD, Grimminger F, Lasch HG. Alveolar surfactant and adult respiratory distress syndrome. Pathogenic role and therapeutic prospects. Clin Invest 1993; 71:177–190.

108. Lachmann B, van Daal G-J. Adult respiratory distress syndrome: animal models. In: Robertson B, van Golde LMG, Batenburg JJ, eds. Pulmonary Surfactant: From Molecular Biology to Clinical Practice. Amsterdam: Elsevier Science Publishers, 1992:635–663.

109. Robertson B. Surfactant inactivation and surfactant replacement in experimental models of ARDS. Acta Anaesthesiol 1991; 35(suppl):22–28.

110. Windsor ACJ. Acute lung injury: what have we learned from animal models? Am J Med Sci 1993; 306:111–116.

111. Cantor JO, ed. Handbook of Animal Models of Pulmonary Disease Boca Raton, FL: CRC Press, 1989.

112. Fine A, Goldstein RH. Animal models of pulmonary fibrosis. In: Crystal RG, West JB, Weibel ER, Barnes PJ I, eds. The Lung: Scientific Foundations. 2nd ed. Philadelphia: Lippincott-Raven, 1997.

113. Gil J, ed. Models of Lung Disease. New York: Marcel Dekker, 1990.

114. Notter RH. Lung Surfactants: Basic Science and Clinical Applications. New York: Marcel Dekker, Inc, 2000.

115. Hunninghake GW, Gadek JE, Kawanami O, Ferrans VJ, Crystal RG. Inflammatory and immune processes in human lung in health and disease: evaluation by bronchoalveolar lavage. Am J Pathol 1979; 97:146–206.

116. Lachmann B, Hallman M, Bergman K-C. Respiratory failure following antilung serum: study on mechanisms associated with surfactant system damage. Exp Lung Res 1987; 12:163–180.

117. Fujita Y, Kogishi K, Suzuki Y. Pulmonary damage induced in mice by a monoclonal antibody to proteins associated with pig pulmonary surfactant. Exp Lung Res 1988; 14:247–260.

118. Suzuki Y, Robertson B, Fujita Y, Grossman G. Respiratory failure in mice caused by a hybridoma making antibodies to the 15kDa surfactant apoprotein. Acta Anaesthesiol Scand 1988; 32:283–289.

119. Scherzer H, Ward PA. Lung injury produced by immune complexes of varying composition. J Immunol 1978; 121:947–952.

120. Pearson DJ, Mentnech MS, Gamble M, Taylor G, Green FHY. Acute pulmonary injury induced by immune complexes. Exp Lung Res 1980; 1: 323–334.

121. Lamm WJ, Albert RK. Surfactant replacement improves lung recoil in rabbit lungs after acid aspiration. Am Rev Respir Dis 1990; 142:1279–1283.

122. Kobayashi T, Ganzuka M, Taniguchi J, Nitta K, Murakami S. Lung lavage and surfactant replacement for hydrochloric acid aspiration in rabbits. Acta Anaesthesiol Scand 1990; 34:216–221.

123. Zucker A, Holm BA, Wood LDH, Crawford G, Ridge K, Sznajder IA. Exogenous surfactant with PEEP reduces pulmonary edema and improves lung function in canine aspiration pneumonitis. J Appl Physiol 1992; 73:679–686.

124. Schlag G, Strohmaier W. Experimental aspiration trauma: comparison of steroid treatment versus exogenous natural surfactant. Exp Lung Res 1993; 19:397–405.

125. Knight PR, Kurek C, Davidson BA, Nader ND, Patel A, Sokolowski J, Notter RH, Holm BA. Acid aspiration increases sensitivity to increased ambient oxygen concentrations. Am J Physiol 2000; 278:L1240–L1247.

126. Nader ND, Knight PR, Bobela I, Davidson BA, Johnson KJ, Morin F. High-dose nitric oxide inhalation increases lung injury after gastric aspiration. Anesthesiology 1999; 91:741–749.

127. Nader-Djalal K, Knight PR, Davidson BA, Johnson K. Hyperoxia exacerbates microvascular injury following acid aspiration. Chest 1997; 112: 1607–1614.

128. Nader-Djalal N, Knight PR, Thusu K, Davidson BA, Holm BA, Johnson KJ, Dandona P. Reactive oxygen species contribute to oxygen-related lung injury after acid aspiration. Anesth Analg 1998; 87:127–133.

129. Sun B, Curstedt T, Robertson B. Exogenous surfactant improves ventilation efficiency and alveolar expansion in rats with meconium aspiration. Am J Respir Crit Care Med 1996; 154:764–770.

130. Cochrane CG, Revak SD, Merritt TA, Schraufstatter U, Hoch RC, Henderson C, Andersson S, Takamori H, Oades ZG. Broncho alveolar lavage with KL4-surfactant in models of meconium aspiration syndrome. Pediatr Res 1998; 44:705–715.

131. Al-Mateen KB, Dailey K, Grimes MM, Gutcher GR. Improved oxygenation with exogenous surfactant administration in experimental meconium aspiration syndrome. Pediatr Pulmonol 1994; 17:75–80.

132. Sun B, Curstedt T, Song GW, Robertson B. Surfactant improves lung function and morphology in newborn rabbits with meconium aspiration. Biol Neonate 1993; 63:96–104.

133. Sun B, Curstedt T, Robertson B. Surfactant inhibition in experimental meconium aspiration. Acta Paediatr 1993; 82:182–189.

134. Paranka MS, Walsh WF, Stancombe BB. Surfactant lavage in a piglet model of meconium aspiration syndrome. Pediatr Res 1992; 31:625–628.

135. Marik PE. Aspiration pneumonitis and aspiration pneumonia. N Engl J Med 2001; 344:665–671.

136. Taeusch HW, Ballard RA, eds. Avery's Diseases of the Newborn. 7th ed. Philadelphia: WB Saunders, 1998.

137. Taussig LM, Landau LI, Le Souef PN, Morgan WJ, Martinez FD, Sly PDE, eds. Pediatric Respiratory Medicine. St Louis: Mosby, 1999.

138. Davidson BA, Knight PR, Helinski JD, Nader ND, Shanley TP, Johnson KJ. The role of tumor necrosis factor alpha in the pathogenesis of aspiration pneumonitis in rats. Anesthesiology 1999; 91:486–499.

139. Folkesson HF, Matthay MA, Hebert C, Broaddus CV. Acid aspiration-induced lung injury in rabbits is mediated by IL-8 dependent mechanisms. J Clin Invest 1995; 96:107–116.

140. Goldman G, Welbourn R, Kobzik L, Valeri CR, Shepro D, Hechtman HB. Tumor necrosis factor-alpha mediates acid aspiration-induced systemic organ injury. Ann Surg 1990; 212:513–520.

141. Knight PR, Druskovich V, Tait AR, Johnson KJ. The role of neutrophils, oxidants and proteases in the pathogenesis of acid pulmonary injury. Anesthesiology 1992; 77:772–778.

142. Knight PR, Rutter T, Tait AR, Coleman E, Johnson KJ. Pathogenesis of gastric particulate lung injury: a comparison and interaction with acidic pneumonitis. Anesth Analg 1993; 77:754–760.

143. Shanley TP, Davidson BA, Nader ND, Bless N, Vasi N, Ward PA, Johnson KJ, Knight PR. The role of macrophage inflammatory protein-2 (MIP-2) in aspiration-induced lung injury. Crit Care Med 2000; 28:2437–2444.

144. Findlay RD, Taeusch HW, Walther FJ. Surfactant replacement therapy for meconium aspiration syndrome. Pediatrics 1996; 97:48–52.

145. Auten RL, Notter RH, Kendig JW, Davis JM, Shapiro DL. Surfactant treatment of full-term newborns with respiratory failure. Pediatrics 1991; 87: 101–107.

146. Lotze A, Mitchell BR, Bulas DI, Zola EM, Shalwitz RA, Gunkel JH. Multicenter study of surfactant (beractant) use in the treatment of term infants with severe respiratory failure. J Pediatr 1998; 132:40–47.

147. Lotze A, Knight GR, Martin GR, Bulas DI, Hull WM, O'Donnell RM, Whitsett JA, Short BL. Improved pulmonary outcome after exogenous surfactant therapy for respiratory failure in term infants requiring extracorporeal membrane oxygenation. J Pediatr 1993; 122:261–268.

148. Braunwald E, Fauci AS, Kasper DL, Hauser SL, Longo DL, Jameson JL, eds. Harrison's Principles of Internal Medicine 15th ed. New York: McGraw-Hill, 2001.

149. Murray JF, Nadel JA, Mason RJ, Boushey HA. Textbook of Respiratory Medicine 3rd ed. New York: WB Saunders, 2000.

150. Hall JB, Schmidt GA, Wood LDH. Principles of Critical Care 2nd ed. New York: McGraw-Hill, 1998.

151. Fletcher MA, McKenna TM, Owens EH, Nadkarni VM. Effects of in vivo pentoxifylline treatment on survival and ex vivo vascular contractility in a rat lipopolysaccharide shock model. Circ Shock 1992; 36:74–80.

152. Lutz C, Carney D, Finck C, Picone A, Gatto L, Paskanik A, Langenbeck E, Nieman G. Aerosolized surfactant improves pulmonary function in endotoxin-induced lung injury. Am J Respir Grit Care Med 1998; 158: 840–845.

153. Lutz CJ, Picone A, Gatto LA, Paskanik A, Landas S, Nieman G. Exogenous surfactant and positive end-expiratory pressure in the treatment of endotoxin-induced lung injury. Crit Care Med 1998; 26:1379–1389.

154. Tashiro K, Li W-Z, Yamada K, Matsumoto Y, Kobayashi T. Surfactant replacement reverses respiratory failure induced by intratracheal endotoxin in rats. Crit Care Med 1995; 23:149–156.

155. Gonzalez PK, Zhuang J, Doctrow SR, Malfroy B, Benson PF, Menconi MJ, Fink MP. Role of oxidant stress in the adult respiratory distress syndrome:

evaluation of a novel antioxidant strategy in a porcine model of endotoxin-induced acute lung injury. Shock 1996; 6:S23–S26.

156. Hoffmann H, Hatherill JR, Crowley J, Harada H, Yonemaru M, Zheng H, Ishizaka A, Raffia TA. Early post-treatment with pentoxifylline or dibutyril cAMP attenuates *Escherichia coli*-induced acute lung injury in guinea pigs. Am Rev Respir Dis 1991; 143:289–293.

157. Pittet J-F, Wiener-Kronish JP, Serokiv V, Matthay MA. Resistance of the alveolar epithelium to injury from septic shock in sheep. Am J Respir Crit Care Med 1995; 151:1093–1100.

158. Oldham KT, Guice KS, Stetson PS, Wolfe RR. Bacteremia-induced suppression of alveolar surfactant production. J Surg Res 1989; 47:397–402.

159. Michie HR, Mangue DR, Spriggs A, Revhaug S, O'Dwyer CA, Dinarello , Carem A, Wolf SM, Wilmore DW. Detection of circulating tumor necrosis factor after endotoxin administration. N Engl J Med 1988; 318:1481–1486.

160. Russo TA, Bartholomew LA, Davidson BA, Helinski JD, Carlino UB, Knight PR, Beers M, Atochina EN, Notter RH, Holm BA. Total extracellular surfactant is increased but abnormal in arat model of Gram-negative bacterial pneumonitis. Am J Physiol 2002; 283:L655–L663.

161. Meyrick B, Brigham KL. Acute effects of *Escherichia coli* endotoxin on the pulmonary microcirculation of anesthesitized sheep. Lab Invest 1990; 62:355–362.

162. Broaddus VC, Boylan AM, Hoeffel JM, Kim KJ, Sadik M, Chuntharapai A, Hebert CA. Neutralization of IL-8 inhibits neutrophil influx in a rabbit model of endotoxin-induced injury. J Immunol 1994; 152:2960–2967.

163. Brigham KL, Meyrick B. Endotoxin and lung injury. Am Rev Respir Dis 1986; 133:913–927.

164. Brigham K, Woolverton WC, Blake CH, Staub NC. Increased sheep lung vascular permeability caused by Pseudomonas bacteremia. J Clin Invest 1974; 54:792–804.

165. Mustard RA, Fusher J, Hayman S, Matlow A, Mullen JBM, Odumeru J, Roomi MW, Schouten BD, Swanson HT. Cardiopulmonary responses to Pseudomonas septicemia in swine: an improved model of the adult respiratory distress syndrome. Lab Anim Sci 1989; 39:37–43.

166. Berger JI, Gibson RL, Redding GI, Standaert TA, Clarke WR, Truog WE. Effect of inhaled nitric oxide during group B streptococcal sepsis in piglets. Am Rev Respir Dis 1993; 147:1080–1086.

167. Sherman MP, Campbell LA, Merritt TA, Long WA, Gunkel JH, Curstedt T, Robertson B. Effect of different surfactants on pulmonary group B streptococcal infection in premature rabbits. J Pediatr 1994; 125:939–947.

168. Eijking EP, van Daal GJ, Tenbrinck R, Luyenduijk A, Sluiters JF, Hannappel E, Lachmann B. Effect of surfactant replacement on *Pneumocystis carinii* pneumonia in rats. Intensive Care Med 1990; 17:475–478.

169. Sheehan PM, Stokes DC, Yeh Y, Hughes WT. Surfactant phospholipids and lavage phospholipase A2 in experimental *Pneumocystis carinii* pneumonia. Am Rev Respir Dis 1986; 134:526–531.

170. Wright TW, Notter RH, Wang Z, Harmsen AG, Gigliotti F. Pulmonary inflammation disrupts surfactant function during *P. carinii* pneumonia. Infect Immun 2001; 69:758–764.

171. Wright TW, Gigliotti F, Finkelstein JN, McBride JT, An CL, Harmsen AG. Immune-mediated inflammation directly impairs pulmonary function, contributing to the pathogenesis of *Pneumocystis carinii* pneumonia. J Clin Invest 1999; 104:1307–1317.

172. Wright TW, Johnston CJ, Harmsen AG, Finkelstein JN. Analysis of cytokine gene expression in the lungs of *Pneumocystis carinii*-infected mice. Am J Respir Cell Mol Biol 1997; 17:491–500.

173. Atochina EN, Beck JM, Scanlon ST, Preston AM, Beers M. *P. carinii* pneumonia alters expression and distribution of lung collectin SP-A and SP-D. J Lab Clin Med 2001; 137:429–439.

174. Atochina EN, Beers MF, Scanlon ST, Preston AM, Beck JM. *P. carinii* induces selective alterations in component expression and biophysical activity of lung surfactant. Am J Physiol 2000; 278:L599–L609.

175. van Daal GJ, Bos JAH, Eijking EP, Gommers D, Hannappel E, Lachmann B. Surfactant replacement therapy improves pulmonary mechanics in end-stage influenza A pneumonia in mice. Am Rev Respir Dis 1992; 145:859–863.

176. van Schaik SM, Vargas I, Welliver RC, Enhorning G. Surfactant dysfunction develops in BALB/c mice infected with respiratory syncytial virus. Pediatr Res 1997; 42:169–173.

177. van Daal GI, Eijking EP, So KL, Fievez RB, Sprenger MJW, van Dam DW, Erdmann W, Lachmann B. Acute respiratory failure during pneumonia indeced by Sendai virus. Adv Exp Med Biol 1992; 316:319–326.

178. van Daal GJ, So KL, Gommers D, Eijking EP, Fievez RB, Sprenger MJ, van Dam DW, Lachmann B. Intratracheal surfactant administration restores gas exchange in experimental adult respiratory distress syndrome associated with viral pneumonia. Anesth Analg 1991; 72:589–595.

179. Malik AB. Pulmonary edema after pancreatitis: role of humoral factors. Circ Shock 1983; 10:71–80.

180. Hall SB, Hyde RW, Notter RH. Changes in subphase surfactant aggregates in rabbits injured by free fatty acid. Am J Respir Crit Care Med 1994; 149:1099–1106.

181. Hall SB, Notter RH, Smith RJ, Hyde RW. Altered function of pulmonary surfactant in fatty acid lung injury. J Appl Physiol 1990; 69:1143–1149.

182. Zelter M, Escudier BJ, Hoeffel JM, Murray JF. Effects of aerosolized artificial surfactant on repeated oleic acid injury in sheep. Am Rev Respir Dis 1990; 141:1014–1019.

183. Shuster D. ARDS: clinical lessons from the oleic acid model of acute lung injury. Am J Respir Crit Care Med 1994; 149:245–260.

184. Shah NS, Nakayama DK, Jacob TD, Nishio I, Imai T, Billiar TR, Exler R, Yousera SA, Motoyama EK, Peitzman AB. Efficacy of inhaled nitric oxide in oleic acid-induced acute lung injury. Crit Care Med 1997; 25:153–158.

185. Zhu GF, Sun B, Niu S, Cai YY, Lin K, Lindwall R, Robertson B. Combined surfactant therapy and inhaled nitric oxide in rabbits with oleic acid-induced

acute respiratory distress syndrome. Am J Respir Crit Care Med 1998; 158:437–443.

186. Ashbaugh DG, Uzawa T. Respiratory and hemodynamic changes after injection of free fatty acids. J Surg Res 1968; 8:417–423.

187. Niewoehner D, Rice K, Sinha A, Wangensteen D. Injurious effects of lysophosphatidylcholine on barrier properties of alveolar epithelium. J Appl Physiol 1987; 63:1979–1986.

188. Hall SB, Lu ZR, Venkitaraman AR, Hyde RW, Notter RH. Inhibition of pulmonary surfactant by oleic acid: mechanisms and characteristics. J Appl Physiol 1992; 72:1708–1716.

189. D'Angio CT, Finkelstein JN. Oxygen regulation in gene expression: a study in opposites [Rev]. Molec Gen Metab 2000; 71:371–380.

190. Clark JM, Lambertsen CJ. Pulmonary oxygen toxicity: a review. Pharmacol Rev 1971; 23:37–133.

191. Deneke SM, Fanburg BL. Normobaric oxygen toxicity of the lung. N Engl J Med 1980; 303:76–86.

192. Roberts RJ, Frank L. Developmental consequences of oxygen toxicity. In: Kacew S, Reasor MJ, eds. Toxicology of the Newborn. New York: Elsevier, 1984:141–171.

193. Bhandari V. Developmental differences in the role of interleukins in hyperoxic lung injury in animal models. Front Biosci 2002; 7:dl624–d1633.

194. Ingbar DH. Mechanisms of repair and remodeling following acute lung injury. Clin Chest Med 2000; 21(3):589–616.

195. Holm BA, Notter RH, Siegle J, Matalon S. Pulmonary physiological and surfactant changes during injury and recovery from hyperoxia. J Appl Physiol 1985; 59:1402–1409.

196. Holm BA, Notter RH, Leary JF, Matalon S. Alveolar epithelial changes in rabbits following a 21 day exposure to 60% O_2. J Appl Physiol 1987; 62: 2230–2236.

197. Loewen GM, Holm BA, Milanowski L, Wild LM, Notter RH, Matalon S. Alveolar hyperoxic injury in rabbits receiving exogenous surfactant. J Appl Physiol 1989; 66:1987–1992.

198. Engstrom PC, Holm BA, Matalon S. Surfactant replacement attenuates the increase in alveolar permeability in hyperoxia. J Appl Physiol 1989; 67: 688–693.

199. Huang YC, Caminiti SP, Fawcett TA, Moon RE, Fracica PJ, Miller FJ, Young SL, Piantadosi CA. Natural surfactant and hyperoxic lung injury in primates. I. Physiology and biochemistry. J Appl Physiol 1994; 76:991–1001.

200. Holm BA, Matalon S, Finkelstein JN, Notter RH. Type II pneumocyte changes during hyperoxic lung injury and recovery. J Appl Physiol 1988; 65:2672–2678.

201. Matalon S, Egan EA. Effects of 100% O_2 breathing on permeability of alveolar epithelium to solute. J Appl Physiol 1981; 50:859–863.

202. Matalon S, Egan EA. Interstitial fluid volumes and albumin spaces in pulmonary oxygen toxicity. J Appl Physiol 1984; 57:1767–1722.

203. Walther FJ, David-Cu R, Lopez SL. Antioxidant-surfactant liposomes mitigate hyperoxic lung injury in premature rabbits. Am J Physiol 1995; 269:L613–L617.

204. Matalon S, Holm BA, Baker RR, Whitfield K, Freeman BA. Characterization of antioxidant activities of pulmonary surfactant mixtures. Biochim Biophys Acta 1990; 1035:121–127.

205. Padmanabhan RV, Gudapaty R, Liener IE, Schwartz BA, Hoidal JR. Protection against pulmonary oxygen toxicity in rats by the intratracheal administration of liposome-encapsulated superoxide dismutase or catalase. Am Rev Respir Dis 1985; 132:164–167.

206. Tanswell A, Freeman B. Liposome-entrapped antioxidant enzymes prevent lethal O_2 toxicity in the newborn rat. J Appl Physiol 1987; 63:347–352.

207. Barnard ML, Baker RR, Matalon S. Mitigation of oxidant injury to lung microvasculature by intratracheal instillation of antioxidant enzymes. Am J Physiol 1993; 265:L340–L345.

208. Walther FJ, Nunex F, David-Cu R, Hill KE. Mitigation of pulmonary oxygen toxicity in rats by intratracheal instillation of polyethylene glycol-conjugated antioxidant enzymes. Pediatr Res 1993; 33:332–335.

209. Adawi A, Zhang Y, Baggs R, Finkelstein J, Phipps R. Disruption of the CD40–CD40 ligand system prevents an oxygen-induced respiratory distress syndrome. Am J Pathol 1998; 152:651–657.

210. Langley SC, Kelly FJ. N-acetylcysteine ameliorates hyperoxic lung injury in the preterm guinea pig. Biochem Pharmacol 1993; 45:841–846.

211. Haagsman HP, White RT, Schilling J, Lau K, Benson BJ, Golden J, Hawgood S, Clements JA. Studies on the structure of lung surfactant protein SP-A. Am J Physiol 1989; 257:L421–L429.

212. Novotny WE, Hudak BB, Matalon S, Holm BA. Hyperoxic lung injury reduces exogenous surfactant clearance in vitro. Am J Respir Crit Care Med 1995; 151:1843–1847.

213. Holm BA, Notter RH. Pulmonary surfactant effects in sublethal hyperoxic lung injury. In: Taylor AE, Matalon S, eds. In: Physiology of Oxygen Radicals. Bethesda, MD: American Physiological Society Press, 1986: 71–86.

214. Brandes ME, Finkelstein JN. The production of alveo-lar macrophage-derived growth-regulating proteins in response to lung injury. Toxicol Lett 1990; 54(l):3–22.

215. D Angio CT, Johnston CJ, Wright TW, Reed CK, Finkelstein JN. Chemokine mRNA alterations in newborn and adult mouse lung during acute hyperoxia. Exp Lung Res 1998; 24(5):685–702.

216. D'Angio CT, Finkelstein JN, Lomonaco MB, Paxhia A, Wright SA, Baggs RB, Notter RH, Ryan RM. Changes in surfactant protein gene expression in a neonatal rabbit model of hyperoxia-induced frbrosis. Am J Physiol 1997; 272(4 Pt l):L720–L730.

217. Coalson JJ, King RJ, Winter VT, Prihoda TJ, Anzueto AR, Peters JI, Johanson WG. O_2- and pneumonia-induced lung injury. I. Pathological and morphometric studies. J Appl Physiol 1989; 67:346–356.

218. King RJ, Coalson JJ, Seidenfeld JJ, Anzueto AR, Smith DB, Peters JI. O_2- and pneumonia-induced lung injury. II. Properties of pulmonary surfactant. J Appl Physiol 1989; 67:357–365.

219. Fracica PJ, Knapp MJ, Piantadosi CA, Takeda K, Fulkerson WJ, Coleman RE, Wolfe WG, Crapo JD. Responses of baboons to prolonged hyperoxia: physiology and qualitative pathology. J Appl Physiol 1991; 71: 2352–2362.

220. Fracica PJ, Knapp MJ, Crapo JD. Patterns of progression and markers of lung injury in rodents and subhuman primates exposed to hyperoxia. Exp Lung Res 1988; 14:869–885.

221. Parsons P, Gillesis M, Moore E, Moore F, Worthen G. Neutrophil response to endotoxin in the adult respiratory distress syndrome: role of CD14. Am J Respir Cell Mol Biol 1995; 13:152–160.

222. Ward JA, Roberts RJ. Effect of hyperoxia on phosphatidylcholine synthesis, secretion, uptake and stability in the newborn rabbit lung. Biochim Biophys Acta 1984; 796:42–50.

223. Ward JA, Roberts RJ. Hyperoxia effects on pulmonary pressure:volume characteristics and lavage surfactant phospholipid in the newborn rabbit. Biol Neonate 1984; 46:139–148.

224. Ward JA, Roberts RJ. Vitamin E inhibition of the effects of hyperoxia on the pulmonary surfactant system of the newborn rabbit. Pediatr Res 1984; 18:329–334.

225. Johnston CJ, Wright TW, Reed CK, Finkelstein JN. Comparison of adult and newborn pulmonary cytokine mRNA expression after hyperoxia. Exp Lung Res 1997; 23(6):537–552.

226. Charafeddine L, DAngio CT, Richards JL, Stripp BR, Finkelstein JN, Orlowski CC, LoMonaco MB, Paxhia A, Ryan RM. Hyperoxia increases keratinocyte growth factor mRNA expression in neonatal rabbit lung. Am J Physiol 1999; 276(1 Pt l):L105–L113.

227. Lachmann B, Robertson B, Vogel J. In vivo lung lavage as an experimental model of the respiratory distress syndrome. Acta Anaesthesiol Scand 1980; 24:231–236.

228. Lachmann B, Fujiwara T, Chida S, Morita T, Konishi M, Nakamura K, Maeta H. Surfactant replacement therapy in experimental adult respiratory distress syndrome (ARDS). In: Cosmi EV, Scarpelli EM, eds. Pulmonary Surfactant System. Amsterdam: Elsevier, 1993:221–235.

229. Kobayashi T, Kataoka H, Ueda T, Murakami S, Takada Y, Kobuko M. Effect of surfactant supplementation and end expiratory pressure in lung-lavaged rabbits. J Appl Physiol 1984; 57:995–1001.

230. Berggren P, Lachmann B, Curstedt T, Grossmann G, Robertson B. Gas exchange and lung morphology after surfactant replacement in experimental adult respiratory distress induced by repeated lung lavage. Acta Anaesthesiol Scand 1986; 30:321–328.

231. Walther FJ, Hernandez-Juviel J, Bruni R, Waring A. Spiking Survanta with synthetic surfactant peptides improves oxygenation in surfactant-deficient rats. Am J Respir Grit Care Med 1997; 156:855–861.

232. Lewis JF, Goffm J, Yue P, McCaig LA, Bjarneson D, Veldhuizen RAW. Evaluation of exogenous surfactant treatment strategies in an adult model of acute lung injury. J Appl Physiol 1996; 80:1156–1164.

233. Balaraman V, Meister J, Ku TL, Sood SL, Tarn E, Killeen J, Uyehara CFT, Egan E, Easa D. Lavage administration of dilute surfactants after acute lung injury in neonatal piglets. Am J Respir Crit Care Med 1998; 158:12–17.

234. van Der Beek J, Plotz F, van Overbeek F, Heikamp A, Beekhuis H, Wildevuur C, Oklen A, Bambang OS. Distribution of exogenous surfactant in rabbits with severe respiratory failure: the effect of volume. Pediatr Res 1993; 34:154–158.

235. Hamer D, Germann P-G, Hauschke D. Effects of rSP-C surfactant on oxygenation and histology in a rat-lung-lavage model of acute lung injury. Am J Respir Crit Care Med 1998; 158:270–278.

236. Walther F, Hernandez-Juviel J, Bruni R, Waring AJ. Protein composition of synthetic surfactant affects gas exchange in surfactant-deficient rats. Pediatr Res 1998; 43:666–673.

237. Moen A, Yu X-Q, Almaas R, Curstedt T, Saugstad OD. Acute effects on systemic circulation after intratracheal instillation of Curosurf or Survanta in surfactant-depleted newborn piglets. Acta Paediatr 1998; 87:297–303.

238. Hamer D, Germann P-G, Hauschke D. Comparison of rSP-C surfactant with natural and synthetic surfactants after late treatment in a rat model of the acute respiratory distress syndrome. Br J Pharmacol 1998; 124:1083–1090.

239. Gommers D, Eijking EP, van't Veen A, Lachmann B. Bronchoalveolar lavage with a diluted surfactant suspension prior to surfactant instillation improves the effectiveness of surfactant therapy in experimental acute respiratory distress syndrome (ARDS). Intensive Care Med 1998; 24:494–500.

240. Ito Y, Gofin I, Veldhuizen R, Joseph M, Fjarneson J, McCaig L, Yao L-J, Marcou J, Lewis J. Timing of exogenous surfactant administration in a rabbit model of acute lung injury. J Appl Physiol 1996; 80:1357–1364.

241. Krause MF, Lienhart H-G, Haberstroh J, Hoebn T, Shulte-Monting J, Leititis JU. Effect of inhaled nitric oxide on intrapulmonary right-to-left shunting in two rabbit models of saline lavage-induced surfactant deficiency and meconium instillation. Eur J Pediatr 1998; 157:410–415.

242. Gommers D, Hartog A, van't Veen A, Lachmann B. Improved oxygenation by nitric oxide is enhanced by prior lung reaeration with surfactant, rather than positive end-expiratory pressure, in lung-lavaged rabbits. Crit Care Med 1997; 25:1868–1873.

243. Kunc L, Kuncova R, Holusa R, Soldan F. Physical properties and biochemistry of lung surfactant following vagotomy. Respiration 1978; 35:192–197.

244. Berry D, Hcegami M, Jobe A. Respiratory distress and surfactant inhibition following vagotomy in rabbits. J Appl Physiol 1986; 61:1741–1748.

245. Crittenden DJ, Beckman DL. Traumatic head injury and pulmonary damage. J Trauma 1982; 22:766–769.

246. Ducker TB, Simmonds RL. Increased intracranial pressure and pulmonary edema. II. The hemodynamic response of dogs and monkeys to increase intracranial pressure. J Neurosurg 1968; 28:118–123.

247. Goldenberg VE, Buckingham S, Sommers SC. Pulmonary alveolar lesions in vagotomized rats. Lab Invest 1967; 16:693–705.

248. Lewis JF, Ikegami M, Jobe AH. Altered surfactant function and metabolism in rabbits with acute lung injury. J Appl Physiol 1990; 69:2303–2310.

249. Harris JD, Jackson F, Moxley MA, Longmore WJ. Effect of exogenous surfactant instillation on experimental acute lung injury. J Appl Physiol 1989; 66:1846–1851.

250. Lewis JF, Ikegami M, Jobe AH. Metabolism of exogenously administered surfactant in the acutely injured lungs of adult rabbits. Am Rev Respir Dis 1992; 145:19–23.

251. Lewis J, Ikegami M, Higuchi R, Jobe A, Absolom D. Nebulized vs instilled exogenous surfactant in an adult lung injury model. J Appl Physiol 1991; 71:1270–1276.

252. Ueda T, Dcegami M. Change in properties of exogenous surfactant in injured rabbit lung. Am J Respir Crit Care Med 1996; 153:1844–1849.

253. Ryan RM, Morris RE, Rice WR, Ciraolo G, Whitsett JA. Binding and uptake of pulmonary surfactant protein (SP)-A by pulmonary type II epithelial cells. J Histochem Cytochem 1989; 37:429–440.

254. Ryan SF, Barrett CR, Liau DF. Nitrosourethane induced lung injury. In: Cantor JO, ed. Handbook of Animal Models of Pulmonary Disease. Boca Raton, FL: CRC Press, 1989:67–106.

255. Cosset JM, Socie G, Dubray B, Girinsky T, Fourquet A, Gluckman E. Single dose versus fractionated total body irradiation before bone marrow transplantation: radiobiological and clinical considerations. Int J Radiat Oncol Biol Phys 1994; 30(2):477–492.

256. Penney DP, Siemann DW, Rubin P, Maltby K. Morphological correlates of fractionated radiation of the mouse lung: early and late effects. Int J Radiat Oncol Biol Phys 1994; 29(4):789–804.

257. Byhardt RW, Martin L, Pajak TF, Shin KII, Emami B, Cox JD. The influence of field size and other treat-ment factors on pulmonary toxicity following hyperfractionated irradiation for inoperable non-small cell lung cancer (NSCLC)—analysis of a radiation therapy oncology group (RTOG) protocol. Int J Radiat Oncol Biol Phys 1993; 27(3):537–544.

258. Rezvani M, Hopewell JW. The response of the pig lungto fractionated doses of X rays. Br J Radiol 1990; 63(745):41–50.

259. Awwad HK, el Badawy S, el Ghamrawy K, el Mongy M, Rizk S. Late tissue reactions after single-fraction sequential half-body irradiation (HBI) in patients with non-Hodgkin's lymphomas. Int J Radiat Oncol Biol Phys 1990; 19(5): 1229–1232.

260. Kozubek S, Vodvarka P. Late effects of fractionated irradiation of normal tissue. Neoplasma 1984; 31(2):203–212.

261. Adamson IY, Bowden DH. Endothelial injury and repair in radiation-induced pulmonary fibrosis. Am J Pathol 1983; 112:224–230.

262. Penney DP, Siemann DW, Rubin P, Shapiro DL, Finkelstein J, Cooper RA Jr. Morphologic changes reflecting early and late effects of irradiation of the distal lung of the mouse: a review. Scan Electron Microsc 1982; 4:413–425.

263. Coggle JE, Lambert BE, Moores SR. Radiation effects in the lung. Environ Health Perspect 1986; 70:261–291.

264. Dubravsky NB, Dubrawsky C, Jampolis S, Mason K, Hunter N, Withers HR. Long-term effects of pulmonary damage in mice on lung weight, compliance, hydroxyproline content and formation of metastases. Br J Radiol 1981; 54(648):1075–1080.

265. Rubin P, Finkelstein JN, Siemann DW, Shapiro DL, Van Houtte P, Penney DP. Predictive biochemical assays for late radiation effects. Int J Radiat Oncol Biol Phys 1986; 12(4):469–476.

266. McBride WH. Cytokine cascades in late normal tissue radiation responses. Int J Radiat Oncol Biol Phys 1995; 33(1):233–234.

267. Franko AJ, Sharplin J. Development of fibrosis after lung irradiation in relation to inflammation and lung function in a mouse strain prone to fibrosis. Radiat Res 1994; 140(3):347–355.

268. Panos RJ, Bak PM, Simonet WS, Rubin JS, Smith LJ. Intratracheal instillation of keratinocyte growth factor decreases hyperoxia-induced mortality in rats. J Clin Invest 1995; 96(4):2026–2033.

269. Johnston CJ, Williams JP, Okunieff P, Finkelstein JN. Radiation-induced pulmonary fibrosis: examination of chemokine and chemokine receptor families. Radiat Res 2002; 157(3):256–265.

270. Rubin P, Finkelstein J, Shapiro D. Molecular biology mechanisms in the radiation induction of pulmonary injury syndromes: interrelationship between the alveolar macrophage and the septal fibroblast. Int J Radiat Oncol Biol Phys 1992; 24(1):93–101.

271. Rubin P, Johnston CJ, Williams JP, McDonald S, Finkelstein JN. A perpetual cascade of cytokines postirradiation leads to pulmonary fibrosis. Int J Radiat Oncol Biol Phys 1995; 33(1):99–109.

272. Asada K, Ogushi F, Tani K, Maniwa K, Ichikawa W, Endo T, Haung L, Nishioka Y, Sone S, Ogura T. The role of cell-associated interleukin-1 in bleomycin-induced pulmonary fibrosis. Tokushima J Exp Med 1996; 43(3–4): 79–86.

273. Beetz A, Messer G, Oppel T, van Beuningen D, Peter RU, Kind P. Induction of interleukin 6 by ionizing radiation in a human epithelial cell line: control by corticosteroids. Int J Radiat Biol 1997; 72(1):33–43.

274. Behrends IL, Peter RU, Hintermeier-Knabe R, Eissner G, Holler E, Bornkamm GW, Caughman SW, Degitz K. Ionizing radiation induces human intercellular adhesion molecule-1 in vitro. J Invest Dermatol 1994; 103(5): 726–730.

275. Buttner C, Skupin A, Reimann T, Rieber EP, Unteregger G, Geyer P, Frank KH. Local production of interleukin-4 during radiation-induced pneumonitis and pulmonary fibrosis in rats: macrophages as a prominent source of interleukin-4. Am J Respir Cell Mol Biol 1997; 17(3):315–325.

276. Chang CM, Limanni A, Baker WH, Dobson ME, Kalinich JF, Patchen ML. Sublethal gamma irradiation increases IL-1 alpha, IL-6, and TNF-alpha mRNA levels in murine hematopoietic tissues. J Interferon Cytokine Res 1997; 17(9):567–572.

277. Chen Y, Williams J, Ding I, Hemady E, Liu W, Smudzin T, Finkelstein JN, Rubin P, Okunieff P. Radiation pneumonitis and early circulatory cytokine markers. Semin Radiat Oncol 2002; 12(1, suppl 1):26–33.

278. Fedorocko P, Egyed A, Vacek A. Irradiation induces increased production of haemopoietic and proinflammatory cytokines in the mouse lung. Int J Radiat Biol 2002; 78(4):305–313.

279. Haveman J, Geerdink AG, Rodermond HM. TNF, IL-1 and IL-6 in circulating blood after total-body and localized irradiation in rats. Oncol Rep 1998; 5(3):679–683.

280. Hosoi Y, Miyachi H, Matsumoto Y, Enomoto A, Nakagawa K, Suzuki N, Ono T. Induction of interleukin-1beta and interleukin-6 mRNA by low doses of ionizing radiation in macrophages. Int J Cancer 2001; 96(5):270–276.

281. O'Brien-Ladner A, Nelson ME, Kimler BF, Wesselius LJ. Release of interleukin-1 by human alveolar macrophages after in vitro irradiation. Radiat Res 1993; 136(1):37–41.

282. Roberts CM, Foulcher E, Zaunders JJ, Bryant DH, Freund J, Cairns D, Penny R, Morgan GW, Breit SN. Radiation pneumonitis: a possible lymphocyte-mediated hypersensitivity reaction. Ann Intern Med 1993; 118(9): 696–700.

283. Martin C, Romero S, Sanchez-Paya J, Massuti B, Arriero JM, Hernandez L. Bilateral lymphocytic alveolitis: a common reaction after unilateral thoracic irradiation. Eur Respir J 1999; 13(4):727–732.

284. Van Haecke P, Vansteenkiste J, Paridaens R, Van der Schueren E, Demedts M. Chronic lymphocytic alveolitis with migrating pulmonary infiltrates after localized chest wall irradiation. Acta Clin Belg 1998; 53(1):39–43.

285. Gibson PG, Bryant DH, Morgan GW, Yeates M, Fernandez V, Penny R, Breit SN. Radiation-induced lung injury: a hypersensitivity pneumonitis? Ann Intern Med 1988; 109(4):288–291.

286. Adawi A, Zhang Y, Baggs R, Rubin P, Williams J, Finkelstein JN, Phipps R. Blockage of CD40–CD40 ligand interac-tions protects against radiation-induced pulmonary inflammation and fibrosis. Clin Immunol Immunopath 1998; 89:222–230.

287. Johnston CJ, Stripp BR, Piedbeouf B, Wright TW, Mango GW, Reed CK, Finkelstein JN. Inflammatory and epithelial responses in mouse strains that differ in sensitivity to hyperoxic injury. Exp Lung Res 1998; 24(2):189–202.

288. Thornton SC, Walsh BJ, Bennett S, Robbins JM, Foulcher E, Morgan GW, Penny R, Breit SN. Both in vitro and in vivo irradiations are associated with induction of macrophage-derived fibroblast growth factors. Clin Exp Immunol 1996; 103(1):67–73.

289. Fulkerson WJ Jr, Gockerman JP. Pulmonary disease induced by drugs. In: Fishman AP, ed. Pulmonary Diseases Disorders. 2nd ed. New York, NY: Mcgraw-Hill Book Company, 1988:793–811.

290. Adamson IY, Bowden DH. The pathogenesis of bleomycm-induced pulmonary fibrosis in mice. Am J Pathol 1974; 77:185–197.

291. Idell S, James KK, Giles C, Fair DS, Thrall RS. Abnormalities of pathways of fibrin turnover in lung lavage of rats with oleic acid and bleomycin-induced lung injury support alveolar fibrin deposition. Am J Pathol 1989; 135: 387–399.

292. Snider GL, Celli BR, Goldstein RH, O'Brien JJ, Lucey EC. Chronic interstitial pulmonary fibrosis produced in hampsters by endotracheal bleomycin:

lung volumes, volume–pressure relations, carbon monoxide uptake, and arterial blood gas studies. Am Rev Respir Dis 1978; 117:289–297.

293. Snider GL, Hayes JA, Korthy AL. Chronic interstitial pulmonary fibrosis produced in hampsters by endotracheal bleomycin: pathology and stereology. Am Rev Respir Dis 1978; 117:1099–1108.

294. McCullough B, Collins JF. Bleomycin-induced diffuse interstitial pulmonary fibrosis in baboons. J Clin Invest 1978; 61:79–88.

295. Imlay JA, Linn S. DNA damage and oxygen radical toxicity. Science 1988; 240(4857):1302–1309.

296. Gille JJ, Joenje H. Cell culture models for oxidative stress: superoxide and hydrogen peroxide versus normobaric hyperoxia. Mutat Res 1992; 275(3–6):405–414.

297. Michiels C, Raes M, Toussaint O, Remade J. Importance of Se-glutathione peroxidase, catalase, and Cu/Zn-SOD for cell survival against oxidative stress. Free Radic Biol Med 1994; 17(3):235–248.

298. Raffray M, Cohen GM. Apoptosis and necrosis in toxicology: a continuum or distinct modes of cell death? Pharmacol Ther 1997; 75(3):153–177.

299. Wispe JR, Warner BB, Clark JC, Dey CR, Neuman J, Glasser SW, Crapo JD, Chang LY, Whitsett JA. Human Mn-superoxide dismutase in pulmonary epithelial cells of transgenic mice confers protection from oxygen injury. J Biol Chem 1992; 267(33):23937–23941.

300. Asikainen TM, Huang TT, Taskinen E, Levonen AL, Carlson E, Lapatto R, Epstein CJ, Raivio KO. Increased sensitivity of homozygous Sod2 mutant mice to oxygen toxicity. Free Radic Biol Med 2002; 32(2):175–186.

301. Das KC, Guo XL, White CW. Induction of thioredoxin and thioredoxin reductase gene expression in lungs of newborn primates by oxygen. Am J Physiol 1999; 276(3 Pt l):L530–L539.

302. Das KC, Pahl PM, Guo XL, White CW. Induction of peroxiredoxin gene expression by oxygen in lungs of newborn primates. Am J Respir Cell Mol Biol 2001; 25(2):226–232.

303. Otterbein LE, Kolls JK, Mantell LL, Cook JL, Alam J, Choi AM. Exogenous administration of heme oxygenase-1 by gene transfer provides protection against hyperoxia-induced lung injury. J Clin Invest 1999; 103(7):1047–1054.

304. Gille JJ, van Berkel CG, Joenje H. Mechanism of hyperoxia-induced chromosomal breakage in Chinese hamster cells. Environ Mol Mutagen 1993; 22(4):264–270.

305. Jyonouchi H, Sun S, Abiru T, Chareancholvanich S, Ingbar DH. The effects of hyperoxic injury and antioxidant vitamins on death and proliferation of human small airway epithelial cells. Am J Respir Cell Mol Biol 1998; 19(3):426–436.

306. Lee PJ, Alam J, Wiegand GW, Choi AM. Overexpression of heme oxygenase-1 in human pulmonary epithelial cells results in cell growth arrest and increased resistance to hyperoxia. Proc Natl Acad Sci USA 1996; 93(19):10393–10398.

307. Otterbein LE, Choi AM. Heme oxygenase: colors of defense against cellular stress. Am J Physiol Lung Cell Mol Physiol 2000; 279(6):L1029–L1037.

308. Holm BA, Hudak BB, Keicher L, Cavanaugh C, Baker RR, Matalon S. Mechanisms of oxidant-induced damage to type II pneumocyte phospholipid

metabolism and protection with PEG-catalase. Am J Physiol 1991; 261:C751–C757.

309. Gilbert D, Gerschman R, Cohen J, Sherwood W. The influence of high oxygen pressures on the viscosity of solutions of sodium desoxyribonucleic acid and of sodium algenate. J Am Chem Soc 1957; 79:5677–5680.

310. Cadenas E, Davies KJ. Mitochondrial free radical generation, oxidative stress, and aging. Free Radical Biol Med 2000; 29(3–4):222–230.

311. Joenje H. Genetic toxicology of oxygen. Mutat Res 1989; 219(4):193–208.

312. Zweier JL, Duke SS, Kuppusamy P, Sylvester JT, Gabrielson EW. Electron paramagnetic resonance evidence that cellular oxygen toxicity is caused by the generation of superoxide and hydroxyl free radicals. FEBS Lett 1989; 252(1–2):12–16.

313. Benitez-Bribiesca L, Sanchez-Suarez P. Oxidative damage, bleomycm, and gamma radiation induce different types of DNA strand breaks in normal lymphocytes and thymocytes. A comet assay study. Ann N Y Acad Sci 1999; 887:133–149.

314. Gille JJ, van Berkel CG, Mullaart E, Vijg J, Joenje H. Effects of lethal exposure to hyperoxia and to hydrogen peroxide on NAD(H) and ATP pools in Chinese hamster ovary cells. Mutat Res 1989; 214(1):89–96.

315. Gille JJ, Joenje H. Chromosomal instability and progressive loss of chromosomes in HeLa cells during adaptation to hyperoxic growth conditions. Mutat Res 1989; 219(4):225–230.

316. Hudak BB, Tufariello J, Sokolowski J, Maloney C, Holm BA. Inhibition of poly (ADP-ribose) polymerase preserves surfactant synthesis after hydrogen peroxide exposure. Am J Physiol 1995; 269:L59–L64.

317. Patel A, Sokolowski J, Knight P, Davidson BA, Holm BA. Halothane potentiation of H_2O_2-induced inhibition of surfactant synthesis: the role of type II cell energy status. Anesth Analg 2002; 94:943–947.

318. Dizdaroglu, M. Measurement of radiation-induced damage to DNA at the molecular level. Int J Radiat Biol 1992; 61(2):175–183.

319. Burcham PC. Genotoxic lipid peroxidation products: their DNA damaging properties and role in formation of endogenous DNA adducts. Mutagenesis 1998; 13(3):287–305.

320. Cleveland L. The whole life cycle of the chromosomes and their coiling systems. Trans Am Phil Soc 1949; 39:1–100.

321. Conger A, Fairchild L. Breakage of chromosomes by oxygen. Proc Natl Acad Sci (USA) 1952; 38:289–299.

322. Gille JI, van Berkel CG, Joenje H. Mutagenicity of metabolic oxygen radicals in mammalian cell cultures. Carcinogenesis 1994; 15(12):2695–2699.

323. Gille JJ, van Berkel CG, Joenje H. Effect of iron chelators on the cytotoxic and genotoxic action of hyperoxia in Chinese hamster ovary cells. Mutat Res 1992; 275(1):31–39.

324. Cacciuttolo MA, Trinh L, Lumpkin JA, Rao G. Hyperoxia induces DNA damage in mammalian cells. Free Radical Biol Med 1993; 14(3):267–276.

325. Rancourt RC, Hayes DD, Chess PR, Keng PC, O'Reilly MA. Growth arrest in Gl protects against oxygen-induced DNA damage and cell death. J Cell Physiol 2002; 193(1):26–36.

326. Olive PL, Banath JP. Induction and rejoining of radiation-induced DNA single-strand breaks: "tail moment" as a function of position in the cell cycle. Mutat Res 1993; 294(3):275–283.

327. O'Reilly MA. DNA damage and cell cycle checkpoints in hyperoxic lung injury: braking to facilitate repair. Am J Physiol 2001; 281(2):L291–L305.

328. Kazzaz JA, Xu J, Palaia TA, Mantell L, Fein AM, Horowitz S. Cellular oxygen toxicity. Oxidant injury without apoptosis. J Biol Chem 1996; 271(25):15182–15186.

329. Rancourt RC, Staversky RJ, Keng PC, O'Reilly AM. Hyperoxia inhibits proliferation of MvlLu epithelial cells independent of TGF-beta signaling. Am J Physiol 1999; 277(6 Pt 1):L1172–1178.

330. Barazzone C, Horowitz S, Donati YR, Rodriguez I, Piguet PF. Oxygen toxicity in mouse lung: pathways to cell death. Am J Respir Cell Mol Biol 1998; 19(4):573–581.

331. Mc Grath-Morrow SA, Stahl J. Apoptosis in neonatal murine lung exposed to hyperoxia. Am J Respir Cell Mol Biol 2001; 25(2):150–155.

332. O'Reilly MA, Staversky RJ, Stripp BR, Finkelstein JN. Exposure to hyperoxia induces p53 expression in mouse lung epithelium. Am J Respir Cell Mol Biol 1998; 18(1):43–50.

333. Waxman AB, Einarsson O, Seres T, Knickelbein RG, Warshaw JB, Johnston R, Homer RH, Elias JA. Targeted lung expression of interleukin-11 enhances murine tolerance of 100% oxygen and diminishes hyperoxia-induced DNA fragmentation. J Clin Invest 1998; 101(9):1970–1982.

334. O'Reilly MA, Staversky RJ, Huyck HL, Watkins RH, LoMonaco MB, D'Angio CT, Baggs RB, Maniscalco WM, Pryhuber GS. Bcl-2 family gene expression during severe hyperoxia induced lung injury. Lab Invest 2000; 80(12):1845–1854.

335. Lu Y, Parkyn L, Otterbein LE, Kureishi Y, Walsh K, Ray A, Ray P. Activated Akt protects the lung from oxidant-induced injury and delays death of mice. J Exp Med 2001; 193(4):545–549.

336. Auten RL, Whorton MH, Mason SN. Blocking neutrophil influx reduces DNA damage in hyperoxia-exposed newborn rat lung. Am J Respir Cell Mol Biol 2002; 26(4):391–397.

337. Ansari B, Coates PJ, Greenstein BD, Hall PA. In situ end-labelling detects DNA strand breaks in apoptosis and other physiological and pathological states. J Pathol 1993; 170(1):1–8.

338. Grasl-Kraupp B, Ruttkay-Nedecky B, Koudelka H, Bukowska K, Bursch W, Schulte-Hermann R. In situ detection of fragmented DNA (TUNEL assay) fails to discriminate among apoptosis, necrosis, and autolytic cell death: a cautionary note. Hepatology 1995; 21(5):1465–1468.

339. Evans MJ, Bils RF. Identification of cells labeled with tritiated thymidme in the pulmonary alveolar walls of the mouse. Am Rev Respir Dis 1969; 100(3):372–378.

340. Evans MJ, Hackney JD, Bils RF. Effects of a high concentration of oxygen on cell renewal in the pulmonary alveoli. Aerospace Med 1969; 40(12): 1365–1368.

341. Northway WH Jr, Rosan RC, Porter DY. Pulmonary disease following respirator therapy of hyaline-membrane disease. Bronchopulmonary dysplasia. N Engl J Med 1967; 276(7):357–368.

342. Eber E, Zach MS. Long term sequelae of bronchopulmonary dysplasia (chronic lung disease of infancy). Thorax 2001; 56(4):317–323.

343. Coalson JJ, Kuehl TJ, Escobedo MB, Hilliard JL, Smith F, Meredith K, Null DM Jr, Walsh W, Johnson D, Robotham JL. A baboon model of bronchopulmonary dysplasia. II. Pathologic features. Exp Mol Pathol 1982; 37(3): 335–350.

344. Coalson JJ, Winter VT, Siler-Khodr T, Yoder BA. Neonatal chronic lung disease in extremely immature baboons. Am J Respir Crit Care Med 1999; 160(4):1333–1346.

345. Maniscalco WM, Watkins RH, O'Reilly MA, Shea CP. Increased epithelial cell proliferation in very premature baboons with chronic lung disease. Am J Physiol Lung Cell Mol Physiol 2002; 283(5):L991–L1001.

346. Maniscalco WM, Watkins RH, Pryhuber GS, Bhatt A, Shea C, Huyck H. Angiogenic factors and alveolar vasculature: development and alterations by injury in very premature baboons. Am J Physiol Lung Cell Mol Physiol 2002; 282(4):L811–L823.

347. Massaro D, Teich N, Maxwell S, Massaro GD, Whitney P. Postnatal development of alveoli. Regulation and evidence for a critical period in rats. J Clin Invest 1985; 76(4):1297–1305.

348. Ten Have-Opbroek AA. The development of the lung in mammals: an analysis of concepts and findings. Am J Anat 1981; 162(3):201–219.

349. Warner BB, Stuart LA, Papes RA, Wispe JR. Functional and pathological effects of prolonged hyperoxia in neonatal mice. Am J Physiol 1998; 275(1Pt):L110 L117.

350. el-Deiry WS, Tokino T, Velculescu VE, Levy DB, Parsons R, Trent JM, Lin D, Mercer WE, Kinzler KW, Vogelstein B. WAF1, a potential mediator of p53 tumor suppression. Cell 1993; 75(4):817–825.

351. O'Reilly MA, Staversky RJ, Watkins RH, Maniscalco WM. Accumulation of p21(Cipl/WAFl) during hyperoxic lung injury in mice. Am J Respir Cell Mol Biol 1998; 19(5):777–785.

352. McGrath SA. Induction of p21WAF/CIPl during hyperoxia. Am J Respir Cell Mol Biol 1998; 18(2):179–187.

353. O'Reilly MA, Staversky RJ, Watkins RH, Reed CK, de Mesy Jensen KL, Finkelstein JN, Keng PC. The cyclin-dependent kinase inhibitor p21 protects the lung from oxidative stress. Am J Respir Cell Mol Biol 2001; 24:703–710.

354. Rueckert RR, Mueller GC. Effect of oxygen tension on HeLa cell growth. Cancer Res 1960; 20:944–949.

355. Clement A, Edeas M, Chadelat K, Brody JS. Inhibition of lung epithelial cell proliferation by hyperoxia. Posttranscriptional regulation of proliferation-related genes. J Clin Invest 1992; 90(5):1812–1818.

356. Corroyer S, Maitre B, Cazals V, Clement A. Altered regulation of Gl cyclins in oxidant-induced growth arrest of lung alveolar epithelial cells. Accumulation of inactive cyclin E-DCK2 complexes. J Biol Chem 1996; 271(41):25117–25125.

357. Xiong Y, Zhang H, Beach D. Subunit rearrangement of the cyclin-dependent kinases is associated with cellular transformation. Genes Dev 1993; 7(8): 1572–1583.

358. O'Reilly MA, Staversky RJ, Flanders KC, Johnston CJ, Finkelstein JN. Temporal changes in expression of TGF-beta isoforms in mouse lung exposed to oxygen. Am J Physiol 1997; 272(1 Pt l):L60–L67.

359. Rancourt RC, Keng PC, Helt CE, O'Reilly MA. The role of p21 Cipl/WAFl in growth of epithelial cells exposed to hyperoxia. Am J Physiol 2001; 280(24 Pt 4):L617–L626.

360. Helt CE, Rancourt RC, Staversky RJ, O'Reilly MA. p53-Dependent induction of p21 Cipl/Wafl/Sdil protects against oxygen-induced toxicity. Toxicol Sci 2001; 63(2):214–222.

361. Pryhuber GS, O'Brien DP, Baggs R, Phipps R, Huyck H, Sanz I, Nahm MH. Ablation of tumor necrosis factor receptor type I (p55) alters oxygen-induced lung injury. Am J Physiol Lung Cell Mol Physiol 2000; 278(5):L1082–L1090.

362. Buckley S, Barsky L, Driscoll B, Weinberg K, Anderson KD, Warburton D. Apoptosis and DNA damage in type 2 alveolar epithelial cells cultured from hyperoxic rats. Am J Physiol 1998; 274(5 Pt 1):L714–L720.

363. Ward NS, Waxman AB, Homer PJ, Mantell LL, Einarsson O, Du Y, Elias JA. Interleukin-6-induced protection in hyperoxic acute lung injury. Am J Respir Cell Mol Biol 2000; 22(5):535–542.

364. Buckley S, Driscoll B, Barskyl L, Weinberg K, Anderson K, Warburton D. ERK activation protects against DNA damage and apoptosis in hyperoxic rat AEC2. Am J Physiol 1999; 277:L159–L166.

365. Petrache I, Choi ME, Otterbein LE, Chin BY, Mantell LL, Horowitz S, Choi AM. Mitogen-activated protein kinase pathway mediates hyperoxia-induced apoptosis in cultured macrophage cells. Am J Physiol 1999; 277(3 Pt 1): L589–L595.

366. Budinger GR, Tso M, McClintock DS, Dean DA, Sznajder JI, Chandel NS. Hyperoxia-induced apoptosis does not require mitochondrial reactive oxygen species and is regulated by Bcl-2 proteins. J Biol Chem 2002; 277(18): 15654–15660.

367. Wang Z, Schwan AL, Lairson LL, O'Donnell JS, Byrne GF, Foye A, Holm BA, Notter RH. Surface activity of a synthetic lung surfactant containing a phospholipase-resistant phosphonolipid analog of dipalmitoyl phosphatidyl-choline. Am J Physiol 2003; 285:L550–L559.

368. Phillips PG, Birnby L, Di Bernardo LA, Ryan TJ, Tsan MF. Hyperoxia increases plasminogen activator activity of cultured endothelial cells. Am J Physiol 1992; 262(1 Pt l):L21–L31.

369. Matalon S, Holm BA, Notter RH. Mitigation of pulmonary hyperoxic injury by administration of exogenous surfactant. J Appl Physiol 1987; 62:756–761.

370. Matalon S, Holm BA, Loewen GM, Baker RR, Notter RH. Sublethal hyperoxic injury to the alveolar epithelium and the pulmonary surfactant system. Exp Lung Res 1988; 14:1021–1033.

371. Holm BA, Notter RH, Finkelstein JH. Surface property changes from interactions of albumin with natural lung surfactant and extracted lung lipids. Chem Phys Lipids 1985; 38:287–298.

11

Genetically Modified Mouse Models of Lung Injury and Repair

BARRY R. STRIPP, ADAM GIANGRECO, and SUSAN D. REYNOLDS

Department of Environmental and Occupational Health, University of Pittsburgh, Pittsburgh, Pennsylvania, U.S.A.

I. Overview

This chapter discusses the rapidly evolving area of genetically modified mouse models and their application to the understanding of basic mechanisms of lung injury and repair. The development of methods to manipulate the mammalian genome has provided significant opportunities for the advancement of basic science research, agriculture, and biotechnology. As described in this chapter, genetically modified mice are variants of the species generated through introduction of stable genetic alterations into germline DNA. These alterations may either result from the random insertion of new DNA sequences, known as transgenes, or the introduction of site-specific insertions and/or deletions. Genetically altered mice provide a unique tool allowing researchers to bridge the gap between carefully designed in vitro studies and classical in vivo models. Current state-of-the-art approaches in the development of transgenic and knockout mouse models allow precise dissection of gene function in the context of the most complicated of biological systems, the whole animal. However, a number of factors including the design of transgenes and targeting vectors, screening of founder mice, and variations in background can significantly impact the phenotype associated with a genetic modification. It is essential to take these factors into account in developing and utilizing transgenic mouse models in basic research. Due to the importance of experimental and genetic characterizations in establishing mouse models, the first half of this chapter summarizes selected approaches relevant for subsequent interpretation of phenotype [technical details for producing transgenic mice are not emphasized due to their in-depth coverage in other published texts (e.g., see Refs. 1, 2)]. The latter half of the chapter focuses on the use of specific genetically modified mouse models in analyzing mechanisms of lung injury and repair. Further discussion of cell and animal models used in studying lung injury and inhalation toxicology is provided in Chapters 10 and 12.

II. Basic Methodology for Modification of the Mouse Genome: Transgenic Mice

Transgenic mice can be generated by multiple approaches including retroviral gene transfer into male spermatagonia (3), preimplantation embryos (4,5), or embryonic stem cells (6), or direct microinjection of DNA into fertilized mouse eggs (7–9). Difficulties with retrovirus-mediated transgenesis, such as a lack of reproducible transgene expression and limitations in the ability to use cell type-specific promoters (4,10), have led to the general acceptance of DNA microinjection as the method of choice for generation of transgenic mice. Injection of heterologous DNA sequences into the male pronucleus results in stable maintenance through random insertion into genomic DNA with a typical frequency of 5–30%. Factors influencing the efficiency of transgenesis, transgene expression, and phenotypic outcomes are discussed below. Application of specific transgenic models to the understanding of lung injury and repair is detailed later in the chapter.

A. Transgene Design: Basic Components

Even though transgenic models have been established using nonexpressed transgenes, the vast majority of transgenic mice are established with the goal of altering the temporal and/or spatial expression pattern of genes to better define their roles in developmental and physiological processes. Discussion here focuses exclusively on studies involving transgenes designed to achieve ectopic expression of linked sequences. Basic components of transgenes that are critical for their expression once integrated into the mouse genome include elements regulating transcription of coding sequences within the transgene, intronic sequences for processing the resulting transcript, and a polyadenylation sequence that directs transcriptional termination and polyadenylation (Fig. 1).

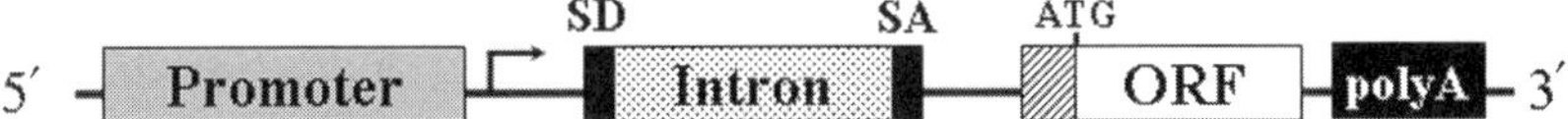

Figure 1 Basic components of a transgene. A transgene represented by the horizontal line is typically assembled from modules consisting of a transcriptional regulatory element frequently termed a promoter, RNA processing signals that include an intron and termination/polyadenylation signal (polyA), and an open reading frame (ORF). The transcriptional start site is indicated by the bent arrow and the translation initiation codon (ATG) is indicated by the vertical line. The promoter provides both the minimal sequence elements necessary for assembly of the basal transcriptional complex as well as those required for tissue-specific, cell type-specific, temporally regulated or ubiquitous expression of linked sequences. The intron and polyA signal which enhance transgene expression via mechanisms involving message stabilization and appropriate processing can be native to the gene of interest or a cassette derived from other genes such as beta-globin or human growth hormone. In the latter case, the intron cassette which contains a splice donor (SD) at the 5'-end and a splice acceptor (SA) at the 3'-end is frequently placed upstream of the gene of interest, although a downstream position is also functional. The sequence of interest which is composed of untranslated sequences at the 5'-end (hatched box) and coding sequences can be either a cDNA or a genomic sequence.

Transcriptional Regulatory Elements

Transcriptional regulatory elements (TREs or promoters) can be broadly categorized based upon the specificity with which they direct expression of linked sequences within cells and tissues of the mouse. Of greatest utility for studies in the lung are promoters capable of conferring either reliable cell type-specific expression or truly ubiquitous ectopic expression of transgene sequences.

Cell type-specific promoters for expression of transgenes within the lung. Of the many different cell types represented within the lung, cells of the pulmonary epithelium and to a lesser extent endothelial cells and smooth muscle cells have been targets for ectopic expression through transgenesis. However, only pulmonary epithelial cells can be specifically targeted in a tissue-specific fashion due to the availability of promoter elements for lung-specific genes whose expression is regulated at the level of gene transcription. Examples of lung epithelial cell-specific promoter elements include the 3.7-kb human surfactant protein-C (hSP-C) gene promoter (11,12) and the 2.4-kb rat Clara cell 10 kDa secretory protein (rCC10 or rCCSP) gene promoter (13,14). For both hSP-C and rCCSP promoter elements, linked genes are expressed in a spatial and temporal pattern that is similar but not identical to that of the corresponding endogenous mouse SP-C and CCSP genes. Transgenic mice harboring the reporter gene chloramphenicol acetyl-transferase (CAT) under the control of either the hSP-C or the rCCSP promoters exhibit earlier developmental onset and a loss of lineage-restricted expression of transgene sequences relative to that of their endogenous counterparts SP-C and CCSP, respectively (12–16). Differences between endogenous SP-C and CCSP gene expression and transgenes under the regulation of the corresponding promoters can be overcome when species-appropriate promoters are used for transgene expression (e.g., Refs. 12,13,17), demonstrating the importance of subtle species differences in organization of promoter elements for appropriate transgene expression in the mouse pulmonary epithelium. Other cell type-specific promoters that have been used to investigate aspects of lung development or function, but whose expression is not limited to the lung, include those that specify expression within endothelial cells (18), within airway epithelial cells (19), and within vascular smooth muscle cells (20).

Ubiquitous promoters. Even though a large number of promoter elements have been examined for their ability to confer broad tissue expression of linked genes in transgenic mice, in most cases, their expression is not ubiquitous. Moreover, methods used to define expression patterns achieved using various promoter elements have often employed reporter genes whose expression is monitored through analysis of tissue homogenates. Due to the diversity of either resident or migratory cells within the lung, derivatives of which have origins from all embryonic germ layers, identification of promoters conferring ubiquitous expression requires detailed localization of transgene expression at the cellular level. Using these criteria to assess expression patterns conferred by promoter elements, two have been identified that confer ubiquitous expression, the hybrid chicken β-actin promoter/CMV enhancer (referred to as CAG) (21) and promoter elements from the ROSA26 locus (6,22). However, among transgenic lines generated using either CAG or ROSA26 promoters to drive reporter gene expression, significant line-to-line variability can occur as a result of integration site effects (also termed position effects) on promoter specificity as described later.

RNA Processing Signals

Signals encoded within genomic DNA that are critical for the appropriate expression of most genes transcribed by RNA polymerase II include splice donor and acceptor sequences that specify interaction of the primary transcript with small nuclear ribonuclear protein complexes for the removal of intronic sequences, and a polyadenylation signal that specifies transcriptional termination and polyadenylation. Introns and their associated splice signals serve important functions in the eukaryotic genome by allowing "exon shuffling," the process whereby gene duplication and exon reassortment results in the creation of new genes. Early studies involving the generation of transgenic mice indicated that introns were not absolutely required for transgene expression (for review, see Refs. 9,23). However, research by Brinster et al. (24,25) provided evidence that use of intact genes with natural introns or, failing that, inclusion of introns upstream of the open reading frame, invariably resulted in improved levels of transgene expression. Interpretation of these experiments was complicated by the fact that placement of intronic sequences at sites other than the 5'-untranslated region resulted in truncation of protein coding sequences that may have led to altered translation with associated changes in mRNA stability. The consensus that emerged from these studies was that efficient expression of transgenes was more likely to occur if introns were included in design of the transgene, that the optimal positioning of the intron was within the 5'-untranslated portion of the mRNA coding sequence, and that no differences were observed between three different introns in their ability to enhance transgene expression. Due to limitations in the amount of DNA that can be practically manipulated and maintained within bacterial plasmids (the most commonly used vehicle for engineering transgene sequences), the majority of transgenes are composed of hybrid minigenes in which heterologous introns are placed in the 5'-untranslated region of cDNAs. However, development over the past 10 years of methods to manipulate large elements of genomic DNA in either yeast or bacteria and use them for the production of transgenic mice has provided new possibilities for the design of transgenes capable of reproducible and efficient expression as detailed later.

The other required component of expression transgenes is sequences specifying transcriptional termination and polyadenylation of nascent transcripts, commonly referred to as the polyadenylation signal. These sequences are frequently provided through cloned polyadenylation signals derived from native genes (25), the advantage of which is that these sequences also retain elements from the 3'-untranslated portion of the mRNA coding sequence that may contribute to stabilization of the transgene mRNA.

Translational Control

The use of either cDNA or genomic DNA sequences that include protein coding information typically involves inclusion of natural translational initiation codons. Translation begins with the assembly of ribosomes at the 5'-end of the mRNA molecule, after which the ribosome scans along the mRNA for initiation of translation usually at the first AUG codon that is encountered. However, careful analysis of this initiation process has revealed that the sequence context of initiation codons contribute to their efficient recognition by the ribosome and correct translational initiation (26). In addition to sequences immediately surrounding the initiation codon sequences, those located more distantly from the AUG codon within the 5'-untranslated region of the mRNA can also influence translational efficiency, presumably as a result of the ease with which this region forms stable secondary structures (27,28). Other factors that can influence the efficiency with which transgene-derived mRNAs are translated include cryptic initiation codons, present within the multiple cloning sites of many bacterial vectors (such as those containing *Sph*I and *Nco*I restriction sites), presence of which may interfere with efficient recognition of the desired initiation codon.

B. Practical Considerations in the Generation and Characterization of Transgenic Mice

Studies by Palmiter and Brinster in the 1980s detailed optimal conditions for DNA microinjection that are the basis for current methods employed for the generation of transgenic mice (8,9). For an extensive compendium of methods and associated background material relevant to the generation of transgenic mice, the reader is directed to two excellent texts, one by Hogan et al. (1) and another by Pinkert (2).

Genetic Background of Injected Embryos

Two principal factors influence the selection of the background mouse strain used for the generation of transgenic mice. Firstly, from a purely technical perspective, selection of inbred mouse strains vs. hybrids has a dramatic influence on efficiency (8). Hybrid embryos have desirable characteristics that improve the efficiency of injection, such as larger pronuclei and reduced lysis following injection. Moreover, hybrid parents generate larger numbers of embryos suitable for microinjection, and the resulting F2 generation hybrid embryos develop into adults that exhibit more robust reproductive performance. These desirable characteristics of hybrid embryos accounted for many transgenic mice being made in either F1 or F2 hybrid genetic backgrounds, typically of crosses between C57Bl/6 and CBA, C57Bl/6 and C3H/HeJ, or C3H/HeJ and DBA/2J (1).

The second factor that influences selection of a mouse strain for the generation of transgenic mice is other genetic influences that may have the potential to impact overall phenotype associated with expression of a transgene or penetrance of this trait among progeny of a single cross. Distinct mouse strains exhibit varying degrees of genetic dissimilarity that results in unpredictable, and in some cases quite dramatic, influences on either steady-state physiology or responsiveness to various environmental stimuli. This fact is highlighted by the exploitation of these genetic differences in the mapping of loci contributing to defined traits such as lung cancer (29), airway responsiveness (30,31), and pollutant susceptibility (32,33). For this reason, the use of embryos derived from inbred mouse strains has become increasingly popular for the generation of transgenic mice. Commonly used mouse strains include FVB/n and C57Bl/6, each of which have unique strengths that must be weighed in deciding the optimal background for introduction of a transgene. The FVB/n strain was developed at the

National Institute of Health as an inbred derivative of the outbred strain, Swiss. Advantages of the FVB/n over other inbred mouse strains were robust breeding performance and the development of large pronuclei (34). In contrast, the C57Bl/6 strain, despite the disadvantages of poor breeding performance and more fragile embryos that are susceptible to lysis, has the advantage of being a relatively well-characterized mouse strain due to extensive use in studies of toxicology, immunobiology, and mouse genetics.

Transgene Insertion: Influence of Time, Location, and Copy Number

Transgenes injected into the mouse embryo are maintained through nonspecific insertion of one to over one hundred copies of the transgene organized in a head-to-tail array within the genome. Transgenic mice that are established are termed "founder" mice, and are considered hemizygous for the transgene locus. Even though this process is thought to be random, areas of active gene transcription and ongoing DNA replication prior to cell division are likely to be hot-spots for transgene insertion.

Mosaicism

Insertion of transgene sequences within chromosomal locations that have just undergone DNA replication within the one cell embryo or at later stages in embryogenesis results in generation of mosaic founders. Under these conditions, the contribution of transgene-bearing cells to either somatic or germline cells is dictated by the stage at which integration occurred. As a consequence, mosaic founder mice typically transmit the transgene to their progeny with a non-Mendelian inheritance pattern. Provided that the F1 progeny from a mosaic founder are viable and fertile, transgenes are transmitted through successive generations in a normal Mendelian fashion. Mice mosaic for transgenes whose expression confers a lethal phenotype have the potential to be of considerable value due to the rescue of the embryo by transgene negative cells. One such example is a line of transgenic mice in which the diphtheria toxin-A chain was expressed under the control of the mouse CCSP promoter (Fig. 2). Whereas the majority of founder mice exhibited a neonatal lethal phenotype, one founder mouse was generated exhibiting a mosaic distribution of transgene-expressing cells within the conducting airway epithelium (Stripp BR, Mango GW, Reynolds SD, unpublished data). Similar observations have been made among transgenic mice expressing a dominant negative form of the KGFRII receptor under the regulatory control of the human SP-C promoter (35). A second form of mosaicism can be observed among female mice in which transgene sequences insert within the X-chromosome; random X-chromosome inactivation results in mosaic expression of transgene sequences among somatic cells of female, but not male, members of the line (36).

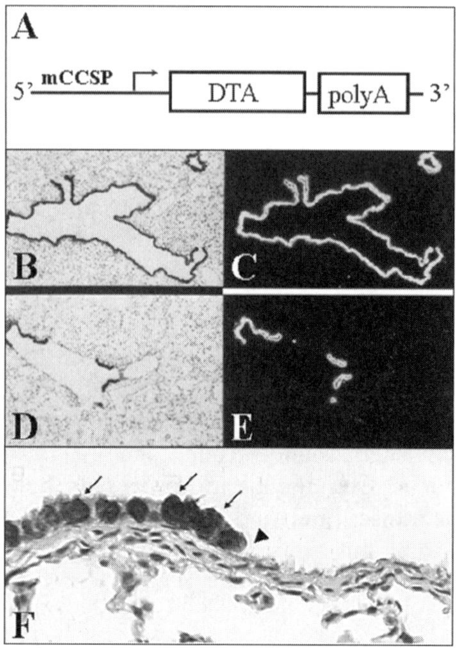

Figure 2 DTA transgenic mouse-mosaic expression of CCSP. (A) The CCSP-DTA transgene was composed of the 2.1 kb mouse CCSP promoter (mCCSP), the diphtheria toxin-A chain (DTA) coding sequence, and an SV40 polyadenylation sequence (polyA). The transcriptional start site is indicated by the bent arrow. (B–E) In situ hybridization analysis of CCSP mRNA in wild-type (B and C) and DTA transgenic (D and E) mice. CCSP message was detected by in situ hybridization using [^{35}S]-labeled antisense riboprobes and autoradiography. Sections were counter-stained with hematoxylin. Bright field photomicrographs in B and D illustrate tissue morphology and the distribution of autoradiographic grains (black). Dark field photomicrographs in C and E demonstrate the distribution of autoradiographic grains (white). Note the uniform expression of CCSP in the wild-type airway epithelium and the contrasting patchy distribution of this mRNA in the airway of the DTA transgenic mouse. (F) Immunohistochemical analysis of CCSP protein in the airway of the DTA transgenic mouse. CCSP immunopositive cells were detected using standard immunohistochemical techniques and are dark grey (arrows). Sections were counter-stained with hematoxylin and nuclei are light grey. Note the sharp demarcation between the CCSP immunopositive and CCSP immunonegative regions (arrowhead).

Multiple integration sites

Using standard procedures for the generation of transgenic mice, the frequency of transgenesis is 5–30% among embryos (injected with nonlethal transgenes) that survive to adulthood. Founder mice identified among progeny typically harbor single integration sites that are transmitted in a

Mendelian fashion. Either mosaicism (discussed above) or multiple integration events can lead to non-Mendelian transmission patterns among progeny resulting from back-cross to a transgene negative mate of the parental strain. The occurrence of multiple integration events is proportional to the transgenesis rate with frequencies of 25% resulting in a population in which approximately 6% (i.e., 25% of the transgene positive group) exhibit multiple integration events. Identification of founder mice with multiple integration sites is typically achieved through analysis of progeny from a back-cross with a transgene negative mate. Founders with single sites of transgene integration will yield 50% transmission of transgene DNA to progeny (1:1 ratio of transgenic:nontransgenic progeny), whereas two integrations will yield 75% transmission (1:2:1 ratio of 2 insertion sites:1 insertion site:nontransgenic progeny). Segregation of integration sites can be readily achieved by analysis of copy number and is critical for establishment of stable lines of mice and appropriate interpretation of the phenotype conferred by transgene expression at each integration site.

Integration site effects

Many factors unique to a transgene and the site at which it is integrated contribute to its regulation. The stimulatory influence of neighboring DNA sequences on qualitative and quantitative expression of transgenes can be demonstrated by experiments involving the use of enhancer-trap strategies for the identification and characterization of transcriptional regulatory sequences. In one such study, expression of the *E. coli* LacZ reporter gene under regulation of the H2-K^b promoter was unexpectedly limited to type II cells within one line of transgenic mice, an outcome that was attributed to integration site-dependent enhancer effects on promoter specificity (37). Similar experiments by Korn et al. (38) have identified numerous loci with distinct influences on the expression of an enhancer-trap LacZ reporter gene. Even though far less dramatic, position effects have been shown to have qualitative influences on promoter sequences commonly used to direct transgene expression to lung cells. As discussed earlier, the 3.7-kb human SP-C promoter exhibits line-to-line variability in the relative contribution of type II and Clara cells to the total transgene-expressing population (12). In contrast, line-to-line variability in the specificity of the rat and mouse CCSP promoters has not been observed although significant quantitative differences in the expression of linked genes among transgenic lines has been reported (13,17).

Mechanisms contributing to integration site effects on transgene expression include insertion within a genomic locus that is incompatible with efficient promoter function and use of promoter elements that lack appropriate regulatory signals to provide insulation from neighboring genomic influences (39–41). Satisfying either of these factors often results in levels of transgene expression more similar to that of the endogenous gene from which the promoter was derived. This effect has been demonstrated for a number of intact genes and minigenes, resulting in the identification of cis-acting DNA sequences capable of conferring position-independent expression, known as locus control regions (LCRs) (41–46). Precise mapping of LCRs within a variety of genes has led to a number of studies designed to determine whether these elements confer position-independence to heterologous promoters in transgenic mice. Results of these experiments appear to be mixed (47–50).

Other factors with potential to influence transgene expression include condensation of multimerized transgene sequences into heterochromatin (51). Even though there is some evidence for this process, factors contributing to condensation of transgene loci into heterochromatin may be more complex, possibly involving hypermethylation of transgene DNA containing bacterial DNA sequences (52,53).

Copy number

Pronuclear injection of transgene DNA into a mouse embryo is followed by multimerization of transgene sequences through intracellular ligation and random integration of multimers carrying varying numbers of transgene copies into a single site within the genome. As such, transgene copy number is defined as the number of transgene units contained within a single integration site. Even though many transgenes exhibit a position-dependent pattern of expression in transgenic mice, there is typically no clear relationship between transgene copy number and expression levels (1,9). The exception to this rule is for transgenes containing functional locus control regions, for which position-independent, copy number-dependent expression of transgene sequences is the norm (44). Despite these general principles, subtle copy number influences can be demonstrated when the transgene locus of hemizygous line is bred to homozygosity. For example, such effects can be observed using coat color as a measure of gene expression among transgenic mice harboring a tyrosinase minigene (36).

Transgene copy number is commonly determined during characterization of a transgenic line and is a critical parameter for both the segregation of multiple integration sites and establishment of homozygous transgenic lines. Copy number is determined by comparison of hybridization signal intensity on genomic Southern blots of DNA from transgene positive mice with that of a transgene negative individual that has been doped with 0.5–200 transgene equivalents per genome equivalent. Using this method, it is possible to determine copy number to within 10% of actual, an accuracy that easily allows the distinction of homozygous vs. hemizygous members of a line and typically allows segregation of multiple transgene insertion loci. Copy number standards are also a critical control when employing either polymerase chain reaction (PCR) or Southern blot assays for the identification of founder lines; not only does this provide an appreciation of transgene copy number (this must be verified among later generations due to potential for mosaicism and multiple integrations), but it serves as a measure of assay sensitivity helping to ensure that low copy number transgenes (i.e., 0.5 copies per genome for a single copy transgene and lower for mosaic lines harboring a single copy transgene) are detected.

C. Technological Improvements in Transgenic Mouse Models

Two major technical advances have occurred that greatly enhance the potential of transgenic mice to provide valuable insights into in vivo mechanisms of lung development and disease. These advances involve the development of methods for conditional regulation of transgene expression and for the manipulation of large genomic clones to allow more reliable and reproducible expression of transgenes.

Conditional Regulation of Transgene Expression

Temporal regulation of gene expression is a key factor governing appropriate orchestration of lung development, responses to lung injury and repair, and homeostatic mechanisms associated with maintenance and normal aging of the steady-state lung. Even though tissue-specific promoter elements have the potential to restrict transgene expression to a limited number of cell types within the mouse, standard transgene constructs described earlier lack the ability to fine tune the temporal pattern of transgene expression. Inappropriate temporal regulation of transgene expression and the downstream consequences of these genetic changes make it difficult or impossible to understand mechanisms leading to an observed phenotype, particularly in adulthood. The most dramatic example of this is observed when the consequences of transgene expression lead to embryonic lethality. However, even subtle developmental changes in cellular and molecular responses that result from ectopic transgene expression may lead to transgene-independent changes in physiological responses. As such, unregulated transgene expression provides only indirect clues into functions for the ectopically expressed gene, making it difficult to definitively establish the precise role of the gene of interest in processes of development, disease, and homeostasis. A number of strategies for conditional transgene activation and repression have been developed in an attempt to overcome these difficulties (reviewed in Ref. 54). These include use of promoter elements from genes whose expression is naturally activated under the regulation of environmental cues, such as the metallothionein (55), cytochrome P450 1A1 (56), or heat-shock protein (57) genes, in addition to novel regulatory systems using ligand-regulated hybrid transcription factors (58–61). Regulated transgenic approaches exploiting the tetracycline, ecdysone, or antiprogesterone (RU486) systems are in many ways analogous and this general strategy has received broad acceptance as the preferred approach for conditional transgene activation.

Tetracycline-based system for conditional regulation of transgene expression. An evolving series of strategies exploiting elements from the *E. coli* tetracycline (Tet) operon were initially developed by Gossen and Bujard (58) for regulated expression of genes in eukaryotic cells. Regulation of the tet operon in *E. coli* is achieved through binding of the tet repressor (tetR) to its cognate cis-element, the tet operator (tetO), resulting in blockade of transcriptional initiation at tetO. Transcriptional repression is reversed in the presence of tetracycline due to specific binding of this compound by tetR and dissociation of the tetracyclin/tetR complex from tetO. Gossen and Bujard (58) generated a potent transcriptional activator specific for tetO elements by fusion of tetO with the transcriptional activation domain of Herpes virus VP16 protein. This hybrid protein, termed tet-trans activator (tTA), was stably transfected into eukaryotic cells and its activity tested using a luciferase reporter gene under the regulation of tetO and a minimal cytomegalovirus (CMV) promoter (Fig. 3). Using this system, HeLa cell lines were established in which luciferase expression could be induced up to 100,000-fold through removal of doxycycline (a more stable and less toxic tetracycline derivative) from culture media (58). Similarly, dramatic induction of gene expression was observed in certain tissues of bitransgenic mice harboring tTA coding sequences under control of the CMV immediate early promoter/enhancer and either the tetO-luciferase or tetO-LacZ reporter genes (59). Since validation of this approach, a variety of modifications have been introduced through manipulation of bacterial tetR sequences. An important advance was the generation of mutant forms of tTA in which the doxycycline dependency of the tetR component was reversed, giving rise to the reverse tTA (rtTA, Fig. 4) (62). More recently, strategies have been developed to overcome doxycycline-independent leakiness of the rtTA system through generation of either tT repressor (tTR) constructs (Fig. 5) (63) or through functional selection in yeast of mutants capable of optimal doxycycline-induction in eukaryotic cells (64). Application of these methods for analysis of pulmonary epithelial cell plasticity is described in more detail later.

Use of Large Genomic Clones to Overcome Positional Effects on Transgene Expression

The inability to insulate transgenes from integration site influences represents one of the more significant hurdles that must be overcome in the establishment of transgenic mouse models. As discussed earlier, locus control regions that function to insulate genes from neighboring DNA were initially described for the globin locus and more recently for other genes. However, in most cases, the identification and characterization of cis-acting

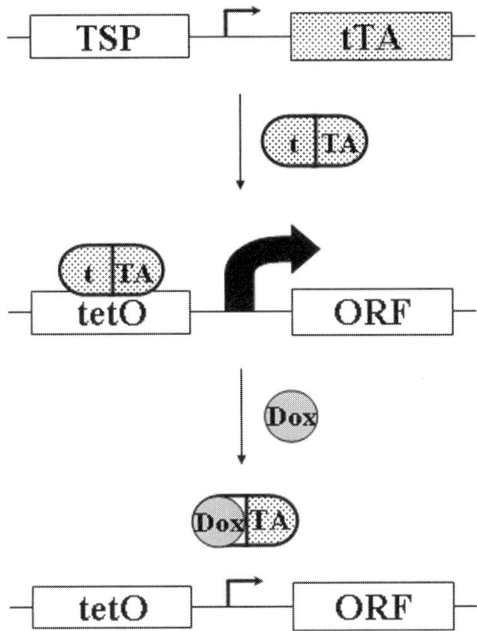

Figure 3 Tet system: the tet-trans activator. Regulated expression of transgenes in eukaryotic cells was originally achieved using cis- and trans-elements derived from the *E. coli* tet operon. The first component of this two transgene system utilized a tissue-specific promoter (TSP) to regulate expression of the tet-trans activator (tTA) a fusion of the tet repressor derived from *E. coli* and the potent transcriptional activation domain of the Herpes simplex virus VP16 protein. The second component of this system utilized the tet operator (tetO) and a minimal CMV promoter to regulate expression of an open reading frame (ORF). In cells or mice harboring both transgenes, the constitutively active tTA interacts specifically with tetO resulting in expression of the downstream ORF (represented by the bold arrow). Addition of the tetracycline derivative doxycyclin (dox) resulted in formation of a dox–tTA complex, dissociation of the complex from tetO, and downregulation of ORF gene expression.

transcriptional regulatory elements associated with genes have been largely confined to the analysis of elements conferring tissue-specific gene regulation, with relatively little emphasis put on the identification and characterization of LCRs. This is particularly true for studies investigating mechanisms of lung gene regulation, as elements that confer position-independent regulation of genes expressed within the pulmonary epithelium have yet to be defined (reviewed in Refs. 65–68).

Two strategies can be employed to overcome these difficulties. One approach uses gene targeting to introduce new gene sequences downstream from endogenous promoter elements, while the other involves use of large

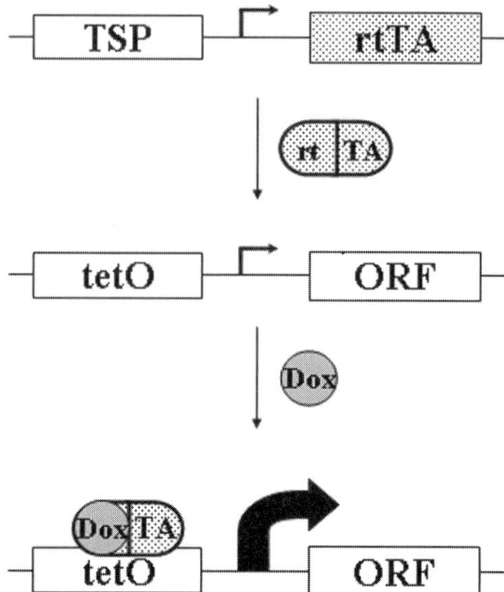

Figure 4   Tet system: the reverse tet-trans activator. Mutagenesis of the tet repressor, tetR, and selection of variants that were activated by doxycyclin resulted in generation of the reverse tet-trans activator (rtTA). In contrast with the system depicted in Fig. 3, expression of rtTA regulated by a tissue-specific promoter (TSP) results in generation of rtTA protein that does not bind DNA. However, addition of doxycyclin (dox) results in the formation of a dox–rtTA complex that interacts specifically with the tet operator (tetO) on a second transgene activating expression of the downstream open reading frame (ORF). Transcription is indicated by the bold arrow.

genomic fragments that can be propagated in either yeast or bacteria as artificial chromosomes (YAC and BAC, respectively) to generate transgenic mice (reviewed in Ref. 69). Precedent for the former strategy comes from gene targeting studies, which frequently involve introduction of a reporter gene to trace gene expression within heterozygous or homozygous knockout mice. However, functional expression of heterologous genes through insertion of these sequences downstream of endogenous promoters has not been widely adopted due to the potential for a confounding phenotype associated with the heterozygous null mutation introduced at the insertion site. In contrast, growing number of laboratories have begin to use YACs and BACs for the generation of transgenic mice.

Transgenic mice using yeast artificial chromosomes.   Yeast artificial chromosomes are linear DNA molecules that include chromosomal DNA sequences allowing their maintenance as a stable episomal element within yeast cells (70). YAC vectors have the largest cloning capacity of any vector systems for the propagation of heterologous DNA sequences, with typical

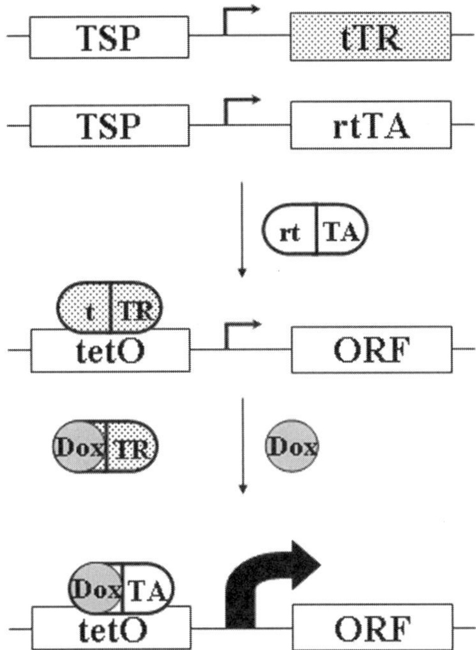

Figure 5 Tet system: tet-trans repressor. In order to overcome difficulties associated with leakiness of the rtTA system, transgenes allowing tet-trans repressor (tTR)-mediated repression of tetO regulated genes have been developed. In this system tTR, fusion between a mutant tet repressor and a strong transcriptional repressor the KRAB-AB domain of the Kid-1 protein is regulated by either tissue-specific (TSP) or ubiquitous promoters. Expression of this transgene results in generation of tTR which interacts specifically with the tet operator (tetO) on a second transgene and represses expression of a downstream open reading frame (ORF). In the presence of doxycyclin (dox), tTR binding to tetO is destabilized resulting in vacancy of the tetO sequence. Simultaneously, the reverse tet-trans activator (rtTA) provided by a third transgene is activated through binding of dox, associates with tetO, and activates expression of the downstream ORF (indicated by the bold arrow).

insert sizes ranging from 100 to 1 Mb. Schedl et al. (71) first demonstrated that a 35-kb YAC containing the tyrosinase gene could be stably introduced into the mouse germline following pronuclear DNA microinjection into mouse embryos. Moreover, both the 35-kb transgene and a much larger 250-kb YAC transgene were functional as assessed by their ability to complement the albino phenotype of a recipient mouse strain (71,72). A number of other laboratories simultaneously developed mouse lines harboring transgenes composed of an 85-kb YAC clone of the human immunoglobulin heavy chain locus (73), either 150-kb (46) or 248-kb (74) YAC clones of the beta-globin locus, and a 650-kb YAC clone of the amyloid precursor protein gene (75). In each case, expression was reported to show similar qualitative and quantitative expression patterns to that shown for the corresponding endogenous gene, suggesting that appropriate elements had been included within each transgene to insulate the transcriptional unit from insertion site influences. The value of YAC transgenic mice as models of human disease are further highlighted by the demonstration that exon 9 skipping alleles of the human CFTR gene, retain this splice defect when the entire CFTR gene is incorporated into the mouse genome as a YAC transgene (76). However, several drawbacks of using YAC clones for the generation of transgenic mice include: (1) the requirement for specialized techniques for the manipulation and isolation of YAC DNA, (2) YAC DNA sequences have a high propensity for rearrangement at the time of integration, and (3) vector DNA sequences are cointroduced with genomic sequences contained within the YAC.

Transgenic mice using bacterial artificial chromosomes. Bacterial and P1 artificial chromosomes (BAC and PAC, respectively) can each accommodate a maximum of 300 kb of heterologous sequence, yet differ in the method of their generation and their copy number. Bacterial artificial chromosomes are derived from the *E. coli* F-factor and hence are propagated as large circular plasmids that are maintained at low copy number (77). Like YACs, BACs have sufficient capacity to carry the largest genes in their entirety as well as sufficient flanking DNA to capture neighboring LCRs and distantly located enhancer elements. The large capacity of BACs allows for the generation of transgenes capable of position-independent, copy number-dependent expression such as that obtained for BACs containing beta-globin and apolipoprotein B genes (78,79). Not surprisingly, BAC transgenes for alpha-globin and apolipoprotein B that lack LCRs revert to a pattern of transgene expression that is dependent upon integration site (79,80).

An important advantage of BACs over YACs is their relative stability and ease of manipulation. A number of methods have been developed for the genetic manipulation of sequences contained within BAC vectors including the introduction of nested deletions (81), recA-assisted restriction endonuclease modification (79), recombinogenic insertion of heterologous DNA sequences (82), and vector linearization using either bacteriophage lambda terminase (83) or Cre-lox (84). Even though methods now exist for the routine elimination of bacterial plasmid DNA from BAC clones prior to microinjection, the integration of linearized BAC clones containing both vector and insert sequences does not appear to interfere with transgene expression. Moreover, residual vector DNA provides a sequence tag to distinguish transgene from endogenous gene sequences in the event that mouse genomic sequences are being reintroduced into the mouse germline (69).

III. Basic Methodology for Modification of the Mouse Genome: Site-Specific Genetic Modification

The demonstration in 1984 that mouse embryonic stem (ES) cells retain their ability to contribute to the germline following introduction into a recipient blastocyst (85) paved the way for approaches allowing site-specific modifications of the ES cell genome. Embryonic stem cells originate from pluripotent cells within the inner cell mass of the developing embryo and ES cell lines can be established from an outgrowth of these cells following in vitro culture of blastocysts (86,87). Conditions for maintenance of ES cells in vitro have been carefully defined (1,88) and represent a critical parameter for the maintenance of pluripotency. Culture conditions typically use media with additives such as leukemic inhibitory factor (LIF) with ES cells commonly cultured on either immortalized or primary embryonic fibroblasts feeder layers. Measures to screen for and avoid contamination with mycoplasma are absolutely required for the establishment of ES cell lines capable of colonizing recipient lastocysts (1).

Initial validation of methods for homologous targeting of the mouse genome took advantage of the X-linked hypoxanthine-guanine phosphoribosyl transferase (HPRT) gene due to the ability of this gene to impose either positive (hypoxanthine, aminopterin, thymidine [HAT]-containing media) or negative (6-thioguanine-containing media) selection for male ES cells expressing a functional gene (89,90). Thomas and Capecchi (79), in addition to targeting a naturally selectable gene, greatly enriched for homologous targeting events at the HPRT locus by including an expression cassette for a second selectable marker, neomycin phosphotransferase (neo^r). A number of parameters were identified in these and other early targeting experiments that have potential to greatly influence the efficiency and outcome of homologous targeting in ES cells.

A. Design of Vectors for Homologous Targeting of Genes Within ES Cells

Important considerations in the design of targeting experiments are the type of targeting vector to be used, length of genomic DNA included within targeting vectors, strain-derivation of genomic DNA sequences, selective pressure applied to enrich for cells with homologous targeting events and the influence of inserted DNA sequences on expression of neighboring genes. These issues are discussed in more detail below. The reader is referred to the comprehensive texts of Hogan et al. (1) and Pinkert (2) for details regarding methodology.

Replacement and Insertion Targeting Vectors

Two general types of targeting vectors, replacement vectors (otherwise known as omega-type vectors) and insertion vectors (otherwise known as o-type vectors), can be used for the modification of gene sequences in cultured ES cells (Figs. 6 and 7). Replacement vectors are constructed with "arms" of homology that flank a selectable gene and typically result in either the insertional disruption and/or deletion of gene sequences through a process that requires a double crossover event (Fig. 6). In contrast, insertion vectors undergo a single crossover recombinational event that results in duplication of sequences common to both the targeting vector and insertion site, coupled with insertion of nonhomologous sequences including both a selectable marker and vector DNA sequences (Fig. 7). Practical features of replacement and insertion vectors that should be considered in the selection of either approach are the efficiency of targeting and the goal of the desired targeting event. In comparisons made in conjunction with single selectable markers, insertion vectors have been found to target homologous loci with greater efficiency than replacement vectors (89,91). However, insertion vectors can result in the generation of hypomorphic alleles rather

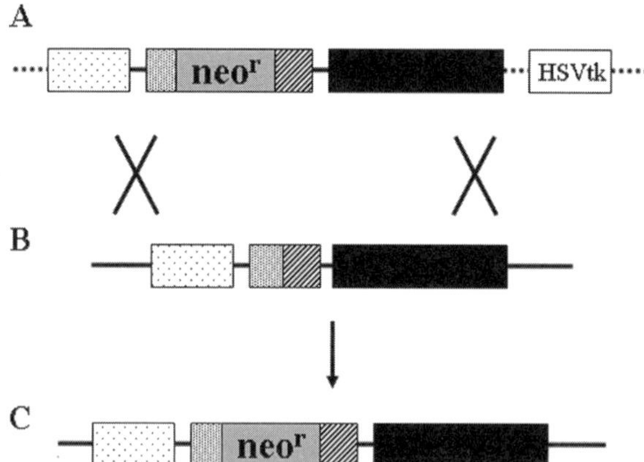

Figure 6   Replacement targeting vector. Replacement vectors (A) are composed of short (light and dark stippled boxes) and long (hatched and black boxes) homology arms separated by a positive selectable marker that is typically the neomycin phosphotransferase gene (neo^r) regulated by the phosphoglycerate kinase promoter. A negative selectable marker such as HSVtk also regulated by the phosphoglycerate kinase promoter is placed outside the homologous sequence and is surrounded by vector sequence (broken line). Homologous recombination between the replacement vector and the endogenous locus (B) involves two crossover events (large X) and results in disruption of the endogenous gene through insertion of neo^r and elimination of the HSVtk cassette (C). Disruption of the gene through sequence deletion and insertion of neo^r is also a commonly used alternative strategy (not shown).

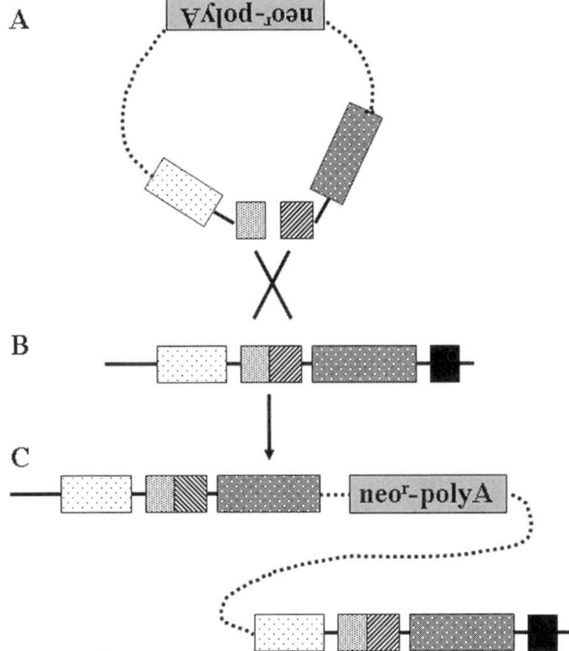

Figure 7 Insertional targeting vector. This type of targeting vector is composed of variable lengths of homologous gene sequence that typically includes one or more introns and a positive selectable marker such as the neomycin phosphotransferase gene (neo^r) regulated by the phosphoglycerate kinase promoter. Vector sequence (broken line) separates the regions of homology and neo^r. Homologous recombination between the insertional vector (A) and the endogenous gene (B) involves a single crossover event (large X) and results in placement of the neo^r cassette and vector sequence between a tandem duplication of common sequences (C). Gene expression is disrupted through truncation and/or aberrant splicing of the primary transcript leading to decreases message stability and/or introduction of frame-shift mutations.

than the desired null allele (92,93), a consideration that has led to the use of replacement vectors for generation of most knockout mice. Finally, insertion vectors are well suited for the generation of subtle genetic alterations such as point mutations (discussed below), an application that is not possible using replacement vectors. Regardless of vector type, use of homology regions that are as closely matched as possible (preferably isogenic) between targeting vector and the specific substrain from which ES cells are derived has been shown to influence targeting efficiency. This effect is most likely dependent upon locus, and the extent to which different chromosomal regions have diverged between mouse strains (94). More difficult to assess has been the influence of the extent of homology between targeting vector and target locus on the efficiency of homologous recombination. A consensus from empirical observations is that greater homology leads to more efficient targeting. However, this trend is locus and even construct-dependent, and may exhibit a threshold beyond which no further increases in efficiency are observed (89,94–96). In addition to influences on efficiency, the extent of homology used within targeting vectors impacts the fidelity of recombination, which is reduced with shorter homology regions (97,98).

Selectable Markers for Enrichment of Homologous Targeting Events

The ability to enrich a population of ES cells that have undergone homologous recombination with a targeting vector is an indispensable strategy employed in all gene targeting experiments. Stable maintenance of the targeting vector within the ES cell genome occurs by random (nonhomologous) integration with a frequency of approximately 10^{-3} and by homologous recombination at a frequency of between 10^{-5} and 10^{-7} (88). As such, selection strategies are necessary to enrich both the population of cells carrying the targeting vector (through either random or homologous insertion) and those having undergone homologous recombination. Homologous targeting of genes, such as the HPRT locus, that themselves confer a selective advantage, can be selected for or against by appropriate culture conditions (89,90). However, no such selective advantage is conferred by the vast majority of homologous targeting events unless appropriate selectable markers are incorporated into homologous sequences within the targeting vector (Figs. 6 and 7). A variety of such genes have now been identified and include the prokaryotic neo^r gene (99) which provides resistance to the antibiotic G418. Typically, neo^r is incorporated into the homologous sequence and as such allows selection of cells harboring insertions that are the result of either random or homologous recombination. Further enrichment of cells in which the targeting sequence has been stably maintained through homologous recombination can be achieved using negative selection against random integration events (100) (Fig. 6). A variety of negative selector genes have been used including the Herpes simplex virus thymidine kinase (HSVtk) gene (101), expression of which confers sensitivity to ganciclovir (GCV), and the catalytic "A" chain of diphtheria toxin, which is directly cytotoxic (101). Importantly, negative selector genes can only be used in combination with replacement-type targeting vectors as this strategy takes advantage of the fact that homologous recombination events (but not random insertion events) result in loss of a negative selector located outside of the homology region. Regardless of the selection strategy, promoter elements capable of directing gene expression in a wide variety of genomic locations must be used to regulate the selectable marker. Based upon empirical observations, the phosphoglycerate kinase (PGK) promoter is utilized in most gene targeting experiments (reviewed in Ref. 88).

Introduction of Subtle Modifications to Gene Structure and/or Function

Even though the majority of gene targeting experiments are performed with the goal of generating a null allele for a specific gene, in some cases, more subtle modifications are required for establishment of animal models of human disease or in the analysis of gene structure and function. Two basic methods have been developed that allow the introduction of subtle modifications, such as point mutations, within the genome of ES cells. A method referred to as "tag and exchange" was first described by Askew et al. (102). This approach involves initial targeting of a locus using a replacement vector carrying both a positive and a negative selectable marker. Following positive selection of cells harboring the targeted allele, a "correcting" vector carrying a point mutation is introduced. Recombination of this sequence with the targeted locus results in introduction of the point mutation and elimination of the negative selectable marker. ES cells harboring the recombined allele are then enriched by negative selection. Use of this approach by Askew et al. (102) allowed the development of mice harboring point mutations within the alpha 2 subunit of Na/K-ATPase. A second method for introducing subtle modifications into the mouse germline, termed the "hit-and-run" method, was developed by Hasty et al. (99). In this case, an insertion-type vector was used that harbored a point mutation within the homologous sequence and both a positive (neo) and a negative (HSVtk) selectable marker within the plasmid sequence. Homologous recombination and positive selection resulted in enrichment of ES cells bearing a tandem duplication and both selectable markers. A subsequent intramolecular homologous recombination resulted in resolution of the duplication through deletion of either the endogenous or the mutated sequence. ES cells bearing the recombined allele were obtained using the negativeselectable marker (99). A concern involving point mutations introduced using this strategy is the potential for random mutations at the target locus due to aberrations in the process of homologous recombination (103). This can be largely overcome by careful design and the inclusion of sufficiently large stretches of homology within targeting vectors (97,98). Despite the development of methods for introducing subtle modifications in the mouse genome, such approaches have been employed infrequently relative to the generation of null alleles.

B. Characterization of Targeted Modifications

Methods used for manipulation of ES cells, selection of cell lines harboring targeted modifications, and establishment of stable mouse lines capable of transmitting the modified allele through the germline have been described in detail elsewhere (88) and are not discussed in depth here. However, a number of parameters must be carefully considered in order to attribute a particular phenotype to the intended genetic modification introduced into ES cells. These include the potential for unintended genetic alterations to the target locus, the influence of genetic background on phenotypic outcomes, and the impact of aberrant developmental outcomes may have on interpretation of a phenotype in adult mice.

Validation of Modified Loci in ES Cells

Careful evaluation of the targeted genetic locus is required to ensure that unintended local rearrangements have not occurred in ES cells. Aberrant recombinational events can occur when using replacement-type vectors if one arm of homology is too short. This design flaw results in random insertion of the short homology arm after the initial homologous recombination event mediated by the longer arm of homology. Targeting vectors harboring a short arm of homology are typically used when PCR-based screening assays are used to identify clones of homologously targeted ES cells. This problem can be largely overcome throughcareful consideration of homology regions used in the design of targeting vectors. However, homologously targeted ES cell lines identified initially by PCR must also be carefully evaluated by Southern analysis of both the 5′- and 3′-ends of the insertion site to confirm the fidelity of recombination and the absence of unintended modifications to the locus.

Establishment of Mouse Lines

Once ES cell lines that harbor the desired genetic modification are identified, ES cell/embryo chimeras are generated for transmission of the genetic modification through the germline. Embryonic stem cells, which are typically derived from either agouti or chinchilla coat colored lines of the 129 strain, are injected into the blastocoel cavity of a developing embryo with black coat color, typically a C57Bl/6 strain mouse embryo. Following reintroduction into the uterus of a foster mother, host and ES-derived cells randomly contribute to the developing embryo resulting in the establishment of a chimera. Those in which the targeted ES cell has contributed to the germline (germline chimeras) are identified through a back-cross of the chimera to a mouse strain with black coat color, typically C57Bl/6, with subsequent evaluation of progeny for transmission of agouti (ES cell-derived) coat color genes.

A common problem encountered in the phenotypic analysis of mice harboring targeted genetic modifications results from the strategy used for establishment of mouse lines from ES cell chimeras. Progeny resulting from crosses between germline chimeras and C57Bl/6 mates are screened through visual inspection of coat color to identify those receiving one haploid genome equivalent from ES cell-derived germline, with subsequent genotypic analysis to identify mice harboring the modified allele. Among this F1 generation, mice heterozygous for the mutant allele are hybrid for 129 and C57Bl/6 genetic backgrounds. Heterozygous F1 hybrids are then typically intercrossed for the establishment of F2 generation hybrids in which the mutant allele segregates with a typical Mendelian 1:2:1 pattern of homozygous wild-type, heterozygous, and homozygous mutant geno-types. Phenotypic analysis of homozygous mutant mice generated using this strategy is subject to the same caveats as those discussed earlier since the genetic background of these mice is a hybrid of the 129 and C57Bl/6 strains. The resulting inability to control for differences in genetic make-up among homozygous mutant 129/C57Bl/6 hybrid lines and wild-type control mice has lead to a corresponding inability to unequivocally attribute phenotypic outcomes to the specific genetic modification introduced into the germline. These difficulties can be overcome through breeding germline chimeras with strain-matched mates resulting in establishment of F1 pro-geny harboring a heterozygous mutant allele on a pure-bred background (for example, see Ref. 104). An alternative strategy for eliminating genetic diversity between hybrid mouse lines harboring targeted modifications and their corresponding wild-type controls is the generation of congenic mutant lines. Such lines are established through repeated back-crossing of the mutant strain to the desired inbred strain with selection for the modified allele at each generation (105). This procedure must be repeated for at least 10 generations unless microsatellite markers are used to identify progeny with greater contributions of the desired inbred background at each genera-tion, a method referred to as "speed congenics" (106). Although the paren-tal strain used for back-crosses is frequently used as a wild-type control, congenic lines harboring the wild-type 129 allele are the preferred (but still not perfect) control strains.

A final caveat in the appropriate selection of wild-type controls in gene targeting experiments is the existence of multiple 129 substrains, some of which exhibit significantly greater polymorphism than the majority due presumably to their accidental genetic contamination (107). The use of microsatellite markers to document the degree of genetic similarity (107) provides a tool to better match genetic backgrounds of ES cell lines and breeding stock used for establishment of mouse lines.

C. Secondary Phenotypic Consequences of Targeted Gene Modifications

The generation of mice homozygous for a targeted null allele has the pot-ential to result in embryonic lethality or systemic abnormalities that may confound interpretation of a phenotype within a specific cell or tissue type. These difficulties have been overcome through the development of chromosomal engineering approaches that allow conditional gene inactivation (108,109). This approach takes advantage of systems from either bacteria or yeast that result in site-specific recombination between two DNA elements of appropriate sequence. The two systems most widely used for these purposes include the Cre recombinase/*LoxP* target DNA sequence from P1 bacteriophage (110,111) and the Flp recombinase/*FRT* target DNA sequence from yeast (112,113). However, additional recombinases, such as bacteriophage PhiC31 integrase and Anabena XisA, with distinct recombinase target sequences (RTS) are also being identified and characterized (114). In each case, RTS are recognized as substrate for recombination resulting in either excision or inversion of intervening sequences depending upon whether pair-wise RTS elements are organized as direct or inverted repeats, respectively (Fig. 8). The initial strategy for chromosome engineering using the Cre/LoxP system was developed and validated by Gu et al. (115) for conditional ablation of the DNA polymerase beta gene in T-cells. The strategy involved homologous targeting of the desired locus by placement of a floxed (flanked by LoxP elements) neo^r selectable marker within a silent portion of the gene (such as an intron) or flanking DNA, and positioning of a third LoxP element within a downstream intron (Fig. 8A). Following targeting of the locus, the floxed neo^r cassette, which could potentially alter the normal expression pattern of the targeted gene, was deleted through transient expression of Cre recombinase and selection for the appropriate recombinational event. This targeting strategy yields a floxed allele in which careful placement of *LoxP* sequences results in a silent phenotype until the floxed element is excised through Cre-mediated recombination (Fig. 8A). More recently, the challenging step of excising the positive selectable marker to create the floxed allele of interest has been simplified by using the Cre/*LoxP* and Flp/*FRT* recombinase systems in conjunction with transgenic lines allowing germline excision of floxed sequences (116,117). Targeting using a positive selectable marker flanked by *FRT* sequences and appropriately positioned LoxP elements allows the desired floxed allele to be created by breeding heterozygous targeted mice with a germline Flp deletor mouse strain (Fig. 8B). Regardless of the mechanism used for establishing a floxed allele in a target gene, the temporal and spatial selectivity of inactivation through recombinase excision is dependent on the parallel establishment of transgenic lines in which the cognate recombinase is placed under control of tissue-specific promoters.

Ligand-Regulated Recombinases

As discussed above, the development of methods for conditional gene inactivation through use of site-specific recombinases has considerable potential. Major advances in this technology have come through development of systems allowing precise regulation of recombinase activity or gene expression. One example of such an approach discussed earlier is the use of

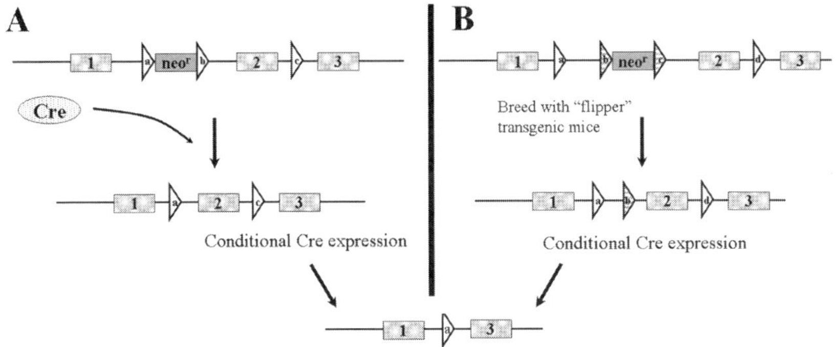

Figure 8　Strategies for conditional gene inactivation. (A) Cre recombinase-mediated generation of a null allele. Homologous recombination in ES cells was utilized to generate a floxed allele in which a neo cassette (neo^r) bordered by sequence recognition sites specific to Cre recombinase (*LoxP*, triangles a and b) in parallel orientation were placed within an intron and a third *LoxP* site (triangle c), also in parallel orientation was placed downstream of the coding sequence to be deleted (box 2). Appropriately targeted ES cells were transiently transfected with Cre recombinase (Cre) and cells that had undergone deletion of the neo cassette via recombination between *LoxP* sites a and b were selected and used to generate transgenic mice. A null allele was generated by breeding these mice with a second transgenic line harboring a transgene providing tissue-specific or conditional expression of Cre recombinase. Recombination between *LoxP* sites a and c resulted in deletion of box 2 and retention of a single *LoxP* site (triangle a) within the null allele. (B) Combined use of Cre and Flp recombinases to generate a null allele. A targeting allele was created in which a neo cassette flanked by sequence recognition sites specific to Flp recombinase (FRT) in parallel orientation (triangles b and c) and a single upstream *LoxP* site (triangle a) was placed within an intron. A second *LoxP* site (triangle d) was placed downstream of the sequence to be deleted (box 2). Appropriately targeted ES cells were selected and used to generate transgenic mice. Breeding of these mice with "flipper" mice, a transgenic line that expresses Flp recombinase in the germline resulted in deletion of the neo cassette via Flp-mediated recombination utilizing the *FRT* sites (triangles b and c). A null allele was generated by breeding these mice with Cre transgenic mice as detailed in (A). Recombination between the two *LoxP* sites (triangles a and d) resulted in deletion of the floxed box 2 and generation of a null allele that retained a single *LoxP* site (triangle a).

transgenic mice with doxycycline-responsive expression of Cre recombinase. Recombinase activity itself can also be regulated while tissue specificity is defined by promoter elements used for Cre expression (118–120). A caveat to this approach for conditional gene inactivation is the unpredictable efficiency with which recombination occurs among Cre-expressing cells. Possible factors that influence recombination efficiency include the conformation of the chromatin in which the RTS are located, proliferative status of the cell, and the level of Cre expression within target cell types.

IV. Lung Injury Applications

Discussion in the remainder of the chapter focuses on selected advances in understanding cellular and molecular mechanisms of lung injury and repair gained through studies in various transgenic and knockout mouse models. Particular emphasis is on the pulmonary epithelium (alveolar and airway), which serves a number of critical biological functions including the clearance and metabolism of inhaled environmental agents, the maintenance of gas exchange, the regulation of lung fluid balance, and the effectiveness of repair following injury (121). Alterations in the numbers and functions of epithelial cells play significant roles in the progression and severity of lung disease and injury (122,123). For example, changes in airway epithelial cell number can involve transient or persistent hyperplasias such as squamous cell, neuroendocrine cell, basal cell, and secretory cell hyperplasia. These changes to the conducting airway epithelium have been associated with an increased risk for the development of both small cell and nonsmall cell lung cancers (124–129). Despite a clear association between chronic airway injury/repair and maintenance or progression of lung disease, the complex nature of the cellular responses to lung injury has only recently begun to be elucidated. These advances have been made in large part with the help of carefully designed transgenic and knockout mouse models to dissect cell and molecular mechanisms of lung injury and repair.

A. Cellular Injury as a Determinant of Airway Repair

Several cell types present in the airways of the adult lung have been shown to have the capacity to proliferate, and in some cases to possess a differentiation potential greater than that required simply for self-renewal. Using thymidine analogs to label S-phase cells of the steady-state rodent lung, the proliferative fraction of airway epithelial cells is in the range of 0.2–1% of total (130). Basal cells and either serous or nonciliated Clara cells account for 70–80% of this proliferative fraction in epithelia of tracheal and bronchial airways (131–133). However, nonciliated Clara cells represent the predominant proliferative epithelial cell type of bronchiolar airways, with minimal, if any, proliferation of basal cells due to their scarcity at this anatomic location (130,134–136).

Manipulation of Cell-Selective Injury for Identification
of Epithelial Stem Cells

Identification of specific roles for distinct progenitor cell populations in maintenance and renewal of various epithelia has typically employed cell-type specific ablation mediated by chemical toxicants or transgenic expression of bacterial toxins (137), cytotoxic viral proteins (17,138–141), or receptors for immunotoxins (142). Progenitor cell populations were originally identified in rodents exposed to the oxidant pollutants O_3, NO_2, and O_2 to promote rapid turnover and renewal of the epithelium (131,143–146). Under these conditions, nonciliated Clara cells are the principal progenitor cell in the bronchiolar epithelium, accounting for >90% of proliferating cells (143). Interestingly basal cells, which account for 28% of proliferating cells in proximal airways of the steady-state lung, account for only 5% of proliferating cells in oxidant injured lung (131,143).

The identity and location of other regenerative airway epithelial cell populations within airways that serve to replenish depleted progenitor cell pools have been determined through selective Clara cell depletion using either chemical or transgenic approaches. Chemical ablation studies exploited the cellular selectivity of the xenobiotic pollutant naphthalene, which is metabolized to a cytotoxic epoxide specifically within Clara cells (147,148). Epithelial renewal in mice following naphthalene-mediated Clara cell ablation initiates at focal sites within airways, a finding that was consistent with depletion of progenitor cells and activation of a latent stem cell pool (149,150). Regenerative foci within bronchioles and a subset of terminal bronchioles were associated with clusters of PNEC organized into neuroepithelial bodies (NEB) (17,151,152). Pulse-labeling studies demonstrated the existence of two mitotic cell types within the NEB microenvironment, Clara cell secretory protein (CCSP)-expressing cells (CE) and Calcitonin gene-related peptide-expressing pulmonary neuroendocrine (PNE) cells (17). Continuous labeling with tritiated thymidine followed by a long (45–100 days) chase period demonstrated that PNE and a subpopulation of CE cells exhibited long-term label-retention, a property of stem cell pools located within other regenerative epithelia (141). Taken together, these studies support the notion that cells contained within the NEB microenvironment of the conducting airway maintain a population of regenerative cells with many properties of tissue-specific stem cells.

While studies using a naphthalene-mediated ablation strategy to deplete progenitor populations suggest the existence of an airway stem cell, they do not define whether PNE cells and/or a population of NEB-associated, pollutant-resistant CE cells might comprise the putative stem cell pool. This question has been addressed using a transgenic mouse model allowing conditional ablation of all CE cell populations to define roles for CE and PNE cells in airway renewal (140,153). A transgene was prepared that placed the procytotoxic HSVtk gene under regulation of the 2.1-kb mouse CCSP promoter (153). Use of the mouse CCSP promoter allowed expression of HSVtk specifically within CE cells distributed throughout the conducting airway epithelium (140,153). Chronic or acute treatment of transgene positive mice with GCV resulted in a greater than 95% decrease in the expression of the Clara cell-specific CCSP and CYP450-2F2 mRNAs and an approximately 95% depletion of CCSP expressing cells. Gancyclovir treatment did not affect the number of ciliated cells in bronchi indicating that this transgenic model of airway injury results in selective ablation of the CE population.

Distinct aspects of the cellular response of airways to CE cell depletion can also be addressed by delivery of GCV. For example, chronic GCV-treatment of CCtk mice has been utilized to investigate the regenerative capacity of PNE and other non-CE cell populations (153). Under these conditions, proliferation among residual airway cells was limited to the CGRP-expressing PNE cell population, and was associated with an increase in the total number of NEB and in the number of PNE cells per NEB. Through use of this continuous ablation model, it was possible to demonstrate that PNEC function autonomously as a self-renewing progenitor population and ruled out earlier speculation that Clara cell proliferation was a prerequisite for PNEC hyperplasia (153). This model did not, however, allow assessment of the differentiation potential of proliferating PNE cells. Through use of the same transgenic mouse model with acute exposure to GCV, it was possible to determine whether PNE cells had the capacity for replenishment of CE and other airway lineages (140). The acute exposure regimen resulted in selective ablation of existing CE cells, while allowing survival of nascent CE cells produced as a consequence of the proliferation and differentiation of PNE cells. Thus, the ability of non-CE cells to restore the CE cell population could be assessed. Airways of mice exposed to GCV for 1 day and recovered in the absence of GCV for 10 days showed intense proliferation of PNE cells with increased cellularity of NEBs, confirming an association between severe Clara cell injury and development of PNEC hyperplasia. However, no regenerating foci of CE cells were detected within the NEB microenvironment, demonstrating that PNE cells failed to restore the depleted CE cell lineage (140). Coupling the findings from this transgenic mouse model with those from naphthalene injury studies suggested that NEBs harbor a population of variant CE cells with many properties common to stem cells of other regenerative epithelia (140).

B. Cell Cycle Control in the Lung

The cell cycle, or the ordered series of events resulting in the generation of two nascent daughter cells from an originating parent, is a process controlled by expression of cyclin proteins and cyclin-dependent kinases. These proteins in turn regulate aspects of DNA synthesis during distinct "phases" of cellular proliferation. In addition to these basic components, a large number of accessory proteins are involved in sequence proofreading, cell cycle arrest/DNA repair, and the orchestration of chromosomal division during mitosis (for a comprehensive review of the cell cycle, see Refs. 154, 155). These networks of interacting proteins facilitate the two major functions of the cell cycle, cell proliferation following injury and prevention of inappropriate mitosis that may result in cancer (156). While numerous in vitro studies have identified proteins involved in regulation of cell proliferation during lung injury/repair or carcinogenesis, these models cannot approximate the actual events occurring within a complex organ such as the lung. It is therefore not surprising that studies of lung cell cycle regulation have increasingly used transgenic and knockout animal technology to address these complex biological questions in vivo.

Targeted Deletion of Cell Cycle Checkpoint Genes

Cellular proliferation is regulated via cell cycle arrest at two phase-transition checkpoints, the G1/S and G2/M transition borders (154,155). In vitro studies have identified several critical proteins that regulate G1/S arrest including p53, members of the Cip/Kip (p21, p27, and p57) family, and the INK4 (p15 p16, p18, p19) family of proteins. Similarly, multiple mechanisms regulate the G2/M transition and include inhibition of cdc25 phosphorylation (157), p53-dependent degradation of cyclin B (158), and activation of GADD45-binding cyclin-dependent kinase 1 (159,160). Gene targeting in ES cells has been used to generate mice bearing null alleles for a variety of the cell cycle regulatory genes including p53, $p21^{Cip1/WAF1}$, p27, p57, $p16^{Ink4/ARF}$, and GADD45 (161–168). The majority of these knockout mice display distinct phenotypes with multiorgan abnormalities resulting from inappropriate cell cycle control. However, only a small number of these strains exhibit an identified phenotype within the lung. Mice bearing a targeted deletion in the G1 phase cyclin-dependent kinase inhibitor $p21^{Cip1/WAF1}$ exhibit increased mortality following exposure to hyperoxia. This phenotype has been attributed to a lack of appropriate cell cycle arrest in type 2 pneumocytes (160). Interestingly, $p53^{-/-}$ mice exposed to hyperoxia for a similar length of time do not demonstrate this phenotype (159,169). This finding, coupled with the observation that p21 levels are increased in lungs of $p53^{-/-}$ mice following hyperoxia exposure, indicates that p21-mediated G1 arrest may function independently of p53 activation (160). The paucity of other lung phenotypes among knockout mouse models with defects in known cell cycle regulatory genes is likely to stem from the fact that the lung is predominately a quiescent organ in healthy adults and/or the existence of redundant mechanisms regulating cell cycle in the developing and mature lung.

Oncogene-Mediated Neoplasia in the Lung

The low mitotic index of the normal lung presents a difficult model for the study of in vivo cell cycle inhibition; however, this same property provides an ideal environment for the study of genes whose presence results in enhanced cellular proliferation, neoplasia, and carcinogenesis. Such genes, termed oncogenes, are either mutated forms of endogenous genes or exogenous genes introduced through exposure to viruses (156). Dysregulation of either the expression or activity of oncogenes leads to a hyperproliferative state through sequestration and activation of the target cell's endogenous proliferative machinery. While the fundamental aspects of oncogene activity are well understood, the specific cell types in which this neoplastic transformation occurs in the lung are poorly defined. Oncogene-mediated neoplasia in the lung is associated with disturbed gene regulation, a consequence of which may be presented as either promiscuous expression of multilineage markers at one extreme vs. expression of a poorly differentiated phenotype with no definitive lineage-specific markers at the other extreme (170–173). Genetically modified mouse models have been employed in order to define mechanisms and cellular origins of lung neoplasms.

Transgenic and knockin approaches have been used for the constitutive overexpression of oncogenes such as simian virus 40 large T antigen (SV40-TAg), viral c-Harvey-ras (v-H-ras), and Kirsten-ras (K-ras) within the lung (174–178). Studies of SV40-TAg have used both the human surfactant protein C (SP-C) promoter and murine CCSP promoter to target cell-specific expression of this oncogene to alveolar type 2 cells or airway Clara cells, respectively (174,177–185). In each case, the resulting adenocarcinomas contained a mixture of airway and alveolar phenotypes, with tumor burdens reaching life-threatening levels by several months of age. Two possible explanations have been offered to explain the apparent heterogeneity of cellular phenotypes within tumors derived from these transgenic lines. First, both the SP-C and CC10 promoters are activated early in lung development prior to lineage commitment (185), leading to the possibility that phenotypic heterogeneity among tumors is a reflection of the phenotype of cells at the time of immortalization. The alternative possibility is that tumor formation results from frequent, concomitant neoplasia within numerous adjoining subsets of differentiated epithelial cells (174). Support for the former possibility stems from the observation that transgenic animals expressing v-H-ras under control of the neuroendocrine cell-specific calcitonin promoter exhibit multiple neoplastic lesions that represent multiple cellular lineages including neuroendocrine, type 2 pneumocyte, and Clara cells (176). Even though these transgenic models have served as a valuable source of immortalized cell lines for in vitro studies, they are of limited value in modeling lung cancer in humans due to the constitutive nature of oncogene expression during the process of lung development, and broad expression within a large population of poorly differentiated precursor cells.

Although there are questions about the relevance of mouse models with constitutive oncogene overexpression in the modeling of human lung cancer, novel transgenic and knockout approaches have recently been developed that overcome many of these caveats (185,186). These new mouse models use three distinct technologies to specifically control for both the onset and incidence of K-ras transgene expression throughout the lung. The first of these involves the generation of a modified allele of the endogenous K-ras gene using a modification of the "hit-and-run" strategy for introduction of point mutations into the ES cell (184,185) (Fig. 9A). A neomycin resistance gene construct flanked by mutated K-ras (G12D) is inserted into the K-ras locus of the mouse ES cells by homologous recombination using an insertion-type vector ("hit"). When mouse lines are established from ES cells carrying this modification, random somatic recombination between adjacent repeats of the K-ras gene is found to be sufficient to trigger expression of a mutant K-ras within the endogenous locus ("run"). As such, tumors arise spontaneously in this mouse model through the stochastic activation of mutant K-ras, a process which occurs with low frequency among many somatic tissues (186). Another strength of this model is that the use of knockin technology ensures that mutated K-ras sequences are expressed at levels similar to that of the wild-type allele. Results of this "hit-and-run" model indicate that the majority of lung tumors arising from random mutations to the K-ras allele express markers of alveolar epithelial cell differentiation, suggesting that they may have been derived from alveolar type 2 cells (187). While this model is a significant improvement over previous transgenic and knockin systems, it remains difficult to control the frequency, developmental onset, or cellular specificity of recombination events.

A second method used to study roles for mutated K-ras in lung neoplasia involves bitransgenic mice in which oncogene expression within specified cell lineages is induced in the presence of doxycycline (187). This methodology not only allows for selective temporal and spatial activation of the K-ras mutation but also provides a mechanism to investigate the consequences of gene inactivation following tumor initiation. While the cellular specificity and incidence of transgene expression reflects the relaxed cellular specificity common with heterologous promoter systems (principally alveolar type 2 pneumocyte expression using a rat CCSP promoter), results reveal progressive alveolar tumorigenesis following administration of doxycycline (188). In particular, continuous administration of doxycycline yields large, alveolar-derived adenomas after two months of treatment identical to those described using the "hit-and-run" system (187). Removal of doxycycline leads to a decrease in K-ras transcript abundance accompanied by rapid tumor regression via apoptosis over several weeks (188). Data from this study support a critical role for sustained expression of mutant K-ras in progressive lung alveolar carcinoma. In addition, the coupling of each of these two genetic models (doxycycline and hit-and-run) with a pre-existing system for cell cycle dysregulation ($p53^{-/-}$ mouse) results in an increased rate of tumor growth and more rapid onset on animal morbidity (187,188). This finding enforces previous observations that many cell cycle regulatory genes may be important in lung, but that their significance will not be evident through studies performed in the absence of promitogenic stimuli.

Finally, two groups have reported temporal regulation of mutant K-ras expression through the use of adenovirus-mediated Cre recombinase (Fig. 9C) (189,190). In this model system, a floxed polyadenylation (transcriptional terminator or STOP) signal cassette positioned upstream of mutant K-ras blocks transcription of the proto-oncogene located within either the endogenous locus (knockin) or downstream of a β-actin promoter-regulated transgene. Following intratracheal administration of adeno-viral-Cre recombinase, the floxed STOP cassette is excised allowing expression of mutant K-ras within those cells that undergo recombination. Results of each of these studies closely resemble those described above for both the "hit-and-run" and doxycycline regulable K-ras expression systems, yet have the advantage that the tissue specificity of K-ras activation is defined by the local administration of Cre-expressing adenovirus. Cre-mediated recombination occurs among all lung epithelial compartments

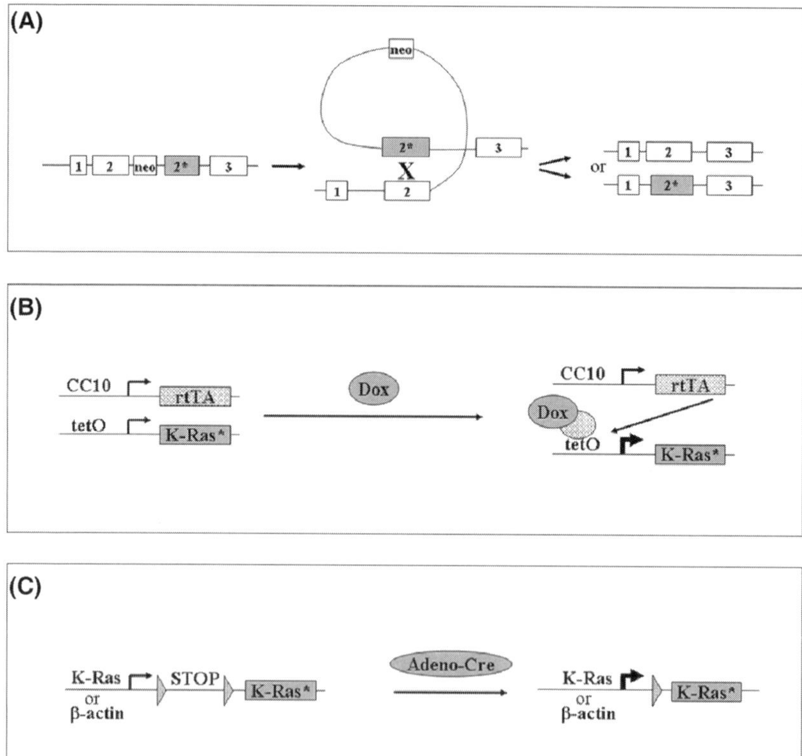

Figure 9   (*Caption on facing page*)

and results in predominately alveolar-type adenocarcinomas (189). These mouse models provide additional evidence that mutatins leading to activation of K-ras lead principally to the development of type 2 cell-derived lung neoplasms. However, classification of tumor origin is still dependent upon retrospective analysis based upon tumor phenotype, thus precluding definitive identification of tumor precursor cells. Application of lineage tagging approaches that have been developed to characterize lineage relationships in the developing and repairing lung may provide definitive identification of precursor cell types for various lung neoplasms.

C. Differentiation Potential of Lung Epithelial Cells During Repair

An understanding of mechanisms responsible for epithelial renewal and restoration of a fully functional epithelium is critical to understanding the pathogenesis of these chronic airway diseases. As discussed previously, Clara cells have been well characterized as a self-renewing progenitor population and as a progenitor for ciliated cells (131,143). Moreover, studies investigating epithelial renewal following progenitor cell depletion suggest

---

Figure 9 (*Facing page*) Strategies for selective expression of oncogenes. Panel A: "Hit-and-run" conditional allele. The K-ras locus was targeted to generate an allele in which a neo cassette (neo, see Fig. 8) and a mutated K-ras exon 2 (box 2*) were located downstream of the wild-type exon 2 (box 2). Rare intramolecular homologous recombination involving a single crossover (large X) resulted in elimination of either the wild-type exon 2 or the mutant exon 2. Panel B: Use of the tet-on system to activate expression of a mutant K-ras in adult mice. Bitransgenic mice were generated by breeding monotransgenic mice harboring a reverse tet-transcriptional activator (rtTA) regulated by the rat CC10 (CC10) promoter or a mutant form of K-ras (K-ras*) regulated by the tet operator (tetO). Systemic treatment of bitransgenic mice with doxycyclin (dox) resulted in association of a dox/rtTA complex with tetO and activation of K-ras* gene expression. Panel C: Use of Cre recombinase to temporally regulate expression of a mutant K-ras. Two systems have been developed to permit Cre-regulated expression of a mutant K-ras gene. In the first of these, the endogenous K-ras gene was silenced through targeting of the locus with a cassette composed of a strong transcriptional stop signal (STOP) bordered by sequence recognition sites specific to Cre recombinase (*LoxP*, triangles) and a downstream mutant K-ras open reading frame (K-ras*). An alternative approach utilized transgenic mice harboring the same transcriptionally silent K-ras* allele under regulation of the β-actin promoter. Animals were instilled with an adenovirus that expressed Cre recombinase and K-ras* gene expression was activated through Cre recombinase-mediated excision of the "STOP" sequence and juxtaposition of the promoter and downstream K-ras* reading frame. The model systems presented in Panels B and C allow temporally regulated activation of proto-oncogene expression where as that presented in Panel A takes advantage of a stochastic process that occurs throughout the life of the animal.

that stem cells with a CCSP-expressing molecular- and a pollutant-resistant functional phenotype reside within distinct microenvironments within the bronchiolar epithelium (17). The contribution made by focal populations of stem cells in epithelial maintenance is poorly understood. However, clonal expansion of branchpoint-associated p53 mutant cells in a chronically injured (smoker's) lung (191) leads to the suggestion that repopulation of the airway epithelium by a small population of progenitor cells can result in fixation of a mutant cell genotype. Similarly, chronic injury and focal repair of the airway in the asthmatic lung may contribute to fixation of a variant cell phenotype(s) and a resultant alteration of the airway microenvironment. The following sections will discuss transgenic and knockout mouse models that have been used to define intrinsic and extrinsic mechanisms regulating epithelial cell differentiation.

Lineage Tagging Approaches to Define Differentiation Potential

Transgenic approaches have been utilized for in vivo lineage tracing with the goal of defining cellular differentiation potential. Typically, these systems utilize two components: a genomic recombination substrate (RS) allele and a system for delivering an activated recombinase to a specific cell type in a temporally regulated manner. Even though any site-specific recombinase system can theoretically be applied to the strategies described below, the Cre/*LoxP* system has been used exclusively in lineage tracing experiments. Using these approaches, a typical recombination substrate is composed of a ubiquitous promoter, a "floxed" transcriptional termination (polyadenylation) signal bordered by 34 bp *LoxP* recombinase recognition sites, and a downstream reporter gene (Fig. 10). Expression of the native transgeneterminates within the floxed cassette while recombinase-mediated excision (see below) of the floxed sequence results in activation of the downstream reporter. When coupled with an appropriate strategy for conditional activation of Cre recombinase, lineage tags can be introduced into target cells according to the specificity and timing of recombinase activation.

Systems utilizing ligand-regulation of Cre recombinase to achieve temporal control of its activity have not been used to assess lineage relationships in the lung, but has been successfully applied to the introduction of lineage tags within other organ systems including skin (192–194), intestine (195,196) and the developing central nervous system (197,198). An alternative strategy that has been employed for temporal activation of Cre recombinase activity is the use of the tet system to achieve temporal regulation of Cre expression. This approach has been applied, for example, to analyze cell lineage relationships in the developing lung through expression of rtTA under the control of the human SP-C promoter with subsequent dox regulation of a tetO-Cre transgene (199) (Fig. 10). Cre-mediated recombination of the "black and blue" ZAP RS transgene

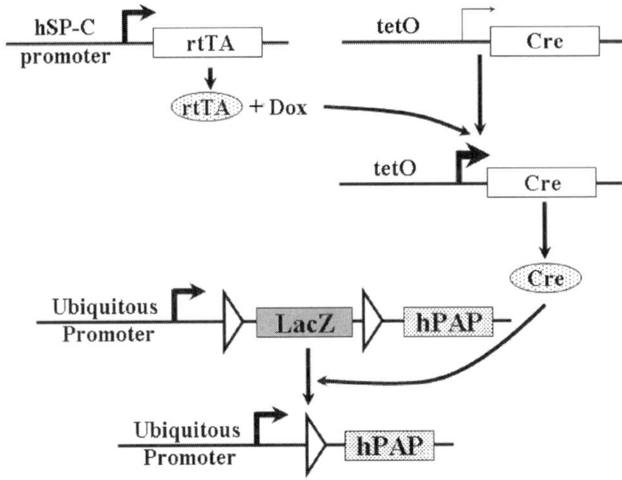

Figure 10 Tet-regulated expression of Cre recombinase for introduction of lineage tags in the developing mouse lung. This strategy for lineage tagging involved use of three independent transgenes that were bred to establish tripple-transgene positive mice. Transgene 1: 3.7-kb human SP-C promoter (hSP-C) driving expression of reverse tet-trans activator (rtTA); transgene 2: Cre recombinase (Cre) under the regulatory control of the tetO minimal promoter; transgene 3: recombination substrate transgene composed of a floxed LacZ reporter (see Figs. 8 and 9) under the control of a ubiquitous promoter element with a downstream human placental alkaline phosphatase (hPAP) reporter gene. Administration of doxycycline (dox) results in potent transactivation of Cre expression and subsequent excision of LacZ reporter gene sequences from the recombination substrate. Excision of the floxed LacZ reporter gene places hPAP under the regulatory control of the ubiquitous promoter, thus introducing a permanent genetic tag in the cell type defined by the hSP-C promoter and the lineage derived from this tagged cell. (Adapted from Ref. 202.)

resulted in deletion of a floxed LacZ reporter gene (blue) and activation of the downstream human placental alkaline phosphatase (black) reporter. Lineage tagged cells in this system were recognized by histochemical detection of alkaline phosphatase. Alternatively, substitution of the recombination substrate with the ZEG RS transgene resulted in excision of the floxed LacZ reporter gene and activation of a downstream enhanced green fluorescent protein reporter gene (199). In this latter case, tagged cells were recognized by direct detection of the fluorescent protein or through immunohistochemical staining. Using either of these reporter systems, continuous treatment of tritransgenic dams with dox from embryonic day (E) 6.5 to E3.5, E14.5, E15.5, E16.5, or postnatal day 5 resulted in tagging of nearly all epithelial cells of the conducting airway and a subset of epithelial cells in the trachea and bronchi

(199). Recombination was strictly dox-dependent prior to E15.5 although rare dox-independent recombination was noted at all time points after E16.5. Recombination efficiency decreased following birth and was nearly undetectable in the steady-state mature lung. The inducible nature of this system was demonstrated by a 48 hr treatment of dams with dox (embryonic day 16.5–18.5) and assessment of Cre recombinase mRNA and protein distribution at the end of the induction period and following a 48- or 96-hr chase period. The narrow window of induction resulted in a high level of recombination, while withdrawal of dox was associated with a marked reduction in the number of Cre-expressing cells at 48 hr and an absence of Cre expression by 96 hr (199). Results of these experiments indicate that the tet-on system can be used to effectively delineate lineage relationships in the embryonic lung.

Extrinsic Regulation of Epithelial Cell Phenotype:
Cytokine Regulation

Even though the regenerative capacity of pulmonary epithelial cells is a critical determinant of effective repair, mechanisms regulating epithelial cell differentiation are central to the restoration of airway homeostasis and perturbation of this process may lead to establishment of chronic lung disease. Due to the complex cytokine and growth factor milieu that exists in the injured/repairing lung, the impact that acute or chronic changes in cytokine and/or growth factor expression has on the restoration of functional epithelial cell types has been an area of intense investigation.

The role played by Th2 cytokines in development of mucous cell metaplasia and mucus hypersecretion has been investigated through analysis of transgenic mice that constitutively overexpress interleukin (IL) -4 (200), IL-5 (201) IL-9 (202), and IL-13 (203) specifically within the lung. These studies have made extensive use of the rat CC10 promoter [also referred to as the CCSP promoter (13)] to direct interleukin gene expression predominantly in Clara cells of the airway epithelium. Unchallenged transgene positive mice exhibit a profound regulation of Clara cell phenotype characterized by hyperplasia of acidic and neutral mucous positive cells in the upper airway, mucous cell metaplasia in the lower airways, and a drastic reduction in the number of CCSP mRNA-expressing cells (200–202). Ultrastructural examination of airway epithelial cells from CC10-IL-4 transgenic mice demonstrated accumulation of vacuoles containing homogenous low-density material in the apical region of nonciliated cells and an absence of electron dense secretory granules characteristic of normal Clara cells (204). Transgenic overexpression of IL-4 induced the primary pulmonary mucin gene MUC5AC but not MUC2 and was associated with accumulation of glycoproteins in the bronchoalveolar lavage (204). A similar analysis of mucin gene expression in CC10-IL-9 transgenic mice demonstrated upregulation of both MUC5AC and MUC2 gene expression as well as increased levels of these proteins in the bronchoalveolar lavage of unstimulated animals (205). Inflammation characterized predominantly by accumulation of eosinophils and lymphocytes was reported for all strains of mice that express Th2 cytokines constitutively in the airway epithelium. Mast cell hyperplasia was noted in IL-9 transgenic mice and increased numbers of macrophages and neutrophils were reported in IL-13 transgenic mice. Other pathological changes to airways of these mice included subepithelial fibrosis and bronchial hyper-responsiveness which were observed in IL-5, IL-9, and IL-13 transgenic mice. In contrast, mice that constitutively express IL-5 (206,207), IL-9 (208,209), or IL-13 (210) in nonpulmonary tissues exhibit lung pathology only after antigen challenge suggesting that high circulating levels of Th2 cytokines are insufficient to initiate mucous cell metaplasia (MCM) or other pathologic changes associated with mucosecretory diseases. Results of these studies indicate that pulmonary-specific expression of individual Th2 cytokines is sufficient for the establishment of mucous cell hyperplasia and that this results in altered gene expression in Clara cells, cellular accumulation of glycoconjugate, and hypersecretion of mucus into the airway lumen.

Temporal Aspects of Mucosecretory Disease

The complex characteristics of mucosecretory diseases are thought to stem both from defects in lung development (211,212) as well as alterations to lung homeostasis associated with chronic injury and repair. Although the morphological and functional alterations associated with mucus hypersecretion are similar in mucosecretory diseases of pediatric and adult patients, the mechanisms leading to this pathology may be distinct: clearly MCM in cystic fibrosis and in childhood asthma represents a functional alteration within the developing lung while similar airway pathology in chronic bronchitis and COPD is a modification of the mature and/or aging lung. Finally, an understanding of the pathway leading to mucus hypersecretion in COPD may be complicated by functional alterations to the alveolar compartment associated with emphysema. The temporal aspects of disease establishment as well as acute exacerbation of symptoms have been difficult to model using CC10 promoter regulated transgenes due to activation of gene expression early in lung development (16), constitutive high level expression in the mature airway epithelium (13), and caveats resulting from persistent low-level activity of the rat CC10 promoter in alveolar type 2 cells (13). However, development of regulable transgene alleles (108,109) and application of these systems for modeling of pulmonary disease has led to segregation of the effects of cytokines on alveolar development and induction of the asthmatic phenotype.

This technology was first applied to issues of pulmonary biology by Elias and colleagues (213,214), who noted that CC10-regulated expression of IL-11 (an IL-6-like cytokine) in the airway epithelium resulted in peribronchiolar aggregations of mononuclear cells, airway remodeling with subepithelial fibrosis, airway hyper-reactivity, and enlarged alveoli. Following ovalbumin sensitization and challenge, eosinophilic and lymphocytic inflammation and Th2 cytokine levels were lower in CC10-IL-11 mice relative to similarly challenged transgene negative littermate controls, although transgenic expression of IL-11 did not alter mucus hypersecretion or expression of MUC5AC (215). These results suggested that distinct mechanisms regulate the development of various aspects of airway pathology in asthma, particularly MCM, mucus hypersecretion and eosinophil recruitment. However, interpretation of these results was complicated by the complex phenotype of steady-state mice. In order to dissociate the developmentally dependent and independent components of this model, bitransgenic mice bearing a rat CC10 promoter-regulated reverse tetracycline transactivator (rtTA) transgene (CC10-rtTA) and a polymeric tetracycline operator (tet-O), minimal CMV promoter-regulated human IL-11 (tetO-IL-11) were generated (216). Transgene expression was induced during gestation, the postnatal period, or in adults by continuous administration of doxycyclin in the drinking water and resulted in maximal expression of IL-11 mRNA and protein within 6 days. Withdrawal of doxycyclin resulted in a greater than 80% decrease in IL-11 message and protein within 24 hr. Results of this study demonstrated that alveolar enlargement in CC10-IL11 mice was the result of IL-11-mediated abnormalities in lung growth and differentiation while airway remodeling and inflammation are independent of the developmental effects of IL-11 (214). A similar strategy was applied to analysis of IL-9-mediated effects and demonstrated that developmental abnormalities do not contribute to IL-9-induced eosinophilia and mucus production (217).

In contrast with the previously mentioned regulable systems where doxycyclin-independent expression of the CC10-regulated transgene was either minimal or nill, leaky expression of IL-13 in CC10-rtTA + tetO-IL-13 bitransgenic mice has been shown to result in a demonstrable phenotype characterized by lung inflammation, MCM, and increasedexpression of chemokine, matrix metalloprotease (MMP), and cathepsin mRNAs as well as increases in alveolar size and lung volume (218). The key position of IL-13 in the hierarchy of Th2 cytokines is likely to account for the sensitivity of the lung to low level IL-13 expression (219,220). In order to suppress baseline activity of the CC10-rtTA transgene, a tet-regulated transcriptional silencer (tTS) was utilized in combination with the CC10-rtTA and tetO-IL-13 transgenes (221). The tet-trans silencer is a fusion protein composed of the Tet repressor and a strong transcriptional repressor, the KRAB-AB domain of the Kid-1 protein. In the absence of doxycyclin, tTS is active and binds to tet-O, thus repressing expression of IL-13. Conversely, addition of doxycyclin to the system results in dissociation of tTS and association of rtTA with tetO, resulting in activation of IL-13 gene expression. In tritransgenic mice, basal expression of

IL-13 was similar to that of transgene negative and monotransgenic mice and the morphological, physiological, and molecular abnormalities associated with leaky IL-13 gene expression were abrogated (221). Treatment of tritransgenic mice with doxycyclin from birth to one month of age resulted in high levels of IL-13 protein in the bronchoalveolar lavage with molecular and cellular phenotypes similar to mice with constitutive IL-13 expression. This approach suggested that the phenotype associated with transient lung IL-13 expression is not a result of altered lung development, although IL-13 may impact postnatal differentiation of the alveolar compartment (221). This tritransgenic system has the potential to model the episodic nature of asthma, since doxycyclin can be administered and withdrawn at various intervals.

Cytokine Hierarchy and Segregation Disease Characteristics

Studies of constitutive and regulable transgenic mice indicate that Th2 cytokines play a critical role in the initiation of MCM. However, these studies have not determined whether this effect is due to direct action of each cytokine on airway epithelial cells, the result of signaling cascades among the Th2 cytokines, or perhaps the result of unidentified factorsproduced by an intermediate cell types such as smooth muscle cells, or lymphocytes, eosinophils, mast cells that are recruited to the airway. A significant hurdle to identification of the central mediator of the asthmatic phenotype has been the complex feedback loops that exist between Th2 cytokines. This difficulty was overcome by Cohn et al. (222,223), who developed a method for in vitro differentiation of antigen-specific T-cells and adoptive transfer of these cells into wild-type or genetically modified hosts. In order to address the role of IL-5 and eosinophils in development of MCM, ovalbumin-specific IL-5$^{-/-}$ Th2 cells were generated in vitro and adoptively transferred to IL-5$^{-/-}$ mice (222). Extensive mucus staining of airways was observed in these mice although eosinophilia and mast cell recruitment was abolished. These data demonstrate that IL-5, eosinophils, and mast cells are not necessary for development of MCM. A similar experiment utilizing adoptive transfer of IL-4$^{-/-}$ Th2 cells has demonstrated that IL-4 is not necessary for MCM (224), suggesting that another cytokine such as IL-13 may stimulate mucus production. Analysis of MCM in mice mutant in various components of the IL-4/IL-13 signal transduction pathway including knockouts of the common chain of the IL-4 receptor [IL-4Rα and signal transducer and activator of transcription 6 (STAT6) (225–227)] confirmed the essential nature of this pathway in development of MCM. Interestingly, the development of eosinophilia and airway hyper-responsiveness was not affected by STAT6 deficiency although this effect was modulated by genetic background (225–227). These data further support the conclusion that the development of MCM is independent of eosinophils and their products, and that altered function of the mesenchymal compartment is not essential for mucus production (228). Similarly, IL-13 has been found to stimulate accumulation of mucus in RAG$^{-/-}$ mice, indicating that this process can occur in the absence of both B- and T-lymphocytes (229). These results suggest that IL-13 is a central regulator of metaplastic changes in the transition to the mucus producing phenotype, and that these alterations can occur in the absence of cellular infiltrates associated with asthma such as eosinophils, mast cells, B- and T-lymphocytes, or alterations in airway fibroblasts.

Cellular Target of IL-13

Direct stimulation of mucus production by IL-13 in primary cultures of human bronchial epithelial cells (205,229) led to the suggestion that IL-13 initiates mucous cell metaplasia through a direct activity on airway epithelial cells. This hypothesis was tested by a combination of knockout and transgenic technology in which STAT6 expression was limited to Clara cells through breeding STAT6$^{-/-}$ mice with a transgenic line in which the human STAT6 cDNA was regulated by the rat CC10 promoter (Epi-hSTAT6) resulting in constitutive overexpression of STAT6 exclusively in airway epithelial cells. In order to overcome deficiencies in production of IL-13 secreting Th2 cells in STAT6 knockout mice, the STAT6$^{-/-}$; Epi-hSTAT6 mice were bred with the CC10-IL13 mice to generate Epi-hSTAT6;CC10-IL-13;STAT$^{+/-}$ bitransgenic/heterozygotic mice that overexpressed IL-13 and STAT6 in the airway, but were deficient in expression of STAT6 in all other cell types and tissues (230). Mucus production in these mice was similar to that observed in IL-13;STAT6 heterozygotes indicating that IL-13 acts directly on Clara cells via the STAT6 pathway to alter gene expression and stimulate mucin production. Interestingly, airway hyper-responsiveness was not altered by the absence of STAT6 in mesenchymal cells, suggesting that the airway may serve as an intermediate in the development of airway hyper-reactivity. It has also been reported that IL-13 (and IL-4) are profibrogenic factors for human bronchial fibroblasts and promoted the transition of fibroblasts to contractile myofibroblasts in the presence of TGF-β (231). An intermediary role for resident airway epithelial cells in the induction of airway hyper-responsiveness is supported by the observation that Th2 cytokines rapidly cause changes in airway resistance in the absence of inflammation (230). These results suggest that IL-13 acts directly on airway epithelial cells to initiate cellular and molecular changes leading to hypersecretion of mucus as well as changes in the mesenchymal compartment that result in increased airway reactivity.

Analysis of human airways and those of antigen sensitized and challenged rodents indicate that the initial phase of MCM represents a gain-of-function in which Clara cells express both lineage markers and nascent glycoconjugate. Studies in IL-13 transgenic mice in combination with in vitro stimulation of Clara-like cell lines indicate that IL-13 directly affects expression of mucin genes themselves as well as components of the secretory pathway including MUC5 (232), and additional genes of unknown function (http://baygenomics.ucsf.edu, http://pgadata.cnmcresearch.org). However, asthma and COPD are also associated with a decrease in the number of CCSP-expressing cells and reductions in serum and bronchoalveolar lavage CCSP levels suggestive of a secondary loss-of-function within the Clara cell. Factors regulating this response have not been delineated although it is known that Th1 cytokines influence expression of CCSP (186,233,234). Studies by Cohn et al. (223,235) using adoptive transfer of antigen-specific Th2 and Th1 cells into wild-type mice indicate that Th1 cells block the mucus-inducing activity of Th2 cells downstream of Th2 cytokine production. Similar analysis in $IFN_\gamma{}^{-/-}$ mice suggests that this activity is mediated by IFNγ acting at the level of the airway epithelial cell (226). These data lead to the hypothesis that Th2-dominated inflammation in the airway perturbs a delicate balance between alternative Clara cell phenotypes which predisposes and/or perpetuates molecular changes leading the MCM.

V. Summary

As detailed in this chapter, genetically modified mouse models are increasingly used in basic research applications, and are widely studied in dissecting mechanisms of lung injury and repair. Current genetic technology permits the systematic development of transgenic and knockout mouse models that are invaluable in studying gene-specific events in the whole animal. A variety of applications using such models in mechanistic studies of lung injury, inflammation, and repair have been illustrated in this chapter. The productive use of transgenic mouse models requires the careful design of transgenes and targeting vectors, comprehensive screening of founder mice, and detailed assessments of genetic background, since these factors have the potential to significantly impact the resulting phenotype and its responses to lung injury. In addition, because many of the genetic signaling interactions and compensatory responses of complex mammalian organisms remain unknown, transgenic mouse models can partly reflect biochemical and cellular changes other than those directly associated with the deletion or alteration of the specific targeted gene or gene product.

First generation transgenic and knockout approaches have highlighted the complexity of intracellular, extracellular, and molecular interactions in the lungs and other organs. Unregulated perturbation of lung gene expression in mice sometimes yields unpredictable phenotypic results that can be misinterpreted. However, the evolution of genetic technologies to include conditional regulatory approaches provides a means to perturb lung gene expression in a precisely controlled manner that more closely recapitulates the dynamic nature of lung injury and repair. Importantly, these strategies can be used to study mechanisms of lung injury and repair in adult animal models that are not confounded by developmental anomalies resulting from constitutive alterations in lung gene expression.

The growing sophistication of genome engineering provides unprecedented opportunities to understand in vivo cell and molecular mechanisms contributing to the maintenance or perturbation of pulmonary homeostasis. Conversely, along with the development of more sophisticated in vivo genetic models comes increased complexity in the design and interpretation of experiments using them. Despite the attendant difficulties of research in genetically modified mouse models, they have clearly redefined the spectrum and specificity of questions that can be addressed in whole animals in vivo. The fundamental information on lung injury and repair that can be gained from such models is difficult if not impossible to obtain from other approaches. Genetic mouse models in principle account for the multiplicity of cell and molecular interactions existing in whole organisms, and allow the effects of individual gene products to be examined with much greater specificity than possible in conventional animal models. At the same time, the utility of data from genetically modified mouse studies is significantly enhanced by integration with mechanistic results obtained in other models. Further details about cell, animal, and inhalation toxicology models used in lung injury research are given in Chapters 10 and 12.

References

1. Hogan B, Beddington R, Constantini F, Lacy E. Manipulating the Mouse Embryo. Cold Spring Harbor Laboratory Press, 1994.
2. Pinkert CA. Transgenic Animal Technology: A Laboratory Handbook Academic Press, 1994.
3. Nagano M, Shinohara T, Avarbock MR, Brinster RL. Retrovirus-mediated gene delivery into male germ line stem cells. FEBS Lett 2000; 475:7–10.
4. Huszar D, Balling R, Kothary R, Magli MC, Hozumi N, Rossant J, Bernstein A. Insertion of a bacterial gene into the mouse germ line using an infectious retrovirus vector. Proc Natl Acad Sci USA 1985; 82:8587–8591.
5. Soriano P, Cone RD, Mulligan RC, Jaenisch R. Tissue-specific and ectopic expression of genes introduced into transgenic mice by retroviruses. Science 1986; 234:1409–1413.
6. Friedrich G, Soriano P. Promoter traps in embryonic stem cells: a genetic screen to identify and mutate developmental genes in mice. Genes Dev 1991; 5:1513–1523.
7. Gordon JW, Scangos GA, Plotkin DJ, Barbosa JA, Ruddle FH. Genetic transformation of mouse embryos by microinjection of purified DNA. Proc Natl Acad Sci USA 1980; 7:7380–7384.
8. Brinster RL, Chen HY, Trumbauer ME, Yagle MK, Palmiter RD. Factors affecting the efficiency of introducing foreign DNA into mice by microinjecting eggs. Proc Natl Acad Sci USA 1985; 82:4438–4442.

9. Palmiter RD, Brinster RL. Germ-line transformation of mice. Annu Rev Genet 1986; 20:465–499.
10. Cherry SR, Biniszkiewicz D, van Parijs L, Baltimore D, Jaenisch R. Retroviral expression in embryonic stem cells and hematopoietic stem cells. Mol Cell Biol 2000; 20:7419–7426.
11. Korfhagen TR, Glasser SW, Wert SE, Bruno MD, Daugherty CC, McNeish JD, Stock JL, Potter SS, Whitsett JA. Cis-acting sequences from a human surfactant protein gene confer pulmonary-specific gene expression in transgenic mice. Proc Natl Acad Sci USA 1990; 87:6122–6126.
12. Glasser SW, Korfhagen TR, Wert SE, Bruno MD, McWilliams KM, Vorbroker DK, Whitsett JA. Genetic element from human surfactant protein SP-C gene confers bronchiolar-alveolar cell specificity in transgenic mice. Am J Physiol 1991; 261:L349–L356.
13. Stripp BR, Sawaya PL, Luse DS, Wikenheiser KA, Wert SE, Huffman JA, Lattier DL, Singh G, Katyal SL, Whitsett JA. Cis-acting elements that confer lung epithelial cell expression of the CC10 gene. J Biol Chem 1992; 267: 14703–14712.
14. Hackett BP, Gitlin JD. Cell-specific expression of a Clara cell secretory protein-human growth hormone gene in the bronchiolar epithelium of transgenic mice. Proc Natl Acad Sci USA 1992; 89:9079–9083.
15. Wert SE, Glasser SW, Korfhagen TR, Whitsett JA. Transcriptional elements from the human SP-C gene direct expression in the primordial respiratory epithelium of transgenic mice. Dev Biol 1993; 156:426–443.
16. Hackett BP, Gitlin JD. 5′ flanking region of the Clara cell secretory protein gene specifies a unique temporal and spatial pattern of gene expression in the developing pulmonary epithelium. Am J Respir Cell Mol Biol 1994; 11: 123–129.
17. Reynolds SD, Giangreco A, Power JHT, Stripp BR. Neuroepithelial bodies of pulmonary airways serve as a reservoir of progenitor cells capable of epithelial regeneration. AmJ Pathol 2000; 156:269–278.
18. Schlaeger TM, Bartunkova S, Lawitts JA, Teichmann G, Risau W, Deutsch U, Sato TN. Uniform vascular-endothelial-cell-specific gene expression in both embryonic and adult transgenic mice. Proc Natl Acad Sci USA 1997; 94: 3058–3063.
19. Chow YH, O'Brodovich H, Plumb J, Wen Y, Sohn KJ, Lu Z, Zhang F, Lukacs GL, Tanswell AK, Hui CC, Buchwald M, Hu J. Development of an epithelium-specific expression cassette with human DNA regulatory elements for transgene expression in lung airways. Proc Natl Acad Sci USA 1997; 94:14695–14700.
20. Millino C, Sarinella F, Tiveron C, Villa A, Sartore S, Ausoni S. Cardiac and smooth muscle cell contribution to the formation of the murine pulmonary veins. Dev Dyn 2000; 218:414–425.
21. Okabe M, Ikawa M, Kominami K, Nakanishi T, Nishimune Y. 'Green mice' as a source of ubiquitous green cells. FEBS Lett 1997; 407:313–319.
22. Kisseberth WC, Brettingen NT, Lohse JK, Sandgren EP. Ubiquitous expression of marker transgenes in mice and rats. Dev Biol 1999; 214:128–138.
23. Jaenisch R. Transgenic animals. Science 1988; 240:1468–1474.

24. Brinster RL, Allen JM, Behringer RR, Gelinas RE, Palmiter RD. Introns increase transcriptional efficiency in transgenic mice. Proc Natl Acad Sci USA 1988; 85:836–840.

25. Palmiter RD, Sandgren EP, Avarbock MR, Allen DD, Brinster RL. Heterologous introns can enhance expression of transgenes in mice. Proc Natl Acad Sci USA 1991; 88:478–482.

26. Kozak M. At least six nucleotides preceding the AUG initiator codon enhance translation in mammalian cells. J Mol Biol 1987; 196:947–950.

27. Kozak M. Features in the 5′ non-coding sequences of rabbit alpha and beta-globin mRNAs that affect translational efficiency. J Mol Biol 1994; 235:95–110.

28. Kozak M. Initiation of translation in prokaryotes and eukaryotes. Gene 1999; 234:187–208.

29. Devereux TR, Kaplan NL. Use of quantitative trait loci to map murine lung tumor susceptibility genes. Exp Lung Res 1998; 24:407–417.

30. Nicolaides NC, Holroyd KJ, Ewart SL, Eleff SM, Kiser MB, Dragwa CR, Sullivan CD, Grasso L, Zhang LY, Messler CJ, Zhou T, Kleeberger SR, Buetow KH, Levitt RC. Interleukin 9: a candidate gene for asthma. Proc Natl Acad Sci USA 1997; 94:13175–13180.

31. De Sanctis GT, Drazen JM. Genetics of native airway responsiveness in mice. Am J Respir Crit Care Med 1997; 156:S82–S88.

32. Prows DR, Shertzer HG, Daly MJ, Sidman CL, Leikauf GD. Genetic analysis of ozone-induced acute lung injury insensitive and resistant strains of mice. Nat Genet 1997; 17:471–474.

33. Kleeberger SR, Levitt RC, Zhang LY, Longphre M, Harkema J, Jedlicka A, Eleff SM, DiSilvestre D, Holroyd KJ. Linkage analysis of susceptibility to ozone-induced lung inflammation in inbred mice. Nat Genet 1997; 17:475–478.

34. Taketo M, Schroeder AC, Mobraaten LE, Gunning KB, Hanten G, Fox RR, Roderick TH, Stewart CL, Lilly F, Hansen CT. FVB/N: an inbred mouse strain preferable for transgenic analyses. Proc Natl Acad Sci USA 1991; 88:2065–2069.

35. Peters K, Werner S, Liao X, Wert S, Whitsett J, Williams L. Targeted expression of a dominant negative FGF receptor blocks branching morphogenesis and epithelial differentiation of the mouse lung. EMBO J 1994; 13:3296–3301.

36. Overbeek P. Factors affecting transgenic animal production. In: Pinkert CA, ed. Transgenic Animal Technology: a laboratory Handbook. Academic Press Inc, 1994.

37. Hansbrough JR, Fine SM, Gordon JI. A transgenic mouse model for studying the lineage relationships and differentiation program of type II pneumocytes at various stages of lung development. J Biol Chem 1993; 268: 9762–9770.

38. Korn R, Schoor M, Neuhaus H, Henseling U, Soininen R, Zachgo J, Gossler A. Enhancer trap integrations in mouse embryonic stem cells give rise to staining patterns in chimaeric embryos with a high frequency and detect endogenous genes. Mech Dev 1992; 39:95–109.

39. Feng YQ, Lorincz MC, Fiering S, Greally JM, Bouhassira EE. Position effects are influenced by the orientation of a transgene with respect to flanking chromatin. Mol Cell Biol 2001; 21:298–309.

40. Eszterhas SK, Bouhassira EE, Martin DI, Fiering S. Transcriptional interference by independently regulated genes occurs in any relative arrangement of the genes and is influenced by chromosomal integration position. Mol Cell Biol 2002; 22:469–479.

41. Bonifer C, Yannoutsos N, Kruger G, Grosveld F, Sippel AE. Dissection of the locus control function located on the chicken lysozyme gene domain in transgenic mice. Nucleic Acids Res 1994; 22:4202–4210.

42. Bonifer C, Huber MC, Jagle U, Faust N, Sippel AE. Prerequisites for tissue specific and position independent expression of a gene locus in transgenic mice. J Mol Med 1996; 74:663–671.

43. Caterina JJ, Ryan TM, Pawlik KM, Palmiter RD, Brinster RL, Behringer RR, Townes TM. Human beta-globin locus control region: analysis of the $5'$ DNase I hypersensitive site HS 2 in transgenic mice. Proc Natl Acad Sci USA 1991; 88:1626–1630.

44. Reitman M, Lee E, Westphal H, Felsenfeld G. Site-independent expression of the chicken beta A-globin gene in transgenic mice. Nature 1990; 348:749–752.

45. Fraser P, Pruzina S, Antoniou M, Grosveld F. Each hypersensitive site of the human beta-globin locus control region confers a different developmental pattern of expression on the globin genes. Genes Dev 1993; 7:106–113.

46. Gaensler KM, Kitamura M, Kan YW. Germ-line transmission and developmental regulation of a 150-kb yeast artificial chromosome containing the human beta-globin locus in transgenic mice. Proc Natl Acad Sci USA 1993; 90:11381–11385.

47. McKnight RA, Spencer M, Wall RJ, Hennighausen L. Severe position effects imposed on a 1 kb mouse when acidic protein gene promoter are overcome by heterologous matrix attachment regions. Mol Reprod Dev 1996; 44:179–184.

48. Guy LG, Kothary R, DeRepentigny Y, Delvoye N, Ellis J, Wall L. The beta-globin locus control region enhances transcription of but does not confer position-independent expression onto the lacZ gene in transgenic mice. EMBO J 1996; 15:3713–3721.

49. Makarova O, Gorneva G, Wu F, Farutin V, Villeponteau B, Poliani L, Fink D, Levine M. Incorporation of nuclear matrix attachment regions into the herpes simplex virus type 1 genome does not induce long-term expression of a foreign gene during latency. Gene Ther 1996; 3:829–833.

50. Emery DW, Yannaki E, Tubb J, Stamatoyannopoulos G. A chromatin insulator protects retrovirus vectors from chromosomal position effects. Proc Natl Acad Sci USA 2000; 97:9150–9155.

51. Henikoff S. Conspiracy of silence among repeated transgenes. Bioessays 1998; 20:532–535.

52. Cohen-Tannoudji M, Vandormael-Pournin S, Drezen J, Mercier P, Babinet C, Morello D. LacZ sequences prevent regulated expression of housekeeping genes. Mech Dev 2000; 90:29–39.

53. You YH, Halangoda A, Buettner V, Hill K, Sommer S, Pfeifer G. Methylation of CpG dinucleotides in the lacI gene of the big blue transgenic mouse. Mutat Res 1998; 420:55–65.

54. DeMayo FJ, Tsai SY. Targeted gene regulation and gene ablation [Review] [78 refs]. Trends Endocrinol Metab 2001; 12:348–353.

55. Palmiter RD, Norstedt G, Gelinas RE, Hammer RE, Brinster RL. Metallothionein-human GH fusion genes stimulate growth of mice. Science 1983; 222:809–814.

56. Campbell SJ, Carlotti F, Hall PA, Clark AJ, Wolf CR. Regulation of the CYP1A1 promoter in transgenic mice: an exquisitely sensitive on-off system for cell specific gene regulation. J Cell Sci 1996; 109:2619–2625.

57. Kothary R, Clapoff S, Darling S, Perry MD, Moran LA, Rossant J. Inducible expression of an hsp68-lacZ hybrid gene in transgenic mice. Dev Suppl 1989; 105:707–714.

58. Gossen M, Bujard H. Tight control of gene expression in mammalian cells by tetracycline-responsive promoters. Proc Natl Acad Sci USA 1992; 89: 5547–5551.

59. Furth PA, St Onge L, Boger H, Gruss P, Gossen M, Kistner A, Bujard H, Hennighausen L. Temporal control of gene expression in transgenic mice by a tetracycline-responsive promoter. Proc Natl Acad Sci USA 1994; 91: 9302–9306.

60. No D, Yao TP, Evans RM. Ecdysone-inducible gene expression in mammalian cells and transgenic mice. Proc Natl Acad Sci USA 1996; 93:3346–3351.

61. Zhao B, Chua SS, Burcin MM, Reynolds SD, Stripp BR, Edwards RA, Finegold MJ, Tsai SY, DeMayo FJ. Phenotypic consequences of lung-specific inducible expression of FGF-3. Proc Natl Acad Sci USA 2001; 98:5898–5903.

62. Gossen M, Freundlieb S, Bender G, Muller G, Hillen W, Bujard H. Transcriptional activation by tetracyclines in mammalian cells. Science 1995; 268:1766–1769.

63. Freundlieb S, Schirra-Muller C, Bujard H. A tetracycline controlled activation/repression system with increased potential for gene transfer into mammalian cells. J Gene Med 1999; 1:4–12.

64. Urlinger S, Baron U, Thellmann M, Hasan MT, Bujard H, Hillen W. Exploring the sequence space for tetracycline-dependent transcriptional activators: novel mutations yield expanded range and sensitivity. Proc Natl Acad Sci USA 2000; 97:7963–7968.

65. Stripp BR, Whitsett JA, Lattier DL. Strategies for analysis of gene expression: pulmonary surfactant proteins. Am J Physiol 1990; 259:L185–L197.

66. Korfhagen TR, Glasser SW, Stripp BR. Regulation of gene expression in the lung. Curr Opin Pediatr 1994; 6:255–261.

67. Whitsett JA, Glasser SW. Regulation of surfactant protein gene transcription. Biochim Biophys Acta 1998; 1408:303–311.

68. Costa RH, Kalinichenko VV, Lim L. Transcription factors in mouse lung development and function. Am J Physiol 2001; 280:L823–L838.

69. Giraldo P, Montoliu L. Size matters: use of YACs, BACs and PACs in transgenic animals. Transgenic Res 2001; 10:83–103.

70. Burke DT, Carle GF, Olson MV. Cloning of large segments of exogenous DNA into yeast by means of artificial chromosome vectors. Science 1987; 236:806–812.

71. Schedl A, Beermann F, Thies E, Montoliu L, Kelsey G, Schutz G. Transgenic mice generated by pronuclear injection of a yeast artificial chromosome. Nucleic Acids Res 1992; 20:3073–3077.

72. Schedl A, Montoliu L, Kelsey G, Schutz G. A yeast artificial chromosome covering the tyrosinase gene confers copy number-dependent expression in transgenic mice. Nature 1993; 362:258–261.
73. Choi TK, Hollenbach PW, Pearson BE, Ueda RM, Weddell GN, Kurahara CG, Woodhouse CS, Kay RM, Loring JF. Transgenic mice containing a human heavy chain immunoglobulin gene fragment cloned in a yeast artificial chromosome. Nat Genet 1993; 4:117–123.
74. Peterson KR, Clegg CH, Huxley C, Josephson BM, Haugen HS, Furukawa T, Stamatoyannopoulos G. Transgenic mice containing a 248-kb yeast artificial chromosome carrying the human beta-globin locus display proper developmental control of human globin genes. Proc Natl Acad Sci USA 1993; 90:7593–7597.
75. Lamb BT, Sisodia SS, Lawler AM, Slunt HH, Kitt CA, Kearns WG, Pearson PL, Price DL, Gearhart JD. Introduction and expression of the 400 kilobase amyloid precursor protein gene in transgenic mice. Nat Genet 1993; 5:22–30.
76. Manson A, Huxley C. Skipping of exon 9 of human CFTR in YAC-transgenic mice. Genomics 2001; 77:127–134.
77. Shizuya H, Birren B, Kim UJ, Mancino V, Slepak T, Tachiiri Y, Simon M. Cloning and stable maintenance of 300-kilobase-pair fragments of human DNA in Escherichia coli using an F-factor-based vector. Proc Natl Acad Sci USA 1992; 89:8794–8797.
78. Huang Y, Liu DP, Wu L, Li TC, Wu M, Feng DX, Liang CC. Proper developmental control of human globin genes reproduced by transgenic mice containing a 160-kb BAC carrying the human beta-globin locus. Blood Cells Mol Dis 2000; 26:598–610.
79. Nielsen LB, Kahn D, Duell T, Weier HU, Taylor S, Young SG. Apolipoprotein B gene expression in a series of human apolipoprotein B transgenic mice generated with recA-assisted restriction endonuclease cleavage-modified bacterial artificial chromosomes. An intestine-specific enhancer element is located between 54 and 62 kilobases 5′ to the structural gene. J Biol Chem 1998; 273:21800–21807.
80. Feng DX, Liu DP, Huang Y, Wu L, Li TC, Wu M, Tang XB, Liang CC. The expression of human alpha-like globin genes in transgenic mice mediated by bacterial artificial chromosome. Proc Natl Acad Sci USA 2001; 98:15073–15077.
81. Chatterjee PK, Yarnall DP, Haneline SA, Godlevski MM, Thornber SJ, Robinson PS, Davies HE, White NJ, Riley JH, Shepherd NS. Direct sequencing of bacterial and P1 artificial chromosome-nested deletions for identifying position-specific single-nucleotide polymorphisms. Proc Natl Acad Sci USA 1999; 96:13276–13281.
82. Lee EC, Yu D, Martinez de Velasco J, Tessarollo L, Swing DA, Court DL, Jenkins NA, Copeland NG. A highly efficient Escherichia coli-based chromosome engineering system adapted for recombinogenic targeting and subcloning of BAC DNA. Genomics 2001; 73:56–65.
83. Chrast R, Scott HS, Antonarakis SE. Linearization and purification of BAC DNA for the development of transgenic mice. Transgenic Res 1999; 8:147–150.

84. Mullins LJ, Kotelevtseva N, Boyd AC, Mullins JJ. Efficient Cre-lox linearisation of BACs: applications to physical mapping and generation of transgenic animals. Nucleic Acids Res 1997; 25:2539–2540.

85. Bradley A, Evans M, Kaufman MH, Robertson E. Formation of germ-line chimaeras from embryo-derived teratocarcinoma cell lines. Nature 1984; 309:255–256.

86. Evans MJ, Kaufman MH. Establishment in culture of pluripotential cells from mouse embryos. Nature 1981; 292:154–156.

87. Martin GR. Isolation of a pluripotent cell line from early mouse embryos cultured in medium conditioned by teratocarcinoma stem cells. Proc Natl Acad Sci USA 1981; 78:7634–7638.

88. Doetschman, T. Gene transfer in embryonic stem cells. In: Pinkert CA, ed. Transgenic Animal Technology: A laboratory Handbook. Academic Press Inc, 1994.

89. Thomas KR, Capecchi MR. Site-directed mutagenesis by gene targeting in mouse embryo-derived stem cells. Cell 1987; 5:503–512.

90. Doetschman T, Gregg RG, Maeda N, Hooper ML, Melton DW, Thompson S, Smithies O. Targetted correction of a mutant HPRT gene in mouse embryonic stem cells. Nature 1987; 330:576–578.

91. Hasty P, Rivera-Perez J, Chang C, Bradley A. Target frequency and integration pattern for insertion and replacement vectors in embryonic stem cells. Mol Cell Biol 1991; 11:4509–4517.

92. Moens CB, Auerbach AB, Conlon RA, Joyner AL, Rossant J. A targeted mutation reveals a role for N-myc in branching morphogenesis in the embryonic mouse lung. Genes Dev 1992; 6:691–704.

93. Moens CB, Stanton BR, Parada LF, Rossant J. Defects in heart and lung development in compound heterozygotes for two different targeted mutations at the N-myc locus. Dev Suppl 1993; 11:485–499.

94. Deng C, Capecchi MR. Reexamination of gene targeting frequency as a function of the extent of homology between the targeting vector and the target locus. Mol Cell Biol 1992; 12:3365–3371.

95. Hasty P, Rivera-Perez J, Bradley A. The length of homology required for gene targeting in embryonic stem cells. Mol Cell Biol 1991; 11:5586–5591.

96. Zhang H, Hasty P, Bradley A. Targeting frequency for deletion vectors in embryonic stem cells. Mol Cell Biol 1994; 14:2404–2410.

97. Zheng H, Hasty P, Brenneman MA, Grompe M, Gibbs RA, Wilson JH, Bradley A. Fidelity of targeted recombination in human fibroblasts and murine embryonic stem cells. Proc Natl Acad Sci USA 1991; 88:8067–8071.

98. Thomas KR, Deng C, Capecchi MR. High-fidelity gene targeting in embryonic stem cells by using sequence replacement vectors. Mol Cell Biol 1992; 12:2919–2923.

99. Hasty P, Ramirez-Solis R, Krumlauf R, Bradley A. Introduction of a subtle mutation into the Hox-2.6 locus in embryonic stem cells. Nature 1991; 350:243–246.

100. Mansour SL, Thomas KR, Capecchi MR. Disruption of the proto-oncogene int-2 in mouse embryo-derived stem cells: a general strategy for targeting mutations to non-selectable genes. Nature 1988; 336:348–352.

101. McCarrick JW III, Parnes JR, Seong RH, Solter D, Knowles BB. Positive-negative selection gene targeting with the diphtheria toxin A-chain gene in mouse embryonic stem cells. Transgenic Res 1993; 2:183–190.

102. Askew GR, Doetschman T, Lingrel JB. Site-directedpoint mutations in embryonic stem cells: a gene-targeting tag-and-exchange strategy. Mol Cell Biol 1993; 13:4115–4124.

103. Thomas KR, Capecchi MR. Introduction of homologous DNA sequences into mammalian cells induces mutations in the cognate gene. Nature 1986; 324:34–38.

104. Stripp BR, Lund J, Mango GW, Doyen KC, Johnston C, Hultenby K, Nord M, Whitsett JA. Clara cell secretory protein: a determinant of PCB bioaccumulation in mammals. Am J Physiol 1996; 271:L656–L664.

105. Snell GD. Congenic resistant strains of mice. In: Morse HC, ed. Origins of Inbred Mice. Academic Press, 1978:119–155.

106. Wakeland E, Morel L, Achey K, Yui M, Longmate J. Speed congenics: a classic technique in the fast lane (relatively speaking). Immunol Today 1997; 18:472–477.

107. Simpson EM, Linder CC, Sargent EE, Davisson MT, Mobraaten LE, Sharp JJ. Genetic variation among 129 substrains and its importance for targeted mutagenesis in mice. Nat Genet 1997; 16:19–27.

108. Rajewsky K, Gu H, Kuhn R, Betz UA, Muller W, Roes J, Schwenk F. Conditional gene targeting. J Clin Invest 1996; 98:600–603.

109. Yu Y, Bradley A. Engineering chromosomal rearrangements in mice. Nat Rev Genet 2001; 2:780–790.

110. Lakso M, Sauer B, Mosinger B Jr, Lee EJ, Manning RW, Yu SH, Mulder KL, Westphal H. Targeted oncogene activation by site-specific recombination in transgenic mice. Proc Natl Acad Sci USA 1992; 89:6232–6236.

111. Sauer B. Inducible gene targeting in mice using the Cre/lox system. Methods 1998; 14:381–392.

112. Dymecki SM. Flp recombinase promotes site-specific DNA recombination in embryonic stem cells and transgenic mice. Proc Natl Acad Sci USA 1996; 93:6191–6196.

113. Buchholz F, Angrand PO, Stewart AF. Improved properties of FLP recombinase evolved by cycling mutagenesis [see comments]. Nat Biotechnol 1998; 16:657–662.

114. Andreas S, Schwenk F, Kuter-Luks B, Faust N, Kuhn R. Enhanced efficiency through nuclear localization signal fusion on phage PhiC31-integrase: activity comparison with Cre and FLPe recombinase in mammalian cells. Nucleic Acids Res 2002; 30:2299–2306.

115. Gu H, Marth JD, Orban PC, Mossmann H, Rajewsky K. Deletion of a DNA polymerase beta gene segment in T cells using cell type-specific gene targeting [see comments]. Science 1994; 265:103–106.

116. Farley FW, Soriano P, Steffen LS, Dymecki SM. Widespread recombinase expression using FLPeR (flipper) mice. Genesis J Genet Dev 2000; 28:106–110.

117. Schwenk F, Baron U, Rajewsky K. A cre-transgenic mouse strain for the ubiquitous deletion of loxP-flanked gene segments including deletion in germ cells. Nucleic Acids Res 1995; 23:5080–5081.

118. Feil R, Brocard J, Mascrez B, LeMeur M, Metzger D, Chambon P. Ligand-activated site-specific recombination in mice. Proc Natl Acad Sci USA 1996; 93:10887–10890.

119. Kellendonk C, Tronche F, Monaghan AP, Angrand PO, Stewart F, Schutz G. Regulation of Cre recombinase activity by the synthetic steroid RU 486. Nucleic Acids Res 1996; 24:1404–1411.

120. Indra AK, Warot X, Brocard J, Bornert JM, Xiao JH, Chambon P, Metzger D. Temporally-controlled site-specific mutagenesis in the basal layer of the epidermis: comparison of the recombinase activity of the tamoxifen-inducible Cre-ER(T) and Cre-ER(T2) recombinases. Nucleic Acids Res 1999; 27: 4324–4327.

121. Rennard SI, Romberger DJ, Sisson JH, Von Essen SG, Rubinstein I, Robbins RA, Spurzem JR. Airway epithelial cells: functional roles in airway disease. Am J Respir Crit Care Med 1994; 150:S27–S30.

122. Carter PM, Heinly TL, Yates SW, Lieberman PL. Asthma: the irreversible airways disease. J Investig Allergol Clin Immunol 1997; 7:566–571.

123. Frampton MW, Morrow PE, Torres A, Voter KZ, Whitin JC, Cox C, Speers DM, Tsai Y, Utell MJ. Effects of ozone on normal and potentially sensitive human subjects. Part II: airway inflammation and responsiveness to ozone in nonsmokers and smokers. Research Report-Health Effects Institute 1997; 78:39–72.

124. Nakanishi K, Hiroi S, Kawai T, Suzuki M, Torikata C. Argyrophilic nucleolar-organizer region counts and DNA status in bronchioloalveolar epithelial hyperplasia and adenocarcinoma of the lung. Hum Pathol 1998; 29:235–239.

125. Betticher DC, Heighway J, Thatcher N, Hasleton PS. Abnormal expression of CCND1 and RB1 in resection margin epithelia of lung cancer patients. Br J Cancer 1997; 75:1761–1768.

126. Smith AL, Hung J, Walker L, Rogers TE, Vuitch F, Lee E, Gazear AF. Extensive areas of aneuploidy are present in the respiratory epithelium of lung cancer patients. Br J Cancer 1996; 73:203–209.

127. Agapitos E, Molo F, Tomatis L, Katsouyanni K, Lipworth L, Delsedime L, Kalandidi A, Karakatsani A, Riboli E, Saracci R, Trichopoulos D. Epithelial, possibly precancerous, lesions of the lung in relation to smoking, passive smoking, and socio-demographic variables. Scan J Soc Med 1996; 24: 259–263.

128. Crowell RE, Gilliland FD, Temes RT, Harms HJ, Neft RE, Heaphy E, Auckley DH, Crooks LA, Jordan SW, Samet JM, Lechner JF, Belinsky SA. Detection of trisomy 7 in nonmalignbant bronchial epithelium from lung cancer patients and individuals at risk for lung cancer. Cancer Epidemiol Biomarkers Prev 1996; 5:631–637.

129. Trichopoulos D, Mollo F, Tomatis L, Agapitos E, Delsedime L, Zavitsanos X, Kalandidi A, Katsouyanni K, Riboli, E and Saracci R. Active and passive smoking and pathological indicators of lung cancer risk in an autopsy study. JAMA 1992; 268:1697–1701.

130. Ayers MM, Jeffrey PK. Proliferation and differentiation in mammalian airway epithelium. Eur Respir J 1988; 1:58–80.

131. Evans MJ, Shami SG, Cabral-Anderson LJ, Dekker NP. Role of nonciliated Clara cells in renewal of the bronchiolar epithelium of rats exposed to NO2. Am J Pathol 1986; 123:126–133.

132. Breuer R, Zajicek G, Christensen TG, Lucey EC, Snider GL. Cell kinetics of normal adult hamster bronchial epithelium in the steady state. Am J Respir Cell Mol Biol 1990; 2:51–58.

133. Donnelly GM, Haack DG, Heird CS. Tracheal epithelium: cell kinetics and differentiation in normal rat tissue. Cell Tissue Kinet 1982; 15:119–130.

134. Plopper CG, Nishio SJ, Alley JL, Kass P, Hyde MD. The role of the nonciliated bronchiolar epithelial (Clara) cell as the progenitor cell during bronchiolar epithelial differentiation in the perinatal rabbit lung. Am J Respir Cell Mol Biol 1992; 7:606–613.

135. Singh G, Katyal SL. Clara cells Clara cell 10 kD protein (CC10). Am J Respir Cell Mol Biol 1997; 17:141–143.

136. Boers JEA, Ambergen W, Thunnissen BF. Number and proliferation of basal and parabasal cells in normal human airway epithelium. Am J Respir Crit Care Med 1998; 157:2000–2006.

137. Saito M, Iwawaki T, Taya C, Yonekawa H, Noda M, Inui Y, Mekada E, Kimata Y, Tsuru A, Kohno K. Diphtheria toxin receptor-mediated conditional and targeted cell ablation in transgenic mice. Nat Biotechnol 2001; 19:746–750.

138. Visnjic D, Kalajzic I, Gronowicz G, Aguila HL, Clark SH, Lichtler AC, Rowe DW. Conditional ablation of the osteoblast lineage in Col2.3deltatk transgenic mice. J Bone Miner Res 2001; 16:2222–2231.

139. Mikola MK, Rahman NA, Paukku TH, Ahtiainen PM, Vaskivuo TE, Tapanainen JS, Poutanen M, Huhtaniemi IT. Gonadal tumors of mice double transgenic for inhibin-alpha promoter-driven simian virus 40 T-antigen and herpes simplex virus thymidine kinase are sensitive to ganciclovir treatment. J Endocrinol 2001; 170:79–90.

140. Hong KU, Reynolds SD, Giangreco A, Hurley CM, Stripp BR. Clara cell secretory protein-expressing cells of the airwayneuroepithelial body microenvironment include a label-retaining subset and are critical for epithelial renewal after progenitor cell depletion. Am J Respir Cell Mol Biol 2001; 24:671–681.

141. Smith CA, Graham CM, Mathers K, Skinner A, Hay AJ, Schroeder C, Thomas DB. Conditional ablation of T-cell development by a novel viral ion channel transgene. Immunology 2002; 105:306–313.

142. Kobayashi T, Kida Y, Kaneko T, Pastan I, Kobayashi K. Efficient ablation by immunotoxin-mediated cell targeting of the cell types that express human interleukin-2 receptor depending on the internal ribosome entry site. J Gene Med 2001; 3:505–510.

143. Evans MJ, Cabral-Anderson LJ, Freeman G. Role of the Clara cell in renewal of the bronchiolar epithelium. Lab Invest 1978; 38:648–655.

144. Creasia DA, Nettesheim P, Kim JCS. Stimulation of DNA synthesis in the lungs of hamsters exposed intermittently to nitrogen dioxide. J Toxicol Environ Health 1977; 2:1173–1181.

145. Lum H, Schwartz LW, Dungworth DL, Tyler SW. A comparative study of cell renewal after exposure to ozone or oxygen. Am Rev Respir Dis 1978; 118: 335–345.

146. Hackett NA. Proliferation of lung and airway cells inducedby nitrogen dioxide. J Toxicol Environ Health 1979; 5:917–928.

147. Chichester CH, Buckpitt AR, Chang A, Plopper CG. Metabolism and cytotoxicity of naphthalene and its metabolites in isolated murine Clara cells. Mol Pharmacol 1994; 45:664–672.

148. Wilson AS, Davis CD, Williams DP, Buckpitt AR, Pirmohamed M, Park BK. Characterisation of the toxic metabolite(s) of naphthalene. Toxicology 1996; 114:233–242.

149. Stripp BR, Maxson KM, Mera R, Singh G. Plasticity of airway cell proliferation and gene expression following acute naphthalene injury. Am J Physiol 1995; 269:L791–L799.

150. Van Winkle LS, Buckpitt AR, Nishio SJ, Isaac JM, Plopper CG. Cellular response in naphthalene-induced Clara cell injury and bronchiolar epithelial repair in mice. Am J Physiol 1995; 269:L800–L818.

151. Stevens TP, McBride JT, Peake JL, Pinkerton KE, Stripp BR. Cell proliferation contributes to PNEC hyperplasia after acute airway injury. Am J Physiol 1997; 272:L486–L493.

152. Giangreco A, Reynolds SD, Stripp BR. Terminal bronchioles harbor a unique airway stem cell population that localizes to the bronchoalveolar duct junction. Am J Pathol 2002; 161:173–182.

153. Reynolds SD, Hong KU, Giangreco A, Mango GW, Guron C, Morimoto Y, Stripp BR. Conditional Clara cell ablation reveals a self-renewing progenitor function of pulmonary neuroendocrine cells. Am J Physiol 2000; 278: L1256–L1263.

154. Alberts B, Bray D, Lewis J, Raff M, Roberts K, Watson JD. Molecular Biology of the Cell. 3rd ed. New York, London: Garland Publishing, 1994.

155. Lodish H, Berk A, Zipursky SL, Matsudaira P, Baltimore D, Darnell JE. Molecular Cell Biology. 4th ed. New York: WH Freeman and Co., 1999.

156. Hanahan D, Weinberg RA. The hallmarks of cancer. Cell 2000; 100:57–70.

157. O'Connor PM, Ferris DK, Hoffmann I, Jackman J, Draetta G, Kohn KW. Role of the cdc25C phosphatase in G2 arrest induced by nitrogen mustard. Proc Natl Acad Sci USA 1994; 91:9480–9484.

158. Innocente SA, Abrahamson JL, Cogswell JP, Lee JM. p53 regulates a G2 checkpoint through cyclin B1. Proc Natl Acad Sci USA 1999; 96:2147–2152.

159. O'Reilly MA, Staversky RJ, Watkins RH, Maniscalco WM, Keng PC. p53-independent induction of GADD45 GADD153 in mouse lungs exposed to hyperoxia. Am J Physiol 2000; 278:L552–L559.

160. O'Reilly MA, Staversky RJ, Watkins RH, Reed CK, de Mesy Jensen KL, Finkelstein JN, Keng PC. The cyclin-dependent kinase inhibitor p21 protects the lung from oxidative stress. Am J Respir Cell Mol Biol 2001; 24:703–710.

161. Nakayama K, Ishida N, Shirane M, Inomata A, Inoue T, Shishido N, Horii I, Loh DY, Nakayama K. Mice lacking p27(Kip1) display increased body size, multiple organ hyperplasia, retinal dysplasia, and pituitary tumors. Cell 1996; 85:707–720.

162. Fero ML, Rivkin M, Tasch M, Porter P, Carow CE, Firpo E, Polyak K, Tsai LH, Broudy V, Perlmutter RM, Kaushansky K, Roberts JM. A syndrome of multiorgan hyperplasia with features of gigantism, tumorigenesis, and female sterility in p27 (Kip 1)-deficient mice. Cell 1996; 85:733–744.

163. Kiyokawa H, Kineman RD, Manova-Todorova KO, Soares VC, Hoffman ES, Ono M, Khanam D, Hayday AC, Frohman LA, Koff A. Enhanced growth of mice lacking the cyclin-dependent kinase inhibitor function of p27(Kip1). Cell 1996; 85:721–732.

164. Jacks T, Remington L, Williams BO, Schmitt EM, Halachmi S, Bronson RT, Weinberg RA. Tumor spectrum analysis in p53-mutant mice. Curr Biol 1994; 4:1–7.

165. Donehower LA, Harvey M, Slagle BL, McArthur MJ, Montgomery CA Jr, Butel JS, Bradley A. Mice deficient for p53 are developmentally normal but susceptible to spontaneous tumours. Nature 1992; 356:215–221.

166. Zhang P, Wong C, DePinho RA, Harper JW, Elledge SJ. Cooperation between the Cdk inhibitors p27(KIP1) and p57(KIP2) in the control of tissue growth and development. Genes Dev 1998; 12:3162–3167.

167. Serrano M, Lee H, Chin L, Cordon-Cardo C, Beach D, DePinho RA. Role of the INK4a locus in tumor suppression and cell mortality. Cell 1996; 85:27–37.

168. Hollander MC, Sheikh MS, Bulavin DV, Lundgren K, Augeri-Henmueller L, Shehee R, Molinaro TA, Kim KE, Tolosa E, Ashwell JD, Rosenberg MP, Zhan Q, Fernandez-Salguero PM, Morgan WF, Deng CX, Fornace AJ Jr. Genomic instability in Gadd45a-deficient mice. Nat Genet 1999; 23:176–184.

169. Barazzone C, Horowitz S, Donati YR, Rodriguez I, Piguet PF. Oxygen toxicity in mouse lung: pathways to cell death. AmJ Respir Cell Mol Biol 1998; 19:573–581.

170. Mabry M, Nelkin BD, Falco JP, Barr LF, Baylin SB. Transitions between lung cancer phenotypes-implications for tumor progression. Cancer Cells 1991; 3:53–58.

171. Mizutani Y, Nakajima T, Morinaga S, Gotoh M, Shimosato Y, Akino T, Suzuki A. Immunohistochemical localization of pulmonary surfactant apoproteins in various lung tumors. Special reference to nonmucus producing lung adenocarcinomas. Cancer 1988; 61:532–537.

172. Pujol JL, Simony J, Laurent JC, Richer G, Mary H, Bousquet J, Godard P, Michel FB. Phenotypic heterogeneity studied by immunohistochemistry and aneuploidy in non-small cell lung cancers. Cancer Res 1989; 49:2797–2802.

173. Tischler AS. Small cell carcinoma of the lung: cellular origin and relationship to other neoplasms. Semin Oncol 1978; 5:244–252.

174. Wikenheiser KA, Clark JC, Linnoila RI, Stahlman MT, Whitsett JA. Simian virus 40 large T antigen directed by transcriptional elements of the human surfactant protein C gene produces pulmonary adenocarcinomas in transgenic mice. Cancer Res 1992; 52:5342–5352.

175. Sandmoller A, Halter R, Suske G, Paul D, Beato M. A transgenic mouse model for lung adenocarcinoma. Cell Growth Differ 1995; 6:97–103.

176. Sunday ME, Haley KJ, Sikorski K, Graham SA, Emanuel RL, Zhang F, Mu Q, Shahsafaei A, Hatzis D. Calcitonin drivenv-Ha-ras induces multilineage

pulmonary epithelial hyperplasias and neoplasms. Oncogene 1999; 18: 4336–4347.

177. Linnoila RI, Sahu A, Miki M, Ball DW, DeMayo FJ. Morphometric analysis of CC10-hASH1 transgenic mouse lung:a model for bronchiolization of alveoli and neuroendocrine carcinoma. Exp Lung Res 2000; 26:595–615.

178. DeMayo FJ, Finegold MJ, Hansen TN, Stanley LA, Smith B, Bullock DW. Expression of SV40 T antigen under control of rabbit uteroglobin promoter in transgenic mice. Am J Physiol 1991; 261:L70–L76.

179. Magdaleno SM, Wang G, Jackson KJ, Ray MK, Welty S, Costa RH, DeMayo FJ. Interferon-gamma regulation of Clara cell gene expression: in vivo and in vitro. Am J Physiol 1997; 272:L1142–L1151.

180. Magdaleno SM, Wang G, Mireles VL, Ray MK, Finegold MJ, DeMayo FJ. Cyclin-dependent kinase inhibitor expression in pulmonary Clara cells transformed with SV40 large T antigen in transgenic mice. Cell Growth Differ 1997; 8:145–155.

181. Wuenschell CW, Sunday ME, Singh G, Minoo P, Slavkin HC, Warburton D. Embryonic mouse lung epithelial progenitor cells co-express immunohistochemical markers of diverse mature cell lineages. J Histochem Cytochem 1996; 44:113–123.

182. Warburton D, Wuenschell C, Flores-Delgado G, Anderson K. Commitment and differentiation of lung cell lineages. Biochem Cell Biol 1998; 76:971–995.

183. Berns A. Cancer. Improved mouse models. Nature 2001; 410:1043–1044.

184. Johnson L, Greenbaum D, Cichowski K, Mercer K, Murphy E, Schmitt E, Bronson RT, Umanoff H, Edelmann W, Kucherlapati R, Jacks T. K-ras is an essential gene in the mouse with partial functional overlap with N-ras. Genes Dev 1997; 11:2468–2481.

185. Tuveson DA, Jacks T. Modeling human lung cancer in mice: similarities and shortcomings. Oncogene 1999; 18:5318–5324.

186. Seperack PK, Strobel MC, Corrow DJ, Jenkins NA, Copeland NG. Somatic and germ-line reverse mutation rates of the retrovirus-induced dilute coat-color mutation of DBA mice. Proc Natl Acad Sci USA 1988; 85:189–192.

187. Johnson L, Mercer K, Greenbaum D, Bronson RT, Crowley D, Tuveson DA, Jacks T. Somatic activation of the K-rasoncogene causes early onset lung cancer in mice. Nature 2001; 410:1111–1116.

188. Fisher GH, Wellen SL, Klimstra D, Lenczowski JM, Tichelaar JW, Lizak MJ, Whitsett JA, Koretsky A, Varmus HE. Induction and apoptotic regression of lung adenocarcinomas by regulation of a K-Ras transgene in the presence and absence of tumor suppressor genes. Genes Dev 2001; 15:3249–3262.

189. Meuwissen R, Linn SC, van der Valk M, Mooi WJ, Berns A. Mouse model for lung tumorigenesis through Cre/lox controlled sporadic activation of the K-Ras oncogene. Oncogene 2001; 20:6551–6558.

190. Jackson EL, Willis N, Mercer K, Bronson RT, Crowley D, Montoya R, Jacks T, Tuveson DA. Analysis of lung tumor initiation and progression using conditional expression of oncogenic K-ras. Genes Dev 2001; 15:3243–3248.

191. Franklin WA, Gazdar AF, Haney J, Wistuba II, La Rosa FG, Kennedy T, Ritchey DM, Miller YE. Widely dispersed p53 mutation in respiratory epithe-

lium. A novel mechanism for field carcinogenesis. J Clin Invest 1997; 100: 2133–2137.

192. Zheng B, Zhang Z, Black CM, de Crombrugghe B, Denton CP. Ligand-dependent genetic recombination in fibroblasts : a potentially powerful technique for investigating gene function in fibrosis. Am J Pathol 2002; 160: 1609–1617.

193. Liang L, Bickenbach JR. Somatic epidermal stem cells can produce multiple cell lineages during development. Stem Cells 2002; 20:21–31.

194. Merrill BJ, Gat U, DasGupta R, Fuchs E. Tcf3 and Lef1 regulate lineage differentiation of multipotent stem cells in skin. Genes Dev 2001; 15:1688–1705.

195. Nomura S, Esumi H, Job C, Tan SS. Lineage and clonal development of gastric glands. Dev Biol 1998; 204:124–135.

196. Garabedian EM, Roberts LJ, McNevin MS, Gordon JI. Examining the role of Paneth cells in the small intestine by lineage ablation in transgenic mice. J Biol Chem 1997; 272:23729–23740.

197. Belachew S, Yuan X, Gallo V. Unraveling oligodendrocyte origin and function by cell-specific transgenesis. Dev Neurosci 2001; 23:287–298.

198. Kaneko Y, Sakakibara S, Imai T, Suzuki A, Nakamura Y, Sawamoto K, Ogawa Y, Toyama Y, Miyata T, Okano H. Musashi1: an evolutionally conserved marker for CNS progenitor cells including neural stem cells. Dev Neurosci 2000; 22:139–153.

199. Perl AK, Wert SE, Nagy A, Lobe CG, Whitsett JA. Early restriction of peripheral and proximal cell lineages during formation of the lung. Proc Natl Acad Sci USA 2002; 99:10482–10487.

200. Jian-Vora, S, Wert SE, Teneamm UA, Randin JA, Witsett JA. Interleukin-4 alters epithelial cell differentiation and surfactant homeostasis in the postnatal mouse lung. Am J Respir Cell Mol Biol 1997; 17:541–551.

201. Lee J, McGarry MP, Farmer SC, Denzler KL, Larson KA, Carrigan PE, Grenneise IE, Horton MA, Haezku A, Gelfand EW, Leikauf GD, Lee NA. Interleukin-5 expression in the lung epithelium of transgenic mice leads to pulmonary changes pathognomonic of asthma. J Exp Med 1997; 185:2143–2156.

202. Temann UA, Geba GP, Rankin JA, Flavell RA. Expression of interleukin 9 in the lungs of transgenic mice causes airway inflammation, mast cell hyperplasia, and bronchial hyperresponsiveness. J Exp Med 1998; 188:1307–1320.

203. Zhu Z, Homer RJ, Wang Z, Chen Q, Geba GP, Wang J, Zhang Y, Elias JA. Pulmonary expression of interleukin-13 causes inflammation, mucus hypersecretion, subepithelial fibrosis, physiologic abnormalities, and eotaxin production. J Clin Invest 1999; 103:779–788.

204. Temann UA, Prasad B, Gallup MW, Basbaum C, Ho SB, Flavell RA, Rankin JA. A novel role for murine IL-4 in vivo: induction of MUC5AC gene expression and mucin hypersecretion. Am J Respir Cell Mol Biol 1997; 16:471–478.

205. Louahed J, Toda M, Jen J, Hamid Q, Renauld JC, Levitt RC, Nicolaides NC. Interleukin-9 upregulates mucus expression in the airways [see comments]. Am J Respir Cell Mol Biol 2000; 22:649–656.

206. Iwamoto T, Takatsu K. Evaluation of airway hyperreactivity in interleukin-5 transgenic mice. Int Arch Allergy Immunol 1995; 108(suppl 1):28–30.

207. Lefort J, Bachelet CM, Leduc D, Vargaftig BB. Effect of antigen provocation of IL-5 transgenic mice on eosinophil mobilization and bronchial hyper-responsiveness. J Allergy Clin Immunol 1996; 97:788–799.

208. Renauld JC, van der Lugt N, Vink A, van Roon M, Godfraind C, Warnier G, Merz H, Feller A, Berns A, Van Snick J. Thymic lymphomas in interleukin 9 transgenic mice. Oncogene 1994; 9:1327–1332.

209. McLane MP, Haczku A, van de Rijn M, Weiss C, Ferrante V, MacDonald D, Renauld JC, Nicolaides NC, Holroyd KJ, Levitt RC. Interleukin-9 promotes allergen-induced eosinophilic inflammation and airway hyperresponsiveness in transgenic mice. Am J Respir Cell Mol Biol 1998; 1:713–720.

210. Fallon PG, Emson CL, Smith P, McKenzie AN. IL-13 overexpression predisposes to anaphylaxis following antigen sensitization. J Immunol 2001; 166: 2712–2716.

211. Holgate ST, Davies DE, Lackie PM, Wilson SJ, Puddicombe SM, Lordan JL. Epithelial-mesenchymal interactions in the pathogenesis of asthma. J Allergy Clin Immunol 2000; 105:193–204.

212. Holgate ST, Lackie PM, Howarth PH, Roche WR, Puddicombe SM, Richter A, Wilson SJ, Holloway JW, Davies DE. Invited lecture: activation of the epithelial mesenchymal trophic unit in the pathogenesis of asthma. Int Arch Allergy Immunol 2001; 124:253–258.

213. Tang W, Geba GP, Zheng T, Ray P, Homer RJ, Kuhn C III, Flavell RA, Elias JA. Targeted expression of IL-11 in the murine airway causes lymphocytic inflammation, bronchial remodeling, and airways obstruction. J Clin Invest 1996; 98: 2845–2853.

214. Ray P, Tang W, Wang P, Homer R, Kuhn C III, Flavell RA, Elias JA. Regulated overexpression of interleukin 11 in the lung. Use to dissociate development-dependent and independentphenotypes. J Clin Invest 1997; 100: 2501–2511.

215. Wang J, Homer RJ, Hong L, Cohn L, Lee CG, Jung S, Elias JA. IL-11 selectively inhibits aeroallergen-induced pulmonary eosinophilia and Th2 cytokine production. J Immunol 2000; 165:2222–2231.

216. Ray P, Tang W, Wang P, Homer R, Kuhn C III, Flavell RA, Elias JA. Regulated overexpression of interleukin 11 in the lung. Use to dissociate development-dependent and -independent phenotypes. J Clin Invest 1997; 100: 2501–2511.

217. Temann UA, Ray P, Flavell RA. Pulmonary overexpression of IL-9 induces Th2 cytokine expression, leading to immune pathology. J Clin Invest 2002; 109:29–39.

218. Zheng T, Zhu Z, Wang Z, Homer RJ, Ma B, Riese RJ Jr, Chapman HA Jr, Shapiro SD, Elias JA. Inducible targeting of IL-13 to the adult lung causes matrix metalloproteinase- and cathepsin-dependent emphysema. J Clin Invest 2000; 106:1081–1093.

219. Grunig G, Warnock M, Wakil AE, Venkayya R, Brombacher F, Rennick DM, Sheppard D, Mohrs M, Donaldson DD, Locksley RM, Corry DB. Requirement for IL-13 independently of IL-4 in experimental asthma. Science 1998; 282:2261–2263.

220. Wills-Karp M, Luyimbazi J, Xu X, Schofield B, Neben TY, Karp CL, Donaldson DD. Interleukin-13: central mediator of allergic asthma. Science 1998; 282:2258–2261.

221. Zhu Z, Ma B, Homer RJ, Zheng T, Elias JA. Use of the tetracycline-controlled transcriptional silencer (tTS) to eliminate transgene leak in inducible overexpression transgenic mice. J Biol Chem 2001; 276:25222–25229.

222. Cohn L, Homer RJ, MacLeod H, Mohrs M, Brombacher F, Bottomly K. Th2-induced airway mucus production is dependent on IL-4Ralpha, but not on eosinophils. J Immunol 1999; 162:6178–6183.

223. Cohn L, Homer RJ, Niu N, Bottomly K. T helper 1 cells and interferon gamma regulate allergic airway inflammation and mucus production. J Exp Med 1999; 190:1309–1318.

224. Cohn L, Tepper JS, Bottomly K. IL-4-independent induction of airway hyperresponsiveness by Th2, but not Th1, cells. J Immunol 1998; 161: 3813–3816.

225. Kuperman D, Schofield B, Wills-Karp M, Grusby M. Signal transducer and activator of transcription factor 6 (STAT6)-deficient mice are protected from antigen-induced airway hyperresponsiveness and mucus production. J Exp Med 1998; 187:939–948.

226. Akimoto T, Numata F, Tamura M, Takata Y, Higashida N, Tadashi T, Takeda K, Akira S. Abrogation of bronchial eosinophilic inflammation and airway hyperreactivity in signal transducers and activators of transcription (STAT)6-deficient mice. J Exp Med 1998; 187:1537–1542.

227. Tomkinson A Kanehiro A, Rabinovitch N, Joetham A, Ciesliwicz G, Gelfand EW. The failure of STAT6-deficient mice to develop airway eosinophilia and airway hyper responsiveness is overcome by interleukin-5. Am J Respir Crit Care Med 1999; 160:1283–1291.

228. Grunig G, Warnock M, Wakil AE, Venkayya R, Brombacher F, Rennick DM, Sheppard D, Mohrs M, Donaldson DD, Locksley RM, Corry DB. Requirement for IL-13 independently of IL-4 in experimental asthma. Science 1998; 282:2261–2263.

229. Laoukili J, Perret E, Willems T, Minty A, Parthoens E, Houcine O, Coste A, Jorissen M, Marano F, Caput D, Tournier F. IL-13 alters mucociliary differentiation and ciliary beating of human respiratory epithelial cells. J Clin Invest 2001; 108:1817–1824.

230. Venkayya R, Lam M, Willkom M, Grunig G, Corry DB, Erle DJ. The Th2 lymphocyte products IL-4 and IL-13 rapidly induce airway hyperresponsiveness through direct effects on resident airway cells. Am J Respir Cell Mol Biol 2002; 26:202–208.

231. Richter A, Puddicombe SM, Lordan JL, Bucchieri F, Wilson SJ, Djukanovic R, Dent G, Holgate ST, Davies DE. The contribution of interleukin (IL)-4 and IL-13 to the epithelial-mesenchymal trophic unit in asthma. Am J Respir Cell Mol Biol 2001; 25:385–391.

232. Zuhdi Alimam M, Piazza FM, Selby DM, Letwin N, Huang L, Rose MC. Muc-5/5ac mucin messenger RNA and protein expression is a marker of goblet cell metaplasia in murine airways. Am J Respir Cell Mol Biol 2000; 22:253–260.

233. Dierynck I, Bernard A, Roels H, DeLey M. Potent inhibition of both human interferon-g production and biologic activity by the Clara cell protein CC16. Am J Respir Cell Mol Biol 1995; 12:205–210.

234. Yao XL, Ikezolo T, Cowan M, Logun C, Angus CW, Shelhamer JH. Interferon-gamma stimulates human Clara cell secretory protein production by human airway epithelial cells. Am J Physiol 1998; 274:L864–L869.

235. Cohn L, Herrick C, Niu N, Homer R, Bottomly K. IL-4 promotes airway eosinophilia by suppressing IFN-gamma production: defining a novel role for IFN-gamma in the regulation of allergic airway inflammation. J Immunol 2001; 166:2760–2767.

12

Inhalation Toxicology: Methods and Models

DANIEL L. COSTA

*Pulmonary Toxicology Branch, Experimental Toxicology Division,
National Health and Environmental Research Laboratory,
Research Triangle Park, North Carolina, U.S.A.*

I. Overview

Modern-day inhalation toxicology merges the principles and technologies of airflow and aerosol engineering with lung biology, and is inclusive of the rapid advances occurring in cell and molecular biology. This chapter approaches the broad area of inhalation toxicology from several perspectives: the relationships between lung structure and function that exist across species; the essential principles of inhalation exposure design and methodology; the determinants of exposure–dose of gaseous and particulate inhalants (deposition and clearance); and the use of animal and cell models as analogs for inhalant-induced acute and chronic lung injury in humans. The inhalation toxicology models and methods emphasized here extend coverage on acute and chronic lung injury in prior chapters to assess inhalation exposure risks and aid the development of therapeutic interventions for related pulmonary injury and disease. Inhalation toxicology is more than simply putting an animal in a box and exposing it to a concentration of gaseous or particulate inhalant to yield an effect. It requires the considered application of exposure technology and predictive dosimetry to design a study that mimics, as best can be, the likely human exposure scenario.

This quest for "relevance" does not exclude the use of injurious high concentrations of a toxicant, but rather puts that exposure into the context of a risk assessment paradigm. There are striking similarities as well as differences in the structure and function of human and laboratory rodent lungs, and how they handle intrusive inhalant particles and gases. These similarities and differences must be appreciated for credible extrapolation of mechanistic experimental studies to real-world human health questions. The spectrum of applications for inhalation toxicology ranges from hazard identification in safety testing to hypothesis generation and testing regarding mechanisms of toxicant injury and disease pathogenesis. By integrating animal inhalation data with human clinical studies, of our understanding of lung injury from toxic inhalants has advanced considerably. Among the classic toxic inhalants, the large, integrated database of ozone toxicology has provided the biomedical and risk community with a model to mimic health research strategies for other toxic inhalants as described in this chapter. Subsequent chapters give details on therapies for clinical acute and chronic lung injury and disease, including conditions caused by toxic inhalation or environmental exposure.

II. Introduction

The lungs have nearly four times the surface area interfacing the environment compared to the combined surface area of the gastrointestinal tract and skin. With so much of the organ exposed to the outside world, the lungs are unique in being both positionally vulnerable to direct inhalant injury and serving as the primary portal for toxicant entry into the organism. Thus, it is not surprising that there has long been interest in how to deliver defined airborne toxicant challenges reproducibly to the respiratory tracts of both human subjects and animals. Where an inhalant deposits along the respiratory tract, and whether the cells populating that region are sensitive to that inhalant, have much to do with the overall impact a given toxicant has on the lung. Some chemicals (usually highly lipid soluble gases and vapors like N_2O or the lighter organics) may pass virtually unnoticed through the lung and into the blood, and become distributed systemically. When the atmospheric source is removed, these gases partition away from the body and leave in expired air. Frequently, however, many inhalants—be they gases, vapors, or particles—that have entered the lung do not pass unnoticed, but rather exert some effect, ranging from a compensatory reflex (e.g., altered ventilation, cell metabolism, or mucus secretion perhaps due to irritancy) to overt cellular or tissue injury. Some chemicals may insidiously alter metabolism in specific cells, like naphthalene induction of cytochrome P_{450} in the Clara cell (1), without overt effect. When followed by another inhalant such as ozone (O_3), however, the impact is magnified beyond that of either substance alone and may be localized to specific regions of the respiratory tract. Similarly, a low level exposure encountered once may impart little effect, but over the long term may demonstrate the property of "chronicity." When extended or repeated over time with some periodicity, the impact of a toxicant exposure may result in altered cell proliferation or metabolism (e.g., antioxidants) and thereby as with naphthalene potentially affect other responses or functions. In the end, anything that interferes with the basic function of the lung tissues or cells or the exchange of O_2 and CO_2 across the air–blood barrier can even affect the well-being of the entire organism.

The discipline of inhalation toxicology has evolved from an interplay and union of basic engineering principles of airflow dynamics and lung biology. The need for some fundamental understanding and facility with engineering is a clear advantage in the development and operation of exposure models. However, it is generally underappreciated that those engineering principles also describe airflow through pipes (airways), compressibility and elasticity (expansion and contraction of the lung parenchyma), and the mixing of gases by diffusion. Moreover, these principles were essential evolutionary determinants of lung structure and biology. Thus, the efficient (least energy demanding) movement of air into and out of the lung and the unimpeded diffusion of O_2 and CO_2 at the air–blood alveolar interface uniquely determined the evolution of mammalian lung function and biology. As such, lung design is essentially normative, where lung function and structure are linked mathematically across species, from the smallest shrew to the largest whale ($\sim$7 orders of magnitude) (Fig. 1A, B) (2,3). It should follow then that potentially toxic inhalants would affect the lung in an animal model largely as in the human exposure–response situation. Likewise, one might expect that the cellular and biochemical attributes of the lung tissues and cells should function in this conceptual framework. But clearly these analogies are imperfect, and there is variation in how various biological processes have evolved to ensure appropriate respiration for a given species in a given environment. This variation, not surprisingly, has significant implications on response outcomes, and naturally the interpretation thereof. Nevertheless, it is the fundamental mammalian biology of the lung that allows the toxicologist to study responses to environmental stressors in a standardized rodent species for the purposes of understanding and predicting potential human health impacts.

III. Structure/Function Relationships of the Respiratory System

A. Basic Anatomy

When air moves from the ambient environment into the respiratory tract, it passes through several structurally distinct regions beginning with the convoluted passages of the nose, transitioning through the oropharynx

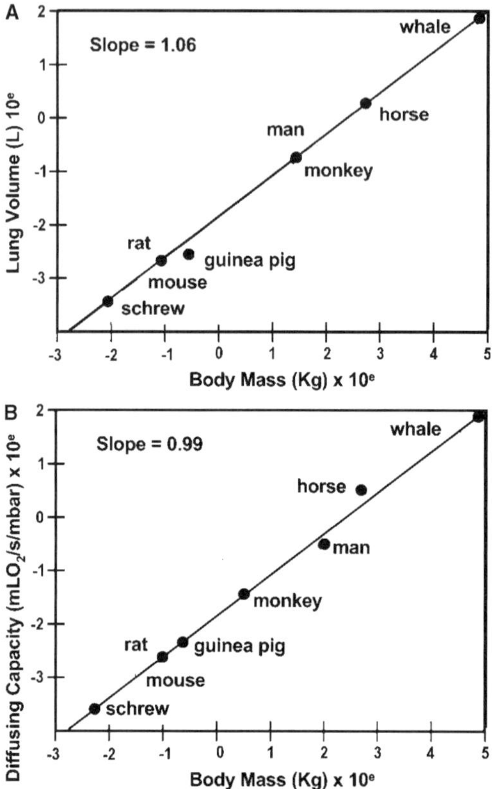

Figure 1   Interspecies correlation of lung function and structure. Allometric plots across mammals of widely different body size: (A) mean lung volume to mean body mass and (B) mean pulmonary diffusing capacity to body mass. Plots modified from combined data published by Gehr et al. (2) and Weibel (3) showing the mathematical linkage between lung structure and function necessary to maintain adequate gas-exchange to meet the oxidative needs of mammals.

and glottal regions through the bronchus to a tree of bifurcating airways of ever decreasing diameter, ending in millions of grape-like clusters of alveolar sacs where actual gas-exchange takes place. More than 45 cell types have been identified from the nose to the alveoli, making the respiratory system one of the most structurally and functionally complex organs of the body. For simplicity of description, however, convention has divided the respiratory tract into three regions: (i) the nasopharynx, (ii) the tracheobronchial tree, and (iii) the pulmonary or alveolar region. These three regions are often used in discussion of models to distinguish regional deposition or for ease in designating areas of impact of a given inhalant.

In adult humans and some larger animal species (e.g., dogs, monkeys), air can enter the respiratory tract through either or both the nose and mouth. In humans, breathing is generally through the nose, but nasal congestion or deformity, exercise or lung disease may accentuate the oral route simply as a path of least resistance. In contrast, human infants are obligate nasal breathers, until growth renders the oropharynx open enough to maintain flow from either port. Rodents are obligate nasal breathers throughout life, and even in the extreme (e.g., heat or exercise), they cannot adequately ventilate via the mouth due to structural limitations. The gross structure of the nose differs significantly across species and has several evolutionary pressures. One finds that the ratio of the nasal internal surface area to the chamber volume (SA/VOL) varies inversely with body size thereby bringing inspired air into closer contact with nasal tissues of small mammals (4). Lining the nasal passages are several epithelial subtypes including cuboidal and columnar epithelia in the areas proximal to the nares, stratified squamous epithelium in the vestibule, and over the major surface of the main nasal chamber, a mix of ciliated pseudostratified and respiratory epithelia, and goblet cells. The percentage coverage of any one type is species-dependent, but notably, the olfactory epithelium and associated neurosensory cells, which occupy the dorsoposterior wall surface, can range from as much as 58% of the SA in the rat to only 8% in the human (3), perhaps reflecting the teleological importance of olfaction in many small mammals. As the olfactory epithelium contains a significant complement of P_{450}- associated enzymatic activity, it often may exhibit injury to inhalants that involve metabolic activation, an outcome frequently overlooked (5). During inhalation, the nasal tissues, which function to humidify and warm the incoming air, also provide physical, antimicrobial, and chemical (e.g., antioxidant) targets to incoming substances, so effects to these tissues should not be unexpected (6). The nose recently has gained special prominence to the inhalation toxicology community as the damage to nasal epithelium by an inhalant has come to be appreciated as potentially predictive of lung epithelial injury. Though the risk model continues to evolve with technology and appropriate toxicity models involving the nose and lungs, indices of nasal injury have been instrumental in determining reference concentrations (RfC) limits for a limited number of toxic inhalants (e.g., methylmethacrylate) (7).

The tracheobronchial airways provide relatively low resistance conduits to deliver air to the pulmonary region of the respiratory system. From the singular trachea, the airways bifurcate repeatedly creating an arborized distribution of small conducting bronchioles, of which none has any systemic gas-exchange function. As one proceeds along a given pathway toward the alveoli, airway diameters decrease, with each bifurcation such that after 15–26 divisions (depending on animal species), the total cross-sectional area of the collective airways increases in a trumpet-like fashion (Fig. 2). The result is a dramatic slowing of the linear velocity (and flow

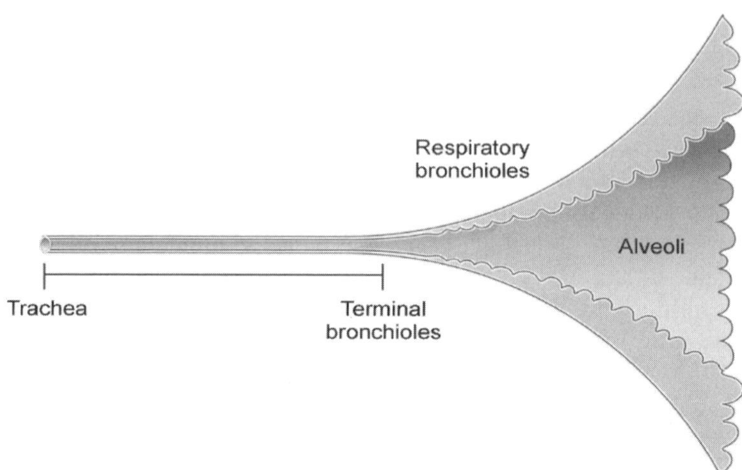

Figure 2 Relative cross-sectional areas of different regions of the lungs. The "trumpeting" lung shown schematically in this figure represents relative cross-sectional areas from the trachea to the alveolar region. The area of the airways including the terminal/respiratory bronchioles is only about 5% of that of the total lung.

in any given bronchiole) with minimal drag or resistance. In the smallest terminal/respiratory bronchioles and alveolar ducts, gas molecules move by simple diffusion along concentration gradients.

The geometric pattern of airway branching differs between primates and other species (Fig. 3). Erect primates have a branching pattern that is nearly symmetric. In other words, each airway bifurcates into two smaller "daughter" branches of similar diameter and at approximately equal angles. In contrast, most other animals (quadrupeds, including rodents) have a monopodial branching pattern resembling that of a pine tree with unequal sized daughter branches coming off a more prominent conduit (8). Obviously, this contrast in branching has implications regarding airflow dynamics and, of course, gas and particle distribution when comparing species. However, if one recalls the evolutionary drive of lung development—delivery and distribution of air into the deep lung for gas-exchange—it becomes apparent that there is a functional consistency of lung architecture across species. This concept can be seen in the allometric association between body size and lung function as seen in Fig. 1 A, B.

In humans, the surface of the large airways is populated by ciliated columnar epithelium, brush, and basal cells, along with scattered glycoprotein-secreting goblet cells (~9%). Subsets of subepithelial glands in the larger airways secrete the bulk of the viscous mucus and more aqueous serous fluid that combines to form the mucus coating of the airway surface.

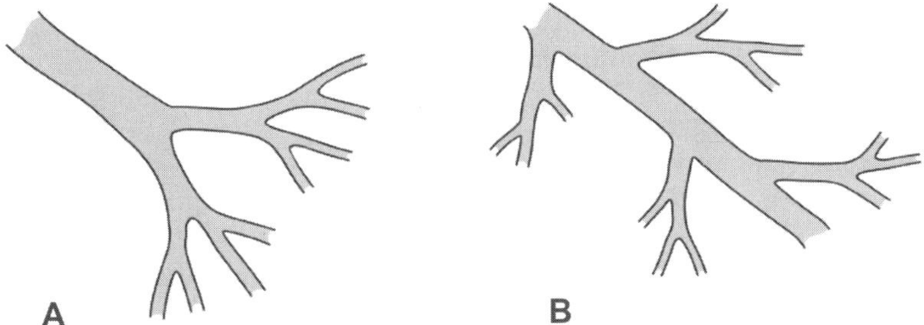

Figure 3 Comparison schematic of the airway branching pattern in primates (symmetric) and rodent (monopodial) lungs.

This bilayer of mucus at the surface with the serous underlayer is of variable thickness and completeness, but is continuously pushed up the airway to the glottis by the synchronous beating of cilia—this functional unit is often referred to as the mucociliary escalator. The distribution of mucus-secreting and ciliated cells decreases as one moves peripherally along the airways, as does the physical thickness of the cell layer and its mucous coat. Other cuboidal cells, primarily Clara cells, which appear to have several functions including metabolism of bioactive compounds, increase in number distally along the airway (9, 10). Despite the generic similarity of the airways and the basic component cell types along the airways across species, the distribution of the cell populations can differ considerably. For example, rodents have few if any goblet cells in the trachea and conducting airways (unless proliferation is stimulated by chronic irritancy—see below). Rats have a substantial number (20–27%) of serous cells in their larger airways, in contrast to the mouse and hamster, which have essentially none. Rather, the latter two species have Clara cells extending from the bronchi to the smaller bronchioles. In fact, the Clara cell in the mouse comprises more than 40% of the tracheal cell population. Hence metabolic functions of the airways across species may differ considerably—not unimportant when one considers the metabolism of carcinogens.

The portion of the lung involved in actual respiration (gas-exchange) is the so-called pulmonary region. The functional unit of this region of lung is the acinus, which includes the terminal bronchiole and its more distal respiratory bronchioles (the smallest bronchioles, defined by their variable number of alveolar out-pockets), alveolar ducts, as well as the alveoli themselves. The rodent, in contrast to the human, has no respiratory bronchioles per se, and thus the basic "ventilatory unit" extends distally from the bronchiolar–alveolar duct (so-called BAD) junction. The adult human lung has about 400 million alveoli originating from about 28,000 respiratory bronchioles, while the rat lung has 10% the number of end airways and ~10 million alveoli (11). This distinction between rodents and primates becomes important when one considers that many pollutants (notably cigarette smoke, but also ozone) induce lung lesions within the respiratory bronchioles and the transition area into the alveolar ducts. However, in studies of chronic lung lesions (e.g., ozone) in the rodent, the lesions are found in the transition-zone analog region, the BAD—the difference being that the respiratory bronchiole component is absent (12, 13).

The acinus of the lung contains a transitional zone, where the columnar cells of the airways are replaced by sparsely ciliated columnar and more cuboidal-shaped cells, including abundant Clara and a few Type II cells (11). The Type II cell is considered an alveolar cell that is metabolically active, secreting the surfactant that coats the entire acinus surface that is so critical to stabilizing alveoli—reducing surface tension and thereby preventing their collapse. The alveolar ducts are actually virtual airways with no definitive structure as they result from the expanded grape-like clusters of alveoli within each acinus. The epithelium of the alveolar structures themselves is a very thin, smooth cell known as the Type I cell, which expands to cover a wide surface area. This cell appears to not be metabolically active having derived from progenitor Type II cells that rim the alveolus (about 3 cells in the rat in contrast to 51 in the human). Only 2–3 Type I cells make up the surface of a given alveoli in the rat where in the human about 32 surprisingly similar-sized Type I cells are required to line a single alveolus. The collective alveolar surface represents about 90–95% of the respiratory tract surface area. As the site of gas-exchange, this 1 μm thick air–blood interface is formed from the fusion of the basement membranes of the alveolar Type I and the juxtaposed endothelial cells of the pulmonary capillary bed. Its thickness is surprisingly consistent across species, as defined by the physics of passive diffusion of O_2 and CO_2. Built on a framework of collagen and elastic fibers interlaced with a complex glycoproteinaceous ground substance, the lung is capable of expanding and retracting repeatedly through a lifetime with only a slight loss of elasticity.

Within the lumen of each alveolus are one or more mononuclear phagocytic cells, called alveolar macrophages (14). These cells comprise an important part of pulmonary host defense as they patrol the alveolus and engulf foreign microorganisms or particles that, due to their aerodynamic size, have evaded physical capture in the airways and deposited in the distal lung beyond the bronchioles and the reaches of the mucociliary escalator. These cells, when satiated with their phagocytized bounty, migrate upstream via the small airways to be cleared by the continuously moving mucociliary escalator of the larger airways, eventually to be swallowed. A smaller fraction of the macrophages may move into the lymphatic system between alveolar cells ending in the lymph nodes (a process thought to function in immunological presentation and sensitization). Under certain circumstances, macrophages (e.g., silica exposure) may mediate lung injury if activated, damaged, or at death when they may release potent oxidants, cytokine, and other mediators that can activate or damage other pulmonary cells (71). Nevertheless, the ultimate task of the macrophage is to rid the body of foreign substances or microbes that reach the fragile and sterile surface of the alveolus.

B. Basic Lung Function

The lung is appropriately designed for gas-exchange (15). To this end, air moves convectively through the airways and diffuses into the alveolar spaces (ventilation), while blood perfuses the parenchymal tissues through the pulmonary capillary bed interfacing the alveoli (perfusion) to allow O_2 and CO_2 exchange across the membranous air–blood barrier (diffusion). As straightforward as these processes may appear, the coordinated interfacing of blood and air and ready diffusion of gases ultimately determines the quality of life, indeed the survival, of the animal. When ventilation/perfusion is asynchronous, mismatched, or otherwise impeded, the animal must expend more energy to achieve adequate gas-exchange by ventilating more alveolar units to reach those that have a blood interface. Fortunately, the lung is designed with significant "functional reserve" and "compensation" ensuring its ability to adapt to a wide range of physiologic (exercise), environmental (altitude) stresses, and even moderate disease. But, by the same token, this reserve may hide insidious disease slowly eroding lung function in areas of the lungs (i.e., small airways) that are not easily assessed by standard methods.

Basic principles of respiration exist across a spectrum of animal species (see Refs. 16–21 for detailed review and discussion of pulmonary physiology and lung function testing). Normal tidal breathing is highly standardized, but unique variations exist to ensure adequate ventilation in some high mountain species or diving mammals. However, the basic process is stereotypic. The sealed thorax that encloses the lungs maintains a slightly negative intrathoracic pressure that keeps the lungs slightly expanded at rest. Thus, there is a volume of air that cannot be exhaled— the residual volume. Inspiration begins when signals from the central nervous system, originating in the breathing center of the medulla, stimulate the phrenic nerve to initiate contraction of the diaphragm and intercostal muscles of the rib cage. With contraction of the diaphragm, the intrathoracic pressure becomes slightly more negative. The virtual space between the thoracic wall and the lung pleura transmits this negative pressure to the compliant lung, which simply follows the chest wall along, transmitting the decreased intra-alveolar pressure such that air flows from high (atmospheric) pressure into the nose or mouth and into the more rarified airspace of the airways and lung lobes. After a brief end-inspiratory pause, pacing neurons also located in the medulla, having integrated vagus nerve-mediated signals from proprioceptors in the deep lung, terminate the inspiratory signal and the diaphragm relaxes along with the muscle and tissues of the thoracic wall. Gravitational and elastic recoil of the lung tissues forces the inspired air to now leave the lung. This cyclic process is energy-conserved and is tightly regulated via O_2, CO_2, and H^+ receptors in the aorta and carotid artery, as well as directly in the brain (via unique CO_2 receptors behind the blood–brain barrier). With muscular exercise or other systemic oxidative demands, the volume of air and frequency of breathing will increase to ensure appropriate gas-exchange to meet metabolic needs. When the lung is diseased, this compensation may be restricted by cardiopulmonary mechanics or it may be too energy demanding (e.g., fatigue resulting from efforts to overcome loss of lung elastic recoil or airway obstruction).

In the clinical setting, respiratory disorders typically appear as disturbing symptoms (e.g., wheeze, shortness of breath) and/or limitations to normal activities (e.g., fatigue). These complaints derive from impairments in cardiopulmonary function, which in many cases can be objectively assessed using an array of lung function testing methods. Because the first signs of pulmonary problems arise from complaints of functional limitations, one might argue that function, not underlying pathology, ultimately defines the seriousness of lung disease, at least in the eyes of the subject (17). However, impaired function generally is an outcome of pathogenic processes that damage large or small airways (e.g., asthma and emphysema) or initiate lung remodeling (e.g., fibrosis). Not surprisingly, therefore, a spectrum of lung function parameters derived from tests to evaluate specific attributes of respiration or functional "limits" has arisen as noninvasive tools to assess the presence and seriousness of disease. Of course, one would think that the direct measurement of O_2 and CO_2 in the blood would give a direct indication of the adequacy of respiration. Unfortunately, dynamic blood gas changes or fluctuating demands render conventional methods very insensitive except in acute respiratory stress or in severe disease. Ventilatory adjustments over time often go unnoticed but are sufficient to compensate and reestablish normal blood gas values.

Other assessment tests characterize the lung as to its static and dynamic properties providing a mechanical evaluation of lung performance and efficiency. These tests may include measures of lung volume apportionment under resting conditions, elasticity of lung tissue, large and small airway mechanics, and basic diffusion competence of the air–blood barrier—all of which are important in maintaining adequate ventilation, which of course impacts the homeostasis of blood gas values. The physiologic basis for these tests has been discussed in numerous texts (e.g., 18,19). Application of lung function tests is well standardized for human clinical assessments (20), and despite some methodological differences, largely due to the need for subject cooperation, most of these tests can be conducted on laboratory animals to garner analogous measures. To obtain such "cooperation" in animal testing, anesthesia is induced and the procedures are largely controlled by the operator (21).

Among the many parameters measured by lung function tests, lung volumes stand prominently as the most frequently reported feature. Volume measures vary from basic static apportionment of the total volume of the lung, but they may also be defined as a volume measured over a fixed time or as the result of a maximum effort. The static volume of the lung when fully inflated is defined as the total lung capacity (TLC), and that volume of air that can be completely exhaled is termed the vital capacity (VC). Not surprisingly, the air left in the lung that cannot be exhaled once a VC is expired is the residual volume (RV = TLC–VC). Perhaps most frequently measured in the clinic, however, is the forced expiratory volume in 1 sec (FEV$_1$), which is achieved by maximal forced expiration from TLC to RV. The FEV$_1$ provides an indirect index of small airway function based on the concept that forced expiration adds a transmural pressure load to the small airways, which if damaged have lost their structural integrity and collapse prematurely, thereby decreasing the FEV$_1$ value. Another notable volume is the forced VC, which is often used in ratio with the FEV$_1$ (as FEV$_1$/FVC); when below 80%, it suggests obstructive disease. The functional residual volume (FRC) is the volume of the lung at the end of a relaxed expiration of a normal tidal breath or volume (V_T). While less often measured in clinics, it represents a relaxation volume where there is balance between the elastic forces trying to collapse the lung within the thorax and the thoracic cage pulling outward. This volume is important is sustaining a partially inflated lung that is more easily (energy conservative) inflated and deflated with each breath. These lung volumes are well established for human subjects and are published as standardized nomograms based on gender, age, height, and weight (20).

When applied to laboratory animal studies, one finds that analogs of these volumes and measures can be determined under conditions of anesthesia and tracheal intubation. The TLC often is defined at ~30 cm H$_2$O positively applied airway pressure (P_{ao}), and –20 cm H$_2$O P_{ao} defines RV, which thus provides a VC by difference for that pressure range. When the airway of the anesthetized animal is exposed to 30 cm H$_2$O P_{ao} to achieve TLC and is rapidly exposed to a more forceful negative P_{ao} (–40 cm H$_2$O P_{ao}), a forced expiratory maneuver can be generated analogous to the FEV—except in this case the time period for analysis would be much smaller (~0.2 sec instead of 1 sec). Alternatively, specific flows along the FEV curve can be compared between the treated animal groups to those of a control group. Many publications have utilized these methods and their relevance to human extrapolation has also been evaluated (21,22).

During normal tidal breathing, one can relate temporally the pressures that drive the breath to its time-specific volume and flow to compute basic measures of mechanics (lung airway resistance—R_L or R_{ao} and dynamic lung tissue/small airway compliance—C_{dyn}). Lung mechanics are of greatest interest when there is concern for airway diseases such as asthma, or when an irritant that can trigger bronchoconstriction challenges the lung. In either case, the bronchial tubes have narrowed and resistance to airflow increases. When airway constriction occurs deep into the lung or is attended by edema in the lung tissue, the lung's ability to expand (compliance) decreases. The added work effort to the breathing cycle may compound the response and cause respiratory distress. The measurement of airway resistance can also be used to establish the presence of baseline bronchoconstriction as might exist in active asthma, and frequently is measured as part of a dose-dependent agonist-induced challenge to the airways to ascertain overall sensitivity of the airway to various irritants—a condition common in asthmatics. The measurement of lung mechanics in laboratory animals is commonly applied to studies of animal models of allergic airways disease (e.g., as an analog to asthma), and has long been used to assess the intrinsic irritancy of various inhalants (23).

Because most impairments to lung function in humans reside in the airways, measurement of the diffusion competency of the lung is less frequently assessed in humans. A defect in the blood–air barrier due to thickening of the alveolar interstitium (e.g., edema or fibrosis—see below) or due to damage to the capillary bed will impair the diffusion of oxygen through the alveolar–capillary membrane. Likewise mismatching of ventilation and perfusion due to these conditions may be the proximate functional abnormality. Lastly, a loss of surface area of the lung such as occurs in severe emphysema would also impair overall diffusion capacity for oxygen (DL_{O2}). The DL_{O2} can be approximated by introducing a defined, small quantity of carbon monoxide (CO), which molecularly has a diffusion constant similar to that of O_2 and binds vigorously to hemoglobin, into the breathing air of an individual, and computing an index of diffusion from the disappearance of the gas from alveolar gas samples over time. There are various specific methods for determining the DL_{CO} in humans, and likewise in experimental animals (21,24).

In the animal toxicology laboratory, the advantage of lung function assessments over standard histopathological evaluation is the nonterminal nature of the measurements and their implicit integration as indices of whole lung integrity. At the same time, the functional parameter may not be explicit for subtle underlying pathology because of its integrative nature and the large functional reserve inherent to the lung. Thus, it is not too surprising that the relative sensitivity of lung function vs. conventional histological methods has been mixed. However, judicious use of function testing methodologies especially in applications where one might expect analogous human responses (e.g., irritant atmospheres) or lung impairments due to small airway disease after chronic exposures can aid in the assessment of toxicant impacts to humans and their quality of life as well as identifying and characterizing organic disease.

IV. Empirical Studies of Inhaled Toxicants
A. Principles of Study Design and Toxicity Testing

The primary objective of any empirical inhalation study is the acquisition of data appropriate and useful in assessing health risk. These data should provide either a basic dose–response relationship or represent a relevant exposure paradigm that will yield generic mechanistic or mode of action information that can refine extrapolations across doses or species. Because inhalation toxicology often furnishes the core information used to assess the potential toxicity of commercial chemicals or products that are likely inhalants, regulatory agencies have established guidelines to ensure standardization of study conduct and its derived data. These guidelines are published (25–27) by agencies like the USEPA, under authority of specific legislation such as the Federal Insecticide, Fungicide, and Rodenticide Act (FIFRA) and the Toxic Substances Control Act (TSCA), to formalize the study designs used for acute, subchronic, and chronic inhalation exposure evaluations, including those addressing carcinogenicity. Analogously, acute inhalation guidelines have been drafted by the Organization for Co-operation and Economic Development (OECD) (http://www.oecd. org/dataoecd/47/29/2765785.pdf) in an attempt to harmonize procedures internationally to meet modern-day economies.

While details on standardized testing procedures are not the focus of this chapter, they will be briefly outlined here, as they remain a major focus for many inhalation toxicology facilities. Although the respiratory system is often the target organ of interest, any chemical that might enter the body via the lungs with potential systemic impact requires evaluation via an inhalation study. Such "toxicity testing" frequently is based on the need for specific information to address fundamental safety questions, as might be indicated in labeling or safety warnings. Acute inhalation tests have the longest history for such applications and although they often involve death and/or overt clinical toxicity, refinements have been made to limit the number of animals used to define toxicity levels (e.g., the "Limit Test"). Usually, a standard acute exposure dose–response scenario comprising multiple concentrations delivered a single time to the test species followed by a period of postexposure observation (usually 14 days). With appropriate statistical estimation of an LC_{50} and comparison with other toxicants of similar toxicity, basic labeling requirements can generally be fulfilled. Histopathology is a major end point for most acute toxicity studies as part of an initial assessment that will be used to determine target organs affected and exposure design for longer-term studies. For health concerns regarding multiple exposures or over a longer time frame, subchronic inhalation studies of at least four exposure levels (one as a control) may follow. These studies are conducted over 90 calendar days (usually 6–8 hr/day, 5 exposures/week). Determination of a no-observable-adverse-effect level (NOAEL) in these studies is important for assessing risk (e.g., RfC determinations), and for estimating exposure concentrations that can be used in chronic bioassays of 2 years duration—as required for carcinogenicity testing. Lastly, chronic inhalation studies, like the subchronic studies, involve four exposure concentrations (one elicits evidence of toxicity, and one does not with another dose in between plus control) and extend over nearly the lifetime of the rodent test species (2 years). Assessments focus on long-term multiorgan pathology and oncogenicity of the chemical of concern. There may be various permutations of these basic study designs to address reproductive and other specific systemic effects, some of which may require periods of clean air post exposure to assess reversibility. The selection of exposure concentrations to sufficiently challenge the test animals, and the appropriateness of certain toxicant specifics, such as particle size in the case of particulate materials, is usually defined within the published guidelines. End points range from death to clinical behaviors, pathology, and in some cases specific biochemical tests depending on the material and its potential use. More information can be found on the internet web sites (e.g., www.epa.gov/docs/ OPPTS_Harmonized/870_Health_Effects_ Test_ Guidelines/Drafts/870– 1350.pdf for Acute Inhalation Toxicity Testing with Histopathology; 870–3465.pdf for subchronic testing, etc.).

B. Investigatory Animal Studies

In contrast to the relatively strict guidelines described above for mandated inhalation toxicity testing, investigatory research of suspected toxic inhalants to elucidate low-concentration or specific scenario effects or to explore mechanisms might have a wide range of designs depending on the study objective or hypothesis. This diversity of design has given investigators the flexibility to tackle questions creatively, yet often cross-study comparisons and integration of data are made more difficult due to the lack of standardization. Even when a toxic inhalant such as the air pollutant O_3 has a wealth of published study data, it can be difficult to sort through the multiple exposure parameters to define a toxic or effective concentration, or to ascertain the relevance of specific mode of action findings (28). Animal studies may have specific nuances that are overlooked in their design, conduct of the exposures, and/or end point selection and interpretation. For example, exposures of rodents should ideally be done with the animals singly caged to avoid clustering and distortion of the actual exposure–dose, especially in the case of reactive gases and particles. Further emphasizing this point are many published studies attempting to address exposure effects in suckling neonates that have reported quite varied effects, leaving the reader to wonder if the differences reside in delivered dose or some other variable. Another factor that can impart variability in exposure-responses relates to whether food and water were provided during the exposure. Most would agree exposures of more than 2 hr should have water available to minimize dehydration stress, but food can confound exposures, especially with reactive or organic gases that can be absorbed or otherwise interact with the food. The result may lead to and exposure "sink" or food spoilage. Prolonged fasting of rodents, on the other hand, affects some baseline metabolic capabilities. And more insidiously, many toxicants can alter normal thermoregulatory control in rodents during and even after exposure (29) with resultant systemic implications (e.g., changes in perfusion or temperature-related metabolic rates). There is evidence to suggest that this hypothermic response is in fact a protective, compensatory reflex to decrease ventilation, metabolism and otherwise minimize dose and injury. Only just recently, this unique rodent attribute (not found in humans) has been realized as a qualitative consideration that should be incorporated in evaluating dose–health outcomes utilized in risk assessments (Jarabek—NCEA/EPA—personal communication). Lastly, some investigators would also argue that the nocturnal rodent should be exposed during its equivalent period of wakefulness and activity (i.e., the dark-phase) (30). This period is also when the diurnal body temperature cycle is at its peak in rodents and when food is consumed and endogenous antioxidants are highest. There is no consensus on this approach as it can be problematic technically and practically, which in part accounts for the fact it has not been widely adopted. Those who do nighttime exposures (30), however, often report greater sensitivity of their animal models. In summary then, the design of any exposure study should be the product of deliberate consideration of the variables that can be controlled in the context of the objectives of the study.

C. Controlled Human Studies

The use of the human as the "ideal" experimental animal for studies of inhalants with potential health concerns obviously avoids the uncertainties of extrapolation associated with nonhuman animal models. Issues of dose or diurnal conflict often inherent in animal studies are also likely to be minimized. Perhaps the most important attribute of a study conducted in human volunteers is that the data can be interpreted in the context of the wealth of available information from basic clinical medicine concerning relevant biomarkers and implications as to outcomes. On the other hand, the heterogeneity of the human population, the limited number of subjects and expense of doing human studies, and notably, the obvious ethical limits to study-related risks impart significant limitations to experimental use of humans. Nevertheless, human study data remain the "gold-standard," and deservedly receive priority consideration in any health assessment of inhaled toxicants.

Empirical inhalation exposure studies in humans are limited to acute and sometimes subacute scenarios. Single event exposures, and if deemed "safe" a limited number of repeated challenges, with a toxicant (such as O_3) at a level likely to be encountered in the ambient environment can be imposed in a controlled manner with relative safety to acquire response data directly relevant to the population (31). Responses are generally contrasted with sham exposures in the same individuals. Unlike most animal studies that use separate study groups of control and toxicant exposure, human studies typically use the same subject as its own control. Randomized, crossover designs are used to minimize problems with the order of challenge and the variability inherent among individuals arising from genetics or lifestyle differences. Historically, physiologic end points such as lung function have been primary pulmonary outcomes (32), but over the last 10 or 15 years, procedures shown to have minimal risk, such as bronchoalveolar or nasal lavage, have become common practice in well-equipped and experienced human study facilities associated with teaching hospitals (33). Indeed, bronchoscopy methods now allow biopsy of airway epithelium from the nose to the level of the segmental airways (third or fourth bifurcation). Bronchoscopy and biopsy procedures have even been performed with moderately asthmatic subjects (34). These newer sampling methods have opened doors for investigatory hypothesis-driven research as they are amenable to the refined molecular probes now available, and provide insight into the underlying biology that may or may not be reflected in lung function changes. Effects at the microlevel can then be linked to more targeted dosimetry and perhaps elucidate cell and subcellular linkages to clinical outcomes. While humans can only be exposed over a short period, these cellular/molecular changes may also signal or suggest potential longer-term outcomes that would not be attainable otherwise, bearing in mind, that the safety of the human subject remains paramount and any study must assure minimal adverse risk and full reversibility of any effects.

Recent interest in identifying potentially susceptible groups and what factors underlie responsiveness to a toxicant has led investigators to include some at-risk groups. Subjects with diseases such as asthma, COPD, or even cardiac disease have been studied successfully with selected air pollutants—e.g., NO_2 and CO (35,36). While the safety limits of such studies must be much more restrictive than with healthy volunteers, certain modestly invasive procedures such as bronchoscopy and biopsy have been performed in asthmatic subjects (34). When linked to studies with animal models, coherent findings can yield fundamental mechanistic data that strengthens the credibility and utility of extrapolation models as well as link to possible longer-term or chronic outcomes. Animal models, as discussed in more detail below, often provide unique opportunities to address specific susceptibility issues not approachable directly in human studies.

V. Inhalation Exposure Methods
A. Exposure Systems and Approaches

There are many detailed texts (27,37) and reviews (38,39) of inhalation exposure technology, and this chapter only summarizes salient principles and potential pitfalls. The basic system generally comprises five components that must function is a coordinated manner: the exposure chamber; the generation device for the inhalant of interest; the dilution units; the contaminant monitors; and lastly the exhaust system. Most inhalation exposure operations in use are dynamic, where air flows continuously through the system. As static chambers are used typically for special applications (e.g., pharmacokinetic studies, radionuclides, etc.), only the dynamic prototype system will be discussed here.

The heart of an inhalation system is the exposure chamber itself. These come in various sizes and shapes (depending on exposure subjects and numbers being exposed), but importantly the chamber must be designed to distribute the incoming air as evenly as possible throughout the chamber. Moreover, there must be assurance that the exposed animals do not significantly offset the toxicant concentration or the heat balance, ammonia level, and/or humidity of the chamber. Generally, the larger the chamber, the better the distribution and less artifactual influence of the subjects and caging (animals). The critical objective, of course, is that the breathing zone of the subject(s) must have a consistent and reproducible microenvironment vis a vis the concentration of airborne material. In the case of human exposures, when generally only one person is being exposed at a time, the "nose-to-nose" distribution in the chamber is not a factor, and with the subject remaining stationary or in one place, the exposure concentration can be calibrated to the breathing zone of that individual. If exercise (treadmill or ergometer) is involved, then the constancy of the breathing zone concentration can become of concern because of local airflow eddies associated with movement, vigorous breathing, or equipment. Diffusion plates at the chamber inflow point and on occasion, fans, generally can remedy or ease distribution problems. Some less elaborate human systems employ head chambers, face-masks/domes, or mouthpieces to deliver the inhalant. Each brings its own set of problems such as restraint-related discomfort, heat or water vapor build-up, or inhalant distribution or losses. The reactivity of the delivery system or chamber material with the inhalant to be studied is likewise important, though it is often overlooked. Inhalants like O_3 may be delivered into the chamber, but this gas reacts with virtually anything it touches—especially fabrics and conduit/chamber walls. Typically, there is no mass-balance between what is introduced and what is measured because of these system losses. Pre-exposure of an empty chamber to "kill" or saturate sites of loss at the walls can reduce this problem. Statically charged particles may also be lost to the system and conduits if not properly neutralized by passing them through a diffusion tube with a shielded alpha emitter like Kr^{85} to bring them to Boltzmann neutrality.

In the case of animal exposures, it is preferable to expose the animals singly in compartments or cages to avoid huddling. The distribution of the inhalant across the chamber in the breathing zone of all the animals must be ascertained and should vary (by convention) no more than 5% for gases and vapors and 15% for aerosols. Adequate ventilation of the chamber nominally requires at least 15 air volume changes per hour to provide turnover of air to meet the gas-exchange and heat dissipation of the animals when loaded to 5% v/v of the chamber volume. Stainless steel dissipates heat better than Plexiglas and therefore this 5% value would need to be lower in the latter case. On the other hand, animal exposures conducted with animals in nose-only or head-only tubes extending into a manifold are less dependent on this 5% rule since the animal body mass is external to the system. In this case, the adequacy of the air face-velocity and flow past the nose of the animal to ensure that rebreathing of expired air does not occur is the critical concern. A rule-of-thumb of $3\times$ the minute volume for each animal in the manifold can be used to estimate the overall flow needs, but ideally the system should be empirically evaluated for each unique system arrangement. The downside of nose-only approaches is the stress to the animals (confinement and lack of water), the need for training of the animals, and heat build-up in plastic restrainer tubes.

Ideally, any exposure chamber (human or animal) should reach concentration equilibrium as fast as possible. Theoretically, the up- and down-phase of the contaminant in the system are mirror-images of each other, such that the integrated exposure approximates a square-wave from turn-on to -off (Fig. 4). However, it is often desirable to achieve a stable, predetermined chamber concentration rapidly. This is achieved by increasing the turnover rate of the system. The nominal computation of this time to equilibrium relationship is given by the simplified formula:

$$t_{C_{95}} = 3 \times [\text{chamber volume/flow}]$$

where C_{95} is 95% of the desired concentration value and the chamber turnover is computed by dividing the chamber volume (L) by the flow rate (L/min). The result of the computation is the time to 95% of the target concentration in minutes. Clearly, the faster the turnover the faster the rise time to equilibrium.

This leads to the second component of the exposure system, inhalant generation. There are many methods of inhalant generation depending on the nature of the material, gas, solid, or liquid, but each has its special set of potential problems that are detailed in other texts (40). In the case of gases, compressed supply cylinders can provide a metered flow of the test inhalant, or in the case of a vapor from a liquid phase at room temperature, the material may be vaporized by any one of several means (e.g., nebulization/evaporation, gentle heating if chemically stable, etc.). Aerosols, on the

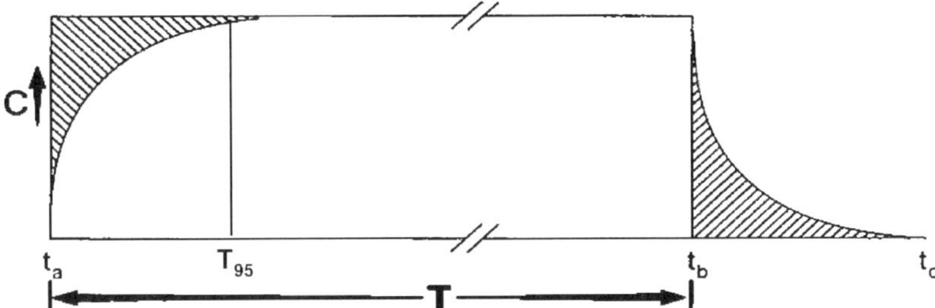

Figure 4 Schematic representation of the build-up, steady state, and blow-down of airborne material generated into a dynamic inhalation chamber. The rate of increase and decrease in concentration is dependent on the turnover rate of the chamber (see text). The T_{95} point is that point when the equilibrium target concentration is 95% achieved. The area under the build-up curve and the blow-down curve theoretically sum to the square wave equivalent of that time period. Therefore the exposure period is reasonably estimated as the integrated area from start-up (t_a) to turn-off (t_b) point.

other hand, offer more of a challenge since they do not disperse as easily into the air as do gases. Liquid aerosols may be nebulized or atomized, while solid particles can be resuspended into the air from a bulk source by various dust feeders (e.g., Wright), jet mills, or fluidized bed generators. Special systems that generate particles by less conventional methods, e.g., electrical discharge across anodes composed of the test material, can impose oxidants or static charges as noted above that may require special treatment or handling. The goal with any aerosol generation system is to obtain an appropriately sized inhalable particle. For humans, particles up to 10–15 μm may be used, though many toxicity questions generally reside with small (< 5 μm) particles. In the case of rodents, inhalability requires particles generally less than 3 μm and preferably less than 1 μm to obtain reasonable deep lung deposition (see the discussion of particle deposition and clearance below). Obviously, the particle size may be part of the hypothesis being tested so specific size ranges may be targeted as desired. In any case, the gases and aerosols generated usually require dilution with clean air before introduction into the chamber. This third component of the exposure system must mix and disperse the inhalant sometimes with an in-line mixing system to assure that the exposure airflow into the chamber is evenly mixed and is of controlled humidity ($\sim$50%) and temperature (70–75 °F). Sometimes diffuser plates or even fans in the inlet system aid in this mixing. It is important that the dilution gas be free of ambient contaminants that may confound the inhalant effects. In-line ventilation air system scrubbers (e.g., water-sprays with driers, activated charcoal, and permanganate-based Purofil^R) and HEPA filters designed for a wide-range of airflows and volumes are available to ensure the removal of ambient pollutants like CO, ozone, nitric and sulfur oxides, and particulate matter (PM). Cogeneration of both gases and aerosols raises potentially unique problems related to their in-chamber interactions (due to their respective reactivities), which may or may not be desirable. Hence, inhalation exposure studies must be well thought out to minimize insidious problems and confounding.

The fourth component of the exposure system is appropriate atmospheric sampling and monitoring methodology to measure the inhalant of interest (41). These systems range from classic collection by impingement systems using trapping buffers or on filters to the latest real-time sophisticated photometric and laser systems. Sampling strategies often must be adapted to the system in use, but the critical factor is measuring as close to breathing zone as possible without disturbing the chamber airflow dynamics. This is relatively straightforward for gases and vapors so long as sampling does not disturb the concentration in the breathing zone. In the case of aerosols, sampling must be appropriate to minimize distortion of the particle characteristics (humidity, temperature, etc.). Critical to any aerosol measurement is the size distribution as well as the mass concentration. In some cases, particle number per unit volume is also an important parameter—especially with the smallest particles often referred to as ultrafines (diameters < 0.1 μm).

Lastly, the exposure system requires an air-cleaning and exhaust system. At first glance, it would appear that this component is least important, but in reality the exhaust is really an extension of the dilution system and balances flows such that the chamber is maintained slightly negative to the atmosphere to ensure that leaks are into and not out of the chamber. The chamber exhaust, because it is contaminated, must also be cleaned before release into the ambient air (usually through a facility exhaust hood or duct). Removing the contaminants involves similar air-cleaning engineering strategies applied to the inlet dilution air but sometimes must be more rigorous since the contamination is likely higher than the ambient air source cleaned and conditioned for dilution. Thus to appropriately and safely operate an exposure facility for animal or human exposures, a combination of disciplines is required—from chemistry to engineering. While there are many sources of information, the novice should avail him/herself of expertise to establish a reliable and safe system for empirical study of toxic inhalants.

B. In Vitro Approaches

Inhalation studies implicitly involve a breathing organism. However, the need to address mechanistic questions has motivated the development of novel in vitro exposure systems to deliver various airborne toxicants to excised lungs or tissues and cells in culture (42,43) (also see Chapter 10). Several cell types isolated from the lung either as an individual type (e.g., macrophage) or a mixture of cells types (e.g., tracheal cells) have been studied in isolation. Some primary cell types have been treated to become "immortalized" cell lines, offering the possibility of greater cell accessibility. Usually these studies involve dissolution of the toxicant in an appropriate buffer or media that is then placed on the culture for a given duration. While this approach has yielded many published reports, newer culture systems have been devised that allow cultured and isolated cells to be exposed to airborne materials with the goal of achieving somewhat more relevance. These systems may incorporate rocking plates that cyclically expose underling cultures as the apical fluid rocks away (44), or they may use transwell plates that have an exposed air surface that is fed by media from a basal well, mimicking to some extent a lung or airway interface (43,45). The transwell technology is a significant advance for studies with lung tissue/cell cultures since surface buffer layer systems are inherently confounded by problems with dissolution and distribution of the toxicants, as well as culture cell hypoxia when compared to in vivo respiratory tract cells normally exposed to the air. Empirical exposure to gases or vapor, while potentially affected by the requisite high humidity and temperature of the chamber, is generally straightforward and has been successfully achieved with several inhalants (e.g., O_3) (43,46). However, aerosol exposures in vitro are more easily distorted by chamber-environmental factors, which make more problematic the challenge of particle delivery and distribution to cells. Recently, however, a system has been described that appears to have overcome the primary problem of particle distribution to cultures grown at the air–liquid interface (47). This system is complex technically (e.g., drying cells), and has to date had limited distribution, but it offers promise for future work with particle exposures to single cell and cocultures that are amenable to transwell culture procedures.

The isolated perfused lung as an in vitro organ procedure has been used for many years to evaluate dosimetry and mechanistic biology questions with inhalants (42). Typically these so-called "hanging-lung" preparations are contained within a thorax-like enclosure with a pump or diaphragm that permits simulated respiration. With this arrangement, gaseous inhalants can be introduced to the trachea or airway from a reservoir or a breathing chamber into which the gas has been generated. To date, these ex vivo systems have had virtually no use with particles (except instilled particles or particles infused in the perfusate) because of problems with dose administration and distribution.

C. Estimating Dose with Inhalation Exposures

The most frequently used metric for administered "dose" for an inhalation study is the characterization of the exposure conditions—concentration, duration, and number of exposures. However, dose and exposure are not synonymous. Frequently, a nominal "dose" is attributed to the product of "concentration $\times$ exposure time" or "$C \times T$" based on the classic interrelationship between these parameters described by Haber for war-gases around the time of WWI (48). Haber's contention was that relative war-gas potency could be ascribed to $C \times T$—there was a proportional dose relationship between $C \times T$ and lethality. Thereafter, this concept evolved as a means of comparing the toxicity of an inhalant over varying concentrations and durations and was applied to end points other than lethality—conditions where the relationship often breaks-down (49). While some investigators continue to argue its relevancy (under some defined limits and mathematical treatments it has been found to be useful in predicting toxicity (50)), it is clear that this simple algebraic concept of dose is very limited if not misleading (49,51).

To derive a better estimate of dose, it is now appreciated that ventilation (minute volume) and the fractional uptake of the inhalant interact to determine what actually deposits on the respiratory tract surface. In a strict modeling sense, minute ventilation is also a simplification since airflows and volume per breath are important dose-determining parameters, but it serves well as an estimate of air breathed into the whole respiratory tract. Fractional uptake, while obviously tied to the exposed subject, is more dependent on the physical chemistry of the gas (e.g., solubility in water/organic) and, in the case of particles, on the mean aerodynamic size and distribution, although water solubility is also an important factor. Sophisticated theoretical models have been developed to refine (see below) estimates of total, regional, and local tissue dose for inhalants, but typically a dose-value for an inhalation study is considered "advanced" when there have been physiologic measures of ventilation during exposure that can be combined with the exposure metrics. Thus one could compute a dose as: $D = C \times T \times V_{min}$. An estimate of fractional uptake or deposition efficiency can refine this estimate even more.

VI. Deposition and Clearance of Environmental Inhalants

For ease of presentation, the terms deposition and clearance will be used to describe the processes of transfer of inhaled material from the airstream to the surface of the airways and conversely the removal of material from the airway surface, respectively. While there are some similarities in these processes regardless of whether the inhaled material is in gaseous or particulate form, there are obviously significant differences as described below.

A. Gases and Vapors

To a physical chemist, gases and vapors are readily distinguishable. Vapors are materials that have a relatively high vaporization temperature and thus can exist in both liquid and gaseous states simultaneously at room temperature. A good example is water, but there are also many low molecular weight organic substances (e.g., formaldehyde, hexane) that coexist as liquid and gas at room temperature (if only temporarily). Gases, on the other hand, have relatively low vaporization temperatures and thus exist entirely in a gaseous state except when cooled to very low temperatures or subjected to high pressures (e.g., oxygen, sulfur dioxide, etc.). However, the principles determining the uptake of gases and vapors by the respiratory tract are exactly the same. These principles lie in the physical/chemical attributes of the gas, thermodynamic equilibrium, and the dynamics of diffusion and subsequent chemical reaction. On the side of the host, uptake efficiency may be influenced by individual airway anatomy and physiology, inclusive of airflow rates, tidal breath volumes, and residency times (end-inspiratory pauses or breath-holding), blood perfusion of airway and lung tissues, and even airway fluid thickness and tissue metabolism (52,53).

The uptake of a gas by airway lining fluids generally follows Henry's Law as it applies to aqueous media, whereby the movement of gas molecules from the air phase into an aqueous interface is based on the concentration gradient and the solubility of the gas in water. Net diffusion into the airway fluids continues until thermodynamic equilibrium is achieved. Depending on gas solubility, equilibrium may or may not be achieved depending on the "residency" of the gas at the site of uptake during the breathing cycle—hence the importance of airflow in this process (54,55). Similarly, if the absorbed gas is cleared from the airway lining fluid rapidly due to chemical reaction or perfusion-mediated dispersal of the absorbed gas molecules (56), the net driving force from the gas phase may always be positive into the fluid even if solubility is low. If the absorbed gas reacts with airway fluid or tissue molecules (as in the case of formaldehyde binding to tissue macromolecules (57), the absorptive process may exhibit an irreversible "sink" effect. On the other hand, when the concentration of the gas in the airstream dips below the equilibrium concentration, the gas absorbed into the airway fluids, blood, and other extracellular fluid compartments may reverse and diffuse back into the air phase. Thus, while the absorption of gases and vapors along the respiratory tract is largely governed by their respective water solubilities, it is clear that this determinant is somewhat of an oversimplification, as there are several modifying factors that may be of significance depending on the specific gas, its interaction with fluid and tissue reactants, and the physiology of the host.

The uptake of a gas, in terms of either the total respiratory tract or regional dose, can be greatly influenced by the anatomical route of exposure. The convoluted passages of the nose and its high surface to volume ratio make it particularly efficient in absorbing water-soluble gases. A viscous, yet aqueous mucus layer and the relatively high, subepithelial vascular perfusion of the nose add to its overall efficiency. In rodents, which are obligate nasal breathers and have a highly convoluted airway structure, nasal absorption is very high for water-soluble gases such HF (58), formaldehyde (59), and SO_2 (60). However, humans and dogs, for example, which can also breathe via the mouth, may introduce a higher concentration into the trachea during oral breathing (54). Furthermore, exercise, which increases airflow and thereby reduces the interface residence-time between the gas and airway fluid surface, can also result in deeper penetration of the inspired water-soluble gas. In the case of gases that are relatively water-insoluble, penetration into the deep lung is much more likely. Gases like N_2 and O_2 equilibrate easily with airway fluids due to their relatively low solubilities and penetrate to the periphery of the lung (obviously important for O_2 that must reach the alveoli to diffuse into the plasma and red blood cells). Pollutant gases of low water solubility (e.g., NO_2 and O_3) can absorb or react in the nose and along the respiratory tract, but because they penetrate to the deep lung where there is an extraordinarily high tissue surface-volume ratio and low convective flow (hence high residence time) their dose to that region can be very high (61,62). The fact that a gas reacts with the lining layer of the end airway and alveoli also will contribute to its effective dose to that region.

The clearance of gases from the respiratory tract varies as per the same properties as absorption. Poorly soluble, nonreactive gases simply desorb back into the expiratory airstream. Water-soluble gases may be excreted in the urine as the ionic forms to which they convert when absorbed (e.g., SO_2 to HSO_3^-) (54). Similarly, gases that react with macromolecules or are metabolized may also be excreted as water-soluble conjugates of small proteins (5) or otherwise recycled in anabolic processes. Many organic vapors that slowly partition from the air into the blood and fatty tissues of the body eventually partition back into the expired breath as the parent molecule or may be converted by metabolism into excretable forms.

B. Particles (Aerosols)

The deposition of solid or liquid particles in the respiratory tract is dependent on many of the same factors as gas deposition with one notable *critically* different determinant, particle size. Because of variability in particle shape and composition, and thus density, particles are typically defined in the context of their aerodynamic behavior rather than their visual dimensions. Thus, particles or aerosols have come to be aerodynamically standardized to a solid, spherical shape with a density of one (1 g/mL). This standardization allows aerosols to be compared, especially when it comes to deposition within the respiratory tract. Inhaled environmental particles are typically polydispersed, encompassing a spectrum of sizes that can be aerodynamically represented as a log-normal distribution of mass vs. log of aerodynamic diameter (63). When sampled with a system that uses aerodynamic "cut-points" to collect aerosols on filters that are subsequently weighed, the distribution of mass yields a peak value that defines the mass median aerodynamic diameter (i.e., MMAD). The MMAD indicates that one half the mass of the distribution lies above this size and one half the mass lies below. Statistically, one can arrive at a numeric representation of the distribution (σ_g) that describes the polydispersity of the distribution by plotting the cumulative frequency vs. the MMAD to get a nominal straight-line. The σ_g can be computed from this plot as:

$$\sigma_g = \text{size at freq. } 84.1\%/\text{size at freq. } 50\%$$
$$\text{or size at freq. } 50\%/\text{size at freq. } 15.9\%$$

When σ_g is less than 1.2, the distribution is generally considered monodisperse—of one nominal size with a very narrow distribution. The MMAD and the σ_g are conventional for defining aerosols generally encountered in the environment or workplace, which are typically polydisperse. When particles become exceedingly small and have no appreciable mass, and they cannot be defined by mass-based aerodynamics, their scale for interactions approaches the mean-free path between molecules of air and the deposition properties of particles and gases converge. These particles are best described by their electrical mobility in a field that can be converted into a count median diameter (CMD) with a corresponding number count per unit volume rather than a mass. Particles in this size range are often referred to as ultrafines (see below).

Aerosols deposit by five basic mechanisms arising from their aerodynamic (MMAD) or physical dimensions. These are represented schematically in Fig. 5.

1. *Impaction* is the primary mechanism of deposition for particles > 1.0 μm, and becomes increasingly dominant as size increases. Impaction occurs in the nose within its convolutions and on nasal hairs, and for particles that make it past the nose, impaction occurs on the airways especially at branching points along the tracheobronchial tree. Increased breathing rate and depth, which increase airflow, also increase impaction.

2. *Interception* is a process similar to impaction, but relates to fibrous aerosols, with a length to diameter aspect ratio > 3:1. When long fibers are inhaled, they have a tendency to spear the airway wall when moving through branching angles. This probability increases with increasing fiber length as fibers tend to travel nearly parallel to the airstream, but overall the probability for deposition is largely determined by the fiber diameter.

3. Those particles between 0.5 μm and 5 μm in size that penetrate into the smaller bronchi and bronchioles where air velocity slows considerably are significantly affected by gravity and succumb to the process of *sedimentation*. As the dynamic forces that held the particles in the airstream begin to wane, the particles will settle dependent upon their aerodynamic

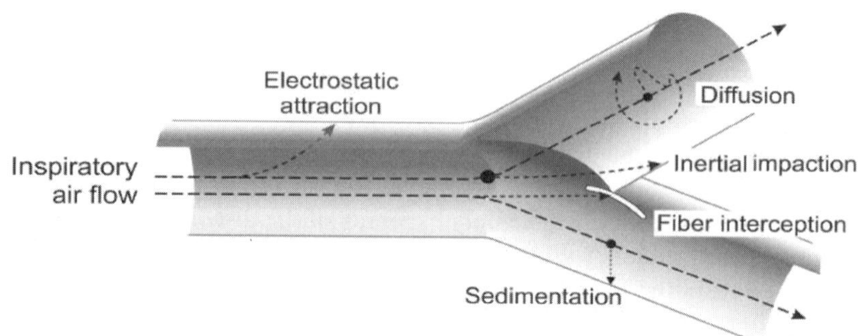

Figure 5 Schematic representation of major pulmonary deposition mechanisms for PM. Five major mechanisms are involved in particle deposition in the lungs (see text for details).

sizes at a constant, terminal velocity defined by Stoke's Law. Thus, as might be expected, sedimentation increases with residence time in the airway or lung and, conversely, decreases with increasing breathing rate which effectively decreases residence time.

4.   Particles in the submicron range, especially < 0.1 μm, can be affected by the constant bombardment of air molecules as the aerosols slip between and among the surrounding gas molecules—a process termed *Brownian motion*. This diffusionary process displaces the particles randomly and they deposit on the airways, especially when convective flow is low and residence time is extended. Deposition can be high in the smallest bronchioles since the displacement distances to the walls are relatively short, but in regions where turbulence is high, ultrafine deposition can also occur due to Brownian motion as the particles are continuously brought close to the walls. Therefore, ultrafine deposition can also be significant throughout the respiratory tract.

5.   While generally considered the least important factor in physiologic deposition of most environmental aerosols, *electrical charges* on smaller particles (often freshly generated by high temperatures or attrition) can impart influential attractive forces. Charged particles are most likely encountered in industrial settings, but charges on environmental particles are typically neutralized over time by other charged ions (e.g., ammonium or chloride ion) or water.

The deposition of polydisperse environmental particles from an aerosol cloud can distribute throughout the respiratory tract depending on the MMAD and σ_g. Where the particles deposit may have implications for potential effects and the predominance of one method of clearance over another (5) (see below). Moreover, the deposition profile can be affected by the composition of the aerosol. A hygroscopic aerosol, like many environmental aerosols containing sulfates and nitrates, can absorb water upon inhalation, and grow potentially by a factor of two or more (63,64). Thus, particles may end up in the nasopharynx or large airways that might otherwise theoretically deposit more peripherally.

As with gases, respiratory tract anatomy and physiology can have a significant impact on deposition. During resting tidal breathing, each inspired breath is only about twice the functional dead space of the airways, but with exercise, each breath volume can increase two- to three-fold with a complementary increase in breathing frequency. Moreover, with exercise breathing shifts from mostly nasal to mostly oral because of less airflow resistance in the mouth. The result is a substantial increase in airflow velocity that augments impaction of inspired particles, while the large inspiratory volumes carry the particles deeper into the lung extending the zone of convective flow into the airways normally dominated by low flows. This could disturb the regional processes of sedimentation and diffusion. Obviously, any narrowing in the airways (such as in asthma and bronchitis) would have the effect of increasing air velocities and enhancing impaction. In contrast, breath-holding can enhance deposition especially of mid-sized particles by increasing residence times and the time available for settling. Thus, there may be a spectrum of deposition profiles and potential health outcomes resulting from the interplay of these physical and biological factors, making deposition or health predictions complex.

A large body of evidence and related modeling has been developed for deposition in the human lung (e.g., ICRP Task Group on Lung Dynamics) (65). If one examines the modeled (66) representation for the human (Fig. 6A), one clearly sees a nadir in the deposition profile at about 0.3–0.5 μm, where the size range of particles is most abundant in nonpolluted air. One can see in Fig. 6B for the rodent lung (66) that the qualitative profile of deposition is quite similar to that of the human. This similarity illustrates further that the environmental forces that dictated the evolutionary development of the mammalian lung (as discussed above) were likewise effective to minimize particle deposition across species.

However similar they may be, comparing the specific deposition profiles of rodents with those of the human raises questions that point to potentially important distinctions. For example, the basic airway structure of the rodent lung, monopodial vs. dichotomous branching in the human, can have a significant impact on aerosol deposition at the bifurcations. With dichotomous branching where two daughter branches split from the parent at about the same angle of incidence, inspirational airflow is focused on the center-point of the angle with the creation of a localized "hot-spot" for impaction. Hot-spots on the upstream sides of the airway wall also theoretically occur during expiration by complex processes due to the merging airflows and local eddies. In contrast, the monopodial pattern has a main flow continuing along the main airway trunk with relatively less ridge-deposition

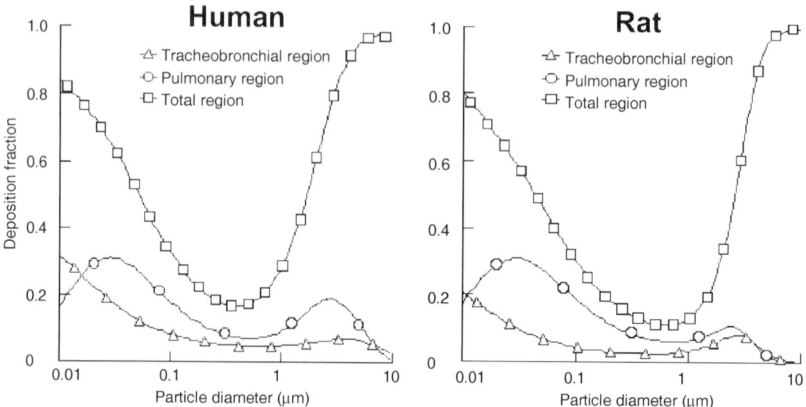

Figure 6 Particle deposition profiles for the human and the rat. Particle deposition profiles were modeled at tidal volumes of: 625 ml-human and 2.1 ml-rat at breathing frequencies of: 12 min^{-1} and 102 min^{-1}. (From Ref. 66.)

at the daughter or tributary split. Thus, deposition at these bifurcation points (apart form other influential factors) is higher in the human than the rodent model. This could have important implications in the microtoxicology and extrapolation of effects of a given particulate inhalant. Nevertheless, some generalizations can be made attempting to incorporate the many factors affecting deposition and differences between species. After adjusting for lung and body size as well as ventilation differences, a rodent and a human breathing the same atmosphere of aerosols for the same duration, the rodent (or relatively smaller animal) will have a greater dose per unit lung or body weight than the human. It has been estimated that for a 1 μm particle, the rat total lung dose will be about five- to 10-fold that of the human (27). If computed on the basis of lung surface area and distributed regional dose, the rat/human dose ratio could be up to 30-fold for the deep lung (66). Whether this accounts for hot-spot differences is speculation at this point, but the issue merits investigation. Theoretical models have estimated hot spots to exceed the average dose by a factor of five or more (67).

Clearance of deposited particles from the lung is essential for host defense. This multifaceted process probably evolved to rid the body of infectious organisms, but it has proven generally effective for inanimate invaders of the lung as well. It is probably safe to assume that the faster foreign materials are removed from the respiratory tract the lesser chance of injury or toxic outcomes. Generally, the specific mechanisms involved in clearance of particles differ by the region of deposition. The mechanisms involve the collaborative efforts of both physical and biological processes. Large particles that deposit in the nose and throat may induce choking, coughing, or sneezing as fundamental physical methods of expulsion of particles from the airways, as mediated by mechanical receptors in the nasopharynx. This reflex is most prominent in large mammals and does not exist in the rodent. The teleological explanation for this difference is not readily apparent, but may relate to a limit on the size of particles that can be rapidly accelerated with small volumes of air and lower maximal expiratory pressures in rodents with highly compliant (low muscle mass) chest walls. However, the removal of most environmental particles that penetrate the respiratory tract typically involves more subtle methods.

Nasal clearance of insoluble particles generally involves the movement of mucus posteriorly toward the throat carrying the particles that are eventually swallowed or spit up. This clearance of mucus to the throat from the medial and posterior regions of the nose usually occurs in a matter of minutes as flow is continuous and can be stimulated by particles themselves. If the particles are water-soluble, they may clear within the mucus gel or sol layers or via the blood perfusing the nasal subepithelium. Recently, attention has again been drawn to the olfactory region of the nose where additional evidence of translocation of particle-related metal ions via the olfactory nerve to the brain has been observed (68). Whether insoluble particles, especially ultrafines, can undergo similar transport is uncertain. In contrast, particles deposited in the anterior regions are usually wiped or blown clear through the nares.

Tracheobronchial clearance involves particles that have deposited on the airways lined with ciliated epithelium and surface fluid secreted from goblet cells and mucous/serous glands. The pattern of clearance of insoluble particles up the ciliary escalator is generally thought to be spiral in nature moving a few to several mm/min up the airways to the pharynx and then swallowed for discharge by the GI tract. There is debate as to whether the mucous layer is a continuous layer or is patchy, but there is nevertheless sufficient continuity to ensure fluid movement up the airways (69). A thin monolayer of surfactant is now thought to line the airway surface, which aids the movement of particle-laden macrophages from the deep lung along the airways (70). Some macrophages appear to have the responsibility to patrol the airway surface in their pursuit of particles and microorganisms. Typically, tracheobronchial clearance is defined functionally as that amount cleared in the first ~24 hr after deposition. Particles retained longer are thought to be more peripheral in the alveoli or the smallest end airways where mucus clearance is less effective (63). Particles in the deep lung clear most slowly, and may be described with two or three temporal phases. Alveolar macrophages in the alveoli have an important role in deep lung/alveolar clearance. The estimated clearance time mediated by macrophages is thought to be somewhere between 2 and 6 weeks (71), and may involve mechanisms whereby macrophage and epithelium-derived mediators recruit more macrophages from interstitial pools or the blood to assist in particle removal. The macrophages with their engulfed particulate material may move to the mucociliary escalator for removal as described or, less frequently, migrate through the lung surface into underlying lymphatic vessels and on to lymph tissues. Some particles have exceedingly long clearance times up to many months, and in some cases (often with high exposures as in coal miners) the clearance may be effectively nil, with sequestering of particles within the lung tissues (72). Some argue that ultrafine particles, in particular, may readily migrate into the lung interstitium and either remain there or penetrate farther to the blood to distribute throughout the body (73). While particles have been found in many systemic tissues in humans who have incurred high/long-term exposures in the workplace, evidence that ultrafines carry special significance to health because of potential migration remains uncertain.

In healthy animal models, clearance of particles deposited in the lungs and airways is qualitatively similar to that of the human, but the speed of clearance after a single exposure is very different, usually much faster (Fig. 7) (74). The primary nonspecific host clearance processes prevail:

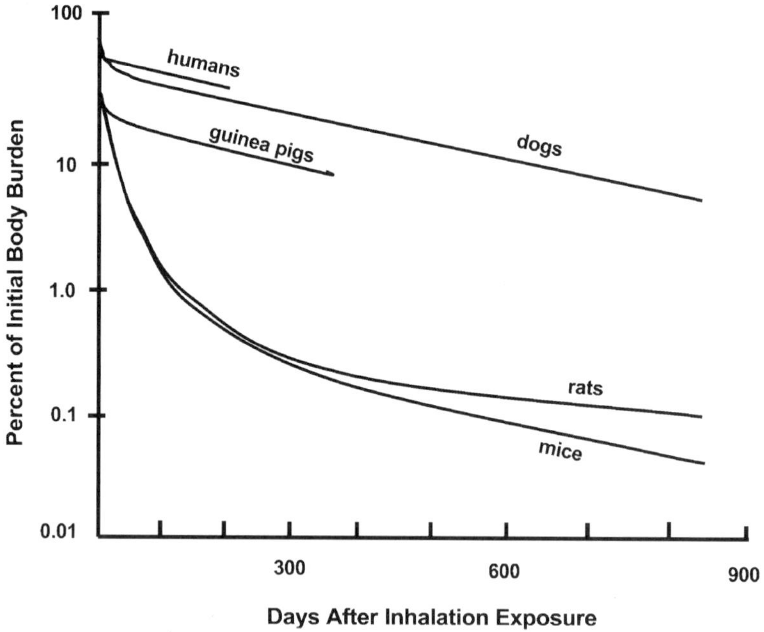

Figure 7 Pulmonary clearance kinetics following aluminosilicate particle exposure. Clearance kinetics is shown after a single exposure to 1.5 μm ^{134}Cs-labeled fused aluminosilicate particles in three laboratory rodents, the dog, and the human. Early clearance (days) is similar across these species, but is dramatically different long term.

mucociliary transport and macrophage engulfment (63). There is some debate as to the degree to which very small particles may move across the epithelium and be sequestered within the lung tissue or move via lymph transport to lymphoid tissues (72), but clearly the bulk of deposited particles are removed from the respiratory surface and cleared. When exposures are repeated, especially at relatively high concentrations as might be encountered in a dusty trade for the human or a chronic exposure protocol in experimental animals, species differences may be amplified or emerge unique. Humans in historically dusty trades, such as coal mining, have been found to have substantial quantities of sequestered particles within the lung tissues themselves, and though pathology results from the dose and inherent toxicity of the dust, the "load" of material is somewhat surprisingly less important to the disease outcome (75). The rat, on the other hand, which is the most frequently used rodent model for chronic inhalation studies, responds quite differently to inhaled particles in circumstances when deposition rate exceeds clearance, a condition sometimes referred to as "overload." Pulmonary overload of poorly soluble particles (PSPs) in the rat results in substantial intralumen accumulation of particles that appear to initiate pathophysiologic processes distinct from that of the human and, indeed, the mouse and hamster as well, which merely accumulate the particles without significant pathology. Theories have been proposed suggesting an important and distinct role for chronic oxidant injury and stimulation of epithelial cells and septal fibroblasts leading to fibrosis and even cancer, but the root mechanistic distinction of why the rat seems so different from other species remains uncertain (76). Thus, an appreciation of the importance of deposition rate and clearance kinetics in test animals relative to these processes in the human should be apparent if one is to reasonably relate findings from the laboratory to the human scenario.

VII. Respiratory Tract Injury

A. Acute Lung Injury

Each of the many cell types of the airways and lungs has a unique function(s) to ensure efficient gas-exchange. It is not surprising that their varied structure, function, and inherent sensitivities coupled with their distribution along the respiratory tree determine their differential risk from an inhalant. Moreover, some cells, like the alveolar macrophage, may mediate "toxic communications" among neighboring cells as in the case of silica (71). Often not appreciated is the intimate relationship of alveolar cells with the pulmonary vasculature and its circulating components that may complicate the response or transmit its impact systemically. Earlier chapters in this text have covered in substantial detail the array of contributors and processes involved in lung injury and inflammation. The goal here is to introduce the basic concepts and overall process of inhalation injury, and the subsequent cellular and mediator responses to the initial stimulus or damage. It is useful to appreciate at the outset that at the cellular level, any number of stimuli, from activation of cell-surface receptors to overt damage to the cell membrane, may trigger a response. Moreover, a response from any given cell type should not be considered alone since it has evolved within a complex matrix of cells that communicate in a variety of ways with the primary goal—however teleological it may be—to protect the lung and its basic function, or secondarily to compensate or aid in repair. Hence the magnitude of response is likely to be a composite of true injury, "damage control," and the initial steps in a repair process. This is not to say that any of these processes cannot go awry, such as in parenchymal fibrosis, but merely to emphasize that "response" per se is rarely monotonic.

Figure 8 schematically shows the spectrum of lung responses to toxic inhalant injury. Injury that results in cell death and overt pathology is easily identified and can be characterized as "adverse." However, inhalants may cause changes that can be measured (i.e., responses), but are reversible or are within physiologic or biologic limits. For example, a gas may trigger an irritant reflex and this may yield sensation or pain through nerve endings and receptors strategically scattered along the airways. This sensation may alter breathing and in the case of the standardized mouse bioassay (ASTM-E981-84) (77,78) can be used to quantify relative irritant potency. But, in

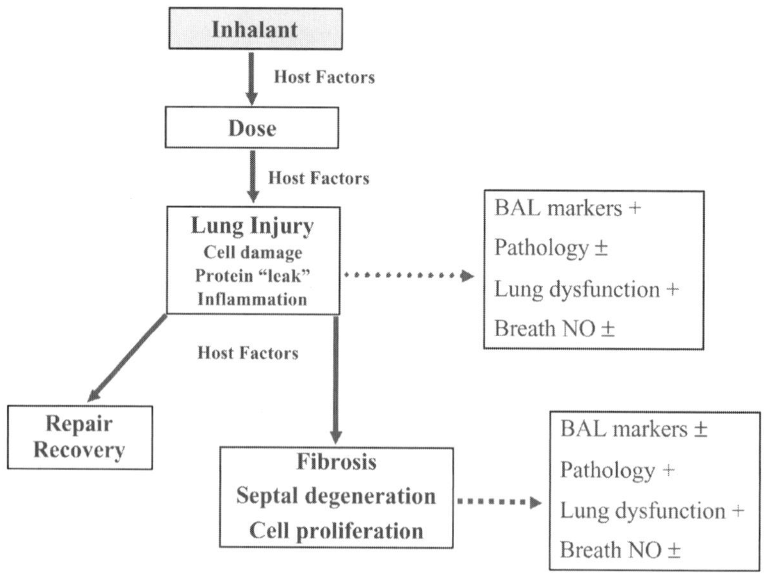

Figure 8   Response cascade of a given host (human or animal model) exposed to a toxic inhalant.

fact, one finds that the alteration of breathing can limit further exposure and thus dose, and the likelihood of damage or injury (79). Obviously, at high concentrations this reflex may be overwhelmed and cells will be damaged, become necrotic or be forced into early senescence and apoptosis, eroding the barrier separating the airspaces from the blood. Hence, permeability may increase (i.e., a "leak") and plasma proteins and other relatively small molecules, including water (as a result of osmosis), will move into the interstitium and eventually into the airspaces. If the damage is sufficiently severe, patent edema may result with respiratory distress and perhaps even death. Sometimes the damage may be followed by significant lung remodeling as has been observed with survivors of the Bhopal, India, tragedy with the accidental release of the highly irritant, hydrolytic gas, methylisocyanate (MIC) (80). However, early in an exposure, even with a highly toxic, alkylating gas like phosgene that chemically disrupts the macromolecular structure of the cell membrane and kills airway cells, one sees that the alveolar–capillary "leak" that occurs almost immediately actually worsens more slowly or deaccelerates over a period of 30–60 min (81). Thus, there appears to be some control or compensation to injury almost immediately—in fact this may reflect an initial part of the repair phase since repeated exposures the next day and even a week later are much less damaging. Other direct acting toxic irritants like ozone show a similar pattern of response (82).

While the edemagenic response to ozone resembles that of phosgene or other corrosive gases (e.g., MIC), it differs significantly in its mode of action. Ozone is believed to react with lung surface fluids and perhaps cell membranes, specifically attacking double bonds in unsaturated lipids (e.g., arachidonate) to initiate a cascade of propagating free radical reactions that further damage the membrane and cell. These bioactive molecules may take a while to fully elicit their damage as they accumulate over time. Products of these reactions (peroxides and carbonyls) are active in eliciting inflammation in the lung via the prostaglandin and leukotriene networks to further magnify and disseminate the stimulus. With the debris of damaged cells and a wide variety of mediators (e.g., cytokines, chemokines, etc.) released from airway epithelium, macrophages and other lung matrix cells accumulate and the response also includes the activation of various cell-surface adhesion molecules (i.e., integrins) on the vascular and respiratory surface. These adhesion molecules are essential to the migration of inflammatory cells from the pulmonary interstitial pool and circulation into the lung (83). Obviously this process, as described, is overly simplified, and indeed there are nuances to each response in kind and degree depending on the toxicant, extent of injury, and model being studied, but clinically the injury phase of the response is largely stereotyped.

Often, the inflammatory response is taken as an adverse response that can be quantified. The number of inflammatory cells can be counted and tracked over time as the syndrome progresses. The argument would be that inflammation with its activated cells releasing oxidants, peroxidases, and elastases inflicts further damage to the lung tissues (83). However, studies have been conducted where the influx of the primary inflammatory cell, the polymorphonuclear neutrophil (PMN), has been suppressed or removed, only to find that the damage due to a toxicant like ozone was in fact worse than when the inflammatory cell was present (84). Thus, the cells despite their armamentarium of bioactive mediators may have an essential repair or modulatory role. Likewise, some of the interleukins, specifically IL-6 and IL-11, once thought to be proinflammatory may have anti-inflammatory potential, either alone or depending on their networked interaction with other mediators (85,86). Many of the specifics of these mediators and their respective roles are discussed in greater detail elsewhere in this text and one should not get the illusion that these processes are easily dissected or well understood. The use of various transgenic and knockout models (e.g., for IL-6 and ozone) as discussed above have proven quite useful in elucidating certain attributes of these mediators, but the likelihood that one cytokine or mediator is pre-eminent in these events is unlikely (87,88).

Further complicating understanding of these events is an underappreciation of the fundamental concept of the dose–response relationship. Not surprisingly, this has a high probability of impact in empirical animal toxicology where typical exposure concentrations are often well above those encountered in the ambient world in an effort to establish clear and consistent responses. However, in the case of ozone, for example, it has been found that certain cytokine responses, such as IL-1 and TNFα, induced by high concentrations (>1 ppm) of ozone, cannot be detected at lower exposure levels. These proinflammatory cytokines are highly expressed in silica-treated animals and in humans with acute respiratory distress who exhibit marked edematous inflammation, and both are thought to have important roles in remodeling of the lung and fibrosis. Hence, some investigators logically contend a similar scenario results from an ozone exposure. However, long-term inhalation studies find only minor end-airway remodeling even above ambient ozone levels, and the above cytokines are not found in humans acutely exposed to ozone. On the other hand, techniques may simply be lacking in appropriate sensitivity and thus be incapable of detecting cytokines which are secreted and act very locally. When there is an apparent divergence of data from animal studies and those gathered in humans, some argue that the animal data may be misleading. However, differences may simply be a dose-related. For example, other cytokines like IL-6 and IL-8 analogs are in fact found at the lower exposure levels in both species and are believed to play modulatory roles in inflammation. Hence, extrapolation from animal species to the human will always be complex as dose–response relationships often exhibit species dependency. Specific issues involved in the extrapolation of animal data to humans are discussed in more detail later.

Acute lung injury in experimental laboratory animals was once entirely defined in terms of observable pathology (e.g., cellular desquamation, granulocyte accumulation in the alveolar lumen, eosinophilic staining in the alveolar space indicative of edema proteins, or other gross analogs such as lung wet to dry weight or hemorrhage). The need for more sensitive markers of injury that might be more closely tied to the mode of action of toxicants acting directly on the lung has pressured toxicologists to develop alternative assessment approaches. Although first used in the 1930s as a therapy, it was later reasoned that sterile saline infused directly into the lungs via the airways could largely be retrieved (~60–80%), and that repeated infusions of the same or multiple aliquots of saline could yield a representative sampling of cells and lipoproteinaceous molecules from the alveolar and airway surface for analysis. This procedure, termed bronchoalveolar lavage (BAL), has been used diagnostically and even therapeutically in humans (89), generally localizing the procedure to a small portion or lobe of the lung to preserve adequate gas-exchange for the subject. The method gained interest by pulmonary toxicologists as a tool that paralleled its human application and one that enhanced assessment sensitivity. In small laboratory rodents, the procedure is usually conducted at study termination and most often involves lavage of the entire lung (90), although some investigators have refined the procedure to limit the lavage to one lobe, preserving other lobes for either pathology or cell/molecular methods.

BAL methodology is now used widely as a relatively sensitive tool to obtain quantifiable evidence of acute lung injury and inflammation in inhalation studies. Its use with more chronic conditions is more selective (being applied more to mechanistic questions than disease pathogenesis) since studies with BAL have shown that under repeated exposure scenarios, many indices of injury and inflammation wane as lung lesions evolve (32,90) (see below). Although BAL fluid assays are often limited to quantifying total extracted cells, ratios of the cell subpopulations (often using the PMN as the hallmark of inflammation) and markers of alveolar–capillary leak (albumin or total protein—markers of plasma infiltration) and cell damage/death (lactate dehydrogenase, LDH), there are in fact many biochemical markers that can be measured to help characterize the nature of the toxic action (91). Table 1 lists several common cellular and biochemical indicators that have been measured in BAL to address lung injury from inhaled toxicants. While many other more focused markers are useful in dissecting the mode of action of a toxicant, the use of BAL and the straightforward assays of inflammatory cell profiles and BAL fluid protein have been proposed by the EPA in new inhalation guidelines to assess hazardous air pollutants as complementary and sensitive indicators to pathological assessments (92).

Table 1 Selected Generic BALF Markers of Lung Injury and Inflammation[a]

BALF indicator	Interpretation
Cell differentials	Total cells (subgroups by number or %)
Macrophages	Nonspecific exposure marker
Neutrophils (PMN)	Classic inflammation, injury marker
Lymphocytes or eosinophils	Immune or allergy markers
Sloughed cells	Detached cells—airway cell damage/death
Total protein	General injury marker; plasma/airway proteins
Albumin	Plasma "leak"—deep lung injury
LDH (lactate dehydrogenase)	Indicator of cell damage; plasma leak
NAG (*N*-acetylglucosaminidase)	Indicator of macrophage activation

[a]Other indicators (e.g., antioxidants, mucins, cytokines, eicosanoids, etc.) can also be measured (90,91,122).

B. Chronic Lung Injury/Disease

The impact of any single exposure to a toxicant may be reversible or irreversible. In most cases (barring inhalants that may be carcinogenic), reversibility is highly dependent on concentration (i.e., dose) or degree of injury. It stands to reason that the greater the injury, the less likely there will be complete repair. The lung is well equipped to handle most challenges from the outside ambient environment. It has a complex array of host defense capabilities: autonomic ventilatory reflexes to minimize dose, nonspecific clearance mechanisms of particulate material, antimicrobial immune-agents and cells, tissue and lung lining antioxidants, and relatively robust epithelial repair processes. However, when exposure to a toxicant is repeated, these defenses may be impaired or overwhelmed. Indeed, sometimes these processes can even "unwittingly" mediate long-term destruction or disease (e.g., macrophage-mediated silica toxicity). When the airway or lung surface epithelium is damaged with resultant cell death, progenitor cells differentiate to replace these dead or sloughed cells. Generally, this turnover is faster than normal cell turnover kinetics and is frequently driven by various chemokine stimuli from mediators such as TNFα, TGFβ, or other growth factors (93). Conceptually, this constant bathing of the epithelium and underlying matrix by growth-promoting agents sets the stage for cell proliferation beyond normal replacement of dead or dying cells. These cells may have altered morphology and biochemistry (e.g., heightened antioxidant metabolism) to compensate for the repeated challenge. In fact, with continued stimuli, interstitial fibroblasts may be prompted to synthesize and secrete more collagenous material, analogous to scarring, as part of the repair or strengthening of the lung or airway matrix. The end result may be thickened epithelium and interstitial fibrosis, which depending on its extent may have functional implications. This pattern of response has been seen with chronic ozone exposure where end-airway squamous epithelium is replaced by more cuboidal cells and end-airway fibrosis, with impairment of small airway function (12). When the challenge is removed, there typically is some reversal of the effect, but the completeness of the process is uncertain. In some cases, the lesions may even be progressive when the challenge is removed (e.g., MIC, $O_3 + NO_2$) (94,95).

It is frequently difficult to predict the outcome of long-term repeated exposures in experimental settings. The actual exposure scenario itself can often dictate the biological outcome. If exposure is continuous (24 hr/day and 7 days/week) vs. daily repeated (4–12 hr/day and 5–7 days/week), one can quickly determine that the extent of injury is not simply a product of $C \times T$ (concentration × time). Lack of "recovery" time between exposures has repair implications and may also have impacts on behavior of the study animals (e.g., suppressed food consumption under continuous exposure conditions), which may have implications on overall health as well as repair capabilities (96). The conventional thinking (in keeping with the traditional concept of dose–response) is that more exposure should yield more severe effects. Indeed, this is in part the basis of the chronic inhalation exposure guidelines of 6 hr/day, 5 days/week, for 24 months. However, several studies have shown that exposures that are intermittent may be more likely to have long-term implications than continual repeated exposures. For many toxic inhalants, especially the oxidant and irritant gases, even a single exposure may impart a condition of protection (adaptation or acclimatization) such that subsequent exposures have less acute effect. If exposure is curtailed for a period of time (usually a few weeks), the susceptibility returns (down-regulation of antioxidant metabolism has been suggested in some cases or loss of resistant cell proliferation), such that another exposure induces acute injury with its cascade of destructive or tissue-stimulating mediators. In the case of ozone, periodic and intermittent exposures have been shown to be more fibroproliferative in rodents and even in monkeys (97,98). The message then may be that more exposure (in terms of time or frequency of repetition) is not always better for evoking effects or studying mechanisms of chronic disease. Periodic or episodic exposures induce repeated acute responses that may sculpt the ultimate lesion. In fact, as one tries to address human health questions, one finds that the human exposure scenario is intermittent, periodic, or episodic, and perhaps it is appropriate that experimental exposure models should attempt to address these more relevant exposure attributes.

C. Extrapolation of Animal Data to the Human Situation

Perhaps the most important, yet least appreciated challenge of inhalation toxicology is the translation of the data obtained from animals to a form that can address specific questions related to human health. Extrapolation is the process of relating such empirical study findings in experimental animals to real-world human scenarios and outcomes. The value of any study conducted in an animal model is enhanced when it has been conducted in a manner consistent with extrapolation concepts. The alternative limits the data to qualitative comparisons and speculation. Achieving fully quantitative extrapolation, while a laudable goal, is rarely easy. Pitfalls lie in the selection of the test species, dosimetry, and the exposure scenario. The development of new sophisticated molecular assays and refined biologic as well as dosimetry models have brought about new thinking and improvements in study design. The first consideration is that of the animal model—even if limited to rodent species. The selection of a species or strain as a toxicological model should involve more than a consideration of cost and convenience. Whenever possible, effects that are homologous (i.e., same end points or mode of action) between the study species and the human should guide selection of the test species or how differences can be accounted for in analysis. For example, if responses to an upper airway irritant (e.g., SO_2 or formaldehyde) are of interest, the guinea pig with its labile and reactive bronchoconstrictive reflex should be selected over the rat, which is not particularly responsive to sensory irritants. By contrast, certain strains of rats (Wistar and Sprague–Dawley) exhibit a clear neutrophilic response to deep lung irritants such as O_3 that resembles the human response, while others do not (F-344) (43). Other innate differences in sensitivity among species may relate to differences in lung structure, specific regionally based cell metabolism or polymorphisms, or overall defenses (e.g., antioxidants) (99,100). When such nuances are unclear or unknown, the replication of responses in multiple species builds confidence in the finding as being the product of conserved mechanisms across species, and therefore strengthens its relevance to the human.

An essential part of extrapolating responses from species to species is the relative dosimetry of the pollutant along the respiratory tract. Significant advances in studies of the distribution of gaseous and particulate pollutants have been made through the use of empirical and mathematical models, the latter of which incorporate parameters of respiratory anatomy and physiology, aerodynamics, and physical chemistry into predictions of deposition and retention. Empirical models combined with theoretical models aid in relating animal toxicity data to humans and help refine the study of injury mechanisms with better estimates of target dose. Figure 9 illustrates the application of such an approach to the reactive gas ozone

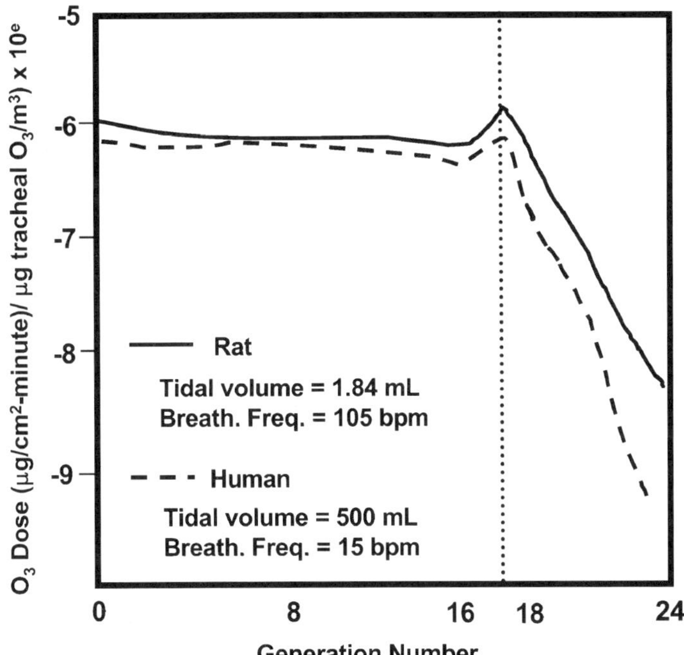

Figure 9 Theoretical uptake curves for ozone in a resting human and a rat. The calculated curves are normalized to the concentration of ozone in inspired air. Airway generation refers to airway branch numbered from the trachea = 0. (From Ref. 101.)

in the human and the rat (101) analogous to that represented for particles in Fig. 6. Anatomic differences between the species clearly affect the deposition of both gases and particles, but the qualitative and to a large extent quantitative similarities in deposition profiles are noteworthy. This is not surprising if one argues teleologically that the lungs of each species evolved with similar functional demands (i.e., O_2–CO_2 exchange, blood acid/base balance), mechanical impediments, and environmental stresses. One needs only a cursory review of the comparative lung physiology literature to appreciate the allometric consistency of the mammalian respiratory tract to meet the challenge of breathing air. This design coherency has provided the essential rationale for the use of animal models for the study of air pollutants.

Susceptible subpopulations that may show exaggerated responsiveness to a pollutant deserve special mention. The existence of hyper-responsive individuals and groups is well accepted among those who study toxic inhalants, although little is actually known about the host traits that make certain individuals more responsive than others. This appreciation for sensitive populations is embedded in testing guidelines and risk paradigms where use of the most sensitive species in the testing process is mandated and mathematical adjustments (safety factors) are included in standard setting. Perhaps best known is the specific mandate in the Clean Air Act where reasonable protection of susceptible groups is forefront in the promulgation of National Ambient Air Quality Standards. There have always been certain definable subgroups that are assumed to be susceptible, including children, the elderly, and those with a pre-existing disease (e.g., asthma, cardiovascular disease, lung disease). In some cases, susceptibility may reside in some innate (genetic) or acquired condition (inflammation), while in other cases it may relate more to the loss of functional reserve or ability to compensate—perhaps altering a response threshold. The lack of detailed data defining susceptible groups for potentially toxic inhalants likely lies in the difficulty in ethically conducting studies in humans who may be at higher risk and recruiting such individuals on a volunteer basis. However, inroads into this issue have been made in recent years, in part because more precise definitions of potential risk factors allow researchers to design studies to examine host attributes at less severe stages of impairment, and also because of the development of more appropriate animal models of disease or dysfunction. Hence, studies in both animals and human subjects are being devised specifically to investigate the roles of diet (e.g., antioxidant content), exercise (as it relates to dosimetry), age, gender, and genetics (e.g., that may relate to a definable genotype, species, or in humans, race). In addition, studies in human subjects with mild asthma or heart–lung disease have been conducted to address the degree of sensitivity these compromised groups exhibit. Analogously, animal models with imposed cardiopulmonary impairments are being used more and more to address the same basic questions (102).

Recent advances in molecular biology can provide tools to bioengineer mice (and occasionally rats) with virtually any trait that is under the control of identifiable genes (Chapter 11). Transgenic and knockout models thereby can express desired traits derived from other animals or even humans, or they can be made devoid of specific traits to isolate the specific impact of that trait on the animal's responsivity to a toxic challenge. These animal models add to the natural mutants that have been inbred historically to purify a desired genotype expressing a specific phenotype, ideally one that is analogous to that of the human (103,104). Natural mutant and bioengineered transgenic and knockout rodent models provide unparalleled potential to examine specific genetic susceptibility factors involved in response. Current technology can also target genes for specific expression in the lung (e.g., linked to a specific cell such as the Clara cell or to a cell product—surfactant protein C [SP-C]). In some cases (conditional trangenics), the model can be established with a control gene that an investigator can use to toggle the gene of interest on or off using a pharmacological or chemical pre/postchallenge. This allows the dissection of underlying mechanisms under very controlled scenarios that avoid the problems of having a gene inappropriately active or inactive through all life-stages.

A major emphasis of studies using genetically modified mouse models has been on mechanisms associated with disease pathogenesis (105,106). Among the most popular use of knockout and transgenic mice in lung studies has been to examine inflammatory cytokines and associated products in asthma, as many of these mediators are under the control of individual genes (e.g.,107,108). Clearly, genetically modified mice are ideally suited for the study of mechanisms where a specific mediator-based hypothesis can be tested as it relates to an impaired function, pathology, or altered inflammatory pattern. When such models are derived to exhibit a desired pathology or disease due to a genetic defect—for example, defects of lung structure or growth, which result by adulthood in diseases like emphysema or fibrosis—they may serve as a surrogate of the human condition (109).

The use of genetically modified animal models in inhalation toxicology has lagged behind that of basic science and toxicology in general. The reasons for this are unclear and may relate to the difficulties in conducting these studies and in incorporating such data into conventional risk assessment paradigms. However, with recent interest in potentially susceptible groups, there has been a definitive upswing in the use of pharmacologically or naturally altered as well as bioengineered animals (102) and the desire to more closely link mechanistic profiles to basic human biology. Ozone has frequently been the test pollutant in these new studies since more is known about O_3 and its effects in humans than any other air pollutant. Frequently, these studies address aspects of inflammation and antioxidant capacity relative to challenge by O_3 or other oxidants (110,111), but with the current interest in particulate matter (PM) health effects, these and other models are being redirected; for example, strain differences and acid coated PM (112); hypertranferrinemic mice and metal-rich PM (113); and metallothionein-null mice and mercury vapor (114).

D. Ozone as a Prototype Toxic Inhalant

Ozone is the prominent oxidant in photochemical smog, due to its inherent bioreactivity and the fact that current urban ambient concentrations elicit overt pulmonary effects in humans and animal models (115). These effects include functional, biochemical, immunological, and even morphological alterations (reviewed in 116). Because of its low water solubility, a substantial portion of inhaled ozone penetrates deep into the lung, but its reactivity is such that about 17% and 40% are scrubbed by the nasopharynx of resting rats and humans, respectively (61,62). It is unclear why scrubbing is higher in humans than rodents, but these findings are reproducible. Interestingly, mouth scrubbing does not differ from nasal scrubbing. Nevertheless, regardless of species, the region of the lung that is predicted to have the greatest O_3 deposition (dose per surface area) is the acinar region from the terminal bronchioles to the opening of the alveolar ducts, sometimes referred to as the proximal alveolar region (52). Because O_3 penetration increases with increased tidal volume and flow rate, exercise increases the dose to the target area. Using $^{18}O_3$ (a nonradioactive isotope of oxygen), Hatch et al. (117) have correlated the dose to the distal lung with the degree of damage to the lung (as determined by BAL protein) from humans who exercised (intermittent 15 min periods for 2 hr) while exposed to 0.4 ppm. The response in humans after exposure at $3\times$ resting ventilation was similar to that in resting rats exposed for the same length of time to 2.0 ppm. It should be clear that exercise is an important factor with O_3, and likely is with any inhalant, and thus needs to be considered before making cross-species or study comparisons.

Animal studies indicate that the acute morphological response to O_3 involves epithelial cell injury along the respiratory tract. The pattern of injury parallels the dosimetry profile with the majority of damage occurring in the deep lung as indicated above. Ciliated cells along the larger airways also appear to be sensitive to O_3, while Clara cells and mucus-secreting cells are the least sensitive. Studies in the rat nose indicate that O_3 also is an effective mucus secretagogue. In the distal lung, the Type 1 epithelium is very sensitive to O_3, in contrast to the Type 2 cell, which serves as its progenitor. The Type 2 cell is more active metabolically and has a high antioxidant profile. Ultrastructural damage can be observed in rats after a few hours at 0.2 ppm, but sloughing of cells generally requires concentrations above 0.8 ppm. Reversal of injury occurs within a couple days with no apparent residual pathology. When a bronchoscope is used to examine the human bronchus after O_3 exposure, the airways appear "sunburned," which reverses readily as does the damage in rodents. What is uncertain is the impact of repeated "sunburning" of the airways.

The mechanisms by which O_3 causes cellular injury have been studied using cellular as well as cell-free systems. As a powerful oxidant, O_3 will extract electrons from any accessible macromolecule. The surface fluid lining the respiratory tract and cell membranes that underlie the lining fluid contain a significant quantity of mono- and polyunsaturated fatty acids (PUFA) either free or as part of the lipoprotein structures of the cell membrane. The carbon double bonds within fatty acids have a labile, unpaired electron that is easily attacked by O_3 to form an ozonide. Ozonides progress through less stable zwitterions or trioxolane (depending on the presence of water) that recombine or decompose primarily to lipohydroperoxides, aldehydes, and hydrogen peroxide. These events are thought to initiate the propagation of lipid-radicals that attack other cell membranes and free macromolecules.

Evidence of free radical-related damage in vivo includes mea surements of breath pentane and ethane and tissue measurements of diene-conjugates. The resultant oxidation of bioactive membrane constituents (e.g., arachidonate) and cellular debris is believed to promote inflammation. Associated cytokines (e.g., IL-6/8 and others) are transiently released from epithelial cells and free macrophages to mediate early responses and initiate repair. Koren et al. (118) have reported that humans exhibit an eight-fold increase in PMNs and two-fold increase in protein in BAL fluid 18-h after a 2-h exposure to 0.4 ppm ozone with exercise. Inflammation markers did not correlate well with functional impairment among the individuals tested. Arachidonate metabolism products, including the prostaglandins PGE_2 and $PGF_{2\alpha}$ and thromboxane B_2, have also been seen to increase in human BAL fluid after 0.4 ppm ozone for 2-h (119). Interestingly, pretreatment with the anti-inflammatory agents indomethecin and ibuprofen (cyclooxygenase inhibitors) decreased the pulmonary function deficit and PGE_2, but not other indicators of cell injury and vascular leak. Sensitivity to O_3 appears to have a genetic element as studies in inbred stains of mice have shown that O_3-induced pulmonary neutrophilia and permeability are governed by a single gene linked to the Toll4 locus (endotoxin sensitivity) (111). Similarly, studies with rats have linked O_3 sensitivity (as well as acrolein and chlorine) to salt-induced hypertension (120,121). It is expected that advances in genetic mapping and molecular biology will yield significant information on the nature of O_3 susceptibility in humans as they have in test animals. When animal data on O_3 sensitivity are combined with information on exposure and dosimetry, it is found that interspecies comparisons can indeed be made and interpreted in a meaningful manner. The integration of human, animal, and model data with this prototypic toxicant sets a paradigm that can be used for other inhaled toxicants that may not be amenable to comprehensive or direct study in humans.

VIII. Summary

Inhalation toxicology is unique among the toxicological sciences in its blend of a broad base of basic and applied sciences from mechanical and aerodynamic engineering to the most detailed molecular biology. This discipline naturally focuses on the respiratory tract as a complex structural target with substantial cellular diversity, but of necessity includes the inherant role of the lungs as a portal to the body. Ambient air contains predominately N_2 and O_2 and a trace of CO_2, along with water vapor. The mammalian lungs evolved to maximize the efficacy of O_2/CO_2 exchange between these inspired gases and pulmonary capillary blood. Allometric studies of the mammalian lungs show clearly that this organ system is designed around principles of matching gas-exchange with oxidative need while minimizing associated respiratory work (16). Pulmonary cell types and their functions are analogous across mammalian species, and despite differences in distribution and population density to meet unique needs, their collective function is to ensure respiratory homeostasis. This consistency of design and biology secures the basic relevancy of using small laboratory animal models in studying the mechanisms and pathophysiology of human lung injury and disease related to toxic inhalants.

An overriding factor in inhalation toxicology emphasized in this chapter is how study design, exposure levels, and animal models affect the relevancy of interpretations for human disease. This is not to negate the importance and impact of the wide range of toxicological studies that have been performed with high-level inhalant exposures over the last four decades. Inhalation toxicology studies of this kind serve as valuable screening or predictive evaluations of potential toxicity, and in this setting, high concentrations of a particular inhalant may be necessary to reveal end points as dramatic as death. Such studies not only help address issues of safety or accidental high dose exposures, but also can be used to generate hypotheses for further research on the mechanistic basis of the observed responses. At the same time, it is crucial to remember that a basic objective of the discipline of inhalation toxicology is to acquire information from known linkages and tenets of lung biology and clinical medicine that relate to human health and disease.

Recent advances in inhalation toxicology and cell and molecular biology enhance the potential to assess toxic effects homologous to those in humans, and open the door to more accurate evaluations of human exposure and health risks. Novel methods utilizing small samples are now frequently able to relate responses at the molecular level to improve understanding of the generic toxicology of an inhalant. Also, the sensitivity of available inhalation toxicology methods has increased, allowing low ambient-like exposure scenarios to be used in animal studies and relevant exposure–dose relationships to be derived. The ability of such relationships to define potential long-term health effects hinge on better theoretical deposition and clearance models that allow accurate interpolations between animal species at the physical and chemical level. The collective merging of methodological advances in inhalation toxicology described in this chapter strengthens mechanistic interpretations involving the underlying biology and physiology, and enhances relevance for human disease. Animal and cell models in inhalation toxicology necessarily overlap conceptually with those used in studying other forms of inflammatory lung injury (e.g., cell, animal, and transgenic models in Chapters 10 and 11). Remaining chapters in this book detail a variety of therapeutic interventions for acute and chronic lung injury derived from mechanistic understanding gained in basic research in animal, cell, and inhalation models.

Acknowledgments

The research and information described in this article have been reviewed by the National Health and Environmental Effects Research Laboratory, U.S. Environmental Protection Agency, and approved for publication. Approval does not signify that the contents necessarily reflect the views and the policies of the Agency nor does mention of trade names or commercial products constitute endorsement or recommendation for use.

References

1. West JA, Pakehham G, Morin D, Fleschner CA, Buckpitt AR, Plopper CG. Inhaled naphthalene causes dose-dependent Clara cell cytotoxicity in mice but not in rats. Toxicol Appl Pharmacol 2001; 173(2):114–119.

2. Gehr P, Mwangi DK, Ammann A, Maloiy GM, Taylor CR, Weibel ER. Design of the mammalian respiratory system. V. Scaling morphometric pulmonary diffusing capacity to body mass: wild and domestic mammals. Respir Physiol 1981; 44(1):61–86.

3. Weibel ER. Scaling of structural and functional variables in the respiratory system. Ann Rev Physiol 1987; 49:147–59.

4. Harkema JR. Epithelial cells of the nasal passages. Chapter 3. In: Parent RA, ed. Comparative Biology of the Normal Lung. Boca Raton: CRC Press, 1991:27–36.

5. Jaskot RH, Costa DL. Toxicity of an anthraquinone violet dye mixture following inhalation exposure, intratracheal instillation, or gavage. Funda Appl Toxicol 1994; 22(1):103–112.

6. Hatch GE. Comparative biochemistry of airway lining fluid. Chapter 33. In: Parent RA, ed. Comparative Biology of the Normal Lung. Boca Raton: CRC Press, 1991:617–632.

7. Jarabek AM, Segal SA. Noncancer toxicity of inhaled toxic air pollutants: available approaches for risk assessment and risk management. In: Patrick DR, ed. Toxic Air Pollution Handbook. New York: Van Nostrand Reinhold, 1994:100–132.

8. McBride JT. Architecture of the tracheobronchial tree. Chapter 5. In: Parent RA, ed. Comparative Biology of the Normal Lung. Boca Raton: CRC Press, 1991:49–61.

9. Mariassy AT. Epithelial cells of trachea and bronchi. Chapter 6. In: Parent RA, ed. Comparative Biology of the Normal Lung. Boca Raton: CRC Press, 1991:63–76.

10. Plopper CG, Hyde DM. Epithelial cells in bronchioles. Chapter 8. In: Parent RA, ed. Comparative Biology of the Normal Lung. Boca Raton: CRC Press, 1991:85–92.

11. Mercer RR, Crapo JD. Architecture of the acinus. Chapter 10. In: Parent RA, ed. Comparative Biology of the Normal Lung. Boca Raton: CRC Press, 1991:109–120.

12. Chang L, Huang Y, Stockstill BL, Graham JA, Grose EC, Menache MG, Miller FJ, Costa DL, Crapo JD. Epithelial injury and interstitial fibrosis in the proximal alveolar regions of rats chronically exposed to a simulated pattern of urban ambient ozone. Toxicol Appl Pharmacol 1992; 115:241–252.

13. Costa DL, Tepper JS, Stevens MA, Watkinson WP, Doerfler DL, Gelzleichter TR, Last JA. Restrictive lung disease in rats chronically exposed to an urban profile of ozone. Am J Resp Crit Care Med 1995; 151:1512–1518.

14. Valberg PA, Blanchard JD. Pulmonary macrophage physiology, origin, motility, endocytosis. Chapter 36. In: Parent RA, ed. Comparative Biology of the Normal Lung. Boca Raton: CRC Press, 1991:681–724.

15. Weibel ER. Scaling of functional and structural variables in the respiratory system. Ann Rev Physiol 1987; 49:147–159.

16. Costa DL, Tepper JS, Raub JA. Interpretations and limitations of pulmonary function testing in small laboratory animals. In: Parent RA, ed. Comparative Biology of the Normal Lung. Boca Raton: CRC Press, 1991:367–399.

17. Macklem PT, Permutt S, eds. The Lung in Transition Between Health and Disease. New York: Marcel Dekker, 1979:389–398.

18. West JB. Respiration Physiology—The Essentials. Baltimore: Williams & Wilkins, 1979:86–113.

19. Fishman AP, ed. Fishman's Pulmonary Diseases and Disorders 3rd ed. New York: McGraw-Hill, 1998.

20. American Thoracic Society. Lung function testing: selection of reference values and interpretative strategies. Amer Lung Assoc 1991; (http://www.thoracic.org/adobe/statements/lftvalue1-17.pdf).

21. Costa DL, Tepper JS. Approaches to lung function assessment in small mammals. In: Gardner DE, Crapo JD, Massaro EJ, eds. Toxicology of the Lung. 1988:147–174.

22. Mauderly JL. Ventilation, lung volumes, and lung mechanics of young adult and old Syrian hamsters. Exper Aging Res 1979; 5(6):497–508.

23. Lambert AL, Winsett DW, Costa DL, Selgrade MK, Gilmour MI. Transfer of allergic airway responses with serum and lymphocytes from rats sensitized to dust mite. Am J Respir Crit Care Med 1998; 157(6 Pt 1):1991–1999.

24. Crapo JD, Crapo RO. Comparison of total lung diffusion capacity and the membrane component of diffusion capacity as determined by physiologic and morphometric techniques. Respir Physiol 1983; 51(2):183–194.

25. Morrow PE, Mermelstein R. Chronic inhalation toxicity studies. In: Mohr U, ed. Inhalation Toxicology: The Design and Interpretation of Inhalation Studies and Their Use in Risk Assessment. ILSI Monograph. New York: Springer-Verlag, 1988:103–118.

26. Phalen RF. Regulations and Guidelines. In: Phalen RF, ed. Inhalation Studies: Foundations and Techniques. Boca Raton: CRC Press, 1984:243–256.

27. Kennedy GL, Valentine R. Inhalation toxicology. In: Hayes AW, ed. Principles and Methods of Toxicology. 3rd ed. New York: Raven Press, 1994: 805–838.

28. U.S. Environmental Protection Agency. Air Quality Criteria for Ozone and Related Photochemical Oxidants. Washington DC: Office of Research and Development, 1996; EPA-600/P-93/004bF.

29. Watkinson WP, Campen MJ, Nolan JP, Costa DL. Cardiovascular and systemic responses to inhaled pollutants in rodents: effects of ozone and particulate matter [Review]. Environ Health Perspect 2001; 109(suppl 4):539–546.

30. Tyler WS, Tyler NK, Last JA, Barstow TJ, Magliano DJ, Hinds DM. Effects of ozone on lung and somatic growth. Pair fed rats after ozone exposure and recovery periods. Toxicology 1987; 46(1):1–20.

31. Folinsbee LJ, Hazuca MJ. Time course of response to ozone exposure in healthy adult females. Inhal Toxicol 2000; 12(3):151–167.

32. Devlin RB, McDonnell WF, Mann R, Becker S, House DE, Schreinemachers D, Koren HS. Exposure of humans to ambient levels of ozone for 6.6 hours causes cellular and biochemical changes in the lung. Am J Respir Cell Mol Biol 1991; 4(1):72–81.

33. Koren HS, Devlin RB. Human upper respiratory tract responses to inhaled pollutants with emphasis on nasal lavage. Ann NY Acad Sci 1992; 641:215–224.

34. Bucchieri F, Puddicombe SM, Lordan JL, Richter A, Buchanan D, Wilson SJ, Ward J, Zummo G, Howarth PH, Djukanovi R, Holgate ST, Davies DE. Asthmatic bronchial epithelium is more susceptible to oxidant-induced apoptosis. Am J Respir Cell Mol Biol 2002; 27(2):179–185.

35. Folinsbee LJ. Does nitrogen dioxide exposure increase airways responsiveness? Toxicol Ind Health 1992; 8(5):273–283.

36. Sheps DS, Herbst MC, Hinderliter AL, Adams KF, Ekelund LG, O'Neil JJ, Goldstein GM, Bromberg PA, Dalton JL, Ballenger MN. Production of arrhythmias by elevated carboxyhemoglobin in patients with coronary artery disease. Ann Intern Med 1990; 113(5):343–351.

37. Phalen R. Methods in Inhalation Toxicology. Boca Raton: CRC Press, 1996.

38. Drew RT. Inhalation toxicology—a status report. Appl Indust Hyg 1987; 2:213–217.

39. Gardner DE, Kennedy GL. Methodologies and technology for animal inhalation toxicology studies. In: Garner DE, Crapo JD, McClellan RO, eds. Toxicology of the Lung. 2nd ed. New York: Raven Press, 1993:1–30.

40. Ledbetter AD, Killough PM, Hudson GF. A low-sample-consumption dry-particulate aerosol generator for use in nose-only inhalation exposures. Inhal Toxicol 1998; 10:239–251.

41. Hollander W. Exposure facilities and aerosol generation and characterization for inhalation experiments. In: Mohr U, ed. Inhalation Toxicology: The Design and Interpretation of Inhalation Studies and Their Use in Risk Assessment. ILSI Monograph. New York: Springer-Verlag, 1988:67–86.

42. Postlethwait EM, Joad JP, Hyde DM, Schelegle ES, Bric JM, Weir AJ, Putney LF, Wong VJ, Velsor LW, Plopper CG. Three-dimensional mapping of ozone-induced acute cytotoxicity in tracheobronchial airways of isolated perfused rat lung. Am J Respir Cell Mol Biol 2000; 22(2):191–199.

43. Dye JA, Madden MC, Richards JH, Lehmann JR, Devlin RB, Costa DL. Ozone effects on airway responsiveness, lung injury, and inflammation. Comparative rat strain and in vivo/in vitro investigations. Inhal Toxicol 1999; 11(11):1015–1040.

44. Rasmussen RE. In vitro systems for exposure of lung cells to NO_2 and O_3. J Toxicol Environ Health 1984; 13(2–3):397–411.

45. Ritter D, Knebel JW, Aufderheide M. In vitro exposure of isolated cells to native gaseous compounds—development and validation of an optimized system for human lung cells. Exp Toxicol Pathol 2001; 53(5):373–386.
46. Devlin RB, McKinnon KP, Noah T, Becker S, Koren HS. Ozone-induced release of cytokines and fibronectin by alveolar macrophages and airway epithelial cells. Am J Physiol 1994; 266(6 Pt 1):L612–L619.
47. Knebel JW, Ritter D, Hoffmann K, Lödding H, Windt H, Koch W, Aufderheide M. Development and validation of a semiautomatic system for generation and deposition of sprays on isolated cells of the respiratory tract. Toxicol Methods 2001; 11:161–171.
48. Witschi H. Some notes on the history of Haber's law. Toxicol Sci 1999; 50(2):164–168.
49. Evans MV, Boyes WK, Simmons JE, Litton DK, Easterling MR. A comparison of Haber's rule at different ages using a physiologically based pharmacokinetic (PBPK) model for chloroform in rats. Toxicology 2002; 176(1–2): 11–23.
50. Highfill J, Costa DL. Statistical response models for ozone exposure: their generality when applied to human spirometric and animal permeability functions of the lung. J Air Waste Manag Assoc 1995; 45(2):95–102.
51. Gelzleichter TR, Witschi H, Last JA. Concentration–response relationships of rat lungs to exposure to oxidant air pollutants: a critical test of Haber's Law for ozone and nitrogen dioxide. Toxicol Appl Pharmacol 1992; 112(1):73–80.
52. Overton JH, Graham RC. Simulation of the uptake of a reactive gas in a rat respiratory tract model with an asymmetric tracheobronchial region patterned on complete conducting airway cast data. Comput Biomed Res 1995; 28(3):171–190.
53. Stott WT, McKenna MJ. The comparative absorption and excretion of chemical vapors by the upper, lower, and intact respiratory tract of rats. Funda Appl Toxicol 1984; 4(4):594–602.
54. Yokoyama E, Frank NR. Respiratory uptake of ozone in dogs. Arch Environ Health 1972; 25:132–138.
55. Brain JD. The uptake of inhaled gases by the nose. Ann Otol Rhinol Laryngol 1970; 79(3):529–539.
56. Morris JB. Overview of upper respiratory tract vapor uptake studies. Inhal Toxicol 2001; 13(5):335–345.
57. Bogdanffy MS, Morgan PH, Starr TB, Morgan KT. Binding of formaldehyde to human and rat nasal mucus and bovine serum. Toxicol Lett 1987; 38(1–2):145–154.
58. Morris JB, Smith FA. Regional deposition and absorption of inhaled hydrogen fluoride in the rat. Toxicol Appl Pharmacol 1982; 62(1):81–89.
59. Overton JH, Kimbell JS, Miller FJ. Dosimetry modeling of inhaled formaldehyde: the human respiratory tract. Toxicol Sci 2001; 64(1):122–134.
60. Amdur MO. 1974 Cummings memorial lecture: the long road from Donora. Am Ind Hyg Assoc J 1974; 35:589–597.

61. Gerrity TR, Weaver RA, Bernsten J, House DE, O'Neil JJ. Extrathoracic and intrathoracic removal of ozone in tidal breathing humans. J Appl Physiol 1988; 65:393–400.

62. Hatch GE, Slade R, Harris LP, McDonnell WF, Devlin RB, Koren HS, Costa DL, McKee J. Ozone dose and effect in humans and rats: a comparison using oxygen-18 labeling and bronchoalveolar lavage. Am J Respir Crit Care Med 1994; 150:676–683.

63. Foster WM. Deposition and clearance of inhaled particles. Chapter 14. In: Samet Air Pollution and Health. 1999:295–324.

64. Kim CS. Methods of calculating lung delivery and deposition of aerosol particles. Respir Care 2000; 45(6):695–711.

65. Morrow PE, Bates DV, Fish BR, Hatch TF, Mercer TT. Deposition and retention models for internal dosimetry of the human respiratory tract (Report of the International Commission on Radiological Protection (ICRP) Task Group on Lung Dynamics). Health Physics 1964; 12:173–207.

66. Asgharian B, Miller FJ, Subramaniam RP. Dosimetry software to predict deposition in humans and rats. CIIT Activities 1999; 19(3):1–12 March (http://libpc.ciit.org//Activities/1999/V19N3.pdf).

67. Martonen TB, Katz I. Deposition patterns of polydisperse aerosols within human lungs. J Aerosol Med 1993; 6:251–264.

68. Brenneman KA, Wong BA, Buccellato MA, Costa ER, Gross EA, Dorman DC. Direct olfactory transport of inhaled manganese (^{54}MnCl$_2$) to the rat brain: toxicokinetic investigations in a unilateral nasal occlusion model. Toxicol Appl Pharmacol 2000; 169(3):238–248.

69. Van As A. Pulmonary airway clearance mechanisms: a reappraisal. Am Rev Respir Dis 1977; 115(5):721–726.

70. Gehr P, Green FH, Geiser M, Im Hof V, Lee MM, Schurch S. Airway surfactant, a primary defense barrier: mechanical and immunological aspects. J Aerosol Med 1996; 9(2):163–181.

71. Yuen IS, Hartsky MA, Snajdr SI, Warheit DB. Time course of chemotactic factor generation and neutrophil recruitment in the lungs of dust-exposed rats. Am J Respir Cell Mol Biol 1996; 15(2):268–274.

72. Nikula KJ, Avila KJ, Griffith WC, Mauderly JL. Sites of particle retention and lung tissue responses to chronically inhaled diesel exhaust and coal dust in rats and cynomolgus monkeys. Environ Health Perspect 1997; 105(suppl 5):1231–1234.

73. Nemmar A, Hoet PH, Vanquickenborne B, Dinsdale D, Thomeer M, Hoylaerts MF, Vanbilloen H, Mortelmans L, Nemery B. Passage of inhaled particles into the blood circulation in humans. Circulation 2002; 105(4):411–414.

74. Snipes MB. Long-term retention and clearance of particles inhaled by mammalian species. CRC Critical Rev Toxicol 1989; 20:175–211.

75. Ruckley VA, Gauld SJ, Chapman JS, Davis JM, Douglas AN, Fernie JM, Jacobsen M, Lamb D. Emphysema and dust exposure in a group of coal workers. Am Rev Respir Dis 1984; 129(4):528–532.

76. ILSI Report. The relevance of the rat lung response to particle overload for human risk assessment: a workshop consensus report. ILSI Sponsored Workshop, March, 1998 In: Olin SS, ed. Inhal Toxicol 2000; 12:101–117.

77. ASTM. 'Standard test method for estimating sensory irritancy of airborne chemicals, Designation: E981–84.' 'American Society for Testing and Materials', Philadelphia, 1984.

78. Tepper JS, Costa DL. Will the mouse bioassay for estimating sensory irritancy of airborne chemicals (ASTM E981–84) be useful for evaluation of indoor air chemicals? Indoor Environ 1992; 1:367–372.

79. Schelegle ES, Alfaro MF, Putney L, Stovall M, Tyler N, Hyde DM. Effect of C-fiber-mediated, ozone-induced rapid shallow breathing on airway epithelial injury in rats. J Appl Physiol 2001; 91(4):1611–1618.

80. Dhara VR, Dhara R, Acquilla SD, Cullinan P. Personal exposure and long-term health effects in survivors of the union carbide disaster at Bhopal. Environ Health Perspect 2002; 110(5):487–500.

81. Hatch GE, Kodavanti U, Costa DL, Dreher KL, Slade R. An injury-time integral model for extrapolating from acute to chronic effects of phosgene. Toxicol Indust Health 2002; 17:285–293.

82. van Bree L, Dormans JA, Boere AJ, Rombout PJ. Time study on development and repair of lung injury following ozone exposure in rats. Inhal Toxicol 2001; 13(8):703–718.

83. Ward PA. Role of complement, chemokines, and regulatory cytokines in acute lung injury. Ann NY Acad Sci 1996; 796:104–112.

84. Cheek JM, McDonald RJ, Rapalyea L, Tarkington BK, Hyde DM. Neutrophils enhance removal of ozone-injured alveolar epithelial cells in vitro. Am J Physiol 1995; 269(4 Pt 1):L527–L535.

85. Meng ZH, Dyer K, Billiar TR, Tweardy DJ. Distinct effects of systemic infusion of G-CSF vs. IL-6 on lung and liver inflammation and injury in hemorrhagic shock. Shock 2000; 14(1):41–48.

86. Sheridan BC, Dinarello CA, Meldrum DR, Fullerton DA, Selzman CH, McIntyre RC Jr. Interleukin-11 attenuates pulmonary inflammation and vasomotor dysfunction in endotoxin-induced lung injury. Am J Physiol 1999; 277(5 Pt 1):L861–L867.

87. McKinney WJ, Jaskot RH, Richards JH, Costa DL, Dreher KL. Cytokine mediation of ozone-induced pulmonary adaptation. Am J Respir Cell Mol Biol 1998; 18(5):696–705.

88. Yu M, Zheng X, Witschi H, Pinkerton KE. The role of interleukin-6 in pulmonary inflammation and injury induced by exposure to environmental air pollutants. Toxicol Sci 2002; 68(2):488–497.

89. Ewig S, Torres A. Flexible bronchoscopy in nosocomial pneumonia. Clin Chest Med 2001; 22(2):263–279.

90. Henderson RF, Mauderly JL, Pickrell JA, Hahn FF, Muhle H, Rebar AH. Comparative study of bronchoalveolar lavage fluid: effects of species, age, and method of lavage. Exp Lung Res 1987; 13:329–342.

91. Henderson RF. Use of bronchoalveolar lavage to detect lung damage. In: Gardner DE, Crapo JD, Massaro EJ, eds. Toxicology of the Lung. 1988:239–268.

92. Federal Register Document. August 15, 1997 (Volume 62, Number 158) pp. 3819–43864. Part III Environmental Protection Agency 40 CFR Part 799,

Toxic Substances Control Act Test Guidelines; Final Rule (http://www.epa. gov/fedrgstr/EPA-TOX/1997/August/Day-15/t21413.htm).
93. Kuwano K, Hagimoto N, Hara N. Molecular mechanisms of pulmonary fibrosis and current treatment. Curr Mol Med 2001; 1(5):551–573.
94. Stevens MA, Fitzgerald S, Menache MG, Graham JA, Costa DL, Bucher JR. Functional airway obstruction in male F-344 rats exposed to methyl isocyanate (MIC). Environ Health Perspect 1987; 72: 89–94.
95. Farman CA, Watkins K, van Hoozen B, Last JA, Witschi H, Pinkerton KE. Centriacinar remodeling and sustained procollagen gene expression after exposure to ozone and nitrogen dioxide. Am J Respir Cell Mol Biol 1999; 20(2):303–311.
96. Tyler WS, Tyler NK, Last JA, Barstow TJ, Magliano DJ, Hinds DM. Effects of ozone on lung and somatic growth. Pair fed rats after ozone exposure and recovery periods. Toxicol 1987; 46(1):1–20.
97. Schwartz LW, Dungworth DL, Mustafa MG, Tarkington BK, Tyler WS. Pulmonary responses of rats to ambient levels of ozone: effects of 7-day intermittent or continuous exposure. Lab Invest 1976; 34(6):565–578.
98. Tyler WS, Tyler NK, Last JA, Gillespie MJ, Barstow TJ. Comparison of daily and seasonal exposures of young monkeys to ozone. Toxicol 1988; 50(2): 131–144.
99. Paige RC, Plopper CG. Acute and chronic effects of ozone in animal models. In:Holgate ST, Samet JM, Koren H, Maynard RL, eds. Air Pollution and Health. London: Academic Press, 1999:531–557.
100. Slade R, Stead AG, Graham JA, Hatch GE. Comparison of lung antioxidant levels in humans and laboratory animals. Am Rev Respir Dis 1985; 131: 742–746.
101. Miller F, Overton J, Graham R. Respiratory deposition of inhaled reactive gases. Chapter 8. In: McClellon RO, Henderson R, eds. Concepts in Inhalation Toxicology. Washington, DC: Hemisphere Press, 1989:229–247.
102. Kodavanti UP, Costa DL, Bromberg P. Rodent models of cardiopulmonary disease: their potential applicability in studies of air pollutant susceptibility. Environ Health Perspect 1998; 106(suppl 1):111–130.
103. Ho YS. Transgenic models for the study of lung biology and disease. Am J Physiol 266 Lung Cell Mol Physiol 1994; 10:L319–L353.
104. Glasser SW, Korfhagen TR, Wert S, et al. Transgenic models for study of pulmonary development and disease. Am J Physiol 267 Lung Cell Mol Physiol 1994; 11:L489–L497.
105. Recio L. Transgeneic animal models and their application in mechanistically based toxicology research. CIIT Activities 1995; 15(10):1–7.
106. Suga T, Kurabayashi M, Sando Y, Ohyama Y, Maeno T, Maeno Y, Aizawa H, Matsumura Y, Kuwaki T, Kuro-O M, Nabeshima Y, Nagai R. Disruption of the klotho gene causes pulmonary emphysema in mice. Am J Respirat Cell Mol Biol 2000; 22:26–33.
107. Kakuyama M, Ahluwalia A, Rodrigo J, Vallance P. Cholingergic contraction is altered in nNOS knockouts: cooperative modulation of neural bronchoconstriction by NOS and COX. Am J Respirat Crit Care Med 1999; 160: 2072–2078.

108. Kuhn III C, Homer RJ, Zhu Z, Ward N, Flavell RA, Geba GP, Elias JA. Airway hyperresponsiveness and air obstruction in transgenic mice: morphologic correlates in mice overexpressingIL-11 and IL-6 in the lung. Am J Respir Cell Mol Biol 2000; 22:289–295.

109. O'Donnell MD, O'Conner CM, FitzGerald MX. Ultrastructure of lung elastin and collagen in mouse models of spontaneous emphysema. Matrix Biol 2000; 18(4):357–360.

110. Johnston CJ, finkelstein JN, Oberdorster G, et al. Clara cell secretory protein-deficient mice differ from wild-type mice in inflammatory chemokine expression to oxygen and ozone, but not to endotoxin. Exp Lung Res 1999; 25(1):7–21.

111. Kleeberger SR, Reddy S, Zhang LY, Cho HY, Jedlicka AE. Genetic susceptibility to ozone-induced lung hyperpermeability. Role of toll-like receptor 4. Am J Respir Cell Mol Bio 2000; 22(5):620–627.

112. Ohtsuka Y, Clarke RW, Mitzner W, Brunson K, Jakab GJ, Kleeberger SR. Interstrain variation in murine susceptibility to inhaled acid-coated particles. Am J Physiol Lung Cell Mol Physiol 2000; 278(3):L469–L476.

113. Ghio AJ, Carter JD, Richards JH, Crissman KM, Bobb HH, Yang F. Diminished injury in hypertranferrinemic mice after exposure to a metal-rich particle. Am J Physiol Lung Cell Mol Physiol 2000; 278(5):L1051–L1061.

114. Yoshida M, Satoh M, Shimada A, Yamamoto E, Yasutake A, Tohyama C. Pulmonary toxicity caused by acute exposure to mercury vapor is enhanced in metallothionein-null mice. Life Sci 1999; 64(20):1861–1867.

115. Lippmann M. Health effects of ozone. A critical review. JAPCA 1989; 39(5):672–695.

116. Bascom R, Bromberg PA, Costa DL, Devlin R, Dockery DW, Frampton MW, Lambert W, Samet JM, Speizer FE, Utell M. State of the art: Health effects of outdoor air pollution. Part I. Am J Respir Crit Care Med 1996; 153:3–50.

117. Hatch GE, Slade R, Harris LP, McDonnell WF, Devlin RB, Koren HS, Costa DL, McKee J. Ozone dose and effect in humans and rats: a comparison using oxygen-18 labeling and bronchoalveolar lavage. J Resp Crit Care Med 1994; 150(3):676–683.

118. Koren HS, Devlin RB, Graham DE, Mann R, McGee MP, Horstman DH, Kozumbo WJ, Becker S, House DE, McDonnell WF. Ozone-induced inflammation in the lower airways of human subjects. Am Rev Respir Dis 1989; 139:407–415.

119. Seltzer J, Bigby BG, Stulbarg M, Holtzman MJ, Nadel JA, Ueki IF, Leikauf GD, Goetzl EJ, Boushey HA. O_3-induced change in bronchial reactivity to methacholine and airway inflammation in humans. J Appl Physiol 1986; 60:1321–1326.

120. Costa DL, Schafrank SH, Wehner RW, Jellett E. Alveolar permeability to protein in rats differentially sensitive to ozone. J Appl Toxicol 1985; 5(3):182–186.

121. Kutzman RS, Wehner RW, Haber SB. The impact of inhaled acrolein on hypertension-sensitive and resistant rats. J Environ Pathol Toxicol Oncol 1986; 6(5–6):97–108.

122. Grigg J, Venge P. Inflammatory markers of outcome. Europ Respir J 1996; 21(suppl 2):16s–21s.

13

Ventilation Therapies and Strategies for Acute Lung Injury

C. C. DOS SANTOS and A. S. SLUTSKY

Department of Critical Care Medicine, St. Michael's Hospital and Interdepartmental Division of Critical Care, Department of Medicine, University of Toronto, Toronto, Ontario, Canada

I. Overview

This chapter reviews and discusses ventilation therapies for clinical acute lung injury (ALI) and the acute respiratory distress syndrome (ARDS). Emphasis is on the concept of ventilator induced lung injury (VILI), and how it can be minimized or prevented by specific ventilation strategies. Acute pulmonary injury from mechanical ventilation in humans is indistinguishable from injury caused by many other processes associated with acute respiratory failure and ARDS. In order to treat the severe hypoxemia present in patients with ALI/ARDS, mechanical ventilation is generally required. However, added lung injury from ventilation therapy can have a considerable negative impact on the morbidity and mortality of affected patients. The concept that mechanical ventilation per se is injurious to the lungs, and that it can generate and exacerbate local and systemic inflammatory responses, has led to a reassessment of ventilation strategies for patients with ALI/ARDS as detailed in this chapter. The aims of lung protective ventilation strategies are twofold: (1) to limit the injurious effect of mechanical forces on the lung itself; and (2) to modulate or prevent the development of a systemic inflammatory response. This chapter highlights experimental and clinical evidence in support of the *biotrauma* theory of lung injury and multiorgan failure in ALI/ARDS, and how it impacts current thinking on lung protective ventilation strategies. Discussion includes the unique properties of the injured lung, and their relevance for the pathophysiology of VILI. In addition, the clinical literature on different ventilatory strategies is reviewed in detail in terms of their effectiveness in improving the outcomes of patients with ALI/ARDS while protecting the lungs from iatrogenic injury.

II. Introduction

The concept that lung injury can result from mechanical ventilation is not new, and has been appreciated by basic and clinical researchers for decades. More recently, a significant ARDS network clinical trial on ventilation in critically ill patients (1) has underscored the importance of VILI as a clinically significant side effect of mechanical ventilation. In addition, a complementary clinical study (2) has demonstrated that protective ventilation strategies are associated with a reduction in markers of inflammation, among them proinflammatory cytokines. These studies, in conjunction with experimental data from in vivo and ex vivo lung injury models, provide compelling evidence for the so-called *biotrauma* hypothesis. This hypothesis states that, even in the absence of overt ultrastructural damage, lung injury from mechanical ventilation can result from excessive release of proinflammatory mediators and overactivation of the immune system. From this perspective, the lung is an immuno-modulatory organ, and can be an active participant in the development of multiorgan failure (MOF) that is frequently found to be present in patients with sepsis or ALI/ARDS.

Although the syndrome of ARDS has been described for over 35 years (3), it still represents a significant therapeutic challenge for the clinical intensivist. Part of the difficulty in developing effective therapies for ALI/ARDS relates to the heterogeneous etiologies of this clinical syndrome, the complex nature of the underlying lung injury pathophysiology, and imprecisions in clinical definitions. Over the past decade, major changes in thinking with regards to ventilatory strategies for ALI/ARDS have occurred. These have primarily come about as a result of enhanced understanding of pulmonary pathology and the dynamic interaction between the lung and the ventilator.

The primary objective of traditional strategies of mechanical ventilation has been to maintain normal levels of oxygen (O_2) and carbon dioxide (CO_2) in the blood, and/or to decrease the energy costs of breathing. In most patients, there is little doubt that volume-cycled or pressure limited modes of conventional mechanical ventilation (CMV) are effective in maintaining arterial oxygenation and providing the time to institute specific therapies to restore pulmonary structure and function. However, in severely injured lungs, elevated dead space and reduced lung compliance may overwhelm the ability of conventional ventilation strategies to cope with the increased work of breathing. Traditional approaches to mechanical ventilation in patients with ALI/ARDS have relied on large tidal volumes to compensate for increased dead space, thus allowing arterial partial pressure of CO_2 ($PaCO_2$) to be maintained at normal levels. Over a number of years, however, evidence from animal and human studies has made it clear that this approach to the management of ALI/ARDS contributes to the unacceptably high mortality rates of affected patients (4,5).

Details about the pathophysiology and clinical presentation of ALI/ARDS have been given in earlier chapters (e.g., Chapter 3). At the center of clinical ALI/ARDS is a sudden change in pulmonary function, apparent as "stiff" (noncompliant) lungs with an inability to support gas exchange. This functional injury is distinguished histologically as diffuse alveolar damage (6). Although severe hypoxemia represents the clinical hallmark of ARDS, patients die more frequently from associated conditions such as MOF and sepsis than they do from intractable respiratory failure (7). It has been postulated that mechanical ventilation per se may contribute to this phenomenon by worsening the severity and extent of lung injury, which ultimately generates a progressive systemic inflammatory response and subsequent MOF (8,9).

Patients with ALI/ARDS have lungs that seem to be exquisitely sensitive to mechanical forces. The realization that mechanical ventilation may cause or exacerbate ALI, and that injurious ventilatory regimens are more deleterious when applied to previously injured lungs (10), has had a substantial impact on current thinking about ventilation therapy in ALI/ARDS. A new era of ventilatory management began in the 1990s with reports that protective ventilatory strategies limit the mechanical insult to the lungs (11). The intricate and dynamic relationship between mechanical forces and pathophysiological proccesses in injured lungs makes mechanical ventilation dictated by two major considerations: (1) the pathophysiological properties of the already injured lungs themselves; and (2) the knowledge that ventilatory strategies differ in the degree to which they exacerbate or propagate acute lung injury. A summary of ventilatory strategies available for the management of patients with ALI/ARDS is given in Table 1. Subsequent sections of the chapter explore the nature of the complex relationships between ventilation and injury, and develop a biological rationale to explain current thinking underlying ventilation strategies in patients with ALI/ARDS.

Table 1 Ventilatory Options in ALI/ARDS

Ventilatory options in ALI/ARDS	Physiological principle	Clinical references
Non-invasive positive pressure ventilation	Uses a tight fitting mask as an alternative interface between the patient and the ventilator to avoid the complications of endotracheal intubation.	Refs. 12–14
Proportional-assist ventilation	This mode of positive pressure ventilation varies directly with patient effort. The inspiratory assistance can be customized to the elastance and resistant properties of each patient's respiratory system.	Refs. 15–16
Small tidal volume ventilation	Use of tidal volumes of 6 ml/kg (predicted body weight) has been shown to improve outcomes in patients with ARDS, presumably because it protects the lung from further ventilator induced injury.	Refs. 1, 17–20
Positive end expiratory pressure (PEEP)	PEEP reduces intra-pulmonary shunt and improves arterial oxygenation, thus allowing for arterial oxygenation at a lower inspired fraction of oxygen. PEEP is also presumed to prevent injurious mechanical forces that occur from ventilation with atelectasis at end-expiration.	Refs. 18, 21–23
Lung-recruitment maneuvers (LRMs)	Recruitment maneuvers are thought to reexpand collapsed lung tissue. Thus minimizing the mechanical injury from ventilating collapsed alveoli.	Refs. 24–28
Prone position	Prone position is thought to prevent VILI by promoting a more uniform distribution of tidal volume and by recruiting dorsal lung regions, preventing repeated opening and closing of small airways or excessive mechanical stress at the margins between well aerated and actelectatic lung units.	Refs. 29–32

High frequency ventilation (HFV)	HFV relies on small tidal volumes at high frequencies to achieve to main lung protective goals: preventing overdistention and ventilating with atelectasis at end-expiration). High frequency oscillation (HFO), additionally, decouples oxygenation from carbon dioxide removal, thus allowing for the maintenance of arterial $PaCO_2$ during oxygenation.	Refs. 33–36
Inhaled nitric oxide (iNO)	NO inhalation dilates pulmonary vessels perfusing aerated lung units, diverting blood from poorly ventilated or shunt areas. Based on these properties, NO has been utilized to treat severe hypoxemia and pulmonary hypertension in ALI/ARDS patients.	Refs. 37–43 and see Chapters 8, 17, and 19
Inverse-ratio ventilation	Inverse ratio ventilation is thought to recruit and stabilize atelectatic alveoli by extending the duration of inspiration and shortening the expiratory time. This technique may improve the shunt and arterial oxygenation obviating the need for higher PEEPS	Refs. 44,45
Surfactant replacement therapy	Exogenous surfactant therapy may benefit patients with ALI/ARDS by antagonizing surfactant dysfunction and improving alveolar ventilation and stability. Associated benefits may include decreases in the pro-inflammatory cytokine production and reduced oxidative injury.	Refs. 46–48 and see Chapter 15
Extra-corporeal gas exchange (ECMO)	ECMO is a consideration in those patients who despite maximum therapy experience refractory hypoxemia. Extracorporeal carbon dioxide removal has been developed as an alternative to minimize the complications from ECMO.	Refs. 49–50
Liquid ventilation	Filing the alveoli with a liquid solution can eliminate surface tension. By using a filing solution that has a high oxygen carrying capacity it is possible to maintain gas exchange during liquid ventilation.	Refs. 51–56

III. Background and Rationale Underlying Ventilatory Strategies in ARDS/ALI

ARDS/ALI represents a significant burden of illness in the intensive care unit setting. Results from the King county lung injury project have estimated the incidence of clinical ALI to be 70 per 10^5 persons/year (57). This is four to five times higher than previous assessments (58,59). Recently, an international utilization review reported that acute respiratory failure accounted for 66% of the indications for mechanical ventilation in major intensive care units (60). Several investigators have evaluated the prevalence of ARDS among hypoxemic patients requiring mechanical ventilation, and have found that these account for up to 20% of all ICU admissions (58).

Reported mortality rates for ARDS remain extremely high at 30–60% (58,59). Current studies comparing recent and historical data have demonstrated an improved outcome with an approximate 65% survival rate in certain patient subgroups. Rubenfeld et al. (57) observed that mortality, risk factors distribution, and ratio of ALI patients to acute respiratory failure were similar to the findings from previous studies (of 988 patients, 745 had ARDS). Because most patients who die with this syndrome do not succumb from their local disease (hypoxemia), alternative explanations invoking iatrogenic injury from mechanical ventilation have been generated to help explain this phenomenon. Two important concepts have been formulated from this observation: (i) mechanical ventilation is in itself injurious to the lungs of patients with ARDS; and (ii) this injury is not confined to the lungs alone, and may contribute to the systemic inflammatory response ultimately responsible for the morbidity and mortality in many patients.

A. Biological Susceptibility of the Injured Lungs

In ARDS/ALI the functional injury is distinguished histologically as diffuse alveolar damage (61). Structural changes in the alveolo-capillary unit lead to loss of integrity of the alveolo-capillary membrane and subsequent disruption of the endothelial barrier. Exudative pulmonary edema ensues as a result of increased vascular permeability, leading to ventilation/perfusion abnormalities and an inability to support gas exchange. In later stages of ALI/ARDS, fibrosis and abnormal remodeling become apparent. Pulmonary pathology in ALI/ARDS is often nonhomogeneous in distribution, but overall is characterized by a reduction in functional alveolar units. Evidence of significant loss of lung volume, compounded by the heterogeneous distribution of inflammatory changes, has shed new light into the concept of VILI (62–64). Along with marked overall reduction in lung volumes ("baby lung"), alveoli in uninjured regions are highly susceptible to overdistension, while other alveoli in injured parts of the lung are collapsed (atelectatic).

Recent experiments using in vivo videomicroscopy have demonstrated that in the normal lungs, volume changes during tidal ventilation are not associated with simple linear, balloon-like expansion and contraction of alveoli. Rather, average alveolar surface areas, and consequently alveolar volume, can change relatively little during significant portions of the tidal breathing cycle (65). Much of the change in lung volume is accommodated either by the elastic properties of the respiratory bronchioles or by the recruitment of new populations of acini. This structural design prevents shear stress injury in the normal lung during tidal ventilation. In contrast, injured lungs have a continuum of alveolar mechanics characterized by three types of alveoli–normal alveoli (type I), alveoli that exhibit greater changes in shape and size with ventilation but do not collapse (type II), and alveoli that totally collapse at end expiration and "pop" open rapidly during inspiration (Type III). Ventilation in injured lungs is characterized by a larger than normal change in alveolar area ($>5000\,\mu m^2$). Moreover, it appears that many injured alveoli do not change volume until a critical airway pressure is reached, at which point they rapidly "pop" open or closed (65).

In acutely injured lungs, alveolar size at peak inspiration can be doubled or more compared to uninjured lungs. Alveolar overdistension occurs even at relatively conservative tidal volumes of 10 mL/kg, and is broadened in scope by the fact that alveoli gain structural support from an anatomical arrangement in an interconnected network. Structural support (interdependence), combined with the surface tension-lowering properties of surfactant, provides important stability to the alveoli. However, the acinus is only structurally sound if alveoli remain inflated. Collapse of an alveolus causes shear stress not only on its own walls, but also on those of adjacent alveoli (65). Mead et al. (66) examined the distribution of pressure during tidal inflation in a model of heterogeneous lung injury. In this model, inflated lungs could be exposed to stresses up to 140 cm H_2O when the trans-pulmonary pressure was only 30 cm H_2O. These stresses were generated by shear force due to: (a) the recruitment of atelectatic areas surrounded by normal alveoli; and (b) the overdistension of alveoli adjacent to atelectatic zones or to the pleura (66). Injured lungs are much more susceptible to damage by shear stress resulting from alveolar collapse and overdistention (or derecruitment–recruitment). This concept has been postulated to play a role in the development of VILI (4,5,67).

B. Injurious Nature of the Ventilator and Ventilator Induced Lung Injury

To date the consensus is that four basic mechanisms contribute to the pathophysiology of VILI (5):

1. *Barotrauma*: This form of VILI is characterized by dramatic clinical manifestations of extra-alveolar air due to gross injury caused by overdistention during mechanical ventilation (68).

2. *Volutrauma*: This is a more subtle form of injury caused by increases in lung volume. In this form of VILI, high end-inspiratory lung stretch has been documented to cause diffuse alveolar damage, pulmonary edema, increased fluid filtration, and changes in alveolo-capillary membrane permeability (9).

3. *Atelectrauma*: In addition to lung injury caused by overdistention, a large body of evidence suggests that ventilation at low lung volumes is also harmful. In this model, the shear stress secondary to repetitive opening/collapse of distal airways (recruitment–derecruitment) and other mechanisms (e.g., regional hypoxia) contributes to lung injury (67).

4. *Biotrauma*: By altering both the pattern and magnitude of stretch, mechanical ventilation may lead to alterations in gene expression and/or cellular metabolism ultimately leading to the development of an overwhelming inflammatory response (8,69,70). This type of injury may occur even in the absence of overt ultrastructural damage.

C. Relation of Mechanical Forces to the Development of MOF in ARDS

Excessive cyclic motion produced by certain modes of mechanical ventilation has been shown to lead to the induction, synthesis, and release of cytokines and inflammatory mediators from the lung (71,72). In addition, mechanical forces generated by injurious ventilatory strategies are able to alter the expression of genes known to modulate pulmonary inflammatory responses (Fig. 1) (71,73). The role of mechanical forces in coordinating pulmonary cellular responses is well recognized as described in earlier chapters (e.g., Chapter 2 on Lung development and growth). Studies in vitro and in vivo have found that both the pattern and the degree of mechanical stretch are important in determining cellular responses (74,75). The postulate is therefore that by altering both the pattern and magnitude of stretch, mechanical ventilation may lead to alterations in gene expression or/and cellular metabolism (71,73).

As noted in the previous section, the term *biotrauma* has been proposed to describe the process by which mechanical stress produced by mechanical ventilation leads to up regulation of an inflammatory response (8,69), as evidenced by neutrophil infiltration in the lungs and increased levels of host inflammatory mediators in bronchoalveolar lavage (BAL). Recent work suggests that in addition to acting locally, these proinflammatory mediators may escape the confines of the lung to either generate or propagate a systemic inflammatory reaction associated with VILI (76,77). It is thought that this systemic inflammatory response, which occurs as compartmentalization of the local pulmonary response is lost, may be a significant contributor to MOF. Also relevant for this process is the

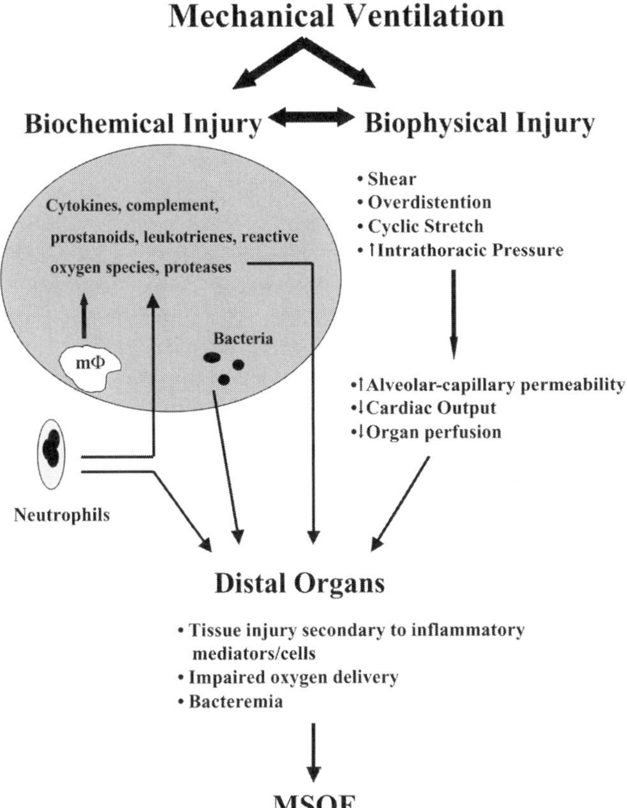

Figure 1 Schematic representation of the postulated mechanisms whereby mechanical ventilation may contribute to multisystem organ failure (MSOF). (Adapted with permission from Ref. 69.)

effectiveness, or lack of effectiveness, of the compensatory systemic anti-inflammatory response initiated in an attempt to down regulate and attenuate the proinflammatory response.

Loss of appropriate immune modulation, or persistent inflammatory injury, appears to be involved in the inability of organisms to bring about resolution of the proinflammatory response and ultimately death (8,69). In an animal model, Chiumello et al. (77) examined the hypothesis that injurious ventilatory strategies [large tidal volume (V_T) and/or low positive end-expiratory pressure (PEEP)] would increase release of inflammatory mediators into the lung and into the systemic circulation (Fig. 2). This group showed that injurious ventilatory strategies are associated with the release of cytokines into the systemic circulation (Fig. 3). Data from Haitsma et al. (76) also suggest that cytokines may leak from the systemic

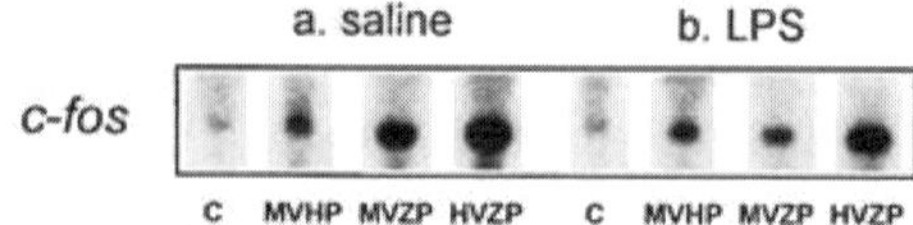

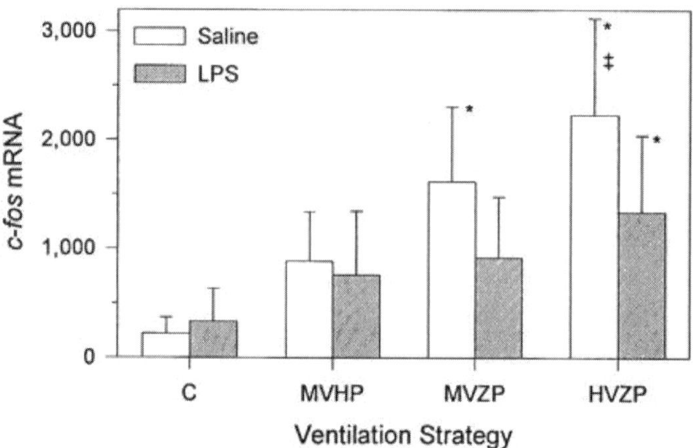

Figure 2 Increased expression of c-fos, in an ex vivo lung injury model, by Northern blot analysis. Fifty-five Sprague–Dawley rats were randomized to either intravenous saline or lipopolysaccharide (LPS). After 50 min of spontaneous respiration, the lungs were excised and randomized to 2 hr of ventilation with one of four strategies: (a) control (C), tidal volume $(V_T) = 7\,cc/kg$, positive end-expiratory pressure (PEEP) $= 3$ cm H_2O; (b) moderate volume, high PEEP (MVHP), $V_T = 15\,cc/kg$; PEEP $= 10$ cm H_2O; (c) moderate volume, zero PEEP (MVZP), $V_T = 15\,cc/kg$, PEEP $= 0$; or (d) high volume, zero PEEP (HVZP), $V_T = 40\,cc/kg$, PEEP $= 0$. Ventilation with zero PEEP (MVZP, HVZP) resulted in significant reductions in lung compliance. Zero PEEP in combination with high volume ventilation (HVZP) had a synergistic effect on cytokine levels (data not shown) and the expression of c-fos. (Reprinted with permission from Ref. 71.)

circulation into the alveolar space possibly explaining how patients with sepsis may develop secondary ARDS. In addition, ventilatory models, which allow end-expiratory collapse can induce bacterial translocation from the lung to the systemic circulation when very high tidal volumes are used (79,80); even strategies that use relatively normal tidal volumes can induce endotoxin translocation from the lung to the systemic circulation (61). Endotoxin translocation is associated with worse outcome in this model (Fig. 4). Moreover, in a recently presented experimental study, the use of lung protective strategies with low tidal volume delayed bacteremia and consequently presumably could affect the onset of MOF (81).

There is clinical evidence in support of this model for the development of MOF in ventilated ARDS patients. Ranieri et al. (2) demonstrated that the concentrations of proinflammatory cytokines in both BAL fluid and plasma could be decreased in patients ventilated with a lung protective strategy. In a prospective randomized trial, this group randomized patients with ARDS to receive conventional ventilation strategy (to keep $PaCO_2$ between 35 and 40 mmHg) or a lung protective strategy using a tidal volume and PEEP level based on individual pressure volume curves (2). Patients in the conventional group had an increase in both systemic and lung lavage concentrations of inflammatory cytokines. Thirty-six hours after randomization, inflammatory mediators were significantly lower in the lung-protective group (2). In another publication, the same group showed that the level of inflammatory mediators correlated with the incidence of MOF in ARDS patients (82). Further evidence in support of biotrauma comes from the ARDS/Net trial (1). In this study, the plasma level of interleukin-6 was lower in the intervention arm in comparison with the control group (1). Consequently, lung-protection strategies may achieve their benefit through reduction in the systemic release of inflammatory mediators and the frequency and severity of MOF. Moreover, preliminary evidence in animals has shown that ventilation strategies may affect levels of anti-inflammatory, even in perfectly normal lungs (83).

Convincing evidence in support for the immuno-modulatory role of the lung in VILI has been recently published by Stuber et al. (84). In this study, mechanical ventilation was changed transiently from a lung protective strategy with PEEP of 15 cm H_2O and a V_T of 5 mL/kg of predicted body weight to a more conventional strategy with PEEP of 5 cm H_2O and V_T of 12 mL/kg predicted body weight for a period of 6 hr. The levels of inflammatory mediators (IL-1β, IL-1RA, IL-6, IL-10, and TNF-α) in the plasma of all patients were measured at varying intervals before, during, and after the intervention (note that each patient is their own control). Switching to CMV was associated with a higher PaO_2 and a marked increase in measured plasma cytokines. Similarly, BAL cytokine levels were also markedly elevated by CMV. Not only are nonprotective strategies associated with higher mortality, higher incidence of MOF, and higher proinflammatory mediators, but also a decrease in anti-inflammatory mediators in preliminary animal experiments (84).

IV. Lung Protective Ventilatory Strategies

The clinical importance of lung protective ventilatory strategies was recently confirmed, when the results of the acute respiratory distress network (ARDS network) trial demonstrated a 22% relative risk (RR) reduction in 180-day mortality rates favoring a low tidal volume group

(6 mL/kg of predicted body weight) vs. a conventional ventilatory strategy group (12 mL/kg) (1). Based on the data reported in the NIH trial, the attributable mortality of VILI may be in the range of nine per cent (absolute risk reduction in mortality between the high- and low-volume ventilatory strategies). This sobering thought underscores both the vital importance of VILI in determining patient outcome and the importance of current and future research in determining the clinically appropriate choice of ventilatory strategy in the management of ventilated patients. Table 1 given earlier summarizes the rationale and most significant references pertaining to common strategies of lung protection in ARDS patients.

The principles of limiting VILI are illustrated by the examination of the pressure–volume curve (P–V curve) of the lung. Matamis et al. (85) used bedside determinations of the P–V curve to characterize the abnormalities in respiratory system mechanics in patients with ARDS. With pressure plotted on the x-axis and volume on the y-axis the curve has a sigmoidal

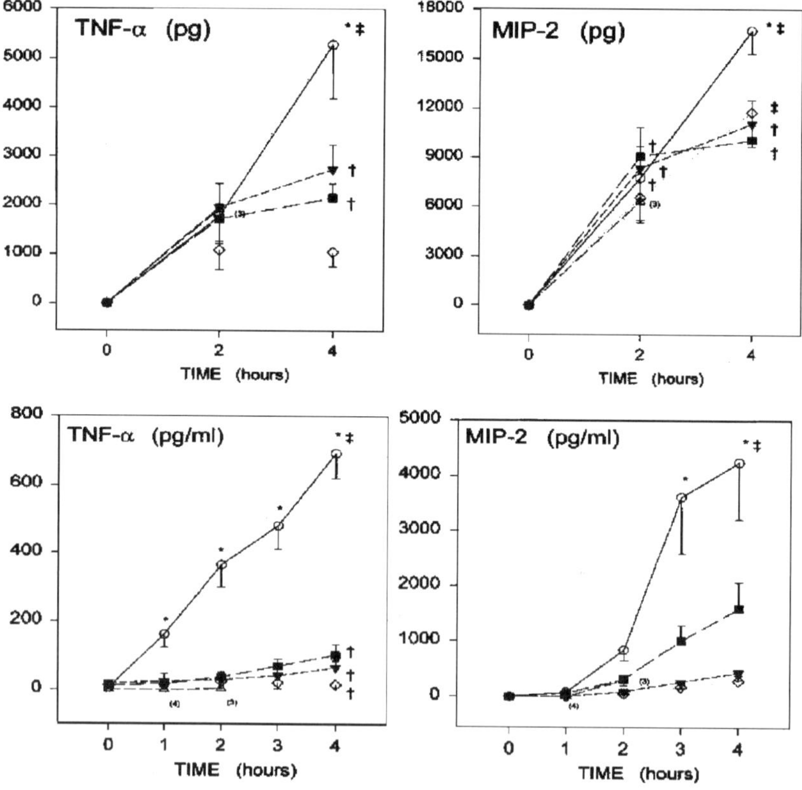

Figure 3   (*Caption on facing page*)

shape, which tends to flatten above and below the bends, defining the upper and lower inflection points, respectively. Initial concepts were that end-inspiratory stretch above the upper inflection point might lead to alveolar overdistention. As well, allowing end-expiratory pressure to fall below the lower inflection point would cause alveoli to collapse and re-open repeatedly (86) (Fig. 5). There are many caveats to this simple model of recruitment, since it is clear that recruitment continues to take place all along the linear portion of the P–V curve beyond the upper and lower inflection points (4).

In general, strategies to limit VILI include avoiding both overdistention and derecruitment, as well as limiting exposure to high oxygen concentrations. Prolonged exposure to high levels of oxygen may cause lung injury through the formation of free radicals and superoxide (see Chapter 7 for further details on the roles of oxidants and antioxidants in lung injury). Moreover, hyperoxia has been associated with absorption atelectasis and myocardial dysfunction (87). There are three main approaches to lung protective ventilatory strategies. The first is based on limiting pulmonary overdistention, by reducing lung volumes during mechanical ventilation. The second relies on "permissive hypercapnia." This strategy, often used in conjunction with limiting tidal volume and airway pressures, is based

---

Figure 3 (*Facing page*) Leakage of cytokines into bronchoalveolar lavage (BAL) fluid and serum of animals treated with an injurious ventilatory strategy. Lung injury was induced in 40 anesthetized paralyzed Sprague–Dawley rats by hydrochloric acid instillation (pH 1.5, 2.5 mL/kg). Rats were then randomized into five groups ($n = 8$): (1) high-volume zero PEEP (HVZP): V_T, 16 mL/kg; (2) high-volume PEEP (HVP): V_T, 16 mL/kg, PEEP, 5 cm H_2O; (3) low-volume zero PEEP (LVZP): V_T, 9 mL/kg; (4) low-volume PEEP (LVP): V_T, 9 mL/kg, PEEP, 5 cm H_2O; (5) same settings as (4) plus a recruitment maneuver performed every hour (LVPR). Respiratory rate was adjusted to maintain normocapnia and fraction of inspired oxygen (FiO$_2$) was 1. Cytokine concentrations [tumor necrosis factor-alpha (TNF-alpha) and macrophage inflammatory protein-2 (MIP-2)] were measured by ELISA. All animals in the LVZP group died before the end of the experiment. After 4 hr of ventilation, the HVZP group had similar lung fluid TNF-alpha concentrations compared with the HVP group: 1861 ± 333 vs. 1259 ± 189 pg/mL; and much higher serum concentrations: 692 ± 74 vs. 102 ± 31 pg/mL ($p < 0.05$). An identical pattern was found for MIP-2. (a) Mean BAL absolute quantity of cytokine (calculated as volume of lung fluid aspirated times cytokine concentration). $^*p<0.05$ vs. all other groups at 4 hr; $^\dagger p<0.05$ vs. time 0; $^\ddagger p<0.05$ vs time 0 and 2 hr. Data are expressed as mean ± SEM; number of animals in brackets. (b) Mean serum cytokine levels during experiment. $^*p<0.05$ vs. all other groups at same time point; $^\dagger p<0.05$ vs. time 0; $^\ddagger p<0.05$ vs. all time points; $\S p<0.05$ vs. time 0 and 1 hr. Data are expressed as mean ± SEM; number of animals in brackets. Symbols: ○ = high volume, zero PEEP (HVZP); ■ = high volume, PEEP (HVP); Δ = low volume, zero PEEP (LVZP); ▼ = low volume, PEEP (LVP); ◆ = low volume, PEEP + recruitment (LVPR). (Reprinted with permission from Ref. 77.)

on the concept that hypercapnia is well tolerated and should be allowed to increase as lung distension is decreased. Thirdly, an "open lung" strategy, which focuses on the use of recruitment maneuvers and PEEP to open alveoli and keep them opened at a safe level, thus avoiding both overdisten-

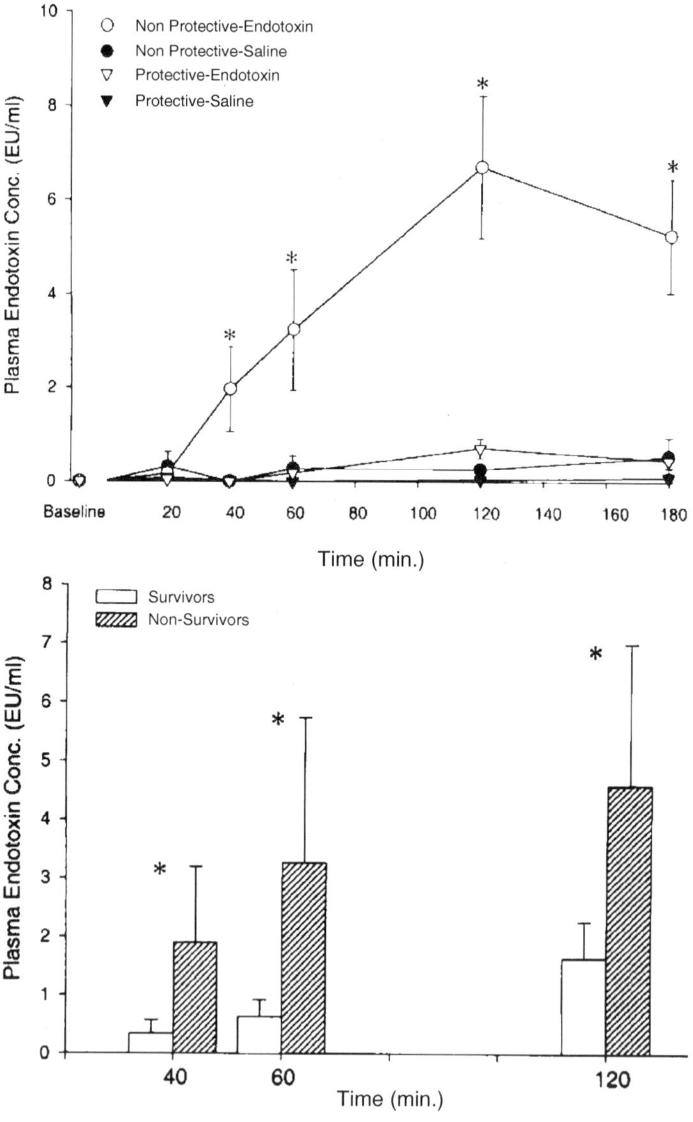

Figure 4   (*Caption on facing page*)

tion and shear stress from repeated opening and closing of the alveoli (Table 1).

A. Limiting Pulmonary Overdistension—Reducing Lung Volumes

Pressure Control vs. Volume Control

A decade ago, an editorial by Marini and Kelsen (88) emphasized the need for prospective control trials comparing pressure control (PC) and volume control (VC) ventilation at fixed transalveolar pressures in ARDS patients. Since then, three prospective randomized trails comparing PCV and VCV were published. Lessard et al. (89) compared nine patients with ARDS treated with either PCV or VCV, while keeping both the level of ventilation and PEEP constant. This group found no difference in respiratory mechanics, hemodynamics, or gas exchange parameters between the two groups. Rappaport et al. (90) prospectively compared early application of PCV and VCV in 27 patients with acute hypoxic respiratory failure and found that PCV was associated with a more rapid increase in static compliance and fewer days of mechanical ventilation in patients who survived and were extubated.

Esteban et al. (91) carried out a multicenter randomized trial of 79 ARDS patients ventilated with either PCV ($n = 37$) or VCV ($n = 42$). In both instances, inspiratory plateau pressures were limited to 35 cm H_2O. The main finding of this study was that, decreasing either tidal volume on VCV, or inspiratory pressure on PCV, to reduce inspiratory plateau pressures did not independently influence mortality. Moreover, this group found that the mortality of ARDS patients was strongly associated with the development of MOF and that neither strategy is particularly better at preventing this complication. One of the key issues in these trials is that they were

---

Figure 4 (*Facing page*) The effects of protective (V_T 5 mL kg^{-1}, PEEP 10–12.5 cm H_2O) vs. nonprotective (V_T 12 mL kg^{-1}, PEEP zero) ventilatory strategy on translocation of endotracheally instilled endotoxin. Anesthetized New Zealand white rabbits were subjected to saline lung lavage, and 32 were randomized to one of four groups: PS (protective ventilation + instilled saline); PE (protective ventilation + instilled endotoxin); NS (nonprotective ventilation + instilled saline); NE (nonprotective ventilation + instilled endotoxin), and ventilated for 3 hr. Plasma endotoxin levels increased significantly in the NE group, and remained low and unchanged in the other groups. (a) Plasma endotoxin concentration vs. time. In the interval 40–180 min after randomization, endotoxin concentration was significantly higher in NE vs. all other groups (*$p < 0.05$). Concentration was unchanged throughout the experiment in all other groups; (b) Plasma endotoxin concentration was significantly higher in eventual nonsurvivors than survivors, at 40, 60, and 120 min after randomization (*$p < 0.05$). (Reprinted with permission from Ref. 78.)

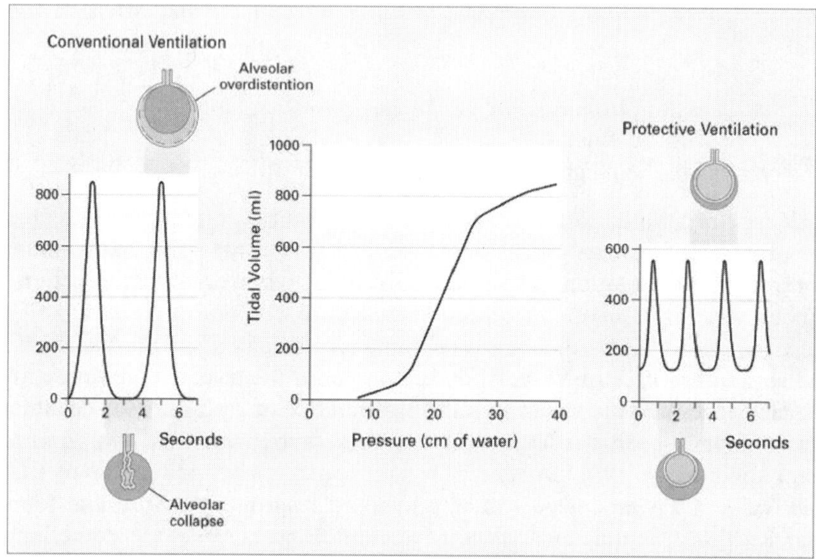

Figure 5 Respiratory pressure–volume curves and the effects of traditional as compared with protective ventilation in a 70 kg patient with ARDS. The lower and upper inflection points of the inspiratory pressure–volume curve (center) are at 14 and 26 cm of H_2O, respectively. With conventional ventilation, when V_T is at 12 mL/kg and zero end-expiratory pressure (left), alveoli collapse at the end of expiration. Generation of shear forces during mechanical ventilation may tear alveolar lining, and attaining and end-inspiratory volume higher than the upper inflection point causes alveolar overdistension. The panel on the right contrasts what happens in protective lung ventilation with tidal volumes limited at 6 mL/kg and addition of PEEP. In this strategy the end-inspiratory volume remains below the upper inflection point and alveolar collapse is prevented at end-expiration, consequently limiting the effects of shear forces during mechanical ventilation. (Reprinted with permission from Ref. 86.)

underpowered; consequently, no definitive conclusions regarding the significance of controlling pressure vs. volume may be drawn.

Pressure and Volume Limited Ventilation

In 1990, Hickling et al. (11) published the first human trial using small tidal volumes (V_T) to ventilate ARDS patients. In this study, intubated patients in the surgical intensive care unit were randomly assigned to a conventional ventilation strategy ($V_T = 12$ mL/kg, $n = 56$) or a low tidal volume strategy ($V_T = 6$ mL/kg, $n = 47$). The incidence of pulmonary infection, and duration of intubation and length of stay, tended to be lower and shorter for non-neurosurgical and noncardiac surgical patients randomized to low V_T, suggesting that morbidity may be decreased. This group noted that the use of low V_T was associated with a statistically significant but clinically irrelevant decrease in oxygenation. This small study marked the beginning of the use of lung protective ventilatory strategies in ARDS.

Since then, conflicting results have been obtained from five randomized controlled trials (RCTs) evaluating similar pressure and volume limited ventilation (PVLV) strategies in ALI patients where mortality was the primary end-point (1,17–20,92) (Table 2). Of these, the best-powered study was the ARDS network trial (1) that examined 861 patients randomly assigned to PVLV (V_T 6 mL/kg predicted body weight; plateau pressure < 30cm H_2O) or conventional ventilation (V_T 12 mL/kg predicted body weight; plateau pressure < 50cm H_2O) (Fig. 4). In this study, PVLV was associated with a mortality reduction from 39.8% in the control group to 31% in the experimental group (RR 0.75; 95% CI 0.62–0.91). Where the trial by Amato et al. (18) also showed a mortality benefit in the group treated with low tidal volumes, three earlier trials exploring the role of this ventilation strategy did not find a change in mortality benefit (17,19,20).

It is difficult to reconcile the discrepancies in the results of the ARDS/Net study with earlier clinical trials evaluating a lung volume restriction strategy but there are a number of possibilities: (i) the method of determining predicted body weight (and hence tidal volume) was different from earlier trials; (ii) patients in the low tidal volume groups had high respiratory rates that may have contributed to significant auto-PEEP, in turn leading to improved alveolar patency or recruitment; (iii) the use of bicarbonate to correct respiratory acidosis may have reduced the need for dialysis and/or potential detrimental effects of hypercapnic acidosis; and (iv) the difference in tidal volume (and airway pressures) between control and the treatment groups was greater than in the other trials, hence increasing the signal/noise ratio.

A meta-analysis published by the Cochrane database system review (93) included the five trials of low tidal volume ventilation in Table 2, which involved a total of 1202 patients. The test for heterogeneity gave a *p* value of 0.12. Ventilation with lower V_T was associated with a decreased mortality at the end of the follow up period for each trial: 216/605 (35.7%) vs. 249/597 (41.7%), RR 0.85 (CI 0.74–0.98). The effect of the intervention however, was not statistically significant when a random effects model was used: RR 0.91 (CI 0.72–1.14). Mortality at day 28 was significantly reduced by lung-protective ventilation: RR 0.74 (CI 0.61–0.88). Nevertheless, the comparison between low and conventional V_T was not significantly different if a plateau pressure less than or equal to 31 cm H_2O in control group was used: RR 1.13 (CI 0.88–1.45). This group felt there was insufficient evidence about morbidity and long-term outcomes to make any generalized statements about the benefits of this strategy. Their primary conclusion was that clinical heterogeneity, such as different lengths of follow up and

Table 2 Clinical Trials of Lung-Protective Ventilation in ARDS

Study	No. of patients	Target V_T		Mean V_T achieved (mL/kg)		Adjusted V_T in CMV group[a]	
		PLV	CMV	PLV	CMV	MBW	PBW
Stewart et al. (17)	120	≤ 8	10–15	6.8	10.1[e]	10.2	12.2
		(IBW[a] mL/kg)					
Brower et al. (19)	52	5–8	10–12	7.3	10.2	8.2	10.2
		(PBW mL/kg)					
Brochard et al. (20)	116	6–10	10–15	7.4	10.7[e]	9.4	11.3
		(DBW[g] mL/kg)					
Amato et al. (18)	53	≤ 6	12	387 mL	738 mL	—	
		(MBW mL/kg)					
ARDS/Net (1)	861	6	12	6.5	11.4	9.8	11.8
		(PBW mL/kg)					

PLV: Protective lung ventilation.
CMV: Conventional mechanical ventilation.
Adjusted V_T: Please see Ref. 92.
[a]Values based on mean V_T as reported.
[b]MBW: Measured body weight.
[c]PBW: Predicted body weight: male PBW (kg) $= 50 + 2.3$ [(height in inches)-60];
  female PBW (kg) $= 45.5 + 2.3$ height (in inches)-60.
[d]IBW: Ideal body weight IBW $= 25 \times$ Height (in m)^2.
[e]Mean values at day 7.
[f]Average daily mean values.
[g]DBW: Dry body weight. DBW $=$ measured weight minus estimated gain from water and
  salt retention.

Target pressure (cm H_2O)		Mean pressure achieved (cm H_2O)		PEEP (cm H_2O)		Primary outcome measures	Results (%)	
PLV	CMV	PLV	CMV	PLV	CMV		PLV	CMV
P_{peak}		P_{peak}		9.6	8.0^e	In-hospital mortality	50	47
≤ 30	50	24.3	33.5					
		$P_{plateau}$ 20.0	28.6^e					
$P_{plateau}$		24.9	30.6^f	Numbers not given		Several	50	46
< 30	45–55							
$P_{plateau}$		24.5	30.5^e	9.6	8.5^e	60 day mortality	46.6	37.9
≤ 25	≤ 60							
P_{peak}		P_{peak}		13.2	9.3	28 day mortality	38	71
20–40	no limit	24.0	45.5				($p < 0.001$)	
		$P_{plateau}$ 23.9	37.8					
P_{peak}		26	37	8.1	9.1	Death	31.0	39.8
< 30	50						($p = 0.007$)	

higher plateau pressure in control arms in two of the trials make the interpretation of the combined results difficult (see Table 2 for details). Consequently, although mortality is significantly reduced at day 28, the effects on long-term mortality are uncertain. Therefore, although the possibility of a clinically relevant benefit cannot be excluded, they felt there was insufficient evidence that low V_T ventilation is beneficial in patients where hypercapnia is potentially harmful (93).

Especially controversial is the study by Amato et al. (18) evaluating PVLV strategies in the management of ARDS. This study has opened the door to a variety of interesting questions about the ventilatory management of ARDS patients. Specifically, this study alludes to the importance of maintaining an "open lung" strategy. This group randomly assigned 53 patients to either CMV or to an experimental intervention that combined a strategy employing a lung recruitment maneuver (LRM), and the use of high PEEP based on the use of the pressure–volume group. The LRM consisted of a 40 sec sustained inflation at 35–40 cm H_2O. To determine the level of PEEP for patients in the experimental arm, they constructed static P–V curves, identified the lower inflection point on the inflation limb, and set PEEP at 2 cm H_2O above this point, using, on average, 16 cm H_2O. This procedure was performed once per patient on the day of randomization to determine PEEP for the duration of mechanical ventilation. Theinvestigators observed quicker recovery of lung function (PaO_2/FiO_2 ratio; lung compliance) and a statistically significant reduction in 28-day mortality (11/29 (38%); deaths in experimental patients, 17/24 (71%) in controls, RR 0.53; 95% CI 0.31–0.91) for patients exposed to the experimental strategy. Although the positive results associated with this experimental ventilation strategy may be attributed in part to PVLV, this study has been criticized for the high mortality rate (exceeding 60%) in the control arm, and the high rate of pneumothoraces in the treatment arm (42%).

Of note, PVLV is not devoid of complications. Limiting tidal volumes can result in progressive alveolar collapse, a reduction in FRC, higher oxygen requirements, and elevation in PCO_2. Thus, the gains achieved by avoiding overdistention injury must be balanced by an increase in shear injury (if more lung units collapse and re-open) and oxygen toxicity, in addition to potential adverse effects of hypercapnia. One possible deleterious effect of hypercapnia in ALI is acute renal failure as suggested by laboratory studies as well as a significant increase in the use of dialysis in an RCT of PVLV (22% vs. 8%; RR 2.75; $p = 0.05$) (26).

B. Permissive Hypercapnia

In the study by Hickling et al. (11), the increase in partial pressure of CO_2 due to the decrease in minute ventilation was not corrected. Patients were allowed to remain hypercapnic. Fifty patients with severe ARDS with a "lung injury score" greater than or equal to 2.5 and a mean PaO_2/FiO_2 ratio of 94 were managed in this manner. The mean maximum $PaCO_2$ was 62 mmHg, the highest being 129 mmHg. The results showed that the hospital mortality was significantly lower than that predicted by Apache II (16% vs. 39.6%, $p<0.001$). Two important concepts arise from this work: (1) limiting tidal volumes may improve patient outcome and (2) allowing for respiratory acidosis may not be harmful to patients. In fact, later studies suggested that respiratory acidosis modulates VILI (94,95). Broccard et al. (96) perfused 21 isolated sets of normal rabbit lungs, ventilated them for 20 min [pressure controlled ventilation (PCV) = 15 cm H_2O] with an inspired CO_2 fraction adjusted for the partial pressure of CO_2 in the perfusate (PCO_2 congruent with 40 mmHg). The lungs ventilated with an injurious strategy and randomized to hypercapnia (PCO_2 70–100 mmHg) or normocapnia (PCO_2 40 mmHg) in lungs ventilated using an injurious ventilatory strategy. This group found that respiratory acidosis attenuated the effects of VILI in this model (96). In an intact animal model of VILI, hypercapnic acidosis was reported to be protective (97).

The mechanisms by which hypercapnic acidosis seems to protect against ALI is unclear. Several possible mechanisms have been proposed (94): (a) physiological pH is necessary for Na/H exchanger activation, and this activation is in turn required for tissue injury. Acid pH may protect the lungs via inhibition of the Na/H exchanger; (b) hypercapnic acidosis increases the production of cAMP by cerebral microvascular cells. These cyclic nucleotides have been shown to protect against pulmonary ischemia reperfusion; and (3) increased xanthine oxidase (XO) activity in cardiac muscle augments membrane permeability to calcium and may potentiate ischemic injury. Also, XO is an important enzyme in the generation of free radicals. Inhibition of XO by hypercapnic acidosis may be one of the main mechanisms by which hypercapnic acidosis reduces tissue injury (98).

Because CO_2 equilibrates rapidly across cell membranes, Laffey et al. (94) hypothesized that hypercapnic acidosis would afford greater protection than metabolic acidosis, and that buffering the hypercapnic acidosis would attenuate its protective effect. In a perfused rabbit lung model of ischemia–reperfusion injury this group demonstrated that despite comparable injury, pulmonary artery pressure elevation was less with buffered hypercapnia vs. control. In vitro XO activity depended on pH, not PCO_2. This group concluded that: (1) hypercapnic acidosis and metabolic acidosis are protective, but hypercapnic acidosis is the most protective; (2) buffering hypercapnic acidosis attenuates its protection and causes pulmonary vasodilation and (3) because metabolic acidosis and hypercapnic acidosis similarly inhibit in vitro XO activity, the differential effects cannot be explained solely on the basis of extracellular XO activity (94).

To date, there are no adult clinical trials addressing specifically the use of hypercapnia. However, one trial in children points to the clinical safety of this treatment strategy. Mariani et al. (95) looked at whether a ventilatory strategy of permissive hypercapnia reduces the duration of assisted ventilation in surfactant-treated preterm infants. Forty-nine infants were randomized during the first 24 hr of age to a permissive hypercapnia group ($PaCO_2$ 45–55 mmHg) or to a normocapnia group ($PaCO_2$ 35–45 mmHg). The primary outcome measure was the total number of days on assisted ventilation. The total number of days on assisted ventilation, expressed as median (25–75th percentiles), was 2.5 (1.5–11.5) in the permissive hypercapnia group and 9.5 (2.0–22.5) in the normocapnia group. The number of patients on assisted ventilation, during the first 96 hr after randomization, was lower in the permissive hypercapnia group. There were no differences in mortality, air leaks, intraventricular hemorrhage, periventricular leukomalacia, retinopathy of prematurity, or patent ductus arteriosus. This was a small study, carried out in a very specific population. Although it demonstrated that permissive hypercapnia is likely feasible and safe, little can be said regarding how this therapy may benefit adults with ARDS.

Based on the lung-protection ventilation trials with permissive hypercapnia it has been inferred that permissive hypercapnia may be a beneficial strategy in the management of patients with ARDS. Three of the studies with a combined total of 288 patients did not demonstrate an advantage from using a protective ventilation strategy (17,19,20). Two of these studies targeted a $PaCO_2$ between 30–45 mmHg (17,19) instead of incorporating permissive hypercapnia into their protective ventilatory strategy. In Brochard et al. (20) different V_T and plateau pressures resulted in different $PaCO_2$ (59.5 $\pm$ 15.0 vs. 41.3 $\pm$ 7.6 mmHg, $p < 0.001$) and pH (7.28 $\pm$ 0.09 vs. 7.4 $\pm$ 0.09, $p < 0.001$). This difference however, did not translate to changes in clinical outcomes. Of the trials that showed mortality benefit in the PVLV group, the ARDS network trial used bicarbonate infusions to buffer the hypercapnic acidosis: $PaCO_2$ (40 vs. 35 mmHg) (1); while in the trial by Amato et al. (18) the $PaCO_2$ was markedly different between the conventional and the low V_T group (33 and 55 mmHg, respectively). For patients who manifest severe ARDS, Kopp et al. (99) suggest that these two level I studies demonstrating that the use of a protective ventilation strategy has a mortality benefit justifies a certain flexibility in varying degrees of hypercapnia.

Although it was previously thought that permissive hypercapnia has few serious side effects, this is not yet certain. Carvalho et al. (100) analyzed the hemodynamic impact of implementing a strategy of permissive hypercapnia and PEEP optimization in ARDS patients and found that in 48 young patients included in the study, there was an immediate hyperdynamic response. Increased cardiac output, decreased systemic vascular resistance and increased pulmonary vascular resistance were documented. This effect dissipated within 36 hr of persistent hypercapnia. In the study by Stewart et al. (17) one of the concerns raised in the low tidal volume group was the higher incidence of renal failure ($PaCO_2$ 45.7 mmHg in

CMV group vs. 54.4 mmHg in the low V_T group). Although systemic effects seem generally tolerated by many critically ill patients, subsets such as those with ischemic heart disease, left or right heart failure, pulmonary hypertension, or cranial injury, may be at higher risk.

In permissive hypercapnia, elevated $PaCO_2$ and the tolerance to it is thought to result from reduced mechanical stretch. However, there are data in the literature suggesting that deliberately elevating CO_2 (therapeutic hypercapnia) may decrease lung injury. Laffey et al. (101) studied an in vivo model of lung ischemia–reperfusion, in which rabbits were randomized to either ventilation with standard eucapnic settings or hypercapnic settings. Hypercapnia was associated with preservation of lung mechanics, attenuation of protein leakage, reduction in pulmonary edema, and improved oxygenation (101). In the therapeutic hypercapnia group, mean BALF-TNF-alpha levels were 3.5% of control levels ($p < 0.01$), and mean 8-isoprostane levels were 30% of control levels ($p = 0.02$). Further analysis also demonstrated reduced lung tissue nitrotyrosine, indicating attenuation of tissue nitration. Future trials are required to determine the clinical benefit of induced hypercapnia.

C. "Open Lung" Strategies
The Role of Positive End-Expiratory Pressure

Strategies that recruit the lung (PEEP, LRMs and prone position) have been thought to improve outcome in patients with ARDS. Initially this was thought to be related to their ability to increase PO_2. Recently however, it has become apparent from animal models that their putative beneficial effect is likely related to their role in limiting VILI. Presumably, this is because they aid in achieving oxygenation/ventilation in the "safe-zone" of the P–V curve and hence reduce exposure to injurious mechanical forces (102).

One of the first studies to examine the role of PEEP in effectively "splinting" open the lung was described in 1963 (103). Since then, many studies have looked at different strategies that aid in maintaining lung volume; collectively they have been termed "open lung" strategies. The application of PEEP is one of the ways in which the lung can be maintained in an open state. This approach involves applying PEEP above an ill-defined, and ever-changing, "critical closing pressure," thus maintaining the lung open. Direct evidence that PEEP maintains alveolar recruitment in ventilated ARDS patients has been provided by CT scan imaging of patient lungs at different levels of PEEP (104–108). In controlled animal studies, the use of PEEP has been shown to prevent VILI (109). These data have been confirmed in the results of clinical case series (110) and physiologic studies (111). In these studies, the use of PEEP increased lung volumes and improved lung compliance, allowing ventilation at lower airway pressures, thus attenuating VILI.

Two RCTs have evaluated a role for PEEP in patients with early ALI. In one study 92 patients were assigned to conventional ventilation using PEEP of zero or 10 cm H_2O (22). There was no apparent effect on the rate of progression of ALI to ARDS (RR 0.92; 95% CI 0.43–2.0), but there were trends toward greater 72 hr recovery from ALI (RR 1.6; 95% CI 0.91–3.0), a lower incidence of major air leaks in patients ventilated with PEEP (RR 0.86; 95% CI 0.53–1.4), and lower mortality (RR 0.79; 95% CI 0.41–1.5). In a related study Weigelt et al. (23) randomly assigned patients with high risk of ARDS to "early" PEEP (immediate PEEP at 5 cm H_2O) or "late" PEEP (applied only when required to correct hypoxemia of $PaO_2 < 60$ mmHg). The investigators reported a lower incidence of ARDS (RR 0.38; 95% CI 0.18–0.77) and fewer pulmonary deaths (RR 0.37; 95% CI 0.12–1.1) with early PEEP. Therefore, both studies support the use of PEEP in ALI; however, neither study demonstrated a significant decrease in mortality and the levels of PEEP used in the "high" PEEP group would now be considered to be relatively low.

A low tidal volume can induce alveolar derecruitment in patients with ALI/ARDS. Also, PEEP is intended as a strategy aimed at limiting derecruitment. One of the questions that arise in ALI/ARDS patients is whether derecruitment results from the decrease in V_T or from a reduction in end-inspiratory plateau pressure. Richard et al. (112) have explored whether there is any benefit in raising the level of PEEP while maintaining a constant plateau pressure. This was a prospective cross-over study of 15 patients. Three ventilation settings were tested: PEEP at the lower inflection point with 6 mL/kg tidal volume, PEEP at the lower inflection point with 10 mL/kg tidal volume, and high PEEP with tidal volume at 6 mL/kg, keeping the plateau pressure constant. The P–V curves at zero PEEP and at set PEEP were recorded, and recruitment was calculated as the volume difference between both curves for pressures ranging from 15 to 30 cm H_2O. This group found that a low V_T with high PEEP strategy led to a marked improvement in recruitment and oxygenation. Consequently, at a given plateau pressure (i.e., similar end-inspiratory distension), lowering V_T and increasing PEEP increase recruitment (112).

There are, however, side effects to the use of PEEP, primarily when plateau pressure is allowed to rise above a critical limit of 35 cm H_2O (113). In a study involving six patients with ALI, the use of PEEP of 13 cm H_2O resulted in the recruitment of nonaerated portions of the lung with a gain of 320 mL in volume, but three patients were believed to have overdistention of already aerated portions of lung with an excess volume of 288 mL (114). It has been suggested that about 30% of patients with ALI do not benefit from PEEP or have a fall in the partial pressure of oxygen (115–117). With the patient in supine position PEEP generally recruits the regions of the lung closest to the apex and sternum (as opposed to the dependent zones most affected by ARDS) (115). Patients who have a primary etiology for their ARDS (pulmonary cause) do not seem to respond to LRMs as well, when compared with patients with secondary ARDS (nonpulmonary cause) (118). Moreover, PEEP may have important hemodynamic side effects, primarily hypotension.

Recent studies have also demonstrated that a high respiratory rate induces intrinsic PEEP. In a recent publication, de Durante et al. (119) tested the hypothesis that the increased respiratory rate used in the ARDS-Net lower V_T strategy might have led to intrinsic PEEPi, raising total PEEP [PEEP (total)]. In this study, 10 patients with ARDS were ventilated using the ARDSNet lower V_T protocol. Respiratory rate was then reduced (10–15 breaths/min) to obtain a V_T of 12 mL/kg (ARDSNet traditional V_T). The PEEP on the ventilator (PEEP (nominal): 10.1 ± 0.7 cm H_2O), FiO_2 (0.7 ± 0.1), and minute ventilation (VE: 12.4 ± 1.7 L/min) were set using the ARDSNet protocol and maintained constant during the two ventilatory strategies. Values of airway pressure at end-expiration of a regular breath [PEEP (external)] and 3–5 sec after the onset of an end-expiratory occlusion [PEEP (total)] were measured. The PEEPi was calculated by subtracting PEEP (external) from PEEP (total). The PEEP (total) and PEEPi were, respectively, 16.3 ± 2.9 and 5.8 ± 3.0 cm H_2O during the lower V_T strategy and 11.7 ± 0.9 and 1.4 ± 1.0 cm H_2O during the traditional V_T strategy $(p < 0.01)$ (119). Other studies have confirmed that respiratory rates at or above 30 breaths/min can be responsible for asubstantial level of intrinsic PEEP. This is primarily due to shorting in the expiratory time and gas trapping (120).

Clinically, one of the major problems is how best to evaluate alveolar recruitment at the bedside (see Ref. 121). Moreover, there is no consensus as to what level of PEEP should be used. Use of the P–V curve has been suggested to guide the clinician in setting PEEP—once the lower inflection point is known, PEEP is set at least 2 cm H_2O above that value (122). This may not necessarily be the best strategy for a variety of reasons: (i) recruitment occurs throughout the compliant portion of the P–V curve; (ii) the measurement of the static P–V curve may not reflect its dynamic variations during the ventilatory cycle; and (iii) calculating the P–V curve is logistically difficult, technically demanding and may be associated with risks to the patient. Moreover, it is a great oversimplification to assume that the lower bend in the P–V curve signals the level of PEEP necessary to prevent end-expiratory collapse and that pressures above the upper bend signal alveolar overdistension (123). The relationship between the shape of the P–V curve and events at the alveolar level is confounded by numerous factors and is the subject on ongoing research and debate. In spite of this controversy, in practice, the consensus of studies of pulmonary P–V behavior and compliance suggests the use of higher levels of PEEP than had been advocated previously. For example, a level of PEEP higher than that considered in traditional strategies (perhaps as high as 20 cm H_2O) is believed to help maintain alveolar recruitment for many patients with severe ALI/ARDS (124). Barbas et al. (125) recently stratified 53 of the patients included in the trial by Amato et al. (18) into quartiles, according to PEEP levels, and found that PEEP levels greater than 12 cm H_2O and especially greater than 16 cm H_2O improved the survival rates in this population.

Due to the absence of appropriate prospective control trials (only one level II study, and level V evidence) demonstrating the benefits of PEEP, a recent evidence-based review of ARDS gave PEEP a grade C recommendation for its use (99). Furthermore, despite encouraging preliminary data in both animals and humans, the ARDS network reported early discontinuation of the "ALVEOLI" study. This study was designed to address the use of higher PEEP levels in ARDS. All patients were ventilated using the ARDS network protocol of low tidal volume (6 mL/kg) ventilation. The groups were randomized to receive either high PEEP or low PEEP. Over 500 patients were included in the study and it was terminated early because of therapeutic futility (126); however, there were significant imbalances in age and P/F ratio that made interpretation of the data difficult.

Lung Recruitment Maneuvers

Another strategy to increase pulmonary functional residual capacity (FRC) is to use periodic LRMs. Mead and Collier (127) were the first to show in 1959 that without periodic inflations there was a progressive fall in compliance during prolonged mechanical ventilation. The idea is that intermittent inflations help maintain lung volume by preventing a progressive alveolar collapse (see Refs. 128,129) for a comprehensive physiologic review of alveolar recruitment). In the past, recruitment maneuvers was largely viewed as a method for increasing oxygenation, and reducing FiO_2. More recently, these have been seen as methods that can be used to minimize VILI, by reducing the recruitment/derecruitment cycle that is generated during tidal ventilation. Much of the literature on recruitment maneuvers focuses on their use during high frequency ventilation (HFV). Evidence of their use during CMV is limited.

A common approach to performing recruitment maneuvers involves the application of moderately increased levels of pressure (e.g., 35–50 cm H_2O) for relatively short periods of time (in the range of 15–40 sec), the goal being to open atelectatic alveoli and to stabilize them against collapsing with each respiratory cycle—thus reversing derecruitment and the deterioration in compliance (130). Shorter inspiratory times do not seem to be enough to recruit more alveolar units (131). Theoretically, once these units are open, their mechanical properties change so that they may remain open for an undetermined period of time. A key issue, however, is thatsufficient PEEP is required to maintain alveolar recruitment (132).

Animal studies appear to support the use of LRMs for the prevention of VILI (133,134). LRMs have been found to produce physiologic benefits in anesthesia-induced atelectasis (135), and in the setting of high-frequency oscillation in pediatric respiratory failure (136). Bond et al. (130) followed the respiratory system compliance in rabbits after recruitment maneuvers during conventional ventilation. This group noted an improvement in compliance with a recruitment maneuver when ventilating with low V_T (7 mL/kg), at any level of PEEP. Moreover, Engelmann et al. (26) observed significant improvements in oxygenation in 13 patients with ARDS by increasing the peak inspiratory pressure by 10 cm H_2O every 3 min to a mean pressure of 61 cm H_2O (26). Lapinsky et al. (27) observed similar improvements in oxygen saturation in seven patients with ARDS.

Complications during the procedure include transient mild oxyhemoglobin desaturation and hypotension. In a recent study in humans, the effect of a LRM on oxygenation over four hours in 12 critically ill patients with severe ALI was evaluated. In this study, Lapinsky et al. (27) individualized the inflation pressure by utilizing the lesser of (i) 45 cm H_2O, and (ii) the peak pressure at 12 mL/kg tidal volume, and maintained the inflation pressures (which varied from 30 to 45 mm H_2O) for 20 sec. In these patients, there was a modest fall in arterial oxygen saturation (SaO_2) (mean 2%) and a modest fall in blood pressure at the end of the LRM, followed by a mean rise in SaO_2 by 6% within 5 min ($p < 0.001$). In 8 of the 12 patients, this improvement lasted for at least 4 hr. In the remaining four patients, a repeat LRM increased SaO_2 again, and the effect was sustained in three patients with the use of higher PEEP (27).

Despite encouraging preliminary data, recent findings do not support the routine use of LRMs to improve oxygenation acutely in patients with ALI. Damasceno et al. (137) and Lim et al. (138) demonstrated the lack of PaO_2/lung volume improvement after the use of a variety of different strategies to recruit the lung. Meade et al. (28) confirmed these findings in 28 patients with moderate to severe ARDS. Preliminary data from this group showed that of those individuals who were randomized to the recruitment maneuver arm, five developed ventilator dysynchrony, four appeared uncomfortable, two became hypotensive and four developed pneumothoraces within 24 hr. Consequently, given the accumulating evidence indicating the lack of benefit of the maneuver and its possible side effects, the routine use of recruitment maneuvers for ARDS patients on conventional ventilators cannot be recommended. However, given the impressive animal data, and given the paucity of human data addressing LRMs, further studies are clearly needed.

Prone Positioning in ARDS

Most patients with ARDS have an increase in the partial pressure of oxygen when they are changed from the supine to the prone position. By decreasing the compressive force acting on the dorsal lung area, prone position decreases dependent pleural pressure, increases dependent transpulmonary pressure, and consequently, may recruit the dorsal lung into participating in gas exchange (138). Pappert et al. (31) confirmed the effect of prone position on lung recruitment in patients with ARDS. Using the multiple inert gas elimination technique they demonstrated that the improvement in PaO_2 in the prone position was the result of a reduction in pulmonary shunt blood flow and an increase in blood flow to regions that have normal ventilation–perfusion ratios. Other theories regarding the mechanism of improved oxygenation in the prone position include increase in end-expiratory lung volume (140) and alterations in chest wall mechanics (141).

Renewed interest in prone position for lung recruitment in ARDS has come about due to observations made by Langer et al. (142) and Gattinoni (30,143) that in some patients with ARDS, proning resulted in a decrease of CT scan densities in dorsal lung regions and improvements in oxygenation. However, studies have shown that not all patients respond with a marked increase in PaO_2 when they are placed in the prone position (144,145). Response rates in these studies range from 60 to 100%. The variation in response rates may relate to the amount of recruitable tissue or the etiology of the ARDS (146,147). In general, responders show an immediate improvement in oxygenation (within the first 10 min). Gattinoni et al. (29) recently published the results of a large (300 patients) multicenter control trial of the effects of prone position in patients with ARDS. This study showed that there was no significant difference in mortality between patients randomly assigned to placement in the prone position and those assigned to conventional treatment. One explanation for the negative result despite the improved oxygenation in the prone position arm of the study may relate to the duration of therapy. Patients were placed prone for 7.0 hr per day. Thus, patients may have been exposed to the deleterious effects of injurious ventilation the other 70% of the time each day (37). The authors also limited the study to 10 days, which may be too short a period for any significant long-term benefits to occur. Despite these discouraging results, post hoc analysis showed that placing patients in the prone position reduced mortality at day 10 in the quartile of patients who were the most ill (32). It must be emphasized that the present belief is that placing patients in the prone position is beneficial from the outcomes point of view because of its ability to decrease the effects of VILI. However, the results of the trial of Gattinoni et al. (29) underscore the need for further investigation of the role of prone positioning for longer periods of time in the most severely affected ARDS patients.

V. High Frequency Ventilation

Although no longer a "new" strategy, high frequency ventilation has recently gained much attention as a potential lung-protective strategy and currently represents an exciting and expanding area of critical care medicine. As described above, there is a substantial body of animal and human data demonstrating that recruitment of lung units and maintenance of recruited lung by an adequate PEEP is an important intervention in preventing VILI (71,77,96,136,146). However, PEEP has side effects, and herein lies the intrinsic theoretical advantage of HFV modes (112,147–149). The basic aim of HFV is to secure adequate gas exchange with small V_T—less than the anatomical dead space (V_D)—delivered at a high respiratory frequency (f); in this way it may be possible to limit the overdistention that occurs with conventional ventilation, while at the same time limiting end-expiratory collapse. HFOV appears to be well suited to the goals of lung protection. The tidal volumes used are usually very small and hence can prevent the lung from overdistention. In addition, by adjusting the bias flow rate, mean airway pressure can be set well above the alveolar closing volume. Because tidal volumes and pressure swings are small, the risk of going above or below the upper and lower inflection points are low. Moreover, with the addition of recruitment maneuvers and better gas mixing within the lung, oxygenation is often improved (102,147).

The usual approaches used to deliver mechanical ventilation attempt to approximate the normal bulk flow of gas as occurs during spontaneous respiration by delivering relatively large tidal volumes at low respiratory rates (150). Using this strategy, gas transport occurs by convection in the conducting airways, and by molecular diffusion in the alveolar region. In order for effective alveolar ventilation (V_A) to occur in this setting, V_T must exceed V_D (151).

$$[V_A = f(V_T - V_D)], \text{ when } V_T > V_D$$

Nearly 80 years ago, Henderson et al. (152) proposed the concept that adequate ventilation could be achieved with tidal volumes less than the dead space. Their observations were made based on breathing patterns of panting dogs. Their hypothesis was that during inspiration, a parabolic cone might reach all the way into the alveolar zone, hence bringing fresh gas to the alveoli—this later became known as the "Henderson spike" (153). Currently, the term HFV encompasses a number of ventilatory strategies that employ respiratory frequencies in excess of normal physiologic respiratory rates (60–3000 breaths/min), with V_T that are near or less than the anatomical dead-space. Figure 6 depicts the spectrum of ventilatory strategies based on frequency of ventilation. McCulloch et al. (136) have proposed that there are two main categories of HFV modes depending on their mechanisms of expiration (111,136): (1) HFV-passive (HFV-P), where

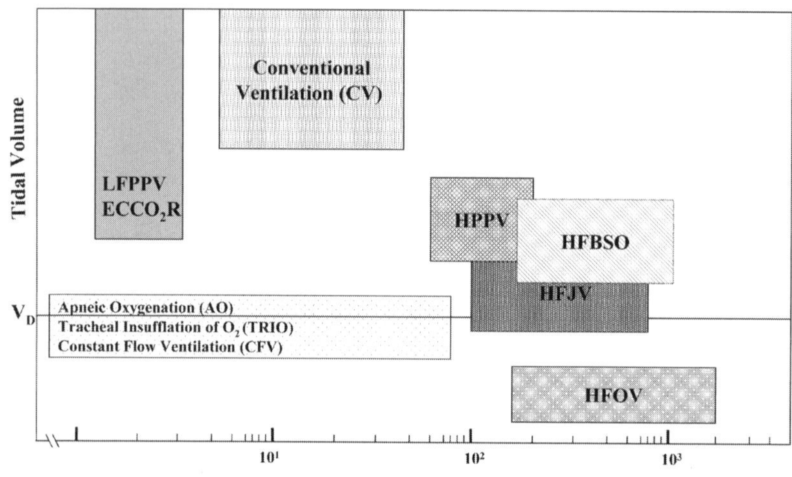

Figure 6 Schematic representation of different modes of high frequency mechanical ventilation. (Reprinted with permission from Ref. 154.)

expiration relies solely on the passive recoil of the chest wall and lung; and (2) HFV-active (HFV-A), where expiration is an active process. The HFV-P devices include those used for high-frequency positive-pressure ventilation (HFPPV) and high-frequency jet ventilation (HFJV); and high-frequency oscillation (HFO) is the mode of choice in HFV-A. Figure 6 provides an overview of HFV modes. Gas transport mechanisms in HFV are detailed further in Ref. 154.

The elegance of the HFOV setup is that it allows for "decoupling" of oxygenation and ventilation (133). Alveolar ventilation, and thus CO_2 elimination, are dependent on the frequency and V_T but are relatively independent of lung volume. In contrast, as with other types of HFV, oxygenation during HFOV is proportional to mean airway pressure and lung volume. Mean airway pressure and thus oxygenation can be manipulated by changing the flow of gas into and out of the ventilator circuit (adjusting the bias flow) (27,76). Three principal mechanisms to explain gas transport in situations in which $V_T < V_D$ have been proposed: (a) diffusion; (b) convection (direct alveolar ventilation by bulk flow, streaming, and pendelluft); and (c) augmented transport (combined effects of mechanisms 1 and 2) (for futher details see Refs. 153, 154).

Current data on HFV suggest that this ventilatory mode can both facilitate gas exchange and protect the lung from mechanical injury. In addition, as evidence of reduction in mechanical injury, a number of studies have shown a decrease in markers of inflammation (59,155,156). Kawano et al. (157) found increased neutrophil activation in animals treated with CMV rather than HFV. Imai et al. (145) demonstrated a decrease in BAL levels of several inflammatory mediators including platelet aggregating factor (PAF), thromboxane and 6-keto-prostaglandin in animals ventilated using a HFV mode. Moreover, Takata et al. (158) demonstrated that CMV was not only associated with progressive hypoxemia, decreased lung compliance, increased neutrophils in BAL fluid, and increased hyaline membrane formation, but it also led to an increase in intra-alveolar gene expression for tumor necrosis factor-alpha (TNF-α) compared to HFV. Specifically for HFV modes, current data in patients seems to support the evidence obtained in animals (8). Animal studies have also shown that the advantage of HFV over CMV becomes more apparent when mean airway pressures are kept above opening pressures (136,146,159,160).

Despite the compelling physiological evidence in support of the utility of HFV in ARDS, the advantages of this mode of ventilation have not yet been borne out in clinical trials in adults. Also, HFV has been shown to be as effective, but not superior to CMV in maintaining oxygenation and ventilation, and no mortality benefit has been observed in published adult studies to date (see Ref. 161 for a review on HFV trials). Herridge et al. (162) published a critical assessment of the clinical trial data using HFV in adults. This group identified major problems with both the physiological premises and study design of the trials currently available, which might partially explain current results. These included the fact that: (i) initial trials used low-pressure/low-volume strategies when it is now known that this strategy may worsen lung injury due to atelectrauma (163); (ii) recruitment maneuvers were rarely used (164,165); (iii) no trials used HFV as an initial ventilation strategy and it is now known that that mechanisms responsible for VILI occur within hours of initiation of mechanical ventilation (84,164); (iv) some trials used HFV as a salvage strategy; (v) sample sizes were too small and the trials were hence underpowered; (vi) trials did not agree on clinical endpoints or magnitudes of benefit; and (vii) some trials were actually case series, which provide a much lower level of evaluation.

The published clinical experience in adults includes several case series of HFOV employed as rescue therapy for patients failing CMV (35,102,166). Fort et al. (35) have published the largest study involving the use of HFOV in adults. Their results show a significant reduction in mean oxygen index (OI) [OI = inspired fraction of oxygen (FiO_2) × mean airway pressure (P_{AW}) × 100/PaO_2] and an increase in PaO_2/FiO_2 over the first 48 hr of HFOV therapy. Mortality in the HFOV group of patients was 53%. Initial OI greater than 47 and a greater number of days on CMV prior to switching to HFOV was being associated with decreased chance of survival. Although the reported mortality rate seems high in the population of patients failing CMV, exaggerated mortality rates in this group are likely. Two additional studies on HFOV have recently been published. Chiche et al. (33), in abstract form only, documented the course of 24 patients who were failing CMV and were treated with HFO using a lung recruitment strategy. The investigators divided their cohort into survivors and nonsurvivors and showed improvement in oxygenation in the survivor group. Similar to the Fort study, they found that survival was associated with a shorter time on CMV prior to initiation of HFOV. Mehta et al. (34) described 24 adult patients with severe hypoxemia who were treated with HFOV after varying periods on CMV. The P_{AW} was initially set 5 cm H_2O greater than P_{AW} during CMV, and was subsequently titrated to maintain an oxygen saturation between 88 and 93% and $FiO_2 \leq 0.6$. Investigators found improvements in OI and P/F ratio over the first seven hours and early institution of HFOV appeared to be advantageous. Derdak et al. (36) have recently completed a RCT of 148 adults. The 30-day mortality was 37% in the HFOV group and 52% in the CMV group ($p = 0.102$). Further randomized trials examining HFO in conjunction with an open lung strategy, as an early intervention in the management of ARDS are currently underway.

VI. Adjuncts to Mechanical Ventilation

Details on pharmacologic and other forms of lung injury therapy are covered in following Chapters 14–19. However, several examples are summarized here of agents and interventions utilized along with mechanical ventilation in patients with ALI/ARDS.

A. Nitric Oxide

Nitric oxide (NO) is a potent vasodilator. Inhalation of NO dilates pulmonary vessels perfusing aerated lung units, diverting blood from poorly ventilated or shunt areas. Given these properties, it has the potential to be of benefit in the treatment of severe hypoxemia and pulmonary hypertension in ALI/ARDS patients (167). These properties could allow for a more protective ventilatory strategy, reduction in FiO_2, potentially leading to a reduction in VILI. Rossaint et al.'s initial description (37) of a reduction in venous admixture in nine patients with ARDS was very promising.

In the pediatric literature, NO has been shown to reduce the need for extracorporeal membrane oxygenation (ECMO) in both persistent pulmonary hypertension of the newborn and respiratory failure of the newborn (168,169). In contrast, three prospective randomized trials were not able to show a survival benefit or a reduction in the duration of mechanical ventilation with iNO therapy (38–40). Dellinger et al. (38) studied 177 patients with ARDS who were randomized to placebo or one of five doses of inhaled NO (iNO). Despite initial improvement in venous admixture in the iNO group, no mortality benefits were observed after 72 hr compared to placebo. Moreover, only 60% of the patients in the iNO group responded to the therapy (defined as a >20% increase in PaO_2). Surprisingly, 25% of the patients had a positive response to the placebo. Lundin et al. (41) performed a large randomized multicenter control trial enrolling only patients who had ARDS and who responded acutely to iNO. A total of 180 patients were randomized to either iNO or placebo. There was no difference neither in 30-day mortality (40% in controls and 44% for iNO), nor did iNO significantly reverse ALI. Analysis of the data from this trial did suggest that the likelihood of developing severe ARDS was smaller in the iNO group ($p < 0.05$). The validity of this study is restricted because of major changes in study design after the inclusion of the first 40 patients, and discontinuation after 268 patients. The results of a further prospective randomized controlled clinical trial have been published only in abstract form (42).

At present, most ICUs use iNO in patients with refractory hypoxemia and who are in extremis, although there is no current evidence to support the use of iNO as "salvage" therapy. Dupont et al. (43) recently performed a 2-year multicenter retrospective analysis of all consecutive ARDS patients in whom iNO was tried to determine if the response to iNO as salvage therapy was an independent factor for survival. This group found that the efficacy of iNO in improving oxygenation was moderate and difficult to predict, response to NO inhalation was not associated with prognosis, and treatment of ARDS with iNO did not influence intensive care unit survival.

One possible explanation for the failure of recent studies to demonstrate a mortality benefit with iNO—despite clear evidence of improved physiological parameters—is that NO has no effect on the underlying pathophysiology driving the acute respiratory inflammatory reaction. Cuthbertson et al. (170) randomized 32 ARDS patients who were responsive to iNO (increase in their PaO_2/FiO_2 ratio $\geq 25\%$) to receive mechanical ventilation with or without iNO. Patients were followed for 30 days or until death, and BAL was performed at 0, 24, and 72 hr. Nitric oxide activity was measured spectrophotometrically, and myeloperoxidase, elastase, interleukin-8, and leukotrienes were measured in the BAL fluid by enzyme immunoassay. Nitric oxide synthase activity decreased significantly and total nitrite increased in patients on iNO. Other markers of inflammation in BAL fluid did not change, suggesting that iNO has no effect on several markers of the inflammatory response. It is also important to note that addressing hypoxemia may not necessarily improve outcome. In fact, in the ARDS/Net trial the higher tidal volume group (that had a higher mortality rate) had higher PaO_2/FiO_2 ratios in the first few days of treatment (1).

Recent evidence suggests that there may be a potential role for iNO as an adjunct to other therapies for ARDS in those patients with right heart impairment. Rialp et al. (171) studied eight primary and seven secondary ARDS patients and compared their response to iNO. This group found that only the patients who had primarily pulmonary cause for their ARDS responded to iNO. This study was not designed to look at morbidity and mortality outcomes. Although prospective randomized clinical trials have shown a benefit of inhaled NO in the pediatric population (168,169), differences in the origin of hypoxic failure and in the neonatal circulation means this data cannot be extrapolated to adults. Consequently, since all level I studies show a lack of positive effects on either mortality or other relevant clinical outcome measures (grade A), iNO cannot be recommended for routine use in adults with ARDS. However, because of the grade II physiological data indicating that inhaled NO can improve oxygenation parameters and reduce the need for extracorporeal membrane oxygenation, the Cochrane library has given iNO a grade C recommendation for use in potentially life threatening hypoxemia (172).

B. Surfactant

Surfactant function is grossly altered in patients with ALI/ARDS (173) (see Chapters 9 and 15 for details). The composition of both surfactant phospholipids and associated proteins can be affected by injury to type II pneumocytes, and the surface activity of alveolar surfactant can be greatly decreased by interactions with plasma proteins or other inhibitory substances in edema fluid. Other injury-induced substances like phospholipases, oxygen radicals, and peroxinitrates can interact chemically with lung surfactant and impair its activity. In addition to effects on surface activity, changes in surfactant proteins (SP)-A and D during lung injury can compromise their important host-defense activites (174). Finally, the proportion of less active small surfactant aggregates (SA) is markedly increased over superior functioning large aggregates (LA) in lung injury. The surface tension-lowering ability of surfactant recovered from the BAL fluid of patients with ARDS has been shown to be markedly reduced.

Ventilation therapy is directly relevant to some of the factors affecting surfactant dysfunction in lung injury. When patients are mechanically ventilated, the levels of PEEP and tidal volume utilized determine alveolar surface area. Ventilator strategies that allow for smaller changes in alveolar surface area, for example, tend to preserve surfactant in its LA form. In addition, ventilator strategies that reduce permeability injury to the alveolar endothelial/epithelial barrier can decrease high molecular weight pulmonary edema and its content of inhibitory proteins. Also, by reducing inflammation associated with VILI, protective ventilation strategies decrease the production of inflammatory substances (reactive oxygen and nitrogen species, lytic phospholipases and proteases) that can interact with and alter lung surfactant components.

Exogenous surfactant therapy is a proven and life saving intervention in premature infants with the respiratory distress syndrome (RDS) and in term neonates with ALI/ARDS from meconium aspiration (Chapter 15). Despite encouraging animal experiments and positive initial human trials, only three large randomized clinical trials have evaluated the use of exogenous surfactant in adults with ARDS. The first, and largest with 725 patients, involved a synthetic preparation (Exosurf) that does not contain any surfactant-associated protein. This aerosolized preparation did not decrease mortality in adults with sepsis-associated ARDS (46). A second study using a natural bovine surfactant preparation (Survanta), which contains SP-C but has very low amounts of SP-B, showed more promising results (47). This preparation was instilled intratracheally and improved outcome in the study group. In a recent small phase II clinical trial, a recombinant SP-C based surfactant (Venticute) instilled tracheally was associated with an increase in ventilator-free days and decrease in mortality (48). However, the results of a larger phase III trial evaluating this surfactant in patients with ARDS has been reported at scientific meetings and has shown no benefit (47).

The variable outcomes in current surfactant trials in adults with ARDS relate, at least in part, to the surfactant preparations and delivery modes used. The relative activity of lung surfactant drugs varies significantly, particularly in basic science assessments, and many of the most active available exogenous surfactants have not been evaluated in adults with ALI/ARDS (Chapter 15). In order to be effective in treating ALI/ARDS, exogenous surfactants need to have the highest possible activity and resistance to dysfunction. Exosurf, for example, has much lower surface activity in vitro and less physiological activity compared to animal-derived preparations of native surfactant lipids and hydrophobic proteins. In addition to activity issues, the delivery of adequate amounts of exogenous surfactant to injured, inflamed lungs in ALI/ARDS is challenging. In the Exosurf study (46), only a very small proportion of the aerosolized surfactant actually reached the alveoli. Even when instilled intratracheally, exogenous surfactant may distribute unevenly to less injured areas in patients with nonuniform lung injury. The timing and dosage of administered exogenous surfactant may also strongly influence patient responses. Modes of mechanical ventilation that preserve adequate lung recruitment tend to conserve exogenous surfactant in an intact form and are associated with a prolonged duration of response (175).

C. Partial Liquid Ventilation

Partial liquid ventilation (PLV), in which conventional gas ventilation is superimposed on lungs partially filled with liquid perfluorocarbon, is an interesting adjunctive strategy during mechanical ventilatory support for ARDS patients. In 1966, Clark and Gollan (176) introduced the concept that lungs could be ventilated using organic liquids. Subsequently, Kylstra et al. (177) described the first successful maintenance of a dog in a hyperbaric chamber using normal saline as the ventilating fluid. Since then, the introduction of perfluorocarbons as oxygen carrying liquids has made liquid ventilation a feasible option in patients with ARDS. Perfluorocarbons have a high oxygen carrying capacity (about 50/100 mL) (178). The first demonstration that PLV was able to maintain gas exchange in animals was documented by Fuhrman et al. (179). Although total liquid ventilation (TLV) may one day indeed become a clinical reality, most of the recent effort has been focused on developing the technique of PLV. The rationale for using PLV includes enhancing lung recruitment, improving gas exchange and lung compliance and minimizing VILI. In addition PLV is much easier to apply than TLV.

Animal studies of PLV have shown improvements in gas exchange (180–184), with concomitant reduction in intrapulmonary shunt fraction (181–184), enhancement in pulmonary compliance (180–183), increase in end-expiratory lung volumes (185), and reduction in morphometric and histologic evidence of lung injury (182). Also, PLV may alter lung perfusion patterns (183). Consequently, PLV may exert its putative beneficial effects by improving recruitment of consolidated and atelectatic dependent alveoli, thus reducing shunt and improving ventilation–perfusion mismatch. In addition, some perfluorocarbons may attenuate increases in pulmonary capillary permeability (186) and limit lung water accumulation (164). Recent studies have reported a reduction in proinflammatory markers in PLV treated lungs (184,187,188).

Clinical experience with PLV has not echoed the encouraging results seen in animal experiments (51,52). Phase I/II trials have been performed to assess the safety and efficacy of PLV in children, preterm infants, full-term newborns with respiratory failure (52–54), and adults with ARDS (55). Most recently, the adult PLV study group published the results of a pilot study to further evaluate the safety and potential efficacy of PVL in adults with ARDS (56). This was a prospective, nonblinded, controlled, randomized study carried out in 18 centers comparing a CMV strategy with PLV. Ninety patients with ARDS were enrolled in the study. The major finding of this study was a reduction in progression of ARDS in the PLV group. No differences in gas exchange, pulmonary function, ventilator-free days, or outcomes were observed. However, subgroup analysis showed that, in patients who were 55 years of age or less, discontinuation of mechanical ventilation occurred more rapidly and there was a trend toward an increase in the 28-day ventilator-free days in the PLV group when compared to the CMV group.

Amongst the adverse events, included were increased in incidence of hypoxia, bradycardia, and respiratory acidosis (56). The same group had previously shown that in adults, no improvement in pulmonary compliance could be documented (55). Other adverse events included decrease in cardiac output, hypotension, hyperbilirubinemia, pneumothorax, dyspnea, and rash (55). In the most recent study by Hirschl et al. (56) no difference in the P/F ratio was detected between the PLV and the CMV study group. The investigators did not find differences in other parameters of gas exchange, ventilation, or pulmonary function. However, the V_T in the study ranged from 4.1–16.1 mL/kg (mean = 8.4–9.8 mL/kg across all time points) in patients in the CMV group and 3.1–17.9 mL/kg of predicted body weight (mean 9.1–10.9 mL/kg across all time points) in patients in the PLV group. No attempt to control V_T or end inspiratory pressure (EIP) was made except that EIP was maintained below 45 cm H_2O. No between-group differences in EIP and V_T were noted. Average PEEP in both groups was about 11 and the average $PaCO_2$ was 45 in the CMV group and 39 in the PVL group. This study was conducted between July 1995 and August of 1996, and the strategies used reflect the evidence available 6–7 years ago. Future studies will likely incorporate low-volume ventilation strategies, as well as open lung approaches to the use of PLV. A large randomized clinical trial comparing PLV with two doses of liquid to a conventional strategy was recently reported at the ATS meeting. In this study, the PLV group had no better outcome than the control group (American Thoracic Society Meeting, Atlanta, GA, U.S.A. 2002, Ref. 189); this study however, has not yet been published.

D. Extracorporeal Membrane Oxygenation

In 1885 Von Frey and Gruber (190) published the first report of a device to oxygenate blood extracorporally for perfusion of isolated organs. Subsequently, the development of heart–lung machines for open-heart surgery was the major impetus for the development of "membrane oxygenators" (191). Impro-vement in membranes permitted successful application of ECMO in adults. In 1972, Hill et al. (192) reported the survival of a 24-year old polytraumatized patient with ARDS who had been treated with ECMO during the acute phase of the disease. Subsequently, Bartlett et al. (193) reported the first newborn treated with ECMO who survived. The first RCT exploring the use of ECMO for the treatment of severe ARDS was published in 1979 (194). This study tested venoarterial ECMO vs. conventional therapy in adults with severe ARDS. The mortality rates documented were as high as 90% and not significantly different from those in the conventional group. The major problem with this strategy was bleeding secondary to coagulopathy.

The idea that ECMO could be used as a protective ventilatory strategy was introduced by Kolobow et al. (195). This group reasoned that this technique could be used to prevent further damage to the diseased lungs by reducing their motion (pulmonary rest). This could be achieved by the application of only a few ventilator breaths with low V_T and low peak inspiratory pressures. In this technique of low frequency positive pressure ventilation (LFPPV), oxygenation was achieved through a nearly motionless lung via apneic oxygenation, and carbon dioxide was cleared through the artificial lung—extracorporeal carbon dioxide removal ($ECCO_2$-R). Because gas exchange could be achieved using low extracorporeal blood flows (20–30% of cardiac output), venovenous bypass techniques, instead of arteriovenous ones could be used. Therefore, less side effects in terms of coagulopathy and detriment to red blood cells occurred. Using this technique, Gattinoni et al. (49) reported survival rates of up to 49% in adults with severe ARDS.

Encouraging results led to a RCT. In 1994, Morris et al. (50) reported the results of an RCT comparing $ECCO_2$-R and pressure-controlled inverse ratio ventilation (pcCMV-IRV) for the treatment of severe ARDS. In this study, computerized protocols generated around-the-clock instructions for management of ventilatory parameters to assure equivalent intensity of care for patients randomized to the new therapy limb and those randomized to the control, mechanical ventilation limb. Forty patients with severe ARDS who met the ECMO entry criteria were randomized. The main outcome measure was survival at 30 days after randomization. Survival was not significantly different in the 19 mechanical ventilation (42%) and 21 new therapy (extracorporeal) (33%) patients ($p = 0.8$). All deaths occurred within 30 days of randomization. Overall patient survival was 38% (15 of 40) and was about four times that expected from historical data ($p = 0.0002$). Extracorporeal treatment group survival was not significantly different from other published survival rates after extracorporeal CO_2 removal. The mechanical ventilation patient group survival was significantly higher than the 12% derived from published data ($p = 0.0001$). In the study, the protocol controlled care 86% of the time. Intensity of care required to maintain arterial oxygenation was similar in both groups (2.6 and 2.6 PEEP changes/day; 4.3 and 5.0 FiO_2 changes/day). This group concluded that there was no significant difference in survival between the mechanical ventilation and the extracorporeal CO_2 removal groups, and that extracorporeal support, as a therapy for ARDS, could not be recommended (50).

Several explanations have been offered to clarify why Morris's trial did not result in better survival rates in the ECMO group. Habashi et al. (196) pointed out that the ventilatory management in the ECMO group was not uniform and may have altered patient outcome. The first half of the patients had peak airway pressures controlled while the in the latter half, tidal volumes were controlled. In fact, peak inspiratory pressures were higher than the recommended maximum in both groups, suggesting that significant VILI may have contributed to the poor outcome in this study (197). Moreover, the ECMO methodology used in Morris's trial may not have been optimized and may not have reflected modern standards of practice (198,199). The unusually high blood loss complication rate associated with the ECMO therapy was considered to be an indication of an out-dated strategy without heparin-coated equipment. The use of new heparinized tubings and membrane oxygenators that limit the bleeding complications from ECMO enable the use of this technique for patients in extremis. European working groups have collected data from more than 850 adult ARDS patients treated with ECMO and observed a survival rate greater than 50% (200). Despite the fact that 2 RCTs failed to show an advantage of ECMO over conventional strategies, the improved ECMO strategies, with advanced protocols like the ones used by European groups, may show promise.

VII. Caveats: The Concept of Primary vs. Secondary ARDS

The American–European consensus conference defined two pathogenic processes leading to ARDS: a *direct* ("primary" or "pulmonary") insult that directly affects lung parenchyma and an *indirect* ("secondary" or "extrapulmonary") insult that results from an acute systemic inflammatory reaction (201) (Fig. 7). This distinction has been supported by the study of Gattinoni

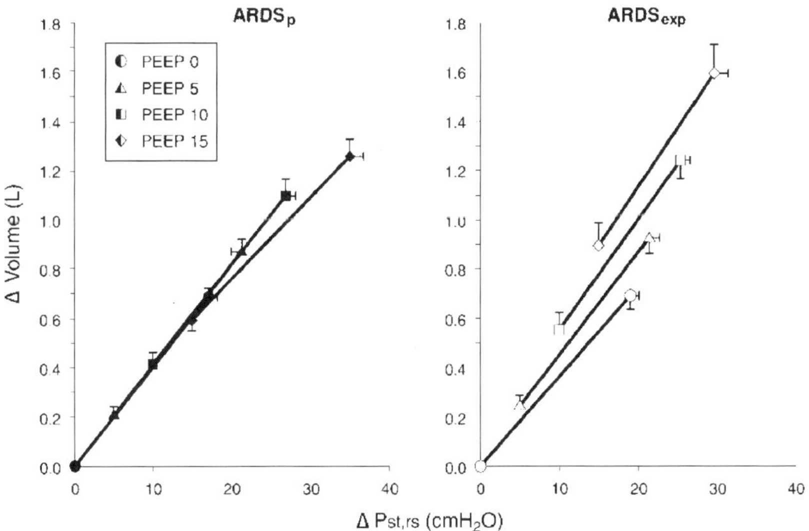

Figure 7 Pressure–volume (P–V) relationships as a function of PEEP in patients with ARDS caused by pulmonary and extrapulmonary disease. (Group 1, left panel) patients with ARDS secondary to pulmonary disease. (Group 2, right panel) patients with ARDS in association with extrapulmonary disease. As shown, in Group 1, the P–V relationships follow systematically the same line, with a slope decreasing at 15 cm H$_2$O (i.e., decreased compliance), whereas the P–V relationships of Group 2 patients are shifted upwards as a function of PEEP (i.e., at the same pressure of volume is greater at higher PEEP, suggesting recruitment). The slope of P–V relationship increases with PEEP, indicating the compliance improvement. Data are presented as mean ± standard error. (Reprinted from Ref. 164.)

et al. (118) reporting differences in the underlying pathology, respiratory mechanics, and response to PEEP in patients with ARDS in the context of the primary and secondary forms of this syndrome (118). In terms of pathophysiology, the current hypothesis is that a direct insult would primarily affect the pulmonary epithelium, causing activation of macrophages and subsequently the inflammatory network. Conversely, in the case of an indirect stimulus, endothelial damage predominates. Changes in the integrity of the endothelial cell membrane cause vasoactive pulmonary edema and consolidation with the generation of an inflammatory response. This putative difference in injury mechanisms may explain some of the differences reported for primary and secondary ARDS. However, it should also be noted that not all studies find differences between primary and secondary ARDS, and that in many cases it is difficult to definitively distinguish between these two conditions in patients.

The most important consequence of different respiratory mechanics in intrapulmonary vs. extrapulmonary ARDS would be that applied airway pressure (i.e., distending pressure) may need to be higher in intrapulmonary compared to extrapulmonary ARDS. Moreover, the potential for alveolar recruitment may be greater in extrapulmonary causes of ARDS. It this were the case, the beneficial effects of recruitment maneuvers (with a given airway pressure) in improving oxygenation would be greater in the secondary ARDS group, since these patients would be more likely to attain a transpulmonary pressure sufficient for lung opening.

These observations seem to be supported by at least some animal experiments. For example, Kloot et al. (202) compared three different experimental models of lung injury during recruitment maneuvers, and found that greater alveolar recruitment occurred in models of secondary ARDS compared to primary ARDS. However, Puybasset et al. (203) found a similar response to PEEP in alveolar recruitment and oxygenation in patients with intrapulmonary or extrapulmonary ARDS. This finding could be explained by the existence of specific differences in the study population and/or the ventilatory and clinical management utilized. Another explanation is that results in the clinical study may include confounding effects from coexisting insults, i.e., direct injury to the lungs (for example pneumonia) and secondary inflammatory mediator induced injury from an extrapulmonary stimulus (for example sepsis).

Two recent trials have attempted to divide patients according to the etiology of their ARDS. Rialp et al. (171) studied eight primary and seven secondary ARDS patients and their response to NO and prone position. Lim et al. (204) examined at 31 primary and 16 secondary ARDS patients and their response to the prone position. Both studies confirmed that primary pulmonary ARDS patients do not respond to recruitment maneuvers as markedly (but they have a more pronounced response to NO). Desai et al. (205) have attempted to reproduce Gattinoni's findings that primary and secondary ARDS have different CT scan patterns. They observed that the typical appearances on CT were independent of the cause of ARDS (odds ratio, 8.9; 95% CI 1.8, 44.2; $p < 0.01$). Foci of nondependent intense parenchymal opacification were more extensive in primary ARDS rather than secondary ARDS, but this finding was ascribable to differences in time to CT (after intubation) between pulmonary and extrapulmonary ARDS. They concluded that the differentiation between primary and secondary ARDS can, with some caveats, be based on whether the CT appearances are typical or atypical of ARDS, but not on any individual CT pattern in isolation.

To understand whether clinically differentiating primary vs. secondary ARDS made a difference in terms of the ventilatory strategy of choice, Eisner et al. (206) examined the relative efficacy of low V_T mechanical ventilation among 902 patients with different clinical risk factors for ALI/ARDS who participated in ARDS network randomized controlled trials. This group found that the clinical risk factor for ALI/ARDS was associated with substantial variation in mortality. Despite these differences in mortality, there was no evidence that the efficacy of the low V_T strategy varied by clinical risk factor ($p = 0.76$, for interaction between ventilator group and risk factor). Visual inspection of the data suggested that only individuals with ARDS secondary to aspiration may not have benefited from low tidal volume ventilation (this was not statistically significant). There was also no evidence of differential efficacy of low V_T ventilation in the other study outcomes: proportion of patients achieving unassisted breathing, ventilator-free days, or development of nonpulmonary organ failure. Controlling for demographic and clinical covariates did not appreciably affect these results. After reclassifying the clinical risk factors as pulmonary vs. nonpulmonary predisposing conditions, and infection-related vs. noninfection-related conditions, there was still no evidence that the efficacy of low V_T ventilation differed among clinical risk factor subgroups. They thus concluded that, there was no evidence that the efficacy of the low V_T ventilation strategy differed among clinical risk factor subgroups for ALI/ARDS. However, the study was not designed or powered to detect a difference between primary or secondary ARDS. Given the methodological concerns, the more clinically relevant question is what is the likelihood that this strategy would benefit any ARDS patient. Using Bayesian subset analysis, it was calculated that there was a 75% chance that this strategy would benefit patients in different ARDS risk factor groups.

VIII. Summary

Effective ventilation strategies for the management of patients with ALI/ARDS begin with the recognition and understanding of the concept of VILI. The existence of this phenomenon was apparent in the early finding that high levels of PEEP resulted in a high incidence of pneumothoraces (barotrauma) (207). Twenty-five years of subsequent research in animal models of lung injury, coupled with clinical trials in lung-injured patients, greatly enhanced understanding about the importance of VILI. This work culminated in the year 2000 with the first successful large trial of protective low tidal volume ventilation in patients with ALI/ARDS (1). A remarkable finding of this trial, and of another related clinical study (2,111), was that protective ventilation strategies were associated with reduced markers of inflammation, including proinflammatory cytokines. This association between reduced inflammation and improved patient outcomes (e.g., mortality) was more apparent than traditional parameters used to judge the efficacy of ventilation strategies such as oxygenation and pulmonary mechanics. The finding that protective ventilation strategies reduce or attenuate pulmonary inflammation supports the notion that *biotrauma* (as opposed to barotrauma alone) is important in determining ultimate outcomes in ventilated patients with ALI/ARDS.

Prior to the emergence of the biotrauma hypothesis, barotrauma, volutrauma and atelectrauma were considered the principal causes of VILI. Uhlig (208) has recently suggested that there are four principal mechanisms that can promote VILI: (1) ventilation, especially with high ventilation pressures with zero PEEP, can cause stress failure of cell membranes and damage the pulmonary epithelial and endothelial barriers. The resulting cellular injury and necrosis leads to the liberation of inflammatory mediators that stimulate intact cells to produce additional inflammation; (2) stress failure and epithelial/endothelial cell injury not only increases local inflammatory mediator production, but also causes loss of compartmentalization with spread of inflammatory mediators and bacteria throughout the body; (3) less injurious ventilation strategies that do not cause frank tissue destruction can also elicit the release of mediators, by activation of stretch-stimulated signaling cascades (mechanotransduction); and (4) ventilation with increasing positive airway pressures raises intravascular pressures in the pulmonary circulation and increases vascular shear stress, both of which are known stimuli affecting endothelial cells and altering their function. In the clinical setting, all of these forces may coexist and interact in producing VILI.

In addition to the important roles of ventilation-associated mechanical forces on inflammatory lung injury and patient outcomes, clinical studies in ALI/ARDS are subject to a multitude of unrelated variables. Specific ventilatory strategies are assessed in the context of these multiple determinants of disease, making it more difficult to isolate the efficacy of ventilation therapy alone. The multifactorial etiologies of ALI/ARDS, the heterogeneity of the affected patients, and the broad variations in supportive care used in critically ill patients, are additional possible confounders in clinical studies. To date, lung protective ventilation strategies that may be beneficial in patients with ALI/ARDS include:

1. Limiting pulmonary overdistension through the use of low tidal volumes and end-inspiratory volumes during ventilation;
2. Allowing for hypercapnic acidosis during ventilation (permissive hypercapnia); and
3. Minimizing FRC by relying on lung re-expansion strategies, primarily increasing PEEP, LRM and HFO (with somewhat less evidence for these compared to the above).

Other agents and interventions are also used as adjuncts to mechanical ventilation therapy in patients with ALI/ARDS. Examples described in this chapter that are under discussion for use in ALI/ARDS include iNO, surfactant replacement, ECMO, and PLV. The latter may become more important if and when gene therapy becomes available for ALI, since it could also have utility as a system for gene delivery. The efficacy of ECMO, particularly in adults with ALI/ARDS, remains unclear. The severity of side effects combined with minimal evidence in support of improved efficacy has limited the interest of clinical intensivists in this strategy. Nevertheless, if vascular side effects can be abrogated with newer technology, there may be a resurgence of interest in this technique for the most severe cases of ARDS. A variety of additional therapeutic interventions for ALI/ARDS are detailed in Chapters 14–19.

The optimization of ventilation therapies for ALI/ARDS is an ongoing process. This area of clinical medicine is now being entered by molecular and cell biologists, and a new comprehension of its problems and solutions is arising. Studies of population genetics and disease susceptibility will most certainly lead to attempts to individualize ventilation therapy and management in the future. Moreover, the use of polydimensional approaches in critical care medicine, coupled with technological advances and improved basic science understanding of the pathophysiology of ALI/ARDS, will also affect the role of the mechanical ventilator in the future. How all the pieces of the puzzle will ultimately fit together in terms of therapeutic development is unclear. However, the ventilator is likely to remain for many years an integral part of the life support provided to patients with ALI/ARDS, and understanding how best to use this technology to improve patient survival with minimal associated lung injury will remain crucial for clinicians and basic science investigators.

References

1. The Acute Respiratory Distress Syndrome Network. Ventilation with lower tidal volumes as compared with traditional tidal volumes for acute lung injury and the acute respiratory distress syndrome. N Engl J Med 2000; 342(18):1301–1308.
2. Ranieri VM, Suter PM, Tortorella C, De Tullio R, Dayer JM, Brienza A, et al. Effect of mechanical ventilation on inflammatory mediators in patients with

acute respiratory distress syndrome: a randomized controlled trial. JAMA 1999; 282(1):54–61.

3. Ashbaugh DG, Bigelow DB, Petty TL, Levine BE. Acute respiratory distress in adults. Lancet 1967; 2(7511):319–323.

4. Dreyfuss D, Saumon G. Ventilator-induced lung injury: lessons from experimental studies. Am J Respir Crit Care Med 1998; 157(1):294–323.

5. Slutsky AS. Lung injury caused by mechanical ventilation. Chest 1999; 116(suppl 1):9S–15S.

6. Ware LB, Matthay MA. The acute respiratory distress syndrome. N Engl J Med 2000; 342(18):1334–1349.

7. Montgomery AB, Stager MA, Carrico CJ, Hudson LD. Causes of mortality in patients with the adult respiratory distress syndrome. Am Rev Respir Dis 1985; 132(3):485–489.

8. Tremblay Lorraine N, Slutsky Arthur S. Ventilator-induced injury: from Barotrauma to Biotrauma. Proc Assoc Am Phys 1998; 110(6):482–488.

9. Dreyfuss D, Saumon G. From ventilator-induced lung injury to multiple organ dysfunction? Intensive Care Med 1998; 24(2):102–104.

10. Dreyfuss D, Soler P, Saumon G. Mechanical ventilation-induced pulmonary edema. Interaction with previous lung alterations. Am J Respir Crit Care Med 1995; 151(5):1568–1575.

11. Hickling KG, Henderson SJ, Jackson R. Low mortality associated with low volume pressure limited ventilation with permissive hypercapnia in severe adult respiratory distress syndrome. Intensive Care Med 1990; 16(6): 372–377.

12. Antonelli M, Conti G, Rocco M, Bufi M, De Blasi RA, Vivino G, et al. A comparison of noninvasive positive-pressure ventilation and conventional mechanical ventilation in patients with acute respiratory failure. N Engl J Med 1998; 339(7):429–435.

13. Brochard L, Mancebo J, Wysocki M, Lofaso F, Conti G, Rauss A, et al. Noninvasive ventilation for acute exacerbations of chronic obstructive pulmonary disease. N Engl J Med 1995; 333(13):817–822.

14. Confalonieri M, Potena A, Carbone G, Porta RD, Tolley EA, Umberto MG. Acute respiratory failure in patients with severe community-acquired pneumonia. A prospective randomized evaluation of noninvasive ventilation. Am J Respir Crit Care Med 1999; 160(5 Pt 1):1585–1591.

15. Younes M, Puddy A, Roberts D, Light RB, Quesada A, Taylor K, et al. Proportional assist ventilation. Results of an initial clinical trial. Am Rev Respir Dis 1992; 145(1):121–129.

16. Younes M. Proportional assist ventilation, a new approach to ventilatory support theory. Am Rev Respir Dis 1992; 145(1):114–120.

17. Stewart TE, Meade MO, Cook DJ, Granton JT, Hodder RV, Lapinsky SE, et al. Evaluation of a ventilation strategy to prevent barotrauma in patients at high risk for acute respiratory distress syndrome. Pressure and volume-limited ventilation strategy group. N Engl J Med 1998; 338(6):355–361.

18. Amato MB, Barbas CS, Medeiros DM, Magaldi RB, Schettino GP, Lorenzi-Filho G, et al. Effect of a protective-ventilation strategy on mortality in the acute respiratory distress syndrome. N Engl J Med 1998; 338(6):347–354.

19. Brower RG, Shanholtz CB, Fessler HE, Shade DM, White P Jr, Wiener CM, et al. Prospective, randomized, controlled clinical trial comparing traditional vs. reduced tidal volume ventilation in acute respiratory distress syndrome patients. Crit Care Med 1999; 27:1492–1498.

20. Brochard L, Roudot-Thoraval F, Roupie E, Delclaux C, Chastre J, Fernandez-Mondejar E, et al. Tidal volume reduction for prevention of ventilator-induced lung injury in acute respiratory distress syndrome. The multicenter trail group on tidal volume reduction in ARDS. Am J Respir Crit Care Med 1998; 158(6):1831–1838.

21. Weisman IM, Rinaldo JE, Rogers RM. Current concepts: positive end-expiratory pressure in adult respiratory failure. N Engl J Med 1982; 307(22):1381–1384.

22. Pepe PE, Hudson LD, Carrico CJ. Early application of positive end-expiratory pressure in patients at risk for the adult respiratory-distress syndrome. N Engl J Med 1984; 311(5):281–286.

23. Weigelt JA, Mitchell RA, Snyder WH III. Early positive end-expiratory pressure in the adult respiratory distress syndrome. Arch Surg 1979; 114(4):497–501.

24. Pelosi P, Cadringher P, Bottino N, Panigada M, Carrieri F, Riva E, et al. Sigh in acute respiratory distress syndrome. Am J Respir Crit Care Med 1999; 159(3):872–880.

25. Hickling KG. The pressure–volume curve is greatly modified by recruitment. A mathematical model of ARDS lungs. Am J Respir Crit Care Med 1998; 158(1):194–202.

26. Engelmann L, Lachmann B, Petros S, Bohm S, Pilz U. ARDS: dramatic rise in arterial PO_2 with the "open lung" approach. Crit Care 1997(suppl):P54.

27. Lapinsky SE, Aubin M, Mehta S, Boiteau P, Slutsky AS. Safety and efficacy of a sustained inflation for alveolar recruitment in adults with respiratory failure. Intensive Care Med 1999; 25(11):1297–1301.

28. Meade MO, Guyatt GH, Cook DJ, Lapinsky SE, Hand L, Griffith L, et al. Physiologic randomized pilot study of a lung recruitment maneuver in acute lung injury. Am J Respir Crit Care Med 2002; 165(8):A683.

29. Gattinoni L, Tognoni G, Pesenti A, Taccone P, Mascheroni D, Labarta V, et al. Effect of prone positioning on the survival of patients with acute respiratory failure. N Engl J Med 2001; 345(8):568–573.

30. Gattinoni L, Pelosi P, Vitale G, Pesenti A, D'Andrea L, Mascheroni D. Body position changes redistribute lung computed-tomographic density in patients with acute respi-ratory failure. Anesthesiology 1991; 74(1):15–23.

31. Pappert D, Rossaint R, Slama K, Gruning T, Falke KJ. Influence of positioning on ventilation–perfusion relationships in severe adult respiratory distress syndrome. Chest 1994; 106(5):1511–1516.

32. Slutsky AS. The acute respiratory distress syndrome, mechanical ventilation, and the prone position. N Engl J Med 2001; 345(8):610–612.

33. Chiche JD, Boukef R, Laurent I, et al. High-frequency oscillatory ventilation (HFOV) improves oxygenation in patients with severe ARDS. Am J Respir Crit Care Med 2000; 161:A48.

34. Mehta S, Lapinsky SE, Hallett DC, Merker D, Groll RJ, Cooper AB, et al. Prospective trial of high-frequency oscillation in adults with acute respiratory distress syndrome. Crit Care Med 2001; 29(7):1360–1369.

35. Fort P, Farmer C, Westerman J, Johannigman J, Beninati W, Dolan S, et al. High-frequency oscillatory ventilation for adult respiratory distress syndrome—a pilot study. Crit Care Med 1997; 25(6):937–947.

36. Derdak S, Mehta S, Stewart TE, Smith T, Rogers M, Buchman TG, et al. Multicenter oscillatory ventilation for acute respiratory distress syndrome trial (MOAT) study investigators. High-frequency oscillatory ventilation for acute respiratory distress syndrome in adults: a randomized, controlled trial. Am J Respir Crit Care Med 2002; 166(6):801–808.

37. Rossaint R, Falke KJ, Lopez F, Slama K, Pison U, Zapol WM. Inhaled nitric oxide for the adult respiratory distress syndrome. N Engl J Med 1993; 328(6):399–405.

38. Dellinger RP, Zimmerman JL, Taylor RW, Straube RC, Hauser DL, Criner GJ, et al. Effects of inhaled nitric oxide in patients with acute respiratory distress syndrome: results of a randomized phase II trial. Inhaled nitric oxide in ARDS study group. Crit Care Med 1998; 26(1):15–23.

39. Michael JR, Barton RG, Saffle JR, Mone M, Markewitz BA, Hillier K, et al. Inhaled nitric oxide vs. conventional therapy: effect on oxygenation in ARDS. Am J Respir Crit Care Med 1998; 157(5 Pt 1):1372–1380.

40. Troncy E, Collet JP, Shapiro S, Guimond JG, Blair L, Ducruet T, et al. Inhaled nitric oxide in acute respiratory distress syndrome: a pilot randomized controlled study. Am J Respir Crit Care Med 1998; 157(5 Pt 1):1483–1488.

41. Lundin S, Mang H, Smithies M, Stenqvist O, Frostell C. Inhalation of nitric oxide in acute lung injury: results of a European multicentre study. The European study group of inhaled nitric oxide. Intensive Care Med 1999; 25(9):911–919.

42. Group d'Etude sur le NO inhale au cours de l'ARDS. Inhaled NO in ARDS: presentation of a double blind randomized multicentric study. Am J Respir Crit Care Med 1996; 153:A590.

43. Dupont H, Le Corre F, Fierobe L, Cheval C, Moine P, Timsit JF. Efficiency of inhaled nitric oxide as rescue therapy during severe ARDS: survival and factors associated with the first response. J Crit Care 1999; 14(3):107–113.

44. Cole AG, Weller SF, Sykes MK. Inverse ratio ventilation compared with PEEP in adult respiratory failure. Intensive Care Med 1984; 10(5): 227–232.

45. Shanholtz C, Brower R. Should inverse ratio ventilation be used in adult respiratory distress syndrome? Am J Respir Crit Care Med 1994; 149(5): 1354–1358.

46. Anzueto A, Baughman RP, Guntupalli KK, Weg JG, Wiedemann HP, Raventos AA, et al. Aerosolized surfactant in adults with sepsis-induced acute respiratory distress syndrome. Exosurf acute respiratory distress syndrome sepsis study group. N Engl J Med 1996; 334(22):1417–1421.

47. Spragg RLJ. Treatment of ARDS with rSP-C surfactant. Am J Respir Crit Care Med 2001; 161:A47.

48. Gregory TJ, Steinberg KP, Spragg R, Gadek JE, Hyers TM, Longmore WJ, et al. Bovine surfactant therapy for patients with acute respiratory distress syndrome. Am J Respir Crit Care Med 1997; 155(4):1309–1315.

49. Gattinoni L, Pesenti A, Mascheroni D, Marcolin R, Fumagalli R, Rossi F, et al. Low-frequency positive-pressure ventilation with extracorporeal CO_2 removal in severe acute respiratory failure. JAMA 1986; 256(7):881–886.

50. Morris AH, Wallace CJ, Menlove RL, Clemmer TP, Orme JF Jr, Weaver LK, et al. Randomized clinical trial of pressure-controlled inverse ratio ventilation and extracorporeal CO_2 removal for adult respiratory distress syndrome. Am J Respir Crit Care Med 1994; 149(2 Pt 1):295–305.

51. Hirschl RB, Pranikoff T, Wise C, Overbeck MC, Gauger P, Schreiner RJ, et al. Initial experience with partial liquid ventilation in adult patients with the acute respiratory distress syndrome. JAMA 1996; 275(5):383–389.

52. Leach CL, Greenspan JS, Rubenstein SD, Shaffer TH, Wolfson MR, Jackson JC, et al. Partial liquid ventilation with perflubron in premature infants with severe respiratory distress syndrome. The liquivent study group. N Engl J Med 1996; 335(11):761–767.

53. Hirschl RB, Pranikoff T, Gauger P, Schreiner RJ, Dechert R, Bartlett RH. Liquid ventilation in adults, children, and full-term neonates. Lancet 1995; 346(8984):1201–1202.

54. Gauger PG, Pranikoff T, Schreiner RJ, Moler FW, Hirschl RB. Initial experience with partial liquid ventilation in pediatric patients with the acute respiratory distress syndrome. Crit Care Med 1996; 24(1):16–22.

55. Hirschl RB, Conrad S, Kaiser R, Zwischenberger JB, Bartlett RH, Booth F, et al. Partial liquid ventilation in adult patients with ARDS: a multicenter phase I–II trial. Adult PLV study group. Ann Surg 1998; 228(5): 692–700.

56. Hirschl RB, Croce M, Gore D, Wiedemann H, Davis K, Zwischenberger J, et al. Prospective, randomized, controlled pilot study of partial liquid ventilation in adult acute respiratory distress syndrome. Am J Respir Crit Care Med 2002; 165(6):781–787.

57. Rubenfeld GD, Caldwell EC MDSK, Hudson LD. The incidence of acute lung injury (ALI) in the US: results of the King county lung injury project. Am J Respir Crit Care Med 2002; 165(8):A219.

58. Roupie E, Lepage E, Wysocki M, Fagon JY, Chastre J, Dreyfuss D, et al. Prevalence, etiologies and outcome of the acute respiratory distress syndrome among hypoxemic ventilated patients. SRLF collaborative group on mechanical ventilation. Societe de reanimation de langue francaise. Intensive Care Med 1999; 25(9):920–929.

59. Luhr OR, Antonsen K, Karlsson M, Aardal S, Thorsteinsson A, Frostell CG, et al. Incidence and mortality after acute respiratory failure and acute respiratory distress syndrome in Sweden, Denmark, and Iceland. The ARF study group. Am J Respir Crit Care Med 1999; 159(6):1849–1861.

60. Esteban A, Anzueto A, Alia I, Gordo F, Apezteguia C, Palizas F, et al. How is mechanical ventilation employed in the intensive care unit? An international utilization review. Am J Respir Crit Care Med 2000; 161(5): 1450–1458.

61. Murphy DB, Cregg N, Tremblay L, Engelberts D, Laffey JG, Slutsky AS, et al. Adverse ventilatory strategy causes pulmonary-to-systemic translocation of endotoxin. Am J Respir Crit Care Med 2000; 162(1):27–33.

62. Gattinoni L, Presenti A, Torresin A, Baglioni S, Rivolta M, Rossi F, et al. Adult respiratory distress syndrome profiles by computed tomography. J Thorac Imaging 1986; 1(3):25–30.

63. Gattinoni L, Pelosi P, Pesenti A, Brazzi L, Vitale G, Moretto A, et al. CT scan in ARDS: clinical and physiopathological insights. Acta Anaesthesiol Scand Suppl 1991; 95:87–94.

64. Gattinoni L, Bombino M, Pelosi P, Lissoni A, Pesenti A, Fumagalli R, et al. Lung structure and function in different stages of severe adult respiratory distress syndrome. JAMA 1994; 271(22):1772–1779.

65. Schiller HJ, McCann UG, Carney DE, Gatto LA, Steinberg JM, Nieman GF. Altered alveolar mechanics in the acutely injured lung. Crit Care Med 2001; 29(5):1049–1055.

66. Mead J, Takishima T, Leith D. Stress distribution in lungs: a model of pulmonary elasticity. J Appl Physiol 1970; 28(5):596–608.

67. Muscedere JG, Mullen JB, Gan K, Slutsky AS. Tidal ventilation at low airway pressures can augment lung injury. Am J Respir Crit Care Med 1994; 149(5):1327–1334.

68. Macklin CC. Transport of air along sheaths of pulmonic blood vessels from alveoli to mediastinum. Arch Intern Med 1939; 64(913):926.

69. Slutsky AS, Tremblay LN. Multiple system organ failure. Is mechanical ventilation a contributing factor? Am J Respir Crit Care Med 1998; 157(6 Pt 1):1721–1725.

70. Kamm RD, Stutsky AS, Drazen JM. High-frequency ventilation. Crit Rev Biomed Eng 1984; 9(4):347–379.

71. Tremblay L, Valenza F, Ribeiro SP, Li J, Slutsky AS. Injurious ventilatory strategies increase cytokines and c-fos mRNA expression in an isolated rat lung model. J Clin Invest 1997; 99(5):944–952.

72. von Bethmann AN, Brasch F, Nusing R, Vogt K, Volk HD, Muller KM, et al. Hyperventilation induces release of cytokines from perfused mouse lung. Am J Respir Crit Care Med 1998; 157(1):263–272.

73. Dos Santos CC, Slutsky AS. Invited review: mechanisms of ventilator-induced lung injury: a perspective. J Appl Physiol 2000; 89(4):1645–1655.

74. Liu M, Post M. Invited review: mechanochemical signal transduction in the fetal lung. J Appl Physiol 2000; 89(5):2078–2084.

75. Liu M, Tanswell AK, Post M. Mechanical force-induced signal transduction in lung cells. Am J Physiol 1999; 277(4 Pt 1):L667–L683.

76. Haitsma JJ, Uhlig S, Goggel R, Verbrugge SJ, Lachmann U, Lachmann B. Ventilator-induced lung injury leads to loss of alveolar and systemic compartmentalization of tumornecrosis factor-alpha. Intensive Care Med 2000; 26(10):1515–1522.

77. Chiumello D, Pristine G, Slutsky AS. Mechanical ventilation affects local and systemic cytokines in an animal model of acute respiratory distress syndrome. Am J Respir Crit Care Med 1999; 160(1):109–116.

78. Murphy DB, Cregg N, Tremblay L, Engelberts D, Laffey JG, Slutsky AS, Romaschin A, Kavanagh BP. Adverse ventilatory strategy causes pulmonary-to-systemic translocation of endotoxin. Am J Respir Crit Care Med 2000; 162(1):27–33.

79. Verbrugge SJ, Sorm V, van't Veen A, Mouton JW, Gommers D, Lachmann B. Lung overinflation without positive end-expiratory pressure promotes bacteremia after experimental *Klebsiella pneumoniae* inoculation. Intensive Care Med 1998; 24(2):172–177.

80. Nahum A, Hoyt J, Schmitz L, Moody J, Shapiro R, Marini JJ. Effect of mechanical ventilation strategy on dissemination of intratracheally instilled *Escherichia coli* in dogs. Crit Care Med 1997; 25(10):1733–1743.

81. Savel RH, Yao EC, Gropper MA. Protective effects of low tidal volume entilation in a rabbit model of *Pseudomonas aeruginosa*-induced acute lung injury. Crit Care Med 2001; 29(2):392–398.

82. Ranieri VM, Giunta F, Suter PM, Slutsky AS. Mechanical ventilation as a mediator of multisystem organ failure in acute respiratory distress syndrome. JAMA 2000; 284(1):43–44.

83. Vreugdenhil HA, Heijnen CJ, Plotz FB, Zijlstra J, Jansen NJ, Haitsma JJ, Lachmann B, Van Vught AJ. Mechanical ventilation of healthy rats suppresses peripheral immune function. Eur J Respir J 2004; ; 284(1):122–128.

84. Stuber F, Wriggle H, Schroeder S, Wetegrove S, Zinserling J, Hoeft A, Putensen C. Kinetic and reversibility of mechanical ventilation-associated pulmonary and systemic inflammatory response in patients with acute lung injury. Intensive Care Med 2002; 28(7):834–841.

85. Matamis D, Lemaire F, Harf A, Brun-Buisson C, Ansquer JC, Atlan G. Total respiratory pressure–volume curves in the adult respiratory distress syndrome. Chest 1984; 86(1):58–66.

86. Tobin MJ. Advances in mechanical ventilation. N Engl J Med 2001; 344(26):1986–1996.

87. Bryan CL, Jenkinson SG. Oxygen toxicity. Clin Chest Med 1988; 9(1):141–152.

88. Marini JJ, Kelsen SG. Re-targeting ventilatory objectives in adult respiratory distress syndrome. New treatment prospects—persistent questions. Am Rev Respir Dis 1992; 146(1):2–3.

89. Lessard MR, Guerot E, Lorino H, Lemaire F, Brochard L. Effects of pressure-controlled with different I:E ratios vs. volume-controlled ventilation on respiratory mechanics, gas exchange, and hemodynamics in patients with adult respiratory distress syndrome. Anesthesiology 1994; 80(5):983–991.

90. Rappaport SH, Shpiner R, Yoshihara G, Wright J, Chang P, Abraham E. Randomized, prospective trial of pressure-limited vs. volume-controlled ventilation in severe respiratory failure. Crit Care Med 1994; 22(1):22–32.

91. Esteban A, Alia I, Gordo F, de Pablo R, Suarez J, Gonzalez G, et al. Prospective randomized trial comparing pressure-controlled ventilation and volume-controlled ventilation in ARDS. For the Spanish lung failure collaborative group. Chest 2000; 117(6):1690–1696.

92. Thompson BT, Hayden D, Matthay MA, Brower R, Parsons PE. Clinicians' approaches to mechanical ventilation in acute lung injury and ARDS. Chest 2001; 120(5):1622–1627.

93. Petrucci N, Iacovelli W. Ventilation with lower tidal volumes vs. traditional tidal volumes in adults for acute lung injury and acute respiratory distress syndrome. Cochrane Database Syst Rev 2003; (3):CD003844.

94. Laffey JG, Engelberts D, Kavanagh BP. Buffering hypercapnic acidosis worsens acute lung injury. Am J Respir Crit Care Med 2000; 161(1):141–146.

95. Mariani G, Cifuentes J, Carlo WA. Randomized trial of permissive hypercapnia in preterm infants. Pediatrics 1999; 104(5 Pt 1):1082–1088.

96. Broccard AF, Hotchkiss JR, Vannay C, Markert M, Sauty A, Feihl F, et al. Protective effects of hypercapnic acidosis on ventilator-induced lung injury. Am J Respir Crit Care Med 2001; 164(5):802–806.

97. Sinclair SE, Lamm WJE, Hlastala MP. Hypercapnic acidosis reduces the severity of ventilator-induced lung injury in vivo. Am J Respir Crit Care Med 2002; 165(8):A784.

98. Shibata K, Cregg N, Engelberts D, Takeuchi A, Fedorko L, Kavanagh BP. Hypercapnic acidosis may attenuate acute lung injury by inhibition of endogenous xanthine oxidase. Am J Respir Crit Care Med 1998; 158(5 Pt 1): 1578–1584.

99. Kopp R, Kuhlen R, Max M, Rossaint R. Evidence-based medicine in the therapy of the acute respiratory distress syndrome. Intensive Care Med 2002; 28(3):244–255.

100. Carvalho CR, Barbas CS, Medeiros DM, Magaldi RB, Lorenzi FG, Kairalla RA, et al. Temporal hemodynamic effects of permissive hypercapnia associated with ideal PEEP in ARDS. Am J Respir Crit Care Med 1997; 156(5):1458–1466.

101. Laffey JG, Tanaka M, Engelberts D, Luo X, Yuan S, Tanswell AK, et al. Therapeutic hypercapnia reduces pulmonary and systemic injury following in vivo lung reperfusion. Am J Respir Crit Care Med 2000; 162(6):2287–2294.

102. Froese AB. High-frequency oscillatory ventilation for adult respiratory distress syndrome: let's get it right this time! Crit Care Med 1997; 25(6):906–908.

103. Bendixen HH, Hedley-Whyte J, Laver MB. Improved oxygenation in surgical patients during anesthesia with controlled ventilation. N Engl J Med 1963; 263:991–996.

104. Gattinoni L, Mascheroni D, Torresin A, Marcolin R, Fumagalli R, Vesconi S, et al. Morphological response to positive end expiratory pressure in acute respiratory failure. Computerized tomography study. Intensive Care Med 1986; 12(3):137–142.

105. Gattinoni L, Pesenti A, Baglioni S, Vitale G, Rivolta M, Pelosi P. Inflammatory pulmonary edema and positive end-expiratory pressure: correlations between imaging and physiologic studies. J Thorac Imaging 1988; 3(3):59–64.

106. Gattinoni L, Pesenti A, Bombino M, Baglioni S, Rivolta M, Rossi F, et al. Relationships between lung computed tomographic density, gas exchange, and PEEP in acute respiratory failure. Anesthesiology 1988; 69(6): 824–832.

107. Gattinoni L, D'Andrea L, Pelosi P, Vitale G, Pesenti A, Fumagalli R. Regional effects and mechanism of positive end-expiratory pressure in early adult respiratory distress syndrome. JAMA 1993; 269(16):2122–2127.

108. Gattinoni L, Pelosi P, Crotti S, Valenza F. Effects of positive end-expiratory pressure on regional distribution of tidal volume and recruitment in adult respiratory distress syndrome. Am J Respir Crit Care Med 1995; 151(6):1807–1814.

109. Ruiz-Bailen M, Fernandez-Mondejar E, Hurtado-Ruiz B, Colmenero-Ruiz M, Rivera-Fernandez R, Guerrero-Lopez F, et al. Immediate application of positive-end expiratorypressure is more effective than delayed positive-end expiratory pressure to reduce extravascular lung water. Crit Care Med 1999; 27(2):380–384.

110. DiRusso SM, Nelson LD, Safcsak K, Miller RS. Survival in patients with severe adult respiratory distress syndrome treated with high-level positive end-expiratory pressure. Crit Care Med 1995; 23(9):1485–1496.

111. Ranieri VM, Mascia L, Fiore T, Bruno F, Brienza A, Giuliani R. Cardiorespiratory effects of positive end-expiratory pressure during progressive tidal volume reduction (permissive hypercapnia) in patients with acute respiratory distress syndrome. Anesthesiology 1995; 83(4):710–720.

112. Richard JC, Brochard L, Vandelet P, Breton L, Maggiore SM, Jonson B, et al. Respective effects of end-expiratory and end-inspiratory pressures on alveolar recruitment in acute lung injury. Crit Care Med 2003; 31(1):89–92.

113. Boussarsar M, Thierry G, Jaber S, Roudot-Thoraval F, Lemaire F, Brochard L. Relationship between ventilatory settings and barotrauma in the acute respiratory distress syndrome. Intensive Care Med 2002; 28(4):406–413.

114. Vieira SR, Puybasset L, Richecoeur J, Lu Q, Cluzel P, Gusman PB, et al. A lung computed tomographic assessment of positive end-expiratory pressure-induced lung overdistension. Am J Respir Crit Care Med 1998; 158(5 Pt 1):1571–1577.

115. Puybasset L, Cluzel P, Chao N, Slutsky AS, Coriat P, Rouby JJ. A computed tomography scan assessment of regional lung volume in acute lung injury. The CT scan ARDS study group. Am J Respir Crit Care Med 1998; 158(5 Pt 1):1644–1655.

116. Horton WG, Cheney FW. Variability of effect of positive end expiratory pressure. Arch Surg 1975; 110(4):395–398.

117. Kanarek DJ, Shannon DC. Adverse effect of positive end-expiratory pressure on pulmonary perfusion and arterial oxygenation. Am Rev Respir Dis 1975; 112(3):457–459.

118. Gattinoni L, Pelosi P, Suter PM, Pedoto A, Vercesi P, Lissoni A. Acute respiratory distress syndrome caused by pulmonary and extrapulmonary disease. Different syndromes? Am J Respir Crit Care Med 1998; 158(1):3–11.

119. de Durante G, del Turco M, Rustichini L, Cosimini P, Giunta F, Hudson LD, et al. ARDSNet lower tidal volume ventilatory strategy may generate intrinsic positive end-expiratory pressure in patients with acute respiratory distress syndrome. Am J Respir Crit Care Med 2002; 165(9):1271–1274.

120. Richard JC, Breton L, Maggiore SM, Vandelet P, Tamion F, Girault C, et al. Influence of respiratory rate on intrinsic positive end-expiratory pressure

(PEEP) in patients with ARDS. Am J Respir Crit Care Med 2002; 165(8):A218.

121. Brochard L. Watching what PEEP really does. Am J Respir Crit Care Med 2001; 163(6):1291–1292.

122. Lee WL, Stewart TE, MacDonald R, Lapinsky S, Banayan D, Hallett D, et al. Safety of pressure–volume curve measurement in acute lung injury and ARDS using a syringe technique. Chest 2002; 121(5):1595–1601.

123. Maggiore SM, Jonson B, Richard JC, Jaber S, Lemaire F, Brochard L. Alveolar derecruitment at decremental positive end-expiratory pressure levels in acute lung injury. Comparison with the lower inflection point, oxygenation, andcompliance. Am J Respir Crit Care Med 2001; 164(5):795–801.

124. Cereda M, Foti G, Musch G, Sparacino ME, Pesenti A. Positive end-expiratory pressure prevents the loss of respiratory compliance during low tidal volume ventilation in acute lung injury patients. Chest 1996; 109(2):480–485.

125. Barbas CSV, Medeiros D, Magaldi RB, Kairalla RA, Carvalho CRR, Amato MBP. High PEEP levels improved survival in ARDS patients. Am J Respir Crit Care Med 2002; 165(8):A218.

126. Brower R. ALVEOLI study—ARDSNet up-date. Presentedat the American Thoracic Society Meeting, Atlanta, U.S.A. May 2002.

127. Mead J, Collier C. Relation of volume history of lungs to respiratory mechanics in anesthetized dogs. J Appl Physiol 1959; 14:669–678.

128. Kacmarek RM. Strategies to optimize alveolar recruitment. Curr Opin Crit Care 2001; 7(1):15–20.

129. Mehta S, Slutsky AS. Mechanical ventilation in acute respiratory distress syndrome: evolving concepts. Monaldi Arch Chest Dis 1998; 53(6):647–653.

130. Bond DM, Froese AB. Volume recruitment maneuvers are less deleterious than persistent low lung volumes in the atelectasis-prone rabbit lung during high-frequency oscillation. Crit Care Med 1993; 21(3):402–412.

131. Pelosi P, Bottino N, Panigada M, Eccher G, Gattinoni L. The sigh in ARDS (acute respiratory distress syndrome). Minerva Anestesiol 1999; 65(5): 313–317.

132. Halter JM, Steinberg JM, Schiller HJ, DaSilva M, Gatto LA, Nieman GF. Positive end-expiratory pressure (PEEP) following recruitment maneuver prevents alveolar recruitment/derecruitment (R/D). Am J Respir Crit Care Med 2002; 165(8):A376.

133. Rimensberger PC, Cox PN, Frndova H, Bryan AC. The open lung during small tidal volume ventilation: concepts of recruitment and "optimal" positive end-expiratory pressure. Crit Care Med 1999; 27(9):1946–1952.

134. Rimensberger PC, Pristine G, Mullen BM, Cox PN, Slutsky AS. Lung recruitment during small tidal volume ventilation allows minimal positive end-expiratory pressure without augmenting lung injury. Crit Care Med 1999; 27(9):1940–1945.

135. Rothen HU, Sporre B, Engberg G, Wegenius G, Hedenstierna G. Re-expansion of atelectasis during general anaesthesia: a computed tomography study. Br J Anaesth 1993; 71(6):788–795.

136. McCulloch PR, Forkert PG, Froese AB. Lung volume maintenance prevents lung injury during high frequency oscillatory ventilation in surfactant-deficient rabbits. Am Rev Respir Dis 1988; 137(5):1185–1192.

137. Damasceno MCP, Silva FL, Lanza FC, Santos M, Beppu OS. Recruitment maneuvers (RM) lack of benefit with high-PEEP. Am J Respir Crit Care Med 2002; 165(8):A682.

138. Lim SC, Hotchkiss JR, Simonson D, Yin P, Adams AB, Dries D, et al. Recruitment maneuvers (RM) methods do not improve PaO_2/lung volume at 15 min post RM in a porcine OAI model. Am J Respir Crit Care Med 2002; 165(8):A683.

139. Albert RK, Leasa D, Sanderson M, Robertson HT, Hlastala MP. The prone position improves arterial oxygenation and reduces shunt in oleic-acid-induced acute lung injury. Am Rev Respir Dis 1987; 135(3):628–633.

140. Douglas WW, Rehder K, Beynen FM, Sessler AD, Marsh HM. Improved oxygenation in patients with acute respiratory failure: the prone position. Am Rev Respir Dis 1977; 115(4):559–566.

141. Pelosi P, Tubiolo D, Mascheroni D, Vicardi P, Crotti S, Valenza F, et al. Effects of the prone position on respiratory mechanics and gas exchange during acute lung injury. Am J Respir Crit Care Med 1998; 157(2):387–393.

142. Langer M, Mascheroni D, Marcolin R, Gattinoni L. The prone position in ARDS patients. A clinical study. Chest 1988; 94(1):103–107.

143. Gattinoni L, Pesenti A, Avalli L, Rossi F, Bombino M. Pressure–volume curve of total respiratory system in acute respiratory failure. Computed tomographic scan study. Am Rev Respir Dis 1987; 136(3):730–736.

144. Mure M, Martling CR, Lindahl SG. Dramatic effect on oxygenation in patients with severe acute lung insufficiency treated in the prone position. Crit Care Med 1997; 25(9):1539–1544.

145. Nakos G, Tsangaris I, Kostanti E, Nathanail C, Lachana A, Koulouras V, et al. Effect of the prone position on patients with hydrostatic pulmonary edema compared with patients with acute respiratory distress syndrome and pulmonary fibrosis. Am J Respir Crit Care Med 2000; 161(2 Pt 1): 360–368.

146. Imai Y, Kawano T, Miyasaka K, Takata M, Imai T, Okuyama K. Inflammatory chemical mediators during conventional ventilation and during high frequency oscillatory ventilation. Am J Respir Crit Care Med 1994; 150(6 Pt 1):1550–1554.

147. Froese AB, Bryan AC. High frequency ventilation. Am Rev Respir Dis 1987; 135(6):1363–1374.

148. Slutsky AS. Barotrauma and alveolar recruitment. Intensive Care Med 1993; 19(7):369–371.

149. Slutsky AS. High frequency ventilation. Intensive Care Med 1991; 17(7): 375–376.

150. Crawford MR. High-frequency ventilation. Anaesth Intensive Care 1986; 14:281–292.

151. Drazen JM, Kamm RD, Slutsky AS. High-frequency ventilation. Physiol Rev 1984; 64(2):505–543.

152. Henderson Y, Chillingsworth F, Whitney J. The respiratory dead space. Am J Physiol 1915; 38:1–19.
153. Slutsky AS, Drazen JM, Kamm R. Alveolar ventilation at high frequencies using tidal volumes smaller than anatomical dead space. Lung Biol Health Dis 1985:137–176.
154. dos Santos CC, Slutsky AS. Overview of high-frequency ventilation modes, clinical rationale, and gas transport mechanisms. Respir Clin North Am 2001; 7(4):549–575.
155. Matsuoka T, Kawano T, Miyasaka K. Role of high-frequency ventilation in surfactant-depleted lung injury as measured by granulocytes. J Appl Physiol 1994; 76(2):539–544.
156. Sugiura M, McCulloch PR, Wren S, Dawson RH, Froese AB. Ventilator pattern influences neutrophil influx and activation in atelectasis-prone rabbit lung. J Appl Physiol 1994; 77(3):1355–1365.
157. Kawano T, Mori S, Cybulsky M, Burger R, Ballin A, Cutz E, et al. Effect of granulocyte depletion in a ventilated surfactant-depleted lung. J Appl Physiol 1987; 62(1):27–33.
158. Takata M, Abe J, Tanaka H, Kitano Y, Doi S, Kohsaka T, et al. Intraalveolar expression of tumor necrosis factor-alpha gene during conventional and high-frequency ventilation. Am J Respir Crit Care Med 1997; 156(1):272–279.
159. Bond DM, McAloon J, Froese AB. Sustained inflations improve respiratory compliance during high- frequency oscillatory ventilation but not during large tidal volume positive-pressure ventilation in rabbits. Crit Care Med 1994; 22(8):1269–1277.
160. Lee WL, Detsky AS, Stewart TE. Lung-protective mechanical ventilation strategies in ARDS. Intensive Care Med 2000; 26(8):1151–1155.
161. Mehta S. High frequency ventilation. Curr Opin Crit Care 2000; 6:38–45.
162. Herridge MS, Slutsky AS, Colditz GA. Has high-frequency ventilation been inappropriately discarded in adult acute respiratory distress syndrome? Crit Care Med 1998; 26(12):2073–2077.
163. Brower RG, Ware LB, Berthiaume Y, Matthay MA. Treatment of ARDS. Chest 2001; 120(4):1347–1367.
164. Pelosi P, Goldner M, McKibben A, Adams A, Eccher G, Caironi P, et al. Recruitment and derecruitment during acute respiratory failure: an experimental study. Am J Respir Crit Care Med 2001; 164(1):122–130.
165. McCann UG, Schiller HJ, Carney DE, Gatto LA, Steinberg JM, Nieman GF. Visual validation of the mechanical stabilizing effects of positive end-expiratory pressure at the alveolar level. J Surg Res 2001; 99(2):335–342.
166. Bryan AC, Froese AB. Reflections on the HIFI trial. Pediatrics 1991; 87(4):565–567.
167. Gerlach H, Rossaint R, Pappert D, Falke KJ. Time-course and dose-response of nitric oxide inhalation for systemic oxygenation and pulmonary hypertension in patients with adult respiratory distress syndrome. Eur J Clin Invest 1993; 23(8):499–502.
168. The neonatal inhaled nitric oxide study group. Inhaled nitric oxide in full-term and nearly full-term infants with hypoxic respiratory failure. N Engl J Med 1997; 336(9):597–604.

169. Clark RH, Kueser TJ, Walker MW, Southgate WM, Huckaby JL, Perez JA, et al. Low-dose nitric oxide therapy for persistent pulmonary hypertension of the newborn. Clinical inhaled nitric oxide research group. N Engl J Med 2000; 342(7):469–474.

170. Cuthbertson BH, Galley HF, Webster NR. Effect of inhaled nitric oxide on key mediators of the inflammatory response in patients with acute lung injury. Crit Care Med 2000; 28(6):1736–1741.

171. Rialp G, Betbese AJ, Perez-Marquez M, Mancebo J. Short-term effects of inhaled nitric oxide and prone position in pulmonary and extrapulmonary acute respiratory distress syndrome. Am J Respir Crit Care Med 2001; 164(2):243–249.

172. Inhaled Nitric Oxide for acute hypoxemis respiratory failure in children and adults. Cochrane Database Syst Rev 2000; 4(CD002787).

173. Jobe AH. Pulmonary surfactant therapy. N Engl J Med 1993; 328(12): 861–868.

174. Notter RH. Lung Surfactants: Basic Science and Clinical Applications. New York: Marcel Dekker, 2000.

175. Ito Y, Veldhuizen RA, Yao LJ, McCaig LA, Bartlett AJ, Lewis JF. Ventilation strategies affect surfactant aggregate conversion in acute lung injury. Am J Respir Crit Care Med 1997; 155(2):493–499.

176. Clark LC, Gollan F. Survival of mammals breathing organic liquids equilibrated with oxygen at atmospheric pressure. Science 1966; 152:1755–1756.

177. Kylstra JA, Paganelli CV, Lanphier EH. Pulmonary gas exchange in dogs ventilated with hyperbarically oxygenated liquid. J Appl Physiol 1966; 21: 177–184.

178. Kacmarek RM. Partial liquid ventilation: is there a niche? Intensive Care Med 2001; 27(1):1–2.

179. Fuhrman BP, Paczan PR, DeFrancisis M. Perfluorocarbon-associated gas exchange. Crit Care Med 1991; 19(5):712–722.

180. Tutuncu AS, Faithfull NS, Lachmann B. Intratracheal perfluorocarbon administration combined with mechanical ventilation in experimental respiratory distress syndrome: dose-dependent improvement of gas exchange. Crit Care Med 1993; 21(7):962–969.

181. Hirschl RB, Tooley R, Parent AC, Johnson K, Bartlett RH. Improvement of gas exchange, pulmonary function, and lung injury with partial liquid ventilation. A study model in a setting of severe respiratory failure. Chest 1995; 108(2):500–508.

182. Quintel M, Heine M, Hirschl RB, Tillmanns R, Wessendorf V. Effects of partial liquid ventilation on lung injury in a model of acute respiratory failure: a histologic and morphometric analysis. Crit Care Med 1998; 26(5):833–843.

183. Hernan LJ, Fuhrman BP, Kaiser RE, Penfil S, Foley C, Papo MC, et al. Perfluorocarbon-associated gas exchange in normal and acid-injured large sheep. Crit Care Med 1996; 24(3):475–481.

184. Papo MC, Paczan PR, Fuhrman BP, Steinhorn DM, Hernan LJ, Leach CL, et al. Perfluorocarbon-associated gas exchange improves oxygenation, lung mechanics, and survival in a model of adult respiratory distress syndrome. Crit Care Med 1996; 24(3):466–474.

185. Gauger PG, Overbeck MC, Chambers SD, Cailipan CI, Hirschl RB. Partial liquid ventilation improves gas exchange and increases EELV in acute lung injury. J Appl Physiol 1998; 84(5):1566–1572.

186. Younger JG, Taqi AS, Till GO, Hirschl RB. Partial liquid ventilation protects lung during resuscitation from shock. J Appl Physiol 1997; 83(5):1666–1670.

187. Rotta AT, Steinhorn DM. Partial liquid ventilation reduces pulmonary neutrophil accumulation in an experimental model of systemic endotoxemia and acute lung injury. Crit Care Med 1998; 26(10):1707–1715.

188. Colton DM, Till GO, Johnson KJ, Dean SB, Bartlett RH, Hirschl RB. Neutrophil accumulation is reduced during partial liquid ventilation. Crit Care Med 1998; 26(10):1716–1724.

189. Wiedemann HP, Kacmarek RM, Lemaire F, Tütüncü AS, Wedel MS, Slutsky AS. Partial liquid ventilation in adult patients with the acute respiratory distress syndrome. In preparation.

190. Von Frey M, Gruber M. Studies on metabolism of isolated organs. A respiration-apparatus for isolated organs (in German). Virchows Arch Physiol 1885; 519:532.

191. Clowes GH, Hopkins AL, Neville WE. An artificial lung dependent upon diffusion of oxygen and carbon dioxide through plastic membranes. J Thorac Cardiovasc Surg 1956; 32:630–637.

192. Hill JD, O'Brien TG, Murray JJ, Dontigny L, Bramson ML, Osborn JJ, et al. Prolonged extracorporeal oxygenationfor acute posttraumatic respiratory failure (shock-lungsyndrome). Use of the Bramson membrane lung. N Engl J Med 1972; 286(12):629–634.

193. Bartlett RH, Gazzaniga AB, Jefferies MR, et al. Extracorporeal membrane oxygenation (ECMO) cardiopulmonary support in infancy. Trans Am Soc Artif Intern Organs 1976; 22:80–93.

194. Zapol WM, Snider MT, Hill JD, Fallat RJ, Bartlett RH, Edmunds LH, et al. Extracorporeal membrane oxygenation in severe acute respiratory failure. A randomized prospective study. JAMA 1979; 242(20):2193–2196.

195. Kolobow T, Gattinoni L, Tomlinson TA, Pierce JE. Control of breathing using an extracorporeal membrane lung. Anesthesiology 1977; 46(2): 138–141.

196. Habashi NM, Borg UR, Reynolds HN. Low blood flow extracorporeal carbon dioxide removal (ECCO2R): a review of the concept and a case report. Intensive Care Med 1995; 21(7):594–597.

197. Brunet F, Mira JP, Dhainaut JF, Dall'ava-Santucci J. Efficacy of low-frequency positive-pressure ventilation-extracorporeal CO_2 removal. Am J Respir Crit Care Med 1995; 151(4):1269–1270.

198. Falke KJ. Randomized clinical trial of pressure-controlled inverse ratio ventilation and extracorporeal CO_2 removal for adult respiratory distress syndrome. Am J Respir Crit Care Med 1997; 156(3 Pt 1):1016–1017.

199. Gattinoni L, Pesenti A, Bombino M, Pelosi P, Brazzi L. Role of extracorporeal circulation in adult respiratoty distress syndrome management New Horiz 1993; 1(4): 603–612.

200. Lewandowski K. Extracorporeal membrane oxygenation for severe acute respiratory failure. Crit Care 2000; 4(3):156–168.

201. Bernard GR, Artigas A, Brigham KL, Carlet J, Falke K, Hudson L, et al. The American–European consensus conference on ARDS. Definitions, mechanisms, relevant outcomes, and clinical trial coordination. Am J Respir Crit Care Med 1994; 149(3 Pt 1):818–824.

202. Kloot TE, Blanch L, Melynne YA, Weinert C, Adams AB, Marini JJ, et al. Recruitment maneuvers in three experimental models of acute lung injury. Effect on lung volume and gas exchange. Am J Respir Crit Care Med 2000; 161(5):1485–1494.

203. Puybasset L, Cluzel P, Gusman P, Grenier P, Preteux F, Rouby JJ. Regional distribution of gas and tissue in acute respiratory distress syndrome. I. Consequences for lung morphology. CT scan ARDS study group. Intensive Care Med 2000; 26(7):857–869.

204. Lim CM, Kim EK, Lee JS, Shim TS, Lee SD, Koh Y, et al. Comparison of the response to the prone position between pulmonary and extrapulmonary acute respiratory distress syndrome. Intensive Care Med 2001; 27(3):477–485.

205. Desai SR, Wells AU, Suntharalingam G, Rubens MB, Evans TW, Hansell DM. Acute respiratory distress syndrome caused by pulmonary and extrapulmonary injury: a comparative CT study. Radiology 2001; 218(3):689–693.

206. Eisner MD, Thompson T, Hudson LD, Luce JM, Hayden D, Schoenfeld D, et al. Efficacy of low tidal volume ventilation in patients with different clinical risk factors for acute lung injury and the acute respiratory distress syndrome. Am J Respir Crit Care Med 2001; 164(2):231–236.

207. Kirby RR, Perry JC, Calderwood HW, Ruiz BC, Lederman DS. Cardiorespiratory effects of high positive end-expiratory pressure. Anesthesiology 1975; 43(5):533–539.

208. Uhlig S. Ventilation-induced lung injury and mechanotransduction: stretching it too far? Am J Physiol Lung Cell Mol Physiol 2002; 282(5):L892–L896.

14

Anti-inflammatory Therapies for Lung Injury

RICHARD PHIPPS, WILLIAM S. BECKETT, JULIA KAUFMAN,
CHRISTINE MARTEY, P. J. SIME, and THOMAS H. THATCHER

*Departments of Medicine and Environmental Medicine, Lung Biology and
Disease Program, University of Rochester School of Medicine,
Rochester, New York, U.S.A.*

I. Overview

This chapter examines anti-inflammatory therapies for respiratory diseases
with a component of acute or chronic lung injury. As detailed in earlier
chapters, a variety of mediators, factors, and pathophysiological pathways
are important in innate pulmonary host defense and inflammatory lung
injury. Basic science understanding has elucidated multiple inflammation-
related molecular processes that might be targeted in treating patients with
pulmonary disease. Since the number of potential anti-inflammatory therapies and strategies is large, discussion in this chapter emphasizes five areas
of lung disease and associated therapeutics—pulmonary infection (pneumonia), asthma, bronchitis, COPD, and fibrosing lung diseases. The utility
of traditional anti-inflammatory medications such as corticosteroids, non-
steroidal anti-inflammatory drugs, and immunosuppressants in treating
these various conditions is described. However, primary importance is
placed on newer treatments or therapeutic strategies that disrupt
immune–immune and immune–structural cell activation, target-specific
proinflammatory mediators, or modulate the effector functions of resident
lung cells. These newer approaches to the therapy of inflammatory lung

injury and disease all derive from basic science understanding and perspectives elucidated in earlier chapters. The specificity and scope of possible anti-inflammatory interventions for pulmonary disease and injury can be expected to become further refined and focused as basic mechanistic understanding improves in the future.

II. Introduction

Inflammation is classically defined as the process whereby white blood cells and regional soluble factors protect the host from invading micro-organisms. This definition emphasizes that inflammation in the lungs and other organs is intended as beneficial for the host. Biologically effective anti-inflammatory agents or interventions must maintain beneficial aspects of the pulmonary inflammatory response, while antagonizing the detrimental effects of overexuberant inflammation. Although the classical view of inflammation as a leukocyte-mediated process involved in defense against micro-organisms has utility, it does not account for the true complexity of the inflammatory response in many organs including the lungs. Symptoms traditionally associated with inflammation include edema, pain, redness, heat, and sometimes loss or reduction of tissue function. While many lung diseases contain elements of these classical features, some, such as lung scarring typified by idiopathic pulmonary fibrosis (IPF), appear to develop without substantial evidence of classical inflammation (1). When discussing inflammatory lung diseases and their therapy, it is thus helpful to broaden the definition of inflammation to include nonclassical processes (Table 1).

From a broad perspective, *inflammation* includes pathological processes occurring in cells and tissues that do not directly involve infiltration of leukocytes and the production of classic mediators. It is now well known that resident lung cells (airway smooth muscle, fibroblasts and

Table 1 Cardinal Features of Classic Pulmonary Inflammation and an Expanded View Useful in Developing Anti-inflammatory Therapies

Classic Inflammation	Expanded View of Inflammation
White blood cell infiltration	May or may not exhibit white blood cell infiltration
Regional production of "pro-inflammatory" mediators and chemokines	Resident lung structural cells as well as leukocytes can produce mediators, cytokines, and products that initiate and contribute to tissue derangement
Reduction or loss of lung function	Reduction or loss of lung function can be directly caused by alterations in the number and/or properties of multiple resident lung cells.

epithelial cells) elaborate and respond to a wide variety of inflammatory mediators and factors that are capable, depending on the circumstances, of causing tissue injury and pain. In many cases, affected lung tissue fails to show classic features of histologically identifiable inflammation (i.e., infiltration of white blood cells). This does not mean, however, that inflammatory processes are not occurring. Fibroblasts, the effector cells in scar formation, can synthesize various cytokines associated with white blood cell recruitment such as IL-8, IL-16, and MCP-1 (2,3). Structural lung cells may also synthesize alternate mediators such as cyclo-oxygenase-2 and prostaglandins, TGF-β, PDGF, and other mediators that evoke fibroblast collagen synthesis and proliferation. Incorporating this into a broader concept of inflammation as in Table 1 identifies multiple pathophysiological targets for "anti-inflammatory" therapies for lung injury. Selected agents that could be used in anti-inflammatory therapies based on current mechanistic understanding are given in Table 2. The use of these and other agents is discussed in the remainder of the chapter in the context of selected pulmonary diseases that include a component of inflammatory injury.

III. Infectious Diseases of the Lung

Pneumonia is the archetypal infective inflammatory disease of the distal airspaces, and is usually the most severe form of respiratory tract infection. Pneumonia is defined as an infection of the distal lung parenchyma, and is the 6th leading cause of death in the United States with an incidence of 4 million cases per year (4). Pneumonia can be categorized in terms of the locale of acquisition as: (a) community-acquired pneumonia (CAP), defined as lower respiratory tract infection within the community or within 72 hr of hospitalization, and (b) nosocomial pneumonia, infection during long hospitalization or institutionalization. Pneumonia can also be classified in terms of the infectious agent (bacterial, viral, fungal) or in terms of the affected patient population. Patient populations particularly susceptible to pneumonia include immune compromised patients (e.g., as a result of neutropenia, HIV/AIDS, or transplant) and patients with cystic fibrosis (CF).

In terms of its distribution in individual patients, pneumonia can affect whole lobes of the lung (lobar pneumonia) or have a more patchy distribution (bronchial pneumonia). A variety of bacterial, viral and fungal pathogens can cause pneumonia. Patients usually exhibit fever, cough (with or without sputum production), shortness of breath, wheezing, pleurisy, and may have signs of consolidation on physical examination. Typically, therapy for pneumonia involves supportive care plus antibiotics for bacterial infection and antifungals for fungal infections. Antiviral therapy may also be given for viral pneumonias, particularly in immune compromised

Table 2 Selected Agents Proposed, on the Basis of Mechanism, as Potential Anti-inflammatory Therapies for Lung Injury

Disease	Current Therapies	Potential Therapies or Targets
Pneumonia	Penicillin	Synthetic antibiotic peptides (defensins)
	Macrolide antibiotics	IFN-γ, Antimicrobial peptides
	Corticosteroids	COX-2 inhibitors (indomethacin, celecoxib)
	Ribavirin	Blocking virulence factors such as bacterial quorum sensing molecules
	Triazoles	NFκB inhibitors
Pneumocystis Carinii Pneumonia	Corticosteroids	Anti-IL-6 targeted therapies
Asthma	Corticosteroids	Anti-TNF-α, anti-IL-2, sIL-4R, anti-IL-5, anti-IgE (omalizumab)
	Leukotriene inhibitors	IL-10, IL-12, PDE4 inhibitors
Bronchitis	Corticosteroids	
Chronic Obstructive Pulmonary Disease	Corticosteroids,	Metalloproteinase inhibitors, adhesion molecule inhibitors, p38 MAPK inhibitors
	PDE inhibitors, e.g. theophyline	PDE4 inhibitors (e.g cilomilast), NFκB inhibitors
Idiopathic Pulmonary Fibrosis	Corticosteroids	Blocking CD40-CD154 pathway with neutralizing antibodies
		Blocking TGF-β and TNF-α pathways with soluble receptors or antibodies against their respective ligands
		Enhancing IFN-γ by administration of IL-7
Sarcoidosis	Corticosteroids	Inhibitors of IL-12 and IL-18

Many of the current anti-inflammatory therapies listed for lung disease are not optimal, and improved mechanistic understanding of inflammation and lung injury identifies a variety of additional agents or targets. Anti-inflammatory therapies for the various pulmonary diseases listed in the table are discussed in the text.

patients. Anti-inflammatory therapies for pneumonia are described below primarily in the context of bacterial pneumonia, but many of the strategies noted are also relevant for viral and fungal pneumonia.

A. Bacterial Pneumonia

The primary bacterial culprits for nosocomial pneumonia are *Staphylococcus pneumoniae* (*S. pneumoniae*) and *Pseudomonas aeruginosa* (*P. aeruginosa*). *P. aeruginosa* and *S. pneumoniae* are ubiquitous pathogens that can cause pneumonia in normal patients but are more commonly found in patients with impaired host defenses (5). Chronic *P. aeruginosa* colonization, for example, is most prevalent in people suffering from bronchiectasis, CF, and HIV/AIDS (6). Poor mucociliary clearance of bacteria from the upper airways is thought to be responsible for the residence and high density of these micro-organisms in the lungs of affected individuals (7). Bacteria such as *Enterobacter, P. cepacia* (*Burkholderia*), *Haemophilus influenzae, E. coli, Klebsiella* and *Proteus* are also capable of causing pneumonia (8,9). In addition, *Chlamydia pneumoniae* and *Mycoplasma pneumoniae* are common causes of pneumonia in normal and HIV infected patients (10). Bacterial pneumonia is a leading cause of morbidity and mortality worldwide. Although broad-spectrum antibiotic regimens have been successful in treating this condition, there are a growing number of multidrug resistant (MDR) bacteria. Several in vivo animal models (*Streptococcus pneumoniae, P. aeruginosa,* and *Klebsiella*) have been developed to better understand innate immunity to pulmonary bacterial infections (11) and development of MDR. The innate inflammatory response is a crucial aspect of pulmonary host defense against invading bacteria, but overexuberant inflammation during the course of pneumonia can cause lung injury. Thus, anti-inflammatory interventions for bacterial pneumonia are highly relevant.

In many cases of pneumonia, host immune responses or prolonged and intensive antibiotic treatment cannot eradicate the bacteria (12). The mucoid form of *P. aeruginosa*, for instance, effectively colonizes the lung and grows in biofilms that have proven impossible to eradicate with antibiotics like penicillin and other beta lactams or fluoroquinolones such as ciprofloxacin (13). Combination therapy with ciprofloxacin and azithromycin, a macrolide antibiotic with anti-inflammatory properties, has been shown to be more effective in killing *P. aeruginosa* embedded in biofilms than ciprofloxacin alone (14,15). In addition, a small study of seven children with CF reported that azithromycin treatment resulted in a small net gain in lung function, with one patient reporting dramatic improvement (16). Macrolide antibiotics may have a role in the treatment of bacterial pneumonia in patients with CF, although they have particular safety concerns including the potential for altered metabolism, decreased effectiveness of DNAse treatment, and altered ion transport (14,17). A number of additional novel anti-inflammatory interventions for bacterial pneumonia are detailed below.

B. Novel Anti-inflammatory Targets in Bacterial Pneumonia

Production of chemokines and cytokines during microbial infection leads to amplification of the inflammatory cycle not only in macrophages, but also in fibroblasts and epithelial cells (18), resulting in the recruitment of additional macrophages, polymorphonuclear neutrophils, and lymphocytes. Overproduction of proinflammatory cytokines also leads to massive activation of the nuclear factor kappa B (NF-κB). Nuclear factor kappa B is a key transcription factor that promotes synthesis of mRNA encoding proinflammatory mediators and cytokines. High levels of NF-κB lead to up-regulation of genes such as IL-6, cyclo-oxygenase-2 (COX-2), and IL-8. Treatment regimens that target down-regulation of NF-κB, such as inhibitors of IκB phosphorylation [glucocorticosteroids (19)] or peptides that block NF-κB translocation to the nucleus [e.g., SN50 peptide (20)], would decrease the proinflammatory effects of NF-κB activation.

As pulmonary infection progresses, anti-inflammatory cytokines may be produced (e.g., IL-10) to localize the inflammatory response within the micro-environment with a final elimination of both inflammation and microbial infection. However, if an individual is incapable of mounting an anti-inflammatory response, then chronic inflammation and abnormal repair may ensue. Patients who are unable to appropriately down-regulate the inflammatory response could, in theory, be treated with anti-inflammatory cytokines like IL-10 in combination with specific antimicrobial therapy. As noted earlier, the challenge in such therapy is to carefully regulate the inflammatory response so that infection is cleared, while overexuberant inflammation is avoided and excessive damage to host lung tissue is prevented. Developing appropriate anti-inflammatory interventions also requires taking into account special features that are present in pulmonary bacterial infections.

Researchers and clinicians have begun to focus on lung damage resulting from inflammation induced by bacterial virulence factors (21). Some of these include cellular factors such as lipopolysaccharide (LPS), mucoid exopolysaccharide (alginate), pili, and leukocidin, as well as extracellular virulence factors secreted by bacteria including exotoxin A, proteases, and exoenzymes S, T, and U (6). Secretion of extracellular virulence factors by bacteria is controlled by quorum-sensing systems signaled by diffusible molecules called acyl homoserine lactones (AHLs). Once AHL concentrations reach a threshold, they stimulate a signaling cascade leading to increased gene transcription. One such AHL is *N*-3-oxo-dodecanoyl homoserine lactone (3O-C$_{12}$-HSL), which has been identified as a proinflammatory agent that induces the expression of IL-8, a neutrophil chemoattractant found at high levels in early *P. aeruginosa* infection of the lungs (22). Furthermore, injection of this compound into the skin of mice results in an increase in COX-2, an enzyme crucial for the conversion of arachidonic acid to prostaglandins (20). This enzyme and its prostaglandin products are responsible, in large part, for edema, inflammatory cellular infiltrates, fever, and pain, all of which are hallmarks of disease progression in patients with pneumonia. It has also been shown in an acute pneumonia mouse model that there is diminished pseudomonal colonization of the lungs in the absence of genes (*lasI*) important for the synthesis of $3O-C_{12}-HSL$ (20). Overall, these studies suggest that compounds which block bacterial AHLs (e.g., antibodies or antagonist analogs) could decrease bacterial colonization of the lungs as well as reduce the production of inflammatory mediators. These studies also suggest that prostaglandin synthesis is another therapeutic target for anti-inflammatory drugs in protecting the lungs from injury during infection. Drugs such as celecoxib and indomethacin, for example, could potentially attenuate escalated prostaglandin synthesis that ensues from elevated levels of COX-2 in the lungs of affected patients.

There are currently a number of anti-inflammatory therapies in clinical trials for treating pulmonary infection in CF patients (sponsored by the CF therapeutics development network). BIIL-284, a drug that blocks neutrophils from responding to the chemoattractant leukotriene B4 (LTB4) is in trials, with the expected result of reducing lung damage caused by large numbers of neutrophils and their activation products (23). Other current Phase I/II trials are focusing on administration of nonsteroidal anti-inflammatory drugs such as piroxicam and ibuprofen which block COX-2 activity. Early results obtained from 145 patients ranging from 5 to 39 years suggest that long-term, high-dose administration of ibuprofen is associated with reduced intravenous antibiotic use and improved nutritional and pulmonary radiographic status (24). Finally, mammalian lung fluid contains a family of small broad-spectrum anionic antimicrobial peptides called defensins (25–27). These peptides have been found to be inactive in high salt environments such as the CF lung, in which chloride levels are elevated due to the malfunction of the cystic fibrosis transmembrane receptor (CFTR) chloride transporter (28–30). Clinical studies are thus currently underway with CF patients to determine whether novel synthetic salt resistant anti-*P. aeruginosa* peptides can decrease lung colonization by this bacterium (15).

As described earlier, antibiotics are typically administered to eradicate bacteria in the lungs of patients with bacterial pneumonia. Common antibiotics used in pneumonia therapy include penicillins, macrolides, cephalosporins, aminoglycosides, fluroquinolones and clindamycin, or various combination treatments, administered orally or occasionally by aerosols (31). If antibiotic therapy is effective in eliminating bacteria, inflammation will be minimized and normal repair can occur. Macrolide antibiotics are particularly interesting in the context of bacterial-induced inflammation since they are one of the few antimicrobials with inherent anti-inflammatory properties. The macrolides are therefore under renewed interest for their ability to modulate the intense host immune response attendant upon microbial invasion (17). Macrolides that have been used to attenuate bacterial infections include erythromycin, azithromycin, clarithromycin, spiramycin (I, II, III), FK 506 (tacrolimus), rapamycin, josamycin, dirithromycin, HMR 3004, and roxithromycin. Macrolides accumulate in leukocytes to concentrations greater than in serum and it is thought that this accumulation alters cellular function (17). Macrolides have been shown to affect IL-8 release with a resulting decrease in neutrophil recruitment, and consequent lowering of cytokine and chemokine production (32).

C. Viral Pneumonia

Viral pneumonia is included in the category of atypical (nonbacterial) pneumonia, and is usually milder than bacterial pneumonia. However, viral pneumonia can prove lethal to immune compromised, chronically ill, or elderly patients. Viruses that lead to a primary manifestation of pneumonia include influenza A and B, respiratory syncytial virus (RSV), parainfluenza, cytomegalovirus (CMV), and adenovirus. Viral pneumonia can also be part of a multisystem syndrome such as measles (Paramyxovirus), varicella-zoster virus, CMV, and herpes simplex virus (HSV) (33). Systemic viremias occur over a period of several days and the adaptive immune response, specifically the actions of cytotoxic T-cells, are the most important host defense that can be mounted. Cytomegalovirus is a particularly lethal type of pneumonia to HIV/AIDS patients and transplant recipients and carries an 85% mortality within this group, due to immunosuppressive properties of this virus (34). The most common viral pathogen leading to pneumonia is influenza A and B (35).

Viral pneumonia, like bacterial pneumonia, involves an innate inflammatory response that seeks to clear the offending micro-organisms. For example, in RSV infection, viremia typically leads to production of various humoral factors such as histamines, leukotriene C4, and virus-specific immunoglobulin E (IgE) (34). Bradykinin and interleukins (IL-1, 6, and 8) are also overexpressed in rhinovirus infections (36). Specific antiviral drugs such as acyclovir (which binds viral DNA polymerase) and ribavirin (which inhibits viral replication) (33,34) can be administered for viral pneumonias, although these drugs are not used in all cases. Currently, anti-inflammatory therapies are not generally administered for viral pneumonias, except macrolide antibiotics when there is combined viral and bacterial pneumonia. However, many of the anti-inflammatory interventions noted earlier for bacterial pneumonia are in principle also relevant for treating viral pneumonia.

D. Fungal Pneumonia

Fungal pneumonia results primarily from opportunistic organisms or endemic infection. Normal individuals can be affected, but fungal pneumonia is most common in patients with congenital lung disease or who are immunocompromised by HIV/AIDS, transplant, or chemotherapy. Fungal organisms capable of causing pneumonia include *Candida albicans*, *Aspergillus* and *Mucorales* species, *Cryptococcus neoformans*, *Histoplasma capsulatum*, and *Coccidioides immitis*. Disease manifestation in fungal pneumonia is similar to bacterial pneumonia, except that patients may develop other manifestations such as hypersensitivity or allergic reactions (e.g., allergic bronchial asthma, allergic bronchopulmonary mycoses), endemic mycoses such as skin plaques and ulcers, and rheumatologic syndromes such as pericarditis and arthritis (37). Typical antifungal agents used in therapy include fluconazole, ketoconazole, and amphotericin B. Triazoles are anti-inflammatory drugs that have been used to treat fungal diseases such as histoplasmosis, but *Aspergillus* species are resistant to this family of compounds (38).

Another fungal-like micro-organism capable of causing pneumonia is *Pneumocystis carinii* (*P. carinii*). The precise classification of this agent is somewhat ambiguous, but it has many of the characteristics of fungi and is discussed in this category here. *P. carinii* was considered a rare pathogen until the outbreak of AIDS in the early 1980s. It is now known to be an important etiological agent in pneumonia, especially in immune compromised patients such as those infected with HIV or treated with long-term corticosteroid or immunosuppressant therapy (39). The host inflammatory response in *P. carinii* pneumonia (PCP) is an important component of lung injury and respiratory impairment in both AIDS and non-AIDS patients (40). For example, higher numbers of neutrophils and higher concentrations of IL-8 in bronchoalveolar lavage (BAL) fluid correlates with decreased survival during PCP (41,42). AIDS patients with PCP who are severely immunosuppressed have higher lung organism burdens, but less inflammation and less pulmonary compromise than non-AIDS patients, who presumably mount a more vigorous inflammatory response (40). Restoration of cell-mediated immunity in AIDS patients following highly active antiretroviral therapies (HAART) can lead to rapid loss of pulmonary function and progression of pre-existing PCP, a condition referred to as immunorestitution disease (43,44). Adjunctive corticosteroid therapy given along with antibiotics is effective in attenuating the degree of pulmonary compromise and reduces the need for intubation (45). Animal studies of novel anti-inflammatory therapies that might further reduce pulmonary complications without impeding clearance of the organism are underway. Preliminary reports suggest that IL-10 and inhibitors of the NF-κB pathway might be productive areas of research (46,47).

IV. Asthma

A. Inflammatory Signaling in Asthma

Asthma is a chronic inflammatory disorder of the airways characterized by hyper-reactivity of airway smooth muscle, excess mucus secretion, edema, and cellular inflammation involving eosinophils, lymphocytes, mast cells, basophils, neutrophils, and macrophages. The most effective treatments currently available are anti-inflammatory agents (corticosteroids, cromolyn, and nedocromil) often combined with bronchodilators (β2-agonists, methylxanthines). However, these treatments are relatively nonspecific, and are often accompanied by side effects that limit the doses that can be used or negatively affect the quality of life (48). Recent advances in understanding of the complex network of inflammatory cells and signals involved in asthma allows more specific therapies targeted to particular inflammatory mediators to be developed. Inflammatory mediators and pathways involved in atopic or allergic asthma are discussed here as an example (Fig. 1).

The allergic response begins with the uptake of an allergen by an antigen-presenting cell, processing of the antigen, and presentation in the context of Class II MHC to CD4+ T helper cell precursors (Th0). When stimulated by antigen, T helper cells (Th1 and Th2) produce cytokines designated as either Th1 cytokines (IL-2, IFN-γ) or Th2 cytokines (IL-4, MCP-1, IL-9, IL-10 and IL-13) (49). Whether an immune response will be more Th1-like or Th2-like depends on several factors including the genotype of the host, the nature of the antigen, the context of exposure, and the specific balance of cytokines present. For example, IL-4 promotes Th2-like immune responses, while IL-12 and IL-18 promote Th1-like responses (50,51). IFN-γ produced by Th1 cells can counteract the effects of IL-4 on Th2 cells (52,53).

Evidence suggests that a Th2 cytokine profile is critical for the development of allergic or atopic asthma (54–57) (Fig. 1). IL-4 and IL-13 promote B-cells to undergo immunoglobulin class switching to produce allergen-specific IgE molecules. IL-4 and IL-9 also recruit and activate mast cells. One critical checkpoint is the engagement of a high-affinity IgE receptor (FcϵRI) on the surface of mast cells by allergen bound to IgE. This results in the release of a number of effector molecules including histamine, proteases, TNF-α, leukotrienes, and prostaglandins, which cause bronchospasm, vascular leakage, edema, and recruitment of other inflammatory cells. Activated mast cells and Th2 cells produce cytokines that recruit eosinophils and neutrophils to the lung, which further contribute to the inflammatory process through the release of additional proinflammatory cytokines, leukotrienes, proteases, and reactive oxygen species. Each step in this complex pathway is a potential target for anti-inflammatory therapies that interfere with the development and maintenance of the chronic inflammation found in allergic asthma. Of course, many cases of

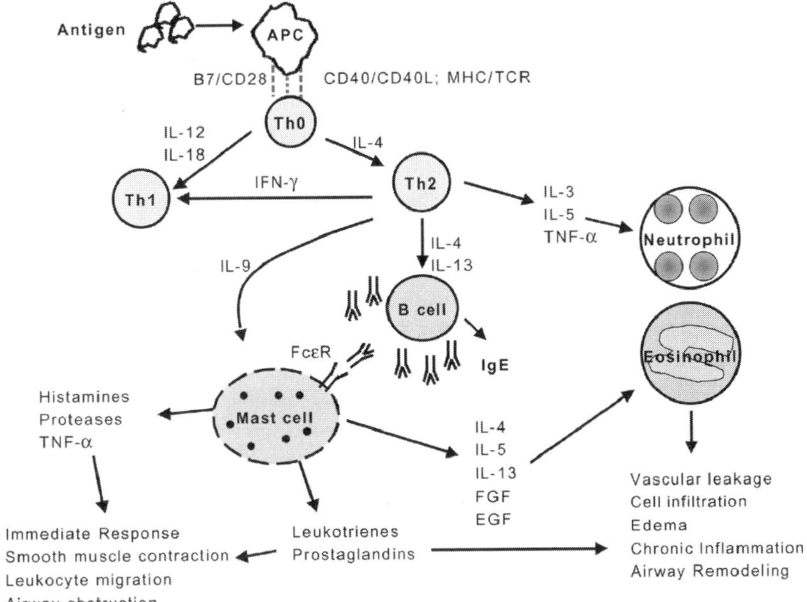

Figure 1 A simplified overview of cytokine signaling pathways in allergic asthma. A complex set of immune-initiated responses contributes to atopic or allergic asthma. Antigens bind to antigen-presenting cells (APC), which interact with CD4+ T helper cell precursors (Th0) to stimulate the release of cytokines. This causes Th1 (type 1) and Th2 (type 2) T helper cells to produce Th1 and Th2 cytokines, which then stimulate downstream events that ultimately affect airway function. All of the mediators and signal pathways illustrated provide potential targets for anti-inflammatory therapy. See text for discussion.

asthma are not associated with known allergies or elevated levels of IgE. However, the inflammatory process is important in all forms of this disease, and many of the mediators involved are likely to be the same.

B. Current Anti-inflammatory Therapies for Asthma

Glucocorticosteroids in many cases offer effective long-term control of asthma symptoms. These drugs suppress the recruitment of airway eosinophils and the release of cytokines and inflammatory mediators, although the mechanism is nonspecific and not thoroughly understood (58,59). Inhalation is the preferred route of administration for corticosteroids in asthma, although systemic corticosteroid treatment may be needed in severely affected patients. Cromolyn and nedocromil also modulate mast cell and eosinophil recruitment and activation, and are effective in reducing asthma symptoms (60). Although corticosteroid therapy remains the mainstay of suppressive anti-inflammatory therapy for asthma, the long-term use of these drugs at high dose has the potential for significant side effects. These include oral candidiasis and dysphonia (with inhaled steroids), and increased appetite and weight gain, fluid retention, loss of bone minerals, suppression of the hypothalamus–pituitary axis, and growth retardation (with systemic glucocorticoids) (61–65).

Leukotrienes are lipid mediators with a wide range of effector functions including constriction of airway smooth muscle, vascular leakage, mucus secretion, and chemoattraction of eosinophils (66,67). Leukotrienes are synthesized from the cell membrane lipid arachidonic acid through the action of the enzyme 5-lipoxygenase (5-LO) and other enzymes, giving rise to the cysteinyl leukotrienes (CysLTs) LTC_4, LTD_4 and LTE_4, and the non-cysteinyl LTB_4. The CysLTs utilize a family of common receptors, CysLT1 and CysLT2. In animal models and patients with asthma, CysLTs promote bronchoconstriction, mucus secretion, and vascular permeability. LTD_4 can stimulate proliferation of airway smooth muscle cells in vitro, suggesting it may also play a role in airway remodeling (68). Cysteinyl leukotriene levels are elevated in BAL and urine of asthma patients following allergen challenge and in aspirin-sensitive asthma patients following exposure to aspirin (69–71). Th2 cytokines drive production of CysLTs by eosinophils in vitro (72,73). Interestingly, corticosteroids do not seem to inhibit CysLT synthesis, suggesting that the anti-inflammatory effects of corticosteroids are mediated through a different pathway (74,75). Thus, drugs that inhibit CysLT activity have been proposed as a useful adjunct to corticosteroids in treating the chronic inflammation underlying asthma.

Two classes of leukotriene inhibitors (LTI) are currently available. Zileuton is an inhibitor of 5-LO and can reduce the production of CysLTs by 70–90%. Montelukast, zafirlukast, and pranlukast are selective inhibitors of the CysLT1 receptor, and act by blocking the effector functions of the CysLTs. In clinical trials, CysLT1 antagonists have been shown to attenuate both the early and late phase asthmatic response, to reduce inflammatory cell accumulation in the airways, and to reduce airway hyper-reactivity (76–79). Leukotriene inhibitors may be effective as monotherapy, particularly in patients with mild asthma (78), and also appear to be useful in steroid-sparing strategies which allow some patients with moderate to severe asthma to significantly reduce their dose of inhaled corticosteroids (ICS) while maintaining asthma control (80–83). Since aspirin inhibits the COX pathway, and shunts arachidonic acid into the 5-LO pathway to produce more CysLTs, it is not surprising that CysLT1 receptor antagonists appear to be useful in treating aspirin-sensitive asthma in some patients (69,84–86). There is as yet no consensus on whether LTIs should be used as a routine adjunct to low-dose ICS in patients with mild asthma, or as an alternative to increasing ICS dose in patients with difficult to control asthma. It is too early to tell whether these drugs have a long-term impact on airway remodeling.

C. New Anti-inflammatory Therapies Under Clinical Evaluation for Asthma

As described earlier, IgE plays a key role in the mediation of allergic inflammation. Binding of allergen plus IgE to the FcεRI receptor on the surface of mast cells results in degranulation, releasing inflammatory mediators that cause bronchospasm, edema, and recruitment of other inflammatory cells (87,88). The importance of allergy in asthma is somewhat controversial in that many adult-onset patients exhibit no detectable allergies and normal levels of serum IgE (89). Nevertheless, IgE is a good therapeutic target for many patients. Omalizumab is a humanized monoclonal antibody that binds the c3 domain of human IgE, preventing IgE from interacting with the FcεRI receptor (90–92). In clinical trials, omalizumab appears to be well tolerated with few side effects. Omalizumab treatment (biweekly intravenous injections) dramatically reduced the level of serum IgE but had only a modest effect in maintaining asthma control during ICS withdrawal (93). However, in more recent trials, monthly subcutaneous injections of omalizumab reduced the need for ICS while improving asthma control, lung function, and selfreported quality of life in patients with moderate to severe asthma who were symptomatic at the start of the study (94). Omalizumab was also effective in reducing steroid use and frequency of exacerbations in pediatric asthma (95). In 2003, omalizumab received FDA approval, and is recommended for treatment of patients with moderate to severe persistent asthma that is not well controlled by traditional therapies (96). It remains to be seen whether blockade of IgE can moderate the natural history of asthma in addition to providing symptomatic relief.

IL-4 is a potential target for therapy of allergic asthma because it is a key cytokine in the development of the allergic response. IL-4 causes B-cells to undergo isotype class switching to produce IgE antibodies and up-regulates IgE receptors on mast cells and basophils. IL-4 also induces expression of vascular cell adhesion molecule 1 (VCAM-1), which promotes recruitment of inflammatory cells to airways (56,97,98). IL-4 along with IL-13 drives T-cell differentiation to the Th2 phenotype, which results in the production of additional cytokines known to promote asthma including IL-5, IL-9 and IL-13 (49,99,100). Blocking the activity of IL-4 should interrupt a number of separate signaling pathways that contribute to asthma. One approach currently being evaluated in clinical trials is the use of a recombinant soluble IL-4 receptor (sIL-4R) that acts as receptor decoy to bind IL-4 and prevent signaling through the IL-4R on inflammatory effector cells (101). A recent study demonstrated the clinical benefits of sIL-4R treatment in patients with moderate asthma who were being treated with ICS. Soluble IL-4 receptor, delivered by nebulizer once per week, preserved lung function following abrupt withdrawal of ICS treatment, while placebo treatment resulted in a decline in forced expiratory volume in one second (FEV_1) and an increase in asthma symptom scores (102). Further studies are needed to determine which inflammatory signaling pathways are being suppressed by sIL-4R and whether sIL-4R may have a long-term effect on preventing airway remodeling.

Eosinophils and their products are believed to play a critical role in the pathogenesis of many forms of asthma. IL-5 is essential for the recruitment, maturation and survival of eosinophils, and is elevated in serum and bronchial biopsies from asthma patients, while inhalation of IL-5 provokes sputum eosinophilia and airway hyper-reactivity (103–107). Thus, IL-5 seems a promising target of anti-inflammatory therapies in asthma. However, two reports of human trials with monoclonal antibodies to IL-5 failed to demonstrate a reduction in the late asthmatic response or airway hyper-reactivity. In these studies, a single dose of anti-IL-5 monoclonal antibody decreased eosinophil numbers in blood and sputum 10–20 fold but did not affect the late asthmatic response, measured as percent change in FEV_1 and change in histamine concentration needed to provoke a 20% reduction in peak flow (PC_{20}) following allergen challenge (108–110). Further research is needed to fully evaluate the potential of eosinophil-specific therapies on asthma outcomes.

Phosphodiesterase type 4 (PDE4) is a key regulator of cyclic AMP levels in immune and inflammatory cells, and PDE4 inhibitors have been shown to reduce neutrophil chemotaxis, activation and degranulation (111), as well as relax smooth muscle cells. Theophylline, a nonspecific phosphodiesterase inhibitor, has long been used in asthma management, but has a narrow therapeutic window along with prominent cardiovascular and central nervous system toxicity (112). A selective PDE4 inhibitor, roflumilast, has anti-inflammatory properties in rat and guinea pig models of allergic airway inflammation (113), and in an early clinical trial was shown to reduce the symptoms of exercise-induced asthma (114).

D. Preclinical Studies of Novel Cytokine-Based Anti-inflammatory Therapy for Asthma

IL-2 is a T-cell autocrine growth factor. Daclizumab is a humanized monoclonal antibody that specifically antagonizes the IL-2 receptor α chain (CD25), which is expressed only on activated T-cells. Daclizumab inhibits cellular immune functions including IL-2-dependent T-cell proliferation and production of both Th1 and Th2 type cytokines (115,116). It also blocks IL-2-dependent signaling (117) and down-regulates IL-2Rα chain expression (118). Daclizumab is effective in reducing the risk of renal allograft transplant rejection (118,119), and is being considered in the treatment of other chronic immune disorders, including asthma and psoriasis (120). Daclizumab would be expected to have a relatively nonspecific anti-inflammatory effect, similar to corticosteroids, in contrast to the relatively allergy-specific effects of omalizumab and sIL-4R. Daclizumab and dexamethasone act synergistically to inhibit T-cell proliferation and cytokine production (116), suggesting that adding daclizumab to corticosteroid therapy may reduce the doses of corticosteroids necessary to provide effective asthma control.

Although IL-10 is often regarded as a pro-Th2 cytokine, it has a number of anti-inflammatory effects that may be important in asthma, including suppression of the eosinophil chemoattractants eotaxin and IL-5 and inhibition of iNOS and COX-2 (121–123). Peripheral blood monocytes and alveolar macrophages from asthma patients produce less IL-10 than normal volunteers (124,125). It has been hypothesized that IL-10 is produced in the late response to allergen and is responsible for down-regulating the inflammatory response of iNOS, COX-2, and other inflammatory chemokines and cytokines (121,126). In fact, oral and mucosal tolerance are associated with increased levels of IL-10 (127,128). Thus, administration of IL-10 might suppress the initial inflammatory response to allergen exposure, an effect that has already been demonstrated in a mouse model of asthma (129). IL-10 has been used to successfully treat patients with inflammatory bowel disease (130), suggesting its anti-inflammatory effects may also be useful in the treatment of asthma.

In the presence of IL-12, T-cells differentiate to a Th1 phenotype. Therefore, therapeutic administration of IL-12 has been suggested as a way of "reprogramming" the predominantly Th2 phenotype associated with asthma (97,126,131). Promising preliminary data include findings that asthma patients and atopic infants produce less IL-12 (132,133), and that administration of IL-12 to allergic mice reduces airway eosinophilia and airway hyper-reactivity (134). The results of a small human study were not promising, however. Administration of recombinant human IL-12 caused a significant reduction in eosinophils in blood and sputum, but had no effect on airway hyper-reactivity as measured by change in FEV_1 and histamine PC_{20} after allergen challenge (135). The results were thus similar to those seen with IL-5 antibodies, except that IL-12 provoked more serious side effects including flu-like symptoms and cardiac arrhythmia.

IL-13, along with IL-4, is one of the key cytokines responsible for driving Th2 responses (97,131). IL-4 and IL-13 have many apparently redundant functions, and the precise contribution of each to asthma pathology is not yet clear. In contrast to IL-4, IL-13 does not support proliferation of T-cells, but may be more important than IL-4 in promoting the effector phase of the allergic response, including mucus hypersecretion and airway hyper-responsiveness (136–138). Thus, it is theoretically possible that blockade of IL-13 might result in a reduction of airway hyper-responsiveness not seen with anti-IL-4 and anti-IL-5 therapies.

TNF-α is an important mediator of many inflammatory processes. Its most important role in asthma may be in up-regulating adhesion molecules that facilitate the recruitment of inflammatory cells into the airway and activating profibrotic mechanisms in the airway epithelium (139,140). Inhaled TNF-α increased methacholine sensitivity and sputum neutrophilia in human subjects (141), while TNF-α receptor antagonists block neutrophil and eosinophil recruitment in animal models of asthma (142). Etanercept is a TNF-α receptor antagonist that has been shown to be effective in treating severe rheumatoid arthritis refractory to standard treatments (143), and is currently under study in patients with mild asthma not requiring corticosteroid treatment.

Finally, increased understanding of the nature of the allergic response has led to renewed interest in immunotherapy to treat patients whose asthma can be traced to a specific antigen trigger. Specific immunotherapy is associated with a decrease in antigen-specific serum IgE, a shift from a Th2 to a Th1-like immune response, and improved symptom control (144,145). However, classical immunotherapy is limited by a lack of standardized extracts for common antigens, lot-to-lot variability, and adverse reactions that can be life-threatening. New strategies combine standardized recombinant antigen preparations with Th1-inducing adjuvants, such as IL-12, IFN-γ and CpG oligodeoxynucleotides, with the goal of creating a vaccine that promotes immune deviation toward a Th1 response and away from the existing allergic Th2 response (92,146,147).

V. Acute and Chronic Bronchitis

Acute bronchitis describes symptomatic inflammatory conditions of the bronchi with prominent cough and mucous expectoration that resolve within days to weeks. In contrast, chronic bronchitis describes airway mucous cell hyperplasia with symptomatic cough and mucous expectoration, but with little airflow obstruction, lasting two or more years. Airway inflammation is present by definition in all forms of bronchitis. Most episodes of acute bronchitis caused by viral infections of the respiratory tract (e.g., rhinovirus) in normal individuals resolve without treatment. More severe acute bronchitis can be caused by inhalation of a broad variety of workplace substances that injure the airways because of their acid, base, or other chemical characteristics. In addition, acute bronchitis can also be superimposed on underlying chronic lung disease and exacerbate its severity. For example, most patients with chronic bronchitis are cigarette smokers, and have some degree of associated chronic obstructive pulmonary disease (COPD). Recurrent episodes of acute bronchitis in patients with severe COPD can produce serious illness, and anti-inflammatory interventions to reduce the frequency or severity of these could markedly improve quality of life. Systemic (oral or intravenous) glucocorticosteroids (e.g., prednisone, prednisolone) given for two weeks in acute episodes of bronchitis in patients with severe underlying COPD may reduce symptom severity or duration, and are often prescribed in combination with other medications in those with advanced disease. Anecdotal evidence also supports the use of a 10-day or longer course of systemic corticosteroids in acute bronchitis caused by inhalation injury due to smoke, strong acids or bases, or other irritating substances after heavy occupational or environmental exposures. However, the full range and potential of anti-inflammatory therapies for bronchitis has not yet been explored.

VI. Chronic Obstructive Pulmonary Disease (COPD)

Chronic obstructive pulmonary disease describes a persistent condition of symptomatic airflow obstruction with underlying pathophysiology of emphysema (loss of alveolar tissue) often in combination with chronic bronchitis. While there is an inflammatory component (148), COPD is primarily a degenerative disease in which the major physiologic impairment is the result of emphysema. Many factors can contribute to the pathogenesis of COPD including: (1) environmental factors (cigarette smoking, viral and bacterial infections, occupational exposures and air pollution, nutritional factors) and (2) genetic factors such as alpha-1 antitrypsin (protease inhibitor) deficiency and the mEH His^{113}/His^{119} haplotype that is associated with decreased function of microsomal epoxide hydrolase (149).

A. Ineffectiveness of Current Anti-inflammatory Therapies for COPD

Anti-inflammatory treatment in COPD has been disappointingly ineffective in treating the underlying disease. Current therapy, while sometimes providing symptomatic relief, does not prolong survival. Glucocorticosteroids are the only anti-inflammatory medications currently in widespread use, and have been used successfully in COPD as a short-course therapy for acute bronchitis episodes in patients with severe disease (described above), for short term treatment in acute deterioration of patients with severe COPD (150), and for chronic treatment in a small subgroup of patients (less than 10%) who have more reversible airflow obstruction and demonstrate a clinical symptomatic response through a therapeutic trial. In these latter patients, the benefits of long-term glucocorticoid therapy must be weighed carefully against the universally experienced adverse effects of such agents. Long-term glucocorticoid treatment in most cases is best accompanied by supplemental calcium, vitamin D, and a bisphosphonate to reduce bone loss.

Inhaled glucocorticosteroids, which may have less severe side effects than systemic drugs, have been studied for use in COPD with relatively little success. Results of clinical studies with inhaled glucocorticoids have shown that: (1) patients with mild COPD who continued to smoke cigarettes experienced a small, one-time increase in lung function but not the desired reduction in the rate of lung function loss (151), and (2) patients with moderate COPD recruited by screening from the general population did not experience clinically significant reductions in acute exacerbations or in the rate of lung function loss (152). Subpopulations who may benefit from inhaled steroids are symptomatic COPD patients with documented spirometric response to ICS or with FEV_1 less than 50% predicted, and repeated exacerbations requiring treatment with antibiotics or oral corticosteroids (153).

Glucocorticoids are potent inhibitors of the transcription factors NF-κB and activator protein 1 (AP-1). Nuclear factor kappa B is activated and stimulates synthesis of IL-6 in both experimental rhinovirus infection of cultured nasal epithelial cells and in natural infection of otherwise healthy adults (154). It is plausible that this pathway could play a role in the acute decompensations that occur in some patients with far-advanced COPD, and appear to be initiated by rhinovirus and other viral respiratory infections. Inhibition of this proposed interaction would require institution of treatment early in the course of community-acquired virus infection in patients with COPD. Also, NF-κB might participate in activation of genes whose products promote the adhesion and extravasation of white blood cells through vessels at sites of inflammation (155). These factors could play a role in the inflammatory component of episodes of infectious exacerbation of COPD (156), though there is as yet relatively little disease-specific information indicating these pathways are important specifically in such exacerbations. The finding of adenovirus DNA in the lungs of many patients with COPD has suggested that interaction of cigarette smoke with chronic adenovirus infection could drive the progression of lung damage occurring in the airways of some actively smoking COPD patients (157).

B. Novel Anti-inflammatory Therapies in COPD

A number of pharmacological agents have been suggested as potential therapies with less toxicity than those in current use against inflammation in COPD (e.g., Table 2). Only a minority of such agents, however, have so far reached human trials. One class of agents for anti-inflammatory therapy in COPD are new phosphodiesterase inhibitors. The nonspecific phosphodiesterase inhibitor theophylline has long been used in COPD to relax smooth muscle, reduce airflow limitation, and improve contractility of the diaphragm. Theophylline provides symptomatic benefit in many patients with COPD, but has a narrow therapeutic window along with prominent cardiovascular and central nervous system toxicity, and it does not alter the long-term course of disease. A number of "second generation" PDE4 inhibitors have been identified which have fewer side effects than earlier PDE4 inhibitors such as rolipram (158). Animal and in vitro studies have shown the potential of these compounds to limit production of inflammatory mediators and lung inflammation in antigen-stimulated rodent models of asthma (but not in models of COPD) (113,159,160). In clinical trials, the selective PDE4 inhibitor cilomilast improved lung function in COPD patients (161,162), and reduced the number of airway tissue inflammatory cells and the production of the neutrophil chemoattractants TNF-α and GM-CSF (163,164).

Mitogen-activated protein (MAP) kinases can play a role in chronic inflammatory conditions including in lung, although a role in COPD has not been specifically defined. Mitogen-activated protein kinases are crucial in pathways and enzyme cascades that lead to production of the proinflammatory cytokines IL-8 and TNF-α, both of which are produced by macrophages, among other cells. The p38 MAP kinase family has four known members (165). Their selective pharmacological inhibition reduced inflammatory prostaglandin release in cultured alveolar cells in a way that suggested their effect was upstream of COX-2 (166). Mitogen-activated protein kinase inhibitors also reduced lipopolysaccharide-stimulated TNF-α mRNA accumulation in vitro in purified human monocytes, and reduced inflammation in animal models of nonpulmonary disease, suggesting the possibility of use for the inflammatory component of COPD (167).

In the genetic form of emphysema caused by alpha-1 antitrypsin deficiency, lack of this major serum inhibitor of serine proteases leads to unopposed action of neutrophil elastase as neutrophils move through lung tissue, resulting in loss of lung elastin and lung alveolar surface. Current attempts to prevent emphysema in patients with this genetic condition include cigarette smoking prevention, and intravenous or inhalation supplementation with recombinant replacement alpha-1 antitrypsin, which can raise serum levels (168,169). This strategy is hoped to retard the progression of disease. In the sense that this replacement therapy opposes the actions of lung neutrophil products (serine proteases), this might be considered a form of anti-inflammatory therapy.

Inhibitors of metalloproteinases or agents that increase their production, such as all-*trans*-retinoic acid (ATRA), have been proposed as potential inhibitors of emphysema (170). Human BAL cells (mostly macrophages) from patients with COPD and other lung diseases express decreased levels of matrix metalloproteinase 9 (MMP-9) and increased levels of the tissue inhibitor of metalloproteinase 1 (TIMP-1) when incubated with ATRA, indicating that this compound can affect the proteinase/antiproteinase ratio (171). In addition, ATRA might have other beneficial effects, since it has been found to promote alveolar formation in rats and to regenerate alveoli in adult rats with elastase-induced emphysema (172). A pilot study of ATRA in human emphysema found no measurable benefit, but since the treatment was well tolerated with few side effects, higher doses, longer treatment, or different dosing schedules might be feasible (173).

VII. Fibrosing Diseases of the Lung (Interstitial Lung Diseases)

Fibrosis or scarring of the lung is a progressive and debilitating pathological condition. Fibroblast hyperplasia, in concert with the deposition of excessive amounts of extracellular matrix components (ECM), leads to thickening of the pulmonary interstitium and a compromised ability for gas exchange. This occurs via a series of overlapping phases that can include coagulation, inflammation, remodeling, and repair. Such phases have similarities to normal wound healing, but in this case, they are abnormal and without resolution. Fibrosis is a seminal feature of a variety of lung disorders that fall into the broad category of interstitial lung diseases (ILD) (also known as restrictive lung diseases). Interstitial lung diseases involve chronic interstitial (and alveolar) inflammation that follows an acute insult to the lungs. Thus, anti-inflammatory therapies are an important focus of current treatments for fibrosis, as well as the subject of ongoing research in this field. However, ILDs often occur in the absence of overt leukocyte infiltration. Rather, lung fibroblasts both produce and respond to inflammatory mediators, giving rise to an expanded definition of inflammation (174). Newer anti-inflammatory strategies that target pulmonary fibroblasts, as well as classical anti-inflammatory therapies, are described below.

A. Interstitial Lung Disease

A variety of etiologies are associated with clinical pulmonary pathology classified under the broad heading of ILD (175) (Chapter 5). Important causes of ILD include occupational and environmental inhalation exposure to silica, asbestos, or other toxic particulates. In addition, inhalation of organic substances such as moldy hay can cause allergic reactions resulting in regional pulmonary fibrosis known as hypersensitivity pneumonitis or extrinsic allergic alveolitis. Other causes of ILD/fibrosis are exposure to drugs and toxins such as radiation and chemotherapeutic agents. Viri, fungi, mycobacterium, and pneumocystis are examples of infectious agents that can lead to ILD and fibrosis. Lung fibrosis can also occur as part of multisystem disorders like collagen vascular diseases, which include systemic sclerosis, rheumatoid arthritis, and systemic lupus erythematosus. In approximately 60% of cases, no underlying cause of ILD can be identified, and these are therefore termed idiopathic pulmonary fibrosis (176). Regardless of cause, patients with ILD suffer from the detrimental effects of limited lung function as a result of tissue fibrosis. Although prognosis varies between individual forms of ILD, there is a limited range of treatments available whose effects vary from patient to patient, and do not offer a great improvement in the quality of life for most patients.

Pulmonary fibrosis in ILD can be viewed as abnormal wound healing in injured tissue. After an initial insult that damages alveolar and airway epithelial cells, healing begins in association with coagulation and an innate acute inflammatory response. These processes often include the recruitment of neutrophils, monocytes, macrophages, and T-cells into the site of injury, followed by the migration and proliferation of fibroblasts/myofibroblasts into the wound along the provisional matrix established via the clotting cascade (177,178). Fibroblasts play a key role in the repair phases of injury. They begin to synthesize collagens and other ECM components necessary to restore tissue integrity. Fibroblasts also are essential in producing enzymes that break down ECM components, which is required for the resolution of scarring and the eventual normalization of tissue function (177,178). Fibroblasts also synthesize many cytokines and chemokines, and participate in pulmonary inflammation as well as repair (179). Thus, fibroblasts coordinate the repair and resolution of scar formation by crosstalk with other resident cells. Dysregulation at any stage of this process may result in the abnormal wound healing that results in fibrosis. Over the last several years, significant progress has been made in understanding the processes, cytokines, chemokines, growth factors, and signaling pathways that contribute to pulmonary inflammation and lead to interstitial fibrosis (e.g., Chapters 3–6). The relative ineffectiveness of current therapies for ILD has led to significant interest in exploiting this improved basic science understanding to develop improved anti-inflammatory interventions.

B. Idiopathic Pulmonary Fibrosis

Idiopathic pulmonary fibrosis is a chronic and progressive disease of unknown etiology. Idiopathic pulmonary fibrosis is one of the most commonly diagnosed ILDs in adults over 50 years of age (176,180). There is no known curative therapy for IPF, and the clinical course of this disease typically progresses to death after respiratory failure. Definitive diagnosis requires histological findings of usual interstitial pneumonia (UIP) in conjunction with exclusion of any other known cause of ILD. The hallmark features of UIP is a heterogeneous pattern of alternating areas of normal lung, inflammation (albeit minimal), fibroproliferation, active fibroblast foci, and dense fibrosis with honeycombing of the lung parenchyma (181). The mortality rate for patients with IPF is appalling, with a median survival time of only 2.8 years (182).

Similar to other fibrosing diseases of the lung, IPF is believed to be associated with chronic inflammation (183). However, at the time of diagnosis, there is relatively little evidence of classical inflammation in most patients. Nonetheless, current treatment strategies are aimed at controlling the "inflammatory response" in hopes of preventing further lung damage/scarring. Treatment options for IPF have remained essentially unchanged over the last 30 years. Corticosteroids, usually prednisone, are still routinely used in therapy (184,185). The current recommended treatment for IPF combines prednisone with cytotoxic immunosuppressive agents, such as cyclophosphamide or azathioprine, and is suggested to be more effective than either single therapy alone (184). Most patients, however, do not improve in response to these anti-inflammatory therapies. Also, the minority of patients that do respond frequently show a transient improvement in lung function but without improved survival or quality of life (184). Not only are current treatment options only marginally effective, they are also associated with many serious side effects.

C. Sarcoidosis

Sarcoidosis is a multisystem ILD of unknown etiology. It is commonly diagnosed in young and middle-aged adults (176,186). Sarcoidosis affects multiple organs, but most commonly involves the lungs. Sarcoidosis is histologically characterized by the appearance of noncaseating epithelioid granulomas. These granulomas consist of epithelioid cells, giant cells, and lymphocytes, predominantly CD4+ T-cells. Sarcoid granulomas may develop fibrotic changes and lead to permanent scarring/fibrosis of the lungs. However, in contrast to IPF, sarcoidosis is often acute and selflimiting, and spontaneous resolution can occur without treatment (187). When pulmonary sarcoidosis is associated with interstitial fibrosis and abnormal and declining lung function, treatment with corticosteroids is usually initiated in an attempt to limit inflammation and potential fibrosis. Oral and ICS have proven to be somewhat beneficial in the relief of respiratory systems and improving radiologic findings in pulmonary sarcoidosis (187). However, little evidence exists for a beneficial effect on long-term lung function. Respiratory symptoms and radiologic findings often reappear within 2 years of discontinuing treatment (176,186). Relapses may be prevented with continuous low-dose corticosteroid treatment; however, the side effects substantially limit their long-term use (186,188).

It has been postulated that the lack of response to corticosteroid treatment in many sarcoid patients is due to more advanced disease associated with irreversible lung damage. It is possible that corticosteroids would be much more effective in early stages of the disease. This is supported by a study published by Pietinalho et al. (188), which shows that treatment of newly detected pulmonary sarcoidosis with the anti-inflammatory steroid prednisone resulted in improvement in lung function in patients with Stage II disease over a 5-year follow-up period. As with IPF, cytotoxic agents have also been used to treat sarcoidosis. These include methotrexate, azathioprine, cyclophosphamide and cyclosporine A (186,189). Although valuable for the treatment of some patients, there is no consensus on the benefits vs. risk of using cytotoxic agents in the treatment of pulmonary sarcoidosis (186).

D. Anti-inflammatory Treatments for ILD/Fibrosis in Current Clinical Trials

The ineffectiveness of standard anti-inflammatory therapies for pulmonary fibrosis has led to the study of alternative approaches that attempt to regulate the activity of the main effector cell in fibrosis, the lung fibroblast. This is achieved either through direct effects on collagen production (colchicine, D-penicillamine, pirfenidone, and IFN-γ), or indirectly by influencing inflammatory signaling pathways (IFN-γ, anti-TNF-α).

Colchicine, an inhibitor of collagen synthesis and secretion, has been evaluated for the treatment of IPF in two studies. Neither colchicine alone, nor prednisone combined with colchicine, resulted in improved clinical outcome (190,191). Pulmonary function continued to decline and median survival was unchanged. The only noted benefits were the fewer side effects of colchicine therapy compared to prednisone. D-penicillamine inhibits collagen accumulation by interfering with collagen crosslinking (192). Although the use of D-penicillamine has produced some benefits in treating systemic sclerosis (193) in humans and in some animal models of IPF (194), it has not provided any significant improvement in the treatment of patients with IPF (191). Another antifibrotic drug, pirfenidone, has been shown to ameliorate bleomycin-induced pulmonary fibrosis in an animal model of IPF (195). It has also provided encouraging results in a Phase II clinical study, which demonstrated that treatment with pirfenidone halted the clinical decline of IPF patients by stabilizing lung function (196).

IFN-γ is a promising antifibrotic therapy as it regulates collagen production by lung fibroblasts, reduces the production and action of the profibrotic cytokine TGF-β, and drives T-cell responses toward the Th1 phenotype and away from the Th2 phenotype closely associated with fibrosis (see Fig. 2). As discussed above, the Th2 phenotype is associated with humoral immunity and allergy, and is marked by production of the cytokines IL-4, IL-5, and IL-13. Evidence is accumulating that the Th2 response is also profibrotic. For example, IL-4 and IL-13 both stimulate lung fibroblasts to produce collagen and other ECM proteins (185,194,197,198). Lung tissues and BAL from patients with IPF have been found to express elevated levels of IL-4, IL-5, and IL-13 (199,200). By driving T-cell responses toward the Th1 phenotype, IFN-γ can reduce the production of profibrotic type 2 cytokines. IFN-γ also directly suppresses deposition of collagen and other ECM proteins by fibroblasts (197). Ziesche et al. (201) reported that IPF patients treated with prednisone plus IFN-γ showed a significant improvement in lung function over those treated with prednisone alone. IFN-γ therapy is currently in Phase III clinical trials for the treatment of IPF (www.Intermune.com).

TNF-α is a proinflammatory cytokine that has been implicated in the pathogenesis of a number of inflammatory diseases including ILD. In

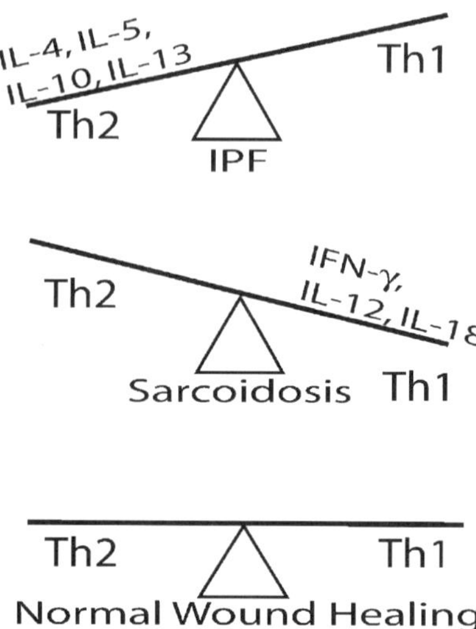

Figure 2   Schematic of the balance of Th 1 (type 1) and Th2 (type 2) cytokines in wound healing and chronic lung disease. An overabundance of either Th1 (type 1) or Th2 (type 2) cytokines can tip the scales from normal wound healing towards development of chronic pulmonary diseases like idiopathic pulmonary fibrosis (IPF) or sarcoidosis. Idiopathic pulmonary fibrosis is characterized by a Th2 cytokine profile, while Sarcoidosis is predominantly a Th1 cytokine dominated disease. See text for details.

animal studies, overexpression of TNF-α induces severe interstitial inflammation and patchy fibrosis (202), while TNF-α neutralizing antibodies and a soluble TNF decoy receptor both attenuate bleomycin-induced fibrosis in animal models (203,204). Increased levels of TNF-α have been found in BAL of patients with sarcoidosis (205,206). Thus, TNF-α is being considered as a target of therapy for sarcoidosis. TNF-α has been a prime therapeutic target in other inflammatory diseases, such as rheumatoid arthritis. Etanercept (a soluble TNF-α receptor fusion protein) and infliximab (an anti-TNF-α antibody) have both been used successfully to treat rheumatoid arthritis (207,208). Pentoxyfylline (POF), a drug that inhibits TNF-α release, has been shown to reduce the exaggerated TNF-α production by alveolar macrophages from sarcoidosis patients in vitro (206). In addition, improvement in lung function has been reported after treatment of sarcoid patients with POF in a small study (209). Both POF and etanercept are in clinical trials to evaluate their effectiveness in the treatment of sarcoidosis (210).

E.   Novel Anti-inflammatory Treatments for ILD

Much more is now known about the complex nature of inflammation and the intercellular communication mechanisms of infiltrating leukocytes and resident lung cells (e.g., airway smooth muscle cells, epithelial cells, fibroblasts) involved in fibrosing ILDs. Although more research is clearly needed, a number of potential candidates for anti-inflammatory therapy for IPF have been identified by animal studies. The CD40–CD40 ligand (CD154) system delivers important regulatory signals to lung fibroblasts (18,179,211,212). For example, blocking CD154 from activating its receptor CD40 has been shown to be useful in substantially blocking inflammation, lung injury, and fibrosis in both ionizing radiation and oxygen-induced mouse models of fibrosis (213,214). Cytosolic phospholipase A2 (cPLA2), a key enzyme for eicosinoid generation, represents another potential therapeutic target. Cytosolic phospholipase A2 knockout mice treated with bleomycin exhibit attenuated inflammation and fibrosis compared to wild type control mice (215). The role of IL-8 in contributing to the pathogenesis of Pseudomonal infection has been discussed above; IL-8 is also elevated in the BAL of IPF patients (216), suggesting therapies targeting this cytokine should be studied in IPF.

TGF-β is proving to be a critical cytokine for lung fibrosis. In animal studies, TGF-β stimulates fibroblasts to produce collagen, and overexpression of TGF-β in the mouse lung induces a fibroproliferative lung disease (217,218). Increased expression of TGF-β1 has been found in the lung tissue of IPF patients (219). A number of strategies to neutralize TGF-β are being explored. Anti-TGF-β antibodies prevent bleomycin-induced fibrosis (220), as does a soluble TGF-β decoy receptor (221). Gene therapy using an adenovirus vector expressing decorin, a naturally occurring inhibitor of TGF-β, in the mouse lung reduces bleomycin-induced fibrosis (222,223).

IL-7, a cytokine that has been shown to enhance IFN-γ production and secretion by T-cells, has also been shown to down-regulate TGF-β production and signaling in pulmonary fibroblasts, and to inhibit lung fibrosis in the mouse bleomycin model (224). Thus, IL-7 may be a potential therapeutic intervention for IPF that would target events upstream of TGF-β. IL-10 has also been studied and some reports indicate its usefulness in controlling bleomycin-induced lung injury (225). However, IL-10 is a Th2 regulatory cytokine that has been shown to inhibit IFN-γ synthesis by T-cells (225), while IFN-γ itself has been shown to be effective in the treatment of IPF (201). This points to the complexity and the redundancy of the cytokine network.

Unlike IPF, pulmonary sarcoidosis is characterized by a Th1 cytokine profile (Fig. 2). T-lymphocytes and BAL cells of patients with sarcoidosis have been shown to have elevated levels of IFN-γ, IL-2, and IL-12 mRNA and protein when compared to normal controls or to their expression of Th2 cytokines (226,227). IL-12 has been shown to play a central role in the skewing of an immune response towards Th1. IL-12 can stimulate IFN-γ production by activated T-cells (228). IL-18, which is increased in BAL of sarcoid patients (229), can synergize with IL-12 to induce IFN-γ

(230). Furthermore, IL-12 induces differentiation of T-cell precursors into Th1 cytokine secreting cells (231). These data provide evidence that sarcoidosis is a Th1-mediated disorder and that progression of this disease may be driven by the dysregulated expression of the Th1 regulatory cytokines IL-12 and IL-18. These studies thus provide a foundation for several possible anti-inflammatory interventions for sarcoidosis. For example, using inhibitors of IL-12 and/or IL-18 may help suppress the predominant Th1 cytokine pattern. IL-10 may also prove to be beneficial, since it is a potent down-regulator of IL-12 production (232) and could skew inflammation towards Th2 so as to restore a proper balance between Th1 and Th2 responses in sarcoidosis.

Expression microarray analysis offers an important new method for identifying added targets of potential relevance for anti-inflammatory therapy in injury-related respiratory disease. Messages that differ significantly in expression between healthy and diseased lung tissue may prove to be important in disease pathogenesis. For example, expression microarray analysis has shown that uteroglobulin (CC10), a small homodimeric protein expressed in lung epithelial mucosa, is significantly down-regulated in patients with IPF, sarcoidosis, asthma, pneumonia, emphysema, and COPD. CC10 may be an important regulator of lung inflammation that could be the subject of future therapeutic interventions (233). Continuing basic research using expression microarray analysis and other new methodologies such as proteomics and bioinformatics should continue to identify molecules and regulatory processes important in pulmonary inflammation and repair that can be exploited in novel anti-inflammatory therapies.

VIII. Summary

An appropriate innate pulmonary inflammatory response is required for clearance of pathogens and initiation of tissue repair following infection or lung injury. However, there are many clinical conditions in which over-exuberant inflammation has pathologic consequences. This chapter has described several important classes of pulmonary disease characterized by dysregulated or persistent inflammatory processes (pneumonia, asthma, bronchitis, COPD, and fibrosing ILDs). All of these diseases contain a component of inflammatory lung injury. Anti-inflammatory therapies for these conditions have been discussed, with an emphasis on the rationale and evidence for novel and emerging treatments.

Pneumonia is marked by a classic inflammatory response, including infiltration of leukocytes and edema, with a resulting loss of lung function. This inflammatory response is required for microbial clearance, but also needs to be selflimiting. In some cases of pneumonia, excessive inflammation occurs, resulting in reduced lung function and increased patient morbidity and mortality. Asthma is also characterized by infiltrating leukocytes, predominantly eosinophils and lymphocytes, but with the additional components of airway smooth muscle hyperplasia and hyper-reactivity, mucus cell hyperplasia, and subepithelial fibrosis. Chronic obstructive pulmonary disease and fibrosing ILDs are associated with chronic inflammation and dysregulation of normal tissue repair. The challenge in each of these diseases is to understand how inflammatory signals and processes contribute specifically to pathology, and to develop anti-inflammatory therapies that antagonize these abnormalities while maintaining the beneficial host defense aspects of the innate inflammatory response.

For many years, the only treatments available for noninfective inflammatory lung diseases were immunosuppressive agents such as the glucocorticosteroids. Advances in basic science understanding of inflammatory cells and signals has led to a second generation of anti-inflammatory therapies which target leukocyte infiltration by inhibiting cells and inflammatory mediators specific to individual disease processes. Some of these therapies are now approved for use, and others are in advanced trials. Researchers have also begun to uncover the role of resident lung cells (fibroblasts, airway smooth muscle, and epithelium) in promoting inflammation. Far from being passive bystanders in a process driven by infiltrating cells, these resident cells actively participate in inflammation by expressing adhesion molecules, chemokines, and cytokines. These cells are also important effectors for pathological lung inflammatory processes including airway hyperreactivity (airway smooth muscle) and fibrosis (fibroblasts). Thus, a third generation of anti-inflammatory drugs is under development which actively targets the proinflammatory role of resident lung cells.

Corticosteroids, especially ICS, remain the most effective treatment for asthma. However, while suppressing the inflammatory response and providing symptomatic relief, these drugs do not treat the underlying causes of asthma and are associated with unwanted side effects. Corticosteroids are also ineffective in most patients with COPD or IPF, which are believed to be inflammatory in nature. Steroid therapy is also contraindicated in infectious diseases, in which immunosuppression can lead to increased organism burden, overwhelming infection, and even death. *P. carinii* pneumonia is an exception to this, in that the host inflammatory response to *P. carinii* is a greater contributor to loss of pulmonary function than the organism itself.

Novel anti-inflammatory therapies for infectious diseases include macrolide antibiotics and inhibitors of bacterial virulence factors. Macrolide antibiotics have both antimicrobial and anti-inflammatory effects, thus offering some control over the negative effects of pulmonary inflammation in pneumonia, particularly in CF patients, without sacrificing pathogen control. In addition to promoting bacterial growth, virulence factors provoke specific inflammatory responses in the host, suggesting that inhibitors of bacterial virulence factors will have multiple therapeutic effects. The anti-inflammatory properties of IL-10 and NF-κB inhibitors may also prove useful, especially in PCP.

Leukotriene inhibitors were the first new therapies for asthma approved in a generation. Leukotrienes are inflammatory mediators produced by infiltrating leukocytes (mainly mast cells and eosinophils), which have direct proinflammatory effects on lung resident cells. Inhibitors that block the production of leukotrienes or antagonize the CysTL1 receptor have proven effective in controlling asthma symptoms, particularly in concert with ICS. Results with antagonists of IgE or inflammatory cytokines important in asthma have been disappointing to date. For example, IgE and IL-4 antagonists, both of which reduce the amount of IgE present in the serum, have only modest effects on lung function in patients with asthma. Similarly, anti-IL-5 monoclonal antibody dramatically reduces the number of infiltrating eosinophils with little effect on airway hyper-reactivity. These results, along with animal studies, demonstrate that leukocyte infiltration can be dissociated from airway hyper-reactivity in asthma. Inflammatory cytokines also directly promote smooth muscle proliferation and mucus hypersecretion. Future improvements in asthma treatment may be obtained by combining antieosinophil or antileukocyte therapies with drugs that reduce smooth muscle proliferation and mucus hypersecretion, or otherwise modulate the activity of resident lung cells.

The role of resident lung cells in chronic pulmonary inflammation and fibrosis is most clearly evident in ILD. There is often little overt leukocyte infiltration in such conditions, while resident fibroblasts respond to inflammatory signals by producing collagen and also express multiple inflammatory cytokines and adhesion molecules. Etanercept and infliximab, TNF-α antagonists, which have been approved for use in rheumatoid arthritis, are being investigated for use in both IPF and asthma. Strategies to neutralize TGF-β have also been promising in animal studies of pulmonary fibrosis. In addition, administration of IFN-γ is being evaluated for use in treating ILD (specifically IPF). IFN-γ not only directly down-regulates production of collagen by fibroblasts, but drives inflammatory responses away from the profibrotic Th2 phenotype. Future progress in anti-inflammatory therapies will depend upon a thorough understanding of leukocyte–leukocyte, leukocyte–resident cell, and resident cell–resident cell signaling, and the relative contribution of each to the different types of pathological lung inflammation.

Acknowledgment

Supported in part by USPHS grants HL078603, EY08976, DE11390, ES01247, HL65208, AI07285, HL66988, the Cystic Fibrosis Foundation (CFF00Z0), and the Philip Morris External Research Program.

References

1. Selman M, King T, Pardo A. Idiopathic pulmonary fibrosis: prevailing and evolving hypotheses about its pathogenesis and implications for therapy. Ann Intern Med 2001; 134(2):136–151.
2. Phipps R. Atherosclerosis: the emerging role of inflammation and the CD40–CD40 ligand system. Proc Natl Acad Sci USA 2000; 97(13):6930–6932.
3. Sempowski G, Rozenblit J, Smith T, Phipps R. Human orbital fibroblasts are activated through CD40 to induce proinflammatory cytokine production. Am J Physiol 1998; 274(3):C707–C714.
4. Marrie TJ. Acute bronchitis and community-acquired pneumonia. In: Fishman AP, ed. Pulmonary Diseases and Disorders. New York: McGraw-Hill, 1998:1985–1996.
5. Tan T. Update on pneumococcal infections of the respiratory tract. Semin Respir Infect 2002; 17(1):3–9.
6. Wilson R, Dowling R. *Pseudomonas aeruginosa* and other related species. Thorax 1998; 53:213–219.
7. Doring G. Cystic fibrosis respiratory infections: interactions between bacteria and host defense. Monaldi Arch Chest Dis 1997; 52(4):363–366.
8. Dinwiddie R. Pathogenesis of lung disease in cystic fibrosis. Respiration 2000; 67(1):3–8.
9. Bartlett M. Update in infectious diseases. Ann Intern Med 2000; 133:285–292.
10. Cunha B. Pneumonias in the compromised host. Infect Dis Clin North Am 2001; 15(2):591–612.
11. Moore T, Standiford T. The role of cytokines in bacterial pneumonia: an inflammatory balancing act. Proc Assoc Am Phys 1998; 110(4):297–305.
12. Hoiby N. Prospects for the prevention and control of pseudomonal infection in children with cystic fibrosis. Paediatr Drugs 2000; 2(6):451–463.
13. Zhanel G, Ennis K, Vercaigne L, Walkty A, Gin A, Embil J, Smith H, Hoban D. A critical review of the fluoroquinolones: focus on respiratory infections. Drugs 2002; 62(1):13–59.
14. Jaffe A, Bush A. Anti-inflammatory effects of macrolides in lung disease. Pediatr Pulmonol 2001; 31(6):464–473.
15. Tonelli MR, Aitken ML. New and emerging therapies for pulmonary complications of cystic fibrosis. Drugs 2001; 61(10):1379–1385.
16. Jaffe A, Francis J, Rosenthal M, Bush A. Long-term azithromycin may improve lung function in children with cystic fibrosis. Lancet 1998; 351(9100):420.
17. Hoyt J, Robbins R. Macrolide antibiotics and pulmonary inflammation. FEMS Microbiol Lett 2001; 205:1–7.
18. Smith RS, Smith TJ, Blieden TM, Phipps RP. Fibroblasts as sentinel cells. Synthesis of chemokines and regulation of inflammation. Am J Pathol 1997; 151(2):317–322.
19. Ware L, Matthay M. The Acute Respiratory Distress Syndrome. N Engl J Med 2000; 342(18):1334–1349.

20. Smith R, Harris S, Phipps R, Iglewski B. The Pseudomonas aeruginosa quorum-sensing molecule *N*-(3-oxododecanoyl) homoserine lactone contributes to virulence and induces inflammation in vivo. J Bacteriol 2002; 184(4):1132–1139.

21. Pearson J, Feldman M, Iglewski B, Prince A. *Pseudomonas aeruginosa* cell-to-cell signaling is required for virulence in a model of acute pulmonary infection. Infect Immun 2000; 68(7):4331–4334.

22. Smith RS, Fedyk ER, Springer TA, Mukaida N, Iglewski HB, Phipps RP. IL-8 production in human lung fibroblasts and epithelial cells activated by the Pseudomonas autoinducer *N*-3-oxododecanoyl homoserine lactone is transcriptionally regulated by NF-kappa B and activator protein-2. J Immunol 2001; 167(1):366–374.

23. Birke FW, Meade CJ, Anderskewitz R, Speck GA, Jennewein HM. In vitro and in vivo pharmacological characterization of BIIL 284, a novel and potent leukotriene B(4) receptor antagonist. J Pharmacol Exp Ther 2001; 297(1): 458–466.

24. Lands LC, Dezateux C, Crighton A. Oral non-steroidal anti-inflammatory drug therapy for cystic fibrosis. In: The Cochrane Library, Issue 4, 2004. Chichester, UK: John Wiley & Sons Ltd.

25. Lehrer RI, Ganz T. Defensins of vertebrate animals. Curr Opin Immunol 2002; 14(1):96–102.

26. Travis SM, Singh PK, Welsh MJ. Antimicrobial peptides and proteins in the innate defense of the airway surface. Curr Opin Immunol 2001; 13(1): 89–95.

27. Travis SM, Anderson NN, Forsyth WR, Espiritu C, Conway BD, Greenberg EP, McCray PB Jr, Lehrer RI, Welsh MJ, Tack BF. Bactericidal activity of mammalian cathelicidin-derived peptides. Infect Immun 2000; 68(5): 2748–2755.

28. Smith JJ, Travis SM, Greenberg EP, Welsh MJ. Cystic fibrosis airway epithelia fail to kill bacteria because of abnormal airway surface fluid. Cell 1996; 85(2):229–236.

29. Yu Q, Lehrer RI, Tam JP. Engineered salt-insensitive alpha-defensins with end-to-end circularized structures. J Biol Chem 2000; 275(6):3943–3949.

30. Goldman MJ, Anderson GM, Stolzenberg ED, Kari UP, Zasloff M, Wilson JM. Human beta-defensin-1 is a salt-sensitive antibiotic in lung that is inactivated in cystic fibrosis. Cell 1997; 88(4):553–560.

31. Smaldone G, Palmer L. Aerosolized antibiotics: current and future. Respir Care 2000; 45(6):667–675.

32. Koyama H, Geddes D. Erythromycin and diffuse panbronchiolitis. Thorax 1997; 52:915–918.

33. Hayden F. Respiratory viral infections. Sci Am Med 1997; 7:1–12.

34. Bartlett J, Breimann R, Mandell L. Community-acquired pneumonia in adults: guidelines for management. The Infect Dis Soc Am Clin Infect Dis 1998; 26(4):811–838.

35. Greenberg SB. Viral infections of the lung and respiratory tract. In: Fishman AP, ed. Pulmonary Diseases and Disorders. New York: McGraw-Hill, 1998: 2333–2346.

36. Johnston SL. Natural and experimental rhinovirus infections of the lower respiratory tract. Am J Respir Crit Care Med. 1995; 152(4 Pt 2):S46–S52.

37. Sugar AM, Olek EA. Aspergillus syndromes, mucormycosis, and pulmonary candidiasis. In: Fishman AP, ed. Pulmonary-Diseases and Disorders. New York: McGraw-Hill, 1998:2265–2287.

38. Wark P, Gibson P. Allergic bronchopulmonary aspergillosis: new concepts of pathogenesis and treatment. Respirology 2001; 6:1–7.

39. Wilkin A, Feinberg J. *Pneumocystis carinii*pneumonia: a clinical review. Am Fam Phys 1999; 60:1699–1714.

40. Sepkowitz KA. Opportunistic infections in patients with and patients without acquired immunodeficiency syndrome. Clin Infect Dis 2002; 34(8): 1098–1107.

41. Mason GR, Hashimoto CH, Dickman PS, Foutty LF, Cobb CJ. Prognostic implications of bronchoalveolar lavage neutrophilia in patients with Pneumocystis carinii pneumonia and AIDS. Am Rev Respir Dis 1989; 139(6): 1336–1342.

42. Benfield TL, Vestbo J, Junge J, Nielsen TL, Jensen AB, Lundgren JD. Prognostic value of interleukin-8 in AIDS-associated *Pneumocystis carinii* pneumonia. Am J Respir Crit Care Med 1995; 151(4):1058–1062.

43. Cheng VC, Yuen KY, Chan WM, Wong SS, Ma ES, Chan RM. Immunorestitution disease involving the innate and adaptive response. Clin Infect Dis 2000; 30(6):882–892.

44. Rodriguez-Rosado R, Soriano V, Dona C, Gonzalez-Lahoz J. Opportunistic infections shortly after beginning highly active antiretroviral therapy. Antiviral Ther 1998; 3(4):229–231.

45. Fishman JA. *Pneumocystis carinii*. In: Fishman AP, ed. Pulmonary Diseases and Disorders. New York: McGraw-Hill, 1998:2313–2331.

46. Hahn PY, Limper AH. *Pneumocystis carinii* beta-glucan stimulation results in alveolar epithelial cell chemokine production via an NF-kappaB dependent pathway. Am J Respir Crit Care Med 2002; 165(8 (Pt 2)):A50.

47. Ruan S, Kolls JK, Shellito JE. Local delivery of the viral IL-10 gene suppresses tissue inflammation in murine P. *carinii* infection. Am J Respir Crit Care Med 2002; 165(8 (Pt 2)):A51.

48. NHLBI. Guidelines for the Diagnosis and Management of Asthma, NIH Publication 1997; 97–4051.

49. Mosmann TR, Coffman RL. TH1 and TH2 cells: different patterns of lymphokine secretion lead to different functional properties. Ann Rev Immunol 1989; 7:145–173.

50. Manetti R, Parronchi P, Giudizi MG, Piccinni MP, Maggi E, Trinchieri G, Romagnani S. Natural killer cell stimulatory factor (interleukin 12 [IL-12]) induces T helper type 1 (Th1)-specific immune responses and inhibits the development of IL-4-producing Th cells. J Exp Med 1993; 177(4): 1199–1204.

51. Marshall JD, Secrist H, DeKruyff RH, Wolf SF, Umetsu DT. IL-12 inhibits the production of IL-4 and IL-10 in allergen-specific human CD4+ T lymphocytes. J Immunol 1995; 155(1):111–117.

52. Hilkens CM, Snijders A, Snijdewint FG, Wierenga EA, Kapsenberg ML. Modulation of T-cell cytokine secretion by accessory cell-derived products. Eur Respir J Suppl 1996; 22:90s–94s.

53. de Vries JE, Carballido JM, Sornasse T, Yssel H. Antagonizing the differentiation and functions of human T helper type 2 cells. Curr Opin Immunol 1995; 7(6):771–778.

54. Ray A, Cohn L. Th2 cells and GATA-3 in asthma: new insights into the regulation of airway inflammation. J Clin Invest 1999; 104(8):985–993.

55. Coffman RL, Carty J. A T cell activity that enhances polyclonal IgE production and its inhibition by interferon-gamma. J Immunol 1986; 136(3):949–954.

56. Renauld JC. New insights into the role of cytokines in asthma. J Clin Pathol 2001; 54(8):577–589.

57. Ricci M, Rossi O, Bertoni M, Matucci A. The importance of Th2-like cells in the pathogenesis of airway allergic inflammation. Clin Exp Allergy 1993; 23(5):360–369.

58. Laitinen LA, Laitinen A, Heino M, Haahtela T. Eosinophilic airway inflammation during exacerbation of asthma and its treatment with inhaled corticosteroid. Am Rev Respir Dis 1991; 143(2):423–427.

59. Barnes PJ, Adcock I. Anti-inflammatory actions of steroids: molecular mechanisms. Trends Pharmacol Sci 1993; 14(12):436–441.

60. Eady RP. The pharmacology of nedocromil sodium. Eur J Respir Dis Suppl 1986; 147:112–119.

61. Kamada AK, Szefler SJ. The safety of inhaled corticosteroid therapy in children. Curr Opin Pediatr 1997; 9(6):585–589.

62. Kamada AK, Szefler SJ, Martin RJ, Boushey HA, Chinchilli VM, Drazen JM, Fish JE, Israel E, Lazarus SC, Lemanske RF. Issues in the use of inhaled glucocorticoids. The Asthma Clinical Research Network. Am J Respir Crit Care Med 1996; 153(6 Pt 1):1739–1748.

63. Toogood JH, Jennings B, Greenway RW, Chuang L. Candidiasis and dysphonia complicating beclomethasone treatment of asthma. J. Allergy Clin Immunol 1980; 65(2):145–153.

64. Toogood JH, Baskerville JC, Markov AE, Hodsman AB, Fraher LJ, Jennings B, Haddad RG, Drost D. Bone mineral density and the risk of fracture in patients receiving long-term inhaled steroid therapy for asthma. J Allergy Clin Immunol 1995; 96(2):157–166.

65. Tabachnik E, Zadik Z. Diurnal cortisol secretion during therapy with inhaled beclomethasone dipropionate in children with asthma. J Pediatr 1991; 118(2):294–297.

66. Dahlen SE, Dahlen B, Kumlin M, Bjorck T, Ihre E, Zetterstrom O. Clinical and experimental studies of leukotrienes as mediators of airway obstruction in humans. Adv Prostaglandin Thromboxane Leukot Res 1994; 22:155–166.

67. Bisgaard, H. Pathophysiology of the cysteinyl leukotrienes and effects of leukotriene receptor antagonists in asthma. Allergy 2001; 56(suppl 66):7–11.

68. Cohen P, Noveral JP, Bhala A, Nunn SE, Herrick DJ, Grunstein MM. Leukotriene D4 facilitates airway smooth muscle cell proliferation via modulation of the IGF axis. Am J Physiol 1995; 269(2 Pt 1):L151–L157.

69.　Sanak M, Sampson AP. Biosynthesis of cysteinyl-leucotrienes in aspirin-intolerant asthma. Clin Exp Allergy 1999; 29(3):306–313.

70.　O'Sullivan S, Roquet A, Dahlen B, Dahlen S, Kumlin M. Urinary excretion of inflammatory mediators during allergen-induced early and late phase asthmatic reactions. Clin Exp Allergy 1998; 28(11):1332–1339.

71.　Kumlin M, Dahlen B, Bjorck T, Zetterstrom O, Granstrom E, Dahlen SE. Urinary excretion of leukotriene E4 and 11-dehydro-thromboxane B2 in response to bronchial provocations with allergen, aspirin, leukotriene D4, and histamine in asthmatics. Am Rev Respir Dis 1992; 146(1):96–103.

72.　Silberstein DS, Owen WF, Gasson JC, DiPersio JF, Golde DW, Bina JC, Soberman R, Austen KF, David JR. Enhancement of human eosinophil cytotoxicity and leukotriene synthesis by biosynthetic (recombinant) granulocyte-macrophage colony-stimulating factor. J Immunol 1986; 137(10): 3290–3294.

73.　Cowburn AS, Holgate ST, Sampson AP. IL-5 increases expression of 5-lipoxygenase-activating protein and translocates 5-lipoxygenase to the nucleus in human blood eosinophils. J Immunol 1999; 163(1):456–465.

74.　Hood PP, Cotter TP, Costello JF, Sampson AP. Effect of intravenous corticosteroid on ex vivo leukotriene generation by blood leucocytes of normal and asthmatic patients. Thorax 1999; 54(12):1075–1082.

75.　Dworski R, Fitzgerald GA, Oates JA, Sheller JR. Effect of oral prednisone on airway inflammatory mediators in atopic asthma. Am J Respir Crit Care Med 1994; 149(4 Pt 1):953–959.

76.　Noonan GP, Williams B, Angner R, Lu S, Knorr B, Reiss TF. Use of oral montelukast in the treatment of asthma. Compr Ther 2001; 27(2):148–155.

77.　Diamant Z, Sampson AP. Anti-inflammatory mechanisms of leukotriene modulators. Clin Exp Allergy 1999; 29(11):1449–1453.

78.　Barnes N, Wei LX, Reiss TF, Leff JA, Shingo S, Yu C, Edelman JM. Analysis of montelukast in mild persistent asthmatic patients with near-normal lung function. Respir Med 2001; 95(5):379–386.

79.　Salvi SS, Krishna MT, Sampson AP, Holgate ST. The anti-inflammatory effects of leukotriene-modifying drugs and their use in asthma. Chest 2001; 119(5):1533–1546.

80.　Tohda Y, Fujimura M, Taniguchi H, Takagi K, Igarashi T, Yasuhara H, Takahashi K, Nakajima S. Leukotriene receptor antagonist, montelukast, can reduce the need for inhaled steroid while maintaining the clinical stability of asthmatic patients. Clin Exp Allergy 2002; 32(8):1180–1186.

81.　Lofdahl CG, Reiss TF, Leff JA, Israel E, Noonan MJ, Finn AF, Seidenberg BC, Capizzi T, Kundu S, Godard P. Randomised, placebo controlled trial of effect of a leukotriene receptor antagonist, montelukast, on tapering inhaled corticosteroids in asthmatic patients. BMJ 1999; 319(7202):87–90.

82.　Laviolette M, Malmstrom K, Lu S, Chervinsky P, Pujet JC, Peszek I, Zhang J, Reiss TF. Montelukast added to inhaled beclomethasone in treatment of asthma. Montelukast/ Beclomethasone Additivity Group. Am J Respir Crit Care Med 1999; 160(6):1862–1868.

83.　Tamaoki J, Kondo M, Sakai N, Nakata J, Takemura H, Nagai A, Takizawa T, Konno K. Leukotriene antagonist prevents exacerbation of asthma during reduction of high-dose inhaled corticosteroid. The Tokyo Joshi-Idai Asthma Research Group. Am J Respir Crit Care Med 1997; 155(4):1235–1240.

84. Volkman JA, Pontikes PJ. Leukotriene modifiers to prevent aspirin-provoked respiratory reactions in asthmatics. Ann Pharmacother 2002; 36(9): 1457–1461.

85. Dahlen SE, Malmstrom K, Nizankowska E, Dahlen B, Kuna P, Kowalski M, Lumry WR, Picado C, Stevenson DD, Bousquet J, Pauwels R, Holgate ST, Shahane A, Zhang J, Reiss TF, Szczeklik A. Improvement of aspirin-intolerant asthma by montelukast, a leukotriene antagonist: a randomized, double-blind, placebo-controlled trial. Am J Respir Crit Care Med 2002; 165(1):9–14.

86. Dahlen B, Nizankowska E, Szczeklik A, Zetterstrom O, Bochenek G, Kumlin M, Mastalerz L, Pinis G, Swanson LJ, Boodhoo TI, Wright S, Dube LM, Dahlen SE. Benefits from adding the 5-lipoxygenase inhibitor zileuton to conventional therapy in aspirin-intolerant asthmatics. Am J Respir Crit Care Med 1998; 157(4 Pt 1):1187–1194.

87. Oettgen HC, Geha RS. IgE regulation and roles in asthma pathogenesis. J Allergy Clin Immunol 2001; 107(3):429–440.

88. Presta L, Shields R, O'Connell L, Lahr S, Porter J, Gorman C, Jardieu P. The binding site on human immunoglobulin E for its high affinity receptor. J Biol Chem 1994; 269(42):26368–26373.

89. Salvi SS, Babu KS. Treatment of allergic asthma with monoclonal anti-IgE antibody. N Engl J Med 2000; 342(17):1292–1293.

90. Boushey HA Jr. Experiences with monoclonal antibody therapy for allergic asthma. J Allergy Clin Immunol 2001; 108(2 suppl):S77-S83.

91. Babu KS, Arshad SH, Holgate ST. Anti-IgE treatment: an update. Allergy 2001; 56(12):1121–1128.

92. Mohapatra SS, San Juan H. Novel immunotherapeutic approaches for the treatment of allergic diseases. Immunol Allerg Clin N Am 2000; 20(3):625–642.

93. Fahy JV, Fleming HE, Wong HH, Liu JT, Su JQ, Reimann J, Fick RB Jr, Boushey HA. The effect of an anti-IgE monoclonal antibody on the early- and late-phase responses to allergen inhalation in asthmatic subjects. Am J Respir Crit Care Med 1997; 155(6):1828–1834.

94. Milgrom H, Fick RB Jr, Su JQ, Reimann JD, Bush RK, Watrous ML, Metzger WJ. Treatment of allergic asthma with monoclonal anti-IgE antibody. rhuMAb-E25 Study Group. antibody. N Engl J Med 1999; 341(26):1966–1973.

95. Milgrom H, Berger W, Nayak A, Gupta N, Pollard S, McAlary M, Taylor AF, Rohane P. Treatment of childhood asthma with anti-immunoglobulin E antibody (omalizumab). Pediatrics 2001; 108(2):E36.

96. Rosenwasser L, Nash D. Incorporating omalizumab into asthma treatment guidelines: consensus panel recommendations. Pharm Therapeut 2003; 28(6):400–410.

97. Barnes PJ. Cytokine modulators as novel therapies for asthma. Ann Rev Pharmacol Toxicol 2002; 42:81–98.

98. Moser R, Fehr J, Bruijnzeel PL. IL-4 controls the selective endothelium-driven transmigration of eosinophils from allergic individuals. J Immunol 1992; 149(4):1432–1438.

99. Shi HZ, Deng JM, Xu H, Nong ZX, Xiao CQ, Liu ZM, Qin SM, Jiang HX, Liu GN, Chen YQ. Effect of inhaled interleukin-4 on airway hyperreactivity in asthmatics. Am J Respir Crit Care 1998; Med 157(6 Pt 1):1818–1821.

100. Seder RA, Paul WE. Acquisition of lymphokine-producing phenotype by CD4+ T cells. Ann Rev Immunol 1994; 12:635–673.

101. Steinke JW, Borish L. Th2 cytokines and asthma. Interleukin-4: its role in the pathogenesis of asthma, and targeting it for asthma treatment with interleukin-4 receptor antagonists. Respir Res 2001; 2(2):66–70.

102. Borish LC, Nelson HS, Corren J, Bensch G, Busse WW, Whitmore JB, Agosti JM. I.R-S.A Group.Efficacy of soluble IL-4 receptor for the treatment of adults with asthma. J Allergy Clin Immunol 2001; 107(6):963–670.

103. Kips JC, Tournoy KG, Pauwels RA. New anti-asthma therapies: suppression of the effect of interleukin (IL)-4 and IL-5. Eur Respir J 2001; 17(3):499–506.

104. Wardlaw AJ, Brightling C, Green R, Woltmann G, Pavord I. Eosinophils in asthma and other allergic diseases. Br Med Bull 2000; 56(4):985–1003.

105. Menzies-Gow A, Robinson DS. Eosinophils, eosinophilic cytokines (interleukin-5), and antieosinophilic therapy in asthma. Curr Opin Pulm Med 2002; 8(1):33–38.

106. Shi HZ, Xiao CQ, Zhong D, Qin SM, Liu Y, Liang GR, Xu H, Chen YQ, Long XM, Xie ZF. Effect of inhaled interleukin-5 on airway hyperreactivity and eosinophilia in asthmatics. Am J Respir Crit Care Med 1998; 157(1):204–209.

107. Shi HZ, Li CQ, Qin SM, Xie ZF, Liu Y. Effect of inhaled interleukin-5 on number and activity of eosinophils in circulation from asthmatics. Clin Immunol 1999; 91(2):163–169.

108. Kips JC, O'Connor BJ, Langley SJ, Woodcock A, Kerstjens HA, Postma DS, Danzig M, Cuss F, Pauwels RA. Effect of SCH55700, a humanized anti-human interleukin-5 antibody, in severe persistent asthma: a pilot study. Am J Respir Crit Care Med 2003; 167(12):1655–1659.

109. Leckie MJ, ten Brinke A, Khan J, Diamant Z, O'Connor BJ, Walls CM, Mathur AK, Cowley HC, Chung KF, Djukanovic R, Hansel TT, Holgate ST, Sterk PJ, Barnes PJ. Effects of an interleukin-5 blocking monoclonal antibody on eosinophils, airway hyper-responsiveness, and the late asthmatic response. Lancet 2000; 356(9248):2144–2148.

110. O'Byrne PM, Inman MD, Parameswaran K. The trials and tribulations of IL-5, eosinophils, and allergic asthma. J Allergy Clin Immunol 2001; 108(4):503–508.

111. Nielson CP, Vestal RE, Sturm RJ, Heaslip R. Effects of selective phosphodiesterase inhibitors on the polymorphonuclear leukocyte respiratory burst. J Allergy Clin Immunol 1996; 86(5):801–808.

112. Spina, D. Theophylline and PDE4 inhibitors in asthma. Curr Opin Pulm Med 2003; 9(1):57–64.

113. Bundschuh DS, Eltze M, Barsig J, Wollin L, Hatzelmann A, Beume R. In vivo efficacy in airway disease models of roflumilast, a novel orally active PDE4 inhibitor. J Pharmacol Exp Ther 2001; 297(1):280–290.

114. Timmer W, Leclerc V, Birraux G, Neuhauser M, Hatzelmann A, Bethke T, Wurst W. The new phosphodiesterase 4 inhibitor roflumilast is efficacious

in exercise-induced asthma and leads to suppression of LPS-stimulated TNF-alpha ex vivo. J Clin Pharmacol 2002; 42(3):297–303.

115. Junghans RP, Waldmann TA, Landolfi NF, Avdalovic NM, Schneider WP, Queen C. Anti-Tac-H, a humanized antibody to the interleukin 2 receptor with new features for immunotherapy in malignant and immune disorders. Cancer Res 1990; 50(5):1495–502.

116. McClellan M, Keller S, Zhao V, Klingbeil C, Vexler VS. Daclizumab inhibits mitogen-stimulated Th1 and Th2 cytokine production from human PBMC. J Allergy Clin Immunol 2002; 109(1):S27.

117. Goebel J, Stevens E, Forrest K, Roszman TL. Daclizumab (Zenapax) inhibits early interleukin-2 receptor signal transduction events. Transpl Immunol 2000; 8(3):153–159.

118. Vincenti F, Kirkman R, Light S, Bumgardner G, Pescovitz M, Halloran P, Neylan J, Wilkinson A, Ekberg H, Gaston R, Backman L, Burdick J. Interleukin-2-receptor blockade with daclizumab to prevent acute rejection in renal transplantation Daclizumab Triple Therapy Study Group. N Engl J Med 1998; 338(3):161–165.

119. Bumgardner GL, Hardie I, Johnson RW, Lin A, Nashan B, Pescovitz MD, Ramos E, Vincenti F. Results of 3-year phase III clinical trials with daclizumab prophylaxis for prevention of acute rejection after renal transplantation. Transplantation 2001; 72(5):839–845.

120. Krueger JG, Walters IB, Miyazawa M, Gilleaudeau P, Hakimi J, Light S, Sherr A, Gottlieb AB. Successful in vivo blockade of CD25 (high-affinity interleukin 2 receptor) on T cells by administration of humanized anti-Tac antibody to patients with psoriasis. J Am Acad Dermatol 2000; 43(3):448–458.

121. Barnes PJ. IL-10: a key regulator of allergic disease. Clin Exp Allergy 2001; 31(5):667–669.

122. Pretolani M, Goldman M. IL-10: a potential therapy for allergic inflammation? Immunol Today 1997; 18(6):277–280.

123. Pretolani M, Goldman M. Cytokines involved in the downregulation of allergic airway inflammation. Res Immunol 1997; 148(1):33–8.

124. Tomita K, Lim S, Hanazawa T, Usmani O, Stirling R, Chung KF, Barnes PJ, Adcock IM. Attenuated production of intracellular IL-10 and IL-12 in monocytes from patients with severe asthma. Clin Immunol 2002; 102(3):258–266.

125. Borish L, Aarons A, Rumbyrt J, Cvietusa P, Negri J, Wenzel S. Interleukin-10 regulation in normal subjects and patients with asthma. J Allergy Clin Immunol 1996; 97(6):1288–1296.

126. Chung F. Anti-inflammatory cytokines in asthma and allergy: interleukin-10, interleukin-12, interferon-gamma. Mediators Inflamm 2001; 10(2):51–59.

127. Zemann B, Schwaerzler C, Griot-Wenk M, Nefzger M, Mayer P, Schneider H, de Weck A, Carballido JM, Liehl E. Oral administration of specific antigens to allergy-prone infant dogs induces IL-10 and TGF-beta expression and prevents allergy in adult life. J Allergy Clin Immunol 2003; 111(5):1069–1075.

128. Akbari O, Stock P, DeKruyff RH, Umetsu DT. Mucosal tolerance and immunity: regulating the development of allergic disease and asthma. Int Arch Allergy Immunol 2003; 130(2):108–118.

129. Zuany-Amorim C, Haile S, Leduc D, Dumarey C, Huerre M, Vargaftig BB, Pretolani M. Interleukin-10 inhibits antigen-induced cellular recruitment into the airways of sensitized mice. J Clin Invest 1995; 95(6):2644–2651.

130. van Deventer SJ, Elson CO, Fedorak RN. Multiple doses of intravenous interleukin 10 in steroid-refractory Crohn's disease. Crohn's Disease Study Group. Gastroenterology 1997; 113(2):383–389.

131. Wills-Karp M. IL-12/IL-13 axis in allergic asthma. J Allergy Clin Immunol 2001; 107(1):9–18.

132. van der Pouw Kraan TC, Boeije LC, de Groot ER, Stapel SO, Snijders A, Kapsenberg ML, van der Zee JS, Aarden LA. Reduced production of IL-12 and IL-12-dependent IFN-gamma release in patients with allergic asthma. J Immunol 1997; 158(11):5560–5565.

133. Prescott SL, Holt PG. Abnormalities in cord blood mononuclear cytokine production as a predictor of later atopic disease in childhood. Clin Exp Allergy 1998; 28(11):1313–1316.

134. Gavett SH, O'Hearn DJ, Li X, Huang SK, Finkelman FD, Wills-Karp M. Interleukin 12 inhibits antigen-induced airway hyperresponsiveness, inflammation, and Th2 cytokine expression in mice. J Exp Med 1995; 182(5): 1527–1536.

135. Bryan SA, O'Connor BJ, Matti S, Leckie MJ, Kanabar V, Khan J, Warrington SJ, Renzetti L, Rames A, Bock JA, Boyce MJ, Hansel TT, Holgate ST, Barnes PJ. Effects of recombinant human interleukin-12 on eosinophils, airway hyper-responsiveness, and the late asthmatic response. Lancet 2000; 356(9248):2149–2153.

136. Moore PE, Church TL, Chism DD, Panettieri RA Jr, Shore SA. IL-13 and IL-4 cause eotaxin release in human airway smooth muscle cells: a role for ERK. Am J Physiol—Lung Cell Mol Physiol 2002; 282(4):L847–L853.

137. Venkayya R, Lam M, Willkom M, Grunig G, Corry DB, Erle DJ. The Th2 lymphocyte products IL-4 and IL-13 rapidly induce airway hyperresponsiveness through direct effects on resident airway cells. Am J Respir Cell Mol Biol 2002; 26(2):202–208.

138. Laoukili J, Perret E, Willems T, Minty A, Parthoens E, Houcine O, Coste A, Jorissen M, Marano F, Caput D, Tournier F. IL-13 alters mucociliary differentiation and ciliary beating of human respiratory epithelial cells. J Clin Invest 2001; 108(12):1817–1824.

139. Thomas PS. Tumour necrosis factor-alpha: the role of this multifunctional cytokine in asthma. Immunol Cell Biol 2001; 79(2):132–140.

140. Lukacs NW, Strieter RM, Chensue SW, Widmer M, Kunkel SL. TNF-alpha mediates recruitment of neutrophils and eosinophils during airway inflammation. J Immunol 1995; 154(10):5411–5417.

141. Thomas PS, Yates DH, Barnes PJ. Tumor necrosis factor-alpha increases airway responsiveness and sputum neutrophilia in normal human subjects. Am J Respir Crit Care Med 1995; 152(1):76–80.

142. Renzetti LM, Paciorek PM, Tannu SA, Rinaldi NC, Tocker JE, Wasserman MA, Gater PR. Pharmacological evidence for tumor necrosis factor as a mediator of allergic inflammation in the airways. J Pharmacol Exp Ther 1996; 278(2):847–853.

143. Feldman M, Taylor P, Paleolog E, Brennan FM, Maini RN. Anti-TNF alpha therapy is useful in rheumatoid arthritis and Crohn's disease: analysis of the mechanism of action predicts utility in other diseases. Transplant Proc 1998; 30(8):4126–4127.

144. Frew AJ, Plummeridge MJ. Alternative agents in asthma. J Allergy Clin Immunol 2001; 108:3–10.

145. Creticos PS. The consideration of immunotherapy in the treatment of allergic asthma. Ann Allergy Asthma Immunol 2001; 87(suppl):13–27.

146. Serebrisky D, Teper AA, Huang CK, Lee SY, Zhang TF, Schofield BH, Kattan M, Sampson HA, Li XM. CpG oligodeoxynucleotides can reverse Th2-associated allergic airway responses and alter the B7.1/B7.2 expression in a murine model of asthma. J Immunol 2000; 165(10):5906–5912.

147. Kumar M, Behera AK, Hu J, Lockey RF, Mohapatra SS. IFN-gamma and IL-12 plasmid DNAs as vaccine adjuvant in a murine model of grass allergy. J Allergy Clin Immunol 2001; 108(3):402–408.

148. Barnes PJ. Chronic obstructive pulmonary disease. N Engl J Med 2000; 343(4):269–280.

149. Sandford AJ, Chagani T, Weir TD, Connett JE, Anthonisen NR, Pare PD. Susceptibility genes for rapid decline of lung function in the lung health study. Am J Respir Crit Care Med 2001; 163(2):469–473.

150. Davies L, Angus RM, Calverley PM. Oral corticosteroids in patients admitted to hospital with exacerbations of chronic obstructive pulmonary disease: a prospective randomised controlled trial. Lancet 1999; 354(9177): 456–460.

151. Pauwels RA, Lofdahl CG, Laitinen LA, Schouten JP, Postma DS, Pride NB, Ohlsson SV. Long-term treatment with inhaled budesonide in persons with mild chronic obstructive pulmonary disease who continue smoking. European Respiratory Society Study on Chronic Obstructive Pulmonary Disease. N Engl J Med 1999; 340(25):1948–1953.

152. Vestbo J, Sorensen T, Lange P, Brix A, Torre P, Viskum K. Long-term effect of inhaled budesonide in mild and moderate chronic obstructive pulmonary disease: a randomised controlled trial. Lancet 1999; 353(9167):1819–1823.

153. Pauwels R. Role of corticosteroids in stable chronic obstructive pulmonary disease. Curr Opin Pulm Med 2001; 7:79–83.

154. Zhu Z, Tang W, Ray A, Wu Y, Einarsson O, Landry ML, Gwaltney J Jr, Elias JA. Rhinovirus stimulation of interleukin-6 in vivo and in vitro. Evidence for nuclear factor kappa B-dependent transcriptional activation. J Clin Invest 1996; 97(2):421–430.

155. Blackwell TS, Blackwell TR, Holden EP, Christman BW, Christman JW. In vivo antioxidant treatment suppresses nuclear factor-kappa B activation and neutrophilic lung inflammation. J Immunol 1996; 157(4):1630–1637.

156. Rahman I, MacNee W. Role of transcription factors in inflammatory lung diseases. Thorax 1998; 53(7):601–612.

157. Keicho N, Elliott WM, Hogg JC, Hayashi S. Adenovirus E1A gene dysregulates ICAM-1 expression in transformed pulmonary epithelial cells. Am J Respir Cell Mol Biol 1997; 16(1):23–30.

158. Dyke HJ, Montana JG. Update on the therapeutic potential of PDE4 inhibitors. Expert Opin Investig Drugs 2002; 11(1):1–13.

159. Hatzelmann A, Schudt C. Anti-inflammatory and immunomodulatory potential of the novel PDE4 inhibitor roflumilast in vitro. J Pharmacol Exp Ther 2001; 297(1):267–279.

160. Billah MM, Cooper N, Minnicozzi M, Warneck J, Wang P, Hey JA, Kreutner W, Rizzo CA, Smith SR, Young S, Chapman RW, Dyke H, Shih NY, Piwinski JJ, Cuss FM, Montana J, Ganguly AK, Egan RW. Pharmacology of *N*-(3,5-dichloro-1-oxido-4-pyridinyl)-8-methoxy-2-(trifluoromethyl)-5-quinoline carboxamide (SCH 351591), a novel, orally active phosphodiesterase 4 inhibitor. J Pharmacol Exp Ther 2002; 302(1):127–137.

161. Sturton G, Fitzgerald M. Phosphodiesterase 4 inhibitors for the treatment of COPD. Chest 2002; 121(5 suppl):192S-196S.

162. Compton C, Gubb J, Nieman R, Edelson J, Amit O, Bakst A, Ayres J, Creemers J, Schultze-Werninghaus G, Brambilla C, Barnes N. Cilomilast, a selective phosphodiesterase-4 inhibitor for treatment of patients with chronic obstructive pulmonary disease: a randomised, dose-ranging study. Lancet 2001; 358:265–270.

163. Profita M, Chiappara G, Mirabella F, Di Giorgi R, Chimenti L, Costanzo G, Riccobono L, Bellia V, Bousquet J, Vignola AM. Effect of cilomilast (Ariflo) on TNF-alpha, IL-8, and GM-CSF release by airway cells of patients with COPD. Thorax 2003; 58(7):573–579.

164. Gamble E, Grootendorst DC, Brightling CE, Troy S, Qui Y, Zhu J, Parker D, Vignola AM, Kroegel C, Morell F, Hansel TT, Rennard SI, Compton C, Ohad A, Tri T, Edelson J, Pavord ID, Rabe KF, Barnes NC, Jeffery PK. Anti-inflammatory effects of the phosphodiesterase 4 inhibitor cilomilast (Ariflo) in COPD. Am J Respir Crit Care Med 2003; 19:19.

165. Lee J, Kumar S, Griswold D, Underwood D, Votta B, Adams J. Inhibition of p38 MAP kinases as a therapeutic strategy. Immunopharmacology 2000; 47:185–201.

166. Newton R, Cambridge L, Hart L, Stevens D, Lindsay M, Barnes P. The MAP kinase inhibitors PDO98059, UO126, and SB203580, inhibit IL1β-dependent PGE2 release via mechanistically distinct processes. Br J Pharmacol 2000; 130:1353–1361.

167. Rutault K, Hazzalin CA, Mahadevan LC. Combinations of ERK and p38 MAPK inhibitors ablate tumor necrosis factor-alpha (TNF-alpha) mRNA induction. Evidence for selective destabilization of TNF-alpha transcripts. J Biol Chem 2001; 276(9):6666–6674.

168. Stockley RA, Bayley DL, Unsal I, Dowson LJ. The effect of augmentation therapy on bronchial inflammation in alpha1-antitrypsin deficiency. Am J Respir Crit Care Med 2002; 165(11):1494–1498.

169. Hubbard RC, Crystal RG. Alpha-1-antitrypsin augmentation therapy for alpha-1-antitrypsin deficiency. Am J Med 1988; 84(6A):52–62.

170. Cawston T, Carrere S, Catterall J, Duggleby R, Elliott S, Shinglton B, Rowan. A. Matrix matalloapreoteinases and TIMPs: properties and implications for the treatment of chronic obstructive pulmonary disease In: Chadwick D

and Goode JA, eds. Chronic Obstructive Pulmonary Disease: Pathogenesis to Treatment. Chichester: John Wiley & Sons, Ltd, 2001:205–228.

171. Frankenberger M, Hauck RW, Frankenberger B, Haussinger K, Maier KL, Heyder J, Ziegler-Heitbrock HW. All trans-retinoic acid selectively down-regulates matrix metalloproteinase-9 (MMP-9) and up-regulates tissue inhibitor of metalloproteinase-1 (TIMP-1) in human bronchoalveolar lavage cells. Mol Med 2001; 7(4):263–270.

172. Massaro GD, Massaro D. Retinoic acid treatment abrogates elastase-induced pulmonary emphysema in rats. Nat Med 1997; 3(6):675–677.

173. Mao JT, Goldin JG, Dermand J, Ibrahim G, Brown MS, Emerick A, McNitt-Gray MF, Gjertson DW, Estrada F, Tashkin DP, Roth MD. A pilot study of all-trans-retinoic acid for the treatment of human emphysema. Am J Respir Crit Care Med 2002; 165(5):718–723.

174. Gauldie J, Strieter RM. Pro: inflammatory mechanisms are a minor component of the pathogenesis of idiopathic pulmonary fibrosis. Con: inflammatory mechanisms are not a minor component of the pathogenesis of idiopathic pulmonary fibrosis. Am J Respir Crit Care Med 2002; 165(9):1205–1206.

175. Raghu G. Interstitial lung disease: a clinical overview and general approach. In: Fishman AP, ed. Pulmonary Dise-ases and Disorders. New York: McGraw-Hill, 1998:1037–1054.

176. Demedts M, Wells AU, Anto JM, Costabel U, Hubbard R, Cullinan P, Slabbynck H, Rizzato G, Poletti V, Verbeken EK, Thomeer MJ, Kokkarinen J, Dalphin JC, Taylor AN. Interstitial lung diseases: an epidemiological overview. Eur Respir J Suppl 2001; 32:2s-16s.

177. Strieter RM, Keane MP. Cytokine biology and the pathogenesis of Interstitial lung disease. In: King TE, ed. New Approaches to Managing Idiopathic Pulmonary Fibrosis. New York: American Thoracic Society, 2000: 27–35.

178. Strieter RM. Mechanisms of pulmonary fibrosis: conference summary. Chest 2001; 120(1 suppl):77S-85S.

179. Kaufman J, Graf BA, Leung EC, Pollock SJ, Koumas L, Reddy SY, Blieden TM, Smith TJ, Phipps RP. Fibroblasts as sentinel cells: role of the CD40–CD40 ligand system in fibroblast activation and lung inflammation and fibrosis. Chest 2001; 120(1 suppl):53S-55S.

180. Lynch JP III, Toews GB. Idiopathic pulmonary fibrosis. In: Fishman AP, ed. Pulmonary Diseases and Disorders. New York: McGraw-Hill, 1998: 1069–1084.

181. American Thoracic Society, European Respiratory Society. Idiopathic pulmonary fibrosis: diagnosis and treatment. International consensus statement. Am J Respir Crit Care Med 2000; 161:646–664.

182. Bjoraker JA, Ryu JH, Edwin MK, Myers JL, Tazelaar HD, Schroeder DR, Offord KP. Prognostic significance of histopathologic subsets in idiopathic pulmonary fibrosis. Am J Respir Crit Care Med 1998; 157(1):199–203.

183. Sime PJ, O'Reilly KM. Fibrosis of the lung and other tissues: new concepts in pathogenesis and treatment. Clin Immunol 2001; 99(3):308–319.

184. Brown KK. Current management of idiopathic pulmonary fibrosis and predictions of outcome. In: King TE, ed. New Approaches to Managing Idiopathic Pulmonary Fibrosis. New York: American Thoracic Society, 2000: 21–26.

185. du Bois RM. Potential future approaches to the treatment of idiopathic pulmonary fibrosis. In: King TE, ed. New Approaches to Managing Idiopathic Pulmonary Fibrosis. New York: American Thoracic Society, 2000: 21–26, 2000:52–57.

186. Joint Statement of the American Thoracic Society (ATS), the European Respiratory Society (ERS) and the World Association of Sarcoidosis and Other Granulomatous Disorders (WASOG) adopted by the ATS Board of Directors and by the ERS Executive Committee, February Statement on sarcoidosis. Am J Respir Crit Care Med 1999; 160(2):736–755.

187. Paramothayan S, Jones PW. Corticosteroid therapy in pulmonary sarcoidosis: a systematic review. JAMA 2002; 287(10):1301–1307.

188. Pietinalho A, Tukiainen P, Haahtela T, Persson T, Selroos O. Oral prednisolone followed by inhaled budesonide in newly diagnosed pulmonary sarcoidosis: a double-blind, placebo-controlled multicenter study. Finnish Pulmonary Sarcoidosis Study Group. Chest 1999; 116(2):424–431.

189. Wyser CP, van Schalkwyk EM, Alheit B, Bardin PG, Joubert JR. Treatment of progressive pulmonary sarcoidosis with cyclosporin A. A randomized controlled trial. Am J Respir Crit Care Med 1997; 156(5):1371–1376.

190. Douglas WW, Ryu JH, Swensen SJ, Offord KP, Schroeder DR, Caron GM, DeRemee RA. Colchicine versus prednisone in the treatment of idiopathic pulmonary fibrosis. A randomized prospective study. Members of the Lung Study Group. Am J Respir Crit Care Med 1998; 158(1):220–225.

191. Selman M, Carrillo G, Salas J, Padilla RP, Perez-Chavira R, Sansores R, Chapela R. Colchicine, d-penicillamine, and prednisone in the treatment of idiopathic pulmonary fibrosis: a controlled clinical trial. Chest 1998; 114(2): 507–512.

192. Herbert CM, Lindberg KA, Jayson MI, Bailey AJ. Biosynthesis and maturation of skin collagen in scleroderma, and effect of D-penicillamine. Lancet 1974; 1(7850):187–192.

193. Steen VD, Medsger TA Jr, Rodnan GP. D-Penicillamine therapy in progressive systemic sclerosis (scleroderma): a retrospective analysis. Ann Intern Med 1982; 97(5):652–659.

194. Fedullo AJ, Karlinsky JB, Snider GL, Goldstein RH. Lung statics and connective tissues after penicillamine in bleomycin-treated hamsters. J Appl Physiol 1980; 49(6):1083–1090.

195. Iyer SN, Wild JS, Schiedt MJ, Hyde DM, Margolin SB, Giri SN. Dietary intake of pirfenidone ameliorates bleomycin-induced lung fibrosis in hamsters. J Lab Clin Med 1995; 125(6):779–785.

196. Raghu G, Johnson WC, Lockhart D, Mageto Y. Treatment of idiopathic pulmonary fibrosis with a new antifibrotic agent, pirfenidone: results of a prospective, open-label Phase II study. Am J Respir Crit Care Med 1999; 159(4 Pt 1):1061–1069.

197. Sempowski GD, Derdak S, Phipps RP. Interleukin-4 and interferon-gamma discordantly regulate collagen biosynthesis by functionally distinct lung fibroblast subsets. J Cell Physiol 1996; 167(2):290–296.

198. Sempowski GD, Beckmann MP, Derdak S, Phipps RP. Subsets of murine lung fibroblasts express membrane-bound and soluble IL-4 receptors. Role of IL-4

in enhancing fibroblast proliferation and collagen synthesis. J Immunol 1994; 152(7):3606–3614.

199. Wallace WA, Ramage EA, Lamb D, Howie SE. A type 2 (Th2-like) pattern of immune response predominates in the pulmonary interstitium of patients with cryptogenic fibrosing alveolitis (CFA). Clin Exp Immunol 1995; 101(3): 436–441.

200. Hancock A, Armstrong L, Gama R, Millar A. Production of interleukin 13 by alveolar macrophages from normal and fibrotic lung. Am J Respir Cell Mol Biol 1998; 18(1):60–65.

201. Ziesche R, Hofbauer E, Wittmann K, Petkov V, Block LH. A preliminary study of long-term treatment with interferon gamma-1b and low-dose prednisolone in patients with idiopathic pulmonary fibrosis. N Engl J Med 1999; 341(17):1264–1269.

202. Sime PJ, Marr RA, Gauldie D, Xing Z, Hewlett BR, Graham FL, Gauldie J. Transfer of tumor necrosis factor-alpha to rat lung induces severe pulmonary inflammation and patchy interstitial fibrogenesis with induction of transforming growth factor-beta1 and myofibroblasts. Am J Pathol 1998; 153(3):825–832.

203. Piguet PF, Vesin C. Treatment by human recombinant soluble TNF receptor of pulmonary fibrosis induced by bleomycin or silica in mice. Eur Respir J 1994; 7(3):515–518.

204. Piguet PF, Collart MA, Grau GE, Kapanci Y, Vassalli P. Tumor necrosis factor/cachectin plays a key role in bleomycin-induced pneumopathy and fibrosis. J Exp Med 1989; 170(3):655–663.

205. Zheng L, Teschler H, Guzman J, Hubner K, Striz I, Costabel U. Alveolar macrophage TNF-alpha release and BAL cell phenotypes in sarcoidosis. Am J Respir Crit Care Med 1995; 152(3):1061–1066.

206. Marques LJ, Zheng L, Poulakis N, Guzman J, Costabel U. Pentoxifylline inhibits TNF-alpha production from human alveolar macrophages. Am J Respir Crit Care Med 1999; 159(2):508–511.

207. Moreland LW, Cohen SB, Baumgartner SW, Tindall EA, Bulpitt K, Martin R, Weinblatt M, Taborn J, Weaver A, Burge DJ, Schiff MH. Long-term safety and efficacy of etanercept in patients with rheumatoid arthritis. J Rheumatol 2001; 28(6):1238–1244.

208. Shergy WJ, Isern RA, Cooley DA, Harshbarger JL, Huffstutter JE, Hughes GM, Spencer-Smith EA, Goldman AL, Roth SH, Toder JS, Warner D, Quinn A, Keenan GF, Schaible TF. Open label study to assess infliximab safety and timing of onset of clinical benefit among patients with rheumatoid arthritis. J Rheumatol 2002; 29(4):667–677.

209. Zabel P, Entzian P, Dalhoff K, Schlaak M. Pentoxifylline in treatment of sarcoidosis. Am J Respir Crit Care Med 1997; 155(5):1665–1669.

210. Moller DR. Treatment of sarcoidosis—from a basic science point of view. J Intern Med 2003; 253(1):31–40.

211. Sempowski GD, Chess PR, Phipps RP. CD40 is a functional activation antigen and B7-independent T cell costimulatory molecule on normal human lung fibroblasts. J Immunol 1997; 158(10):4670–4677.

212. Zhang Y, Cao HJ, Graf B, Meekins H, Smith TJ, Phipps RP. CD40 engagement up-regulates cyclooxygenase-2 expression and prostaglandin E2 production in human lung fibroblasts. J Immunol 1998; 160(3):1053–1057.

213. Adawi A, Zhang Y, Baggs R, Finkelstein J, Phipps RP. Disruption of the CD40–CD40 ligand system prevents an oxygen-induced respiratory distress syndrome. Am J Pathol 1998; 152(3):651–657.

214. Adawi A, Zhang Y, Baggs R, Rubin P, Williams J, Finkelstein J, Phipps RP. Blockade of CD40–CD40 ligand interactions protects against radiation-induced pulmonary inflammation and fibrosis. Clin Immunol Immunopath 1998; 89(3):222–230.

215. Nagase T, Uozumi N, Ishii S, Kita Y, Yamamoto H, Ohga E, Ouchi Y, Shimizu T. A pivotal role of cytosolic phospholipase A(2) in bleomycin-induced pulmonary fibrosis. Nat Med 2002; 8(5):480–484.

216. Lynch JP III, Standiford TJ, Rolfe MW, Kunkel SL, Strieter RM. Neutrophilic alveolitis in idiopathic pulmonary fibrosis. The role of interleukin-8. Am Rev Respir Dis 1992; 145(6):1433–1439.

217. Liu JY, Sime PJ, Wu T, Warshamana GS, Pociask D, Tsai SY, Brody AR. Transforming growth factor-beta(1) overexpression in tumor necrosis factor-alpha receptor knockout mice induces fibroproliferative lung disease. Am J Respir Cell Mol Biol 2001; 25(1):3–7.

218. Gauldie J, Sime PJ, Xing Z, Marr B, Tremblay GM. Transforming growth factor-beta gene transfer to the lung induces myofibroblast presence and pulmonary fibrosis. Curr Top Pathol 1999; 93:35–45.

219. Khalil N, O'Connor RN, Flanders KC, Unruh H. TGF-beta 1, but not TGF-beta 2 or TGF-beta 3, is differentially present in epithelial cells of advanced pulmonary fibrosis: an immunohistochemical study. Am J Respir Cell Mol Biol 1996; 14(2):131–138.

220. Giri SN, Hyde DM, Hollinger MA. Effect of antibody to transforming growth factor beta on bleomycin induced accumulation of lung collagen in mice. Thorax 1993; 48(10):959–966.

221. Wang Q, Wang Y, Hyde DM, Gotwals PJ, Koteliansky VE, Ryan ST, Giri SN. Reduction of bleomycin induced lung fibrosis by transforming growth factor beta soluble receptor in hamsters. Thorax 1999; 54(9):805–812.

222. Kolb M, Margetts PJ, Galt T, Sime PJ, Xing Z, Schmidt M, Gauldie J. Transient transgene expression of decorin in the lung reduces the fibrotic response to bleomycin. Am J Respir Crit Care Med 2001; 163(3 Pt 1):770–777.

223. Kolb M, Margetts PJ, Sime PJ, Gauldie J. Proteoglycans decorin and biglycan differentially modulate TGF-beta-mediated fibrotic responses in the lung. Am J Physiol Lung Cell Mol Physiol 2001; 280(6):L1327–L1334.

224. Huang M, Sharma S, Zhu LX, Keane MP, Luo J, Zhang L, Burdick MD, Lin YQ, Dohadwala M, Gardner B, Batra RK, Strieter RM, Dubinett SM. IL-7 inhibits fibroblast TGF-beta production and signaling in pulmonary fibrosis. J Clin Invest 2002; 109(7):931–937.

225. Arai T, Abe K, Matsuoka H, Yoshida M, Mori M, Goya S, Kida H, Nishino K, Osaki T, Tachibana I, Kaneda Y, Hayashi S. Introduction of the interleukin-10 gene into mice inhibited bleomycin-induced lung injury in vivo. Am J Physiol Lung Cell Mol Physiol 2000; 278(5):L914–L922.

226. Moller DR, Forman JD, Liu MC, Noble PW, Greenlee BM, Vyas P, Holden DA, Forrester JM, Lazarus A, Wysocka M, Trinchieri G, Karp C. Enhanced expression of IL-12 associated with Th1 cytokine profiles in active pulmonary sarcoidosis. J Immunol 1996; 156(12):4952–4960.

227. Bergeron A, Bonay M, Kambouchner M, Lecossier D, Riquet M, Soler P, Hance A, Tazi A. Cytokine patterns in tuberculous and sarcoid granulomas: correlations with histopathologic features of the granulomatous response. J Immunol 1996; 159(6):3034–3043.

228. Trinchieri G. Interleukin-12: a cytokine produced by antigen-presenting cells with immunoregulatory functions in the generation of T-helper cells type 1 and cytotoxic lymphocytes. Blood 1994; 84(12):4008–4027.

229. Shigehara K, Shijubo N, Ohmichi M, Takahashi R, Kon S, Okamura H, Kurimoto M, Hiraga Y, Tatsuno T, Abe S, Sato N. IL-12 and IL-18 are increased and stimulate IFN-gamma production in sarcoid lungs. J Immunol 2001; 166(1):642–649.

230. Yoshimoto T, Takeda K, Tanaka T, Ohkusu K, Kashiwamura S, Okamura H, Akira S, Nakanishi K. IL-12 up-regulates IL-18 receptor expression on T cells, Th1 cells, and B cells: synergism with IL-18 for IFN-gamma production. J Immunol 1998; 161(7):3400–3407.

231. Trinchieri G. Interleukin-12 and its role in the generation of TH1 cells. Immunol Today 1993; 14(7):335–338.

232. D'Andrea A, Aste-Amezaga M, Valiante NM, Ma X, Kubin M, Trinchieri G. Interleukin 10 (IL-10) inhibits human lymphocyte interferon gamma-production by suppressing natural killer cell stimulatory factor/IL-12 synthesis in accessory cells. J Exp Med 1993; 178(3):1041–1048.

233. Pilon AL. Rationale for the development of recombinant human CC10 as a therapeutic for inflammatory and fibrotic disease. Ann NY Acad Sci 2000; 923:280–299.

15

Surfactant Replacement Therapy in Lung Injury

PATRICIA R. CHESS, JACOB N. FINKELSTEIN, BRUCE A. HOLM, and
ROBERT H. NOTTER

*Departments of Pediatrics and Environmental Medicine, University of Rochester, Rochester,
New York, U.S.A., and Departments of Pediatrics and Obstetrics and Gynecology,
State University of New York (SUNY) at Buffalo, Buffalo, New York, U.S.A.*

I. Overview

This chapter examines exogenous surfactant therapy and its utility in mitigating clinical acute lung injury (ALI) and the acute respiratory distress
syndrome (ARDS). Extensive biophysical research indicates that inhibitor-induced surfactant dysfunction in lung injury can be reversed or mitigated by increasing surfactant concentration (Chapter 9). In addition,
research in animal models of ALI/ARDS indicates that surfactant dysfunction in injured lungs in vivo can be improved by exogenous surfactant
administration. Exogenous surfactant therapy is now standard in neonatal
intensive care, and is life-saving in preventing or treating the respiratory distress syndrome (RDS) in premature infants. However, extension of this
therapy to patients with clinical ALI/ARDS is still under investigation.
This chapter details the rationale and current status of exogenous surfactant
therapy in infants, children, and adults with ALI/ARDS. Also emphasized
are factors that complicate surfactant therapy in ALI/ARDS, including the multifaceted pathophysiology of inflammatory lung injury, the
heterogeneity of affected patient populations, and the difficulty of delivering

exogenous surfactant material to alveoli in injured lungs. Differences in activity and inhibition resistance among clinical exogenous surfactants are also detailed, and examples of on-going exogenous surfactant development are described. The possibility of using exogenous surfactant therapy in combination with agents directed against other aspects of inflammatory lung injury is also noted (combined-modality interventions for lung injury are described in detail in Chapter 19).

II. Rationale for Surfactant Therapy in ALI/ARDS

Exogenous surfactant therapy is straightforward in concept: if endogenous surfactant is deficient or becomes dysfunctional, then it can be replaced or supplemented by the delivery of exogenous surface active material to the alveoli (Fig. 1). Exogenous surfactant therapy is by nature acute, and is intended to preserve lung function over the short term while the patient's lungs develop or recover the ability to produce and maintain adequate levels of endogenous surfactant. Although simple in concept, the development of clinically effective exogenous surfactant therapy in premature infants required decades of biophysical and animal model research following the discovery of lung surfactant in the 1950s (1,2). The utility of exogenous surfactant therapy in premature infants is now well documented by an extensive body of literature (e.g., see Refs. 3–6 for review). This chapter deals with the even more difficult challenge of developing effective exogenous surfactant therapy for clinical ALI/ARDS. The rationale for exogenous surfactant therapy in ALI/ARDS is based primarily on the existence of surfactant dysfunction (also called surfactant inactivation or inhibition) in affected patients (Fig. 2). Surfactant deficiency, if present, provides an additional treatment rationale.

Based on current definitions, all patients with ARDS also have clinical ALI (7) (Chapter 3). These syndromes arise in association with acute inflammatory lung injury from a variety of causes in patients ranging in age from infants to adults (Table 1). The most common causes of clinical ALI/ARDS in adults are sepsis and sepsis syndrome, gastric aspiration, shock with multiple transfusions, diffuse pulmonary infection, and mechanical trauma including head injuries (8,9). The most common causes of ALI/ARDS in children include sepsis, near-drowning, hypovolemic shock, and closed space burn injury (10). Common etiologies of lung injury and acute respiratory failure in full-term infants include meconium aspiration, sepsis, or pulmonary infection (10,11). Premature infants are also not immune to pulmonary injury. Acute respiratory failure in premature neonates is typically initiated by surfactant deficiency, but secondary lung injury and surfactant dysfunction can arise in association with hyperoxia, mechanical ventilation, infection, edema from patent ductus arteriosis, or a variety of other factors (Fig. 3).

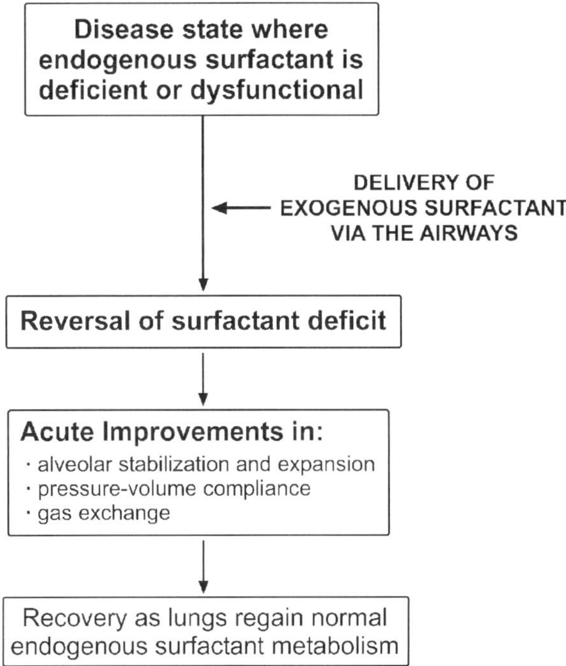

Figure 1 Concept of exogenous surfactant therapy. Exogenous surfactant therapy involves the delivery of surface active material from outside the body into the lungs to overcome a deficiency or dysfunction of endogenous surfactant. Exogenous surfactant therapy is acute in nature, and eventual normalization of endogenous surfactant homeostasis is necessary. Implicit in this therapy is the requirement that the exogenous surfactant used must be functionally active and delivered in adequate amounts to the alveoli.

Mechanisms of surfactant dysfunction during acute pulmonary injury are detailed in Chapter 9 and reviewed in Refs. 3, 12. Alterations in surfactant composition, surface activity, or large aggregate content have been well documented in bronchoalveolar lavage, edema fluid, or tracheal aspirates from patients with ALI/ARDS or other diseases with a component of lung injury (13–25). Biophysical research has shown that the surface activity of lung surfactant can be reduced by injury-related inhibitors including plasma and blood proteins (26–33), meconium (34), cell membrane lipids (28,33,35), fluid free fatty acids (33,36–38), sphingolipids (39), reactive oxidants (36,40–42), and lytic enzymes such as inflammatory proteases (43) and phospholipases (44,45). Surfactant dysfunction from inhibitor-induced interactions has also been demonstrated in multiple animal models of acute inflammatory lung injury (see Refs. 3, 12, 46–49 for review). Importantly, biophysical and animal model studies are consistent in showing that many forms of lung surfactant dysfunction can be reversed or mitigated by raising

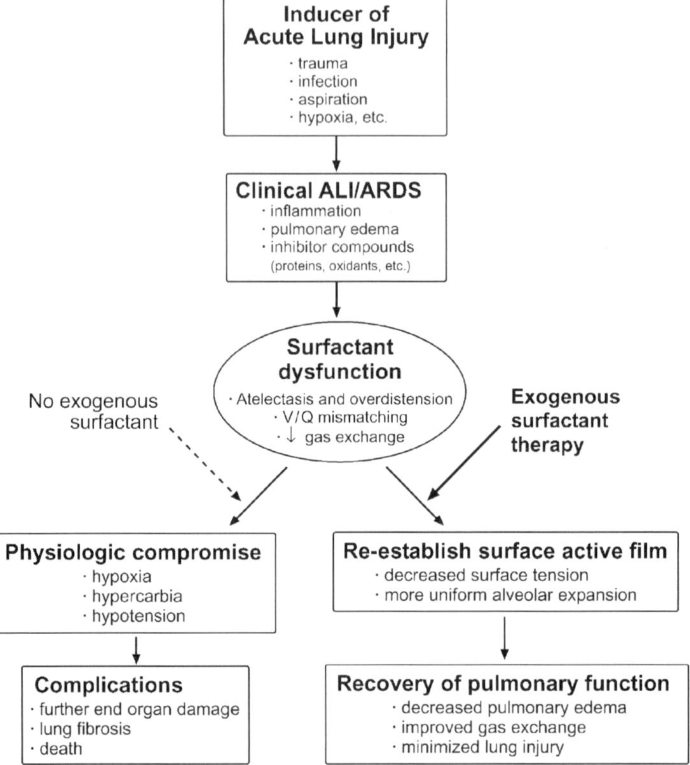

Figure 2 Exogenous surfactant therapy to mitigate surfactant dysfunction in ALI/ARDS. The pathophysiology of acute inflammatory lung injury includes surfactant dysfunction, which contributes to respiratory failure in full-term infants, children, and adults with clinical acute lung injury (ALI) and the acute respiratory distress syndrome (ARDS). Surfactant dysfunction reduces lung volumes and compliance, causes atelectasis and overdistension, increases ventilation/perfusion (V/Q) mismatching, and reduces gas exchange. Surfactant dysfunction in ALI/ARDS can, at least in principle, be ameliorated by exogenous surfactant therapy based on scientific understanding as discussed in this chapter.

surfactant concentration despite the continued presence of inhibitors. Selected animal models of ALI/ARDS in which exogenous surfactant therapy has been shown to improve respiratory function or mechanics are listed in Table 2. Examples of studies of surfactant replacement in the tabulated models are: acid aspiration (50–52), meconium aspiration (53–56), antilung serum (57), bacterial or endotoxin injury (58–63), vagotomy (64), hyperoxia (65–69), in vivo lavage (70–75), *N*-nitroso-*N*-methylurethane (NNNMU) injury (76–78), and viral pneumonia (79,80). In addition to demonstrating that surfactant therapy has significant potential benefits in ALI/ARDS,

Table 1 Clinical Respiratory Distress Syndromes Involving Lung Surfactant Deficiency and/or Dysfunction

Syndrome	Primary process	Patient age	Associated conditions	Predisposing conditions
RDS	Surfactant deficiency	Premature infants	Secondary lung injury; complications of prematurity	Premature birth
ALI/ARDS (direct injury)	Direct toxic injury to lungs	Any age	Associated with the cause of lung injury	Aspiration Inhaled toxic gas Lung contusion Near drowning Pulmonary infection Lung radiation
ALI/ARDS (indirect injury)	Injury through systemic inflammation	Any age	SIRS, MODS, MOF, and less severe multiorgan involvement	Infection/sepsis Cardiopulmonary bypass Drug overdose Blood transfusion Severe trauma, burns Shock Uremia

The pathophysiology of ALI/ARDS generally has a prominent component of surfactant dysfunction (Chapters 3 and 9), and surfactant dysfunction from acquired lung injury can also occur in premature infants with RDS. See text for details.
Abbreviations: RDS, respiratory distress syndrome of premature infants; ALI, clinical acute lung injury; ARDS, acute respiratory distress syndrome; MODS, multiple organ dysfunction syndrome; MOF, multiple organ failure; SIRS, systemic inflammatory response syndrome. Table adapted from Ref. 3.

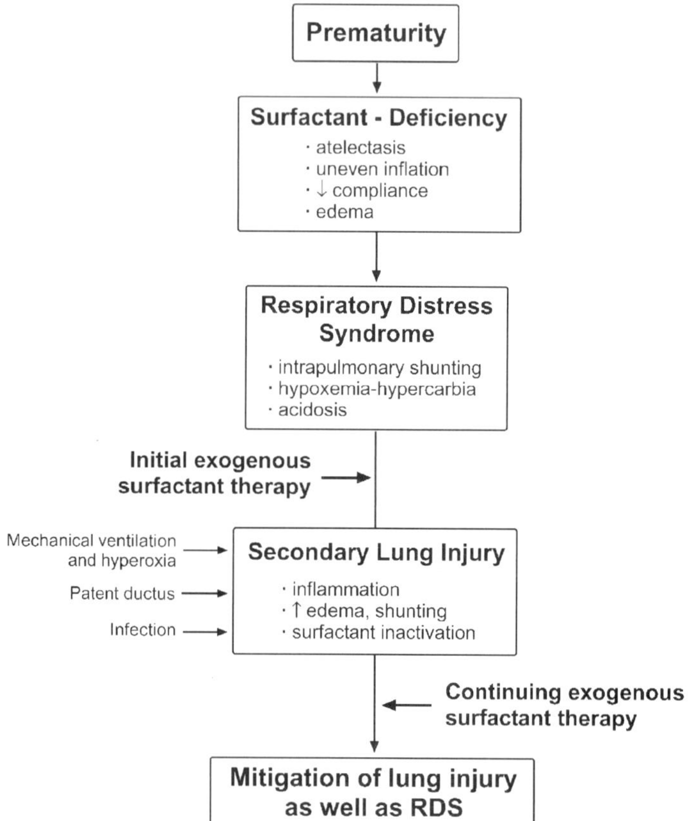

Figure 3 Lung injury with surfactant dysfunction can also occur in premature infants with RDS. Initial surfactant therapy in premature infants primarily targets surfactant deficiency, but the clinical course of RDS can include superimposed lung injury from hyperoxia, mechanical ventilation, sepsis, pulmonary infection, persistent patent ductus arteriosis, and many other predisposing conditions. Lung injury-induced surfactant dysfunction in premature infants can respond to additional or prolonged exogenous surfactant therapy.

animal studies are also important in examining the pulmonary activity of different clinical exogenous surfactants in the context of their composition, surface active properties, and inhibition resistance.

III. Current Clinical Exogenous Surfactants

In order to be effective as therapeutic agents in ALI/ARDS, exogenous surfactants must have high intrinsic surface activity plus the ability to resist

Table 2 Selected Animal Models of ALI/ARDS Shown to Respond to Exogenous Surfactant Therapy

Acid or meconium aspiration
Antilung serum infusion
Bacterial or endotoxin-induced injury
Bilateral vagotomy
Hyperoxic lung injury
In vivo lung lavage
NNNMU-induced lung injury
Viral pneumonia

See text for specific literature citations on exogenous surfactant therapy in the tabulated models. Animal models of ALI/ARDS and surfactant dysfunction are also discussed in Chapters 9 and 10 and are reviewed by Notter (3).
NNNMU is *N*-nitroso-*N*-methylurethane.

inactivation. Clinical exogenous surfactants used worldwide to treat surfactant-related lung disease are listed in Table 3. The table classifies clinical surfactants into three groups: (I) organic solvent extracts of lavaged endogenous lung surfactant from animals; (II) organic solvent extracts of processed animal lung tissue with or without additional synthetic additives; and (III) synthetic preparations not containing animal-derived surfactant

Table 3 Clinical Exogenous Surfactant Drugs Used Worldwide to Treat Surfactant-Related Lung Disease

I. Organic solvent extracts of lavaged animal lung surfactant
  Alveofact
  bLES
  Infasurf (CLSE)
II. Supplemented or unsupplemented organic solvent extracts of processed animal lung tissue
  Curosurf
  Survanta
  Surfactant-TA
III. Synthetic exogenous lung surfactants
  ALEC
  Exosurf
  KL4
  Recombinant SP-C surfactant

Survanta (Abbott/Ross Laboratories), Infasurf (ONY, Inc and Forest Laboratories), and Curosurf (Chesi Farmaceutici and Dey Laboratories) are approved by the Food and Drug Administration (FDA). Exosurf (Glaxo-Wellcome) is also FDA-approved, but is no longer used clinically in the United States. KL4 and recombinant SP-C surfactant are currently being tested clinically, and additional synthetic surfactants are under development. See text for details. (Adapted from Ref. 3.)

material (see Ref. 3 for review). Organic solvent extracts of lavaged alveolar surfactant in Category I contain, in principle, all of the lipid and hydrophobic protein components of endogenous surfactant, although the compositional details of such preparations do vary depending on source and processing. Extracts of homogenized or minced lung tissue are noted separately in Category II because they contain tissue-derived components and require more extensive processing that can substantially alter the content and compositional ratios of surfactant components. For example, the functionally important hydrophobic surfactant protein (SP)-B is reduced to very low levels in Survanta during processing from bovine lung tissue (29,81–83). Compositional differences in clinical exogenous surfactants have important consequences for activity, as detailed later. The two synthetic surfactants in Category III that have been most widely studied in clinical applications to date are Exosurf and artificial lung expanding compound (ALEC). Exosurf is a mixture of dipalmitoyl phosphatidylcholine (DPPC), hexadecanol, and tyloxapol in a weight ratio of 1:0.11:0.075, and ALEC is a 7:3 mixture of DPPC and egg phosphatidylglycerol. These two synthetic surfactants are no longer widely used clinically because of their lower activity relative to Category I and II surfactants. The synthetic exogenous surfactants KL4 and recombinant SP-C surfactant in Table 3 are presently under clinical evaluation, and additional synthetic surfactants are being studied at the basic research level as discussed later in the chapter.

IV. Experience with Surfactant Therapy in ALI/ARDS

Exogenous surfactant therapy has thus far had mixed success in patients with lung injury, particularly in adults with ALI/ARDS. Published studies of exogenous surfactant therapy in term infants, children, and adults with lung injury-associated acute respiratory failure are described below (for additional review see Refs. 3,12,46–48,84).

A. Surfactant Therapy in Term Infants with Lung Injury-Associated Acute Respiratory Failure

The largest experience with surfactant therapy in term infants with lung injury involves meconium aspiration. Fetuses stressed in utero can pass meconium, a thick, tarry substance present in the gastrointestinal tract of all infants. If this material is aspirated before or during delivery, it obstructs and injures the lungs, leading to life-threatening pneumonitis. Meconium has been shown to inhibit the surface activity of lung surfactant in vitro (34,85), and instilled exogenous surfactant can improve lung function in animals with meconium aspiration (53–56). In an initial pilot trial, Auten et al. (86) showed that tracheal instillation of 90 mg/kg calf lung surfactant extract (CLSE, equivalent to Infasurf) substantially improved arterial oxygenation in 14 full-term infants with severe respiratory failure from meconium aspiration or pneumonia (Fig. 4). The observed pattern of rapid, significant improvement in lung function following initial CLSE instillation was similar to that reported in premature infants receiving this preparation in "rescue" therapy for established RDS (87,88). In the study of Auten et al. (86), eight infants received a second dose of CLSE after meeting prospective retreatment criteria, and again had rapid significant improvements in arterial oxygenation. Three infants received a third dose of surfactant and exhibited smaller improvements in gas exchange. All 14 of the term infants studied survived, and none developed air leak complications or chronic lung disease (86). Khammash et al. (89) also reported an uncontrolled study showing acute lung functional improvements after instillation of bLES in 15 of 20 full-term neonates with meconium aspiration.

The utility of exogenous surfactant in term infants with meconium aspiration syndrome was further documented in a subsequent randomized controlled trial by Findlay et al. (90). Infants receiving three doses of Survanta ($n = 20$) had improved oxygenation as well as significant reductions in the incidence of pneumothorax, duration of mechanical ventilation and oxygen therapy, and time of hospitalization compared to control infants given air-placebo (90) (Table 4). Also, fewer surfactant-treated infants

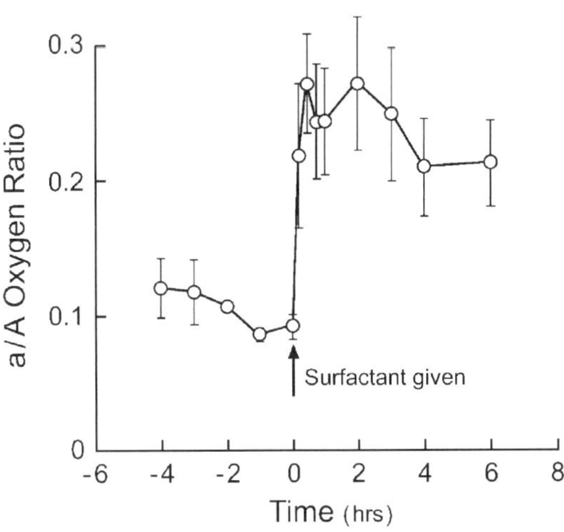

Figure 4 Improved lung function following instillation of Infasurf (CLSE) in full-term infants with respiratory failure. The arterial/alveolar (a/A) oxygen ratio is shown before and after an initial dose of exogenous CLSE (90 mg phospholipid/kg body weight) in 14 term infants with severe respiratory failure from meconium aspiration or pneumonia. Instilled surfactant significantly improved arterial oxygenation. See text for details. (Redrawn from Ref. 86.)

Table 4 Improved Outcomes in Full-Term Infants with Meconium Aspiration Treated with Exogenous Surfactant (Survanta)

Outcome variable	Control group ($n = 20$)	Surfactant-treated ($n = 20$)	P-value
Air leaks	5	0	0.024
Duration of mech vent (d)	10.8 ± 1.3	7.7 ± 0.7	0.047
Duration of O_2 therapy (d)	19.6 ± 2.6	13.0 ± 1.4	0.031
Duration of hospitalization (d)	24.3 ± 2.4	15.9 ± 1.2	0.003
ECMO requirement	6	1	0.037
Mortality <28 d	0	0	NS
Discharge with O_2 therapy	8	6	NS

Surfactant-treated patients received three doses of Survanta (150 mg/kg in 6 mL instilled endotracheally over 20 min for each dose). Initial dose was at <6 hr of age, with others 6 hr apart. Control patients were instilled with air. Data are mean ± SEM from Ref. 90.

required extracorporeal membrane oxygenation (ECMO) (90). Lotze et al. (91) have also reported favorable results using Survanta in a controlled trial in term infants referred for ECMO as a result of severe respiratory failure. Twenty-eight infants treated with four doses of Survanta 150 mg/kg had improved pulmonary mechanics, decreased duration of ECMO treatment, and a lower overall incidence of complications after ECMO compared to a similar number of control infants (91). A subsequent larger multicenter controlled trial by Lotze et al. (92) in 328 term infants with acute respiratory failure also reported significant improvements in respiratory status and the need for ECMO following treatment with Survanta. Meconium aspiration was a prominent cause of respiratory failure in both of these two studies (91,92).

In addition to meconium aspiration in full-term neonates, the utility of exogenous surfactant has also been reported in infants hospitalized for pediatric intensive care for acute respiratory failure in association with severe respiratory syncytial virus (RSV) bronchiolitis (93–95). These results are consistent with findings of abnormal surfactant content and activity in infants with inflammatory lung disease and viral bronchiolitis (23–25). Luchetti et al. (93) reported that 10 infants with RSV bronchiolitis treated with tracheally instilled porcine-derived surfactant (Curosurf, 50 mg/kg body weight) had improved gas exchange and a reduced time on mechanical ventilation and in the pediatric intensive care unit compared to an equal number not treated with exogenous surfactant. A subsequent multicenter controlled trial in 40 infants (20 per group) also found that surfactant therapy with Curosurf improved gas exchange and respiratory mechanics, and shortened the duration of mechanical ventilation and hospitalization, in infants with acute respiratory failure from RSV bronchiolitis (94). Also, Tibby et al. (95) have reported that nine infants with severe RSV bronchiolitis who received two doses of Survanta (100 mg/kg) had a more rapid improvement in oxygenation and ventilation indices in the first 60 hr compared to 10 control infants receiving air-placebo.

B. Clinical Cases Illustrating the Efficacy of Exogenous Surfactant in Full-Term Infants with ALI/ARDS

The consensus of published studies above supports the use of exogenous surfactant therapy in treating lung injury-related acute respiratory failure in infants. The following two cases abstracted from recent patient data at the Neonatal Intensive Care Unit (NICU) at the Children's Hospital at Strong at the University of Rochester, Rochester, NY, illustrate the utility of exogenous surfactant therapy in term infants with ALI/ARDS from meconium aspiration (Baby A) and pulmonary infection (Baby B).

Baby A (female) was the 2675 g product of a 38 4/7-week gestation pregnancy, which was uncomplicated. The mother presented in labor, and had artificial rupture of membranes 4 hr prior to delivery. An amnioinfusion was performed due to persistent fetal heart rate decelerations and the presence of thick meconium. The infant was delivered vaginally, and was suctioned with a Delee catheter on the perineum. The infant was apneic, cyanotic, and hypotonic. She was intubated and the trachea was suctioned for a moderate amount of meconium. The infant developed spontaneous respirations, but had increased work of breathing and a PaO_2 of 53 mm Hg on 100% oxyhood. The infant was intubated and given positive pressure ventilation. Chest x-ray (CXR) revealed evidence of meconium aspiration (Fig. 5A). Blood pressure support was provided with fluid boluses, dopamine, and dobutamine. Follow-up CXR performed at 12 hr of age for progressive hypoxia revealed a coarse interstitial pattern consistent with pneumonitis (Fig. 5B). The infant was changed to high frequency ventilation without improvement. Intratracheal surfactant (Infasurf, 100 mg phospholipid/kg body weight) was administered with significant improvement in work of breathing and PaO_2. CXR demonstrated significant clearing of the lung fields following surfactant instillation (Fig. 5C). The infant was extubated on day 12.

Baby B (female) was the 3896 g product of a 37 6/7-week gestation pregnancy, complicated by maternal pneumonia 6 weeks prior to delivery. The mother presented in active labor, and artificial rupture of membranes was performed without incident 3 hr prior to vaginal delivery. There were no immediate signs of infection, and the infant was taken to the newborn nursery. Over the next few hours, the infant developed hypoxia and a mild increase in the work of breathing. Blood cultures were sent, and the infant was treated in the NICU with antibiotics and supplemental oxygen for presumed pneumonia. By 24 hr of age, the infant had significantly increased work of breathing and hypoxia, with CXR demonstrating diffuse haziness and a left upper lobe infiltrate (Fig. 6A). The infant was intubated with persistence of symptoms, and exogenous

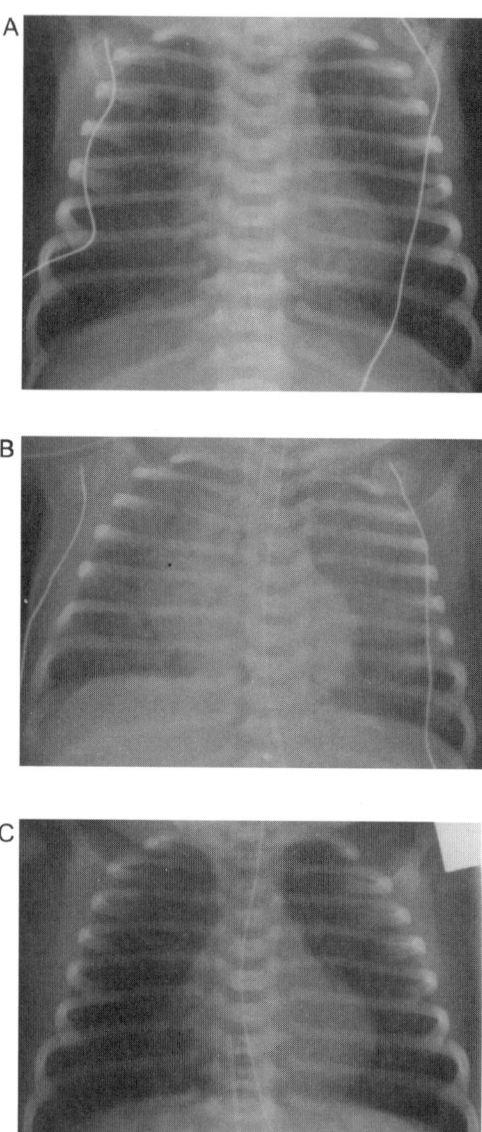

Figure 5 Radiographic changes associated with meconium aspiration and surfactant therapy in a term infant. The initial x-ray reveals a course interstitial pattern (A). The x-ray taken 12 hr later reveals diffuse pneumonitis (B). The x-ray taken 4 hr after treatment with Infasurf 100 mg/kg shows substantial clearing of lung fields (C). The clinical course of the baby is described in Case A in the text.

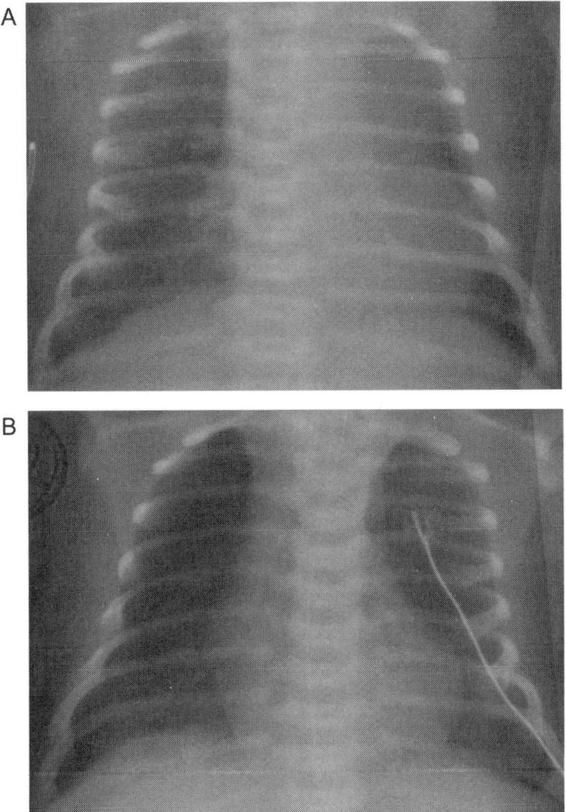

Figure 6 Clearing of pulmonary infiltrates after surfactant therapy in a term neonate with pneumonia. The initial x-ray demonstrates diffuse haziness with left upper lobe infiltrate (A). The x-ray taken 4 hr after receiving Infasurf 100 mg/kg demonstrates significant clearing of lung fields (B). The clinical course of the baby is given in Case B in the text.

surfactant (Infasurf, 100 mg phospholipid/kg body weight) was administered intratracheally (Fig. 6B). The infant had rapid improvements in work of breathing and PaO_2 following surfactant therapy, and was extubated on day 2.

C. Surfactant Therapy in Children with ALI/ARDS or Acute Respiratory Failure

Exogenous surfactant therapy has also been found to be beneficial in improving lung function in children with ALI/ARDS (96,97). In an initial treatment study, Willson et al. (96) showed that instillation of Infasurf 70 mg/kg improved lung function in 24 of 29 children (0.1–16 years of age) with ALI/ARDS in the Pediatric Intensive Care Units at six medical centers. Improvement was defined prospectively as a 25% decrease in oxygenation index (OI = 100×Mean Airway Pressure×FiO$_2$/PaO$_2$). A subsequent randomized controlled trial in 42 children at eight centers demonstrated that patients receiving one or two doses of Infasurf (70 mg/kg instilled intratracheally in four aliquots) had significantly better OI values over the 50 hr post-treatment (97) (Fig. 7). Statistically significant differences in survival were not found in this relatively small study, but several prospectively chosen outcome variables including days of mechanical ventilation and days in the intensive care unit were significantly improved by instillation of Infasurf. Surfactant-treated patients also had a significant increase in "ventilator free days" during the first 14 days of hospitalization and a higher incidence of extubation by 72 hr (97).

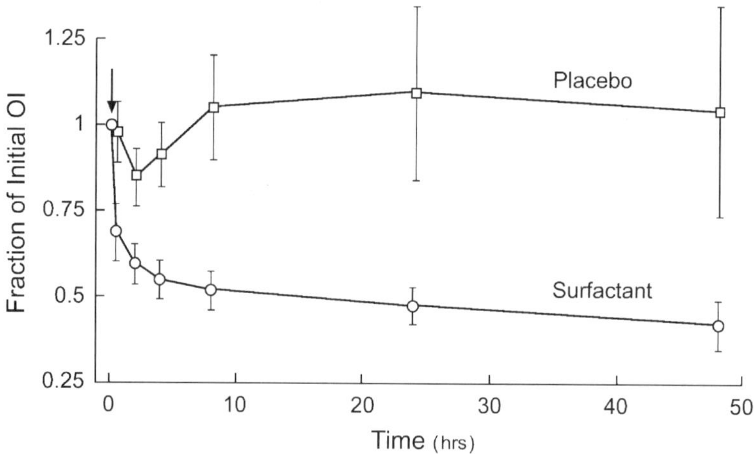

Figure 7 Improvements in oxygenation index (OI) after instillation of Infasurf in children with ARDS-related respiratory failure. Patients ranging in age from 1 day through 18 years in eight pediatric intensive care units were randomized to Infasurf or control groups. Infasurf patients received 80 mL/m^2 body surface (70 mg/kg body weight) by tracheal instillation during hand-ventilation with 100% oxygen (arrow). Control patients received hand-ventilation and 100% oxygen alone. Ten of 21 surfactant-treated patients received a second dose 12 or more hours after the first. Significant improvements were found in lung function in patients receiving exogenous surfactant therapy. OI is defined as 100 ×MAP × FiO$_2$/PaO$_2$, where MAP = mean airway pressure; FiO$_2$ = fraction of inspired oxygen; PaO$_2$ = arterial partial pressure of oxygen. (Data from Ref. 97.)

D. Surfactant Therapy in Adults with ALI/ARDS

Studies of exogenous surfactant therapy in adults with ARDS have thus far not been as successful as in infants and children. Acute improvements in arterial oxygenation have been reported in several small uncontrolled studies following bronchoscopic instillation of Curosurf (98) and Alveofact (99) in adults with ARDS. A larger uncontrolled study from five medical centers has also reported substantial improvements in gas exchange following the bronchoscopic administration of 300 mg/kg Alveofact in 27 severely ill patients with ARDS and septic shock (100). The mortality rate in surfactant-treated patients in this latter study was 44%, all from nonrespiratory causes, compared to a calculated risk of death of 74 ± 3.5% based on the Acute Physiology and Chronic Health Evaluation (APACHE) II scores in enrolled patients at study entry (100). However, results were less successful in a controlled trial by Gregory et al. (101), which investigated the efficacy of Survanta in 59 adults with ARDS following trauma, multiple blood transfusions, aspiration of gastric contents, or sepsis syndrome. Survanta-treated patients ($n = 43$) were randomized in three groups to receive up to eight doses of 50 mg/kg, up to eight doses of 100 mg/kg, or up to four doses of 100 mg/kg (101). The third group had a significantly decreased FiO_2 at 120 hr, but there were no significant differences from control in the other two groups of Survanta-treated patients, and no statistically significant improvements in survival were found (101). In a recent Phase I/II trial in 42 patients with ARDS, treatment with up to four doses of recombinant SP-C surfactant (Venticute, ALTANA Pharma; 25 mg/kg or 50 mg/kg per dose in LOW and HIGH groups) was found to be safe but did not improve lung function over the first 24 hr or the number of ventilator-free days over the first 28 days compared to control patients not receiving surfactant (102). Exogenous surfactant was not detected in lavage fluid obtained at 120 hr in this study (102). In addition, two clinical studies have reported a lack of efficacy of synthetic protein-free surfactants in adult patients with acute respiratory failure (103,104). A small controlled study by Macnaughton et al. (103) in 16 adults found that bronchoscopic instillation of ALEC was ineffective in improving lung function following cardiopulmonary bypass. By far the largest study to date of surfactant therapy in adults found no benefits from the use of aerosolized Exosurf in 725 patients with sepsis-associated ARDS (104). The negative results of this latter study were accompanied by an editorial in the *New England Journal of Medicine* indicating that lung surfactant replacement therapy was ineffective for ARDS (105).

E. Lessons from Prior Research on Exogenous Surfactant Therapy in Premature Infants

A crucial lesson from prior research on exogenous surfactant therapy in premature infants is that meaningful evaluations of this treatment approach in ALI/ARDS require studying the most active surfactant drugs in controlled trials of adequate size. In addition, effective methods of delivery must be used to ensure that adequate amounts of exogenous surfactant actually reach the alveoli. The existence of surfactant deficiency and increased pulmonary surface tension in premature infants with RDS (Hyaline Membrane Disease) was initially recognized in the 1950s (106–109). However, early studies of surfactant replacement therapy with aerosolized synthetic DPPC were unsuccessful in premature infants in the mid-1960s (110,111). These early studies were limited by the misconception that DPPC was equivalent in activity to whole surfactant, as well as by the inability to deliver adequate amounts of surfactant to the alveoli by available aerosol methodology. Nonetheless, because therapy with aerosolized DPPC was not successful, it was erroneously concluded that surfactant therapy in general was ineffective in premature infants and that RDS was primarily a disease of vascular dysfunction rather than surfactant deficiency (110,112). This misunderstanding substantially delayed the development of clinically effective surfactant therapy for premature infants.

The ability of whole surfactant harvested from the lungs of adult animals to improve pulmonary function and mechanics when instilled into the trachea of surfactant-deficient premature animals of the same or different species became well established in basic research during the 1970s (113–122). The understanding that the surface activity of lung surfactant depended on the molecular biophysical interactions of multiple lipid and protein constituents rather than DPPC alone also became appreciated through basic research at this time (123–133). This scientific foundation led to the design and implementation of successful placebo-controlled studies of exogenous surfactant therapy to prevent or treat RDS in premature infants from 1985 through the early 1990s (for review see Refs. 3–6, 134, 135). These clinical studies showed clear improvements in respiratory function and outcomes for premature infants treated with several different exogenous surfactant drugs either by intratracheal instillation at birth (prophylactic therapy) or after a clinical diagnosis of RDS (rescue therapy).

V. Considerations Affecting the Efficacy of Exogenous Surfactant Therapy in ALI/ARDS

Several factors make it challenging to develop effective surfactant therapy for clinical ALI/ARDS. Although patients with ALI/ARDS share common aspects of lung injury pathophysiology, these diagnoses are clinical syndromes that comprise a diverse set of etiologies. The occurrence of ALI/ARDS in a heterogeneous population of patients with varying degrees of lung injury and systemic disease significantly reduces the resolving power of clinical trials of surfactant therapy. In addition, edema and inflammation in patients with acute pulmonary injury make it more difficult to deliver and distribute exogenous surfactant to the alveoli. Despite these complications, exogenous surfactant therapy has been found to have benefits in infants and children with acute respiratory failure and ALI/ARDS as described earlier (86,89–94,96,97). There is a pressing need to improve current treatments for ARDS, since mortality in adults with this severe syndrome remains in the range of 30–50% despite great advances in medical technology and intensive care. Specific considerations relevant for surfactant therapy and its use in ALI/ARDS are discussed below.

A. Methods of Delivery of Exogenous Surfactants to Patients with Lung Injury

The routine method of delivering exogenous surfactants to premature infants with RDS is by intratracheal instillation in saline through an endotracheal tube. Surface active material instilled into the airways has the capacity to rapidly spread and distribute to the periphery of the lung (136–138). Spreading from the central airways towards the alveoli is promoted by surface tension gradients that drive transport from regions of high surfactant concentration to regions of lower surfactant concentration. Typical doses of intratracheal surfactant in premature infants are 100 mg/kg body weight. This represents a significant excess over the amount of surfactant phospholipid needed to cover the surface of the alveolar network with a tightly packed film (~3.1 mg/kg of surfactant phospholipid at a molecular weight of 750 are required to form a monomolecular film at a limiting concentration of 40 Å^2/molecule covering an alveolar surface of 1 m^2/kg body weight (3,139)). Excess instilled exogenous surfactant not lost during distribution through the airways provides a reservoir of material for the alveolar hypophase and interface, and can also be incorporated into endogenous surfactant pools via recycling pathways.

Intratracheal and segmental bronchoscopic instillation are currently the most effective methods of delivering exogenous surfactants to patients with ALI/ARDS. To achieve a comparable dose to premature infants based on body weight or body surface area, much larger total instilled drug amounts and volumes are required. The prototypical "70 kg adult" requires 7 g of exogenous surfactant at a dosage level of 100 mg/kg. This necessitates an instilled volume of 87.5–280 mL at the phospholipid concentrations of current clinical surfactant drugs in saline (25–80 mg/mL). It is obviously important to minimize instilled surfactant volumes in patients with severe respiratory failure as in ALI/ARDS. At the same time, instilled surfactant volume impacts intrapulmonary drug distribution, which is already compromised by edema and inflammation as noted earlier. Studies in animal models of ALI/ARDS have indicated that the distribution of exogenous surfactant can be improved by instilling larger fluid volumes or utilizing associated bronchoalveolar lavage (140–143), but the feasibility and/or utility of these approaches in clinical practice is uncertain. Clinical studies on intratracheal or bronchoscopic instillation of exogenous surfactants in patients with ALI/ARDS have used a range of instilled volumes, with doses as high as 300 mg/kg (100) and as low as 25 mg/kg (102).

An alternative to administering exogenous surfactant drugs by instillation is to deliver them in aerosol form. In theory, aerosolization could significantly reduce required surfactant doses, since delivery can be targeted to the alveoli by controlling particle size. Phospholipid aerosols with stable particle sizes appropriate for alveolar deposition in normal lungs can be formed by ultrasonic or jet nebulization (139,144,145), and exogenous surfactants have been aerosolized to animals and patients with surfactant deficiency or dysfunction (59,73,78,104,146–148). However, the theoretical potential of aerosols to improve alveolar deposition and reduce required surfactant doses has not been replicated in practice. Aerosol technology to date has not been able to deliver exogenous surfactants to the alveoli as effectively as instillation. Another approach to facilitate the delivery and distribution of exogenous surfactants in injured lungs involves the use of specific modes and strategies of mechanical ventilation. For example, studies indicate that the distribution and/or efficacy of instilled exogenous surfactant can be improved by jet ventilation (149,150) and partial liquid ventilation (151–153). Additional mechanism-based research on the impact of specific ventilation methods and strategies on the delivery, distribution, and efficacy of exogenous surfactants is important for optimizing this therapy in ALI/ARDS. The delivery and distribution of surfactant drugs in injured lungs could also potentially be improved by the use of low viscosity formulations to reduce transport resistance after tracheal or bronchoscopic instillation. Whole surfactant and animal-derived exogenous surfactants have complex non-Newtonian, concentration-dependent viscosities that vary significantly among preparations (154,155). For a given surfactant preparation at fixed shear rate, viscosity can be significantly reduced by altering the physical formulation through changes in dispersion methodology, ionic environment, or temperature (154,155).

B. Activity and Inhibition Resistance of Exogenous Surfactant Drugs

One of the most important considerations in the clinical efficacy of surfactant therapy is the relative activity of different exogenous surfactant drugs. Differences in efficacy between clinical exogenous surfactants have been demonstrated in a number of comparison trials in premature infants (156–165). Results of these clinical comparisons indicate that "natural" surfactants derived from animal lungs (Categories I and II in Table 3) have significantly greater efficacy than the protein-free synthetic surfactants Exosurf and ALEC. This is also the conclusion of retrospective meta analyses combining clinical data from multiple surfactant trials (4,5,135,166,167). As noted earlier, several unsuccessful studies of surfactant therapy in adults with ALI/ARDS have utilized these less active protein-free synthetic surfactant drugs (103,104). The hydrophobic surfactant apoproteins are highly active components of endogenous and exogenous lung surfactants. Substituting for these active components in protein-free synthetic surfactants is a challenging task. Addition of mixed bovine SP-B/SP-C to Exosurf greatly improves its surface activity and its physiological efficacy in reversing surfactant-deficient pressure–volume (P–V) mechanics in excised rat lungs (168), indicating that the biochemical components of Exosurf are not equal substitutes for the hydrophobic surfactant apoproteins in activity.

Animal-derived clinical exogenous surfactants themselves also differ substantially in their surface activity and ability to resist inhibitor-induced dysfunction. The consensus of biophysical and animal research indicates that exogenous surfactants based on extracts of lavaged large aggregate endogenous surfactant in Category I of Table 3 have the greatest overall surface and physiological activity. This reflects the fact that these drugs have close compositional analogy to the mix of phospholipids and hydrophobic proteins in active alveolar surfactant. Figure 8 shows data from Ref. 29 on the surface tension lowering ability of several clinical surfactants during dynamic cycling on a pulsating bubble apparatus (37°C, 20 cycles/min, 50% area compression). Suspensions of CLSE (Infasurf) were found to reach the lowest minimum surface tensions at the lowest surfactant concentrations among the preparations studied (Fig. 8). Additional pulsating bubble studies have shown that the synthetic protein-free surfactant Exosurf only reaches minimum surface tensions near 30 mN/m even during prolonged cycling at a high concentration of 10 mg lipid/mL (168). Category I exogenous surfactants such as CLSE and Alveofact also resist inhibition by blood proteins more effectively than exogenous surfactants like Survanta and Curosurf that are processed from lung tissue (29,168) (Fig. 9).

The activity differences between Infasurf and Survanta in Figs. 8 and 9 relate primarily to differences in the content of SP-B in these two preparations (74,81,83). Survanta has an SP-B content by ELISA of only 0.044% by weight relative to phospholipid, while Infasurf has an SP-B content of 0.9% by weight that approaches that of lavaged whole surfactant (83). SP-B is known to be the most active of the hydrophobic surfactant proteins in enhancing the adsorption, dynamic surface activity, and inhibition resistance of phospholipids (83,169–177). The addition of bovine SP-B or synthetic SP-B peptides to Survanta significantly improves its surface and physiological activity towards that of Infasurf and whole surfactant

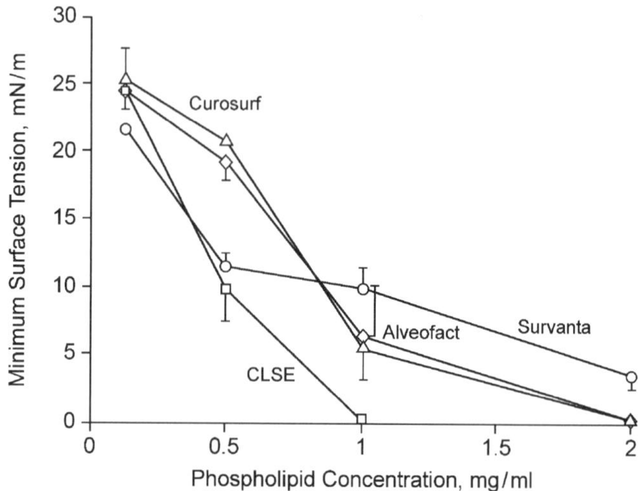

Figure 8 Dynamic surface tension lowering behavior of different clinical exogenous surfactants. Minimum surface tension after 5 min of pulsation in a bubble surfactometer (37 °C, 20 cycles/ min, 50% area compression) is plotted as a function of surfactant concentration for several widely used clinical exogenous surfactants. These exogenous surfactants vary widely in surface activity, with the most active being CLSE (Infasurf) from Category I, Table 3. (Data are redrawn from Ref. 29.)

(74,81,83). Despite its lack of SP-B, other active surfactant components in Survanta allow it to have significant efficacy in some forms of ALI/ARDS as noted earlier (e.g., see Refs. 90–92). Treatment with Survanta has not been found to give substantial improvements in adult patients with ARDS (101), but Category I exogenous surfactants with the complete mix of surfactant lipids and near-endogenous amounts of both SP-B and SP-C may prove to have increased efficacy.

Activity differences between exogenous surfactants in basic research as in Figs. 8 and 9 are generally much larger than those reported in clinical comparison trials of surfactant drugs in premature infants (156–165). One reason for this is that basic science studies can discriminate phenomena at a more mechanistic and detailed level than possible in clinical trials. Patient outcomes in clinical surfactant trials are influenced by multiple variables unrelated to lung surfactant activity. Patient outcomes in surfactant trials can also be affected by secondary phenomena involving drug incorporation into type II cell recycling pathways or combination with small amounts of native surfactant apoproteins in the alveoli (3). Even placebo-controlled studies of surfactant therapy in premature infants typically required substantial numbers of patients to demonstrate improvements in survival and

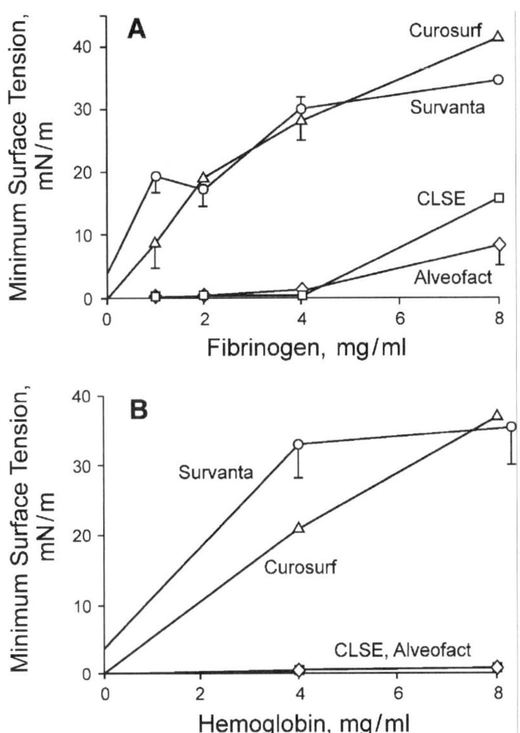

Figure 9 Resistance of clinical exogenous surfactants to inhibition by fibrinogen and hemoglobin. Minimum surface tension after 5 min of pulsation in a bubble surfactometer (37 °C, 20 cycles/min, and 50% area compression) is plotted against the concentration of the inhibitory proteins fibrinogen and hemoglobin. Category I drugs CLSE (Infasurf) and Alveofact from Table 3 reach lower surface tensions in the presence of higher inhibitor concentrations than the other surfactants studied. See text for discussion. Surfactant phospholipid concentration was constant at 2 mg/mL. (Redrawn from Ref. 29.)

other long-term outcomes (as opposed to acute lung functional improvements) (3). This is even more true in clinical studies comparing exogenous surfactant drugs. Consistent, mechanism-based activity differences demonstrated between exogenous surfactants in correlated biochemical, biophysical, and animal research clearly have important relevance for the treatment of patients with ALI/ARDS.

VI. Examples of New Synthetic Surfactants for ALI/ARDS

In addition to investigating the activity and delivery of clinical exogenous surfactants, research is also attempting to develop new synthetic or semisynthetic surfactants for treating lung injury (see Refs. 3, 12, 178–181 for review). Synthetic lung surfactants manufactured under controlled conditions in the laboratory have significant potential advantages in purity, reproducibility, and quality control compared to animal-derived preparations. Moreover, human sequence protein materials can be used in such surfactants, and constituents can be designed to have novel molecular properties like phospholipase resistance. As biological products, animal surfactants have significant batch-to-batch variability that increases the cost and complexity of quality control testing during manufacture. Laboratory-synthesized drugs in principle become increasingly cost-effective after initial development expenses are recovered, and can be produced in unlimited amounts. Synthetic surfactants are also free from concerns about animal pathogens such as prions, and they are not subject to ethnographic considerations affecting the use of bovine- or porcine-derived preparations in some countries. Several important approaches of on-going exogenous surfactant development are outlined below (see Ref. 3 for additional review and discussion of research on synthetic exogenous surfactants).

A. Synthetic Hydrophobic Peptides or Recombinant Hydrophobic Surfactant Apoproteins in Synthetic Exogenous Surfactants

One important strategy for developing new lung surfactants involves the use of synthetic hydrophobic or amphipathic peptides with varying homology to human SP-B or SP-C. An example of an exogenous surfactant based on this approach that is currently under clinical study is KL4 (55,75,182–189) (Table 3). This surfactant drug contains synthetic lipids combined with a 21 amino acid synthetic peptide containing repeating subunits with one lysine (K) and four leucine (L) residues designed roughly to reflect the balance of hydrophobic and hydrophilic residues in native SP-B (185,186,190). More specific human sequence regional and full-length synthetic hydrophobic SP-B and SP-C peptides are also being investigated as components in exogenous surfactants (see Refs. 3, 179–181 for review). For example, synthetic surfactants containing monomer or dimer peptides based on the N-terminal sequence of human SP-B (SP-B$_{1-25}$) have been shown to have significant activity in biophysical and animal model studies (75,180,191–196). In addition to synthetic SP-B and SP-C peptides, recombinant versions of the hydrophobic surfactant apoproteins are also available for use in exogenous surfactants (197–200). Recombinant SP-C surfactant (Table 3, Byk Gulden and ALTANA Pharma AG, Konstanz, Germany) has been the most widely studied preparation of this kind to date (e.g.,Refs.102,201–206). Although exogenous surfactants containing synthetic hydrophobic peptides or recombinant hydrophobic apoproteins are of great interest, current preparations have not been shown to have surface and physiological activities fully equivalent to the most active animal-derived lung surfactants. Continuing basic research to optimize synthetic lipid:peptide compositions and combination methods in conjunction with detailed molecular structure–function investigations is important for developing optimal synthetic preparations of this kind in the future.

B. The Use of Recombinant SP-A or Related Human Sequence SP-A Peptides to Increase Inhibition Resistance in Exogenous Surfactants

SP-A is known to improve several aspects of phospholipid surface activity (207–211), and it acts synergistically with SP-B in facilitating the formation of large surfactant aggregates including tubular myelin (211–214). Although organic solvent extracts of lavaged surfactant that contain only lipids and hydrophobic SP-B/C have very high surface activity, whole surfactant at the same phospholipid concentration has slightly greater activity plus a better ability to resist inhibition by plasma proteins and related substances (see Ref. 3 for review). Addition of purified animal SP-A has been found in several studies to improve the ability of hydrophobic organic solvent surfactant extracts to maintain high surface activity in the presence of plasma proteins (215–217). Because of potential cross-species antigenicity, human sequence SP-A is necessary in exogenous surfactants for clinical use. Both human sequence recombinant SP-A (218–220) and related regional synthetic peptides (221,222) are currently available. Although including recombinant SP-A or related synthetic peptides in exogenous surfactants has the potential to improve inhibition resistance, it would also increase cost and could affect physical and biological properties other than surface tension. SP-A is much more sensitive than the hydrophobic surfactant apoproteins to environmental variables such as heating, which is widely used in sterilizing exogenous surfactant suspensions. Regional SP-A peptides containing only lipid-associated amphipathic domains rather than the whole apoprotein (221) may have less heat-sensitivity. The presence of SP-A in exogenous surfactants could also impact their uptake and recycling by type II cells in vivo.

C. New Phospholipid Constituents to Enhance the Physicochemical Properties to Exogenous Surfactants

Although protein components in exogenous surfactants are extremely important, phospholipid constituents should not be ignored. Essentially all current clinical lung surfactants have substantial contents of DPPC. Although DPPC is the most prevalent phospholipid compound in endogenous surfactant, multiple additional saturated and unsaturated phospholipids are also found (see Ref. 3 for review). These additional glycerophospholipids include non-DPPC phosphatidylcholines as well as anionic phospholipids that make significant contributions to overall surface active behavior. Anionic phospholipids have the potential to interact specifically not only with apoproteins or peptides in endogenous and exogenous surfactants, but also with DPPC based on factors like chain miscibility. Several anionic phospholipids including palmitoyl-oleoyl phosphatidylglycerol (POPG; C16:0,C18:1) and egg-phosphatidylglycerol are utilized in current synthetic clinical surfactants. However, the relative activity of other PG compounds such as dipalmitoyl PG (DPPG, C16:0,C16:0), which has full chain miscibility with DPPC, have not been examined in detail. Mixed chain disaturated PC compounds like palmitoyl-myristoyl-PC and myristoyl-palmitoyl-PC (C16:0,C14:0 isomers), which are found in natural surfactant and have gel-to-liquid crystal transition temperatures slightly below body temperature (223), are additional examples of the many glycerophospholipids that could impact molecular behavior in synthetic exogenous surfactants (3).

Another approach to obtain active new surfactants for use in lung injury involves novel synthetic phospholipid analogs designed to have specific molecular behaviors plus chemical properties like phospholipase-resistance (e.g., see Refs. 224–232). The structure of a diether phosphonate analog of DPPC (designated DEPN-8) is shown in Fig. 10. Diether phosphonolipids such as DEPN-8 lack sites for cleavage by phospholipases A_1, A_2, and D, and are also partially resistant to phospholipase C by virtue

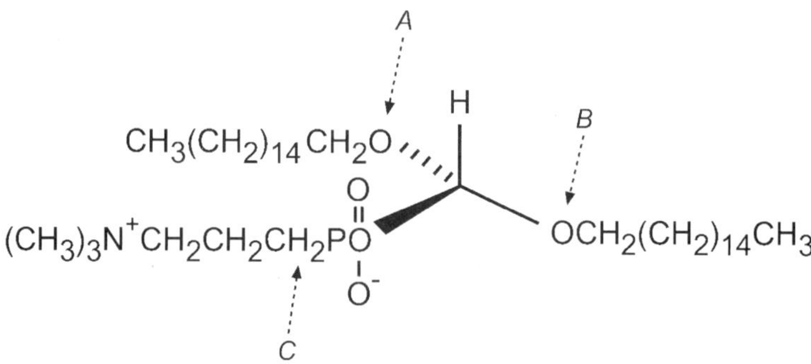

Figure 10 Molecular structure of a diether phosphonolipid analog of DPPC. The racemic form of the analog molecule shown is designated DEPN-8 (225). This analog has two saturated C16:0 chains and a choline group like DPPC, but has ether rather than ester linkages with the glycerol backbone (sites A and B). A methylene group is also substituted for oxygen in the headgroup (site C), making the molecule a phosphonolipid rather than a phospholipid. These substitutions make DEPN-8 more hydrophobic than DPPC. They also make DEPN-8 resistant to most phospholipases, and lead to better molecular spreading and adsorption while maintaining high dynamic surface tension lowering. See text for discussion. (Adapted from Ref. 3.)

of steric and/or chiral considerations (231). Due to its structural modifications, DEPN-8 has significantly better adsorption and film respreading than DPPC, while retaining the ability to reduce surface tension to $<1\,\mathrm{mN/m}$ in dynamically compressed surface films (224–228). The change from ester to ether linkages in DEPN-8 increases hydrophobicity and slightly increases gel to liquid crystal transition temperature relative to DPPC (224,229,230). This disaturated compound thus maintains a high interfacial molecular packing ability that facilitates surface tension lowering during film compression. At the same time, the greater hydrophobicity and more flexible nature of ether bonds compared to ester bonds promotes fatty chain interactions and increases adsorption and film respreading (226,227). The improved spreading and adsorption of DEPN-8 may also be related to the fact that it can form interdigitated as well as normal opposed bilayers (230).

The ability of DEPN-8 and related analogs to resist phospholipase degradation might be particularly beneficial in synthetic exogenous surfactants for use in inflammatory lung injury. Because of its excellent combination of surface tension lowering, adsorption, and spreading, DEPN-8 is highly surface active both as a pure compound and when combined with surfactant apoproteins (228) (Table 5). Moreover, the phospholipase resistance of this analog allows a synthetic surfactant composed of DEPN-8 + 1.5% bovine SP-B/C to retain high surface activity in the presence of phospholipase A_2 (Table 5). Resistance to phospholipase degradation also obviates the production of toxic, inhibitory byproducts like lyso-PC and fluid free fatty acids that themselves can impair surfactant activity in injured lungs. Synthetic exogenous surfactants containing purified sheep SP-B/C combined with DEPnC (DEPN-8) have been reported to improve P–V mechanics in 27-day gestation rabbit fetuses as effectively as a chloroform:methanol extract of sheep surfactant (232). The molecular characteristics of diether analogs potentially affect their metabolism and recycling in vivo. However, diether phospholipids and phosphonolipids have previously been shown to enter surfactant recycling pathways in type II cells (233–235), and they do not have observable short-term pulmonary toxicity in animals (232). Diether analogs are just one example of a spectrum of synthetic phospholipid-like components that could be utilized in future exogenous surfactant development.

VII. Surfactant Therapy in Combinations with Other Agents in ALI/ARDS

To achieve the most significant impact in treating patients with ALI/ARDS, it is logical to attack simultaneously more than one aspect of the complex pathology of lung injury. The use of multiple therapeutic agents

Table 5 Dynamic Surface Activity of Calf Lung Surfactant Extract and Synthetic Phospholipase-Resistant Surfactants with or without Phospholipase A_2

Surfactants	Minimum surface tension (mN/m) at various times of bubble pulsation (min)				
	1	2	5	10	15
DEPN-8	18.3 ± 2.1	12.4 ± 1.3	9.6 ± 1.7	3.0 ± 1.8	<1
DEPN-8 + 1.5% SP	3.0 ± 1.9	1.3 ± 0.6	<1 (3 min)		
CLSE	2.3 ± 1.4	1.0 ± 0.8	<1 (3 min)		
DEPN-8 + 1.5% SP + 0.1 U PLA_2	3.5 ± 1.5	1.2 ± 0.6	<1 (3 min)		
CLSE + 0.1 U PLA_2	19.7 ± 2.2	18.2 ± 1.7	17.2 ± 1.4	15.6 ± 1.3	14.1 ± 2.3

DEPN-8 + 1.5% SP has surface tension lowering equal to highly active CLSE, and maintains this activity in the presence of phospholipase A_2. Minimum surface tension values are on a pulsating bubble surfactometer (37°C, 20 cycles/min, 50% area compression) at a uniform phospholipid or phosphonolipid concentration of 1 mg/mL.

Abbreviations: DEPN-8, synthetic diether analog of DPPC (Fig. 10); CLSE, calf lung surfactant extract; SP, mixed bovine SP-B/SP-C purified from CLSE; PLA_2, phospholipase A_2; U, standard unit of enzyme activity. Percentage of SP in mixtures with DEPN-8 is by weight. (Data from Ref. 228.)

or interventions in a combination approach has the potential to achieve additive or even synergistic benefits to respiratory function and long-term patient outcomes. Aside from surfactant dysfunction, prominent aspects of the pathophysiology of acute pulmonary injury include inflammation, vascular dysfunction, and oxidant injury. Pharmacologic agents targeting these aspects of acute injury, as well as agents directed against chronic lung injury, are detailed in Chapters 14, 16, and 17. Examples of agents that might be synergistic with exogenous surfactant in treating lung injury include anti-inflammatory antibodies or receptor antagonists, antioxidants, and vasoactive drugs such as inhaled nitric oxide (iNO). In addition, ventilation modalities or strategies that reduce ventilator-induced lung injury as described in Chapter 13 may also be additive or synergistic with exogenous surfactant therapy. References 46, 236–257 provide additional review and discussion on agents and interventions for lung injury and sepsis that could potentially be incorporated in combination therapy approaches.

Combined-modality and multiagent therapies for lung injury are discussed in detail in Chapter 19. One relevant example of such an approach involves the use of exogenous surfactant in combination with iNO to improve ventilation/perfusion matching in patients with lung injury. Delivery of iNO has been shown to improve gas exchange in infants and adults with ARDS-related acute respiratory failure when administered as an individual agent (258–266). By selectively dilating the pulmonary vasculature in ventilated lung regions, iNO has potential synergy with exogenous surfactant which recruits and stabilizes alveoli and increases alveolar ventilation. Research in animal models of ALI/ARDS has demonstrated improved oxygenation in response to combination therapy with iNO and exogenous surfactant compared to either agent alone (267–271). NO is highly reactive, and could interact chemically with surfactant at high concentration (272–274). However, no detrimental effects of iNO on lung surfactant activity have been reported at the 5–40 ppm levels used clinically. The potential clinical utility of therapy with iNO and exogenous surfactant is indicated by a case study in three term infants with severe acute respiratory failure consistent with ARDS (275). All three infants had significantly improved arterial oxygenation following treatment with iNO and surfactant (Survanta, 100 mg/kg body weight), and all survived without referral for ECMO or the need for supplemental oxygen (275). These favorable findings support further prospective controlled studies on the efficacy of exogenous surfactant and iNO in combination therapy for ALI/ARDS.

VIII. Summary

Exogenous lung surfactant therapy involves the delivery of surface active material from outside the body to the alveoli to replace or supplement deficient or dysfunctional endogenous surfactant. Exogenous surfactant therapy is largely applicable for acute rather than chronic lung injury, and requires that patients ultimately produce and maintain sufficient amounts of endogenous surfactant within the lungs. This chapter has reviewed and discussed current information about the efficacy of exogenous surfactant therapy in infants, children, and adults with clinical ALI/ARDS. The pathophysiology of lung injury is known to include an important element of surfactant dysfunction. The rationale for exogenous surfactant therapy in ALI/ARDS is strengthened by the observation that many forms of surfactant dysfunction can be mitigated or abolished by raising surfactant concentration, despite the continued presence of compounds that inhibit surface activity. Exogenous surfactant therapy has been shown to have significant benefits in improving respiratory function and/or P–V mechanics in multiple animal models of ALI/ARDS. These animal models include hyperoxia, aspiration of acid or meconium, bilateral vagotomy, antibody-induced lung injury, endotoxin or bacterial-induced injury, influenza-induced pneumonia, NNNMU-induced lung injury, and in vivo lavage with mechanical ventilation (Chapters 9, 10).

The current status of surfactant therapy for ALI/ARDS is much like that existing for RDS in premature infants in the 1980s when systematic clinical studies with surfactant drugs were initially done. The phenomenology of surfactant dysfunction and replacement is well characterized in basic research, and abnormalities in surfactant activity have been extensively documented in patients with ALI/ARDS. Studies in full-term infants with acute respiratory failure from meconium aspiration or infection have shown that tracheal instillation of several exogenous surfactants gives significant improvements in respiratory function and in the severity and duration of required mechanical ventilation. Improvements in gas exchange and respiratory outcomes from exogenous surfactant therapy have also been demonstrated in children with ALI/ARDS. Several pilot studies have reported significant acute lung functional improvements from bronchoscopic instillation of exogenous surfactant in adults with ARDS, but other controlled studies have reported little or no clinical benefit from surfactant therapy. By far, the largest clinical trial of exogenous surfactant therapy in adults with ARDS reported no benefits from aerosolized Exosurf. However, Exosurf is known to have very low biophysical and physiological activity compared to other exogenous surfactants, and aerosolization is currently not as effective as tracheal or bronchoscopic instillation as a delivery method for exogenous surfactant.

Experience from the development of surfactant therapy for RDS in premature infants shows the importance of using active exogenous surfactant drugs and delivering them effectively to the alveoli. Initial attempts at surfactant replacement therapy in premature infants with aerosolized synthetic DPPC in the 1960s were ineffective. This was misinterpreted as indicating that surfactant therapy itself was not applicable in RDS.

Subsequent biophysical and animal research over several decades established the basis of surfactant activity more fully, and led to successful clinical trials of surfactant therapy. Meaningful evaluations of surfactant therapy in ALI/ARDS require testing exogenous surfactants with maximal activity and inhibition resistance that are administered appropriately in controlled studies of adequate size. The consensus of basic research shows that current exogenous surfactants obtained by saline lavage of intact animal lungs have the closest compositional analogy to endogenous surfactant, as well as the greatest surface activity, inhibition resistance, and physiological efficacy in animals. Several of the more active available clinical exogenous surfactants have not yet been well studied in adults with ALI/ARDS. Continuing research is also investigating a number of approaches to develop new synthetic or semisynthetic exogenous surfactants of high activity for possible use in ALI/ARDS.

Tracheal or bronchoscopic instillation are currently the best methods for delivering exogenous surfactants to patients with ALI/ARDS. Divided dosing is typically required, since 50–100 times as much surfactant drug is needed in an adult to achieve a comparable dose to a premature infant based on body weight. Aerosol methods for administering exogenous surfactants are not currently perfected, but advances in nebulizer and particle technology may make this approach more useful in the future. Research also suggests that the delivery and distribution of exogenous surfactant in patients with ALI/ARDS might be facilitated by specialized modes of ventilation such as partial liquid ventilation or jet ventilation. The distribution of instilled exogenous surfactant in patients with lung injury might also be improved by using drug dispersions formulated to have low shear viscosity to minimize transport resistance during transport to the pulmonary periphery.

Even if exogenous surfactant therapy is fully effective in mitigating surfactant dysfunction in patients with ALI/ARDS, improvements in clinical outcomes and survival may be obscured due to remaining elements of inflammation, tissue injury, and multiorgan disease. Future clinical research on surfactant therapy in ALI/ARDS thus needs not only to utilize and deliver the most active exogenous surfactant drugs, but also to examine the efficacy of exogenous surfactant therapy in conjunction with additional agents and interventions that simultaneously target multiple aspects of the pathophysiology of lung injury. Multiagent and combined-modality therapies for inflammatory lung injury are covered in detail in Chapter 19.

Acknowledgment

The financial support of grants HL-56176 and HL-03910 from the National Institutes of Health is gratefully acknowledged.

References

1. Pattle RE. Properties, function, and origin of the alveolar lining layer. Nature 1955; 175:1125–1126.
2. Clements JA. Surface tension of lung extracts. Proc Soc Exp Biol Med 1957; 95:170–172.
3. Notter RH. Lung Surfactants: Basic Science and Clinical Applications. New York: Marcel Dekker, 2000.
4. Soll RF, Merritt TA, Hallman M. Surfactant in the prevention and treatment of respiratory distress syndrome. In: Boynton BR, Carlo WA, Jobe AH, eds. New Therapies for Neonatal Respiratory Failure. New York: Cambridge University Press, 1994:49–80.
5. Soll RF. Surfactant therapy in the USA: trials and current routines. Biol Neonate 1997; 71:1–7.
6. Jobe AH. Pulmonary surfactant therapy. N Engl J Med 1993; 328:861–868.
7. Bernard GR, Artigas A, Brigham KL, Carlet J, Falke K, Hudson L, Lamy M, Legall JR, Morris A, Spragg R. The American–European Consensus Conference on ARDS: definitions, mechanisms, relevant outcomes, and clinical trial coordination. Am J Respir Crit Care Med 1994; 149:818–824.
8. Kumar V, Cotran RS, Robbins SL. Basic Pathology. 6th ed. Philadelphia: WB Saunders, 1997.
9. Hall JB, Schmidt GA, Wood LDH. Principles of Critical Care. 2nd ed. New York: McGraw Hill, 1998.
10. Taussig LM, Landau LI, Le Souef PN, Morgan WJ, Martinez FD, Sly PDE. Pediatric Respiratory Medicine. St. Louis: Mosby, 1999..
11. Taeusch HW, Ballard RA. Avery's Diseases of the Newborn. 7th ed. Philadelphia: WB Saunders, 1998.
12. Notter RH, Wang Z. Pulmonary surfactant: physical chemistry, physiology and replacement. Rev Chem Eng 1997; 13:1–118.
13. Petty T, Reiss O, Paul G, Silvers G, Elkins N. Characteristics of pulmonary surfactant in adult respiratory distress syndrome associated with trauma and shock. Am Rev Respir Dis 1977; 115:531–536.
14. Hallman M, Spragg R, Harrell JH, Moser KM, Gluck L. Evidence of lung surfactant abnormality in respiratory failure. J Clin Invest 1982; 70:673–683.
15. Seeger W, Pison U, Buchhorn R, Obestacke U, Joka T. Surfactant abnormalities and adult respiratory failure. Lung 1990; 168(suppl):891–902.
16. Pison U, Seeger W, Buchhorn R, Joka T, Brand M, Obertacke U, Neuhof H, Schmit-Neuerberg K. Surfactant abnormalities in patients with respiratory failure after multiple trauma. Am Rev Respir Dis 1989; 140:1033–1039.
17. Gregory TJ, Longmore WJ, Moxley MA, Whitsett JA, Reed CR, Fowler AA, Hudson LD, Maunder RJ, Crim C, Hyers TM. Surfactant chemical composition and biophysical activity in acute respiratory distress syndrome. J Clin Invest 1991; 88:1976–1981.
18. Günther A, Siebert C, Schmidt R, Ziegle S, Grimminger F, Yabut M, Temmesfeld B, Walmrath D, Morr H, Seeger W. Surfactant alterations in severe pneumonia, acute respiratory distress syndrome, and cardiogenic lung edema. Am J Respir Crit Care Med 1996; 153:176–184.

19. Veldhuizen R, McCaig L, Akino T, Lewis J. Pulmonary surfactant subfractions in patients with the acute respiratory distress syndrome. Am J Respir Crit Care Med 1995; 152:1867–1871.

20. Griese M. Pulmonary surfactant in health and human lung diseases: state of the art. Eur Respir J 1999; 13:1455–1476.

21. Mander A, Langton-Hewer S, Bernhard W, Warner JO, Postle AD. Altered phospholipid composition and aggregate structure of lung surfactant is associated with impaired lung function in young children with respiratory infections. Am J Respir Cell Mol Biol 2002; 27:714–721.

22. Schmidt R, Meier U, Markart P, Grimminger F, Velcovsky HG, Morr H, Seeger W, Gunther A. Altered fatty acid composition of lung surfactant phospholipids in interstitial lung disease. Am J Physiol 2002; 283:L1079–L1085.

23. Skelton R, Holland P, Darowski M, Chetcuti P, Morgan L, Harwood J. Abnormal surfactant composition and activity in severe bronchiolitis. Acta Paediatr 1999; 88:942–946.

24. LeVine AM, Lotze A, Stanley S, Stroud C, O'Donnell R, Whitsett J, Pollack MM. Surfactant content in children with inflammatory lung disease. Crit Care Med 1996; 24:1062–1067.

25. Dargaville PA, South M, McDougall PN. Surfactant abnormalities in infants with severe viral bronchiolitis. Arch Dis Child 1996; 75:133–136.

26. Holm BA, Notter RH, Finkelstein JH. Surface property changes from interactions of albumin with natural lung surfactant and extracted lung lipids. Chem Phys Lipids 1985; 38:287–298.

27. Seeger W, Stohr G, Wolf HRD, Neuhof H. Alteration of surfactant function due to protein leakage: special interaction with fibrin monomer. J Appl Physiol 1985; 58:326–338.

28. Holm BA, Notter RH. Effects of hemoglobin and cell membrane lipids on pulmonary surfactant activity. J Appl Physiol 1987; 63:1434–1442.

29. Seeger W, Grube C, Günther A, Schmidt R. Surfactant inhibition by plasma proteins: differential sensitivity of various surfactant preparations. Eur Respir J 1993; 6:971–977.

30. Holm BA, Enhorning G, Notter RH. A biophysical mechanism by which plasma proteins inhibit lung surfactant activity. Chem Phys Lipids 1988; 49:49–55.

31. Fuchimukai T, Fujiwara T, Takahashi A, Enhorning G. Artificial pulmonary surfactant inhibited by proteins. J Appl Physiol 1987; 62:429–437.

32. Keough KWM, Parsons CS, Tweeddale MG. Interactions between plasma proteins and pulmonary surfactant: pulsating bubble studies. Can J Physiol Pharmacol 1989; 67:663–668.

33. Wang Z, Notter RH. Additivity of protein and non-protein inhibitors of lung surfactant activity. Am J Respir Crit Care Med 1998; 158:28–35.

34. Moses D, Holm BA, Spitale P, Liu M, Enhorning G. Inhibition of pulmonary surfactant function by meconium. Am J Obstet Gynecol 1991; 164:477–481.

35. Cockshutt A, Possmayer F. Lysophosphatidylcholine sensitizes lipid extracts of pulmonary surfactant to inhibition by plasma proteins. Biochim Biophys Acta 1991; 1086:63–71.

36. Seeger W, Lepper H, Hellmut RD, Neuhof H. Alteration of alveolar surfactant function after exposure to oxidant stress and to oxygenated and native arachadonic acid in vitro. Biochim Biophys Acta 1985; 835:58–67.
37. Hall SB, Lu ZR, Venkitaraman AR, Hyde RW, Notter RH. Inhibition of pulmonary surfactant by oleic acid: mechanisms and characteristics. J Appl Physiol 1992; 72:1708–1716.
38. Hall SB, Hyde RW, Notter RH. Changes in subphase surfactant aggregates in rabbits injured by free fatty acid. Am J Respir Crit Care Med 1994; 149: 1099–1106.
39. Ryan AJ, McCoy DM, McGowan SE, Salome RG, Mallampalli RK. Alveolar sphingolipids generated in response to TNF-αmodifies surfactant biophysical activity. J Appl Physiol 2003; 94:253–258.
40. Hickman-Davis JM, Fang FC, Nathan C, Shepherd VL, Voelker DR, Wright JR. Lung surfactant and reactive oxygen-nitrogen species: antimicrobial activity and host-pathogen interactions. Am J Physiol 2001; 281:L517–L523.
41. Haddad IY, Ischiropoulos H, Holm BA, Beckman JS, Baker JR, Matalon S. Mechanisms of peroxynitrite-induced injury to pulmonary surfactants. Am J Physiol 1993; 265:L555–L564.
42. Amirkhanian JD, Merritt TA. Inhibitory effects of oxyradicals on surfactant function: utilizing in vitro Fenton reaction. Lung 1998; 176:63–72.
43. Pison U, Tam EK, Caughey GH, Hawgood S. Proteolytic inactivation of dog lung surfactant-associated proteins by neutrophil elastase. Biochim Biophys Acta 1989; 992:251–257.
44. Holm BA, Keicher L, Liu M, Sokolowski J, Enhorning G. Inhibition of pulmonary surfactant function by phospholipases. J Appl Physiol 1991; 71:1–5.
45. Enhorning G, Shumel B, Keicher L, Sokolowski J, Holm BA. Phospholipases introduced into the hypophase affect the surfactant film outlining a bubble. J Appl Physiol 1992; 73:941–945.
46. Notter RH, Apostolakos M, Holm BA, Willson D, Wang Z, Finkelstein JN, Hyde RW. Surfactant therapy and its potential use with other agents in term infants, children and adults with acute lung injury. Perspect Neonatol 2000; 1(4):4–20.
47. Lewis JF, Jobe AH. Surfactant and the adult respiratory distress syndrome. Am Rev Respir Dis 1993; 147:218–233.
48. Seeger W, Günther A, Walmrath HD, Grimminger F, Lasch HG. Alveolar surfactant and adult respiratory distress syndrome. Pathogenic role and therapeutic prospects. Clin Invest 1993; 71:177–190.
49. Lachmann B, van Daal G-J. Adult respiratory distress syndrome: animal models. In: Robertson B, van Golde LMG Batenburg JJ, eds. Pulmonary Surfactant: From Molecular Biology to Clinical Practice. Amsterdam: Elsevier Science Publishers, 1992:635–663.
50. Kobayashi T, Ganzuka M, Taniguchi J, Nitta K, Murakami S. Lung lavage and surfactant replacement for hydrochloric acid aspiration in rabbits. Acta Anaesthesiol Scand 1990; 34:216–221.
51. Zucker A, Holm BA, Wood LDH, Crawford G, Ridge K, Sznajder IA. Exogenous surfactant with PEEP reduces pulmonary edema and improves

lung function in canine aspiration pneumonitis. J Appl Physiol 1992; 73: 679–686.

52. Schlag G, Strohmaier W. Experimental aspiration trauma: comparison of steroid treatment versus exogenous natural surfactant. Exp Lung Res 1993; 19:397–405.

53. Al-Mateen KB, Dailey K, Grimes MM, Gutcher GR. Improved oxygenation with exogenous surfactant administration in experimental meconium aspiration syndrome. Pediatr Pulmonol 1994; 17:75–80.

54. Sun B, Curstedt T, Robertson B. Exogenous surfactant improves ventilation efficiency and alveolar expansion in rats with meconium aspiration. Am J Respir Crit Care Med 1996; 154:764–770.

55. Cochrane CG, Revak SD, Merritt TA, Schraufstatter U, Hoch RC, Henderson C, Andersson S, Takamori H, Oades ZG. Bronchoalveolar lavage with KL4-surfactant in models of meconium aspiration syndrome. Pediatr Res 1998; 44:705–715.

56. Sun B, Curstedt T, Song GW, Robertson B. Surfactant improves lung function and morphology in newborn rabbits with meconium aspiration. Biol Neonate 1993; 63:96–104.

57. Lachmann B, Hallman M, Bergman K-C. Respiratory failure following anti-lung serum: study on mechanisms associated with surfactant system damage. Exp Lung Res 1987; 12:163–180.

58. Nieman G, Gatto L, Paskanik A, Yang B, Fluck R, Picone A. Surfactant replacement in the treatment of sepsis-induced adult respiratory distress syndrome in pigs. Crit Care Med 1996; 24:1025–1033.

59. Lutz C, Carney D, Finck C, Picone A, Gatto L, Paskanik A, Langenbeck E, Nieman G. Aerosolized surfactant improves pulmonary function in endotoxin-induced lung injury. Am J Respir Crit Care Med 1998; 158:840–845.

60. Lutz CJ, Picone A, Gatto LA, Paskanik A, Landas S, Nieman G. Exogenous surfactant and positive end-expiratory pressure in the treatment of endotoxin-induced lung injury. Crit Care Med 1998; 26:1379–1389.

61. Tashiro K, Li W-Z, Yamada K, Matsumoto Y, Kobayashi T. Surfactant replacement reverses respiratory failure induced by intratracheal endotoxin in rats. Crit Care Med 1995; 23:149–156.

62. Eijking EP, van Daal GJ, Tenbrinck R, Luyenduijk A, Sluiters JF, Hannappel E, Lachmann B. Effect of surfactant replacement on *Pneumocystis carinii*pneumonia in rats. Intensive Care Med 1990; 17:475–478.

63. Sherman MP, Campbell LA, Merritt TA, Long WA, Gunkel JH, Curstedt T, Robertson B. Effect of different surfactants on pulmonary group B streptococcal infection in premature rabbits. J Pediatr 1994; 125:939–947.

64. Berry D, Ikegami M, Jobe A. Respiratory distress and surfactant inhibition following vagotomy in rabbits. J Appl Physiol 1986; 61:1741–1748.

65. Matalon S, Holm BA, Notter RH. Mitigation of pulmonary hyperoxic injury by administration of exogenous surfactant. J Appl Physiol 1987; 62:756–761.

66. Loewen GM, Holm BA, Milanowski L, Wild LM, Notter RH, Matalon S. Alveolar hyperoxic injury in rabbits receiving exogenous surfactant. J Appl Physiol 1989; 66:1987–1992.

67. Engstrom PC, Holm BA, Matalon S. Surfactant replacement attenuates the increase in alveolar permeability in hyperoxia. J Appl Physiol 1989; 67:688–693.

68. Matalon S, Holm BA, Loewen GM, Baker RR, Notter RH. Sublethal hyperoxic injury to the alveolar epithelium and the pulmonary surfactant system. Exp Lung Res 1988; 14:1021–1033.

69. Novotny WE, Hudak BB, Matalon S, Holm BA. Hyperoxic lung injury reduces exogenous surfactant clearance in vitro. Am J Respir Crit Care Med 1995; 151:1843–1847.

70. Lachmann B, Fujiwara T, Chida S, Morita T, Konishi M, Nakamura K, Maeta H. Surfactant replacement therapy in experimental adult respiratory distress syndrome (ARDS). In: Cosmi EV, Scarpelli EM, eds. Pulmonary Surfactant System. Amsterdam: Elsevier, 1983:221–235.

71. Kobayashi T, Kataoka H, Ueda T, Murakami S, Takada Y, Kobuko M. Effect of surfactant supplementation and end expiratory pressure in lung-lavaged rabbits. J Appl Physiol 1984; 57:995–1001.

72. Berggren P, Lachmann B, Curstedt T, Grossmann G, Robertson B. Gas exchange and lung morphology after surfactant replacement in experimental adult respiratory distress induced by repeated lung lavage. Acta Anaesthesiol Scand 1986; 30:321–328.

73. Lewis JF, Goffin J, Yue P, McCaig LA, Bjarneson D, Veldhuizen RAW. Evaluation of exogenous surfactant treatment strategies in an adult model of acute lung injury. J Appl Physiol 1996; 80:1156–1164.

74. Walther FJ, Hernandez-Juviel J, Bruni R, Waring A. Spiking Survanta with synthetic surfactant peptides improves oxygenation in surfactant-deficient rats. Am J Respir Crit Care Med 1997; 156:855–861.

75. Walther F, Hernandez-Juviel J, Bruni R, Waring AJ. Protein composition of synthetic surfactant affects gas exchange in surfactant-deficient rats. Pediatr Res 1998; 43:666–673.

76. Harris JD, Jackson F, Moxley MA, Longmore WJ. Effect of exogenous surfactant instillation on experimental acute lung injury. J Appl Physiol 1989; 66:1846–1851.

77. Lewis JF, Ikegami M, Jobe AH. Metabolism of exogenously administered surfactant in the acutely injured lungs of adult rabbits. Am Rev Respir Dis 1992; 145:19–23.

78. Lewis J, Ikegami M, Higuchi R, Jobe A, Absolom D. Nebulized vs. instilled exogenous surfactant in an adult lung injury model. J Appl Physiol 1991; 71:1270–1276.

79. van Daal GJ, So KL, Gommers D, Eijking EP, Fievez RB, Sprenger MJ, van Dam DW, Lachmann B. Intratracheal surfactant administration restores gas exchange in experimental adult respiratory distress syndrome associated with viral pneumonia. Anesth Analg 1991; 72:589–595.

80. van Daal GJ, Bos JAH, Eijking EP, Gommers D, Hannappel E, Lachmann B. Surfactant replacement therapy improves pulmonary mechanics in end-stage influenza A pneumonia in mice. Am Rev Respir Dis 1992; 145: 859–863.

81. Mizuno K, Ikegami M, Chen C-M, Ueda T, Jobe AH. Surfactant protein-B supplementation improves in vivo function of a modified natural surfactant. Pediatr Res 1995; 37:271–276.

82. Hamvas A, Cole FS, deMello DE, Moxley M, Whitsett JA, Colten HR, Nogee LM. Surfactant protein B deficiency: antenatal diagnosis and prospective treatment with surfactant replacement. J Pediatr 1994; 125:356–361.

83. Notter RH, Wang Z, Egan EA, Holm BA. Component-specific surface and physiological activity in bovine-derived lung surfactants. Chem Phys Lipids 2002; 114:21–34.

84. Lewis JF, Brackenbury A. Role of exogenous surfactant in acute lung injury. Crit Care Med 2003; 31(suppl):S324–S328.

85. Clark DA, Nieman GF, Thompson JE, Paskanik AM, Rokhar JE, Bredenberg CE. Surfactant displacement by meconium free fatty acids: an alternative explanation for atelectasis in meconium aspiration syndrome. J Pediatr 1987; 110:765–770.

86. Auten RL, Notter RH, Kendig JW, Davis JM, Shapiro DL. Surfactant treatment of full-term newborns with respiratory failure. Pediatrics 1991; 87: 101–107.

87. Kendig JW, Notter RH, Cox C, Reubens LJ, Davis JM, Maniscalco WM, Sinkin RA, Bartoletti A, Dweck HS, Horgan MJ, Risemberg H, Phelps DL, Shapiro DL. A comparison of surfactant as immediate prophylaxis and as rescue therapy in newborns of less than 30 weeks gestation. N Engl J Med 1991; 324:865–871.

88. Davis JM, Vaness-Meehan K, Notter RH, Bhutani VK, Kendig JW, Shapiro DL. Changes in pulmonary mechanics after the administration of surfactant to infants with respiratory distress syndrome. N Engl J Med 1988; 319: 476–479.

89. Khammash H, Perlman M, Wojtulewicz J, Dunn M. Surfactant therapy in full-term neonates with severe respiratory failure. Pediatrics 1993; 92: 135–139.

90. Findlay RD, Taeusch HW, Walther FJ. Surfactant replacement therapy for meconium aspiration syndrome. Pediatrics 1996; 97:48–52.

91. Lotze A, Knight GR, Martin GR, Bulas DI, Hull WM, O'Donnell RM, Whitsett JA, Short BL. Improved pulmonary outcome after exogenous surfactant therapy for respiratory failure in term infants requiring extracorporeal membrane oxygenation. J Pediatr 1993; 122:261–268.

92. Lotze A, Mitchell BR, Bulas DI, Zola EM, Shalwitz RA, Gunkel JH. Multicenter study of surfactant (beractant) use in the treatment of term infants with severe respiratory failure. J Pediatr 1998; 132:40–47.

93. Luchetti M, Casiraghi G, Valsecchi R, Galassini E, Marraro G. Porcine-derived surfactant treatment of severe bronchiolitis. Acta Anaesthesiol Scand 1998; 42:805–810.

94. Luchetti M, Ferrero F, Gallini C, Natale A, Pigna A, Tortorolo L, Marraro G. Multicenter, randomized, controlled study of porcine surfactant in severe respiratory syncytial virus-induced respiratory failure. Pediatr Crit Care Med 2002; 3:261–268.

95. Tibby SM, Hatherill M, Wright SM, Wilson P, Postle AD, Murdoch IA. Exogenous surfactant supplementation in infants with respiratory syncytial virus bronchiolitis. Am J Respir Crit Care Med 2000; 162:1251–1256.

96. Willson DF, Jiao JH, Bauman LA, Zaritsky A, Craft H, Dockery K, Conrad D, Dalton H. Calf lung surfactant extract in acute hypoxemic respiratory failure in children. Crit Care Med 1996; 24:1316–1322.

97. Willson DF, Bauman LA, Zaritsky A, Dockery K, James RL, Stat M, Conrad D, Craft H, Novotny WE, Egan EA, Dalton H. Instillation of calf lung surfactant extract (calfactant) is beneficial in pediatric acute hypoxemic respiratory failure. Crit Care Med 1999; 27:188–195.

98. Spragg R, Gilliard N, Richman P, Smith R, Hite R, Pappert D, Robertson B, Curstedt T, Strayer D. Acute effects of a single dose of porcine surfactant on patients with the adult respiratory distress syndrome. Chest 1994; 105: 195–202.

99. Walmrath D, Gunther A, Ghofrani HA, Schermuly R, Schnedier T, Grimminger F, Seeger W. Bronchoscopic surfactant administration in patients with severe adult respiratory distress syndrome and sepsis. Am J Respir Crit Care Med 1996; 154:57–62.

100. Walmrath D, Grimminger F, Pappert D, Knothe C, Obertacke U, Benzing A, Gunther A, Schmehl T, Leuchte H, Seeger W. Bronchoscopic administration of bovine natural surfactant in ARDS and septic shock: Impact on gas exchange and haemodynamics. Eur Respir J 2002; 19:805–810.

101. Gregory TJ, Steinberg KP, Spragg R, Gadek JE, Hyers TM, Longmere WJ, Moxley MA, Guang-Zuan CAI, Hite RD, Smith RM, Hudson LD, Crim C, Newton P, Mitchell BR, Gold AJ. Bovine surfactant therapy for patients with acute respiratory distress syndrome. Am J Respir Crit Care Med 1997; 155:109–131.

102. Spragg RG, Lewis JF, Wurst W, Hafner D, Baughman RP, Wewers MD, Marsh JJ. Treatment of acute respiratory distress syndrome with recombinant surfactant protein C surfactant. Am J Respir Crit Care Med 2003; 167: 1562–1566.

103. Macnaughton PD, Evans TW. The effect of exogenous surfactant therapy on lung function following cardiopulmonary bypass. Chest 1994; 105: 421–425.

104. Anzueto A, Baughman RP, Guntupalli KK, Weg JG, Wiedemann HP, Raventos AA, Lemaire F, Long W, Zaccardelli DS, Pattishall EN. Exosurf ARDS Sepsis Study Group. Aerosolized surfactant in adults with sepsis-induced acute respiratory distress syndrome. N Engl J Med 1996; 334:1417–1421.

105. Matthay MA. The acute respiratory distress syndrome (editorial). N Engl J Med 1996; 334:1469–1470.

106. Avery ME, Mead J. Surface properties in relation to atelectasis and hyaline membrane disease. Am J Dis Child 1959; 97:517–523.

107. Gruenwald P. The mechanism of abnormal expansion of the lungs of mature and premature newborn infants. Bull Margaret Hague Maternity Hosp 1955; 8:100–106.

108. Gruenwald P. The significance of pulmonary hyaline membranes in newborn infants. J Am Med Assoc 1958; 166:621–623.

109. Pattle RE. Properties, function and origin of the alveolar lining layer. Proc R Soc (London) Ser B 1958; 148:217–240.
110. Chu J, Clements JA, Cotton EK, Klaus MH, Sweet AY, Tooley WH. Neonatal pulmonary ischemia. Clinical and physiologic studies. Pediatrics 1967; 40: 709–782.
111. Robillard E, Alarie Y, Dagenais-Perusse P, Baril E, Guilbeault A. Microaerosol administration of synthetic β,γ-dipalmitoyl-l-α-lecithin in the respiratory distress syndrome: a preliminary report. Can Med Assoc J 1964; 90:55–57.
112. Chu J, Clements JA, Cotton EK, Klaus MH, Sweet AY, Thomas MA, Tooley WH. The pulmonary hypoperfusion syndrome. Pediatrics 1965; 35:733–742.
113. Enhorning G, Grossman G, Robertson B. Tracheal deposition of surfactant before the first breath. Am Rev Respir Dis 1973; 107:921–927.
114. Enhorning G, Grossman G, Robertson B. Pharyngeal deposition of surfactant in the premature rabbit fetus. Biol Neonate 1973; 22:126–132.
115. Enhorning G, Hill D, Sherwood G, Cutz E, Robertson B, Bryan C. Improved ventilation of prematurely derived primates following tracheal deposition of surfactant. Am J Obstet Gynecol 1978; 132:529–536.
116. Enhorning G, Robertson B. Lung expansion in the premature rabbit fetus after tracheal deposition of surfactant. Pediatrics 1972; 50:58–66.
117. Robertson B, Enhorning G. The alveolar lining of the premature newborn rabbit after pharyngeal deposition of surfactant. Lab Invest 1974; 31:54–59.
118. Adams FH, Towers B, Osher AB, Ikegami M, Fujiwara T, Nozak M. Effect of tracheal instillation of natural surfactant in premature lambs. I. Clinical and autopsy findings. Pediatr Res 1978; 12:841–848.
119. Robertson B. Surfactant substitution: experimental models and clinical applications. Lung 1980; 158:57–68.
120. Notter RH, Shapiro DL. Lung surfactant in an era of replacement therapy. Pediatrics 1981; 68:781–789.
121. Ikegami M, Hesterberg T, Nozaki M, Adams FH. Restoration of lung pressure–volume characteristics with surfactant: comparison of nebulization versus instillation and natural versus synthetic surfactant. Pediatr Res 1977; 11:178–182.
122. Ikegami M, Adams FH, Towers B, Osher AB. The quantity of natural surfactant necessary to prevent the respiratory distress syndrome in premature lambs. Pediatr Res 1980; 14:1082–1085.
123. Enhorning G. Pulsating bubble technique for evaluation of pulmonary surfactant. J Appl Physiol 1977; 43:198–203.
124. Notter R, Taubold R, Finkelstein J. Comparative adsorption of natural lung surfactant, extracted phospholipids, and synthetic phospholipid mixtures. Chem Phys Lipids 1983; 33:67–80.
125. Notter RH. Surface chemistry of pulmonary surfactant: the role of individual components. In:Roberson B, van Golde LMG, Batenburg JJ, eds. Pulmonary Surfactant. Amsterdam: Elsevier Science Publishers, 1984:17–53.
126. Notter RH, Finkelstein JN. Pulmonary surfactant: an interdisciplinary approach. J Appl Physiol 1984; 57:1613–1624.
127. Notter RH, Morrow PE. Pulmonary surfactant: a surface chemistry viewpoint. Ann Biomed Eng 1975; 3:119–159.

128. Possmayer F, Yu S-H, Weber JM, Harding PGR. Pulmonary surfactant. Can J Biochem Cell Biol 1984; 62:1121–1133.
129. Yu SH, Harding PGR, Smith N, Possmayer P. Bovine pulmonary surfactant: chemical composition and physical properties. Lipids 1983; 18:522–529.
130. Yu SH, Possmayer F. Reconstitution of surfactant activity by using the 6 kDa apoprotein associated with pulmonary surfactant. Biochem J 1986; 236: 85–89.
131. Notter RH, Tabak SA, Mavis RD. Surface properties of binary mixtures of some pulmonary surfactant components. J Lipid Res 1980; 21:10–22.
132. Notter RH, Shapiro DL. Lung surfactants for replacement therapy: biochemical, biophysical, and clinical aspects. Clin Perinatol 1987; 14:433–479.
133. Goerke J, Clements JA. Alveolar surface tension and lung surfactant. In: Fishman AP, Mackelroy PT, Mead J Geiger GR, eds. Handbook of Physiology. The Respiratory System. Mechanics of Breathing. Vol. III. Bethesda, MD: American Physiological Society Press,1986:247–261.
134. Shapiro D, Notter R, eds. Surfactant Replacement Therapy. New York: AR Liss, 1989.
135. Kattwinkel J. Surfactant: Evolving issues. Clin Perinatol 1998; 25:17–32.
136. Davis JM, Russ GA, Metlay L, Dickerson B, Greenspan BS. Short-term distribution kinetics in intratracheally administered exogenous lung surfactant. Pediatr Res 1992; 31:445–450.
137. Espinosa FF, Shapiro AH, Fredberg JJ, Kamm RD. Spreading of exogenous surfactant in an airway. J Appl Physiol 1993; 75:2028–2039.
138. Grotberg JB, Halpern D, Jensen OE. Interaction of exogenous and endogenous surfactant: spreading-rate effects. J Appl Physiol 1995; 78:750–756.
139. Marks LB, Notter RH, Oberdoerster G, McBride JT. Ultrasonic and jet aerosolization of phospholipids and the effects on surface activity. Pediatr Res 1984; 17:742–747.
140. Balaraman V, Meister J, Ku TL, Sood SL, Tam E, Killeen J, Uyehara CFT, Egan E, Easa D. Lavage administration of dilute surfactants after acute lung injury in neonatal piglets. Am J Respir Crit Care Med 1998; 158:12–17.
141. Balaraman V, Sood SL, Finn KC, Hashiro G, Uyehara CFT, Easa D. Physiologic response and lung distribution of lavage vs bolus Exosurf in piglets with acute lung injury. Am J Respir Crit Care Med 1996; 153: 1838–1843.
142. Gommers D, Eijking EP, van't Veen A, Lachmann B. Bronchoalveolar lavage with a diluted surfactant suspension prior to surfactant instillation improves the effectiveness of surfactant therapy in experimental acute respiratory distress syndrome (ARDS). Intensive Care Med 1998; 24:494–500.
143. van Der Beek J, Plotz F, van Overbeek F, Heikamp A, Beekhuis H, Wildevuur C, Oklen A, Bambang OS. Distribution of exogenous surfactant in rabbits with severe respiratory failure: the effect of volume. Pediatr Res 1993; 34:154–158.
144. Marks LB, Oberdoerster G, Notter RH. Generation and characterization of aerosols of dispersed surface active phospholipids by ultrasonic and jet nebulization. J Aerosol Sci 1983; 14:683–694.

145. Wojciak JF, Notter RH, Oberdoerster G. Size stability of phosphatidylcholine-phosphatidylglycerol aerosols and a dynamic film compression state from their interfacial impaction. J Colloid Interface Sci 1985; 106:547–557.

146. Dijk PH, Heikamp A, Bambang-Oetomo S. Surfactant nebulization versus instillation during high frequency ventilation in surfactant-deficient rabbits. Pediatr Res 1998; 44:699–704.

147. Ellyett KM, Broadbent RS, Fawcett ER, Campbell AJ. Surfactant aerosol treatment of respiratory distress syndrome in the spontaneously breathing rabbit. Pediatr Res 1996; 39:953–957.

148. Zelter M, Escudier BJ, Hoeffel JM, Murray JF. Effects of aerosolized artificial surfactant on repeated oleic acid injury in sheep. Am Rev Respir Dis 1990; 141:1014–1019.

149. Davis JM, Richter SE, Kendig JW, Notter RH. High frequency jet ventilation and surfactant treatment of newborns in severe respiratory failure. Pediatr Pulmonol 1992; 13:108–112.

150. Davis JM, Notter RH. Lung surfactant replacement for neonatal pathology other than primary respiratory distress syndrome. In: Boynton B, Carlo W, Jobe A, eds. New Therapies for Neonatal Respiratory Failure: A Physiologic Approach. Cambridge: Cambridge University Press, 1994:81–92.

151. Leach CL, Greenspan JS, Rubenstein SD, Shaffer TH, Wolfson MR, Jackson JC, DeLemos R, Fuhrman BP. Partial liquid ventilation with perflubron in premature infants with severe respiratory distress syndrome. N Engl J Med 1996; 335:761–767.

152. Leach CL, Holm BA, Morin FC, Fuhrman BP, Papo MC, Steinhorn D, Hernan LJ. Partial liquid ventilation in premature lambs with respiratory distress syndrome: efficacy and compatibility with exogenous surfactant. J Pediatr 1995; 126:412–420.

153. Chappell SE, Wolfson MR, Shaffer TH. A comparison of surfactant delivery with conventional mechanical ventilation and partial liquid ventilation in meconium aspiration injury. Respiratory Medicine 2001; 95:612–617.

154. King DM, Wang Z, Kendig JW, Palmer HJ, Holm BA, Notter RH. Concentration-dependent, temperature-dependent non-Newtonian viscosity of lung surfactant dispersions. Chem Phys Lipids 2001; 112:11–19.

155. King DM, Wang Z, Palmer HJ, Holm BA, Notter RH. Bulk shear viscosities of endogenous and exogenous lung surfactants. Am J Physiol 2002; 282:L277–L284.

156. Hudak ML, Farrell EE, Rosenberg AA, Jung AL, Auten RL, Durand DJ, Horgan MJ, Buckwald S, Belcastro MR, Donohue PK, Carrion V, Maniscalco WM, Balsan MJ, Torres BA, Miller RR, Jansen RD, Graeber JE, Laskay KM, Matteson EJ, Egan EA, Brody AS, Martin DJ, Riddlesberger MM, Montogomery P, and (21 Center group). A multicenter randomized masked comparison of natural vs synthetic surfactant for the treatment of respiratory distress syndrome. J Pediatr 1996; 128:396–406.

157. Bloom BT, Kattwinkel J, Hall RT, Delmore PM, Egan EA, Trout JR, Malloy MH, Brown DR, Holzman IR, Coghill CH, Carlo WA, Pramanik AK, McCaffree MA, Toubas PL, Laudert S, Gratny LL, Weatherstone KB, Seguin JH, Willett LD, Gutcher GR, Mueller DH, Topper WH, and (13 center

group). Comparison of Infasurf (calf lung surfactant extract) to Survanta (Beractant) in the treatment and prevention of RDS. Pediatrics 1997; 100:31–38.

158. Hudak ML, Martin DJ, Egan EA, Matteson EJ, Cummings J, Jung AL, Kimberlin LV, Auten RL, Rosenberg AA, Asselin JM, Belcastro MR, Donahue PK, Hamm CR, Jansen RD, Brody AS, Riddlesberger MM, Montgomery P, and (10 Center group). A multicenter randomized masked comparison trial of synthetic surfactant versus calf lung surfactant extract in the prevention of neonatal respiratory distress syndrome. Pediatrics 1997; 100:39–50.

159. Horbar JD, Wright LL, Soll RF, Wright EC, Fanaroff AA, Korones SB, Shankaran S, Oh W, Fletcher BD, Bauer CR, and (NIH NICHHD Neonatal Research Network). A multicenter randomized trial comparing two surfactants for the treatment of neonatal respiratory distress syndrome. J Pediatr 1993; 123:757–766.

160. Vermont-Oxford Neonatal Network. A multicenter randomized trial comparing synthetic surfactant with modified bovine surfactant extract in the treatment of neonatal respiratory distress syndrome. Pediatrics 1996; 97:1–6.

161. Rollins M, Jenkins J, Tubman R, Corkey C, Wilson D. Comparison of clinical responses to natural and synthetic surfactants. J Perinat Med 1993; 21: 341–347.

162. Sehgal SS, Ewing CK, Richards T, Taeusch HW. Modified bovine surfactant (Survanta) vs a protein-free surfactant (Exosurf) in the treatment of respiratory distress syndrome in preterm infants: a pilot study. J Natl Med Assoc 1994; 86:46–52.

163. Choukroun ML, Llanas B, Apere H, Fayon M, Galperine RI, Guenard H, Demarquez JL. Pulmonary mechanics in ventilated preterm infants with respiratory distress syndrome after exogenous surfactant administration: A comparison between two surfactant preparations. Pediatr Pulmonol 1994; 18:273–298.

164. Bloom BT, Delmore P, Rose T, Rawlins T. Human and calf lung surfactant: A comparison. Neonat Intensive Care 1993, March/April:31–35.

165. Speer CP, Gefeller O, Groneck P, Laufkotter E, Roll C, Hanssler L, Harms K, Herting E, Boenisch H, Windeler J, Robertson B. Randomised clinical trial of two treatment regimens of natural surfactant preparations in neonatal respiratory distress syndrome. Arch Dis Child 1995; 72:F8–F13.

166. Halliday HL. Overview of clinical trials comparing natural and synthetic surfactants. Biol Neonate 1995; 67(suppl):32–47.

167. Halliday HL. Controversies—synthetic or natural surfactant—the case for natural surfactant. J Perinat Med 1996; 24(5):417–426.

168. Hall SB, Venkitaraman AR, Whitsett JA, Holm BA, Notter RH. Importance of hydrophobic apoproteins as constituents of clinical exogenous surfactants. Am Rev Respir Dis 1992; 145:24–30.

169. Curstedt T, Jornvall H, Robertson B, Bergman T, Berggren P. Two hydrophobic low-molecular-mass protein fractions of pulmonary surfactant: characterization and biophysical activity. Eur J Biochem 1987; 168:255–262.

170. Oosterlaken-Dijksterhuis MA, Haagsman HP, van Golde LM, Demel RA. Characterization of lipid insertion into monomolecular layers mediated by

lung surfactant proteins SP-B and SP-C. Biochemistry 1991; 30: 10965–10971.

171. Oosterlaken-Dijksterhuis MA, Haagsman HP, van Golde LM, Demel RA. Interaction of lipid vesicles with monomolecular layers containing lung surfactant proteins SP-B or SP-C. Biochemistry 1991; 30:8276–8281.

172. Oosterlaken-Dijksterhuis MA, van Eijk M, van Golde LMG, Haagsman HP. Lipid mixing is mediated by the hydrophobic surfactant protein SP-B but not by SP-C. Biochim Biophys Acta 1992; 1110:45–50.

173. Revak SD, Merritt TA, Degryse E, Stefani L, Courtney M, Hallman M, Cochrane CG. The use of human low molecular weight (LMW) apoproteins in the reconstitution of surfactant biological activity. J Clin Invest 1988; 81:826–833.

174. Seeger W, Günther A, Thede C. Differential sensitivity to fibrinogen inhibition of SP-C- vs. SP-B-based surfactants. Am J Physiol 1992; 261: L286–L291.

175. Wang Z, Gurel O, Baatz JE, Notter RH. Differential activity and lack of synergy of lung surfactant proteins SP-B and SP-C in surface-active interactions with phospholipids. J Lipid Res 1996; 37:1749–1760.

176. Yu SH, Possmayer F. Comparative studies on the biophysical activities of the low-molecular-weight hydrophobic proteins purified from bovine pulmonary surfactant. Biochim Biophys Acta 1988; 961:337–350.

177. Wang Z, Baatz JE, Holm BA, Notter RH. Content-dependent activity of lung surfactant protein B (SP-B) in mixtures with lipids. Am J Physiol 2002; 283:L897–L906.

178. Johansson J, Curstedt T, Robertson B. Synthetic protein analogues in artificial surfactants. Acta Paediatr 1996; 85:642–646.

179. Johansson J, Gustafsson M, Zaltash S, Robertson B, Curstedt T. Synthetic surfactant protein analogs. Biol Neonate 1998; 74(suppl):9–14.

180. Walther FJ, Gordon LM, Zasadzinski JM, Sherman MA, Waring AJ. Surfactant protein B and C analogues. Mol Gen Metab 2000; 71:342–351.

181. Robertson B, Johansson J, Curstedt T. Synthetic surfactants to treat neonatal lung disease. Mol Med Today 2000; 6:119–124.

182. Cochrane CG, Revak SD, Merritt TA, Heldt GP, Hallman M, Cunningham MD, Easa D, Pramanik A, Edwards DK, Alberts MS. The efficacy and safety of KL4-surfactant in preterm infants with respiratory distress syndrome. Am J Respir Crit Care Med 1996; 153:404–410.

183. Cochrane CG, Revak SD. Surfactant lavage treatment in a model of respiratory distress syndrome. Chest 1999; 116(suppl):85S–86S.

184. Wiswell TE, Smith RM, Katz LB, Mastroianni L, Wong DY, Willms D, Heard S, Wilson M, Hite RD, Anzueto A, Revak SD, Cochrane CG. Bronchopulmonary segmental lavage with Surfaxin (KL(4)—surfactant) for acute respiratory distress syndrome. Am J Respir Crit Care Med 1999; 160:1188–1195.

185. Cochrane CG, Revak SD. Pulmonary surfactant protein B (SP-B): structure–function relationships. Science 1991; 254:566–568.

186. Cochrane CG, Revak SD. Protein-phospholipid interactions in pulmonary surfactant. Chest 1994; 105:57S–62S.

187. Merritt TA, Kheiter A, Cochrane CG. Positive end-expiratory pressure during KL4 surfactant instillation enhances intrapulmonary distribution in a simian model of respiratory distress syndrome. Pediatr Res 1995; 38:211–217.

188. Revak S, Merritt T, Cochrane C, Heldt G, Alberts M, Anderson D, Kheiter A. Efficacy of synthetic peptide-containing surfactant in the treatment of respiratory distress syndrome in preterm infant rhesus monkeys. Pediatr Res 1996; 39:715–724.

189. Revak SD, Merritt TA, Hallman M, Heldt G, La Polla RJ, Hoey K, Houghten RA, Cohrane CG. The use of synthetic peptides in the formation of biophysically and biologically active surfactants. Pediatr Res 1991; 29: 460–465.

190. Ma J, Koppennol S, Yu H, Zografti G. Effects of a cationic and hydrophobic peptide KL4 on model lung surfactant lipid monolayers. Biophys J 1998; 74:1899–1907.

191. Walther FJ, Hernandez-Juviel JM, Gordon LM, Sherman MA, Waring AJ. Dimeric surfactant protein B peptide SP-B$_{1-25}$in neonatal and acute respiratory distress syndrome. Exp Lung Res 2002; 28:623–640.

192. Walther FJ, Hernandez-Juviel JM, Mercado PE, Gordon LM, Waring AJ. Surfactant with SP-B and SP-C analogs improves lung function in surfactant deficient rats. Biol Neonate 2002; 82:181–187.

193. Gordon LM, Lee KYC, Lipp MM, Zasadzinski JM, Walther FJ, Sherman MA, Waring AJ. Conformational mapping of the N-terminal segment of surfactant protein B in lipid using ^{13}C-enhanced Fourier transform infrared spectroscopy. J Peptide Res 2000; 55:330–347.

194. Gordon LM, Horvath S, Longo ML, Zasadzinski JAN, Taeusch HW, Faull K, Leung C, Waring AJ. Conformation and molecular topography of the N-terminal segment of surfactant protein B in structure-promoting environments. Protein Sci 1996; 5:1662–1675.

195. Gupta M, Hernandez-Juviel JM, Waring AJ, Bruni R, Walther FJ. Comparison of functional efficacy of surfactant protein B analogues in lavaged rats. Eur Respir J 2000; 16:1129–1133.

196. Gupta M, Hernandez-Juviel JM, Waring AJ, Walther FJ. Function and inhibition sensitivity of the N-terminal segment of surfactant protein B (SP-B$_{1-25}$) in preterm rabbits. Thorax 2001; 56:871–876.

197. Yao L-J, Richardson C, Ford C, Mathialagan N, Mackie G, Hammond GL, Harding PG, Possmayer F. Expression of mature pulmonary surfactant-associated protein B (SP-B) in Escherichia coli using truncated human SP-B cDNAs. Biochem Cell Biol 1990; 68:559–566.

198. Schilling JWJ, White RT, Cordell BI, inventors. Recombinant alveolar surfactant protein. Patent USA 4,659,805. 1987 April 21.

199. Hawgood S, Ogawa A, Yukitake K, Schlueter M, Brown C, White T, Buckley D, Lesikar D, Benson B. Lung function in premature rabbits treated with recombinant human surfactant protein-C. Am J Respir Crit Care Med 1996; 154:484–490.

200. Veldhuizen EJA, Batenburg JJ, Vandenbussche G, Putz G, van Golde LMG, Haagsman HP. Production of surfactant protein C in the baculovirus expression system: the information required for correct folding and palmitoylation

of SP-C is contained within the mature sequence. Biochim Biophys Acta 1999; 1416:295–308.

201. Ikegami M, Jobe AH. Surfactant protein-C in ventilated premature lamb lung. Pediatr Res 1998; 44:860–864.

202. Davis AJ, Jobe AH, Hafner D, Ikegami M. Lung function in premature lambs and rabbits treated with a recombinant SP-C surfactant. Am J Respir Crit Care Med 1998; 157:553–559.

203. Lewis J, McCaig L, Hafner D, Spragg R, Veldhuizen R, Kerr C. Dosing and delivery of a recombinant surfactant in lung-injured sheep. Am J Respir Crit Care Med 1999; 159:741–747.

204. Hafner D, Germann P-G, Hauschke D. Effects of rSP-C surfactant on oxygenation and histology in a rat-lung-lavage model of acute lung injury. Am J Respir Crit Care Med 1998; 158:270–278.

205. Spragg RG, Smith RM, Harris K, Lewis JF, Hafner D, Germann P. Effect of recombinant SP-C surfactant in a porcine lavage model of acute lung injury. J Appl Physiol 1999; 88:674–681.

206. Spragg RG, Lewis JF, Rathgeb F, Hafner D, Seeger W. Intratracheal instillation of rSP-C surfactant improves oxygenation in patients with ARDS [abstr]. Am J Respir Crit Care Med 2002; 165:A22.

207. Ross GF, Notter RH, Meuth J, Whitsett JA. Phospholipid binding and biophysical activity of pulmonary surfactant-associated protein SAP-35 and its non-collagenous C-terminal domains. J Biol Chem 1985; 261:14283–14291.

208. Yu SH, Possmayer F. Adsorption, compression, and stability of surface films of natural, lipid extract, and reconstituted pulmonary surfactants. Biochim Biophys Acta 1993; 1167:264–271.

209. Schurch S, Possmayer F, Cheng S, Cockshutt AM. Pulmonary SP-A enhances adsorption and appears to induce surface sorting of lipid extract surfactant Am J Physiol 1992; 263:L210–L218.

210. Taneva S, McEachren T, Stewart J, Keough KM. Pulmonary surfactant protein SP-A with phospholipids in spread monolayers at the air–water interface. Biochemistry 1995; 34:10279–10289.

211. Hawgood S, Benson BJ, Schilling J, Damm D, Clements JA, White RT. Nucleotide and amino acid sequences of pulmonary surfactant protein SP 18 and evidence for cooperation between SP 18 and SP 28–36 in surfactant lipid adsorption. Proc Natl Acad Sci USA 1987; 84:66–70.

212. Suzuki Y, Fujita Y, Kogishi K. Reconstitution of tubular myelin from synthetic lipids and proteins associated with pig lung surfactant. Am Rev Respir Dis 1989; 140:75–81.

213. Williams MC, Hawgood S, Hamilton RL. Changes in lipid structure produced by surfactant proteins SP-A, SP-B, and SP-C. Am J Respir Cell Mol Biol 1991; 5:41–50.

214. Veldhuizen RAW, Hearn SA, Lewis JF, Possmayer F. Surface-area cycling of different surfactant preparations: SP-A and SP-B are essential for large aggregate integrity. Biochem J 1994; 300:519–524.

215. Venkitaraman A, Hall S, Whitsett J, Notter R. Enhancement of biophysical activity of lung surfactant extracts and phospholipid-apoprotein admixtures by surfactant protein A. Chem Phys Lipids 1990; 56:185–194.

216. Cockshutt AM, Weitz J, Possmayer F. Pulmonary surfactant-associated protein A enhances the surface activity of lipid extract surfactant and reverses inhibition by blood proteins in vitro. Biochemistry 1990; 19:8424–8429.

217. Yukitake K, Brown CL, Schlueter MA, Clements JA, Hawgood S. Surfactant apoprotein A modifies the inhibitory effect of plasma proteins on surfactant activity in vivo. Pediatr Res 1995; 37:21–25.

218. Voss T, Eistetter H, Schafer KP, Engel J. Macromolecular organization of natural and recombinant lung surfactant protein SP28–36. Structural homology with the complement factor C1q. J Mol Biol 1988; 201:219–227.

219. Voss T, Melchers K, Scheirle G, Schafer KP. Structural comparison of recombinant pulmonary surfactant protein SP-A derived from two human coding sequences: implications for the chain composition of natural human SP-A. Am J Respir Cell Mol Biol 1991; 4:88–94.

220. Haas C, Voss T, Engel J. Assembly and disulfide rearrangement of recombinant surfactant protein A in vitro. Eur J Biochem 1991; 197:799–803.

221. Walther FJ, David-Cu R, Leung C, Bruni R, Hernandez-Juviel J, Gordon LM, Waring AJ. A synthetic segment of surfactant protein A—structure, in vitro surface activity, and in vivo efficacy. Pediatr Res 1996; 39:938–946.

222. McLean LR, Lewis JE, Hagaman KA, Owen TJ, Jackson RL. Amphipathic alpha-helical peptides based on surfactant apoprotein SP-A. Biochim Biophys Acta 1993; 1166:31–38.

223. Serrallach EN, de Haas GH, Shipley GG. Structure and thermotropic properties of mixed-chain phosphatidylcholine bilayers. Biochemistry 1984; 23: 713–720.

224. Turcotte JG, Sacco AM, Steim JM, Tabak SA, Notter RH. Chemical synthesis and surface properties of an analog of the pulmonary surfactant dipalmitoyl phosphatidylcholine analog. Biochim Biophys Acta 1977; 488:235–248.

225. Turcotte JG, Lin WH, Pivarnik PE, Sacco AM, Bermel MS, Lu Z, Notter RH. Chemical synthesis and surface activity of lung surfactant phospholipid analogs. II. Racemic N-substituted diether phosphonolipids. Biochim Biophys Acta 1991; 1084:1-12.

226. Liu H, Lu RZ, Turcotte JG, Notter RH. Dynamic interfacial properties of surface-excess films of phospholipids and phosphonolipid analogs. I. Effects of pH. J Colloid Interface Sci 1994; 167:378–390.

227. Liu H, Turcotte JG, Notter RH. Dynamic interfacial properties of surface-excess films of phospholipid and phosphonolipid analogs: II. Effects of chain linkage and headgroup structure. J Colloid Interface Sci 1994; 167:391–400.

228. Wang Z, Schwan AL, Lairson LL, O'Donnell JS, Byrne GF, Foye A, Holm BA, Notter RH. Surface activity of a synthetic lung surfactant containing a phospholipase-resistant phosphonolipid analog of dipalmitoyl phosphatidylcholine. Am J Physiol 2003; 285:L550-L559.

229. Liu H, Turcotte JG, Notter RH. Thermotropic behavior of structurally-related phospholipids and phosphonolipid analogs of lung surfactant glycerophospholipids. Langmuir 1995; 11:101–107.

230. Skita V, Chester DW, Oliver CJ, Turcotte JG, Notter RH. Bilayer characteristics of a diether phosphonolipid analog of the major lung surfactant

glycerophospholipid dipalmitoyl phosphatidylcholine. J Lipid Res 1995; 36:1116–1127.

231. Lin WH, Cramer SG, Turcotte JG, Thrall RS. A diether phosphonolipid surfactant analog, DEPN-8, is resistant to phospholipase-C cleavage. Respiration 1997; 64:96–101.

232. Dizon-Co L, Ikegami M, Ueda T, Jobe AH, Lin WH, Turcotte JG, Notter RH, Rider ED. In vivo function of surfactants containing PC analogs. Am J Respir Crit Care Med 1994; 150:918–923.

233. Rider ED, Ikegami M, Jobe AH. Intrapulmonary catabolism of surfactant saturated phosphatidylcholine in rabbits. J Appl Physiol 1990; 69:1856–1862.

234. Rider ED, Pinkerton KE, Jobe AH. Characterization of rabbit lung lysosomes and their role in surfactant dipalmitoylphosphatidylcholine catabolism. J Biol Chem 1991; 266:22522–22528.

235. Rider ED, Ikegami M, Jobe AH. Localization of alveolar surfactant clearance in rabbit lung cells. Am J Physiol 1992; 263:L201–L209.

236. Artigas A, Bernard GR, Carlet J, Dreyfuss D, Gattinoni L, Hudson L, Lamy M, Marini JJ, Matthay MA, Pinsky MR, Spragg R, Suter PM, and (Consensus Committee). The American–European consensus conference on ARDS, Part 2: Ventilatory, pharmacologic, supportive therapy, study design strategies and issues related to recovery and remodeling. Intensive Care Med 1998; 24:378–398.

237. Temmesfeld-Wollbruck B, Walmrath D, Grimminger F, Seeger W. Prevention and therapy of the adult respiratory distress syndrome. Lung 1995; 173: 139–164.

238. Kollef MH, Schuster DP. The acute respiratory distress syndrome. N Engl J Med 1995; 332:27–37.

239. Karima R, Matsumoto S, Higashi H, Matsushima K. The molecular pathogenesis of endotoxin shock and organ failure. Mol Med Today 1999; 5:123–132.

240. Hudson LD. New therapies for ARDS. Chest 1995; 108(suppl):79S–91S.

241. Fulkerson WJ, Macintyre N, Stamler J, Crapo JD. Pathogenesis and treatment of the adult respiratory distress syndrome. Arch Intern Med 1996; 156:29–38.

242. Paulson T, Spear R, Peterson B. New concepts in the treatment of children with acute respiratory failure. J Pediatr 1995; 127:163–175.

243. Ring J, Stidham G. Novel therapies for acute respiratory failure. Pediatr Clin North Am 1994; 41:1325–1363.

244. Sessler C, Bloomfield G, Fowler A. Current concepts of sepsis and acute lung injury. Clin Chest Med 1996; 17:213–235.

245. Weikert LF, Bernard GR. Pharmacology of sepsis. Clin Chest Med 1996; 17:289–305.

246. Berthiaume Y, Lesur O, Dagenais A. Treatment of adult respiratory distress syndrome: Plea for rescue therapy of the alveolar epithelium. Thorax 1999; 54:150–160.

247. Ware LB, Matthay MA. The acute respiratory distress syndrome. N Engl J Med 2000; 342:1334–1348.

248. Thompson BT. Glucocorticoids and acute lung injury. Crit Care Med 2003; 31(suppl):S253–S257.

249. Steinbrook R. How best to ventilate? Trial design and patient safety in studies of the acute respiratory distress syndrome. N Engl J Med 2003; 348: 1393–1401.

250. Sokol J, Jacobs SE, Bohn D. Inhaled nitric oxide for acute hypoxemic respiratory failure in children and adults (update of Cochrane Database Syst Rev 2000; (4):CD002787; PMID: 11034763). Cochrane Database Syst Rev 2003; (1):CD002787..

251. Laterre PF, Wittebole X, Dhainaut JF. Anticoagulant therapy in acute lung injury. Crit Care Med 2003; 31(suppl):S329–S336.

252. Kaisers U, Busch T, Deja M, Donaubauer B, Falke KJ. Selective pulmonary vasodilation in acute respiratory distress syndrome. Crit Care Med 2003; 31(suppl):S337–S342.

253. Derdak S. High-frequency oscillatory ventilation for acute respiratory distress syndrome in adult patients. Crit Care Med 2003; 31(suppl):S317–S323.

254. Marraro G. Innovative practices of ventilatory support with pediatric patients. Pediatr Crit Care Med 2003; 4:8–20.

255. Sime PJ, O'Reilly KMA. Fibrosis of the lung and other tissues: new concepts in pathogenesis and treatment. Clinical Immunology 2001; 99:308–319.

256. Selman M, King TEJ, Pardo A. Idiopathic pulmonary fibrosis: prevailing and evolving hypotheses about its pathogenesis and implications for therapy. Ann Intern Med 2001; 134:136–151.

257. American Thoracic Society, European Respiratory Society, and American College of Chest Physicians. Idiopathic pulmonary fibrosis: diagnosis and treatment. International consensus statement. Am J Respir Crit Care Med 2000; 161:646–664..

258. Young JD, Brampton WJ, Knighton JD, Finfer SR. Inhaled nitric oxide in acute respiratory failure in adults. Br J Anaesth 1994; 73:499–502.

259. Rossaint R, Gerlach H, Schmidt-Ruhnke H, Pappert D, Lewandowski K, Steudel W, Falke K. Efficacy of inhaled nitric oxide in ARDS. Chest 1995; 107:1107–1115.

260. Fierobe L, Brunet F, Dhainaut J-F, Monchi M, Belghith M, Mira J-P, Dallava-Santucci J, Dinh-Xuan A. Effect of inhaled nitric oxide on right ventricular function in adult respiratory distress syndrome. Am J Respir Crit Care Med 1995; 151:1414–1419.

261. Demirakca S, Dotsch J, Knotche C, Magsaam J, Reiter HL, Bauer J, Kuehl PG. Inhaled nitric oxide in neonatal and pediatric acute respiratory distress syndrome: dose response, prolonged inhalation, and weaning. Crit Care Med 1996; 24:1913–1919.

262. Goldman AP, Tasker RC, Hosiasson S, Henrichsen T, Macrae DJ. Early response to inhaled nitric oxide and its relationship to outcome in children with severe hypoxemic respiratory failure. Chest 1997; 112:752–758.

263. Nakagawa TA, Morris A, Gomez RJ, Johnston SJ, Sharkey PT, Zaritsky AL. Dose response to inhaled nitric oxide in pediatric patients with pulmonary hypertension and acute respiratory distress syndrome. J Pediatr 1997; 131:63–69.

264. Dellinger RP, Zimmerman JL, Hyers TM, Taylor RW, Straube RC, Hauser DL, Samask MC, Davis K, Criner GJ, Davis K, Hyers TM, Papadokos P. Inhaled nitric oxide in ARDS: preliminary results of a multicenter clinical trial. Crit Care Med 1996; 24:A29.

265. Dellinger RP, Zimmerman JL, Taylor RW, Straube RC, Hauser DL, Criner GJ, Davis K, Hyers TM, Papadakos P, and (and INO in ARDS Study Group). Effects of inhaled nitric oxide in patients with acute respiratory distress syndrome: results of a randomized phase II trial. Crit Care Med 1998; 26:15–23.

266. Troncy E, Collet JP, Shapiro S, Guimond J-G, Blair L, Ducruet T, Francceur M, Charbonneau M, Blaise G. Inhaled nitric oxide in acute respiratory distress syndrome. A pilot randomized controlled study. Am J Respir Crit Care Med 1998; 157:1483–1488.

267. Karamanoukian HL, Glick PL, Wilcox DL, Rossman JE, Morin FC, Holm BA. Pathophysiology of congenital diaphragmatic hernia VII: inhaled nitric oxide requires exogenous surfactant therapy in the lamb model of CDH. J Pediatr Surg 1995; 30:1–4.

268. Zhu GF, Sun B, Niu S, Cai YY, Lin K, Lindwall R, Robertson B. Combined surfactant therapy and inhaled nitric oxide in rabbits with oleic acid-induced acute respiratory distress syndrome. Am J Respir Crit Care Med 1998; 158:437–443.

269. Gommers D, Hartog A, van't Veen A, Lachmann B. Improved oxygenation by nitric oxide is enhanced by prior lung reaeration with surfactant, rather than positive end-expiratory pressure, in lung-lavaged rabbits. Crit Care Med 1997; 25:1868–1873.

270. Hartog A, Gommers D, van't Veen A, Erdmann W, Lachmann B. Exogenous surfactant and nitric oxide have a synergistic effect in improving gas exchange in experimental ARDS. Adv Exp Med Biol 1997; 428:277–279.

271. Rais-Bahrami K, Rivera O, Seale W, Short B. Effect of nitric oxide in meconium aspiration syndrome after treatment with surfactant. Crit Care Med 1997; 25:1744–1747.

272. Hallman M, Waffarn F, Bry K, Turbow R, Kleinman MT, Mautz WJ, Rasmussen RE, Bhalla DK, Phalen RF. Surfactant dysfunction after inhalation of nitric oxide. J Appl Physiol 1996; 80:2026–2034.

273. Matalon S, DeMarco V, Haddad IY, Myles C, Skimming JW, Schurch S, Cheng S, Cassin S. Inhaled nitric oxide injures the pulmonary surfactant system of lambs in vivo. Am J Physiol 1996; 270:L273-L280.

274. Hallman M, Bry K, Lappalainen U. A mechanism of nitric oxide-induced surfactant dysfunction. J Appl Physiol 1996; 80:2035–2043.

275. Uy IP, Pryhuber GS, Chess PR, Notter RH. Combined-modality therapy with inhaled nitric oxide and exogenous surfactant in term Infants with acute respiratory failure. Pediatr Crit Care Med 2000; 1:107–110.

16

Antioxidant Therapy for Lung Injury

TIINA M. ASIKAINEN and CARL W. WHITE

Hospital for Children and Adolescents, University of Helsinki, Helsinki, Finland, and National Jewish Medical and Research Center, Denver, Colorado, U.S.A.

I. Overview

This chapter discusses therapeutic approaches to mitigate or prevent oxidant-generated pathology in lung injury. Throughout life, lung cells encounter several-fold higher oxygen concentrations than present in utero, and are thus exposed to relative oxidative stress. Furthermore, a number of lung diseases in newborns and older individuals necessitate the administration of higher than atmospheric concentrations of oxygen. Reactive oxygen and nitrogen species have been implicated in the pathogenesis of various forms of lung injury as detailed in earlier chapters (e.g., Chapter 7). In the normal lungs, the activity of reactive oxygen species (ROS) is antagonized by intracellular and extracellular antioxidant substances. The elaborate endogenous antioxidant system includes classical antioxidant enzymes (AOEs), glutathione, and thioredoxin with their associated redox cycles, heme oxygenases, and numerous small molecular weight antioxidants. This chapter considers therapeutic agents that can supplement or substitute for endogenous antioxidants if they are depleted or overwhelmed during lung injury. An ideal antioxidant therapeutic agent, either natural or synthetic, should have good bioavailability, and it should be potent in penetrating to site of action and efficient in scavenging appropriate radical species. The agent should be stable, nontoxic, nonimmunogenic, and preferably inexpensive. Importantly, it should allow essential developmental and healing processes to proceed. A wide variety of antioxidant agents, including classical AOEs, catalytic antioxidants and antibodies, thiol-based antioxidants, vitamins, lazaroids, and novel antioxidant approaches have been investigated in experimental models in vitro and in vivo in an attempt to prevent or ameliorate lung injury. Although research indicates favorable responses to several antioxidant compounds, the usefulness of these agents in the treatment of human lung injury and respiratory disease has yet to be fully explored.

II. Introduction
A. Reactive Oxygen Species

Oxidative stress in tissues is mediated through ROS (e.g., superoxide anion, hydroxyl radical, hydrogen peroxide), which are generated endogenously by several mechanisms under both physiological and pathological conditions (Table 1). The major source of ROS in the lung is the mitochondrial

Table 1 Sources of ROS in the Lung

Endogenous	Source[a]
Localization	
Mitochondrion	Electron transport chain (NADH dehydrogenase, ubiquinone Q-cytochrome b)
Cytosol	XOR
	Transition metals (Fe^{2+}, Cu^{1+})
	"Auto-oxidation" of small molecules
	Riboflavin
Plasma membrane	NADPH oxidase (phagocytic cells[b])
	Cyclo-oxygenase and lipoxygenase (arachidonic acid metabolism)
Endoplasmic reticulum and nuclear membrane	Cytochromes P-450 and b5
Intracellular granules	Myeloperoxidase (neutrophils)
Peroxisomes	Various oxidases (urate oxidase, fatty acyl-CoA oxidase)
Exogenous	
Hyperoxia	
Ozone	
Cigarette smoke	
Fibrogenic material	
Radiation	
Cytotoxic drugs	

[a]NADH, nicotinamide adenine dinucleotide; NADPH, nicotinamide adenine dinucleotide phosphate; XOR, xanthine oxidoreductase.
[b]Possibly also in some nonphagocytic cells (7).
(From Refs. 5 and 6.)

respiratory chain, in which the four-step reduction of molecular oxygen to water is coupled to the vital production of cellular adenosine triphosphate (ATP), i.e., oxidative phosphorylation. Under physiological conditions not more than approximately 1–2% of the oxygen entering the respiratory chain accidentally leaks out as superoxide (1). Under hyperoxic conditions, however, the pulmonary mitochondrial production of superoxide is enhanced in linear relation to oxygen tension (2). At an inhaled oxygen concentration of approximately 60%, the slope of this relationship is increased such that even greater quantities of ROS are formed. The reactivity of superoxide is relatively low, but it is capable of producing more harmful reactants by dismutation into hydrogen peroxide, either spontaneously or several times faster enzymatically through superoxide dismutases (SOD). Superoxide reacts also with nitric oxide to form the very reactive peroxynitrite. Hydrogen peroxide gives rise to the extremely reactive and potentially harmful hydroxyl radical by reacting with transition metals, such as iron or copper in the Fenton reaction, or with superoxide in the metal-catalyzed Haber–Weiss reaction (3). Most reactive oxygen and nitrogen species and their metabolites are capable of initiating harmful chain reactions, causing damage to proteins, lipids, and DNA, i.e., to virtually all components of the cell. However, in light of recent evidence, it appears that cell death following exposure to hyperoxia can also occur without mitochondrial production of ROS (4). Details of the production, chemistry, and biological effects of reactive oxygen and nitrogen species are discussed in Chapter 7.

B. Endogenous Antioxidant Defense Mechanisms

In healthy organisms, protection against the deleterious effects of reactive oxygen and nitrogen species (ROS and RNS, respectively) is achieved by maintaining a delicate balance between oxidants and antioxidants. Therefore, the continuous production of ROS in aerobic organisms has to be met with a similar rate of their consumption by antioxidants. Oxidative stress is defined as an imbalance of the prooxidant/antioxidant equilibrium in favor of the prooxidants. Antioxidants, either enzymatic or nonenzymatic, are substances that prevent the formation of ROS, scavenge them, or repair the damage they cause (8). The most important endogenous antioxidants are listed in Table 2.

Pulmonary Antioxidant Defenses During Ontogenesis

The maturation of the pulmonary surfactant system during the final one-third of term gestation is paralleled by increased expression of AOEs in various mammals (15–18). The late gestational increase in AOE activities has been considered to occur in preparation for birth into an oxygen-rich environment. These findings implicate that preterm neonates may be deficient in antioxidant defenses, and may therefore be exceptionally vulnerable to

Table 2 The Endogenous Antioxidant Defense System

	Location[a]	Function[b]
Enzymatic[c]		
MnSOD	M	Scavenges superoxide
CuZnSOD	C, M	Scavenges superoxide
ECSOD	E	Scavenges superoxide
Catalase	P	Scavenges hydrogen peroxide
GPx	C, E, M, Pl	Scavenges hydrogen peroxide and other peroxides
GR	C	Reduces GSSG back to GSH
γ-GCL	C	Rate-limiting enzyme in GSH synthesis
TrxPx	C, M, P	Scavenges hydrogen peroxide and other peroxides
TrxR	C, M	Reduces Trx-S_2 back to Trx-$(SH)_2$
Heme oxygenase	C	Degrades heme to bilirubin
Nonenzymatic[d]		
GSH	C, E, M, N	Cosubstrate for GPx, direct radical scavenger, conjugation reactions, maintenance of thiol status of proteins, cysteine storage, etc.
Trx	C, M, N	Cosubstrate for TrxPx and ribonucleotide reductase
α-Tocopherol (vitamin E)	BL	Prevents lipid peroxidation
Ascorbate (vitamin C)	C, Pl	Reduces tocopherol radical back to α-tocopherol, direct radical scavenger
Urate, bilirubin, ubiquinol, etc.	Pl	Direct radical scavenger
Metal chelating proteins (transferrin, ferritin, lactoferrin, metallothionein, ceruloplasmin, albumin)	C, Pl	Binding and storage of transition metals and toxic heavy metals

[a]BL, biological lipid phases; C, cytosolic; E, extracellular; M, mitochondrial; N, nuclear; P, peroxisomal; Pl, plasma.

[b]GSSG, oxidized form of glutathione; Trx-S_2, oxidized form of thioredoxin; Trx-$(SH)_2$, reduced form of thioredoxin.

[c]CuZnSOD, copper–zinc superoxide dismutase; ECSOD, extracellular SOD; γ-GCL, gamma glutamate–cysteine ligase (previously called gamma glutamylcysteine synthetase, γ-GCS); GPx, glutathione peroxidase; GR, glutathione reductase; MnSOD, manganese SOD; TrxPx, thioredoxin peroxidase (peroxiredoxin); TrxR, thioredoxin reductase.

[d]GSH, reduced glutathione, Trx, thioredoxin.

(From Refs. 3 and 9–14.)

oxygen-induced lung injury, unless capable of rapidly mounting an antioxidative response when exposed to hyperoxia. Indeed, preterm baboons and rabbits are unable to increase the activities of some AOEs when challenged with hyperoxia, and are consequently more susceptible to oxygen-induced injury (19,20). However, the regulation of pulmonary AOEs in hyperoxia is complex, and differs between animal species and also among different age groups within the same species (21–24). It should be noted that, although there is substantial experimental evidence to link the induction of AOEs, especially that of MnSOD, to development of tolerance to hyperoxia, contradictory results have also been obtained (25,26). Recent studies implicate increased expression of proteins involved in glycolysis and glucose transport (27) and of surfactant proteins (28) in the development of oxygen tolerance.

Results from human studies have shown that catalase is the only pulmonary AOE to increase in activity during ontogenesis and suggest that preterm human neonates are not deficient in some classical pulmonary AOEs as compared with term neonates or adults (29–31). However, preterm human neonates appear not to be able to increase levels of SOD when challenged with hyperoxia (32,33). Furthermore, concentrations of GSH in plasma and bronchoalveolar lavage fluid (BALF) in preterm human infants have been found to be lower than in term infants (34). While the GSH synthetic capacity in several tissues of preterm human neonates appears similar to that of term neonates (35), GSH synthesis in these infants may be impaired due to lack of substrate (36).

III. Rationale for Antioxidant Therapy: Role of Oxidative Stress in Lung Diseases

The rationale for antioxidant therapy is based on the knowledge that increased generation of reactive oxidants plays a significant role in the pathogenesis of a wide variety of lung diseases. In order to fully appreciate the rationale, it is crucial to understand the mechanisms of oxidative lung injury in neonates as well as in older individuals. Mechanisms and mediators contributing to the pathophysiology of acute and chronic lung injury and inflammation have been covered in detail earlier in this book (e.g., Chapters 3–6). The roles of oxidative stress in selected pulmonary diseases in neonates and adults are described below.

A. Oxidative Stress in Respiratory Distress Syndrome and Bronchopulmonary Dysplasia

The human lung is structurally prepared to breathe when the blood–gas barrier has been formed and surfactant synthesis begins. This occurs in the canalicular period, usually after 24 gestational weeks (see Chapter 2 for overview on lung development). Upon transition from placental to pulmonary respiration at birth, lung cells are exposed to approximately sevenfold higher oxygen concentration than in utero. Thus, the newborn lung is exposed to relative oxidative stress. Furthermore, very preterm infants are at risk of developing respiratory distress syndrome (RDS, also called hyaline membrane disease) due to surfactant deficiency, which is characterized by decreased lung volumes and impaired gas exchange resulting in hypoxemia. To provide adequate oxygenation, high inhaled oxygen concentrations are commonly necessary in the treatment of RDS. This oxygen treatment is lifesaving, but also carries associated risks. Hyperoxia, along with volumetric stress or barotrauma from mechanical ventilation, can cause both acute and chronic lung injury in neonates. Acute hyperoxic lung injury increases edema and inflammation in premature infants with RDS, causing more severe acute respiratory failure. In addition, exposure to hyperoxia is a major risk factor for the development of chronic lung injury and bronchopulmonary dysplasia (BPD), also known as chronic lung disease (CLD) of infancy (37).

BPD was initially described as oxygen dependency for over 28 days and persistent increased densities on chest radiographs (38). However, because of improvements in neonatal intensive care, extremely preterm infants survive today, and oxygen dependency for more than 28 days has been found not to be a good criterion for BPD in these babies. Therefore, the definition of BPD has been modified and now includes infants with oxygen dependency at the postmenstrual age of 36 weeks (39). According to the most recent proposal, the severity of BPD is also categorized at the time point of assessment. The incidence of BPD is approximately 30% in infants with birth weights less than 1000 g (37).

The role of oxygen toxicity in the pathogenesis of BPD has been extensively investigated. Studies clearly demonstrate that the histological findings in experimental pulmonary oxygen toxicity are strikingly similar to those seen in BPD (40–43). Typical histopathological findings include endothelial and epithelial cell damage, bronchial smooth muscle hypertrophy, interstitial fibrosis, and simplification of the acinar structure with reduction in total number and surface area of alveoli. The involvement of ROS in the pathogenesis of BPD is further supported by indirect evidence from several human studies (44,45). For example, the amount of lipid peroxidation products is increased in the exhaled gas from very low birth weight premature infants, and the increase directly correlates with a poor outcome (46). Furthermore, protein oxidation products in tracheal aspirates (47) as well as nitrotyrosine levels in plasma samples (48) are elevated, and total glutathione concentrations in BALF are reduced in infants destined to develop BPD (49). Plasma cysteine concentrations and GSH/GSSG ratio are lower in preterm infants receiving oxygen therapy for respiratory distress as compared with neonatal or adult controls (50,51).

B. Oxidative Stress in Persistent Pulmonary Hypertension of the Newborn and Meconium Aspiration Syndrome

Several diseases of term neonates also necessitate treatment with high inhaled oxygen concentrations and resultant oxidative stress. One example is persistent pulmonary hypertension of the newborn (PPHN), which is characterized by high pulmonary vascular resistance leading to severe hypoxemia (52). Another example is the meconium aspiration syndrome (MAS), which usually affects asphyxiated term neonates and leads to a severe respiratory failure. The pathogenetic factors of MAS include direct toxic effects of meconium and the consequent massive inflammatory response (53).

C. Oxidative Stress in the Acute Respiratory Distress Syndrome

Acute respiratory distress syndrome (ARDS), which occurs in both adult and pediatric patients, is associated with a wide variety of precipitating factors such as shock, aspiration, and severe infection (Chapter 3). Also, ARDS, which can have a mortality rate as high as 40–50%, is characterized by neutrophil accumulation, diffuse pulmonary infiltrates, and edema. Increased ROS production, primarily a consequence of inflammatory cell activation and secondarily of oxygen therapy, has been implicated in the pathogenesis ARDS (54). Levels of plasma and alveolar lining fluid antioxidants, such as total glutathione, selenium, α-tocopherol, ascorbate, and β-carotene, have been found to be decreased, and pulmonary nitrotyrosine and plasma malondialdehyde levels to be increased, in patients with ARDS (55–57).

D. Oxidative Stress in Inflammatory and Chronic Obstructive Airway Diseases

Inflammatory cell sequestration and activation with resulting increased production of ROS is a central feature in a number of inflammatory airway diseases. One important example is asthma, which is characterized by reversible airflow obstruction, bronchial hyperresponsiveness, and chronic eosinophilic inflammatory reaction. Airway epithelial cells have been identified as an important source of various cytokines leading to amplification of the inflammatory process with subsequent increased ROS production (58). A pivotal role of ROS in the pathophysiology of asthma is further supported by findings that superoxide generation from bronchoalveolar lavage cells (59) and from blood monocytes (60) is higher in patients with asthma as compared with nonasthmatic patients. Furthermore, reduced SOD activity in bronchoalveolar lavage cells and bronchial epithelial cells of patients with asthma (61,62) perpetuates the increased oxidative stress in asthmatic lung. Interestingly, inhaled corticosteroids, which alleviate the inflammatory reaction, have been found to result in normalization of bronchial epithelial CuZnSOD specific activity (61). A recent study reveals that loss of SOD activity occurs within minutes of an acute asthmatic response to segmental antigen instillation into the lungs of individuals with atopic asthma (63). Another study using gene manipulated mice demonstrated that mice with elevated levels of pulmonary CuZnSOD were resistant to allergen-induced increases in cholinergic reactivity and released less acetylcholine as compared with wild-type controls (64). Levels of extracellular GPx and total glutathione, which represent the first line of antioxidant defense on the airway epithelial surface, are higher in asthmatic airways compared with controls (65,66) suggesting a possible compensatory mechanism.

Oxidative stress from ROS generated by inflammatory cells is also thought to play a central role in the pathogenesis of chronic obstructive pulmonary disease (COPD) (67–69). COPD is characterized by a predominantly neutrophilic inflammation of the airways, and irreversible parenchymal destruction (emphysema) leading to airway obstruction through dynamic collapse and/or compression (67). The inflammatory cell-mediated oxidative stress in the lungs of COPD patients is typically potentiated by cigarette smoke, which is considered to be an important pathogenetic factor of COPD. One puff of cigarette smoke contains approximately 10^{15} radicals (70). Other pathogenic factors of COPD include other inhaled pollutants and protease–antiprotease interactions. Lung epithelial lining fluid GSH has been found to decrease during acute smoking, and to be increased in chronic smokers. The latter finding possibly reflects upregulation of genes involved in GSH synthesis (71). Both increased/unchanged (72) and decreased (73) levels of CuZnSOD and GPx activities have been detected in alveolar macrophages of long-term smokers. In the lungs of cigarette smoke exposed rats, MnSOD expression is increased in bronchial epithelial cells, which normally express low levels of MnSOD (74). Plasma antioxidant capacity is reduced, with increased levels of lipid peroxidation products, in chronic smokers as compared with nonsmokers. Similar changes also have been identified during acute exacerbations of COPD (75).

E. Oxidative Stress in Interstitial Lung Diseases

ROS have also been implicated in the pathogenesis of a wide variety of interstitial lung diseases. For example, alveolar macrophages from patients with fibrotic pulmonary disease generate high levels of superoxide (76). The MnSOD expression has been found to be elevated in granulomas of pulmonary sarcoidosis and allergic alveolitis (77). Furthermore, coordinated increased expression of MnSOD and catalase has been detected in the lungs of patients with chronic interstitial pneumonias and granulomatous lung diseases (78). Inhaled fibrogenic minerals, especially asbestos fibers, generate ROS by direct mechanisms as indicated by oxidation of proteins and DNA, and these effects are further potentiated by the inflammatory reaction caused by the fibers (79). Asbestos inhalation results in increased activities of total SOD, catalase, and GPx in rat lungs (80).

F. Oxidative Stress in Drug-Related Lung Injury

Certain drugs are known to cause a variety of pulmonary reactions ranging from infiltrations and diffuse pneumonia to fibrotic lesions. Such drugs include, for example, antibacterial antibiotics such as nitrofurantoin, and antineoplastic antibiotics (anticancer drugs), such as antimetabolites (methotrexate), alkylating agents (nitrosoureas, e.g., 1,3-bis[2-chloroethyl]-1-nitrosourea, BCNU), and bleomycin. Oxidative stress is involved in the pathogenic activity of many of these substances. Bleomycin-induced pulmonary toxicity, for example, is mediated by redox-cycling oxidation reactions, and is typically potentiated by hyperoxia, radiation, and the presence of iron. Bleomycin appears to be internalized by a receptor-mediated endocytosis mechanism into the cell, where it exerts cytotoxic activity due to DNA strand break generation and lipid peroxidation (81). Moreover, activity of the bleomycin inactivating enzyme, bleomycin hydrolase, is low in the lung, which may add to the pulmonary toxicity of the drug (82).

Environmental toxicants such as insecticides and herbicides can also generate oxidative stress and associated lung disease. Paraquat (1,1'-dimethyl-4,4'-bipyridylium dichloride), a popular herbicide in the past, is known to cause severe lung injury leading to fibrosis. Although paraquat-induced lung damage in humans has been largely overcome by replacement of paraquat with modern herbicides, each year there are a number of cases of lung injury due to intentional swallowing of this substance. Paraquat is also frequently used as a model of lung injury in experimental settings. Toxic effects of paraquat are manifested as swelling and injury to alveolar epithelial cells and Clara cells, which also appear to accumulate the drug by a specific diamine transport process. Paraquat undergoes an NADPH-dependent reduction to form paraquat radical, which, in turn, reacts with molecular oxygen to form superoxide (83).

G. Oxidative Stress in Lung Transplantation

Reperfusion of ischemic tissue (reoxygenation) is an important mechanism of cell injury in lung transplantation. Ischemia–reperfusion results in increased ROS generation through the oxidation of hypoxanthine to xanthine and on to uric acid by the oxidized form of xanthine oxidoreductase (XOR) and/or through neutrophil accumulation in ischemic and reperfused tissue (84). Inhibition of XOR by allopurinol attenuates ischemia–reperfusion related lung injury in experimental models (85). Although endothelial XOR is considered important in mediating ischemia–reperfusion injury in animal models, its role in human lung transplantation remains uncertain because of the very low/undetectable expression of XOR in human lung tissue (86). Furthermore, XOR activity does not appear to be released to the blood stream during human heart–lung transplantation (87). However, pulmonary capillary endothelium may be injured through release of XOR from liver during ischemia (88). Other ROS-producing mechanisms, such as the mitochondrial respiratory chain, also may play a role in ischemia–reperfusion related injury in lung cells (89). The role of inflammatory cells in acute lung injury is discussed in detail earlier in this book (e.g., Chapter 3).

IV. Antioxidant Therapy for Lung Injury

Given the importance of ROS in the pathogenesis of various forms of lung disease, several antioxidants and means of delivery have been studied in order to prevent or ameliorate the severity of pulmonary injury. Potential antioxidant agents include a wide variety of compounds, both natural and synthetic. The most important characteristics of an ideal antioxidant therapeutic agent are listed in Table 3.

A. Antioxidant Enzymes

Considerable effort has been directed toward administration of AOEs in order to prevent or ameliorate oxygen-induced lung injury. The problems encountered in parenteral administration of AOEs include the short plasma half-lives [6–10 min for CuZnSOD, 5–6 hr for MnSOD (90)] and poor penetrance into cells. To improve stability and cell penetration, pharmacological manipulations including liposome encapsulation and polyethylene glycol (PEG) conjugation have been explored. This has proven beneficial in vitro, since lung-derived cells and endothelial cells treated with catalase and

Table 3 Characteristics of an Ideal Antioxidant Therapeutic Agent

---

Good bioavailability
Reaches desired site of action
Potent scavenging of appropriate radical species
Stability
Nontoxic, wide therapeutic window
Nonimmunogenic
Allows important developmental and healing processes to proceed
Inexpensive

CuZnSOD show increases in intracellular AOE activities and are resistant to ROS-mediated injury (91,92). Addition of surfactant protein A to the liposome-encapsulated AOEs further enhances their uptake by type-II alveolar epithelial cells (93).

Several in vivo experiments have also been conducted with varying results. Intravenous or intraperitoneal administration of liposome-encapsulated or PEG-conjugated CuZnSOD and catalase provides protection against oxygen toxicity in rats and rabbits (94–97). Gene and protein engineering of SOD to facilitate targeting of SOD to critical cellular and tissue components also has been investigated in experimental models (98). For example, human CuZnSOD carrying a C-terminal heparin-binding domain binds to heparin-like proteoglycans on the vascular endothelial cell surface, and may thereby protect this sensitive cell type against ROS-induced injury. Intratracheal administration of AOEs, such as MnSOD, CuZnSOD, and catalase has been evaluated in ROS-mediated injury, with promising results in various animal species (99–104). For example, aerosolized MnSOD (3 mg/kg/day) decreases lung edema, increases levels of lung phospholipids and phosphatidylcholine, improves pulmonary hemodynamics, and preserves arterial oxygenation during hyperoxia in adult baboons exposed to 100% oxygen for 96 hr (103). Furthermore, in the same model, a protective effect was seen at the level of alveolar epithelial surface by preservation of type-I alveolar epithelium and integrity of the epithelial cell surface (104). No effect was found with respect to fibroblast hypertrophy, interstitial thickening, or inflammatory cell recruitment to the lung (104). It is noteworthy that intratracheally administered, cationic rhMnSOD was found extracellularly, primarily along the airway and alveolar epithelial surfaces. Therefore, it is possible that it exerts its protective effect by scavenging ROS generated by activated inflammatory cells.

Treatment of human preterm babies with intratracheal recombinant CuZnSOD (2.5 mg/kg or 5 mg/kg rhCuZnSOD every 48 hr, up to seven doses, in a placebo-controlled and randomized study) increases activity of this enzyme in intratracheal fluid, serum, and urine and reduces markers of acute lung injury (neutrophil chemotactic activity, albumin concentration) in tracheal aspirate (105), but, according to preliminary results, does not affect the primary outcomes of death or BPD at the mean age of 28 months corrected age (105). However, administration of CuZnSOD was associated with less severe intraventricular hemorrhage and periventricular leukomalacia.

The ability of lecithinized SOD (phosphatidylcholine, PC-SOD) to ameliorate bleomycin-induced lung injury has been studied in mice with promising results. The PC-SOD at a low dose (1 mg/kg/day) suppressed levels of total cell number and of inflammatory cells and reduced expression of interleukin-1β and of platelet-derived growth factor in BALF of bleomycin-exposed mice (106). Moreover, the degree of lung fibrosis detected by histopathologic examination was less dramatic in PC-SOD treated mice as compared with nontreated mice. Intratracheal, PEG-conjugated catalase has also been shown to attenuate the severity of lung injury in rats chronically exposed to crocidolite asbestos, as estimated by reduced levels of lactic dehydrogenase, protein, and of total and inflammatory cell numbers in BALF, and by decreases in the extent of fibrotic lesions and in the amount of hydroxyproline in the lung (107).

B. Catalytic Antioxidants

To overcome some of the limitations of natural AOEs (limited cell penetration due to large size, short plasma half-life, antigenicity, expense), a number of low molecular weight antioxidants have been developed. Factors such as type of metal center, redox potential, and electrostatic charge act as determinants of the antioxidant potency of these compounds, and the antioxidant activity of some of the new agents exceeds that of the native SOD enzyme (108,109). The three main classes of metal-containing SOD-mimetics include salen, macrocyclic or macrolide, and metalloporphyrin groups. Of these, the metalloporphyrins [tetrakis-(4-benzoic acid) porphyrin (MnTBAP), tetrakis-(N-methyl-2-pyridyl) porphyrin (MnTM-2-PyP), tetrakis-(N-methyl-4-pyridyl) porphyrin (MnTM-4-PyP), β-octabromo-tetrakis-(N-methyl-4-pyridyl) porphyrin (OBTM-4-PyP)] have been studied most extensively in the prevention of ROS-induced injury. The SOD activity of the metalloporphyrins is based on alternate reduction and oxidation of the manganese center [valence changes between Mn(III) and Mn(II)] as occurs in the native MnSOD enzyme. In addition to scavenging superoxide, some of the metalloporphyrins also can scavenge hydrogen peroxide, peroxynitrite, and/or lipid peroxyl radicals (108).

The essential role of MnSOD has been demonstrated with a knockout mouse model (110,111). The phenotype of the homozygous mutant (*Sod2−/−*) is lethal within the first few weeks of life, and the mice die with metabolic acidosis, anemia, and severe cardiac and hepatic complications. Decreased activities of respiratory chain enzymes NADH dehydrogenase and succinate dehydrogenase, as well as the citric acid cycle enzyme aconitase, in several organs, notably including the heart, of *Sod2−/−* mice indicate mitochondrial injury (110,112), and suggest that one important role of MnSOD is to protect the iron-containing enzymes of the citric acid cycle from direct inactivation by superoxide. The survival of *Sod2−/−* mice under physiological conditions has been prolonged with MnTBAP-treatment (113). The MnTBAP has also been shown to protect endothelial cells against paraquat-induced injury (paraquat increases intracellular superoxide levels by redox cycling with cellular diaphorases) (114). Furthermore, inhaled MnTBAP (5 mM) protects mice from paraquat-induced lung injury as assessed by decreases in lactate dehydrogenase protein levels and in the percentage of polymorphonuclear leukocytes in BALF (115). Also, MnTBAP, as well as MnSOD, and CuZnSOD in combination with catalase have been reported to mitigate the inhibitory effect of 50% oxygen on lung branching morphogenesis in mouse lung explants (116). Intraperitoneal MnTBAP (5 mg/kg) also has been found to attenuate bleomycin-induced lung injury in mice, as estimated by reduction in lung hydroxyproline content, attenuation of airway dysfunction, and reduction in the severity of the lung fibrotic response in bleomycin-exposed mice (117). It was recently shown that sickle cell disease-associated episodes of intrahepatic hypoxia-reoxygenation induce the release of XO from the liver into the circulation leading to impaired vascular function through oxidant reactions between XO-produced superoxide and nitric oxide. Further, treatment of aortic vessels with MnTM-2-PyP restored the nitric oxide-dependent vascular function in an experimental sickle cell disease model (118).

An increasing body of evidence indicates that antioxidant therapies may have potential efficacy in inhibiting, or possibly reversing, emphysema due to cigarette smoke exposure or other causes. Recent findings indicate that disruption of vascular endothelial growth factor (VEGF) signaling, either by targeted disruption of VEGF gene expression in mice using a Cre/Lox system (119) or using a specific antagonist of the VEGF receptor, SU5416 (120), can cause emphysema-like changes in rodent lungs. In the latter model, various markers of oxidative stress, such as oxidized proteins, were found, and the macrocyclic MnSOD mimetic agent M40419 (Metaphore) was found to protect against the development of emphysematous changes detected by morphometry, such as increased mean alveolar diameter and mean linear intercept (120). Of great interest, an MnSOD mimetic agent, which is chemically quite different (AEOL 10150, a metalloporphyrin; Incara), also has been found to be effective in preventing the early changes of COPD in a rodent model in which adult animals were exposed to cigarette smoke for approximately 3 months. Airway inflammation and squamous cell metaplasia, macrophage inflammatory protein 2 (MIP-2) in BALF, and intercellular adhesion molecule 1 (ICAM-1) in lung tissue, each earlier markers of smoke-induced lung injury, were substantially decreased by the MnSOD mimetic (121). These findings provide interesting and potentially important information about the role of trophic VEGF stimulation in maintaining the alveolar–capillary unit in adult animals and on the curious possible action of MnSOD or MnSOD mimetics to antagonize the development of emphysema due to various causes.

EUK-8 is a synthetic, low molecular weight salen–manganese complex that exhibits both SOD-like and catalase-like activities. This compound has been studied in a swine model of experimental ARDS, where it could attenuate arterial hypoxemia, pulmonary hypertension, and pulmonary edema (122). Following EUK treatment (10 mg/kg), the level of lipid peroxidation products was decreased in this model.

Synthetic compounds with GPx-like activity have also been invented. The first of these was ebselen [2-phenyl-1, 2-benzisoselenazol-3(2H)-one], a seleno-organic compound. The beneficial effects of ebselen are related not only to its GPx-like activity, but also to its anti-inflammatory actions. For example, the anti-inflammatory effect of ebselen has been studied in a guinea pig asthma model. Ebselen (10–20 mg/kg per orally) was found to attenuate the late asthmatic response following ovalbumin challenge, reduce the number of inflammatory cells in BALF, and inhibit generation of ROS in bronchial epithelial cells. Possible mechanisms for these findings may include suppression of inducible nitric oxide synthase (iNOS) and ROS production in endothelial cells (123). Ebselen also has been found to alleviate lung edema and reduce amount of proinflammatory cytokines and inflammatory cells in BALF in a rat model of sephadex-induced lung injury (124,125). The protective effect of ebselen against ozone-induced lung injury may arise from direct ROS scavenging and enhancement of endogenous AOEs, including MnSOD and CuZnSOD (126). Newer compounds with GPx-like activity include dicyclodextrinyl ditelluride (2-TeCD), whose hydroperoxide removing activity is 46 times greater than that of ebselen. Other improvements include good water solubility, and chemical and biological stability. The 2-TeCD has been found to protect mitochondria against oxidative stress (127).

From the above studies, it can be concluded that catalytic antioxidants, especially metalloporphyrins, satisfy many of the criteria required for an ideal antioxidant therapeutic agent, in that they possess high activity, are stable and potentially nontoxic, and have been shown to protect against ROS-mediated lung injury in experimental models. It should be noted that their actions might be unpredictable due to their ability to react with a wide variety of ROS/RNS. Recent investigation showed for the first time that one of the catalytic antioxidants, a metalloporphyrin AEOL 10113, might have beneficial effects in reducing the risk of pulmonary oxygen toxicity in preterm baboon model of BPD (128). Extensive experimental research is still needed before these compounds can be tested in clinical trials.

C. Thiol-Based Antioxidants

Augmentation of GSH-dependent antioxidant defense has been extensively studied, with the rationale that GSH synthesis may be limited in the preterm neonate (34,36). Administration of GSH as an aerosol increases functional GSH levels in alveolar lining fluid of normal sheep (129). Intravenous GSH prevents the postdelivery decline in plasma cysteine concentrations in the baboon model of prematurity (130). Given that the ability of GSH to cross biological membranes is poor and that systemic administration of cysteine is limited by its instability in plasma (13,131), some studies have concentrated on elucidating the role of cysteine precursors such as *N*-acetyl cysteine (NAC) in preventing ROS-induced lung injury. NAC is a relatively stable, thiol-containing compound, which scavenges radicals directly (132,133) and, perhaps more importantly, can promote GSH synthesis by providing more substrate (134–136). The clinical use of NAC is well established as an antidote in acetaminophen poisoning (137). Lung cells can likely deacetylate NAC in vivo, since an NAC-deacetylating acylase has been found recently in the cell membranes of several organs including the lung (138). Also, NAC has been shown to increase mitochondrial GSH and restore important mitochondrial functions in vivo following genetically or pharmacologically impaired GSH homeostasis (139,140). However, intraperitoneal NAC (400 mg/kg/day) does not prolong the survival of *Sod2* knockout mice in 21 or 50% oxygen (141). Further, NAC has been shown to ameliorate ROS-mediated lung injury and enhance recovery from acute lung injury in animal (142,143) and also human studies (144,145). However, it should be noted that although NAC was found to improve oxygenation and shorten the duration of acute lung injury in human studies, the mortality rate was not changed (144,145). In some studies, NAC has not shown any positive effects in the treatment of ARDS (146). In a Nordic double-blinded multicenter trial, a 6-day course of intravenous NAC (16–32 mg/kg/day) did not prevent BPD or death in extremely low-birth-weight infants (147). Oral and inhaled NAC have been shown to ameliorate bleomycin-induced lung injury in rodents through repression of chemokines and lipid hydroperoxide production, and to cause an increase of BALF–GSH, resulting in the attenuation of subsequent lung fibrosis (148,149). Also, NAC has been tested in prevention of ischemia–reperfusion injury, because GSH is depleted during these conditions. Pretreatment of transplanted lungs with NAC results in two-fold increase of lung GSH content, and prevents, to some degree, the reperfusion injury as assessed by improved wet-to-dry tissue weight ratio and decreased amount of inflammatory cells in BALF (150).

Oral supplementation with another cysteine precursor, L-2-oxothiazolidine-4-carboxylate (OTC), has been found to protect protein-energy malnourished rats against oxygen-induced lung injury, as estimated by improved lung-to-body weight ratios and enhanced pulmonary GSH levels (151). In human ARDS patients OTC repleted red blood cell GSH levels but did not alter mortality (145). In addition, postnatal supplementation of selenium to preterm neonates did not prevent the incidence of BPD (152). In sum, there have been no reproducible trials indicating a beneficial therapeutic effect of NAC or OTC on mortality or long-term outcomes in RDS or ARDS. Although NAC and other reduced thiols are not intrinsically toxic, they are highly susceptible to "auto-oxidation" reactions (153). These reactions are potentiated by the presence of free iron, superoxide, hydrogen peroxide, and/or hydroxyl radicals. All of these may be present in excess in RDS or ARDS. Chelation of iron may help prevent such reactions (153), but iron chelation has had overwhelming deleterious effects in models of RDS (154). Addition of SOD and catalase also can limit or prevent thiol oxidation (153). Thus, their addition to such antioxidant therapies could restore balance and allow a net beneficial effect to be realized.

D. Vitamins

Oral supplementation of vitamin E has been found to be protective against oxygen-mediated lung injury in the rabbit (97), but others have found vitamin E supplementation to be of no therapeutic benefit in adult mice (Rusakow and White, unpublished observation). Oral administration of antioxidants to preterm neonates can be limited by immaturity of the gut and poor bioavailability. Clinical trials using vitamin E to prevent BPD have not shown any positive effects (155,156). Intramuscular high-dose vitamin A administered over a 4-week period slightly decreases the risk of BPD in extremely low-birth-weight infants (157). Vitamin C has been found to be a critical antioxidant in epithelial lining fluid responsible for protection of lung cells against ozone (158).

E. Catalytic Antibodies

Monoclonal antibodies with catalytic groups incorporated into the substrate-binding site, also called abzymes, have been developed recently. Examples of such catalytic antibodies are the selenium-containing monoclonal antibodies 2F3, 3G5, 4A4, and 5C9, which were raised against GSH-derivative and which exhibit high catalytic efficiency for decomposition of hydroperoxides (GPx activity) (159–161). These catalytic antibodies have been shown to protect cardiac mitochondria against oxidative stress, but their in vivo function remains to be elucidated.

F. Lazaroids

Lazaroid U-74389G, and other synthetic 21-aminosteroids, reduce the amount of iron-dependent lipid peroxidation, and have therefore been studied in the prevention of hyperoxic lung injury as well as ischemia–reperfusion injury. In a neonatal rat model of BPD, U-74389G attenuated the formation of lipid peroxidation products and hydroxyl radical formation in lungs and serum, and also had a beneficial effect on inhibition of lung cell proliferation induced by 95% oxygen (162). U-74389G did not, however, either reduce mortality or improve lung wet-to-dry weight ratio (162). Recently the same researchers have found that exposure of newborn rats to a lower concentration of oxygen for a prolonged time (60% oxygen for 14 days) leads to development of pulmonary hypertension with concomitant increase in the level of 8-isoprostane, a marker of lipid peroxidation, as well as up regulation of endothelin-1. The oxygen-induced development of pulmonary hypertension could be blocked by U-74389G (10 mg/kg/day intraperitoneally) (163).

In a canine model of warm ischemia, arterial oxygen saturation and cardiac output were significantly higher, and left pulmonary vascular resistance significantly lower in the U-74389G group as compared with vehicle or methylprednisolone controls 30 min after reperfusion (164). Improved clinical variables were reflected in higher survival rates in the U-74389G-treated group (164). In the rat lung transplantation model, gas exchange function was significantly improved and tissue lipid peroxidation significantly reduced in U-74389G-treated group as compared with no treatment group 60 min after reperfusion (165). These positive effects were seen when U-74389G was administrated either intravenously to both donor and recipient, or as an additive to the University of Wisconsin preservation solution (165). However, mixed results have been obtained from swine model of lung allotransplantation, where intravenous treatment of both the donor and the recipient with another lazaroid compound, U-74006F, resulted in reduction of lipid peroxidation and neutrophil migration in the allograft, but did not reduce posttransplant edema or improve pulmonary hemodynamics (166).

G. Surfactant and Glucocorticoid Therapy

Both surfactant and glucocorticoid therapy have potential effects in terms of mitigating oxidative stress in lung injury. Intratracheal administration of exogenous surfactants clearly decreases the degree of respiratory failure and improves the outcome of premature infants with RDS (37,167), and this therapy may also be beneficial in clinical acute lung injury (ALI) and ARDS (Chapter 15). Although therapeutic responses to exogenous surfactant are largely due to improved surface-active function, some degree of antioxidant activity may also be involved. Natural lung surfactant has both direct and indirect antioxidant effects, which have primarily been attributed to surfactant proteins A (SP-A) and D (SP-D). The direct effects include, for example, protection of surfactant phospholipids and macrophages from oxidative damage through inhibition of lipid peroxidation and oxidative cell injury (168,169). Furthermore, natural lung surfactant also possesses SOD and catalase activity (170). The indirect antioxidant effects are in most part anti-inflammatory in nature and include, for example, downregulation of proinflammatory cytokine response (171) and inhibition of redox-sensitive transcription factor NF-κB and subsequently of metalloproteinase expression (172) in alveolar macrophages. Paradoxical to the antioxidant effects of surfactant proteins, by amplifying inflammatory host defenses against infecting organisms they also may increase production of ROS and RNS. Also, SP-A and D play an important role in adaptive immune responses of the lung (173–175). The inclusion of recombinant human SP-A or related synthetic SP-A peptides in current exogenous surfactants containing only hydrophobic surfactant proteins may enhance their antioxidant activity, but this has not been studied directly.

Another therapeutic intervention that affects oxidant/antioxidant balance is the administration of glucocorticoids or related steroids. The use of antenatal maternal glucocorticoids to enhance pulmonary maturation in the developing fetus has proved beneficial in experimental models (176,177) and human trials (178), and is now routinely integrated in the treatment of impending preterm delivery. In animal models, the beneficial effects of antenatal glucocorticoids may arise not only from the maturational effects on surfactant production, but also from acceleration of maturation of AOEs (179,180). Infants at risk for developing BPD often are also treated with glucocorticoids postnatally. However, this treatment cannot currently be recommended because postnatal administration of glucocorticoids may be associated with central nervous system complications (181). In addition, impaired alveolar septation within the developing lung has been documented in animal models (37). All-*trans* retinoic acid has been found to ameliorate glucocorticoid-induced inhibition of alveolarization in neonatal rodents (182). Prenatal administration of thyrotropin releasing hormone in order to stimulate AOEs and surfactant maturation seemed promising, but, in fact, was associated with severe adverse effects in experimental models (183,184) and in a clinical trial (185).

Despite the beneficial effects of prenatal corticosteroids and exogenous surfactant replacement therapy on survival, high morbidity still persists in very preterm newborns with RDS (186,187). Among the latest modifications in therapy are less aggressive ventilatory strategies, which can decrease barotrauma and secondary inflammatory reactions. Furthermore, 100% oxygen is not automatically used in resuscitation of preterm babies, and use of room air in resuscitation has been evaluated in controlled studies (188,189). Treatment with inhaled nitric oxide has also been found to improve oxygenation and decrease lung neutrophil accumulation in preterm animals and in human neonates with hypoxemic respiratory failure (190). The beneficial effects of nitric oxide may include reduction of neutrophil-associated oxidative stress, although this gas itself contributes an exogenous oxidant burden (Chapter 7).

H. Novel Approaches (Transcription Factors, Signaling Pathways, DNA Repair Mechanisms, Growth Factors)

Genetic predisposition may play a role in the development of RDS (191) and BPD (192) in human infants. The mechanisms behind genetic influence on oxygen toxicity and development of lung injury, however, have been unknown. Recently, the gene for a potent transcription factor NRF2, Nfe2l2 (nuclear factor, erythroid derived 2, like 2 or Nrf2), has been identified as a strong candidate gene for susceptibility to hyperoxia in mice (193). NRF2 plays a central role in the protection against oxidative stress through antioxidant response element (ARE)-mediated transcriptional regulation of various antioxidants and phase 2 enzymes. Genetic inactivation of Nrf2 in mice has been shown to lead to increased susceptibility to hyperoxic lung injury, as estimated by increased pulmonary hyperpermeability and enhanced macrophage inflammation as well as epithelial injury. The NAD(P) H:quinone oxidoreductase 1 and glutathione-*S*-transferase among others have been identified as down stream molecular targets of NRF2 in hyperoxic lung response (194). Another strong candidate gene, Toll-like receptor 4 (Tlr4) on mouse chromosome 4, for ozone susceptibility has recently been identified (195). This gene has also been implicated in innate immunity and endotoxin susceptibility.

Although transcription and growth factors are not understood as "traditional" antioxidants, their action can lead to prevention or repair of ROS-induced damage to DNA or other intracellular constituents, and therefore, they could fulfill the definition of an antioxidant. Enhanced repair of DNA damage (possibly also mitochondrial DNA damage) may enhance cell survival and cell growth potential, irrespective of antioxidant defense status. This could be a factor in pulmonary vascular and lung growth, or lack thereof, in BPD. Apurinic/apyrimidinic endonuclease (APE-1) or APE-1/Ref-1 is a ubiquitous multifunctional protein, which possesses both DNA repair activity and redox regulatory activity. The DNA repair activity of APE-1 occurs through its participation in the excision and replacement of damaged nucleotides in DNA, and it has been shown to be involved in repair of both spontaneous and oxidative damage to cellular DNA. The APE-1/Ref-1 also mediates DNA-binding of a number of redox-sensitive transcription factors, such as AP-1, NF-κB, Pax-5, Pax-8, and HIF-1 (196). Overexpression of yeast apurinic/apyrimidinic endonuclease (APN1) in A549 cells protects these cells against bleomycin, as indicated by reduction of DNA damage and increased cell survival (197). However, overexpression of APE-1/Ref-1 was not shown to be beneficial in an another study using nonpulmonary cell lines (198). Mitochondrial DNA may be even more susceptible to oxidative damage due to less efficient repair mechanisms. Given that various pulmonary cell lines show extensive mtDNA damage following exposure to oxidative stress (199), interventions directed at improving mitochondrial DNA repair in pulmonary epithelial cells could possibly have valuable effects.

As discussed above, hyperoxia damages DNA and other cell constituents through formation of ROS. Available evidence indicates that limiting DNA replication during hyperoxia is protective and enhances cell survival. The pathways by which cells pause proliferation in hyperoxia have recently been described. In hyperoxia, cells appear to increase the expression of the tumor suppressor p53 and its down stream target, the cyclin-dependent kinase inhibitor p21(Cip1/WAF1/Sdi1) (p21), which limits DNA replication by blocking entry from G1 phase into S phase in pulmonary and nonpulmonary cell lines (200,201). Studies using mice lacking p21 and p53 have shown that p21 is, in fact, induced by hyperoxia also in the absence of p53. On the other hand, hyperoxia does not limit DNA replication in p21 deficient mice. Furthermore, the survival of p21 deficient mice is decreased with an associated increased level of apoptotic and necrotic cell death. The authors suggested that p21 protects the lung from oxidative stress, in part, by inhibiting DNA replication and thereby allowing additional time to repair damaged DNA (202). It is noteworthy, however, that even though promoting growth arrest of all lung cells might be protective under hyperoxic conditions, it could also lead to aggravation of the pathology of BPD.

Paradoxical to the protective effect of promoting growth arrest, some growth factors have also been shown to have beneficial effects on repair of the alveolar epithelium in hyperoxia. Upon oxidative insult, there is progressive loss of type-I cells and a reactive hyperplasia of type-II cells, which are progenitor cells of the alveolar epithelium. Keratinocyte growth factor/fibroblast growth factor 7 (KGF-7) has been shown to promote alveolar type-II cell growth in primary culture and alveolar epithelial hyperplasia in vivo. In a rat model of oxygen-induced lung injury, treatment with intratracheal rhKGF (1 or 5 mg/kg) resulted in proliferation of type-II cells, enhanced survival, and alleviation of lung injury as estimated by decreased amount of hemorrhage and exudate (203). It also has been suggested that the protective effect of KGF against oxidative stress may be due to enhanced DNA repair involving tyrosine kinase, protein kinase C, and DNA polymerases (204). According to a recent study, fibroblast-derived KGF inhibits synthesis and secretion of the phosphatidylcholines of pulmonary surfactant in hyperoxia, and thus, could also play a role in the surfactant dysfunction detected in ARDS patients (205). Nevertheless, KGF and possibly other growth factors, such as fibroblast growth factor 10 (FGF-10) and hepatocyte growth factor (HGF), may have therapeutic potential in facilitation of repair of hyperoxia-induced epithelial injury (206).

V. Limitations to Antioxidant Therapy

Although there have been great advances in understanding molecular mechanisms involved in the pathogenesis of various forms of lung injury, difficult questions remain. In order to develop effective antioxidant therapies, it is necessary to identify specific target radicals that are deleterious and mediate disease in a given clinical condition. Currently the direct in vivo measurement of radicals is impossible, and therefore the evidence of ROS as pathogenetic factors in various disease states has been obtained via indirect measurements, i.e., assessments of stable end products resulting from reactions of ROS on various cellular components or added spin traps. Some of the methods widely used in such assessments carry significant "pitfalls" and inaccuracies. Likewise, for successful antioxidant therapy, precise answers are needed to other extremely important questions, such as, what biochemical targets are most in need of protecting, where are they located, when should protection be attempted, and by which specific antioxidant(s) and means of delivery can protection best be achieved?

The goal of optimal antioxidant therapy is to scavenge the excess of harmful radicals without interfering with essential cellular functions. Despite the harmful effects of ROS and other radicals, they also have important physiological roles in, for example, killing of micro-organisms, oxidation of xenobiotics, and regulation of smooth muscle tone (207). ROS also have been recognized as modulators of signal transduction cascades culminating in, for example, regulation of cell growth, proliferation, and differentiation (7,208). The role of ROS in the growth of lung and other target tissues carries significant implications for the use of antioxidants in neonatal therapy (209).

The balance not only between oxidants and antioxidants but also between various antioxidants may be of major importance in protection against ROS-mediated injury. For example, endogenous up regulation of catalase and/or GPx sometimes parallels that of SOD (210,211), suggesting a balancing mechanism in response to increased hydrogen peroxide production. In some studies, overexpression of only one antioxidant pathway, with no adaptive increases in other antioxidant mechanisms, has led to paradoxical adverse effects (212,213). On the other hand, increased levels of several antioxidant pathways associate with successful adaptation to hyperoxia. Furthermore, overexpression of both catalase and SOD protects against hyperoxia in rodent lung in vitro (214) and in vivo (215). Interestingly, in the latter study, overexpression of SOD alone worsened ischemia–reperfusion injury, but concomitant overexpression of catalase prevented this adverse effect (215). Further studies are needed to expand our understanding of which antioxidant, or combination of antioxidants, might have most beneficial effects with minimal untoward effects in given clinical circumstances.

Some studies have shown that clinical factors not directly related to oxidant activity are crucial to the potential success or failure of antioxidant therapy. For example, although intravenous GSH therapy in premature baboons had clinically and biochemically beneficial effects as indicated by normalization of circulating cysteine and glutathione, the alveolar–arterial oxygen gradient was increased indicating in fact worsening oxygenation (130). The ductus arteriosus was patent in all animals studied. Because thiols as well as other antioxidants can have profound effects on nitric oxide metabolism, the authors speculated that the findings were related to changes in pulmonary blood flow through the ductus resulting from generalized pulmonary vasodilation (130). Another example comes from a study where deferoxamine, a widely used iron chelator, was administered to preterm baboons in an attempt to inhibit iron-catalyzed free radical generation and lessen the severity of oxygen-induced pulmonary injury (154). However, sudden death occurred in a large number of deferoxamine-treated animals because of profound, cardiovascular collapse. Although widely used clinically, deferoxamine is not normally used under hyperoxic conditions. Deferoxamine can decrease markedly the reactivation cycle of iron–sulfur cluster-containing enzymes (216), and hyperoxia caused the profound inactivaton of such enzymes in the lung, including aconitase (217) and α-ketoglutarate dehydrogenase (218). Interestingly, impairment of the activity of these enzymes also occurs in homozygous MnSOD knockout mice breathing room air (219), and cardiovascular failure also appears to be the cause of death in these animals (220).

Many natural enzymes have an intracellular site of action, often within specific organelles. At present, antioxidants generally cannot be delivered or expressed precisely where needed. Sometimes the localization of an AOE appears more important than the native form of the enzyme itself since, for example, CuZnSOD targeted into the mitochondria protects against radiation-induced oxidative stress, but MnSOD retained in the cytosol does not (221). Likewise, nuclear overexpression of catalase sensitizes cells to paraquat, whereas peroxisomal, cytosolic, or mitochondrial catalase overexpression protects cells against oxidants (222,223).

Providing immunologically unrecognizable proteins also has yet to be achieved. Protein glycosylation is an important issue in immune recognition or lack thereof. Depending on the species in which the protein is produced, the presence of additional sugar moieties, such as mannose, also may have the capability of activating innate immunity. Gene therapy approaches could circumvent some of these problems. However, at present, such approaches also have potential untoward immunologic side-effects. Although attachment to PEG can diminish some immune responses to foreign proteins, such reactions still exist, at times with important clinical consequences. Furthermore, encapsulation or attachment of antioxidants to various carrier substances may also affect the host-defense mechanisms, such as neutrophil bactericidal activity (224). Although specific targeting of enzymes themselves or liposomes containing them also have been demonstrated in some animal models, to our knowledge no such antioxidant approaches have yet been approved for clinical trials for oxidative lung diseases.

For synthetic antioxidant compounds, inert, nontoxic molecules with established safety profiles are not yet available (although numerous products are in development). Penetration of these molecules into appropriate tissues, cells, and organelles also remains to be established. The reactivities of many of the synthetic and mimetic compounds are not specific for given ROS or RNS. In itself, this is not necessarily a problem, and may cause beneficial effects to be observed in various diseases or disease models. However, because these species can have diverse roles in host defense, signal transduction, gene regulation and expression, and other vital processes, it is also possible that undesirable clinical side-effects may be noted due to these less than specific reactivities. These same considerations also may apply to natural enzymatic scavengers of ROS. For example, with regard to safety and optimal action, there appears to be a "therapeutic window," or optimal range, of dosage for MnSOD in the treatment of ARDS (103) and ischemia–reperfusion related heart injury (225).

With regard to novel antioxidant approaches, various shortcomings remain for each. For modulation of transcription factors, even though there is evidence that their activation could cause global beneficial responses, compounds or approaches to cause specific on/off activation are not currently available. Similarly, immunologically inert agents targeting endotoxin and its components have not been identified. Humans are exquisitely sensitive to endotoxin, which tends to "prime" immune and inflammatory responses and cytokine production. Uncontrolled inflammation induced by endotoxin or other forms of lung injury is known to be counterproductive, but it is not yet clear how or if therapies can effectively antagonize this process for long-term benefits to patients. Concerning modulation or delivery of growth factors or cell survival factors, although such therapies have been found to be of benefit in animal models (KGF; Akt, respectively), their successful application to combat oxidative stress has not been demonstrated in primate models or human disease states. Again, the potentially global actions of such agents or interventions could easily have untoward as well as beneficial clinical effects. Finally, with regard to interventions that could modulate DNA damage, progress in this area simply has not yet progressed sufficiently far that it has been tried in higher mammals or humans for lung disorders related to oxidative stress. Nonetheless, findings in animal models have so far been encouraging, and continuing research progress can be expected.

VI. Summary

Elaborate endogenous pulmonary antioxidant defenses are present to protect the host against deleterious effects of reactive oxidants. Protection is achieved by maintaining a delicate balance between oxidants and antioxidants, and therefore the continuous production of ROS in aerobic organisms has to be met with a similar rate of their consumption by antioxidants. Oxidative stress is defined as an imbalance of the prooxidant / antioxidant equilibrium in favor of the prooxidants. Antioxidants, either enzymatic or nonenzymatic, are substances that prevent the formation of ROS or other oxidants, scavenge them, and/or repair the damage they cause. The intricate endogenous antioxidant system consists of, for example, classical AOEs, glutathione, and thioredoxin with their associated redox cycles, heme oxygenases, and numerous small molecular weight antioxidants (metal chelating proteins, vitamins, urate, etc.).

Throughout postnatal life, the lung is exposed to higher concentrations of oxygen than other organs. Furthermore, a variety of clinical conditions necessitate the administration of supraphysiological concentrations of oxygen, which exposes lung cells to additional oxidative stress. These conditions include, for example, RDS and BPD in premature infants, as well as acute respiratory failure associated with clinical ALI/ARDS in adult and pediatric patients. Additional clinical conditions discussed in this chapter that involve increased oxidative stress include inflammatory airway diseases (asthma, COPD), interstitial lung diseases, drug-related (bleomycin) lung injury, and lung transplantation (ischemia–reperfusion injury). The rationale for antioxidant therapy is based on the belief that affected individuals are deficient in endogenous antioxidant defenses as a consequence of: (i) developmental regulation, and/or (ii) overwhelming oxidative stress from the clinical condition itself or from its treatment.

Because of the importance of ROS in the pathogenesis of various forms of lung injury, a wide variety of antioxidants and means of delivery have been studied in order to prevent or ameliorate the severity of pulmonary damage. The goal of optimal antioxidant therapy is to scavenge the excess of harmful radicals without interfering with essential cellular functions, such as cell growth and differentiation. An ideal antioxidant therapeutic agent should possess several characteristics; it should have: (i) good bioavailability, (ii) potency in penetrating to the critical site(s) of action, (iii) efficiency in scavenging appropriate radical species, (iv) stability, (v) minimal or absent toxicity or immunogenicity, and (vi) low cost. An effective antioxidant must also facilitate or allow essential developmental and healing processes to proceed. So far no antioxidant agent has fulfilled all of these requirements. However, promising results with respect to alleviating the severity of lung injury have been obtained from in vitro and in vivo studies using both natural and synthetic antioxidants such as SOD, catalase, thiols (cysteine precursors, glutathione), catalytic antioxidants and antibodies, and 21-aminosteroids. Results from experimental studies utilizing more novel approaches suggest that modulation of certain transcription factors and signaling pathways, whose activation results in regulation of a variety of antioxidant defenses, might present a powerful way to affect outcomes in oxidative stress. Likewise, accumulating experimental data suggest that enhancing DNA repair mechanisms, promoting growth arrest, and paradoxically, inducing growth factors, may have advantageous effects in the prevention of lung injury. All of these may share enhanced DNA repair as a common pathway.

Some antioxidant agents, such as CuZnSOD, vitamin A and E, selenium, NAC, and GSH, have been studied in controlled human studies with varying results. Although valuable biochemical changes have been achieved, primary outcomes of severity of lung disease or death generally have not been improved. More studies directed at the basic biochemical mechanisms are needed to delineate the therapeutic potential of specific antioxidants in the treatment of human disease. Antioxidant treatment of neonatal lung disorders merits special attention because ROS may exert pivotal functional roles in cell growth and differentiation. Continuing mechanistic research on oxidants and antioxidants and their roles in the pathophysiology of inflammatory lung injury should help identify specific agents or combinations of agents able to mitigate oxidant-induced damage, providing a solid foundation for the development of successful pulmonary antioxidant therapy.

References

1. Turrens JF. Superoxide production by the mitochondrial respiratory chain. Biosci Rep 1997; 17:3–8.
2. Freeman BA, Crapo JD. Hyperoxia increases oxygen radical production in rat lungs and lung mitochondria. J Biol Chem 1981; 256:10986–10992.
3. Halliwell B, Gutteridge JMC. Free Radicals in Biology and Medicine Oxford: Clarendon Press, 1989.
4. Budinger GR, Tso M, McClintock DS, Dean DA, Sznajder JI, Chandel NS. Hyperoxia-induced apoptosis does not require mitochondrial reactive oxygen species and is regulated by Bcl-2 proteins. J Biol Chem 2002; 277: 15654–15660.
5. Kinnula VL, Crapo JD, Raivio KO. Generation and disposal of reactive oxygen metabolites in the lung. Lab Invest 1995; 73:3–19.
6. Freeman BA, Crapo JD. Biology of disease: free radicals and tissue injury. Lab Invest 1982; 47:412–426.
7. Thannickal VJ, Fanburg BL. Reactive oxygen species in cell signaling. Am J Physiol Lung Cell Mol Physiol 2000; 279:L1005–L1028.
8. Sies H. Oxidative stress: from basic research to clinical application. Am J Med 1991; 91:31S–38S.
9. Fridovich I, Freeman B. Antioxidant defenses in the lung. Annu Rev Physiol 1986; 48:693–702.
10. Powis G, Montfort WR. Properties and biological activities of thioredoxins. Annu Rev Pharmacol Toxicol 2001; 41:261–295.
11. Halliwell B. Antioxidant defence mechanisms: from the beginning to the end (of the beginning). Free Radic Res 1999; 31:261–272.
12. Chance B, Sies H, Boveris A. Hydroperoxide metabolism in mammalian organs. Physiol Rev 1979; 59:527–605.

13. Meister A. Glutathione deficiency produced by inhibition of its synthesis, and its reversal; applications in research and therapy. Pharmacol Ther 1991; 51:155–194.

14. Kinnula VL, Crapo JD. Superoxide dismutases in the lung and human lung diseases. Am J Respir Crit Care Med 2003; 167:1600–1619.

15. Hass MA, Massaro D. Developmental regulation of rat lung Cu,Zn-superoxide dismutase. Biochem J 1987; 246:697–703.

16. Rickett GM, Kelly FJ. Developmental expression of antioxidant enzymes in guinea pig lung and liver. Development 1990; 108:331–336.

17. Walther FJ, Wade AB, Warburton D, Forman HJ. Ontogeny of antioxidant enzymes in the fetal lamb lung. Exp Lung Res 1991; 17:39–45.

18. Kim HS, Kang SW, Rhee SG, Clerch LB. Rat lung peroxiredoxins I and II are differentially regulated during development and by hyperoxia. Am J Physiol Lung Cell Mol Physiol 2001; 280:L1212–L1217.

19. Frank L, Sosenko IR. Failure of premature rabbits to increase antioxidant enzymes during hyperoxic exposure: increased susceptibility to pulmonary oxygen toxicity compared with term rabbits. Pediatr Res 1991; 29:292–296.

20. Morton RL, Das KC, Guo XL, Ikle DN, White CW. Effect of oxygen on lung superoxide dismutase activities in premature baboons with bronchopulmonary dysplasia. Am J Physiol Lung Cell Mol Physiol 1999; 276:L64–L74.

21. Frank L. Developmental aspects of experimental pulmonary oxygen toxicity. Free Radic Biol Med 1991; 11:463–494.

22. Yam J, Frank L, Roberts RJ. Oxygen toxicity: comparison of lung biochemical responses in neonatal and adult rats. Pediatr Res 1978; 12:115–119.

23. Sosenko IR, Frank L. Guinea pig lung development: antioxidant enzymes and premature survival in high O_2. Am J Physiol 1987; 252:R693–R698.

24. Chen Y, Whitney PL, Frank L. Comparative responses of premature vs. full-term newborn rats to prolonged hyperoxia. Pediatr Res 1994; 35:233–237.

25. Baker RR, Holm BA, Panus PC, Matalon S. Development of O_2 tolerance in rabbits with no increase in antioxidant enzymes. J Appl Physiol 1989; 66:1679–1684.

26. Kinnula VL, Pietarinen P, Aalto K, Virtanen I, Raivio KO. Mitochondrial superoxide dismutase induction does not protect epithelial cells during oxidant exposure in vitro. Am J Physiol Lung Cell Mol Physiol 1995; 268:L71–L77.

27. Allen CB, Guo XL, White CW. Changes in pulmonary expression of hexokinase and glucose transporter mRNAs in rats adapted to hyperoxia. Am J Physiol Lung Cell Mol Physiol 1998; 274:L320–L329.

28. White CW, Greene KE, Allen CB, Shannon JM. Elevated expression of surfactant proteins in newborn rats during adaptation to hyperoxia. Am J Respir Cell Mol Biol 2001; 25:51–59.

29. McElroy MC, Postle AD, Kelly FJ. Catalase, superoxide dismutase and glutathione peroxidase activities of lung and liver during human development. Biochim Biophys Acta 1992; 15:153–158.

30. Asikainen TM, Raivio KO, Saksela M, Kinnula VL. Expression and developmental profile of antioxidant enzymes in human lung and liver. Am J Respir Cell Mol Biol 1998; 19:942–949.

31. Strange RC, Cotton W, Fryer AA, Drew R, Bradwell AR, Marshall T, Collins MF, Bell J, Hume R. Studies on the expression of Cu, Zn superoxide

dismutase in human tissues during development. Biochim Biophys Acta 1988; 964:260–265.

32. Strange RC, Cotton W, Fryer AA, Jones P, Bell J, Hume R. Lipid peroxidation and expression of copper–zinc and manganese superoxide dismutase in lungs of premature infants with hyaline membrane disease and bronchopulmonary dysplasia. J Lab Clin Med 1990; 116:666–673.

33. Asikainen TM, Heikkilä P, Kaarteenaho-Wiik R, Kinnula VL, Raivio KO. Cell-specific expression of manganese superoxide dismutase protein in the lungs of patients with respiratory distress syndrome, chronic lung disease, or persistent pulmonary hypertension. Pediatr Pulmonol 2001; 32:193–200.

34. Jain A, Mehta T, Auld PA, Rodrigues J, Ward RF, Schwartz MK, Martensson J. Glutathione metabolism in newborns: evidence for glutathione deficiency in plasma, bronchoalveolar lavage fluid, and lymphocytes in prematures. Pediatr Pulmonol 1995; 20:160–166.

35. Levonen AL, Lapatto R, Saksela M, Raivio KO. Expression of gamma-glutamylcysteine synthetase during development. Pediatr Res 2000; 47:266–270.

36. Viña J, Vento M, Garcia-Sala F, Puertes IR, Gasco E, Sastre J, Asensi M, Pallardo FV. L-Cysteine and glutathione metabolism are impaired in premature infants due to cystathionase deficiency. Am J Clin Nutr 1995; 61: 1067–1069.

37. Jobe AH, Bancalari E. Bronchopulmonary dysplasia. Am J Respir Crit Care Med 2001; 163:1723–1729.

38. Northway WJ, Rosan RC, Porter DY. Pulmonary disease following respirator therapy of hyaline-membrane disease. Bronchopulmonary dysplasia. N Engl J Med 1967; 276:357–368.

39. Shennan AT, Dunn MS, Ohlsson A, Lennox K, Hoskins EM. Abnormal pulmonary outcomes in premature infants: prediction from oxygen requirement in the neonatal period. Pediatrics 1988; 82:527–532.

40. deLemos RA, Coalson JJ. The contribution of experimental models to our understanding of the pathogenesis and treatment of bronchopulmonary dysplasia. Clin Perinatol 1992; 19:521–539.

41. Anderson WR, Strickland MB, Tsai SH, Haglin JJ. Light microscopic and ultrastructural study of the adverse effects of oxygen therapy on the neonate lung. Am J Pathol 1973; 73:327–348.

42. Crapo JD. Morphologic changes in pulmonary oxygen toxicity. Annu Rev Physiol 1986; 48:721–731.

43. Margraf LR, Tomashefski JF Jr, Bruce MC, Dahms BB. Morphometric analysis of the lung in bronchopulmonary dysplasia. Am Rev Respir Dis 1991; 143:391–400.

44. Saugstad OD. Chronic lung disease: the role of oxidative stress. Biol Neonate 1998; 1:21–28.

45. Gitto E, Reiter RJ, Karbownik M, Xian-Tan D, Barberi I. Respiratory distress syndrome in the newborn: role of oxidative stress. Intensive Care Med 2001; 27:1116–1123.

46. Pitkänen OM, Hallman M, Andersson SM. Correlation of free oxygen radical-induced lipid peroxidation with outcome in very low birth weight infants. J Pediatr 1990; 116:760–764.

47. Varsila E, Pesonen E, Andersson S. Early protein oxidation in the neonatal lung is related to development of chronic lung disease. Acta Pediatr 1995; 84:1296–1299.

48. Banks BA, Ischiropoulos H, McClelland M, Ballard PL, Ballard RA. Plasma 3-nitrotyrosine is elevated in premature infants who develop bronchopulmonary dysplasia. Pediatrics 1998; 101:870–874.

49. Grigg J, Barber A, Silverman M. Bronchoalveolar lavage fluid glutathione in intubated premature infants. Arch Dis Child 1993; 69:49–51.

50. Smith CV, Hansen TN, Martin NE, McMicken HW, Elliott SJ. Oxidant stress responses in premature infants during exposure to hyperoxia. Pediatr Res 1993; 34:360–365.

51. White CW, Stabler SP, Allen RH, Moreland S, Rosenberg AA. Plasma cysteine concentrations in infants with respiratory distress. J Pediatr 1994; 125:769–777.

52. Levin DL, Heymann MA, Kitterman JA, Gregory GA, Phibbs RH, Rudolph AM. Persistent pulmonary hypertension of the newborn infant. J Pediatr 1976; 89:626–630.

53. Kääpä P. Meconium aspiration syndrome: a role for phospholipase A2 in the pathogenesis? Acta Paediatr 2001; 90:365–367.

54. Chabot F, Mitchell JA, Gutteridge JM, Evans TW. Reactive oxygen species in acute lung injury. Eur Respir J 1998; 11:745–757.

55. Pacht ER, Timerman AP, Lykens MG, Merola AJ. Deficiency of alveolar fluid glutathione in patients with sepsis and the adult respiratory distress syndrome. Chest 1991; 100:1397–1403.

56. Haddad IY, Pataki G, Hu P, Galliani C, Beckman JS, Matalon S. Quantitation of nitrotyrosine levels in lung sections of patients and animals with acute lung injury. J Clin Invest 1994; 94:2407–2413.

57. Metnitz PG, Bartens C, Fischer M, Fridrich P, Steltzer H, Druml W. Antioxidant status in patients with acute respiratory distress syndrome. Intensive Care Med 1999; 25:180–185.

58. Barnes PJ. Pathophysiology of asthma. Br J Clin Pharmacol 1996; 42:3–10.

59. Jarjour NN, Calhoun WJ. Enhanced production of oxygen radicals in asthma. J Lab Clin Med 1994; 123:131–136.

60. Vachier I, Damon M, Le Doucen C, de Paulet AC, Chanez P, Michel FB, Godard P. Increased oxygen species generation in blood monocytes of asthmatic patients. Am Rev Respir Dis 1992; 146:1161–1166.

61. De Raeve HR, Thunnissen FB, Kaneko FT, Guo FH, Lewis M, Kavuru MS, Secic M, Thomassen MJ, Erzurum SC. Decreased Cu, Zn–SOD activity in asthmatic airway epithelium: correction by inhaled corticosteroid in vivo. Am J Physiol Lung Cell Mol Physiol 1997; 272:L148–L154.

62. Smith LJ, Shamsuddin M, Sporn PH, Denenberg M, Anderson J. Reduced superoxide dismutase in lung cells of patients with asthma. Free Radic Biol Med 1997; 22:1301–1307.

63. Comhair SA, Bhathena PR, Dweik RA, Kavuru M, Erzurum SC. Rapid loss of superoxide dismutase activity during antigen-induced asthmatic response. Lancet 2000; 355:624.

64. Larsen GL, White CW, Takeda K, Loader JE, Nguyen DD, Joetham A, Groner Y, Gelfand EW. Mice that overexpress Cu/Zn superoxide dismutase are resistant to allergen-induced changes in airway control. Am J Physiol Lung Cell Mol Physiol 2000; 279:L350–L359.

65. Comhair SA, Bhathena PR, Farver C, Thunnissen FB, Erzurum SC. Extracellular glutathione peroxidase induction in asthmatic lungs: evidence for redox regulation of expression in human airway epithelial cells. FASEB J 2001; 15:70–78.

66. Smith LJ, Houston M, Anderson J. Increased levels of glutathione in bronchoalveolar lavage fluid from patients with asthma. Am Rev Respir Dis 1993; 147:1461–1464.

67. Barnes PJ. Mechanisms in COPD: differences from asthma. Chest 2000; 117:10S–14S.

68. Rahman I, MacNee W. Role of oxidants/antioxidants in smoking-induced lung diseases. Free Radic Biol Med 1996; 21:669–681.

69. Langen RC, Korn SH, Wouters EF. ROS in the local and systemic pathogenesis of COPD. Free Radic Biol Med 2003; 35:226–235.

70. Church DF, Pryor WA. Free-radical chemistry of cigarette smoke and its toxicological implications. Environ Health Perspect 1985; 64:111–126.

71. Rahman I, MacNee W. Lung glutathione and oxidative stress: implications in cigarette smoke-induced airway disease. Am J Physiol Lung Cell Mol Physiol 1999; 277:L1067–L1088.

72. McCusker K, Hoidal J. Selective increase of antioxidant enzyme activity in the alveolar macrophages from cigarette smokers and smoke-exposed hamsters. Am Rev Respir Dis 1990; 141:678–682.

73. Kondo T, Tagami S, Yoshioka A, Nishimura M, Kawakami Y. Current smoking of elderly men reduces antioxidants in alveolar macrophages. Am J Respir Crit Care Med 1994; 149:178–182.

74. Gilks CB, Price K, Wright JL, Churg A. Antioxidant gene expression in rat lung after exposure to cigarette smoke. Am J Pathol 1998; 152:269–278.

75. Rahman I, Morrison D, Donaldson K, MacNee W. Systemic oxidative stress in asthma, COPD, and smokers. Am J Respir Crit Care Med 1996; 154:1055–1060.

76. Strausz J, Muller-Quernheim J, Steppling H, Ferlinz R. Oxygen radical production by alveolar inflammatory cells in idiopathic pulmonary fibrosis. Am Rev Respir Dis 1990; 141:124–128.

77. Lakari E, Pääkkö P, Kinnula VL. Manganese superoxide dismutase, but not Cu–Zn superoxide dismutase, is highly expressed in the granulomas of pulmonary sarcoidosis and extrinsic allergic alveolitis. Am J Respir Crit Care Med 1998; 158:589–596.

78. Lakari E, Pääkkö P, Pietarinen-Runtti P, Kinnula VL. Manganese superoxide dismutase and catalase are coordinately expressed in the alveolar region in chronic interstitial pneumonias and granulomatous diseases of the lung. Am J Respir Crit Care Med 2000; 161:615–621.

79. Kinnula VL. Oxidant and antioxidant mechanisms of lung disease caused by asbestos fibres. Eur Respir J 1999; 14:706–716.

80. Janssen YM, Marsh JP, Absher MP, Hemenway D, Vacek PM, Leslie KO, Borm PJ, Mossman BT. Expression of antioxidant enzymes in rat lungs after inhalation of asbestos or silica. J Biol Chem 1992; 267:10625–10630.

81. Pron G, Mahrour N, Orlowski S, Tounekti O, Poddevin B, Belehradek J Jr, Mir LM. Internalisation of the bleomycin molecules responsible for bleomycin toxicity: a receptor-mediated endocytosis mechanism. Biochem Pharmacol 1999; 57:45–56.

82. Dorr RT. Bleomycin pharmacology: mechanism of action and resistance, and clinical pharmacokinetics. Semin Oncol 1992; 19:3–8.

83. Smith LL. Mechanism of paraquat toxicity in lung and its relevance to treatment. Hum Toxicol 1987; 6:31–36.

84. Saugstad OD. Role of xanthine oxidase and its inhibitor in hypoxia: reoxygenation injury. Pediatrics 1996; 98:103–107.

85. Lynch MJ, Grum CM, Gallagher KP, Bolling SF, Deeb GM, Morganroth ML. Xanthine oxidase inhibition attenuates ischemic-reperfusion lung injury. J Surg Res 1988; 44:538–544.

86. Linder N, Rapola J, Raivio KO. Cellular expression of xanthine oxidoreductase protein in normal human tissues. Lab Invest 1999; 79:967–974.

87. Kinnula VL, Sarnesto A, Heikkilä L, Toivonen H, Mattila S, Raivio KO. Assessment of xanthine oxidase in human lung and lung transplantation. Eur Respir J 1997; 10:676–680.

88. Pesonen EJ, Linder N, Raivio KO, Sarnesto A, Lapatto R, Höckerstedt K, Mäkisalo H, Andersson S. Circulating xanthine oxidase and neutrophil activation during human liver transplantation. Gastroenterology 1998; 114: 1009–1015.

89. Li C, Jackson RM. Reactive species mechanisms of cellular hypoxia-reoxygenation injury. Am J Physiol Cell Physiol 2002; 282:C227–C241.

90. Gorecki M, Beck Y, Hartman JR, Fischer M, Weiss L, Tochner Z, Slavin S, Nimrod A. Recombinant human superoxide dismutases: production and potential therapeutic uses. Free Radic Res Commun 1991; 1:401–410.

91. Freeman BA, Young SL, Crapo JD. Liposome-mediated augmentation of superoxide dismutase in endothelial cells prevents oxygen injury. J Biol Chem 1983; 258:12534–12542.

92. Buckley BJ, Tanswell AK, Freeman BA. Liposome-mediated augmentation of catalase in alveolar type II cells protects against H_2O_2 injury. J Appl Physiol 1987; 63:359–367.

93. Walther FJ, David-Cu R, Supnet MC, Longo ML, Fan BR, Bruni R. Uptake of antioxidants in surfactant liposomes by cultured alveolar type II cells is enhanced by SP-A. Am J Physiol Lung Cell Mol Physiol 1993; 265: L330–L339.

94. Turrens JF, Crapo JD, Freeman BA. Protection against oxygen toxicity by intravenous injection of liposome-entrapped catalase and superoxide dismutase. J Clin Invest 1984; 73:87–95.

95. Tanswell AK, Freeman BA. Liposome-entrapped antioxidant enzymes prevent lethal O_2 toxicity in the newborn rat. J Appl Physiol 1987; 63:347–352.

96. White CW, Jackson JH, Abuchowski A, Kazo GM, Mimmack RF, Berger EM, Freeman BA, McCord JM, Repine JE. Polyethylene glycol-attached

antioxidant enzymes decrease pulmonary oxygen toxicity in rats. J Appl Physiol 1989; 66:584–590.

97. Jacobson JM, Michael JR, Jafri MH, Gurtner GH. Antioxidants and antioxidant enzymes protect against pulmonary oxygen toxicity in the rabbit. J Appl Physiol 1990; 68:1252–1259.

98. Inoue M. Targeting superoxide dismutase by gene and protein engineering. Methods Enzymol 1994; 233:212–221.

99. Padmanabhan RV, Gudapaty R, Liener IE, Schwartz BA, Hoidal JR. Protection against pulmonary oxygen toxicity in rats by the intratracheal administration of liposome-encapsulated superoxide dismutase or catalase. Am Rev Respir Dis 1985; 132:164–167.

100. Davis JM, Rosenfeld WN, Sanders RJ, Gonenne A. Prophylactic effects of recombinant human superoxide dismutase in neonatal lung injury. J Appl Physiol 1993; 74:2234–2241.

101. Walther FJ, Nunez FL, David-Cu R, Hill KE. Mitigation of pulmonary oxygen toxicity in rats by intratracheal instillation of polyethylene glycol-conjugated antioxidant enzymes. Pediatr Res 1993; 33:332–335.

102. Walther FJ, David-Cu R, Lopez SL. Antioxidant-surfactant liposomes mitigate hyperoxic lung injury in premature rabbits. Am J Physiol 1995; 269:L613–L617.

103. Simonson SG, Welty-Wolf KE, Huang YC, Taylor DE, Kantrow SP, Carraway MS, Crapo JD, Piantadosi CA. Aerosolized manganese SOD decreases hyperoxic pulmonary injury in primates. I. Physiology and biochemistry. J Appl Physiol 1997; 83:550–558.

104. Welty-Wolf KE, Simonson SG, Huang YC, Kantrow SP, Carraway MS, Chang LY, Crapo JD, Piantadosi CA. Aerosolized manganese SOD decreases hyperoxic pulmonary injury in primates. II. Morphometric analysis. J Appl Physiol 1997; 83:559–568.

105. Davis JM, Richter SE, Biswas S, Rosenfeld WN, Parton L, Gewolb IH, Parad R, Carlo W, Couser RJ, Baumgart S, Atluru V, Salerno L, Kassem N. Long-term follow-up of premature infants treated with prophylactic, intratracheal recombinant human Cu–Zn superoxide dismutase. J Perinatol 2000; 20:213–216.

106. Tamagawa K, Taooka Y, Maeda A, Hiyama K, Ishioka S, Yamakido M. Inhibitory effects of a lecithinized superoxide dismutase on bleomycin-induced pulmonary fibrosis in mice. Am J Respir Crit Care Med 2000; 161: 1279–1284.

107. Mossman BT, Marsh JP, Sesko A, Hill S, Shatos MA, Doherty J, Petruska J, Adler KB, Hemenway D, Mickey R et al. Inhibition of lung injury, inflammation, and interstitial pulmonary fibrosis by polyethylene glycol-conjugated catalase in a rapid inhalation model of asbestosis. Am Rev Respir Dis 1990; 141:1266–1271.

108. Patel M, Day BJ. Metalloporphyrin class of therapeutic catalytic antioxidants. Trends Pharmacol Sci 1999; 20:359–364.

109. Aston K, Rath N, Naik A, Slomczynska U, Schall OF, Riley DP. Computer-aided design (CAD) of Mn(II) complexes: superoxide dismutase mimetics with catalytic activity exceeding the native enzyme. Inorg Chem 2001; 40:1779–1789.

110. Li Y, Huang TT, Carlson EJ, Melov S, Ursell PC, Olson JL, Noble LJ, Yoshimura MP, Berger C, Chan PH, Wallace DC, Epstein CJ. Dilated cardiomyopathy and neonatal lethality in mutant mice lacking manganese superoxide dismutase. Nat Genet 1995; 11:376–381.

111. Lebovitz RM, Zhang H, Vogel H, Cartwright JJ, Dionne L, Lu N, Huang S, Matzuk MM. Neurodegeneration, myocardial injury, and perinatal death in mitochondrial superoxide diamutase-deficient mice. Proc Natl Acad Sci USA 1996; 93:9782–9787.

112. Melov S, Coskun P, Patel M, Tuinstra R, Cottrell B, Jun AS, Zastawny TH, Dizdaroglu M, Goodman SI, Huang TT, Miziorko H, Epstein CJ, Wallace DC. Mitochondrial disease in superoxide dismutase 2 mutant mice. Proc Natl Acad Sci USA 1999; 96:846–851.

113. Melov S, Schneider JA, Day BJ, Hinerfeld D, Coskun P, Mirra SS, Crapo JD, Wallace DC. A novel neurological phenotype in mice lacking mitochondrial manganese superoxide dismutase. Nat Genet 1998; 18:159–163.

114. Day BJ, Shawen S, Liochev SI, Crapo JD. A metalloporphyrin superoxide dismutase mimetic protects against paraquat-induced endothelial cell injury in vitro. J Pharmacol Exp Ther 1995; 275:1227–1232.

115. Day BJ, Crapo JD. A metalloporphyrin superoxide dismutase mimetic protects against paraquat-induced lung injury in vivo. Toxicol Appl Pharmacol 1996; 140:94–100.

116. Wilborn AM, Evers LB, Canada AT. Oxygen toxicity to the developing lung of the mouse: role of reactive oxygen species. Pediatr Res 1996; 40: 225–232.

117. Oury TD, Thakker K, Menache M, Chang LY, Crapo JD, Day BJ. Attenuation of bleomycin-induced pulmonary fibrosis by a catalytic antioxidant metalloporphyrin. Am J Respir Cell Mol Biol 2001; 25:164–169.

118. Aslan M, Ryan TM, Adler B, Townes TM, Parks DA, Thompson JA, Tousson A, Gladwin MT, Patel RP, Tarpey MM, Batinic-Haberle I, White CR, Freeman BA. Oxygen radical inhibition of nitric oxide-dependent vascular function in sickle cell disease. Proc Natl Acad Sci USA 2001; 98: 15215–15220.

119. Tang K, Wagner PD, Breen EC. Lung-specific inactivation of VEGF in adult mice leads to emphysema like changes. [abstr]. Am J Respir Crit Care Med 2002; 165:8 (part 2 of 2), B54.

120. Tuder RM, Taraseviciene-Stewart L, Flores S, Salvemini D, Voelkel NF. M40419, a superoxide dismutase mimetic, prevents the development of emphysema induced by VEGF receptor blockade [abstr]. Am J Respir Crit Care Med 2002; 165:8 (part 2 of 2), A463.

121. Smith KR, Uyeminami DL, Kodavanti UP, Crapo JD, Chang L-Y, Pinkerton KE. Inhibition of tobacco smoke-induced lung inflammation by a catalytic antioxidant. Free Radic Biol Med. 2002; 15:1106–1114.

122. Gonzalez PK, Zhuang J, Doctrow SR, Malfroy B, Benson PF, Menconi MJ, Fink MP. Role of oxidant stress in the adult respiratory distress syndrome: evaluation of a novel antioxidant strategy in a porcine model of endotoxin-induced acute lung injury. Shock 1996; 6:S23–S26.

123. Zhang M, Nomura A, Uchida Y, Iijima H, Sakamoto T, Iishii Y, Morishima Y, Mochizuki M, Masuyama K, Hirano K, Sekizawa K. Ebselen suppresses late airway responses and airway inflammation in guinea pigs. Free Radic Biol Med 2002; 32:454–464.

124. Cotgreave IA, Johansson U, Westergren G, Moldeus PW, Brattsand R. The anti-inflammatory activity of ebselen but not thiols in experimental alveolitis and bronchiolitis. Agents Actions 1988; 24:313–319.

125. Belvisi MG, Haddad EB, Battram C, Birrell M, Foster M, Webber S. Anti-inflammatory properties of ebselen in a model of sephadex-induced lung inflammation. Eur Respir J 2000; 15:579–581.

126. Ishii Y, Hashimoto K, Hirano K, Morishima Y, Mochizuki M, Masuyama K, Nomura A, Sakamoto T, Uchida Y, Sagai M, Sekizawa K. Ebselen decreases ozone-induced pulmonary inflammation in rats. Lung 2000; 178:225–234.

127. Ren X, Xue Y, Liu J, Zhang K, Zheng J, Luo G, Guo C, Mu Y, Shen J. A novel cyclodextrin-derived tellurium compound with glutathione peroxidase activity. Chem biochem 2002; 3:356–363.

128. Chang LY, Subramaniam M, Yoder BA, Day BJ, Ellison MC, Sunday ME, Crapo JD. A catalytic antioxidant attenuates alveolar structural remodeling in bronchopulmonary dysplasia. Am J Respir Crit Care Med 2003; 167: 57–64.

129. Buhl R, Vogelmeier C, Critenden M, Hubbard RC, Hoyt RF, Wilson EM, Cantin AM, Crystal RG. Augmentation of glutathione in the fluid lining the epithelium of the lower respiratory tract by directly administering glutathione aerosol. Proc Natl Acad Sci USA 1990; 87:4063–4067.

130. Stabler SP, Morton RL, Winski SL, Allen RH, White CW. Effects of parenteral cysteine and glutathione feeding in a baboon model of severe prematurity. Am J Clin Nutr 2000; 72:1548–1557.

131. Anderson ME, Meister A. Intracellular delivery of cysteine. Methods Enzymol 1987; 143:313–325.

132. Aruoma OI, Halliwell B, Hoey BM, Butler J. The antioxidant action of *N*-acetylcysteine: its reaction with hydrogen peroxide, hydroxyl radical, superoxide, and hypochlorous acid. Free Radic Biol Med 1989; 6:593–597.

133. Winterbourn CC, Metodiewa D. Reactivity of biologically important thiol compounds with superoxide and hydrogen peroxide. Free Radic Biol Med 1999; 27:322–328.

134. Moldeus P, Cotgreave IA, Berggren M. Lung protection by a thiol-containing antioxidant: *N*-acetylcysteine. Respiration 1986; 1:31–42.

135. Phelps DT, Deneke SM, Daley DL, Fanburg BL. Elevation of glutathione levels in bovine pulmonary artery endothelial cells by *N*-acetylcysteine. Am J Respir Cell Mol Biol 1992; 7:293–299.

136. Shattuck KE, Rassin DK, Grinnell CD. N-acetylcysteine protects from glutathione depletion in rats exposed to hyperoxia. J Parenter Enteral Nutr 1998; 22:228–233.

137. Vale JA, Proudfoot AT. Paracetamol (acetaminophen) poisoning. Lancet 1995; 346:547–552.

138. Uttamsingh V, Baggs RB, Krenitsky DM, Anders MW. Immunohistochemical localization of the acylases that catalyze the deacetylation of *N*-acetyl-L-

cysteine and haloalkene-derived mercapturates. Drug Metab Dispos 2000; 28:625–632.

139. Traber J, Suter M, Walter P, Richter C. In vivo modulation of total and mitochondrial glutathione in rat liver. Depletion by phorone and rescue by N-acetylcysteine. Biochem Pharmacol 1992; 43:961–964.

140. Will Y, Fischer KA, Horton RA, Kaetzel RS, Brown MK, Hedstrom O, Lieberman MW, Reed DJ. Gamma-glutamyltranspeptidase-deficient knockout mice as a model to study the relationship between glutathione status, mitochondrial function, and cellular function. Hepatology 2000; 32:740–749.

141. Asikainen TM, Huang TT, Taskinen E, Levonen AL, Carlson E, Lapatto R, Epstein CJ, Raivio KO. Increased sensitivity of homozygous Sod2 mutant mice to oxygen toxicity. Free Radic Biol Med 2002; 32:175–186.

142. Langley SC, Kelly FJ. *N*-acetylcysteine ameliorates hyperoxic lung injury in the preterm guinea pig. Biochem Pharmacol 1993; 45:841–846.

143. Davreux CJ, Soric I, Nathens AB, Watson RW, McGilvray ID, Suntres ZE, Shek PN, Rotstein OD. *N*-acetyl cysteine attenuates acute lung injury in the rat. Shock 1997; 8:432–438.

144. Suter PM, Domenighetti G, Schaller MD, Laverriere MC, Ritz R, Perret C. *N*-acetylcysteine enhances recovery from acute lung injury in man. A randomized, double-blind, placebo-controlled clinical study. Chest 1994; 105: 190–194.

145. Bernard GR, Wheeler AP, Arons MM, Morris PE, Paz HL, Russell JA, Wright PE. A trial of antioxidants *N*-acetylcysteine and procysteine in ARDS. The antioxidant in ARDS study group. Chest 1997; 112:164–172.

146. Domenighetti G, Suter PM, Schaller MD, Ritz R, Perret C. Treatment with *N*-acetylcysteine during acute respiratory distress syndrome: a randomized, double-blind, placebo-controlled clinical study. J Crit Care 1997; 12:177–182.

147. Ahola T, Lapatto R, Raivio KO, Selander B, Stigson L, Jonsson B, Jonsbo F, Esberg G, Stovring S, Kjartansson S, Stiris T, Lossius K, Virkola K, Fellman V. *N*-acetylcysteine does not prevent bronchopulmonary dysplasia in immature infants: a randomized controlled trial. J Pediatr 2003; 143:713–719.

148. Cortijo J, Cerda-Nicolas M, Serrano A, Bioque G, Estrela JM, Santangelo F, Esteras A, Llombart-Bosch A, Morcillo EJ. Attenuation by oral *N*-acetylcysteine of bleomycin-induced lung injury in rats. Eur Respir J 2001; 17: 1228–1235.

149. Hagiwara SI, Ishii Y, Kitamura S. Aerosolized administration of *N*-acetylcysteine attenuates lung fibrosis induced by bleomycin in mice. Am J Respir Crit Care Med 2000; 162:225–231.

150. Weinbroum AA, Kluger Y, Abraham RB, Shapira I, Karchevski E, Rudick V. Lung preconditioning with *N*-acetyl-L-cysteine prevents reperfusion injury after liver no flow-reflow: a dose–response study. Transplantation 2001; 71:300–306.

151. Levy MA, Sikorski B, Bray TM. Selective elevation of glutathione levels in target tissues with L-2-oxothiazolidine-4-carboxylate (OTC) protects against hyperoxia-induced lung damage in protein-energy malnourished rats: implications for a new treatment strategy. J Nutr 1998; 128:671–676.

152. Darlow BA, Winterbourn CC, Inder TE, Graham PJ, Harding JE, Weston PJ, Austin NC, Elder DE, Mogridge N, Buss IH, Sluis KB. The effect of selenium supplementation on outcome in very low birth weight infants: a randomized controlled trial. The New Zealand neonatal study group. J Pediatr 2000; 136:473–480.

153. Das KC, Lewis-Molock Y, White CW. Activation of NF-kappa B and elevation of MnSOD gene expression by thiol reducing agents in lung adenocarcinoma (A549) cells. Am J Physiol Lung Cell Mol Physiol 1995; 269: L588–L602.

154. deLemos RA, Roberts RJ, Coalson JJ, deLemos JA, Null DMJ, Gerstmann DR. Toxic effects associated with the administration of deferoxamine in the premature baboon with hyaline membrane disease. Am J Dis Child 1990; 144:915–919.

155. Watts JL, Milner R, Zipursky A, Paes B, Ling E, Gill G, Fletcher B, Rand C. Failure of supplementation with vitamin E to prevent bronchopulmonary dysplasia in infants less than 1500 g birth weight. Eur Respir J 1991; 4: 188–190.

156. Ehrenkranz RA, Ablow RC, Warshaw JB. Effect of vitamin E on the development of oxygen-induced lung injury in neonates. Ann NY Acad Sci 1982; 393:452–466.

157. Tyson JE, Wright LL, Oh W, Kennedy KA, Mele L, Ehrenkranz RA, Stoll BJ, Lemons JA, Stevenson DK, Bauer CR, Korones SB, Fanaroff AA. Vitamin A supplementation for extremely-low-birth-weight infants. National institute of child health and human development neonatal research network. N Engl J Med 1999; 340:1962–1968.

158. Langford SD, Bidani A, Postlethwait EM. Ozone-reactive absorption by pulmonary epithelial lining fluid constituents. Toxicol Appl Pharmacol 1995; 132:122–130.

159. Ding L, Liu Z, Zhu Z, Luo G, Zhao D, Ni J. Biochemical characterization of selenium-containing catalytic antibody as a cytosolic glutathione peroxidase mimic. Biochem J 1998; 332:251–255.

160. Ren X, Gao S, You D, Huang H, Liu Z, Mu Y, Liu J, Zhang Y, Yan G, Luo G, Yang T, Shen J. Cloning and expression of a single-chain catalytic antibody that acts as a glutathione peroxidase mimic with high catalytic efficiency. Biochem J 2001; 359:369–374.

161. Su D, Ren X, You D, Li D, Mu Y, Yan G, Zhang Y, Luo Y, Xue Y, Shen J, Liu Z, Luo G. Generation of three selenium-containing catalytic antibodies with high catalytic efficiency using a novel hapten design method. Arch Biochem Biophys 2001; 395:177–184.

162. Luo X, Sedlackova L, Belcastro R, Cabacungan J, Lye SJ, Tanswell AK. Effect of the 21-aminosteroid U74389G on oxygen-induced free radical production, lipid peroxidation, and inhibition of lung growth in neonatal rats. Pediatr Res 1999; 46:215–223.

163. Jankov RP, Luo X, Cabacungan J, Belcastro R, Frndova H, Lye SJ, Tanswell AK. Endothelin-1 and O_2-mediated pulmonary hypertension in neonatal rats: a role for products of lipid peroxidation. Pediatr Res 2000; 48:289–298.

164. Takeyoshi I, Iwanami K, Kamoshita N, Takahashi T, Kobayashi J, Tomizawa N, Kawashima Y, Matsumoto K, Morishita Y. Effect of lazaroid U-74389G on pulmonary ischemia-reperfusion injury in dogs. J Invest Surg 2001; 14:83–92.

165. Kuwaki K, Komatsu K, Sohma H, Abe T. Lazaroid U74389G ameliorates ischemia-reperfusion injury in the rat lung transplant model. Ann Thorac Cardiovasc Surg 1999; 5:11–17.

166. Hillinger S, Schmid RA, Stammberger U, Boehler A, Schob OM, Zollinger A, Weder W. Donor and recipient treatment with the Lazaroid U-74006F do not improve post-transplant lung function in swine. Eur J Cardiothorac Surg 1999; 15:475–480.

167. Hallman M, Glumoff V, Rämet M. Surfactant in respiratory distress syndrome and lung injury. Comp Biochem Physiol A Mol Integr Physiol 2001; 129:287–294.

168. Bridges JP, Davis HW, Damodarasamy M, Kuroki Y, Howles G, Hui DY, McCormack FX. Pulmonary surfactant proteins A and D are potent endogenous inhibitors of lipid peroxidation and oxidative cellular injury. J Biol Chem 2000; 275:38848–38855.

169. Blanco O, Catala A. Surfactant protein A inhibits the non-enzymatic lipid peroxidation of porcine lung surfactant. Prostaglandins Leukot Essent Fatty Acids 2001; 65:185–190.

170. Matalon S, Holm BA, Baker RR, Whitfield MK, Freeman BA. Characterization of antioxidant activities of pulmonary surfactant mixtures. Biochim Biophys Acta 1990; 1035:121–127.

171. Rosseau S, Hammerl P, Maus U, Gunther A, Seeger W, Grimminger F, Lohmeyer J. Surfactant protein A down-regulates proinflammatory cytokine production evoked by *Candida albicans* in human alveolar macrophages and monocytes. J Immunol 1999; 163:4495–4502.

172. Yoshida M, Korfhagen TR, Whitsett JA. Surfactant protein D regulates NF-kappa B and matrix metalloproteinase production in alveolar macrophages via oxidant-sensitive pathways. J Immunol 2001; 166:7514–7519.

173. McCormack FX, Whitsett JA. The pulmonary collectins, SP-A and SP-D, orchestrate innate immunity in the lung. J Clin Invest 2002; 109:707–712.

174. Crouch E, Wright JR. Surfactant proteins a and d and pulmonary host defense. Annu Rev Physiol 2001; 63:521–554.

175. Mason RJ, Greene K, Voelker DR. Surfactant protein A and surfactant protein D in health and disease. Am J Physiol 1998; 275:L1–L13.

176. Kessler DL, Truog WE, Murphy JH, Palmer S, Standaert TA, Woodrum DE, Hodson WA. Experimental hyaline membrane disease in the premature monkey: effects of antenatal dexamethasone. Am Rev Respir Dis 1982; 126:62–69.

177. Frank L. Prenatal dexamethasone treatment improves survival of newborn rats during prolonged high O_2 exposure. Pediatr Res 1992; 32:215–221.

178. Crowley P. Prophylactic corticosteroids for preterm birth (Cochrane review). Cochrane Database Syst Rev 2000; 2:CD000065.

179. Frank L, Lewis PL, Sosenko IR. Dexamethasone stimulation of fetal rat lung antioxidant enzyme activity in parallel with surfactant stimulation. Pediatrics 1985; 75:569–574.

180. Clerch LB, Iqbal J, Massaro D. Perinatal rat lung catalase gene expression: influence of corticosteroid and hyperoxia. Am J Physiol Lung Cell Mol Physiol 1991; 260:L428–L433.

181. Halliday HL, Ehrenkranz RA. Delayed (>3 weeks) postnatal corticosteroids for chronic lung disease in preterm infants (Cochrane review). Cochrane Database Syst Rev 2001; 2:CD001145.

182. Massaro GD, Massaro D. Retinoic acid treatment partially rescues failed septation in rats and in mice. Am J Physiol Lung Cell Mol Physiol 2000; 278: L955–L960.

183. Rodriguez-Pierce M, Sosenko IR, Frank L. Prenatal thyroid releasing hormone and thyroid releasing hormone plus dexamethasone lessen the survival of newborn rats during prolonged high O_2 exposure. Pediatr Res 1992; 32: 407–411.

184. Chen Y, Whitney PL, Frank L. Negative regulation of antioxidant enzyme gene expression in the developing fetal rat lung by prenatal hormonal treatments. Pediatr Res 1993; 33:171–176.

185. Ballard RA, Ballard PL, Cnaan A, Pinto-Martin J, Davis DJ, Padbury JF, Phibbs RH, Parer JT, Hart MC, Mannino FL, Sawai SK. Antenatal thyrotropin-releasing hormone to prevent lung disease in preterm infants. North American thyrotropin-releasing hormone study group. N Engl J Med 1998; 338:493–498.

186. Eber E, Zach MS. Long term sequelae of bronchopulmonary dysplasia (chronic lung disease of infancy). Thorax 2001; 56:317–323.

187. Van Marter LJ, Allred EN, Leviton A, Pagano M, Parad R, Moore M. Antenatal glucocorticoid treatment does not reduce chronic lung disease among surviving preterm infants. J Pediatr 2001; 138:198–204.

188. Saugstad OD. Resuscitation with room-air or oxygen supplementation. Clin Perinatol 1998; 25:741–756.

189. Vento M, Asensi M, Sastre J, Garcia-Sala F, Viña J. Six years of experience with the use of room air for the resuscitation of asphyxiated newly born term infants. Biol Neonate 2001; 79:261–267.

190. Kinsella JP, Abman SH. Inhaled nitric oxide: current and future uses in neonates. Semin Perinatol 2000; 24:387–395.

191. Haataja R, Marttila R, Uimari P, Löfgren J, Rämet M, Hallman M. Respiratory distress syndrome: evaluation of genetic susceptibility and protection by transmission disequilibrium test. Hum Genet 2001; 109:351–355.

192. Clark DA, Pincus LG, Oliphant M, Hubbell C, Oates RP, Davey FR. HLA-A2 and chronic lung disease in neonates. JAMA 1982; 248:1868–1869.

193. Cho HY, Jedlicka AE, Reddy SP, Zhang LY, Kensler TW, Kleeberger SR. Linkage analysis of susceptibility to hyperoxia. Nrf2 is a candidate gene. Am J Respir Cell Mol Biol 2002; 26:42–51.

194. Cho HY, Jedlicka AE, Reddy SP, Kensler TW, Yamamoto M, Zhang LY, Kleeberger SR. Role of NRF2 in protection against hyperoxic lung injury in mice. Am J Respir Cell Mol Biol 2002; 26:175–182.

195. Kleeberger SR, Reddy S, Zhang LY, Jedlicka AE. Genetic susceptibility to ozone-induced lung hyperpermeability: role of toll-like receptor 4. Am J Respir Cell Mol Biol 2000; 22:620–627.

196. Flaherty DM, Monick MM, Hunninghake GW. AP endonucleases and the many functions of Ref-1. Am J Respir Cell Mol Biol 2001; 25:664–667.

197. He YH II, Wu M, Kobune M, Xu Y, Kelley MR, Martin WJ. Expression of yeast apurinic/apyrimidinic endonuclease (APN1) protects lung epithelial cells from bleomycin toxicity. Am J Respir Cell Mol Biol 2001; 25:692–698.

198. Prieto-Alamo MJ, Laval F. Overexpression of the human HAP1 protein sensitizes cells to the lethal effect of bioreductive drugs. Carcinogenesis 1999; 20:415–419.

199. Grishko V, Solomon M, Wilson GL, LeDoux SP, Gillespie MN. Oxygen radical-induced mitochondrial DNA damage and repair in pulmonary vascular endothelial cell phenotypes. Am J Physiol Lung Cell Mol Physiol 2001; 280:L1300–L1308.

200. Helt CE, Rancourt RC, Staversky RJ, O'Reilly MA. p53-dependent induction of p21(Cip1/WAF1/Sdi1) protects against oxygen-induced toxicity. Toxicol Sci 2001; 63:214–222.

201. Rancourt RC, Keng PC, Helt CE, O'Reilly MA. The role of p21(CIP1/WAF1) in growth of epithelial cells exposed to hyperoxia. Am J Physiol Lung Cell Mol Physiol 2001; 280:L617–L626.

202. O'Reilly MA, Staversky RJ, Watkins RH, Reed CK, de Mesy Jensen KL, Finkelstein JN, Keng PC. The cyclin-dependent kinase inhibitor p21 protects the lung from oxidative stress. Am J Respir Cell Mol Biol 2001; 24:703–710.

203. Panos RJ, Bak PM, Simonet WS, Rubin JS, Smith LJ. Intratracheal instillation of keratinocyte growth factor decreases hyperoxia-induced mortality in rats. J Clin Invest 1995; 96:2026–2033.

204. Wu KI, Pollack N, Panos RJ, Sporn PH, Kamp DW. Keratinocyte growth factor promotes alveolar epithelial cell DNA repair after H_2O_2 exposure. Am J Physiol 1998; 275:L780–L787.

205. Vivekananda J, Awasthi V, Awasthi S, Smith DB, King RJ. Hepatocyte growth factor is elevated in chronic lung injury and inhibits surfactant metabolism. Am J Physiol Lung Cell Mol Physiol 2000; 278:L382–L392.

206. Ware LB, Matthay MA. Keratinocyte and hepatocyte growth factors in the lung: roles in lung development, inflammation, and repair. Am J Physiol Lung Cell Mol Physiol 2002; 282:L924–L940.

207. Bast A, Haenen GR, Doelman CJ. Oxidants and antioxidants: state of the art. Am J Med 1991; 91:2S–13S.

208. Dalton TP, Shertzer HG, Puga A. Regulation of gene expression by reactive oxygen. Annu Rev Pharmacol Toxicol 1999; 39:67–101.

209. Jankov RP, Negus A, Tanswell AK. Antioxidants as therapy in the newborn: some words of caution. Pediatr Res 2001; 50:681–687.

210. White CW, Avraham KB, Shanley PF, Groner Y. Transgenic mice with expression of elevated levels of copper–zinc superoxide dismutase in the lungs are resistant to pulmonary oxygen toxicity. J Clin Invest 1991; 87:2162–2168.

211. Ho YS. Transgenic models for the study of lung biology and disease. Am J Physiol Lung Cell Mol Physiol 1994; 266:L319–L353.

212. Elroy SO, Bernstein Y, Groner Y. Overproduction of human Cu/Zn-superoxide dismutase in transfected cells: extenuation of paraquat-mediated cytotoxicity and enhancement of lipid peroxidation. EMBO J 1986; 5:615–622.

213. de Haan JB, Cristiano F, Iannello R, Bladier C, Kelner MJ, Kola I. Elevation in the ratio of Cu/Zn-superoxide dismutase to glutathione peroxidase activity induces features of cellular senescence and this effect is mediated by hydrogen peroxide. Hum Mol Genet 1996; 5:283–292.

214. Ilizarov AM, Koo HC, Kazzaz JA, Mantell LL, Li Y, Bhapat R, Pollack S, Horowitz S, Davis JM. Overexpression of manganese superoxide dismutase protects lung epithelial cells against oxidant injury. Am J Respir Cell Mol Biol 2001; 24:436–441.

215. Danel C, Erzurum SC, Prayssac P, Eissa NT, Crystal RG, Herve P, Baudet B, Mazmanian M, Lemarchand P. Gene therapy for oxidant injury-related diseases: adenovirus-mediated transfer of superoxide dismutase and catalase cDNAs protects against hyperoxia but not against ischemia–reperfusion lung injury. Hum Gene Ther 1998; 9:1487–1496.

216. Gardner PR, Raineri I, Epstein LB, White CW. Superoxide radical and iron modulate aconitase activity in mammalian cells. J Biol Chem 1995; 270: 13399–13405.

217. Gardner PR, Nguyen DD, White CW. Aconitase is a sensitive and critical target of oxygen poisoning in cultured mammalian cells and in rat lungs. Proc Natl Acad Sci USA 1994; 91:12248–12252.

218. Ahmad S, White CW, Chang LY, Schneider BK, Allen CB. Glutamine protects mitochondrial structure and function in oxygen toxicity. Am J Physiol Lung Cell Mol Physiol 2001; 280:L779–L791.

219. Van Remmen H, Williams MD, Guo Z, Estlack L, Yang H, Carlson EJ, Epstein CJ, Huang TT, Richardson A. Knockout mice heterozygous for Sod2 show alterations in cardiac mitochondrial function and apoptosis. Am J Physiol Heart Circ Physiol 2001; 281:H1422–H1432.

220. Huang TT, Carlson EJ, Kozy HM, Mantha S, Goodman SI, Ursell PC, Epstein CJ. Genetic modification of prenatal lethality and dilated cardiomyopathy in Mn superoxide dismutase mutant mice. Free Radic Biol Med 2001; 31:1101–1110.

221. Wong GH. Protective roles of cytokines against radiation: induction of mitochondrial MnSOD. Biochim Biophys Acta 1995; 1271:205–209.

222. Bai J, Rodriguez AM, Melendez JA, Cederbaum AI. Overexpression of catalase in cytosolic or mitochondrial compartment protects HepG2 cells against oxidative injury. J Biol Chem 1999; 274:26217–26224.

223. Schriner SE, Smith AC, Dang NH, Fukuchi K, Martin GM. Overexpression of wild-type and nuclear-targeted catalase modulates resistance to oxidative stress but does not alter spontaneous mutant frequencies at APRT. Mutat Res 2000; 449:21–31.

224. McDonald RJ, Berger EM, White CW, White JG, Freeman BA, Repine JE. Effect of superoxide dismutase encapsulated in liposomes or conjugated with polyethylene glycol on neutrophil bactericidal activity in vitro and bacterial clearance in vivo. Am Rev Respir Dis 1985; 131:633–637.

225. Nelson SK, Bose SK, McCord JM. The toxicity of high-dose superoxide dismutase suggests that superoxide can both initiate and terminate lipid peroxidation in the reperfused heart. Free Radic Biol Med 1994; 16:195–200.

17

Vascular Therapies in Lung Injury

MAHESH BOMMARAJU, VASANTH H. KUMAR,
SATYAN LAKSHMINRUSIMHA, RITA M. RYAN, and
FREDERICK C. MORIN, III

*Department of Pediatrics, State University of New York (SUNY) at Buffalo,
The Women & Children's Hospital of Buffalo,
Buffalo, New York, U.S.A.*

I. Overview

This chapter details vascular-based therapies for lung injury and associated
acute respiratory failure. Physiological processes contributing to the disruption of pulmonary vascular regulation in lung injury are also described
(Chapter 8 gives additional details on mechanisms and mediators important
in pulmonary vascular dysfunction). During acute injury, the overall balance of vasoconstriction and vasodilation in the lungs is shifted towards
vasoconstriction, leading to ventilation/perfusion (V_A/Q) mismatching,
increased pulmonary vascular resistance (PVR), and pulmonary hypertension (PH). These factors, along with associated decreases in cardiac output,
compromise gas exchange and reduce systemic oxygen delivery. This chapter discusses pharmacologic therapies targeting various aspects of injury-
associated pulmonary vascular pathophysiology. Particular coverage is
devoted to the clinical use of short-acting inhaled vasodilators normally
synthesized by the vascular endothelium: nitric oxide (NO) and prostacyclin
(PGI_2). Therapies utilizing phosphodiesterase (PDE) inhibitors or other

agents that work in concert with NO and PGI_2 are also covered. In addition, the use of selective vasoconstrictors, anticoagulants, and growth factors in the treatment of pulmonary vascular dysfunction is also noted. An important emphasis of discussion is that continuing mechanistic basic research is crucial for improving understanding about regulatory pathways and processes involved in vascular pathology in lung injury to facilitate future therapeutic development.

II. Introduction

Numerous events occur during the dynamic process of injury to disrupt the normal functions of the parenchyma and vasculature of the lungs. As detailed elsewhere in this book, significant advances have occurred in understanding lung injury in general as well as the specific roles of the pulmonary vasculature in its pathophysiology. Clinical acute lung injury (ALI) and the acute respiratory distress syndrome (ARDS) arise from a diverse set of etiologies involving direct and indirect insults to the lungs (Chapter 3). By definition, patients with ALI/ARDS suffer from acute hypoxemic respiratory failure. Noncardiogenic pulmonary edema is an early prominent aspect of pathology, and hemorrhage with fibrin deposition may also occur. The early exudative pathology of ALI/ARDS can also progress through a proliferative phase to more chronic injury with hyaline membrane formation and alveolar consolidation. The severity and persistence of the innate inflammatory response is a major determinant of the progression and outcome of clinical lung injury. A host of mediators produced by pulmonary cells and leukocytic cells are involved in the inflammatory pathophysiology of acute and chronic lung injury (Chapters 3–6) (1).

Inflammation and tissue injury in ALI/ARDS disrupt the normal regulation of the pulmonary circulation (Fig. 1). The overall balance between vasodilation and vasoconstriction within the pulmonary circulation becomes shifted in the direction of vasoconstriction for several reasons. Damage to the pulmonary vascular endothelium results in the loss of endothelium-derived vasodilators. In addition, the inflammatory cascade causes the release of multiple mediators that by themselves, or via the cyclo-oxygenase and lipo-oxygenase pathways, promote vasoconstriction of the pulmonary vascular bed, and at times, inappropriate vasodilation in poorly ventilated lung units. As hypoxic pulmonary vasoconstriction worsens, additional mediators of vasoconstriction are released while mediators of vasodilation are down-regulated. The overall shift towards vasoconstriction in acute injury directly increases PVR. Perivascular edema in association with increased endothelial permeability also increases PVR, and this in turn leads to PH, increased right ventricular (RV) afterload, and decreased cardiac output (Fig. 1) (2).

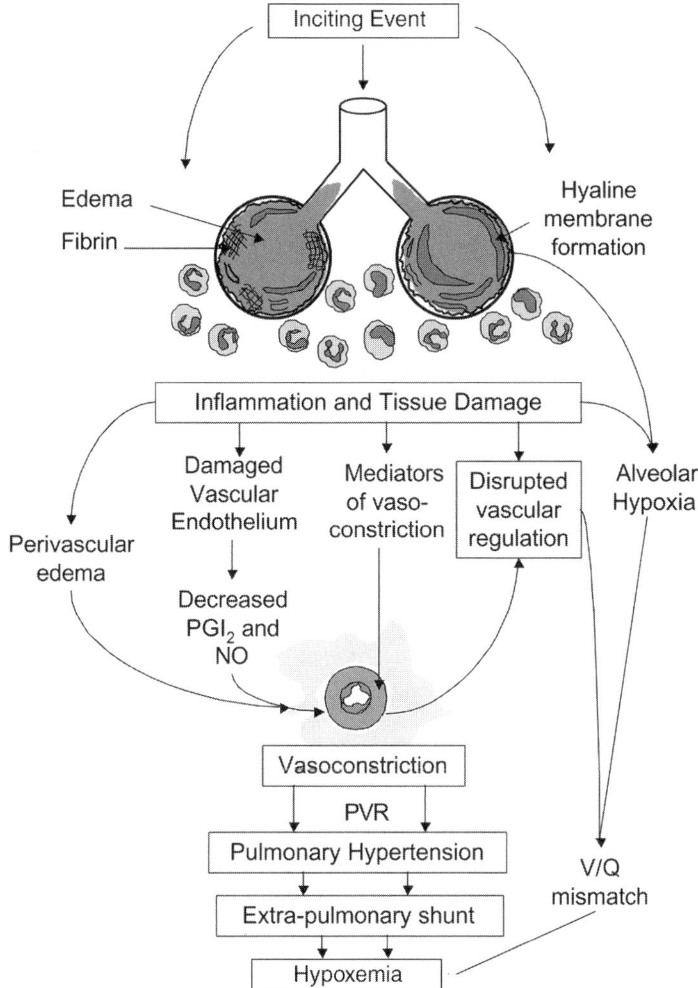

Figure 1 The cascade of events that alter the pulmonary circulation in acute lung injury. A variety of factors affect the pulmonary circulation during acute injury. Inflammation and tissue damage decrease the production of vasodiliatory mediators like nitric oxide (NO) and prostaglandin I_2 (PGI_2 or prostacyclin), while increasing the levels of vasoconstrictive mediators. This leads to increased pulmonary vascular resistance (PVR), pulmonary hypertension, intra-pulmonary shunting (ventilation–perfusion (V_A/Q) mismatching), and hypoxemia. In neonates with lung injury, extra-pulmonary shunting through the ductus arteriosis may also occur. See text for details.

If the inflammatory cascade is sufficiently severe and persistent, it causes chronic as well as acute changes in the pulmonary parenchyma and vasculature. Increased production of vasoconstrictors not only acutely elevates PVR, but also can lead to structural changes in the pulmonary vasculature (3). A decreased ability to release or respond to vasodilators that normally counteract hypertensive stimuli may also augment the severity of PH and accelerate the rate of vascular remodeling (4). Similar pathways are thought to contribute to the development of bronchopulmonary dysplasia (BPD) and subsequent *cor pulmonale* in newborns (5). The inflammatory cascade is implicated early in this disease, and infants with higher levels of amniotic fluid proinflammatory cytokines like interleukin (IL)-1β, IL-6, IL-8, and tumor necrosis factor α (TNFα) are at higher risk to later develop BPD (6). Affected infants have pulmonary vascular abnormalities that include an increase in pulmonary arterial medial smooth muscle thickness and the extension of muscle into smaller, more peripheral arteries (7). Infants who die of BPD have significant changes in the pulmonary vasculature with pathologic evidence of increased muscularization of arterioles. Infants with BPD also have increased muscularization of bronchioles and bronchi (8), which contributes to their reactive airways disease. Abnormal muscularization in the media of intra-acinar pulmonary arteries also occurs in infants with the acute lung disease, persistent pulmonary hypertension of the newborn (PPHN) (9), as well as in animal models of PPHN (10).

Pulmonary vascular dysfunction in lung injury causes decreased systemic oxygen delivery through several mechanisms (Fig. 2). The overall shift towards vasoconstriction in lung injury decreases blood flow through the microcirculation so that gas exchange is reduced. The distribution of pulmonary blood flow is also affected, in that a smaller proportion flows through well-ventilated gas exchange units (acini) relative to poorly ventilated or nonventilated acini. This V_A/Q mismatching (also called intrapulmonary shunting) causes a net desaturation of pulmonary venous blood, resulting in decreased systemic oxygen delivery. In addition, systemic oxygen delivery is decreased in lung injury if cardiac output is reduced by the increased afterload caused by increased PVR and hypertension. Decreases in cardiac output can also cause decreased mixed venous oxygen saturation due to increased tissue extraction.

As described in following sections, vascular-based therapies for lung injury have primarily been directed at counteracting abnormal vascular regulation so as to decrease PVR. The challenge has been to decrease PVR selectively, so that blood flow is increased in well ventilated acini but not in poorly ventilated acini or in the systemic circulation. The most successful strategy has been to use inhaled vasodilators such as NO and PGI$_2$, which have very short half-lives and also function endogenously as local vasodilators. Since these agents act by increasing the synthesis of cyclic nucleotides in vascular smooth muscle, a therapeutic alternative is to increase pulmonary vasodilation by blocking PDE enzymes that clear cyclic nucleotides. Other therapeutic approaches that have had some success in lung injury involve combining a vasodilator with a vasoconstrictor to reduce

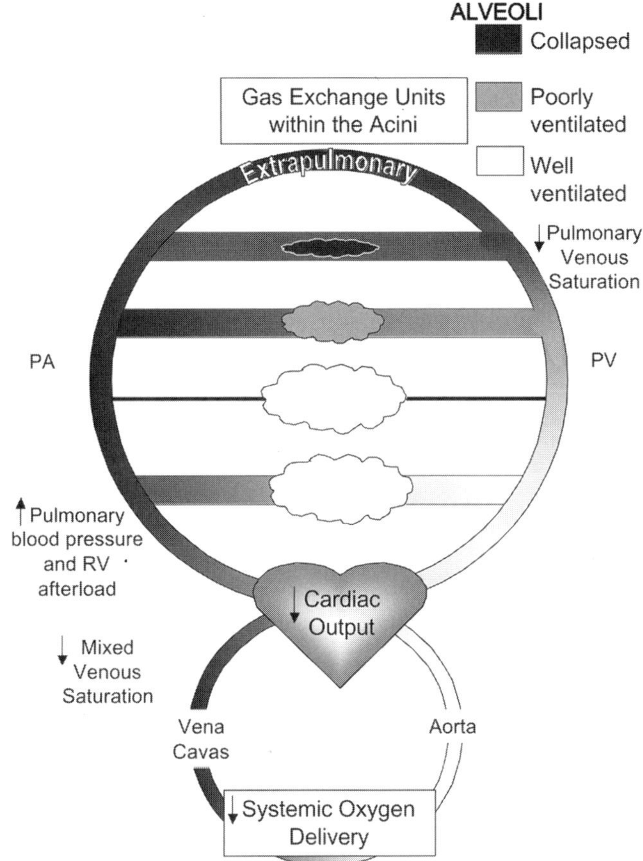

Figure 2 Disruption of pulmonary vascular regulation in lung injury causes decreased systemic oxygen delivery. Nonproductive blood flow through collapsed and poorly ventilated alveoli, as well as reduced blood flow through well-ventilated alveoli, lead to ventilation–perfusion mismatching and a reduced oxygen saturation in pulmonary venous blood. In addition, increased pulmonary vascular resistance and pulmonary hypertension increase the afterload on the right ventricle and decrease cardiac output. Decreases in pulmonary venous saturation and cardiac output both decrease systemic oxygen delivery. Extrapulmonary (ductal) shunting in neonates with lung injury can also contribute to arterial desaturation. PA—pulmonary artery; PV—pulmonary vein; ■—deoxygenated blood; □—oxygenated blood; shades of gray represent intermediate degrees of oxygenation.

blood flow to poorly ventilated acini, or with a lung recruitment strategy to increase the tissue area reached by the inhaled dilator. Additional vascular therapies have targeted coagulation/microthrombosis and the increased permeability of the pulmonary microcirculation during acute injury. Before detailing these therapeutic approaches, the next section describes injury-related alterations of pulmonary vascular regulation.

III. Disruption of Normal Pulmonary Vascular Regulation in Acute Injury

There are a variety of physiologically important biochemical mediators of vasoactivity, including prostaglandins (PGs), NO, leukotrienes, thromboxane, endothelin (ET-1), platelet-derived growth factor (PDGF), and platelet-activating factor (PAF). In addition to having direct vasoactive properties, many of these mediators have regulatory roles and induce or moderate the production of other factors. There are thus significant interactions between these vasomediators and inflammatory mediators involved in innate host defense and lung injury.

A. Increased Vasoconstriction

Arachidonic Acid Metabolites (PGs, Leukotrienes, Thromboxane)

During the innate inflammatory response, arachidonic acid (AA) metabolism generates potent vasoactive substances via the cyclo-oxygenase and lipo-oxygenase pathways resulting in the synthesis of $PGF_{2\alpha}$, thromboxane and leukotrienes that cause pulmonary vasoconstriction in preterm, newborn, or adult animals (11–18). Other PGs such as PGD_2 can be pulmonary dilators or pulmonary constrictors depending on age and physiologic circumstances (19,20).

Other Pulmonary Vasoconstrictors (ET-1, PDGF, PAF)

Hypoxia and other stresses cause pulmonary endothelial cells to regulate vascular tone by releasing several important vasoconstrictors including ET-1, PDGF (21), and PAF. ET-1 is a potent vasoconstrictor (22) as well as a smooth muscle mitogen (23). ET-1 also plays a role in the production of cytokines (24), AA metabolism, and the generation of oxygen free radicals (25). ET-1 production is increased in response to hypoxia (26), and increased ET-1 levels have been demonstrated in adults with primary pulmonary hypertension (PPH) (27) and in infants with PPHN (28). PDGF causes vasoconstriction of pulmonary blood vessels in acute hypoxia (29), and also generates vascular smooth muscle cell (SMC) hyperplasia in chronic hypoxia (30). PAF has been implicated as a significant early mediator of cellular metabolic dysfunction, microvascular leak, and pulmonary vasoconstriction in the acute stages of Gram-negative sepsis (31). Acute systemic sepsis with *Escherichia coli* (*E. coli*) bacteria rapidly causes PH in association with increased PAF, which is also involved in the production of ET-1 and neutrophil activation. When the PAF receptor antagonist WEB 2086 is given to adult rats with *E. coli* bacteremia, both PH and capillary leak are diminished (31). The lung appears to be particularly susceptible to PAF, although this mediator also induces systemic hypotension and tachycardia (32,33).

Loss of Vasodilators

The normal tone of pulmonary vascular smooth muscle involves a balance of vasorelaxation and vasoconstriction. During lung injury, damaged vasodilating mechanisms become inadequate to oppose vasoconstriction (34–37). The principal intracellular mechanisms of pulmonary vasodilation are mediated either through cyclic adenosine $3',5'$-monophosphate (cAMP) or cyclic guanosine $3',5'$-monophosphate (cGMP). cAMP-mediated pulmonary vasodilation has been shown to be dysfunctional in animals with acute pulmonary injury from mesenteric ischemia–reperfusion (38). Impairments in β-adrenergic signal transduction in hypoxia may be involved with dysfunction of cAMP-mediated mechanisms of pulmonary vasodilation (36). Injury-associated decreases in cGMP and NO production also have been shown to lead to vasoconstriction (35,36,39). Loss of endothelium-dependent relaxation in pulmonary vessels, for example, contributes to vasoconstriction and the sustained PH that develops after prolonged exposure to endotoxin (35). In addition to affecting the magnitude and distribution of pulmonary blood flow, PH in concert with elevated vascular permeability also causes pulmonary edema (40).

IV. Vasodilator Therapy in Lung Injury

As described above, the vascular pathophysiology of acute pulmonary injury includes vasospasm and net vasoconstriction, intrapulmonary (and sometimes extrapulmonary) shunting, V_A/Q mismatching, and increased PVR and PH (Figs. 1 and 2). Because of the shift towards overall pulmonary vasoconstriction, an important group of therapies for acute pulmonary injury utilizes pharmacologic delivery of vasodilators. Of particular interest are selective pulmonary vasodilators and delivery methods that can potentially reverse inappropriate vasoconstriction in well ventilated regions of the lungs while having much less effect on poorly ventilated regions or the systemic circulation. The most successful of these agents have been substances such as PGI_2 and NO that are also produced endogenously in normal lungs to maintain low PVR.

A. Intravenous Prostacyclin (PGI₂)

PGI_2 has been used extensively as an acute vasodilator since its discovery by Moncada and Vane in 1976 (41). This compound, a primary cyclo-oxygenase product of AA in vascular tissue, is a potent vasodilator and inhibitor of platelet aggregation (Fig. 3) (41). Studies of cultured cells from the vascular wall indicate that PGI_2 is produced most actively by endothelial cells, and that its synthesis is progressively decreased towards the adventitial surface (42). Experimental and clinical studies have confirmed that PGI_2 is an important mediator in the complex interactions that occur among blood vessels, blood flow, and platelets. The generation of PGI_2 by endothelial cells is thought to be an important physiologic mechanism that protects the vessel wall from excessive contraction and from deposition of platelet aggregates (41,43). PGI_2 is vasodilatory in all vascular beds, and inhibits platelet aggregation and the proliferation of vascular SMCs. The effects of PGI_2 are mediated by stimulation of adenylate cyclase, which causes an increase in cAMP in platelets and vascular SMCs.

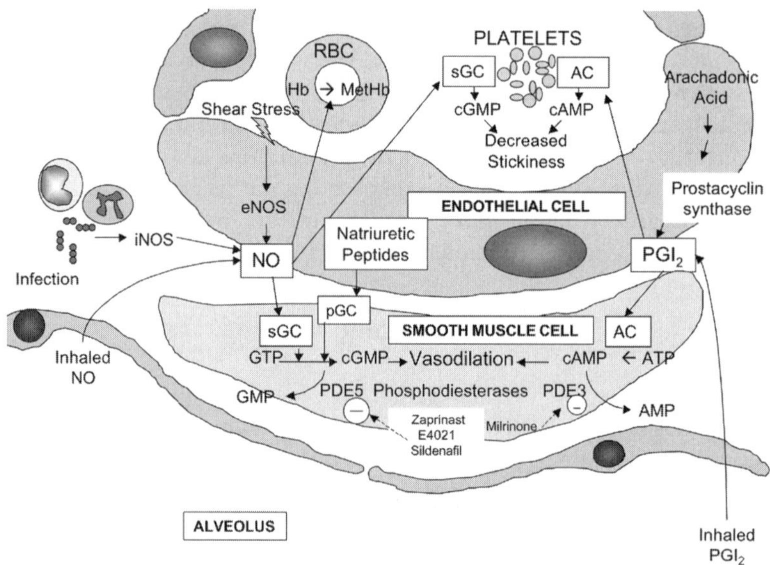

Figure 3 The origin, actions and clearance of selected endogenous and/or inhaled pulmonary vasodilators. The important endogenous pulmonary vasodilators NO, PGI_2 (prostacyclin), and natriuretic peptides act through a variety of interactive biochemical pathways to affect capillary endothelial cells, smooth muscle cells, or other aspects of the pulmonary vasculature. In additon to being present endogenously, NO and PGI_2 can also be delivered as inhaled agents during therapeutic applications. (Hb: hemoglobin; Methb: methemoglobin; sGC: soluble guanylyl cyclase; pGC: particulate guanylyl cyclase; AC: adenyl cylase; eNOS: endothelial nitric oxide synthase; iNOS: inducible nitric oxide synthase; PDE: phosphodiesterase). (−) indicates inhibition.

Intravenous administration of PGI_2 has been used in the acute and chronic therapy of PPH (44–47) in the acute treatment of neonates with PPHN (48–52), and in the acute treatment of adults with ALI/ARDS (53–56). Several centers have used PGI_2 as an investigational agent in acute vasodilator trials in PPH. Such studies have demonstrated the efficacy of PGI_2 in improving symptoms and hemodynamics in the acute, short-term management of patients with this condition (Fig. 4) (44–46,57). PGI_2 also has benefits for long-term patient outcomes in PPH. Higenbottam et al. (47) were the first to report a significant improvement of oxygenation, exercise tolerance, and quality of life following long-term continuous infusion of PGI_2 in a patient with PPH. The beneficial effects of long-term therapy with PGI_2 on hemodynamics and exercise capacity in patients with PPH were subsequently verified in a larger study (58). Long-term PGI_2 infusion may be especially helpful in seriously ill patients awaiting transplantation. Patients have been reported to receive PGI_2 by continuous infusion for almost 10 years with sustained clinical and hemodynamic benefits (59).

Although PGI_2 has been used extensively in treating adults with PPH, some of the first reports of its clinical use were in pediatric patients and newborns with PH (51,60). PGI_2 was first used clinically in a newborn with severe and refractory hypoxemia secondary to pulmonary

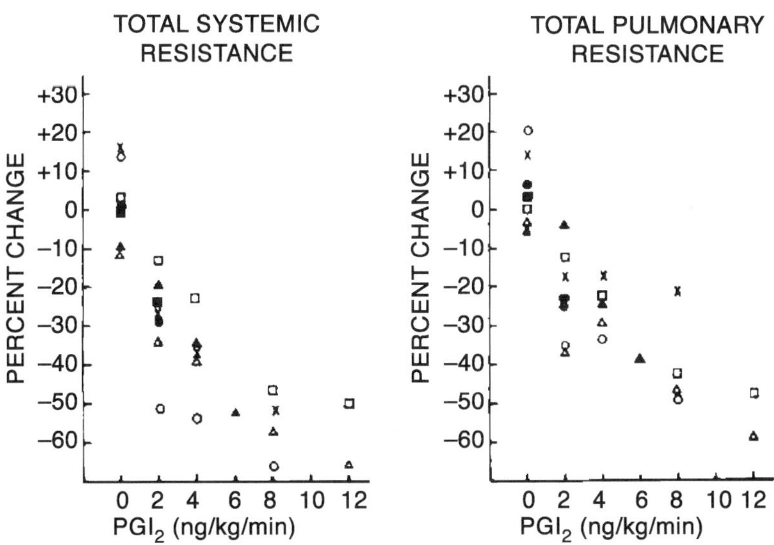

Figure 4 Effects of intravenous prostacyclin (PGI_2) on total systemic and total pulmonary resistance in patients with primary pulmonary hypertension (PPH). Values are percent changes compared with control. The 0 ng/kg/min dose represents the effects of glycine buffer (vehicle). Symbols represent individual patients studied. (From Ref. 57.)

vasoconstriction and PPHN (60). Also, intravenous PGI_2 for 72 hr was able to reverse the right to left shunt in PPHN by decreasing pulmonary artery pressure (PAP) in eight newborns on maximal respiratory and inotropic support, and these infants avoided extracorporeal membrane oxygenation (ECMO) (49). The successful use of intravenous PGI_2 as an acute vasodilator was also reported in a child with severe idiopathic pulmonary arterial hypertension (51). More recently, infusion of TTC-909 (a PGI_2 analog incorporated in lipid microspheres) markedly reduced PAP and PVR in a case study involving an infant with PPH (61).

Short-term infusion of PGI_2 has also been shown to increase cardiac index concomitant with improved right ventricular function when baseline RV ejection fractions were depressed in eight patients with ARDS and increased PAP (62). Since improving oxygen delivery is one of the major goals in managing ALI/ARDS, PGI_2 may be useful to lower PAP in these patients. Unfortunately, the lack of selectivity of PGI_2 when it is given intravenously can lead to generalized dilatation of systemic and pulmonary vessels. This can cause systemic hypotension and, in patients with parenchymal lung disease, perfusion of nonventilated as well as ventilated acini to increase intrapulmonary shunting (Table 1). Two studies have shown that the use of intravenous PGI_2 in ALI/ARDS is limited by its propensity to cause systemic hypotension and increased pulmonary venous admixture (63,64). The study of Rossaint et al. (63), for example, found that systemic PGI_2 infusion reduced PAP, but also increased intrapulmonary shunting and reduced systemic arterial pressure (SAP) in adults with ARDS.

B. Nitric Oxide (NO)

In 1980, Furchgott and Zawadzki (65) demonstrated that the pulmonary vascular endothelium produces a factor that mediates vasodilation of the

Table 1 Probable Effects of Various Pulmonary Vascular Therapies on Cardiac Output, Ventilation–Perfusion Matching, and Systemic Oxygen Delivery

Physiologic parameter	Intravenous dilators	Inhaled dilators	Intravenous constrictors	Intravenous constrictors and inhaled dilators
Cardiac output	– to ↑	– to ↑	– to ↓	–
Ventilation–perfusion matching	↓	↑	↑	↑↑
System oxygen delivery	– to ↓	↑ to ↑↑	↑ to ↓	↑

Unchanged (–); increased (↑); decreased (↓).

vascular smooth muscle. Over the next several years, it was determined that this so-called endothelium-derived relaxing factor (EDRF) was a diffusible, short-lived reactive molecule that induced relaxation by activating smooth muscle soluble guanylate cyclase (sGC) (cf. Fig. 3)(66). EDRF was subsequently identified as NO (67,68). NO is synthesized from the terminal guanidine nitrogen atom of L-arginine through a metabolic pathway mediated by NO synthase (NOS) (69). There are three NOS isoenzymes: endothelial NO synthase (eNOS), inducible NO synthase (iNOS), and neuronal NO synthase (nNOS). eNOS is constitutively expressed in endothelial cells where it is activated by Ca^{2+} in response to endogenous substances such as acetycholine, bradykinin, and substance P (70), and by shear stress (71,72). iNOS is induced in many cell types by proinflammatory cytokines, and is thought to be particularly important in lung injury responses. Once induced, it produces NO at a sustained high rate. The nNOS is constitutively expressed by neurons.

NO relaxes muscular arteries and veins by activating sGC and increasing cGMP (73,74). NO is a free radical that binds to hemoglobin with a very high affinity and also interacts with other molecules including oxygen. Endogenously produced NO is rapidly inactivated and does not cause vasodilation at sites distant from its synthesis (75). Pharmacologically delivered NO also rapidly becomes inactivated in vivo, but has systemic effects of varying degree prior to this depending on its route of administration. Before the clinical use of NO, available pulmonary vasodilators like sodium nitroprusside, PGI_2, isoprenaline, and tolazoline were usually given intravenously. These intravenous agents reduced PAP by causing generalized pulmonary vasodilation, but they also increased perfusion to underventilated areas of the lungs to worsen intrapulmonary shunting and in addition caused systemic hypotension (76) (Table 1). If administered by inhalation, the vasodilatory effects of NO (and other dilators such as PGI_2) are more effectively confined to ventilated regions of the lung. At least in principle, this allows selective improvements in the perfusion of ventilated acini and reductions in intrapulmonary shunting without significant systemic hypotension (Table 1).

Experience with Inhaled Nitric Oxide (iNO) in Adults

Since the first reported beneficial effect of iNO on PH by Pepke-Zaba et al. (76) in 1991, several studies have demonstrated that this agent can reduce PAP without worsening intrapulmonary shunting or inducing systemic hypotension. Rossaint et al. (63) demonstrated that iNO decreased intrapulmonary shunting and improved arterial oxygenation while reducing PAP in patients with ARDS. Also, a large prospective, multicenter double-blind placebo-controlled trial by Dellinger et al. (77) demonstrated an acute improvement in oxygenation within the first few hours in patients with

ARDS who received iNO. These results suggested that iNO might be a major advance in the treatment of PH associated with ALI/ARDS and other causes of hypoxic respiratory failure (78,79).

Despite its clinical benefits in some adults, questions remain about the overall efficacy of iNO, its utility and risks in different subgroups of patients with ALI/ARDS, and the preferred timing and dosing regimens for its use. Thirty to forty percent of adult patients with respiratory failure characterized by increased PAP and hypoxemia fail to respond to iNO (80). Among patients who do respond, the effects of iNO on PH can be transient and most pronounced in the first 24 hr of therapy (81). Also, at high doses of iNO, systemic oxygenation can paradoxically be worsened even though PVR continues to decrease (82). Because of the numerous etiologies and complex pathophysiology of ALI/ARDS, it is not surprising that iNO treatment does not affect all patients equally (83). However, therapy with iNO has not been shown to give significant improvements in mortality in adults with ARDS. Troncy et al. (84) carried out a single center randomized clinical trial of iNO in adult patients with ARDS and concluded that it improved gas exchange but did not affect mortality. Several more recent multicenter clinical trials in adults with ALI/ARDS have also demonstrated improvements in arterial oxygenation but no positive effects on the duration of mechanical ventilation or mortality (77,85,86). From these trials, it appears that although iNO does reduce PAP and improve the matching of ventilation and perfusion in adults with ALI/ARDS, this physiological improvement does not translate into improved survival. The failure of iNO to improve survival in adults with ARDS may in part reflect the fact that many of these patients have multiorgan system failure and a degree of pulmonary injury that is too severe to be reversible. Moreover, the complex pathophysiology of lung injury involves numerous aspects in addition to vascular dysfunction, and combined-modality interventions may be required in order to substantially improve long-term patient outcomes (Chapter 19).

Experience with iNO in Infants and Children

Treatment with iNO has been shown to markedly improve oxygenation in term newborns with acute hypoxic respiratory failure from several causes including PPHN. Basic research understanding of the role of endogenous NO synthesis in the normal transition in the pulmonary circulation at birth (87–89), and studies showing reduced NO synthesis and the benefits of iNO in animal models of PPHN (90–94), laid the foundation for successful clinical therapy for this serious condition in infants. In a randomized controlled trial in infants with severe PPHN, iNO acutely improved systemic oxygenation without causing hypotension, and continued treatment with iNO reduced the need for ECMO (Fig. 5) (95). Another randomized controlled

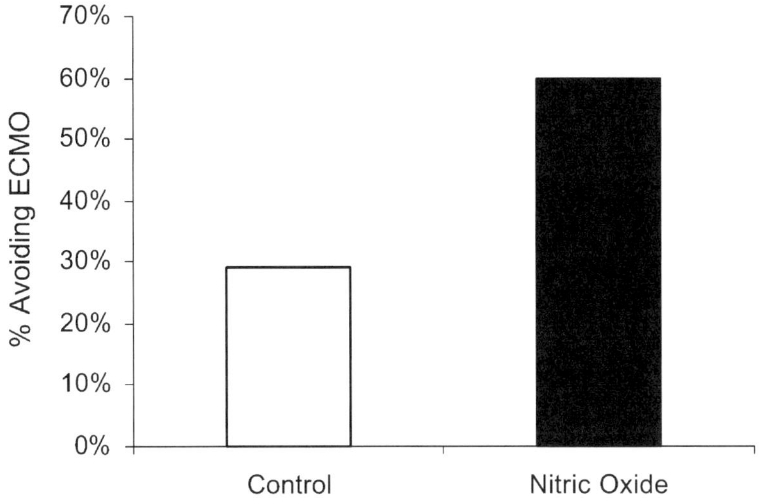

Figure 5 The percentage of newborns with persistent pulmonary hypertension avoiding extracorporeal membrane oxygenation (ECMO) with and without inhaled NO. (From Ref. 95.)

trial demonstrated that treatment with iNO reduced the incidence of death or ECMO in a cohort of full-term and nearly full-term infants with acute hypoxic respiratory failure who did not respond to aggressive conventional therapy (96). Early treatment with iNO at a dose of as little as 5 ppm has been shown to produce both acute and sustained improvements in oxygenation and to reduce the need for ECMO in term infants with PPHN (97,98). Clinical studies also suggest that high frequency oscillatory ventilation (HFOV) plus iNO can be more successful than either intervention alone in treating infants with PPHN (99,100). The Federal Drug Administration (FDA) has approved iNO for use in term infants with PPHN and acute respiratory failure. iNO may be more effective in changing outcomes in these neonates in comparison to adults with ARDS because these young patients have only one primary system failure (pulmonary). In addition, there may be less anatomic damage in the lungs of neonatal patients, particularly those with primary PPHN rather than PPHN in association with significant parenchymal disease or injury (e.g., meconium aspiration syndrome).

Therapy with iNO has also been attempted in premature infants with several lung diseases. Administration of iNO was found to improve oxygenation in preterm infants with chronic lung disease (CLD), without inducing changes in markers of inflammation or oxidative injury (101). iNO has also been reported to be effective alone, or in combination with HFOV, in treating severe respiratory failure secondary to respiratory syncytial virus infection in preterm infants with CLD (102,103). In addition, Peliowski et al. (104) used iNO to treat eight preterm infants with severe respiratory distress in association with maternal premature rupture of membranes and oligohydramnios. Arterial oxygenation was improved in these preterm infants, and required ventilator mean airway pressures were reduced (104).

The iNO has also been shown to improve oxygenation in preterm infants with RDS (105,106). The incidence of intraventricular hemorrhage (IVH) was high in these studies, and there was concern that this might be related to an NO-induced decrease in platelet adhesion or aggregation (Fig. 3) (107,108). However, a larger controlled trial by Kinsella et al. (109) showed that low-dose iNO improved oxygenation but did not increase the risk of intracranial hemorrhage in severely hypoxemic preterm infants. Improvements in survival were not demonstrated, but it was suggested that low-dose iNO decreased the risk of CLD in this patient population (109). Subhedar et al. (110), however, could not demonstrate that iNO prevented CLD in preterm infants. Two abstracts have indicated that iNO improves oxygenation and neurodevelopmental outcomes in preterm infants with RDS (111,112). Several large randomized controlled clinical trials are currently in progress to determine more conclusively if iNO prevents or mitigates CLD in premature newborns either by decreasing required ventilatory support and associated oxygen toxicity and barotrauma, or by modulating inflammation.

Potential Effects of NO on Inflammation

The roles and interactions of NO in the pulmonary inflammatory response are complex and not fully understood. Increased cytokine activity in acute pulmonary injury is known to increase the expression of iNOS, enhancing endogenous NO production (113,114). Cytokines also cause endothelial cells and neutrophils to increase production of superoxide anion (78), which can overwhelm the scavenging capacity of superoxide dismutase (SOD). Superoxide anion reacts avidly with NO to generate other reactive species including peroxynitrite (115–117) (Chapter 7). Peroxynitrite has been found in increased concentrations in the lungs of patients with ARDS (118). Peroxynitrite can impair lung surfactant by lipid peroxidation (119) and apoprotein nitration, as well as poison the mitochondria of alveolar type II cells to reduce surfactant production (120). In addition, peroxynitrite damages the pulmonary arterial endothelium (121). Pharmacologic NO, like endogenous NO, can interact with superoxide anion and produce peroxynitrite. iNO may also stimulate pulmonary macrophages to produce superoxide so as to further stimulate iNOS production (122,123) and inhibit mitochondrial metabolic activity (115,124). Thus, although iNO may initially reduce PVR and intrapulmonary shunting, it may also increase the accumulation of toxic reactive species and metabolites that predispose the pulmonary arterial circulation to later vasoconstriction (78). This may explain why the response to iNO is transient in some patients and why its withdrawal can be followed by rebound hypertension. On the other hand, NO has been shown to inhibit LPS-stimulated cytokine production in human alveolar macrophages from normal volunteers (125). Also, iNO has been found to reduce hydrogen peroxide (H_2O_2) production, adhesion molecule expression, and levels of IL-6 and IL-8 in neutrophils lavaged from patients with ARDS (126). Further research on the interactions of iNO with the inflammatory process will help to define its risks and benefits in therapeutic applications more clearly.

C. Inhaled PGI_2

In analogy with iNO, inhalation of aerosolized PGI_2 has potential advantages in pulmonary selectivity over systemic (intravenous) delivery in treating lung injury (53,127–129) (Table 1). Since aerosolization is involved, particle size distribution becomes an important added variable affecting the pattern of pulmonary delivery. Inhaled aerosols of PGI_2 ($iPGI_2$) and its stable analog Iloprost cause selective pulmonary vasodilation, increased cardiac output, and improved venous and arterial oxygenation in adults with severe PH (128). $iPGI_2$ has also been reported to be at least as effective as iNO in decreasing PH in animals and adult humans (127,130), and selective pulmonary vasodilation from $iPGI_2$ was found to be comparable to iNO in heart transplant candidates with elevated PVR (127). However, aerosolized Iloprost was not as effective as intravenous PGI_2 in long-term administration for treating adults with PH (131).

A number of small studies or case reports indicate that $iPGI_2$ has potential utility in infants and children with PH. $iPGI_2$ was effective in achieving selective acute pulmonary vasodilation in five children with confirmed PH from congenital heart disease (132). $iPGI_2$ also improved oxygenation in four term infants with PPHN who had persistent hypoxemia despite iNO (52). The mean oxygenation index (OI) in these infants was 29 ± 3 at the initiation of treatment with $iPGI_2$, and decreased to a mean of 15 ± 2 within 6 hr without changes in SAP (52). $iPGI_2$ (20–28 ng/kg/min) also significantly improved alveolar–arterial difference and modestly decreased PAP without altering SAP in two neonates with PH (50). In four hypoxic preterm neonates with PH, $iPGI_2$ increased the mean PaO_2/FiO_2 ratio from a mean of 47 to 218 mmHg, with no change in SAP (133). The $iPGI_2$ also significantly improved PaO_2 without affecting SAP in a preterm infant [28-week gestational age] with PPHN (134).

Administering PGI_2 by inhalation may be most important in treating vascular dysfunction in patients who have significant intrapulmonary shunting as a result of injury or disease. Inhalation therapy ensures that the drug preferentially reaches better ventilated acini, where it dilates the vasculature and redistributes blood flow away from nonventilated regions. Several studies have shown that iPGI$_2$ acutely improves oxygenation in patients with ALI/ARDS (53–56,129). Reduced intrapulmonary shunting and oxygenation in these patients suggests better targeting of prostanoid activity to vessels in well ventilated areas. In 16 mechanically ventilated patients with ARDS, individually titrated doses of iNO (17.8 ± 2.7 ppm) and iPGI$_2$ (7.5 ± 2.5 ng/kg/min) selectively dilated pulmonary circulation and facilitated redistribution of blood flow from shunt areas to well-ventilated pulmonary regions with nearly identical efficacy (54). Decreased mean PAP, decreased intrapulmonary right-to-left shunt, and increased PaO$_2$/FiO$_2$ have also been observed in other studies assessing iPGI$_2$ and iNO in patients with ARDS (Fig. 6) (56). Low dose iPGI$_2$ (6.6 ± 3.0 ng/kg/min) also has been found to improve pulmonary hemodynamics and arterial oxygenation in ventilated patients with severe community-acquired pneumonia with no preexisting lung disease (55). In patients with underlying interstitial fibrosis and pneumonia, higher doses of iPGI$_2$ (33 ± 12 ng/kg/min) were needed for induction of pulmonary vasodilation, consistent with the more extensive pulmonary pathology present in these patients (55). These high doses of iPGI$_2$, however, were accompanied by systemic vasodilation and increased intrapulmonary shunt (55).

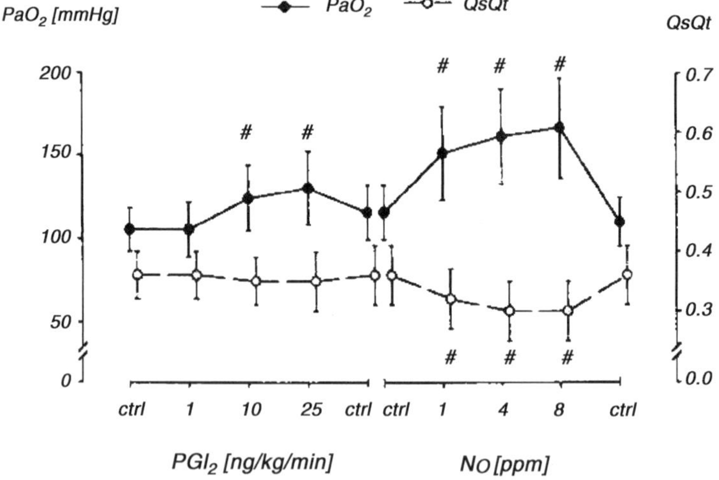

Figure 6 Effects of PGI$_2$-aerosol and inhaled NO on gas exchange. Dose–response curves are depicted for three doses of PGI$_2$-aerosol (1, 10, and 25 ng/kg/min) and three concentrations of inhaled NO (1, 4, and 8 ppm), respectively, compared with control (ctrl) values. Changes in PaO$_2$ and intrapulmonary shunt (QsQt) are indicated. All data are mean ± SEM; $n = 8$ (QsQt, $n = 6$). [#]$p < 0.05$ (vs. control value before administration of NO). (From Ref. 56.)

As in the case of iNO, predicting which patients with ALI/ARDS will respond to PGI_2 is an important issue, and this is only now beginning to be addressed. In a randomized nonprospective interventional study, Domenighetti et al. (135) found a differential response of oxygenation and pulmonary hemodynamics to $iPGI_2$ in 15 mechanically ventilated patients with ARDS of pulmonary vs. extrapulmonary origin. Administration of $iPGI_2$ increased oxygenation in eight patients, all in the extrapulmonary ARDS group. However, $iPGI_2$ was ineffective and even worsened gas exchange in patients in the pulmonary ARDS group (135). Computed tomography density numbers quantitated in Hounsfield Units (HU) were significantly less negative in the pulmonary ARDS group vs. the extrapulmonary ARDS group (–258 ± 16 HU vs. –445 ± 22 HU), consistent with less aeration and a more severe pulmonary pathology in the former. The underlying mechanisms responsible for these findings are not yet known.

D. Inhaled PGE_1

Another potentially useful pulmonary vasodilator is Prostaglandin E_1 (PGE_1). PGE_1 has a pulmonary clearance of approximately 70–80% in first passage, a significant advantage in attaining selective pulmonary vasodilation (136). In an animal model of smoke inhalation injury, inhaled PGE_1 selectively dilated the pulmonary circulation comparably to iNO and $iPGI_2$, although none of these drugs improved gas exchange (137). However, inhaled PGE_1 did improve oxygenation and decrease venous admixture without affecting SAP in patients with severe ALI and multiple organ failure (138). Inhaled PGE_1 has also been reported to generate equivalent responses to iNO in adult patients with ARDS (139).

E. Phosphodiesterase (PDE) Inhibitors

As noted earlier, vasodilation by NO and PGI_2 is mediated by the production of the cyclic nucleotides cGMP and cAMP, respectively. These cyclic nucleotides are cleared via hydrolysis by several families of PDE enzymes (140–142). Some PDE enzymes hydrolyze both cGMP and cAMP, some metabolize only one, and some are activated or inhibited by one of the nucleotides themselves. Because cAMP and cGMP compete for clearance by some PDEs and inhibit the activity of others, it is possible that elevated concentrations of one of these cyclic nucleotides could increase the concentration of the other. Due to the importance of cGMP and cAMP in vasodilation by NO and PGI_2, these PDE inhibitors have been investigated as therapeutic pulmonary vasodilators. In particular, attention has been focused on antagonizing the activity of Type V PDE (PDE_5), which is specific for cGMP (cf. Fig. 3).

Most PDEs including PDE_5 are present in lung tissue and vascular smooth muscle (140–146). PDE_5 is found in large concentrations in lung tissue

(145,146), and is quantitatively a major source of cGMP phosphodiesterase activity in the pulmonary vasculature (144). PDE_5 activity is thought to be important in regulating pulmonary vascular tone in both normal and pathophysiologic states. Type V PDE protein and activity are increased late in fetal life when PVR is markedly elevated, and decreased expression occurs postnatally when PVR is much lower (147). PDE_5 activity but not content is elevated in the lungs of fetal lambs with PH following occlusion of the ductus arteriosus, and blocking its activity dilates the pulmonary circulation of these lambs (148,149). Postnatally, PDE_5 inhibition dilates the pulmonary circulation of newborn lambs (150,151). The PDE_5 inhibition also dilates the pulmonary circulation of older lambs and eNOS deficient mice with PH from acute or chronic hypoxia (152). Selective blockade of PDE_5 activity by E4021 in newborn lambs with PPH from in utero ligation of the ductus arteriosus for 10 days, markedly and selectively dilates the pulmonary circulation and improves gas exchange (153). In humans, PDE_5 inhibition decreases acute hypoxia-induced PH (152,154,155). Oral Sildenafil (Viagra™), a selective PDE_5 inhibitor, potentially and selectively dilates the pulmonary circulation in adults with severe pulmonary arterial hypertension (156). Trials of Sildenafil for the treatment of PPHN are underway.

F. Purinergic Agonists

Adenosine and ATP are purine nucleotides known to dilate the pulmonary and systemic circulations (157). Adenosine acts primarily via P1 purinergic receptors, while ATP acts via P2 purinergic receptors (158). Circulating concentrations of adenosine and ATP rise at birth. These substances cause marked pulmonary vasodilation if infused in the fetus, and if their receptors are blocked the normal decrease in PVR at birth is markedly attenuated (159,160). The vasodilatory actions of adenosine and ATP appear, in part, to involve stimulation of endogenous NO synthesis (161). Intravenous administration of adenosine has been reported to improve oxygenation without significantly increasing SAP in term infants with acute respiratory failure (162). Also, intravenous adenosine has been reported to decrease PVR at least as much as intravenous PGI_2, while having less systemic vascular effect (163). Intravenous infusion of ATP has also been found to selectively dilate the pulmonary circulation in adults with chronic obstructive pulmonary disease (COPD) (164).

V. Anticoagulant Therapy

Occlusion of segments of the pulmonary vasculature by inappropriate coagulation can contribute to the pathophysiology of acute pulmonary injury. Intravascular and extravascular derangements in fibrin deposition and coagulation have been demonstrated in both neonates and adults with ALI/ARDS (165–169). During acute injury, the intrinsic and extrinsic coagulation pathways are activated resulting in fibrin deposition that is further enhanced by impaired fibrinolysis (170). In this process, natural anticoagulant proteins and coagulation inhibitors are rapidly consumed and thought to fall out of balance with proclotting proteins (171). Disseminated intravascular coagulation has been associated with ALI/ARDS, suggesting that microvascular thrombi potentiated by this process contribute to parenchymal tissue injury (172,173). Thrombi can occur in the pulmonary arteries in severe ALI/ARDS, and are associated with increased PVR and increased mortality (168,169). The pulmonary vasculature is also at risk for acute edematous injury in association with intravascular coagulation (174–176).

Clotting abnormalities can be particularly severe in premature infants with lung disease and injury who have reduced levels of clotting factors and platelets compared to older infants and adults (177). Hyaline membranes with a high content of fibrin are a pathologic hallmark of the respiratory distress syndrome (RDS) in premature infants. Fibrinolytic therapy for this condition (also called hyaline membrane disease, HMD) was evaluated in several early studies in premature infants prior to the development of exogenous surfactant therapy. Ambrus et al. (178,179) showed a survival benefit in a small group of premature neonates with RDS who received urokinase activated plasminogen. In a larger study, Ambrus et al. (180) used supplemental intravenous plasminogen at birth vs. placebo and showed less severe HMD and fewer deaths which were confined to the very smallest neonates. However, this treatment approach has not been widely accepted due to the high risk of intracranial and intraventricular hemorrhage in premature infants, and because of the now well-established efficacy of exogenous surfactant therapy. More recently, several natural anticoagulant proteins are at the phase III level of investigation for use in patients with ARDS (181–187). A recently concluded a phase III study on antithrombin III therapy did not demonstrate a statistically significant reduction in mortality (247). However, a study involving human recombinant protein C in patients with sepsis met early efficacy criteria in reducing mortality when compared to the placebo group (248).

VI. Combined Therapies for Vascular Dysfunction
A. Combinations of Vasodilators

It is potentially possible to achieve synergy in vascular therapy by using combinations of agents that work by complementary mechanisms (see Chapter 19 for additional detailed discussion of combination therapies for lung injury). For example, simultaneously giving iNO to increase cGMP synthesis, while blocking PDE_5 to slow cGMP catabolism, could theoretically produce higher concentrations of this cyclic neucleotide and result in greater vasodilation.

Consistent with this, low doses of the cGMP PDE inhibitor Zaprinast markedly enhance the decrease in PVR seen with low doses of iNO in lambs with PPHN (Fig. 7) (188). Similarly, in children receiving iNO for postoperative PH, PDE$_5$ blockade with dipyridamole decreases rebound PH when iNO is discontinued (189). Inhaled milrinone, a cAMP selective PDE-inhibitor, also appears to potentiate and prolong the selective pulmonary vasodilatory effects of iPGI$_2$ in patients with PH and right ventricular failure (190). Compared with iPGI$_2$ or inhaled milrinone alone, the combination of the two gave a more prolonged decrease in PVR and an increase in stroke volume (190). Another combination therapy approach involves the use of agents to simultaneously raise cAMP and cGMP concentrations in pulmonary vascular smooth muscle, and this has been examined in adults with severe PH by stimulating cAMP synthesis with iPGI$_2$ or while inhibiting cGMP clearance with sildenafil (191,192). In both trials (191,192), combined treatment was more effective in decreasing PVR than iPGI$_2$ alone. In one of the studies, the combination was also more effective than iNO alone (192). In contrast, combination therapy with iNO and intravenous PGI$_2$ has not been found to lead to an additive vasodilator effect (193).

B. Combining Intravenous Vasoconstrictors and Inhaled Vasodilators

An important reason for V_A/Q mismatching and arterial hypoxemia in lung injury is nonproductive blood flow to unventilated or poorly ventilated lung

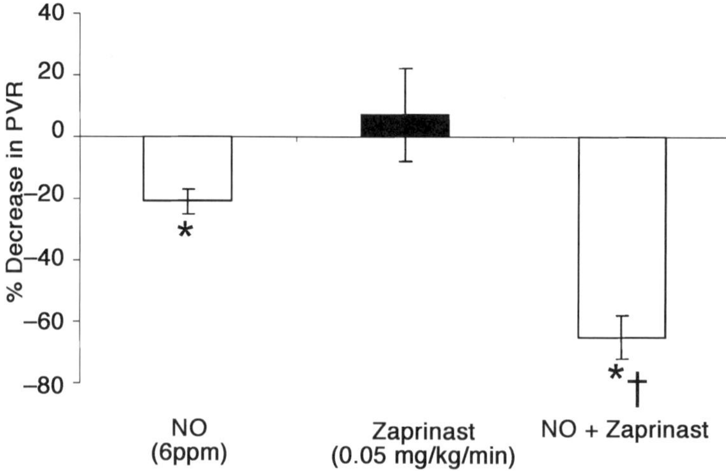

Figure 7   The percentage decrease in pulmonary vascular resistance (PVR) produced by inhaled nitric oxide (NO) alone, Zaprinast alone, and the combination of NO and Zaprinast in newborn lambs with persistent pulmonary hypertension. (From Ref. 188.)

units (194,195). Combination therapies have thus been developed where an inhaled vasodilator is used to enhance blood flow to well-ventilated acini, while blood flow to poorly ventilated acini is reduced by an intravenous vasoconstrictor (Table 1). Almitrine, a peripheral chemoreceptor stimulant with pulmonary vasoconstrictive activity improves oxygenation during hypoxic exercise (196). Almitrine is thought to cause vasoconstriction of pulmonary vessels preferentially in unventilated lung regions, and to divert blood flow to better ventilated areas to reduce intrapulmonary shunting and improve gas exchange (197). However, treatment with intravenous almitrine alone can raise PVR and potentially cause PH and decreased cardiac output. Combining intravenous almitrine with iNO, which has vasodilatory effects in ventilated lung units, has the potential to improve arterial oxygenation without these adverse side effects. Almitrine in combination with iNO reduces intrapulmonary shunting in an in vivo lavage model of acute pulmonary injury (198). In addition, a variety of clinical studies have confirmed the effectiveness of intravenous almitrine and iNO in improving gas exchange and oxygenation in the early phases of ALI/ARDS in adult patients (199–206). In contrast, the combination of intravenous almitrine and $iPGI_2$ did not give additive improvements in gas exchange in animals with ALI (207).

C. Inhaled Vasodilators in Conjunction with Lung Recruitment Strategies

The clinical efficacy of inhaled vasodilators depends on their ability to reach active pulmonary gas exchange tissue. For example, iNO is not effective in improving oxygenation or decreasing PH in infants or newborn lambs with congenital diaphragmatic hernia (CDH), a condition where pulmonary hypoplasia and surfactant deficiency severely limit alveolar expansion (208). However, if lambs with CDH are treated at birth with surfactant or liquid ventilation to improve alveolar recruitment, iNO decreases PVR and PH and improves gas exchange (209). This is consistent with the concept that inhaled vasodilators may be more effective if they are paired with lung recruitment strategies that increase the accessible area of pulmonary gas exchange tissue. A large study of newborns with acute hypoxic respiratory failure found that iNO was more effective when paired with HFOV to improve lung recruitment (99). Therapies involving inhaled vasodilators and lung recruitment strategies (e.g., prone positioning, surfactant therapy, specialized ventilator modalities) are described further in other chapters.

VII. Future Therapies

A. Natriuretic Peptides

Atrial natriuretic peptide (ANP) and brain natriuretic peptide (BNP) are produced by cardiac tissue and have potent natriuretic and vasorelaxant properties (210). The C-type natriuretic peptide (CNP) was initially identified in the central nervous system (211), and later shown to be synthesized and released by endothelial cells (212). Like NO, natriuretic peptides have vascular effects mediated by stimulating the production of cGMP (cf. Fig. 3). However, unlike NO which stimulates sGC, natriuretic peptides act by stimulating a membrane bound particulate guanylate cyclase (pGC) through natriuretic peptide receptors (NPRs). There are three known types of NPRs: NPR-A, NPR-B, and NPR-C. NPR-A and NPR-B receptors are coupled to pGC enzyme activity, while NPR-C receptors are considered to be clearance receptors (213). ANP and BNP act predominately through the NPR-A receptor (214), while CNP is a specific agonist of the NPR-B receptor (215). In pulmonary arteries and veins isolated from fetal lambs, ANP and CNP induce significant vasodilation (216). In addition to mediating pulmonary vasodilatory effects, natriuretic peptides induce diuresis and natriuresis.

In patients with severe lung injury, mean concentrations of plasma ANP have been reported to be significantly higher than in normal subjects (217). Plasma ANP levels were found to decrease in parallel with the improvement of lung injury, and to remain high in patients who did not recover (217). Plasma ANP levels have also been shown to correlate with PAP in patients with ARDS (218,219). Plasma ANP levels correlate positively with urine volume and the fractional excretion of sodium. Elevation of ANP may reflect an adaptive mechanism to remove excess fluid retention and to reduce PH during acute pulmonary injury (218). Circulating BNP levels are also found to be elevated in patients with ALI/ARDS and to correlate with PVR (219). Circulating levels of BNP may be a sensitive humoral marker for the degree of ventricular dysfunction associated with ALI/ARDS (219). Plasma BNP measurements are currently used in many emergency departments as a screening tool to diagnose cardiogenic dyspnea (220,221). In patients on mechanical ventilation for moderate ALI, intravenous infusion of genetic recombinant alpha-human ANP (Carperitide) has been reported to give significant improvements in oxygenation and thoracic compliance (222). The lung injury score and extent of shunting decreased significantly in treated patients, and there was also a significant increase in urine volume after initiating ANP infusion (222). However, iNO has been shown to be more beneficial than intravenous ANP in improving PH associated with severe ARDS (223). In terms of risks, intravenous natriuretic peptides have similar problems with systemic hypotension as other vasodilatory agents delivered by this route, and further research on the feasibility and efficacy of alternate modes of delivery is needed. Also, the efficacy of natriuretic peptide agents may be enhanced in combination therapies where they are used in conjunction with selective inhibitors of natriuretic peptide metabolism.

B. Superoxide Dismutase

Patients with ALI/ARDS are often ventilated with high concentrations of oxygen to maintain adequate systemic oxygenation. Iatrogenic hyperoxia, along with severe tissue inflammation, provides a rich environment for the production of superoxide anions (224) and other oxidative species in the lungs of these patients. The vascular adventitia is also metabolically active during lung injury, and produces additional superoxide (225–227). In addition, therapeutic agents such as iNO can further increase superoxide formation in pulmonary cells (228). As noted earlier in this chapter, superoxide anions not only have direct toxic effects but also can combine with endogenous or pharmacologic NO to form highly reactive peroxynitrite (229). Among its multiple biological effects, peroxynitrite can inhibit prostacyclin synthase so as to promote vasoconstriction (230). By eliminating superoxide and preventing its reaction with NO to form peroxynitrite, SOD has been shown to significantly enhance cGMP production and vasodilatory responses to NO in vitro (231,232).

Animal experiments indicate that intratracheal instillation of recombinant human copper–zinc superoxide dismutase (rhSOD) produces selective dilation of the pulmonary circulation in newborn lambs with PPHN (233). In addition, the combination of rhSOD and iNO has been found to have enhanced pulmonary vascular effects compared to iNO alone (233). In studies in neonatal piglets, prophylactic intratracheal administration of rhSOD 10 min prior to the induction of acute pulmonary injury with instilled endotoxin resulted in increased PaO_2 and lower $PaCO_2$ (234). Intratracheal administration of rhSOD also mitigated inflammatory changes, oxidative damage, and the severity of lung injury from exposure to 100 ppm NO and 90% O_2 in mechanically ventilated newborn piglets (235). However, intravenous administration of SOD after the establishment of acute pulmonary injury was not effective in improving oxygenation in ewes with smoke inhalation (236). Clinical data indicate that the antioxidative system is severely compromised in adult patients with ARDS (237), suggesting potential benefits for antioxidant therapy (Chapters 16, 19). Intratracheal administration of rhSOD in premature babies with RDS is well tolerated (238) and does not have deleterious effects on long-term neurodevelopmental outcome (239). Further human trials are necessary to examine the whether the clinical benefits of iNO in patients with ALI/ARDS are augmented by rhSOD administered intratracheally, by nebulization (240), or by intravenous infusion.

C. Blockade of Vasoconstriction

A number of studies indicate that blockade of the vasoconstrictive effects of thromboxanes, leukotrienes or ETs can be beneficial in animal models of pulmonary disease and injury (Chapter 8). A recent clinical trial has also suggested that an ET-1 receptor antagonist (Bosentan) has beneficial effects in adults with PPH (241). Continuing clinical and basic research will help to further define the effectiveness of this and other approaches to antagonize injury-related pulmonary vasoconstriction.

D. Growth Factors

Patients with lung injury not only must survive acute physiologic derangements of gas exchange and over-exuberant inflammation, but also must recover from injury by repairing damaged tissue. Therapy with agents such as vascular growth factors could potentially facilitate repair and improve long-term outcomes in patients with ALI/ARDS. Lung growth and development is an on-going process in infants and children (Chapter 2), and data suggest that pulmonary blood vessels can grow even in adults following injury. For example, in adult rats after two weeks of *Pseudomonas aeruginosa* infection, airway volume is increased and growth of the vascular compartment has occurred (242). Growth factors such as vascular endothelial growth factor (VEGF) are thought to be highly important in mediating blood vessel proliferation and growth. VEGF is a potent mediator of angiogenesis and endothelial cell proliferation that also significantly increases vascular permeability. In an in vivo model of VEGF overexpression, Kaner et al. (243) demonstrated a dose-dependent increase in lung wet/dry weight ratios, histological pulmonary edema, and increased vascular permeability to albumin. Pretreatment with an adenovirus vector expressing a truncated soluble form of a receptor that cleared VEGF blocked the vascular permeability increase (243). Studies by Thickett et al. (244) suggest that antagonizing excessive VEGF activity could be useful in clinical ALI/ARDS. These investigators examined 40 patients with ARDS, 28 "at-risk" patients, 14 normal patients, and nine ventilated control patients. Plasma VEGF levels were higher in patients with ARDS, higher in ARDS patients with hypotension, and increasing VEGF levels over time were associated with death. Peripheral blood monocytes from ARDS patients spontaneously produced more VEGF. Plasma from the ARDS patients caused increased albumin flux across pulmonary endothelial cell monolayers. This was reduced by half with the addition of a soluble VEGF inhibitor (244).

Although antagonizing excessive VEGF activity during lung injury may be beneficial to vascular permeability, the angiogenic activity of this growth factor may be protective against the development of PH. Partovian et al. (245) studied the effect of adenovirus (Ad) -VEGF to determine if VEGF overexpression would be helpful in mitigating hypoxic PH in rats. Pretreatment with Ad-VEGF two days before a 2-week exposure to 10% oxygen resulted in lower PAP, lower right ventricle weight, and less muscularization of distal vessels. Pretreatment with Ad-VEGF increased eNOS activity in lung tissue and partially restored endothelium-dependent vasodilatation (245). Campbell et al. (246) used cell-based gene transfer and delivered intravenously syngenic SMCs overexpressing VEGF to rats with PH induced by the pulmonary endothelial toxin monocrotaline. VEGF treated animals had less RV hypertension and less RV and vascular hypertrophy. The VEGF treated animals also had less Caspase-3 immunostaining in the endothelium, suggesting that VEGF was protective against endothelial cell apoptosis (246). These studies suggest a potential therapeutic role for angiogenic factors like VEGF in certain forms of PH. However, the potentially positive angiogenic activity of VEGF in lung injury therapy must be balanced against its negative effects in increasing vascular permeability. Further research is necessary to define patient populations appropriate for therapies promoting or antagonizing VEGF activity, as well as to better understand when during lung injury such therapies might be best applied.

VIII. Summary

Vascular tone in the normal lungs depends on a balance of vasodilation and vasoconstriction, and this is disrupted by numerous events during injury. Stimulation of the innate nonadaptive infammatory response leads to the release of multiple vasoactive mediators that by themselves, or via the cyclooxygenase and lipoxygenase pathways, lead to overall vasoconstriction of the pulmonary vascular bed and (at times) inappropriate vasodilation in poorly ventilated gas exchange units. Endogenous vasoactive substances important in pulmonary vascular regulation include PGs, leukotrienes, thromboxane, NO, ET-1, PDGF, and PAF. Arachidonic acid metabolites including $PGF_{2\alpha}$, thromboxane and leukotrienes are potent pulmonary vasoconstrictors, as are ET-1, PDGF, and PAF. Important pulmonary vasodilators include PGI_2 (prostacyclin), NO, and natriuretic peptides such as ANP and CNP. The majority of pulmonary vasodilators act by pathways involving the cyclic neucleotides cGMP or cGMP.

Injury-induced disruptions in pulmonary vascular regulation decrease systemic oxygen delivery by several mechanisms. Overall pulmonary vasoconstriction decreases total microcirculatory blood flow. Intrapulmonary shunting (V_A/Q mismatching) from local vasoconstriction in ventilated acini and inappropriate vasodilation in poorly ventilated acini impairs gas exchange and lowers oxygen saturation of pulmonary venous blood. Pulmonary vasoconstriction increases PVR and causes PH, leading to decreases in cardiac output that further reduce systemic oxygen delivery. In addition, in neonates or patients with intracardiac or arterial connections between the pulmonary and systemic circulations, PH also results in extrapulmonary right to left shunting of blood and lower systemic oxygen delivery. The prevalence and severe physiological consequences of vascular dysfunction makes this aspect of lung injury pathophysiology an important target of clinical therapy.

Most current therapies for vascular dysfunction in lung injury have been directed at counteracting disruptions of pulmonary vascular regulation, particularly those causing increased PVR. The primary goal of such therapies is to selectively decrease vascular resistance so that perfusion increases in well-ventilated but not poorly ventilated lung regions, and systemic hypotension is not induced. The most successful current therapies of this kind have used iNO and PGI_2, which have short biological half-lives and are also produced endogenously by endothelial cells. NO vasodilates by increasing the synthesis of cGMP (via cGC) in vascular smooth muscle, while PGI_2 vasodilates by increasing the synthesis of cAMP in these cells. An alternative approach utilized to enhance pulmonary vasodilation is by blocking PDE enzymes that clear these cyclic nucleotides. Other vascular therapies discussed in this chapter have been combinations of an inhaled pulmonary vasodilator with a selective vasoconstrictor to improve ventilation–perfusion matching in the lungs, or utilizing alveolar recruitment strategies to increase the accessible area of gas exchange tissue reached by an inhaled vasodilator. Therapies directed against coagulation-microthrombosis and permeability increases in the pulmonary circulation are also noted as having potential utility in injured lungs.

Mechanistic understanding of the pathophysiology of lung injury is crucial in developing optimal therapies for vascular dysfunction. For example, mechanistic studies on the importance of endogenous NO synthesis in reducing PVR at birth, along with studies showing reduced NO synthesis and improved gas exchange from iNO in animal models of PPHN, led to the development of clinical iNO therapy for this severe condition. Current vascular-based therapies including the use of iNO have had somewhat limited success in adult patients with ARDS. This may in part be due to the multiple etiologies causing this severe lung injury syndrome, as well as the complex pulmonary and systemic pathology of affected patients. The efficacy of vascular-based therapies with iNO and other agents could be improved if subgroups of patients could be identified who have a high probability of response based on mechanistic understanding of their underlying disease. Also, better understanding of the initial triggers of inflammatory lung injury could lead to earlier detection and intervention before cellular and anatomic damage becomes so severe that no therapy can produce more than modest results. In addition, optimal therapies for ALI/ARDS may require multiagent or combined-modality approaches that combine vascular therapy with agents or interventions that target other aspects of lung injury pathophysiology (Chapter 19).

Acknowledgment

The authors wish to thank Cheryl Krieger for her help in the preparation of this manuscript.

References

1. American Thoracic Society Conference Report. Acute lung injury. Am J Respir Crit Care Med 1998; 158:675–679.
2. Bigatello LM, Zapol WM. New approaches to actue lung injury. Br J Anaesth 1996; 77:99–109.
3. Dzau VJ. Role of endothelium-derived vasoactive substances in the regulation of vascular tone via structural remodeling of blood vessels. In: Ryan U, Rubanyi GM, eds. Endothelial Regulation of Vascular Tone. New York: Marcel Dekker, 1992:331–340.
4. Abman SH, Ivy DD, Ziegler JW, Kinsella JP. Mechanisms of abnormal vasoreactivity in persistent pulmonary hypertension of the newborn infant. J Perinatol 1996; 16:S18–S23.
5. Watterberg KL, Demers LM, Scott SM, Murphy S. Chorioamnionitis and early lung inflammation in infants in whom bronchopulmonary dysplasia develops. Pediatrics 1996; 97:210–215.
6. Yoon BH, Romero R, Jun JK, Park KH. Amniotic fluid cytokines (interleukin-6, tumor necrosis factor-a, interleukin-1b, and interluekin-8) and the risk for the development of bronchopulmonary dysplasia. Am J Obstet Gynecol 1997; 177:825–830.
7. Hislop AA, Haworth SG. Pulmonary vascular damage and the development of cor pulmonale following hylane membrane disease. Pediatr Pulmonol 1990; 9:152–161.
8. Margraf LR, Tomashefski JFJ, Bruce MC, Dahms BB. Morphometric analysis of the lung in bronchopulmonary dysplasia. Am Rev Respir Dis 1991; 143:391–400.
9. Murphy JD, Rabinovitch M, Goldstein JD, Reid LM. The structural basis of persistent pulmonary hypertension of the newborn infant. J Pediatr 1981; 98:962–967.
10. Wild LM, Nickerson PA, Morin FC III. Ligating the ductus arteriosus before birth remodels the pulmonary vasculature of the lamb. Pediatr Res 1989; 25:251–257.
11. Tod ML, Cassin S. Perinatal pulmonary responses to arachidonic acid during normoxia and hypoxia. J Appl Physiol Respirat Environ Exercise Physiol 1984; 57:977–983.
12. Tyler T, Leffler CW, Cassin S. Circulatory responses of perinatal goats to prostaglandin precursors. Prostaglandins Med 1978; 1:213–229.
13. Cassin S, Gause G, Davis T, Riet M, Baker R. Do inhibitors of lipoxygenase and cyclooxygenase block neonatal hypoxic pulmonary vasoconstriction? J Appl Physiol 1989; 66:1779–1784.
14. Printz MP, Skidgel RA, Friedman WF. Studies of pulmonary prostaglandin biosynthetic and catabolic enzymes as factors in ductus arteriosus patency and closure. Evidence for a shift in products with gestational age. Pediatr Res 1984; 18:19–24.
15. Lock JE, Olley PM, Coceani F. Direct pulmonary vascular responses to prostaglandins in the conscious newborn lamb. Am J Physiol 1980; 238:H631–H638.
16. Leffler CW, Tyler T, Cassin S. Responses of pulmonary and systemic circulations of perinatal goats to prostaglandin F_2a^1. Can J Physiol Pharmacol 1979; 57:167–173.

17. Schreiber MD, Heymann MA, Soifer SJ. The differential effects of leuko-triene C4 and D4 on the pulmonary and systemic circulations in newborn lambs. Pediatr Res 1987; 21:176–182.

18. Kadowitz PJ, Lippton DB, McNamara EW, Hyman AL. Action and metabolism of prostaglandins in the pulmonary circulation. In: Oates JA, ed. Prostaglandins and the Cardiovascular System. New York: Raven Press, 1982: 333–356.

19. Soifer SJ, Morin FC III, Heymann MA. Prostaglandin D2 reverses pulmonary hypertension in the newborn lamb. Pediatrics 1982; 100:458–463.

20. Soifer S, Morin FC III, Kaslow D, Heymann M. The developmental effects of prostaglandin D_2 on the pulmonary and systemic circulations in the newborn lamb. J Dev Physiol 1983; 5:237–250.

21. Kourembanas S, McQuillan LP, Leung GK, Faller DV. Nitric oxide regulates the expression of vasoconstrictors and growth factors by vascular endothelium under both normoxia and hypoxia. J Clin Invest 1993; 92:99–104.

22. Yanagisawa M, Kurihara H, Kuimura S, et al. A novel potent vasoconstrictor peptide produced by vascular endothelial cells. Nature 1988; 332:411–415.

23. Komuro I, Kurihara J, Sugiyama T, Takaku F, Yazaki Y. Endothelin stimulates c-fos and c-myc expression and proliferation of vascular smooth muscle cells. FEBS 1988; 238:249–252.

24. Battistini B, Forget MA, Laight D. Potential roles for endothelins in systemic inflammatory response syndrome with a particular relationship to cytokines. Shock 1996; 5:167–183.

25. Nagase T, Fukuchi Y, Jo C, et al. Endothelin-1 stimulates arachidonate 15-lipoxygenase activity and oxygen radical formation in the rat distal lung. Biochem Biophys Res Comm 1990; 168:485–489.

26. Kourembanas S, Marsden PA, McQuillan LP, Faller DV. Hypoxia induces endothelin gene expression and secretion in cultured human endothelium. J Clin Invest 1991; 88:1054–1057.

27. Stewart DJ, Levy RD, Cernacek P, Langleben D. Increased plasma endothelin-1 in pulmonary hypertension: marker or mediator of disease. Ann Intern Med 1991; 114:464–469.

28. Rosenberg AA, Kennaugh J, Koppenhafer SL, Loomis M, Chatfield BA, Abman SH. Elevated immunoreactive endothelin-1 levels in newborn infants with persistent pulmonary hypertension. J Pediatr 1993; 123:109–114.

29. Sachinidis A, Locher R, Hoppe J, Vetter W. The platelet-derived growth factor isomers, PDGF-AA, PDGF-AB and PDGF-BB, induce contraction of vascular smooth muscle cells by different intracellular mechanisms. FEBS 1990; 275:95–98.

30. Kourembanas S, Hannan RL, Faller DV. Oxygen tension regulates the expression of the platelet-derived growth factor-B chain gene humn endothelial cells. J Clin Invest 1990; 86:670–674.

31. Clavijo LC, Carter MB, Matheson PJ, et al. Platelet-activating factor and bacteremia-induced pulmonary hypertension. J Surg Res 2000; 88:173–180.

32. Laurindo FR, Goldstein RE, Davenport NJ, Ezra D, Feuerstein GZ. Mechanisms of hypotension produced by platelet-activating factor. J Appl Physiol 1989; 66:2681–2690.

33. McMurtry IF, Morris KG. Platelet-activating factor causes pulmonary vasodilation in the rat. Am Rev Respir Dis 1986; 134:757–762.

34. Kurrek MM, Zapol WM, Holzmann A, Filippov G, Winkler M, Bloch KD. In vivo lipopolysaccharide pretreatment inhibits cGMP release from the isolated-perfused rat lung. Am J Physiol 1995; 269:L618–624.

35. Spath JA Jr, Sloane PJ, Gee MH, Albertine KH. Loss of endothelium-dependent vasodilation in the pulmonary vessels of sheep after prolonged endotoxin. J Appl Physiol 1994; 76:361–369.

36. McIntyre RC, Banerjee A, Agrafojo J, Fullerton DA. Pulmonary hypertension in acute lung injury is due to impaired vasodilation with intact vascular contractility. J Surg Res 1995; 58:765–770.

37. Fullerton DA, McIntyre RC Jr, Hahn AR, et al. Dysfunction of cGMP-mediated pulmonary vasorelaxation in endotoxin-induced acute lung injury. Am J Physiol 1995; 268:L1029–1035.

38. Fullerton DA, Hahn AR, Koike K, Banerjee A, Harken AH. Intracellular mechanisms of pulmonary vasomotor dysfunction in acute lung injury caused by mesenteric ischemia–reperfusion. Surgery 1993; 114:366–367.

39. Koike K, Moore EE, Moore FA, Kim FJW, Carl VS, Banerjee A. Gut phospholipase A_2 mediates neutrophil priming and lung injury after mesenteric ischemia–reperfusion. Am J Physiol 1995; 268:G397–G403.

40. Erdmann AJ III, Vaughan TR Jr, Brigham KL, Woolverton WC, Staub NC. Effect of increased vascular pressure on lung fluid balance in unanesthetized sheep. Circ Res 1975; 37:271–284.

41. Moncada S, Gryglewski R, Bunting S, Vane JR. An enzyme isolated from arteries transforms prostaglandin endoperoxides to an unstable substance that inhibits platelet aggregation. Nature London 1976; 263:663–665.

42. Moncada S, Herman AG, Higgs EA, Vane JR. Differential formation of prostacyclin (PGX or PGI2) by layers of the arterial wall. An explanation for the anti-thrombotic properties of vascular endothelium. Thromb Res 1977; 11: 323–344.

43. Vane JR, Botting RM. Pharmacodynamic profile of prostacyclin. Am J Cardiol 1995; 75:3A–10A.

44. Groves BM, Rubin LJ, Frosolono MF, Cato AE, Reeves JT. A comparison of the acute hemodynamic effects of prostacyclin and hydralazine in primary pulmonary hypertension. Am Heart J 1985; 110:1200–1204.

45. Scott JP, Higenbottam T, Wallwork J. The acute effect of the synthetic prostacyclin analogue iloprost in primary pulmonary hypertension. Br J Clin Pract 1990; 44:231–234.

46. Barst RJ, Rubin LJ, Long WA, et al. A comparison of continuous intravenous epoporstenol with conventional therapy for primary pulmonary hypertnsion. N Engl J Med 1996; 334:296–301.

47. Higenbottam T, Wheeldon D, Wells F, Wallwork J. Long-term treatment of primary pulmonary hypertension with continuous intravenous epoprostenol (prostacyclin). Lancet 1984; 1:1046–1047.

48. Lock J, Olley P, Coceani F. Direct pulmonary vascular response to prostaglandins in the conscious newborn lamb. Am J Physiol 1980; 238: H631–H638.

49. Eronen M, Pohjavuori M, Andersson S, Pesonen E, Raivio KO. Prostacyclin treatment for persistent pulmonary hypertension of the newborn. Pediatr Cardiol 1997; 18:3–7.

50. Bindl L, Fahnenstich H, Peukert U. Aerosolised prostacyclin for pulmonary hypertension in neonates. Arch Dis Child 1994; 71:F214–F216.

51. Watkins WD, Peterson MB, Crone RK, Shannon DC, Levine L. Prostacyclin and prostaglandin E1 for severe idiopathic pulmonary artery hypertension. Lancet 1980; 1:1083.

52. Kelly LK, Porta F, Steinhorn RH. Inhaled prostacyclin improves oxygenation in infants with PPHN refractory to inhaled nitric oxide. Pediatric Academic Societies 2002 Annual Meeting, Baltimore, MD, May 4–7: 2002.

53. Pappert D, Busch T, Gerlach H, Lewandowski K, Radermacher P, Rossaint R. Aerosolized prostacyclin vs. inhaled nitric oxide in children with severe acute respiratory distress syndrome. Anesthesiology 1995; 82:1507–1511.

54. Walmrath D, Schneider T, Schermuly R, Olschewski H, Grimminger F, Seeger W. Direct comparison of inhaled nitric oxide and aerosolized prostacyclin in acute respiratory distress syndrome. Am J Respir Crit Care Med 1996; 153:991–996.

55. Walmrath D, Schneider T, Pilch J, Schermuly R, Grimminger F, Seeger W. Effects of aerosolized prostacyclin in severe pneumonia. Impact of fibrosis. Am J Respir Crit Care Med 1995; 151:724–730.

56. Zwissler B, Kemming G, Habler O, et al. Inhaled prostacyclin (PGI2) vs. inhaled nitric oxide in adult respiratory distress syndrome. Am J Respir Crit Care Med 1996; 154:1671–1677.

57. Rubin LJ, Groves BM, Reeves JT, Frosolono M, Handel F, Cato AE. Prostacyclin-induced acute pulmonary vasodilation in primary pulmonary hypertension. Circulation 1982; 66:334–338.

58. Barst RJ, Rubin LJ, McGoon MD, Caldwell EJ, Long WA, Levy PS. Survival in primary pulmonary hypertension with long-term continuous intravenous prostacyclin. Ann Intern Med 1994; 121:409–415.

59. Rubin LJ. Primary pulmonary hypertension. N Engl J Med 1997; 336:111–117.

60. Lock J, Olley P, Coceani F, Swyer PR, Rowe RD. Use of prostacyclin in persistent fetal circulation. Lancet 1979; 1:1343.

61. Takigiku K, Shibata T, Yasui K, et al. Treatment of infantile primary pulmonary hypertension by intravenous infusion of lipo-prostaglandin I2 analog. J Pediatr 1997; 130:835–838.

62. Radermacher P, Santak B, Wust HJ, Tarnow J, Falke KJ. Prostacyclin and right ventricular function in patients with pulmonary hypertension associated with ARDS. Intensive Care Med 1990; 16:227–232.

63. Rossaint R, Falke KJ, Lopez F, Slama K, Pison U, Zapol WM. Inhaled nitric oxide for the adult respiratory distress syndrome. N Engl J Med 1993; 328:399–405.

64. Radermacher P, Santak B, Wust HJ, Tarnow J, Falke KJ. Prostacyclin for the treatment of pulmonary hypertension in the adult respiratory distress syndrome: effects on pulmonary capillary pressure and ventilation–perfusion distributions. Anesthesiology 1990; 72:238–244.

65. Furchgott RF, Zawadzki JV. The obligatory role of endothelial cells in the relaxation of arterial smooth muscle. Nature 1980; 288:373–376.

66. Furchgott RF. The 1989 Ulf von Euler lecture. Studies on endothelium-dependent vasodilation and the endothelium-derived relaxing factor. Acta Physiol Scand 1990; 139:257–270.

67. Ignarro LJ, Byrns RE, Bugfa GM, Wood KS. Endothelium-derived relaxing factor from pulmonary artery and vein possesses pharmacologic and chemical properties identical to those of nitric oxide radical. Circ Res 1987; 61: 866–879.

68. Palmer RMJ, Ferrige AG, Moncada SA. Nitric oxide release accounts for the biological activity of endothelium-derived relaxing factor. Nature 1987; 327:524–526.

69. Palmer RM, Ashton DS, Moncada S. Vascular endothelial cells synthesize nitric oxide from L-arginine. Nature 1988; 333:664–666.

70. Bredt DS, Snyder SH. Nitric oxide: a physiologic messenger molecule. Ann Rev Biochem 1994; 63:175–195.

71. Jeremy JY, Nystrom ML, Barradas MA, Mikhailidis DP. Eicosanoids and septicaemia. Prostaglandins Leukot Essent Fatty Acids 1994; 50:287–297.

72. Rubanyi GM, Romero JC, Vanhoutte PM. Flow-induced release of endothelium-derived relaxing factor. Am J Physiol 1986; 250:H1145–H1149.

73. Rapoport RM, Murad F. Agonist-induced endothelium-dependent relaxation in rat thoracic aorta may be mediated through cGMP. Circ Res 1983; 52: 352–357.

74. Ignarro LJ. Biological actions and properties of endothelium-derived nitric oxide formed and released from artery and vein. Circ Res 1989; 65:1–20.

75. Gibson QH, Roughton FJW. The kinetics and equilibria of the reactions of nitric oxide with sheep haemoglobin. J Physiol 1957; 136:507–526.

76. Pepke-Zaba J, Higenbottam TW, Dinh-Xuan AT, Stone D, Wallwork J. Inhaled nitric oxide as a cause of selective pulmonary vasodilation in pulmonary hypertension. Lancet 1991; 338:1173–1174.

77. Dellinger RP, Zimmerman JL, Taylor RW, et al. Effects of inhaled nitric oxide in patients with acute respiratory distress syndrome: results of a randomized phase II trial. Crit Care Med 1998; 26(suppl 1):15–23.

78. Stuart-Smith K, Jeremy JY. Microvessel damage in acute respiratory distress syndrome: the answer may not be NO. BJA: Br J Anaesth 2001; 87:272–279.

79. Kinsella JP, Abman SH. Recent developments in the pathophysiology and treatment of persistent pulmonary hypertension of the newborn. J Pediatr 1995; 126:853–864.

80. Young JD. Inhaled nitric oxide in acute respiratory failure. BJA: Br J Anaesth 1997; 79:695–696.

81. Michael JR, Barton RG, Saffle JR, et al. Inhaled nitric oxide vs. conventional therapy: effect on oxygenation in ARDS. Am J Respir Crit Care Med 1998; 157:1372–1380.

82. Gerlach H, Keh D, Falke J. Inhaled nitric oxide: clinical experience. In: Marini JJ, Evans TW, eds. Update in Intensive Care and Emergency Medicine. Vol. 30. Berlin: Springer-Verlag, 1999:353–369.

83. Payen D. Inhaled nitric oxide and acute lung injury. Clin Chest Med 2000; 21:519–529.

84. Troncy E, Collet JP, Shapiro S, et al. Inhaled nitric oxide in acute respiratory distress syndrome: a pilot randomized controlled study. Am J Respir Crit Care Med 1998; 157:1483–1488.

85. Lundin S, Mang H, Smithies M, Stenqvist O, Frostell C. Inhalation of nitric oxide in acute lung injury: results of a European multicentre study. The European Study Group of Inhaled Nitric Oxide. Intensive Care Med 1999; 25:911–919.

86. Payen D, Vallet B, Geno A. Results of the French prospective multicentric randomized double blind placebo controlled trial on inhaled nitric oxide in ARDS [abstr 647]. Intensive Care Med 1999; 25:S166.

87. Shaul PW, Farrar MA, Zellers TM. Oxygen modulates endothelium-derived relaxing factor production in fetal pulmonary arteries. Am J Physiol Heart circ Physiol 1992; 262:H355–H364.

88. Fineman JR, Wong J, Morin FC III, Wild LM, Soifer SJ. Chronic nitric oxide inhibition in utero produces persistent pulmonary hypertension in newborn lambs. J Clin Invest 1994; 93:2675–2683.

89. Abman SH, Chatfield BA, Hall SL, McMurtry IF. Role of endothelium-derived relaxing factor during transition of pulmonary circulation at birth. Am J Physiol 1990; 259:H1921–H1927.

90. Shaul PW, Yuhanna IS, German Z, Chen Z, Steinhorn RH, Morin FC III. Pulmonary endothelial NO synthase gene expression is decreased in fetal lambs with pulmonary hypertension. Am J Physiol 1997; 272:L1005–L1012.

91. Zayek M, Wild LM, Roberts JD, Morin FC III. Effect of nitric oxide on survival and lung injury in newborn lambs with persistent pulmonary hypertension. J Pediatr 1993; 123:947–952.

92. Zayek M, Cleveland D, Morin FC III. Treatment of persistent pulmonary hypertension in the newborn lamb by inhaled nitric oxide. J Pediatr 1993; 122:743–750.

93. Kinsella JP, Neish SR, Shaffer E, Abman SH. Low-dose inhalation nitric oxide in persistent pulmonary hypertension of the newborn. Lancet 1992; 340:819–820.

94. Roberts JD, Polaner DM, Lang P, Zapol WM. Inhaled nitric oxide in persistent pulmonary hypertension of the newborn. Lancet 1992; 340:818–819.

95. Roberts JD Jr, Fineman JR, Morin FC III, et al. Inhaled nitric oxide and persistent pulmonary hypertension of the newborn. N Engl J Med 1997; 336:605–610.

96. Inhaled nitric oxide in full-term and nearly full-term infants with hypoxic respiratory failure. The neonatal Inhaled Nitric Oxide Study Group. N Engl J Med 1997; 336:597–604.

97. Davidson D, Barefield ES, Kattwinkel J, et al. Inhaled nitric oxide for the early treatment of persistent pulmonary hypertension of the term newborn: a randomized, double-masked, placebo-controlled, dose–response, multicenter study. The I-NO/PPHN study group. Pediatrics 1998; 101:325–334.

98. Clark RH, Kueser TJ, Walker MW, et al. Low-dose nitric oxide therapy for persistent pulmonary hypertension of the newborn. Clinical inhaled nitric oxide research group. N Engl J Med 2000; 342:469–474.

99. Kinsella JP, Truog WE, Walsh WF, et al. Randomized, multicenter trial of inhaled nitric oxide and high- frequency oscillatory ventilation in severe, persistent pulmonary hypertension of the newborn. J Pediatr 1997; 131:55–62.

100. Kinsella JP, Abman SH. Inhaled nitric oxide and high frequency oscillatory ventilation in persistent pulmonary hypertension of the newborn. Eur J Pediatr 1998; 157(suppl 1):S28–S30.

101. Clark PL, Ekekezie II, Kaftan HA, Castor CA, Truog WE. Safety and efficacy of nitric oxide in chronic lung disease. Arch Dis Child Fetal Neonatal Ed 2002; 86:F41–F45.

102. Leclerc F, Riou Y, Martinot A, et al. Inhaled nitric oxide for a severe respiratory syncytial virus infection in an infant with bronchopulmonary dysplasia. Intensive Care Med 1994; 20:511–512.

103. Thompson MW, Bates JN, Klein JM. Treatment of respiratory failure in an infant with bronchopulmonary dysplasia infected with respiratory syncytial virus using inhaled nitric oxide and high frequency ventilation. Acta Paediatr 1995; 84:100–102.

104. Peliowski A, Finer NN, Etches PC, Tierney AJ, Ryan CA. Inhaled nitric oxide for premature infants after prolonged rupture of the membranes. J Pediatr 1995; 126:450–453.

105. Skimming JW, Bender KA, Hutchison AA, Drummond WH. Nitric oxide inhalation in infants with respiratory distress syndrome. J Pediatr 1997; 130:225–230.

106. Meurs KP, Rhine WD, Asselin JM, Durand DJ. Response of premature infants with severe respiratory failure to inhaled nitric oxide. Preemie NO collaborative group. Pediatr Pulmonol 1997; 24:319–323.

107. Radomski MW, Palmer RM, Moncada S. Comparative pharmacology of endothelium-derived relaxing factor, nitric oxide and prostacyclin in platelets. Br J Pharmacol 1987; 92:181–187.

108. Golino P, Cappelli-Bigazzi M, Ambrosio G, et al. Endothelium-derived relaxing factor modulates platelet aggregation in an in vivo model of recurrent platelet activation. Circ Res 1992; 71:1447–1456.

109. Kinsella JP, Walsh WF, Bose CL, et al. Inhaled nitric oxide in premature neonates with severe hypoxaemic respiratory failure: a randomised controlled trial (see comments). Lancet 1999; 354:1061–1065.

110. Subhedar NV, Ryan SW, Shaw NJ. Open randomised controlled trial of inhaled nitric oxide and early dexamethasone in high risk preterm infants. Arch Dis Child 1997; 77:F185–F190.

111. Gin-Mestan KK, Srisuparp P, Carlson AD, Thomas GR, Lee G, Marks JD. Inhaled nitric oxide improves oxygenation in permature infants with RDS: preliminary results of a prospective, randomized trial. Pediatric Academic Societies' 2002 Annual Meeting, Baltimore, MD, May 4–7, 2002.

112. Gin-Mestan KK, Troyke S, Lee G, Hecox KE. Improved neurodevelopmental outcome at one year in premature infants treated with inhaled nitric oxide:

preliminary results of a prospective, randomized trial. Pediatric Academic Societies' 2002 Annual Meeting, Baltimore, MD May 4–7, 2002.

113. Durante W, Schini VB, Kroll MH, et al. Platelets inhibit the induction of nitric oxide synthesis by interleukin-1 beta in vascular smooth muscle cells. Blood 1994; 83:1831–1838.

114. Joly GA, Schini VB, Vanhoutte PM. Balloon injury and interleukin-1 beta induce nitric oxide synthase activity in rat carotid arteries. Circ Res 1992; 71:331–338.

115. Wolin MS, Davidson CA, Kaminski PM, Fayngersh RP, Mohazzab HK. Oxidant-nitric oxide signalling mechanisms in vascular tissue. Biochemistry-Russia 1998; 63:810–816.

116. Gow AJ, Thom SR, Ischiropoulos H. Nitric oxide and peroxynitrite-mediated pulmonary cell death. Am J Physiol 1998; 274:L112–L118.

117. Darley-Usmar V, White R. Disruption of vascular signalling by the reaction of nitric oxide with superoxide: implications for cardiovascular disease. Exp Physiol 1997; 82:305–316.

118. Kooy NW, Royall JA, Ye YZ, Kelly DR, Beckman JS. Evidence for in vivo peroxynitrite production in human acute lung injury. Am J Respir Crit Care Med 1995; 151:1250–1254.

119. Bouhafs RK, Jarstrand C. Interaction between lung surfactant and nitric oxide production by alveolar macrophages stimulated by group B streptococci. Pediatr Pulmonol 2000; 30:106–113.

120. Haddad IY, Zhu S, Crow J, Barefield E, Gadilhe T, Matalon S. Inhibition of alveolar type II cell ATP and surfactant synthesis by nitric oxide. Am J Physiol 1996; 270:L898–L906.

121. Benkusky NA, Lewis SJ, Kooy NW. Attenuation of vascular relaxation after development of tachyphylaxis to peroxynitrite in vivo. Am J Physiol 1998; 275:H501–H508.

122. Weinberger B, Fakhrzadeh L, Heck DE, Laskin JD, Gardner CR, Laskin DL. Inhaled nitric oxide primes lung macrophages to produce reactive oxygen and nitrogen intermediates. Am J Respir Crit Care Med 1998; 158:931–938.

123. Weinberger B, Heck DE, Laskin DL, Laskin JD. Nitric oxide in the lung: therapeutic and cellular mechanisms of action. Pharmacol Ther 1999; 84:401–411.

124. Moncada S. Nitric oxide and cell respiration: physiology and pathology. Verhandelingen–Koninklijke Academie voor Geneeskunde van Belgie 2000; 62:171–181.

125. Thomassen MJ, Buhrow LT, Connors MJ, Kaneko FT, Erzurum SC, Kavuru MS. Nitric oxide inhibits inflammatory cytokine production by human alveolar macrophages. Am J Respir Cell Mol Biol 1997; 17:279–283.

126. Chollet-Martin S, Gatecel C, Kermarrec N, Gougerot-Pocidalo MA, Payen DM. Alveolar neutrophil functions and cytokine levels in patients with the adult respiratory distress syndrome during nitric oxide inhalation. Am J Respir Crit Care Med 1996; 153:985–990.

127. Haraldsson A, Kieler-Jensen N, Nathorst-Westfelt U, Bergh CH, Ricksten SE. Comparison of inhaled nitric oxide and inhaled aerosolized prostacyclin

in the evaluation of heart transplant candidates with elevated pulmonary vascular resistance. Chest 1998; 114:780–786.

128. Olschewski H, Walmrath D, Schermuly R, Ghofrani A, Grimminger F, Seeger W. Aerosolized prostacyclin and iloprost in severe pulmonary hypertension. Ann Intern Med 1996; 124:820–824.

129. Walmrath D, Schneider T, Pilch J, Grimminger F, Seeger W. Aerosolised prostacyclin in adult respiratory distress syndrome. Lancet 1993; 342: 961–962.

130. Zobel G, Dacar D, Rodl S, Friehs I. Inhaled nitric oxide vs. inhaled prostacyclin and intravenous vs. inhaled prostacyclin in acute respiratory failure with pulmonary hypertension in piglets. Pediatr Res 1995; 38:198–204.

131. Schenk P, Petkov V, Madl C, et al. Aerosolized iloprost therapy could not replace long-term IV epoprostenol (prostacyclin) administration in severe pulmonary hypertension. Chest 2001; 119:296–300.

132. Doctor A, Walsh B, Doorley P, Lowson S. Inhaled prostacyclin for acute pulmonary hypertension complicating congenital heart disease. Pediatric Academic Societies' 2002 Annual Meeting, Baltimore, MD, May 4–7, 2002.

133. De Jaegere AP, van den Anker JN. Endotracheal instillation of prostacyclin in preterm infants with persistent pulmonary hypertension. Eur Respir J 1998; 12:932–934.

134. Soditt V, Aring C, Groneck P. Improvement of oxygenation induced by aerosolized prostacyclin in a preterm infant with persistent pulmonary hypertension of the newborn. Intensive Care Med 1997; 23:1275–1278.

135. Domenighetti G, Stricker H, Waldispuehl B. Nebulized prostacyclin (PGI2) in acute respiratory distress syndrome: impact of primary (pulmonary injury) and secondary (extrapulmonary injury) disease on gas exchange response. Crit Care Med 2001; 29:57–62.

136. Moncada S. Eighth Gaddum Memorial Lecture. University of London Institute of Education, December 1980. Biological importance of prostacyclin. Br J Pharmacol 1982; 76:3–31.

137. Booke M, Bradford DW, Hinder F. Inhaled nitric oxide versus nebulized prostaglandin E_1 and nebulized prostacyclin. Appl Cardiovasc Pathophysiol 1997; 6:233–239.

138. Meyer J, Theilmeier G, Van Aken H, et al. Inhaled prostaglandin E1 for treatment of acute lung injury in severe multiple organ failure. Anesth Analg 1998; 86:753–758.

139. Putensen C, Hormann C, Kleinsasser A, Putensen-Himmer G. Cardiopulmonary effects of aerosolized prostaglandin E1 and nitric oxide inhalation in patients with acute respiratory distress syndrome. Am J Respir Crit Care Med 1998; 157:1743–1747.

140. Ahn HS, Crim W, Pitts B, Sybertz EJ. Calcium-calmodulin-stimulated and cyclic-GMP-specific phosphodiesterases. In: Strada SJ, Hidaka H, eds. Advances in Secoral Messenger and Phosphoprotein Research. Vol. 25. New York: Raven Press, 1992:271–288.

141. Sonnenburg WK, Beavo JA. Cyclic GMP and regulation of cyclic nucleotide hydrolysis. Adv Pharmacol 1994; 26:87–114.

142. Thompson WJ. Cyclic nucleotide phosphodiesterases: pharmacology, biochemistry and function. Pharmac Ther 1991; 51:13–33.

143. Murray KJ, England PJ. Inhibitors of cyclic nucleotide phosphodiesterases as therapeutic agents. Biochem Soc Trans 1992; 20:460–464.

144. Rabe KF, Tenor H, Dent G, Schudt C, Nakashima M, Magnussen H. Identification of PDE isozymes in human pulmonary artery and effect of selective PDE inhibitors. Am J Physiol 1994; 266:L536–L543.

145. Thomas M, Francis S, Corbin J. Characterization of a purified bovine lung CGMP-binding cGMP phosphodiesterase. J Biol Chem 1990; 265: 14964–14970.

146. Torphy TJ, Zhou HL, Burman M, Huang LB. Role of cyclic nucleotide phosphodiesterase isozymes in intact canine trachealis. Mol Pharmacol 1991; 39:376–384.

147. Hanson KA, Burns F, Rybalkin SD, Miller JW, Beavo J, Clarke WR. Developmental changes in lung cGMP phosphodiesterase-5 activity, protein, and message. Am J Respir Crit Care Med 1998; 158:279–288.

148. Hanson KA, Ziegler JW, Rybalkin SD, Miller JW, Abman SH, Clarke WR. Chronic pulmonary hypertension increases fetal lung cGMP phosphodiesterase activity. Am J Physiol 1998; 275:L931–L941.

149. Sanchez LS, Bloch KD. Nitric oxide regulates cGMP and cAMP phosphodiesterase enzyme activity and gene expression in rat pulmonary artery smooth muscle cells. Circulation 1999; 100:384.

150. Braner DA, Fineman JR, Chang R, Soifer SJ. M&B 22948, a cGMP phosphodiesterase inhibitor, is a pulmonary vasodilator in lambs. Am J Physiol 1993; 264:H252–H258.

151. Ziegler JW, Ivy DD, Fox JJ, Kinsella JP, Clarke WR, Abman SH. Dipyridamole, a cGMP phosphodiesterase inhibitor, causes pulmonary vasodilation in the ovine fetus. Am J Physiol 1995; 269:H473–H479.

152. Zhao L, Mason NA, Morrell NW, et al. Sildenafil inhibits hypoxia-induced pulmonary hypertension. Circulation 2001; 104:424–428.

153. Dukarm RC, Russell JA, Morin FC III, Perry BJ, Steinhorn RH. The cGMP-specific phosphodiesterase inhibitor E4021 dilates the pulmonary circulation. Am J Respir Crit Care Med 1999; 160:858–865.

154. Ziegler JW, Ivy DD, Wiggins JW, Kinsella JP, Clarke WR, Abman SH. Effects of dipyridamole and inhaled nitric oxide in pediatric patients with pulmonary hypertension. Am J Respir Crit Care Med 1998; 158:1388–1395.

155. Ziegler JW, Ivy DD, Fox JJ, Kinsella JP, Clarke WR, Abman SH. Dipyridamole potentiates pulmonary vasodilation induced by acetylcholine and nitric oxide in the ovine fetus. Am J Respir Crit Care Med 1998; 157:1104–1110.

156. Michelakis E, Tymchak W, Lien D, Webster L, Hashimoto K, Archer S. Oral sildenafil is an effective and specific pulmonary vasodilator in patients with pulmonary arterial hypertension. Circulation 2002; 105:2398–2403.

157. Mentzer RM Jr, Rubio R, Berne RM. Release of adenosine by hypoxic canine lung tissue and its possible role in pulmonary circulation. Am J Physiol 1975; 229:1625–1631.

158. Burnstock G. Overview. Purinergic mechanisms. Ann NY Acad Sci 1990; 603:1–18.

159. Konduri GG, Mital S, Gervasio CT, Rotta AT, Forman K. Purine nucleotides contribute to pulmonary vasodilation caused by birth-related stimuli in the ovine fetus. Am J Physiol 1997; 272:H2377–H2384.

160. Konduri GG, Theodorou AA. Nitro-L-arginine attenuates pulmonary vasodilation caused by adenosine in fetal lambs. Pediatr Res 1992; 31:62A.

161. Konduri GG, Mital S. Adenosine and ATP cause nitric oxide-dependent pulmonary vasodilation in fetal lambs. Biol Neonate 2000; 78:220–229.

162. Konduri GG, Garcia DC, Kazzi NJ, Shankaran S. Adenosine infusion improves oxygenation in term infants with respiratory failure. Pediatrics 1996; 97:295–300.

163. Nootens M, Schrader B, Kaufmann E, Vestal R, Long W, Rich S. Comparative acute effects of adenosine and prostacyclin in primary pulmonary hypertension. Chest 1995; 107:54–57.

164. Gaba SJ, Bourgouin-Karaouni D, Dujols P, Michel FB, Prefaut C. Effects of adenosine triphosphate on pulmonary circulation in chronic obstructive pulmonary disease. ATP: a pulmonary vasoregulator? Am Rev Respir Dis 1986; 134:1140–1144.

165. Schmidt BK. Antithrombin III deficiency in neonatal respiratory distress syndrome. Blood Coagul Fibrinolysis 1994; 5:S13–S17.

166. Bachofen M, Weibel ER. Structural alterations of lung parenchyma in the adult respiratory distress syndrome. Clin Chest Med 1982; 3:35–56.

167. Jackson LK. Idiopathic pulmonary fibrosis. Clin Chest Med 1982; 3:579–592.

168. Zapol WM, Jones R. Vascular components of ARDS. Clinical pulmonary hemodynamics and morphology. Am Rev Respir Dis 1987; 136:471–474.

169. Greene R. Pulmonary vascular obstruction in the adult respiratory distress syndrome. J Thorac Imaging 1986; 1:31–38.

170. Idell S. Extravascular coagulation and fibrin deposition in acute lung injury. New Horizons 1994; 2:566–574.

171. Hite RD, Morris PE. Acute respiratory distress syndrome: pharmacological treatment options in development. Drugs 2001; 61:897–907.

172. Bone RC, Francis PB, Pierce AK. Intravascular coagulation associated with the adult respiratory distress syndrome. Am J Med 1976; 61:585–589.

173. Idell S. Endothelium and disordered fibrin turnover in the injured lung: newly recognized pathways. Crit Care Med 2002; 30:S274–S280.

174. Johnson A, Tahamont MV, Malik AB. Thrombin-induced lung vascular injury. Roles of fibrinogen and fibrinolysis. Am Rev Respir Dis 1983; 128:38–44.

175. Neuhof H, Seeger W, Wolf HR. Generation of mediators by limited proteolysis during blood coagulation and fibrinolysis—its pathogenetic role in the adult respiratory distress syndrome (ARDS). Resuscitation 1986; 14:23–32.

176. Kaplan JE, Malik AB. Thrombin-induced intravascular coagulation: role in vascular injury. Semin Thromb Hemost 1987; 13:398–415.

177. Bell EF. Fluid therapy. In: Sinclair JC, Bracken MB, eds. Effective Care of the Newborn Infant. New York: Oxford University Press, 1992:59–72.

178. Ambrus CM, Weintraub DH, Dunphy D. Studies on hyaline membrane disease. The fibrinolysin system in pathogenesis and therapy. Pediatrics 1963; 32:10–24.

179. Ambrus CM, Weintrallb DH, Ambrus JL. Studies on hyaline membrane disease. 3. Therapeutic trial of urokinase-activated human plasmin. Pediatrics 1966; 38:231–43.

180. Ambrus CM, Choi TS, Cunnanan E, et al. Prevention of hyaline membrane disease with plasminogen. A cooperative study. JAMA 1977; 237:1837–1841.

181. Giudici D, Baudo F, Palareti G, Ravizza A, Ridolfi L, A DA. Antithrombin replacement in patients with sepsis and septic shock. Haematologica 1999; 84:452–460.

182. Inthorn D, Hoffmann JN, Hartl WH, Muhlbayer D, Jochum M. Effect of antithrombin III supplementation on inflammatory response in patients with severe sepsis. Shock. 1998; 10:90–96.

183. Eisele B, Lamy M, Thijs LG, et al. Antithrombin III in patients with severe sepsis. A randomized, placebo-controlled, double-blind multicenter trial plus a meta-analysis on all randomized, placebo-controlled, double-blind trials with antithrombin III in severe sepsis. Intensive Care Med 1998; 24:663–672.

184. Baudo F, Caimi TM, de Cataldo F, et al. Antithrombin III (ATIII) replacement therapy in patients with sepsis and/or postsurgical complications: a controlled double-blind, randomized, multicenter study. Intensive Care Med 1998; 24:336–342.

185. Goldfarb RD, Glock D, Johnson K, et al. Randomized, blinded, placebo-controlled trial of tissue factor pathway inhibitor in porcine septic shock. Shock. 1998; 10:258–264.

186. Randolph MM, White GL, Kosanke SD, et al. Attenuation of tissue thrombosis and hemorrhage by ala-TFPI does not account for its protection against *E. coli*—a comparative study of treated and untreated nonsurviving baboons challenged with LD100 *E. coli*. Thromb Haemost 1998; 79:1048–1053.

187. Carr C, Bild GS, Chang AC, et al. Recombinant E. coli-derived tissue factor pathway inhibitor reduces coagulopathic and lethal effects in the baboon gram-negative model of septic shock. Circ Shock 1994; 44:126–137.

188. Thusu KG, Morin FC III, Russell JA, Steinhorn RH. The cGMP phosphodiesterase inhibitor zaprinast enhances the effect of nitric oxide. Am J Respir Crit Care Med 1995; 152:1605–1610.

189. Ivy DD, Kinsella JP, Ziegler JW, Abman SH. Dipyridamole attenuates rebound pulmonary hypertension after inhaled nitric oxide withdrawal in postoperative congenital heart disease. J Thorac Cardiovasc Surg 1998; 115:875–882.

190. Haraldsson A, Kieler-Jensen N, Ricksten S-E. The additive pulmonary vasodilatory effects of inhaled prostacyclin and inhaled milrinone in postcardiac surgical patients with pulmonary hypertension. Anestha Analg 2001; 93: 1439–1445.

191. Wilkens J, Guth A, König J, et al. Effect of inhaled iloprost plus oral sildenafil in patients with primary pulmonary hypertension. Circulation 2001; 104:1218–1222.

192. Ghofrani HA, Wiedemann R, Rose F, et al. Combination therapy with oral sildenafil and inhaled iloprost for severe pulmonary hypertension. Ann Intern Med 2002; 136:515–522.

193. Sitbon O, Brenot F, Denjean A, et al. Inhaled nitric oxide as a screening vasodilator agent in primary pulmonary hypertension. A dose–response study and comparison with prostacyclin. Am J Respir Crit Care Med 1995; 151:384–389.

194. Ashbaugh D, Bigelow D, Petty T, Levine B. Acute respiratory distress in adults. Lancet 1967; August 12:319–323.
195. Dantzker DR, Brook CJ, Dehart P, Lynch JP, Weg JG. Ventilation–perfusion distributions in the adult respiratory distress syndrome. Am Rev Respir Dis 1979; 120:1039–1052.
196. Naeije R, Melot C, Niset G, Delcroix M, Wagner PD. Mechanisms of improved arterial oxygenation after peripheral chemoreceptor stimulation during hypoxic exercise. J Appl Physiol 1993; 74:1666–1671.
197. Reyes A, Roca J, Rodriquez-Roisin R, Torres A, Ussetti P, Wagner PD. Effect of almitrine on ventilation–perfusion distribution in adult respiratory distress syndrome. Am Rev Respir Dis 1988; 137:1062–1067.
198. Dembinski R, Max M, Lopez F, Kuhlen R, Sunner M, Rossaint R. Effect of inhaled nitric oxide in combination with almitrine on ventilation–perfusion distributions in experimental lung injury. Intensive Care Med 2000; 26:221–228.
199. Papazian L, Bregeon F, Gaillat F, et al. Inhaled NO and almitrine bismesylate in patients with acute respiratory distress syndrome: effect of noradrenalin. Eur Respir J 1999; 14:1283–1289.
200. Wysocki M, Delclaux C, Roupie E, et al. Additive effect on gas exchange of inhaled nitric oxide and intravenous almitrine bismesylate in the adult respiratory distress syndrome. Intensive Care Med 1994; 20:254–259.
201. Lu Q, Mourgeon E, Law-Koune JD, Roche S, Vezinet C. Dose–response curves of inhaled nitric oxide with and without intravenous almitrine in nitric oxide-responding patients with acute respiratory distress syndrome. Anesthesiology 1995; 83:929–943.
202. Jolliet P, Bulpa P, Ritz M, Ricou B, Lopez J, Chevrolet JC. Additive beneficial effects of the prone position, nitric oxide, and almitrine bismesylate on gas exchange and oxygen transport in acute respiratory distress syndrome. Crit Care Med 1997; 25:786–794.
203. B'chir A, Mebazaa A, Losser MR, Romieu M, Payen D. Intravenous almitrine bismesylate reversibly induces lactic acidosis and hepatic dysfunction in patients with acute lung injury. Anesthesiology 1998; 89:823–830.
204. Payen D, Muret J, Beloucif S, Gatecel C. Inhaled nitric oxide, almitrine infusion, or their coadministration as a treatment of severe hypoxemic focal lung lesions. Anesthesiology 1998; 89:1157–1165.
205. Gallart L, Lu Q, Puybasset L, Rao GS, Coriat P, Rouby JJ. Intravenous almitrine combined with inhaled nitric oxide for acute respiratory distress syndrome. Am J Respir Crit Care Med 1998; 158:1770–1777.
206. Gillart T, Bazin JE, Cosserant B, et al. Combined nitric oxide inhalation, prone positioning and almitrine infusion improve oxygenation in severe ARDS. Can J Anaesth 1998; 45:402–409.
207. Dembinski R, Max M, Lopez F, Kuhlen R, Kurth R, Rossaint R. Effect of inhaled prostacyclin in combination with almitrine on ventilation–perfusion distributions in experimental lung injury. Anesthesiology 2001; 94:461–467.
208. Karamanoukian HL, Glick PL, Zayek M, et al. Inhaled nitric oxide in congenital hypoplasia of the lungs due to diaphragmatic hernia or oligohydramnios. Pediatrics 1994; 94:715–718.

209. Wilcox DT, Glick PL, Karamanoukian HL, Leach CL, Morin FC III, Fuhrman BP. Perfluorocarbon associated gas exchange improves pulmonary mechanics, oxygenation, ventilation, and allows nitric oxide delivery in the hypoplastic lung congenital diaphragmatic hernia lamb model. Crit Care Med 1995; 23:1858–1863.

210. Levin ER, Gardner DG, Samson WK. Mechanisms of Disease: Natriuretic peptides. N Engl J Med 1998; 339:321–328.

211. Sudoh T, Minamino N, Kanagawa K, Hisayauki M. C-type natriuretic peptide (CNP): a new member of natriuretic peptide family identified in porcine brain. Biochem Biophys Res Commun 1990; 168:863–870.

212. Suga S, Nakao K, Itoh H, et al. Endothelial production of C-type natriuretic peptide and its marked augmentation by transforming growth factor-beta. Possible existence of "vascular natriuretic peptide system" J Clin Invest 1992; 90:1145–1149.

213. Lewicki JA, Protter AA. Molecular determinants of natriuretic peptide clearance receptor function. In: Samson WK, Levin ER, eds. Contemporary Endocrinology; Natriuretic peptides in Health and Disease. Totowa, NJ: Humana Press, 1997:51–69.

214. Foster DC, Garbers DL, Wedel BJ. The guanylyl cyclase-A receptor. In: Samson WK, Levin ER, eds. Contemporary Endocrinology; Natriuretic peptides in Health and Disease. Totawa, NJ: Humana Press, 1997:21–34.

215. Lowe DG. The guanylyl cyclase-B receptor. In: Samson WK, Levin ER, eds. Contemporary Endocrinology; Natriuretic peptides in Health and Disease. Totowa, NJ: Humana Press, 1997:35–50.

216. Lakshminrusimha S, D'Angelis CA, Russell JA, et al. C-type natriuretic peptide system in fetal ovine pulmonary vasculature. Am J Physiol Lung Cell Mol Physiol 2001; 281:L361–L368.

217. Tanabe M, Ueda M, Endo M, Kitajima M. Effect of acute lung injury and coexisting disorders on plasma concentrations of atrial natriuretic peptide. Crit Care Med 1994; 22:1762–1768.

218. Mitaka C, Hirata Y, Nagura T, Sakanishi N, Tsunoda Y, Amaha K. Plasma alpha-human atrial natriuretic peptide concentration in patients with acute lung injury. Am Rev Respir Dis 1992; 146:43–46.

219. Mitaka C, Hirata Y, Nagura T, Tsunoda Y, Itoh M, Amaha K. Increased plasma concentrations of brain natriuretic peptide in patients with acute lung injury. J Crit Care 1997; 12:66–71.

220. Richards AM, Lainchbury JG, Nicholls MG, Troughton RW, Yandle TG. BNP in hormone-guided treatment of heart failure. Trends Endocrinol Metab 2002; 13:151–155.

221. Nicholls MG, Lainchbury JG, Richards AM, Troughton RW, Yandle TG. Brain natriuretic peptide-guided therapy for heart failure. Ann Med 2001; 33:422–427.

222. Mitaka C, Hirata Y, Nagura T, Tsunoda Y, Amaha K. Beneficial effect of atrial natriuretic peptide on pulmonary gas exchange in patients with acute lung injury. Chest 1998; 114:223–228.

223. Bindels AJ, van der Hoeven JG, Groeneveld PH, Frolich M, Meinders AE. Atrial natriuretic peptide infusion and nitric oxide inhalation in patients with acute respiratory distress syndrome. Crit Care 2001; 5:151–157.

224. Demiryurek AT, Wadsworth RM. Superoxide in the pulmonary circulation. Pharmacol Ther 1999; 84:355–365.

225. Steinhorn RH, Russell JA. Nitric oxide and persistent pulmonary hypertension in the newborn. In: Ignarro LJ, ed. Nitric oxide—Biology and Pathobiology. San Diego CA: Academic Press, 2000:963–981.

226. Steinhorn RH, Morin FC III, Russell JA. The adventitia may be a barrier specific to nitric oxide in rabbit pulmonary artery. J Clin Invest 1994; 94:1883–1888.

227. Wang Y, Coceani F. EDRF in pulmonary resistance vessels from fetal lamb: stimulation by oxygen and bradykinin. Am J Physiol Heart Circ Physiol 1994; 266 :H936–H943.

228. Munzel T, Sayegh H, Freeman BA, Tarpey MM, Harrison DG. Evidence for enhanced vascular superoxide anion production in nitrate tolerance. A novel mechanism underlying tolerance and cross-tolerance. J Clin Invest 1995; 95:187–194.

229. Beckman JS, Beckman TW, Chen J, Marshall PA, Freeman BA. Apparent hydroxyl radical production by peroxynitrite: implications for endothelial injury from nitric oxide and superoxide. Proc Natl Acad Sci U S A 1990; 87:1620–1624.

230. Zou M, Ullrich V. Peroxynitrite formed by simultaneous generation of nitric oxide and superoxide selectively inhibits bovine aortic prostacyclin synthase. FEBS Lett 1996; 382(1–2):101–104.

231. Cherry PD, Omar HA, Farrell KA, Stuart JS, Wolin MS. Superoxide anion inhibits cGMP-associated bovine pulmonary arterial relaxation. Am J Physiol Heart CIRC Physiol 1990; 259 :H1056–H1062.

232. Friebe A, Schultz G, Koesling D. Stimulation of soluble guanylate cyclase by superoxide dismutase is mediated by NO. Biochem J 1998; 335:527–531.

233. Steinhorn RH, Albert G, Swartz DD, Russell JA, Levine CR, Davis JM. Recombinant human superoxide dismutase enhances the effect of inhaled nitric oxide in persistent pulmonary hypertension. Am J Respir Crit Care Med 2001; 164:834–839.

234. Nakamura T, Ogawa Y. Prophylactic effects of recombinant human superoxide dismutase in neonatal lung injury induced by the intratracheal instillation of endotoxin in piglets. Biol Neonate 2001; 80:163–168.

235. Robbins CG, Horowitz S, Merritt TA, et al. Recombinant human superoxide dismutase reduces lung injury caused by inhaled nitric oxide and hyperoxia. Am J Physiol 1997; 272:L903–L907.

236. Bone HG, Sakurai H, Schenarts PJ, Traber LD, Traber DL. Effects of manganese superoxide dismutase, when given after inhalation injury has been established. Crit Care Med 2002; 30:856–860.

237. Metnitz PG, Bartens C, Fischer M, Fridrich P, Stelzner H, Druml W. Antioxidant status in patients with acute respiratory distress syndrome. Intensive Care Med 1999; 25:180–185.

238. Davis JM, Rosenfeld WN, Richter SE, et al. Safety and pharmacokinetics of multiple doses of recombinant human CuZn superoxide dismutase administered intratracheally to premature neonates with respiratory distress syndrome. Pediatrics 1997; 100:24–30.

239. Davis JM, Richter SE, Biswas S, et al. Long-term follow-up of premature infants treated with prophylactic, intratracheal recombinant human CuZn superoxide dismutase. J Perinatol 2000; 20:213–216.

240. Langenback EG, Davis JM, Robbins C, Sahgal N, Perry RJ, Simon SR. Improved pulmonary distribution of recombinant human Cu/Zn superoxide dismutase, using a modified ultrasonic nebulizer. Pediatr Pulmonol 1999; 27:124–129.

241. Rubin LJ, Badesch DB, Barst RJ, et al. Bosentan therapy for pulmonary arterial hypertension. N Engl J Med 2002; 346:896–903.

242. Hopkins N, Cadogan E, Giles S, McLoughlin P. Chronic airway infection leads to angiogenesis in the pulmonary circulation. J Appl Physiol 2001; 91:919–928.

243. Kaner RJ, Ladetto JV, Singh R, Fukuda N, Matthay MA, Crystal RG. Lung overexpression of the vascular endothelial growth factor gene induces pulmonary edema. Am J Respir Cell Mol Biol 2000; 22:657–664.

244. Thickett DR, Armstrong L, Christie SJ, Millar AB. Vascular endothelial growth factor may contribute to increased vascular permeability in acute respiratory distress syndrome. Am J Respir Crit Care Med 2001; 164:1601–1605.

245. Partovian C, Adnot S, Raffestin B, et al. Adenovirus-mediated lung vascular endothelial growth factor overexpression protects against hypoxic pulmonary hypertension in rats. Am J Respir Cell Mol Biol 2000; 23:762–761.

246. Campbell AIM, Zhao Y, Sandhu R, Stewart DJ. Cell-based gene transfer of vascular endothelial growth factor attenuates monocrotaline-induced pulmonary hypertension. Circulation 2001; 104:2242–2248.

247. Warren BL, Eid A, Singer P, Pillay SS, Carl P, Novak I, Chalupa P, Atherstone A, Penzes I, Kubler A, Knaub S, Keinecke HO, Heinrichs H, Schindel F, Juers M, Bone RC, Opal SM. (KyperSept Trial Study Group). Caring for the critically ill patient. High-dose antithrombin III in severe sepsis: a randomized controlled trial. JAMA 2001; 286:1869–1878.

248. Bernard GR, Margolis BD, Shanies HM, Ely EW, Wheeler AP, Levy H, Wong K, Wright TJ. (Extended Evaluation of Recombinant Human Activated Protein C United States Investigators). Extended evalution of recombinant human activated protein C United States Trial (ENHANCE US): a single-arm, phase 3B, muticenter study of drotrecogin alfa (activated) in severe sepsis. Chest 2004; 125:2206–2216.

18

Gene Therapy for Lung Injury

P. J. SIME, R. J. WHITE, M. KOLB, M. HITT, and J. GAULDIE

*Department of Medicine (Division of Pulmonary and Critical Care Medicine),
University of Rochester, Rochester, New York, U.S.A.,
Department of Oncology, Cross Cancer Institute, Edmond, Alberta, Canada, and
Department of Pathology and Molecular Medicine, McMaster University,
Hamilton, Ontario, Canada*

I. Overview

This chapter discusses gene therapy and its use in mitigating pulmonary pathology involving acute or chronic lung injury. Strategies of gene transfer can be directed at genomic integrated long-term (permanent) expression, long-term nonintegrated expression, or short-term nonintegrated expression. Gene therapy is unique among clinical interventions in that it has the potential to generate a prolonged effect at the cellular level that is not subject to pathways of excretion that affect traditional pharmacologic agents. Conversely, gene therapy presents unique challenges in terms of its development and application. This chapter discusses the scope of potential gene-based therapies for lung injury, and the advantages and disadvantages of common delivery systems including viral vectors, liposomes or polymer encapsulation, and naked DNA. Current preclinical research and clinical trials of gene therapy for inflammatory, fibrotic, and immune diseases are reviewed, and specific practical examples of gene therapy are presented. Future directions for this evolving and exciting field are also outlined.

II. Introduction

Rapid advances in understanding the mechanistic pathophysiology of lung injury have identified a number of agents and therapeutic strategies of potential benefit to patients with related pulmonary diseases. However, current clinical therapies for many injury-related pulmonary diseases are far from optimal. Ventilation therapies for injury-associated respiratory failure have been detailed in Chapter 13, and pharmacologic therapies directed against inflammation, surfactant dysfunction, oxidant injury, and vascular dysfunction are discussed in Chapters 14–17 and 19. Pharmacologic therapies for lung injury entail systemic or airway administration of agents seeking to antagonize key effectors of inflammation or other aspects of pathology, or to augment pulmonary defenses. An alternate approach to achieve these goals is pulmonary gene therapy. In principle, delivery of genes to lung tissue allows the controlled transient or prolonged overexpression of protective proteins that can then act at the intracellular and extracellular level to antagonize specific lung injury processes and signaling pathways. The methods used in gene therapy, and current information on the efficacy of this strategy in patients with pulmonary disease, are the primary focus of discussion here.

III. Gene Transfer Approaches

A central issue in gene therapy is the effective delivery and uptake of genetic material by target cells. The accessibility of the lungs to airway delivery makes this organ particularly attractive for gene therapy applications. A number of systems have been used to transfer genes of interest into the lungs, not all directed at therapeutic intervention. Gene transfer to the highly accessible tracheobronchial epithelium is the most straightforward. Gene transfer to the lower bronchioles or the alveolar epithelium is also feasible, depending on factors such as the method of administration (fluid instillation, aerosolized liquid, or particulate powder, etc.), the size of the delivered particles, and the state of the subject. Access to the pulmonary parenchyma relies on absorption through the airway or alveolar epithelium, and is a much more difficult task for targeted gene therapy. The vasculature of the lung can also be accessed, although there are few approaches developed to date that confine this kind of delivery to the lungs when vectors or plasmids are introduced into the circulation. Vascular trapping of ex vivo gene modified cells may have some utility for endothelial gene transfer. Most data to date on pulmonary gene transfer have involved the airway epithelium. However, systems used for all approaches are summarized here to provide a broader spectrum of information.

Transfer of genes falls into three main categories: genomic integrated long-term (permanent) expression, long-term nonintegrated expression, and short-term nonintegrated expression. With appropriate delivery systems, gene transfer should result in cell-specific expression of therapeutic molecules, using targeted vectors and cell-specific promoters. However, there are a number of barriers that present problems for efficient gene transfer to the lung. The mucus lining, surfactant, and glycocalyx all provide natural physical and chemical protection against infections and thus impair access of gene transfer vectors to pulmonary epithelial cells. Moreover, the receptors for many of the virus vectors used to date appear to reside on the basolateral surface of the epithelium and are less available for interaction and subsequent entry of the vector to the cell (1–3). Delivery of therapeutic genes also requires a system able to withstand the hostile environment of a damaged or infected lung with many inflammatory mediators and an abundance of leukocytes and associated degradative contents (4,5). It would be beneficial if the mode of delivery were to be restricted to the lung, such as delivery by bronchoscope or by aerosol inhalation, routes that have already been used for some systems (6–8). Other approaches may need to involve access to the parenchyma through opening of epithelial cell tight junctions using EGTA (9) or delivery in surfactant (10,11). Table 1 summarizes the characteristics of an ideal vector system.

Gene vectors and transfer systems differ in their modes of action and routes of introduction to cells, although all have the capacity to cause expression of the gene of interest as a therapeutic intervention or disease modifier. Recent advances in the design of adenovirus, adeno-associated virus (AAV), poxvirus, retrovirus, lentivirus, and nonviral vectors make it technically feasible to deliver therapeutic genes to lung tissue. However, different vector and transfer systems have specific advantages and limitations. Table 2 summarizes the properties of the various vector systems available, which are described in more detail below.

A. Retroviral Vectors: Murine Leukemia Virus and Lentivirus

Retroviruses (RVs) have been classified into different groups based on biological properties and genome structure (12). Most retroviral gene therapy vectors have been derived from murine leukemia viruses (MLVs), which are mammalian C-type retroviruses. Ecotropic MLVs replicate in murine cells only, while xenotropic MLVs replicate in nonmurine mammalian cells and amphotropic MLVs replicate in both murine and nonmurine cells. Recently, lentiviruses, another subfamily of retroviruses, have gained appeal as gene transfer vectors because of their ability to transduce nondividing cells.

RV particles (12) contain two single-stranded RNA genomes packaged in an enveloped nucleocapsid. This nucleocapsid is composed of structural proteins as well as viral proteins required for proviral DNA

Table 1 Ideal Vector Characteristics for Pulmonary Gene Transfer

High affinity for respiratory epithelial cells
High affinity for pulmonary vascular endothelial cells
Efficient transfer and expression in epithelial or endothelial cells
Nonintegrating or targeted integration to the genome
Controlled or well-described duration of expression
Survives within hostile inflamed tissue
Elicits little or no immune or inflammatory response

synthesis and integration within the cell. A ubiquitous phosphate transporter has been identified as the receptor for amphotropic MLV (13). Primate lentiviruses bind to CD4, one of the chemokine receptors on T-lymphocytes and other cells involved in inflammation and immunity (14). Receptor bind-

Table 2 Comparison of Vector Properties for Gene Transfer

Vector	Gene insert size	Localization and duration	Efficiency of expression	Immuno-genicity
RNA virus				
Retrovirus	8 kb	Nuclear, integrated, long term	Low to moderate	Low
Lentivirus	8 kb	Nuclear, integrated, long term	Low to moderate	Low
DNA virus				
Pox virus	>25 kb	Episomal, transient	High	High
Adenovirus 1st generation	8.3 kb	Episomal, transient	High	Moderate to high
Adenovirus helper dependent	37 kb	Episomal, transient/long	High	Low
Adeno-associated virus	4 kb	Episomal and integrated, long term	Moderate	Low
Nonviral vectors				
Cationic lipids	Unknown	Episomal, transient	Low	Low
Cationic polymers	Unknown	Episomal, transient	Low	Low to moderate
Naked DNA	Unknown	Episomal, transient	Low	Low

ing triggers fusion of the viral and cellular membranes allowing entry of the viral nucleocapsid into the cytoplasm of the host cell. Using a cellular tRNA as primer, the viral reverse transcriptase catalyzes synthesis of double-stranded proviral DNA. Once inside the nucleus, the viral integrase mediates random insertion of proviral DNA into the host chromosome. Although they share many features, the genomic structure of the prototypical lentivirus HIV-1 is more complex than that of MLV (12,15).

B. Murine Leukemia Virus Vectors

Retroviral vector systems based on MLV have been in use for nearly 20 years (16,17). The vector backbone incorporates all of the *cis*-acting elements required for virus production, i.e., the 5′ and 3′ long terminal repeats (LTRs) that include the sequences required for chromosomal integration, the initiation of reverse transcription, and the packaging signal between the 5′ LTR and *gag* coding sequences. With all of the viral coding sequences removed, retroviral vectors can accommodate up to about 8 kilobase (kb) of foreign DNA. High levels of transgene expression can be promoted from the vector LTRs, or from an internal heterologous promoter. Gag, Pol, and Env precursors are supplied by packaging cell lines (termed production in *trans*). The *env* gene is usually derived from an amphotropic virus to increase the vector host range to include both rodents and humans and most useful vectors are grown in human cell lines (18).

RV vectors can transduce a wide variety of cells as long as the cells are proliferating. However, transduction efficiency is typically low, and transgene expression is variable and depends on the number of cells transduced, the strength of the promoter, and whether the chromosome at the site of insertion is in an active configuration (19). Moreover, cells such as alveolar macrophages are able to inactivate retroviruses, making in vivo administration to the lungs questionable (20). To circumvent these problems, most retroviral gene transfer is performed ex vivo, and transduced cells expressing the highest level of transgene are selected and expanded for reintroduction into the host. At best this strategy is cumbersome, and the process of selection and expansion can potentially alter the desired target cell population, e.g., inducing differentiation of stem cells or selecting for a subset of target cells.

The stable integration of retroviral vectors into the host chromosome allows transgene expression to continue indefinitely as long as the promoter stays active. However, chromosomal integration of proviral DNA is accompanied by a risk of insertional mutagenesis. This is countered by an advantage of MLV vectors, which do not induce host immune responses against vector-infected cells, since the vectors are stripped of all viral coding sequences.

C. Lentiviral Vectors

Cis-acting viral sequences carried by lentiviral vectors are similar to those described for MLV vectors (21,22). Functions required for virus production are supplied in *trans*. Studies have shown that all of the accessory genes can be deleted with little loss in transduction efficiency for most cell types (23). In addition, the *Tat* genes are also dispensable if the promoter sequence in the LTR is replaced with that of RSV or the HCMV immediate early gene (24). The current method of choice for high titer lentivirus vector production requires complex cotransfection of a cell line with multiple plasmids. Because this procedure is not amenable to large scale vector production, attempts have been made to generate packaging cell lines (21), but none have been completely successful. Lentiviral vectors can transduce a number of nondividing cell types either in vitro or in vivo, including neurons, retinal cells, liver, and skeletal muscle (25–27), but to date have a low expression capacity in airway cells (28). Although the transduction efficiency is less than that of adenovirus vectors, transgene expression has been observed for months following in vivo lentiviral gene delivery (27,29). Importantly, no inflammation or host immune response against vector-infected cells has been detected.

D. Adeno-Associated Viral Vectors

Adeno-associated virus is a small nonpathogenic DNA virus, which is relatively common based on the prevalence of AAV neutralizing antibodies in the population (30). The AAV virion consists of a 4.7 kb single-stranded linear DNA genome enclosed in a nonenveloped viral capsid (Fig. 1A). Although the host cell receptors for AAV have not been definitively demonstrated, evidence suggests that the AAV type 2 virion, at least, enters the cell by binding to the proteoglycan heparan sulfate, with alpha-v-beta-5 integrin and/or fibroblast growth factor receptor 1 acting as coreceptors (31–33). The virion is transported to the nucleus where the transcriptionally inactive single-stranded genome is converted to a double-stranded template. In the absence of helper virus, AAV generates a latent infection. Rep proteins, which have helicase, ATPase, and site-specific nicking activities, mediate integration of the AAV genome at a specific site in chromosome 19 (34,35), albeit at a low frequency. In the presence of helper virus, which can be adenovirus, herpes simplex virus, or others, a productive AAV infection ensues which requires Rep, helper proteins, and host factors (36).

The recombinant adeno-associated virus (rAAV) vector systems in use today are based on AAV serotype 2 (37,38). Both the *rep* and *cap* genes are deleted from current AAV vectors to allow insertion of transgene expression cassettes up to 4.7 kb in length (Fig. 1B). Because *rep* and *cap* are required for virus production, they must be provided in *trans*. AAV vectors can trans-

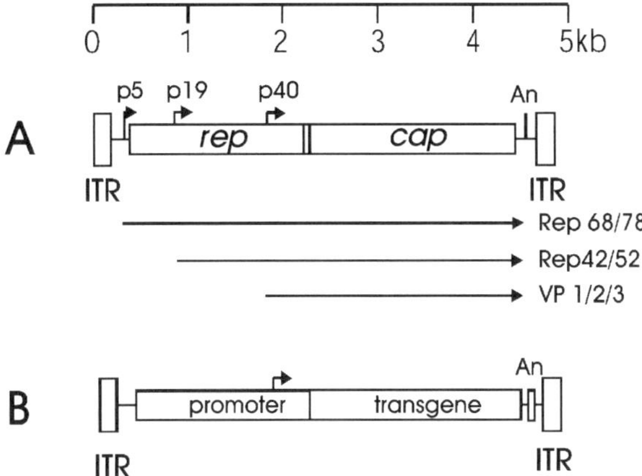

Figure 1 Adeno-associated virus and AAV vector maps. Open boxes at the ends of the genome map indicate the inverted terminal repeats (ITRs). Transcription start sites are indicated by bent arrows above the genome map. The polyadenylation signal is designated An. (A) Map of adeno-associated virus genome and primary transcripts. AAV transcripts are indicated by arrows below the genome map. (B) Map of AAV vector.

duce many different cell types, including both proliferating and non-proliferating cells. Interestingly, greater transduction is obtained in dividing cells than nondividing cells in vitro, while the opposite is true in vivo, although the reasons for this are not totally clear (37). AAV has a high trophism for epithelial cells (39–41) and has shown promise as a vector for therapy of single gene diseases such as cystic fibrosis (CF) because of the capacity for long-term expression (42–44). AAV vectors can integrate into the host chromosome allowing long-term stable gene expression even in proliferating cells. Unlike wild-type AAV, however, this integration is at random sites, since *rep* has been deleted from the recombinant vector, introducing a risk of potential insertional mutagenesis in rAAV-transduced cells. Another disadvantage of AAV as a vector is the high degree of pre-existing immunity to AAV in the population.

E. Adenovirus Vectors

Adenovirus (Ad) is the vector of choice when the objective is to produce high levels of transgene expression in pulmonary epithelium or to transduce the greatest number of cells. Ad vectors are relatively easy to generate, grow to high titers and are quite stable. Ad has a high affinity for gene transfer to pulmonary tissue as epithelial cells represent the primary site for infection and these cells express high levels of the Coxsackie-adenovirus receptor (CAR), required for entry into the cell. The virus itself has been well characterized, having been used extensively for over 20 years as a model for gene regulation, transcription, and RNA processing in mammalian cells. Furthermore, even wild-type Ad is relatively nonpathogenic, producing symptoms similar to a mild case of influenza. The major disadvantage of standard (first generation) Ad vectors is the antiviral immune response induced in the recipient. However, recent modifications in the vector backbone have reduced this immunogenicity, upholding the status of Ad as one of the most useful delivery vehicles available for gene transfer to the lung.

The Ad particle is composed of a 30–40 kb double-stranded linear DNA genome enclosed in a nonenveloped capsid of virally encoded proteins (45) (Fig. 2A). Two of the capsid proteins, fiber and penton base, are involved in viral entry into the host cell. The receptor for Coxsackie-adenovirus, which is expressed on a wide variety of cells, has been identified as one cellular receptor for Ad (46,47), while penton base binds to alpha-v integrins on the host (48), inducing endocytosis of Ad. Inside the cell, the endosomal membrane is disrupted releasing the virus into the cytoplasm. The viral capsid is shed gradually as the virus is transported finally to the nucleus, where the genome remains in an episomal form throughout the processes of transcription, replication, and packaging.

First Generation Ad Vector

Dozens of serotypes of adenovirus have been identified, with Ad type 2 (Ad2) and Ad type 5 (Ad5), being the most commonly used for gene transfer (49,50). Nearly all of early region 1(E1) is deleted from most Ad vectors to prevent virus replication and as a consequence, Ad vectors must be propagated in cell lines which can supply E1 proteins in *trans,* such as the 293 cell line (51). Because E3 is not required for propagation of the virus in vitro, it too is usually deleted from the vector backbone (Fig. 2B). Vectors referred to as "first generation" Ad vectors are lacking only the E1 and E3 regions, and can accept inserts with a maximum size of about 8.3 kb (52).

The transduction efficiency of recombinant Ad vectors for many cell types is quite high, reaching close to 100% for epithelial cells in culture, although in vivo transduction rates of 10–30% are more common. Ad can transduce a wide variety of cell types (and of different species), regardless of the proliferation status of the cells. However, the viral genome remains episomal, and the vector is therefore not stably maintained in proliferating cells. Nonetheless, viral gene expression begins within hours and lasts for up to 10 days at significant detectable levels (53). There has been considerable effort made in attempting to direct the infection of specific cell types by Ad vectors. Antibodies directed to the angiotensin-converting enzyme (ACE) or to CD105 have had some success in targeting the pulmonary

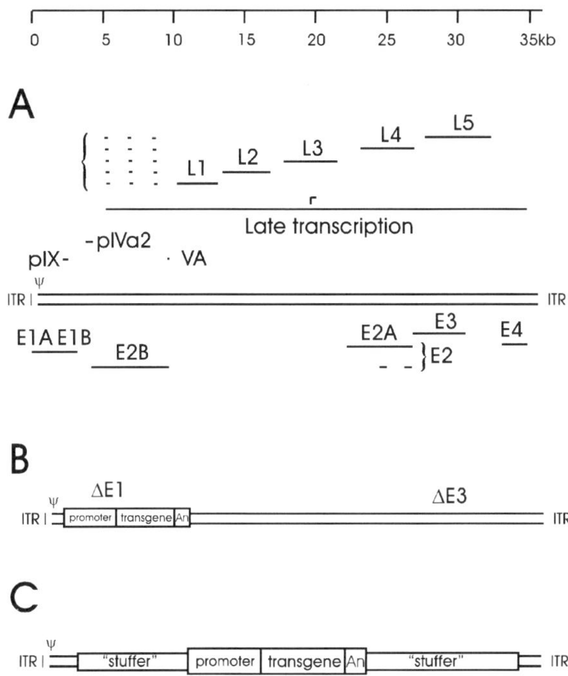

Figure 2 Adenovirus and Ad vector maps. Open boxes at the ends of the genome map indicate the ITRs. The packaging signal is designated by the symbol ψ. (A) Map of Ad5 genome and transcription units. Early region transcripts are indicated by solid arrows below the genome map and intermediate or late transcripts are shown above the genome. The primary major late promoter (MLP) transcript is processed to generate the families of late transcripts (L1–L5) as shown. (B) Map of first generation Ad vector. (C) Map of helper-dependent Ad vector. The sites of early region (E) 1 and 3 deletions are indicated by ΔE1 and ΔE3, respectively. The transgene expression cassette, with the polyadenylation signal designated An, is indicated by open boxes within the genome. The "stuffer" sequence ideally contains no open reading frames.

endothelium (54,55) or engineering fiber domains of the adenovirus to express RGD epitopes (56,57). However, there has been little success in restricting infection and expression to the epithelium by this approach. Vascular restriction might be enhanced by using cell-specific promoters, such as the VEGF receptor (flt-1) in the vector (58,59).

The most serious problem associated with first generation Ad vectors, particularly for long-term gene expression, is the induction of an antiviral immune response in the host (60). This response can be attributed to expression of viral proteins in the transduced cells (61), as well as the viral particle itself (62,63). The result of the host inflammatory response is to limit both the duration of expression and the effectiveness of readministration of the vector (64,65). It is possible by the use of formulation additives such as polyethylene glycol or other fluids, to modulate the effect of the immune response (66,67). However, the fact remains that Ad is a pathogenic organism in humans. As a result, Ad vectors are likely to stimulate a robust host response under many conditions, thus limiting their use to short-term, nonrepeated administration.

Helper-Dependent Ad Vectors

Ad vectors have recently been reported which encode no viral proteins at all, thus minimizing the host immune response against vector-infected cells, while maximizing the cloning capacity (up to 37 kb). The only Ad sequences carried by these vectors are the inverted terminal repeats (ITRs) and the packaging element (Fig. 2C). Because all viral proteins must be provided in *trans* by a helper Ad, these vectors are called helper-dependent Ads (HDAs) or "gutless" Ad vectors (68,69). The major drawbacks with HDAs are the stability of the vectors, and the contamination of vector preparations with helper virus. However, recent developments provide HDAs with helper virus contamination levels as low as 0.01% (70), and have been shown to express high levels of transgene products in vivo for up to a year (71,72), suggesting that indeed the host immune response against vector-infected cells has been eliminated.

F. Poxvirus Vectors

Poxviruses are large enveloped viruses containing a double-stranded linear DNA genome of about 200 kb with a hairpin loop and ITR at each terminus (73). Because poxviruses are transcribed and replicated in the cytoplasm rather than the nucleus, all of the proteins necessary to initiate viral transcription must be present in the virion. Recently, a receptor for the myxoma poxvirus was identified as a chemokine receptor (74), although other receptors almost certainly exist. Early genes are transcribed in the cytoplasm within the virus core. Intermediate genes, coding for factors required for late transcription, are not expressed until after the onset of viral replication. Late transcripts encode predominantly virion proteins. The viral genome and proteins assemble into a core structure which matures to an enveloped infectious form in the cytoplasm. Virus production is highly cytotoxic to the infected cell, in part due to a strong inhibition of host DNA, RNA, and protein synthesis, with the consequence that within a few days after infection the host cell dies.

Vaccinia virus (VV) is the most commonly used recombinant poxviral vector. VV replicates in the host and induces a strong antipoxviral immune response that provides the rationale for its use as a smallpox vaccine. For safety reasons, the attenuated VV strains NYVAC and MVA have been developed by deletion of genes not required for replication in tissue culture or by serial passage in avian cells, respectively (75,76). Neither of these strains, nor the canarypox vector ALVAC (75), replicate significantly in human cells or cause pathology in immunodeficient animal models, although all retain their gene transfer ability (77). Without deleting any of the vector backbone, the maximum insert size of poxviral vectors is about 25 kb (78). Poxviral recombinants can be grown to high titer and are very stable. Like the wild type or attenuated parental viruses, the recombinants can infect many cell types, but infection and transgene expression are accompanied by a vigorous immune response. Because of this strong immunogenicity and the cytotoxicity of poxviruses, these recombinants are primarily useful as vaccine vectors (79) and are not likely to be used for lung gene transfer in vivo.

G. Nonviral Vectors

The potential for nonviral gene therapy was first demonstrated over a decade ago (80). The advantages of nonviral gene transfer are the ease of manufacturing plasmid DNA, the low level of vector-induced immunogenicity, and the increased safety, since no infectious agents are required. An upper limit for the size of DNA that can be transduced by nonviral vectors has not yet been established. The major barriers that must be overcome for efficient nonviral gene transduction are delivery to the target cell, translocation into the cell, and transport to the nucleus. Although progress has been made in overcoming these barriers, the level of expression attainable in vivo still remains low. In addition, plasmid DNA generally remains episomal, resulting in transient expression in dividing cells. There are three major nonviral methods for delivering transgenes to target cells: (1) in a liposomal complex with cationic lipids (lipoplex), (2) in a complex with cationic polymers (polyplex), and (3) by direct administration of naked DNA.

Cationic lipids are positively charged hydrophobic molecules that, after mixing with neutral lipids, spontaneously condense plasmid DNA into lipoplexes. The positively charged lipoplex binds to the negatively charged membrane of the target cell, and the complex is then internalized either by endocytosis (81) or by fusion with the cell membrane. It is not clear exactly how the DNA is transported to the nucleus, but the process probably involves dissociation from the lipid component (82). The plasmid remains episomal in the nucleus, where expression levels are determined to some extent by promoter activity. Dozens of formulations of cationic lipids have been developed for in vitro and in vivo use (83,84). Numerous cell types can be transduced in vivo by lipoplexes, and in the absence of cell proliferation, this transduction can last for weeks (85). It may also be possible to target some cell types, since one particular lipid formulation has been shown to preferentially transduce endothelial cells (86). Lipoplexes are capable of inducing marked inflammatory responses, most likely due to plasmid CpG sequences that activate Toll-like receptors on many cells (87–89). The distribution of lipoplexes within the lungs and their efficiency of inducing gene expression depend on the route of administration and the physicochemical properties of the lipoplex (90). Lipoplex delivery generally leads to transduction of a low percent of cells within the epithelium, but expression begins within 24 hr and lasts for a few days to weeks (91,92). While barriers such as mucus and inflammatory cells represent real issues for lipoplex delivery to the lungs (93), this kind of system has yielded the first extended clinical trials for human lung gene therapy (94,95).

A polyplex is formed when DNA is condensed by cationic polymers, such as polylysine. One advantage of using cationic polymers instead of lipids is the ease with which specific ligands (such as antibodies to specific cell markers) can be incorporated into the polyplex, allowing targeting of specific cell types via ligand–receptor interactions (96–98). Most receptor-targeted polyplexes are internalized by endocytosis, requiring release from the endosome for transduction, but this delivery system has not shown much efficacy in the lungs in vivo (99,100). Substitution of branched polycations such as polyethyleneimine (PEI) for polylysine in the polyplex allows endosomal release and an increase in transduction of three orders of magnitude in vitro (101). The polycation component of the polyplex facilitates transport of the plasmid DNA into the nucleus (82). In vitro transduction efficiencies obtained with polyplexes have been variable, depending on the cell type, ligand, and polycation employed. Although extensive in vivo data have not yet been obtained, in some cases high transient expression levels have been observed (96), particularly in lung tissue (102,103).

Although naked DNA is not taken up by cultured cells, it is clearly capable of transducing cells in vivo (80). The mechanism by which plasmid DNA is taken up by cells and transported to the nucleus is not fully understood (104). In vivo, naked DNA can be introduced into tissue either by direct injection or by particle bombardment in which gold particles are coated with the vector and fired at high velocity into the target tissue (105). Although a high degree of transduction has been obtained in muscle and liver cells, and to a lesser extent in cells in a variety of other tissues (104), efficient gene transfer is dependent on accessibility of the target tissue and would only be considered for ex vivo gene transfer to lung cells. A recent advance has been to use stably transfected mesenchymal cells, such as pulmonary artery smooth muscle cells or pulmonary fibroblasts, which are delivered to the lungs by the internal jugular vein. A significant portion of these stably transfected cells transmigrate through the arteriolar wall to engraft within the pulmonary microcirculation (106,107). Such an approach could be used to deliver genes to modify the nature of the vascular structures within the lung and deliver gene product via the pulmonary circulation.

As apparent from the above discussion, several methods of gene transfer are potentially relevant for pulmonary gene therapy. Each of these gene transfer methods has its own advantages and disadvantages, and efficient and safe in vivo gene transfer for patients remains a continuing challenge in research. The future, however, is bright as gene transfer techniques continue to be refined and developed. The following sections review the use of gene therapy in acute lung injury, in patients with CF where most existing human trials have occurred, and in the treatment of pulmonary fibrosis.

IV. Gene Therapy for Acute Lung Injury

At the present time, gene therapy for acute lung injury remains an unfulfilled but exciting possibility. There are as yet no published reports of gene transfer to humans in the setting of acute lung injury. Thus, discussion here addresses two large areas of animal research in which gene therapy for acute lung injury looks particularly promising: hyperoxia and acute radiation-induced lung injury.

A. Hyperoxia

Endogenous and exogenous reactive oxygen species (ROS) are important in causing epithelial and endothelial damage in a variety of inflammatory human lung diseases. For example, in the systemic inflammatory response syndrome (SIRS), neutrophils elaborate myeloperoxidase and generate superoxide anion to cause "collateral" tissue damage. Also, patients with clinical acute lung injury (ALI) and the acute respiratory distress syndrome (ARDS) are frequently treated with high inspired oxygen concentrations to achieve adequate levels of arterial oxygenation. Since the proximal pulmonary epithelium is readily accessible to gene delivery systems, oxidant-mediated lung injury is an obvious model in which to assess the efficacy of gene therapies directed at augmenting antioxidant levels.

Danel et al. (108) tested the efficacy of intratracheal delivery of two antioxidant systems in animal models of ROS-mediated injury. The principal enzyme for degrading cytosolic superoxide anion (superoxide dismutase, SOD), and that for detoxifying hydrogen peroxide (catalase, CAT), were expressed in adenoviral vectors and delivered to adults rats exposed either to hyperoxia or to ischemia–reperfusion injury. In the normobaric hyperoxia model (100% O_2 for 62 hr, 3 days after intratracheal adenoviral infection), CAT, SOD, or the combination all increased survival markedly (from $\sim$10% in control animals to $\sim$80% in the treated animals). Immunohistochemistry revealed a patchy distribution of the human proteins in epithelial cells of the distal respiratory tract; some areas had contiguous cells with robust staining while other areas had no staining. Cells recovered in bronchoalveolar lavage (BAL) and from lung tissue lysates had high levels of the expressed human enzyme (CAT or SOD) by ELISA. The authors reasonably concluded that the production of antioxidant enzymes induced through adenoviral gene therapy was feasible and functionally significant, and could directly influence survival.

Otterbein et al. (109) tested the efficacy of heme oxygenase-1 (HO-1) using a similar intratracheal gene transfer approach in hyperoxic injury in rats. HO-1 is the inducible form of the enzymatic system that degrades heme into biliverdin IXa, carbon monoxide (CO), and iron. HO-1 is upregulated in response to a variety of physiologic signals, as well as by local and systemic insults including oxidative stress (for review, see Ref. 110). In this well-written study, intratracheal delivery of virus was followed immediately by placement of rats in the hyperoxic chamber (as opposed to waiting for peak levels of enzyme expression) (109). The effect of Ad5-HO-1 expression and hyperoxia were clearly synergistic in generating mRNA expression, which was present in lung lysates as early as 6 hr, peaked at 48 hr, and disappeared by 7 days. Marginally increased levels of HO-1 protein were found in lung lysates from Adβgal controls at 72 hr, but much more impressive elevations of HO-1 protein were present in experimental animals at 72 hr and persisted at intermediate levels for 14 days. Immunohistochemistry revealed very uniform staining for HO-1 protein in the bronchiolar epithelium (109).

In the study of Otterbein et al. (109), the high levels of HO-1 protein induced by gene transfer were associated with significant protection against hyperoxic lung injury assessed in several ways. Pleural effusion volume (a standardized surrogate marker for injury) was reduced by more than 50% in Ad5-HO-1 treated rats at 56 hr. In addition, histology in these animals was preserved at the alveolar level with essentially no visible alveolar edema or hemorrhage and only trivial increases in interstitial cellularity in gene transfer animals. Survival was also markedly better in treated animals: all of the control rats were dead at 66 hr, while 2/3 of the Ad5-HO-1 animals were alive at 96 hr. In additional mechanistic assessments, a robust 75% reduction was found in absolute neutrophil counts in BAL from Ad5-HO-1 animals at 56 hr. The timing of the BAL did not allow the authors to discriminate causality from association, but the observed reduction in neutrophils correlated nicely with the histology (109).

Weng et al. (111) utilized a different approach to pulmonary gene therapy by injecting plasmid HO-1/lipofectin mixtures transcutaneously into the lungs of neonatal mice. The injected mixture included a reporter plasmid encoding the bioluminescent enzyme luciferase under the influence of a bidirectional tetracycline control. Luciferase measurements taken every 24 hr allowed an in vivo assay of the transfection efficiency with reasonable spatial and temporal resolution. This study demonstrated a heterogenous distribution of luminescence over the right lung field that had already peaked when first measured; the intensity was greatest in the right middle lobe where the actual injection was made (111). The luminescence persisted at reasonable levels until day 3 postinjection, slowly falling to background levels by day 7. The same luciferase assay was used to validate the use of the bidirectional tetracycline promoter in vivo: with Tet-On plasmid cotransfection, doxycycline gave a 10-fold increase in bioluminescence, while the converse was true with Tet-Off (111).

Consistent with the findings of Otterbein et al. (109) above, hyperoxia itself was found by Weng et al. (111) to raise HO-1 levels. Transcutaneous injection of plasmid HO-1/lipofectin also increased HO-1 protein as assayed by Western blot in lung lysates, but in contrast to the data with Ad5-HO-1, the combined effects of hyperoxia and plasmid HO-1/lipofectin ipofectin were less than additive (111). Immunohistochemistry at 48 hr after transfection with surfactant protein C was used to show that the production of HO-1 was localized in type II alveolar pneumocytes and (in other sections) vascular smooth muscle. Enzyme activity measurements in right middle lobe lysates showed a convincing increase in transcutaneously transfected animals (about 50%, without exposure to hyperoxia) (111). This contrasts with the findings of Danel et al. (108) as described earlier, who were not able to measure differences in antioxidant enzyme activity in lung lysates after intratracheal adenoviral-mediated delivery of CAT or SOD.

The study of Weng et al. (111) included additional interesting data with regard to traditional protein and lipid markers of oxidative injury. Protein carbonyl measurements in air-exposed transfected animals were threefold higher in the right middle lobe as compared to the left (nontransfected) lung. Hyperoxia increased protein carbonyls in all lung fields as expected; however, the transfected right middle lobe was not protected. Instead, the carbonyl content was about 20% higher than in the left lung. Isoprostanes (as an assay of lipid peroxidation) were predictably increased by hyperoxia in control-transfected animals (111). Again, however, HO-1 expression increased isoprostanes in air-exposed animals and did not protect against lipid peroxidation in 100% oxygen. Data on histopathology and survival were not presented, but the authors commented that type-II pneumocyte expression may be a suboptimal site for HO-1 upregulation (111). This study is important, however, in demonstrating increased enzyme activity (even though histochemistry suggested a restricted distribution of HO-1 expression) and because the luciferase methods illustrate a novel way to assess the spatial and temporal distribution of gene expression in vivo. It would also be interesting to perform the carbonyl and isoprostane experiments in the Otterbein et al. (109) model where survival was so obviously improved.

Factor et al. (112) presented still another gene therapy approach to the problem of hyperoxia. The Na^+–K^+-ATPase on the basolateral membrane of type II pneumocytes is critically important in clearing lung edema fluid both perinatally and in some models of lung injury. These authors created an adenoviral construct expressing either α_1 or β_1 subunits of the rat Na^+–K^+-ATPase. Surfactant and a null vector were used as controls (112). Previous experiments had suggested that provision of the β_1 subunit alone would increase active transport in targeted cells, and the Ad-α_1 subunit group thus served as an additional expressed protein control. Experiments began 1 week after adenoviral infection. Normobaric hyperoxia was administered to a large group of animals and survival was measured at 12-hr intervals for 2 weeks. All 20 Ad-β_1 animals remained alive; survival was 20–40% in control groups, and animals began dying at day 3. Ad-β_1 treated animals had no pleural effusions and remained healthy throughout 64 hr of hyperoxia. In contrast, all of the control animals (including vehicle, vector, and Ad-α_1) were clinically ill and had 5–7 mL bilateral effusions (112).

Although questions about mechanisms of pulmonary gene therapy in hyperoxia clearly remain, the preliminary survival data from three of the articles discussed above are very encouraging (108,109,112). If less inflammatory vectors can be developed, gene therapies such as these might allow clinicians to support ARDS patients with higher oxygen tensions while avoiding hyperoxic injury. It would be very interesting in future research to test such strategies in animals that already have established acute lung injury since that is the most relevant clinical application.

B. Radiation-Induced Injury

Radiation-induced pulmonary injury commonly occurs during the treatment of chest malignancies, and is usually the limiting factor in determining the tolerable dose of treatment. Gene therapy approaches to protect the surrounding lung thus offer the promise of reduced toxicity and increased efficacy for radiation oncology. Since the timing of the injury is known, protective strategies involving gene delivery are plausible even if high-level expression is not quickly achieved.

The protective effects of human manganese superoxide dismutase (MnSOD) expression have been demonstrated in a model of radiation-induced organizing alveolitis by Epperly et al. (113). MnSOD is an isoform of superoxide with some differences from the Cu–ZnSOD form of the enzyme discussed earlier. In particular, MnSOD has a leader sequence targeting mitochondria, and a catalytic site that utilizes a different heavy metal. The study of Epperly et al. (113) extended preliminary data by the same investigators showing that MnSOD overexpression had protective effects in a cell culture model of radiation-induced tissue damage. In the in vivo study, athymic nude (Nu/J) mice were used to eliminate confounding effects associated with inflammation directed against the Ad vectors used (113). Uninfected mice and Adβgal infected mice were used as controls. Animals received 850–950 cGy doses of radiation directed at the thorax 4 days after delivery of the Ad-MnSOD or Adβgal vectors (113).

Nested RT-PCR confirmed the presence of the transgene in whole lung lysates; the same assay confirmed expression specifically in the trachea (dissected separately) and harvested alveolar type II cells (113). In contrast to the study of Danel et al. (108), a significant increase in whole lung SOD activity (both MnSOD and Cu–ZnSOD) was demonstrated in the experimental mice (113). Densitometry analysis showed mRNA increases (normalized to actin) twofold greater than control immediately after irradiation, and more than threefold on day 1 after radiation. An additional large group of similarly treated mice was examined histopathologically at 4 months postradiation. The extent of alveolitis was quantified in seven sections from each of five lobes. Animals receiving the lower radiation dose of 850 cGy did not have substantial alveolitis and MnSOD was thus not found to be beneficial in this group. However, at the higher dose of 950 cGy, many of the control mice had substantial lung injury and animals receiving Ad-MnSOD were significantly protected (8/9) (113).

In additional mechanistic studies, Epperly et al. (113) investigated mRNA levels for transforming growth factor beta (TGFβ), which has previously been shown to incite pulmonary fibrosis when delivered via an adenoviral vector (114). TGFβ levels were increased 5–10-fold in lung lysates from uninfected and Adβgal control mice five to 10-fold on day 1 following radiation, and this effect was completely suppressed in animals with MnSOD overexpression secondary to Ad-MnSOD delivery. Similar but much more modest effects were seen when messages for tumor necrosis factor alpha (TNF-α) and interleukin (IL)-1 were analyzed in mice receiving gene transfer (113).

A second paper by Epperly et al. (115) extended the above work to examine both the mode of transgene delivery and effect of the transgene on tumor killing. This study used C57BL/6J mice in which tumors were produced by 3LL carcinoma cells. Difficulties associated with Ad-associated inflammation were avoided by using lipofectin, which also shortened the time required between gene transfer and radiation treatment to 24 hr. Initial experiments confirmed transgene (MnSOD) expression in whole lysates from portions of lung that were free from tumor, while tumor (from the same lung) did not show transgene expression (115). Survival curves indicated a clear advantage for the group of animals given MnSOD via lipofectin prior to 18 Gy radiation (115). The possibility of a direct effect of MnSOD on the tumor itself was excluded in a separate set of experiments. These animals were treated similarly to establish tumors, MnSOD or empty liposomes were delivered, and irradiation at 18 Gy was performed. Tumor levels of cytokine mRNA at 1 day following irradiation were shown to be unaffected by MnSOD (115). As expected from the prior experiments (113), adjacent lung levels of mRNA for profibrotic signaling (TGF-β3, macrophage migration inhibitory factor, IL-1 β, and IL-1Ra) were increased by irradiation in the animals given empty liposomes (115). Pretreatment with

MnSOD liposomes abrogated this increased message expression at 1 day postirradiation time point.

The increased survival found in MnSOD mice in the study of Epperly et al. (115) indicated that radiation was more effective against the growth of tumor in these animals. Radiation treatment at the level of 18 Gy normally causes fibrosis at time points past 100 days in mice. If the only effect of MnSOD gene therapy was on the development of fibrosis in these animals, a significant difference in survival would not be expected to be present at much earlier times. However, improvements in survival were found by Epperly et al. (115) to appear as early as 2 weeks, and there was an impressive fivefold increase in survival at 60 days. Future experiments will be necessary to evaluate the mechanism of this apparent increase in tumoricidal activity, but both the antifibrotic and potential tumoricidal benefits of gene therapy appear to hold real promise for future human clinical trials.

V.   Gene Therapy for Chronic Lung Injury
A.   Cystic Fibrosis

Cystic fibrosis is a common and serious clinical problem. During the past decade, significant progress has been made in establishing the foundation for gene therapy for this debilitating pulmonary disease. The CF transmembrane regulator (CFTR) protein is normally present on the apical surface of epithelial cells and functions as a crucial chloride channel. The common homozygous mutation (ΔF508) in this gene that causes CF leaves patients without effective chloride transport across the epithelial lining in the lungs, nasal passages, gut, pancreas, liver, and reproductive tract. Progressive obstructive lung disease and repeated pulmonary infection is eventually the cause of death in 80% of patients with CF despite the best supportive care. The respiratory epithelium is easily accessible to gene therapy delivery systems, and in vitro data suggest that functioning CFTR in as few as 10% of epithelial cells is sufficient to restore normal chloride transport (116,117).

In the first small clinical study that looked at functional changes in the airways following gene therapy, Alton et al. (118) randomized 16 patients to receive either placebo lipid or lipid and CFTR (under a cytomegalovirus promoter) via a nebulizer. The patients were relatively healthy at the time of study with an $FEV_1 > 70\%$; they underwent two fiberoptic examinations of the lower airways—one immediately prior to nebulization and the second 48 hr later. During the bronchoscopy, potential differences in a segmental airway and at the carina were measured to assess the functional significance of CFTR delivered by liposomes. Epithelial cells obtained with brushes were also examined by fluorescence microcopy to determine agonist-driven chloride efflux. In separate experiments, scanning electron microscopy was used to assess pseudomonal adherence to epithelial cells obtained at bronchoscopy (118).

Results indicated that the lipid component (presumably) caused airway irritation and symptoms in 75% of both the placebo and CFTR patients (118). However, this was mild and responded to bronchodilators in patients who required treatment. There was a corresponding drop in both FEV_1 and FVC in both groups, but there were no signs of pulmonary inflammation on visual inspection and no differences between bronchial histology in the two groups. Serum C-reactive protein was substantially elevated in the CFTR group compared to lipid placebo. Vector-specific CFTR DNA was detected in cells from the carina and the segmental airways in all eight lipid-CFTR patients. Unfortunately, no corresponding mRNA for CFTR was found in any patient sample. From a functional standpoint, the invasively measured epithelial potential difference increased towards normal with agonist application. This was different than the placebo group, and the investigators estimated that about 25% of the chloride conductance had been restored by gene therapy (118). Fluorescence measurements (ex vivo) of chloride efflux corroborated this result, with a small but statistically significant increase in transport in lipid-CFTR patients. Bacterial adherence measured by scanning EM (again measured ex vivo) was reduced approximately 30% in the CFTR group 48 hr after therapy compared to pretreatment baseline values (118).

In summary, the above initial clinical study demonstrated short-term CFTR expression and some relevant physiological differences both in vivo and in ex vivo samples from treated patients. Moreover, the treatment and invasive studies were generally well tolerated. These findings are an important first step towards larger and more complete studies with repeated administration to assess relevant clinical endpoints. The results also indicate that delivery systems that elicit less inflammation (as assessed by C-reactive protein) may also help to increase the duration of gene expression in future studies.

The utility of a third-generation Ad vector has also been examined in a preliminary dose escalation and toxicity study in humans (119). This study hypothesized that E1/E4 deleted Ad would elicit less of a Th-2 inflammatory response, and be associated with longer transgene expression and less epithelial injury. Eleven adult CF subjects without advanced airway obstruction were given a suspension of virus into a relatively healthy segment of lung (as assessed by CT scan) via fiberoptic bronchoscopy. A prolonged post-treatment monitoring period was used to assess viral shedding via the rectum or nares, virus-induced immunity (out to 90 days), lung function (out to 30 days), and gene expression within airway epithelium of the treated segment (at days 4 and 43 after gene transfer). At the highest dose, two subjects had fever and an infiltrate, the latter of which persisted for 10 days. The highly sensitive Ad focus-forming unit assay, however, detected no viral shedding in any patient. Gene expression in about 1% of bronchial epithelial cells was found in 6/11 patients at day 4 without regard to dose. No expression was found at day 43 (119).

All subjects in this study developed a virus-specific immune response as assayed by lymphoproliferation in an assay performed on peripheral blood (119). In addition, nearly all subjects developed impressive interferon gamma (IFN-γ) responses when lymphocytes collected 2 weeks after exposure were subjected to inactivated adenovirus for 2 days. Virus-stimulated IL-10 production was also up in some cases. Dose of administered vector did not seem to matter in the magnitude of the response. Three of the 11 subjects had pre-existing neutralizing antibodies for adenovirus. The treatment elicited less impressive increases in humoral immunity: only 4/11 patients increased their titers by more than 10-fold. Western blots measuring circulating antibodies against serotype specific adenovirus antibodies did not demonstrate an increase in antibody secretion. These results are important in illustrating that increasing doses of viral vector do not necessarily increase gene expression. Moreover, terminally differentiated epithelium may be somewhat resistant to adenoviral infection from the luminal surface. Cell-mediated immunity remains an important barrier to long-term transgene expression even in E1/E4 deleted adenoviral delivery systems. Conversely, humoral immunity is less likely to present a barrier.

In summary, research on gene therapy in patients with CF and in related experimental models indicates that this approach is promising. Brief but successful CTFR transgene expression has been demonstrated in the lower airways of CF patients, along with some corresponding physiologic differences. The ability to maximize the number of gene-expressing cells, and to limit immune responses associated with gene transfer vectors, will be key factors in determining the ultimate clinical efficacy of gene therapy in patients with this severe inherited disorder.

B. Pulmonary Fibrosis

Pulmonary fibrosis and related interstitial lung diseases are particularly important and serious clinical problems. Patients with fibrotic lung diseases suffer significant morbidity and mortality. Gene transfer strategies have been used experimentally to provide important data on the role of key mediators in the pathogenesis of these serious diseases (120,121). By identifying key mediators and pathways involved in the genesis of the fibrogenic response, gene therapy vectors can ultimately be utilized to deliver genes of proteins able to disrupt these fibrogenic signals. Currently, there have been no human clinical trials of gene therapy for fibrotic lung disease, but there have been a number of promising and exciting animal preclinical studies as discussed below.

Many different forms of lung injury result in a fibrogenic repair process and lead to diseases characterized by pulmonary fibrosis. These include idiopathic pulmonary fibrosis (IPF), sarcoidosis, pneumoconiosis, hypersensitivity pneumonitis, drug and radiation-induced fibroses, and fibrosing alveolitis associated with collagen vascular diseases such as rheumatoid arthritis. Common to all of these diseases are elevations in cytokines such as TGFβ, TNFα, platelet-derived growth factor (PDGF), and connective tissue growth factor (CTGF) (see Chapter 6 for detailed discussion of these cytokines and their activities). In particular, TGFβ appears to be a key fibrogenic cytokine, and is elevated in the lung of patients with fibrotic lung diseases. However, finding an elevation of a particular mediator such as TGFβ does not prove that it is causally involved in generating the observed pathology. Gene transfer with recombinant adenovirus vectors can be used to demonstrate the key role of cytokines such as TGFβ in fibrogenesis. In a study by Sime et al. (114), a virus expressing active TGFβ was used to transfer the gene for this cytokine into the epithelium of the lung. A high level of TGFβ protein was measured both in lavage fluid and lung tissue over the following 14–21 days (114). Overexpressing active TGFβ protein in the lung using this gene transfer technique induced severe and irreversible fibrosis, which had many of the histological features of human IPF including accumulation of fibroblasts, myofibroblasts, and extracellular matrix proteins like collagen (121,122). Adenovector-mediated gene transfer thus provided an excellent tool to study the key role of TGFβ in lung fibrogenesis. Using similar gene transfer techniques, important roles in lung inflammation and fibrosis have also been demonstrated for other cytokines such as TNFα (123), IL-1 (124), granulocyte–macrophage colony-stimulating factor (GM-CSF) (125) and CTGF (126).

Since TGFβ is a key fibrogenic signaling molecule, targeting its activity may provide an excellent new therapeutic strategy for pulmonary fibrosis. Decorin is a small proteoglycan that inhibits active TGFβ by binding to its core protein and preventing ligand–receptor binding (127). A recombinant Ad vector has been engineered by Kolb et al. (128), and used to express decorin core protein in the lungs to test its effects in mitigating bleomycin-induced fibrosis in mice. Administration of the decorin viral vector 2 days before intratracheal administration of bleomycin significantly inhibited the development of fibrosis in this model (128). Interestingly, there was no effect on the inflammatory response. Using a different strategy to block the TGFβ pathway, Nakao et al. (129) engineered an adenovector expressing Smad7, one of several Smad proteins known to be key intracellular signaling molecules for TGFβ-mediated responses. The Smad family comprises both stimulatory and inhibitory members, with Smad7 being inhibitory. When the adenovector expressing Smad7 was administered 12 hr before 7 days subcutaneous infusion of bleomycin, fibrosis was reduced compared to controls (129). These studies highlight the potential efficacy of targeting TGFβ activity in the therapy of fibrotic lung disease.

Another mediator, PDGF, has also been implicated as an important mediator in lung fibrosis. Using a different gene therapy vector, Yoshida et al. (130) targeted the PDGF pathway. They employed an HVJ-liposomal vector expressing the extracellular domain of the PDGFβ receptor to bind PDGF, and were able to reduce collagen accumulation in an animal model of bleomycin-induced fibrosis.

Gene therapy can also potentially be used to augment pulmonary defenses against injury. As discussed earlier in this chapter, HO-1 can mitigate acute lung injury (e.g., see Refs. 109,110). Recently, Tsuburai et al. (131) demonstrated that adenoviral vector overexpression of HO-1 reduced bleomycin-induced pulmonary fibrosis. It is also technically feasible to augment other natural host defenses such as antioxidants using similar gene therapeutic strategies. Perhaps in the future, the greatest impact of gene therapy will come from a combination of strategies, where it is used in conjunction with conventional drugs to target effector molecules or enhance pulmonary defenses. Combination therapies directed at multiple aspects of lung injury pathology are considered in the following chapter (Chapter 19).

VI. Summary

This chapter has discussed the current state of the art in gene delivery and transfer systems, with an emphasis on systems of interest for gene therapy in the lungs. The outcomes of current preclinical and/or clinical studies utilizing gene transfer methods in hyperoxic lung injury, pulmonary irradiation, CF, and fibrotic lung disease have also been described. There are important technical hurdles to overcome before gene therapy can become a reality either for acute or chronic lung disease. However, this field is advancing rapidly with many new exciting developments. Depending on the delivery system and specific application, gene transfer can generate integrated long-term expression, long-term nonintegrated expression, or short-term nonintegrated expression. Pulmonary gene therapy is also influenced by accessibility issues for targeted cells (epithelial, parenchymal, or endothelial), as well as by physical barriers to gene delivery (e.g., the airway mucus lining, extracellular glycocalyx, and cell membrane). Effective delivery of therapeutic genes also requires they withstand the hostile environment of damaged, infected, or inflamed tissue. It may also be desirable to deliver pulmonary gene therapy in ways that restrict it to the lungs.

Available vectors for gene transfer include retroviruses like MLVs and lentiviruses, as well as adenoviruses, adeno-associated viruses, poxvirus, and nonviral vectors. The ideal gene transfer vector has high affinity for and enters targeted cells, and is expressed within the cell either as a nonintegrating entity or after targeted integration into the genome. Effective gene vectors must also be associated with a controlled or well-described duration of expression, survive within hostile inflamed tissue, and elicit little or no immune or inflammatory response. Vector systems for delivering genes to pulmonary cells are improving rapidly, particularly in terms of reducing associated inflammation and enhancing the duration of expression of encoded genes. In addition, experience from current preclinical and clinical research is helping to drive the generation of even more effective vector delivery systems and methods. Gene transfer studies themselves are also helping to elucidate the pathogenetic basis of several aspects of acute and chronic lung diseases.

There is a pressing need to improve current clinical treatments for many forms of injury-related pulmonary pathology. This includes clinical ALI/ARDS, as well as chronic interstitial lung diseases like IPF and a variety of others. In terms of new therapies, available data in animals suggest that gene transfer approaches will be able to achieve at least some benefits in acute lung injury, and application of gene therapy to chronic lung disease also appears feasible in the relatively near future given the rapid pace of developments in this field. Gene therapy offers novel ways of manipulating cellular function that cannot be achieved with standard pharmaceutical approaches. The heavy burden of morbidity and mortality associated with acute and chronic pulmonary disease is a strong driving force for continuing basic science research on gene therapy approaches. Gene transfer has the potential to induce the targeted cellular production of molecules that target key cytokines involved in overexuberant inflammation or to augment pulmonary host defenses. Overall, the future for gene therapy is both challenging and promising.

References

1. Kitson C, Angel B, Judd D, Rothery S, Severs NJ, Dewar A, et al. The extra- and intracellular barriers to lipid and adenovirus-mediated pulmonary gene transfer in native sheep airway epithelium. Gene Ther 1998; 6:534–536.
2. Pickles RJ, Fahrner JA, Petrella JM, Boucher RC, Bergelson JM. Retargeting the Coxsackievirus and adenovirus receptor to the apical surface of polarized epithelial cells reveals the glycocalyz as a barrier to adenovirus-mediated gene transfer. J Virol 2000; 74:6050–6057.
3. Van Heeckeren A, Ferkol T, Tosi M. Effects of bronchopulmonary inflammation induced by pseudomonas aeruginosa on adenovirus-mediated gene transfer to airway epithelial cells in mice. Gene Ther 1998; 5:345–351.
4. Zhang H-G, Zhou T, Yang P, Edwards CKI, Curiel DT, Mountz JD. Inhibition of tumor necrosis factor a decreases inflammation and prolongs adenovirus gene expression in lung and liver. Hum Gene Ther 1998; 9: 1875–1884.

5. Sung RS, Qin L, Bromberg JS. TNFα and IFNγ induced by innate anti-adenoviral immune responses inhibit adenovirus-mediated transgene expression. Mol Ther 2001; 3:757–767.

6. Simon RH, Engelhardt JF, Yang Y, Zepeda M, Weber-Pendleton S, Grossman M, et al. Adenovirus-mediated transfer of the CFTR gene to lung of nonhuman primates: toxicity study. Hum Gene Ther 1993; 4:771–780.

7. Sene C, Bout A, Imler JL, Schultz H, Willemot JM, Hennebel V, Zurcher C, Valerio D, Lamy D, Pavirani A. Aerosol-mediated delivery of recombinant adenovirus to the airways of nonhuman primates. Hum Gene Ther 1995; 6: 1587–1593.

8. Bellon G, Michel-Calemard L, Thouvenot D, Jagneaux V, Poitevin F, Malcus C, et al. Aerosol administration of a recombinant adenovirus expressing CFTR to cystic fibrosis patients: a phase I clinical trial. Hum Gene Ther 1997; 8:15–25.

9. Chu Z, St. George JA, Lukason M, Cheng SH, Scheule RK, Eastman SJ. EGTA enhancement of adenovirus-mediated gene transfer to mouse tracheal epithelium in vivo. Hum Gene Ther 2001; 12:455–467.

10. Factor P, Saldias F, Ridge K, Dumasius V, Zabner J, Jaffe HA, et al. Augmentation of lung liquid clearance via adenovirus-mediated transfer of a Na^+/K^+–ATPase beta 1 subunit gene. J Clin Invest 1998; 102:1421–1430.

11. Factor P, Mendez M, Mutlu G, Dumasius V. Gene transfer to severely injured rat lungs. Mol Ther 2001; 3:S337–S338.

12. Coffin JM. Retroviridae: the viruses and their replication. In: Fields BN, Knipe DM, Howley PM, Chanock RM, Melnick JL, Monath TP, Roizman B, Strauss SE, eds. Fields Virology. 3rd ed Philadelphia, PA: Lippincott-Raven, 1996:1767–1848.

13. Kavanaugh MP, Miller DG, Zhang W, Law W, Kozak SL, Kabat D, Miller AD. Cell-surface receptors for gibbon ape leukemia virus and amphotropic murine retrovirus are inducible sodium-dependent phosphate symporters. Proc Natl Acad Sci USA 1994; 91:7071–7075.

14. Zaitseva M, Blauvelt A, Lee S, Lapham C, Klaus-Kovtun V, Mostowski H, Manischewitz J, Golding H. Expression and function of CCR5 and CXCR4 on human Langerhans cells and macrophages: implications for HIV primary infection. Nat Med 1997; 3:1369–1375.

15. Luciw PA. Human immunodeficiency viruses and their replication. In: Fields BN, Knipe DM, Howley PM, Chanock RM, Melnick JL, Monath TP, Roizman B, Strauss SE, eds. Fields Virology. 3rd ed. Philadelphia, PA: Lippincott-Raven, 1996:1881–1952.

16. Miller AD, Miller DG, Garcia JV, Lynch CM. Use of retroviral vectors for gene transfer and expression. Methods Enzymol 1993; 217:581–599.

17. Yee J-K. Retroviral vectors. In: Friedmann T, ed. The Development of Human Gene Therapy. Cold Spring Harbor, NY: Cold Spring Harbor Laboratory Press, 1999:21–45.

18. Cosset FL, Takeuchi Y, Battini JL, Weiss RA, Collins MK. High-titer packaging cells producing recombinant retroviruses resistant to human serum. J Virol 1995; 69:7430–7436.

19. Engelhardt JF, Yankaskas JR, Wilson JM. In vivo retroviral gene transfer into human bronchial epithelia of xenografts. J Clin Invest 1992; 90:2598–2607.

20. McCray PB, Wang G, Kline JN, Zabner J, Chada S, Jolly DI, et al. Alveolar macrophages inhibit retrovirus-mediated gene transfer to airway epithelia. Hum Gene Ther 1997; 8:1087–1093.

21. Klimatcheva E, Rosenblatt JD, Planelles V. Lentiviral vectors and gene therapy. Front Biosci 1999; 4:D481–D896.

22. Naldini L, Verma I. Lentivirus vectors. In: Friedmann T, ed. The Development of Human Gene Therapy. Cold Spring Harbor: Cold Spring Harbor Laboratory Press, 1999:47–60.

23. Zufferey R, Nagy D, Mandel RJ, Naldini L, Trono D. Multiply attenuated lentiviral vector achieves efficient gene delivery in vivo. Nat Biotechnol 1997; 15:871–875.

24. Dull T, Zufferey R, Kelly M, Mandel RJ, Nguyen M, Trono D, Naldini L. A third-generation lentivirus vector with a conditional packaging system. J Virol 1998; 72:8463–8471.

25. Naldini L, Blomer U, Gage FH, Trono D, Verma IM. Efficient transfer, integration, and sustained long-term expression of the transgene in adult rat brains injected with a lentiviral vector. Proc Natl Acad Sci USA 1996; 93:11382–11388.

26. Miyoshi H, Takahashi M, Gage FH, Verma IM. Stable and efficient gene transfer into the retina using an HIV-based lentiviral vector. Proc Natl Acad Sci USA 1997; 94:10319–10323.

27. Kafri T, Blomer U, Peterson DA, Gage FH, Verma IM. Sustained expression of genes delivered directly into liver and muscle by lentiviral vectors. Nat Genet 1997; 17:314–317.

28. Goldman MJ, Lee PS, Yang JS, Eilson JM. Lentiviral vectors for gene therapy of cystic fibrosis. Hum Gene Ther 1997; 8:2261–2268.

29. Blomer U, Naldini L, Kafri T, Trono D, Verma IM, Gage FH. Highly efficient and sustained gene transfer in adult neurons with a lentivirus vector. J Virol 1997; 71:6641–6649.

30. Blacklow NR, Hoggan MD, Rowe WP. Serologic evidence for human infection with adenovirus-associated viruses. J Natl Cancer Inst 1968; 40:319–327.

31. Summerford C, Samulski RJ. Membrane-associated heparan sulfate proteoglycan is a receptor for adeno-associated virus type 2 virions. J Virol 1998; 72:1438–1445.

32. Summerford C, Bartlett JS, Samulski RJ. AlphaVbeta 5 integrin: a co-receptor for adeno-associated virus type 2 infection. Nat Med 1999; 5:78–82.

33. Qing K, Mah C, Hansen J, Zhou S, Dwarki V, Srivastava A. Human fibroblast growth factor receptor 1 is a co-receptor for infection by adeno-associated virus 2. Nat Med 1999; 5:71–77.

34. Weitzman MD, Kyostio SR, Kotin RM, Owens RA. Adeno-associated virus (AAV) rep proteins mediate complex formation between AAV DNA and its integration site in human DNA. Proc Natl Acad Sci USA 1994; 91: 5808–5812.

35. Linden RM, Winocour E, Berns KI. The recombination signals for adeno-associated virus site-specific integration. Proc Natl Acad Sci USA 1996; 93:7966–7972.

36. Berns KI. Parvoviridae: the viruses and their replication. In: Fields BN, Knipe DM, Howley PM, Chanock RM, Melnick JL, Monath TP, Roizman B, Strauss SE, eds. Fields Virology. 3rd ed. Philadelphia, PA: Lippincott-Raven, 1996:2173–2198.

37. Samulski RJ, Sally M, Muzyczka N. Adeno-associated viral vectors. In: Friedmann T, ed. The Development of Human Gene Therapy. Cold Spring Harbor: Cold Spring Harbor Laboratory Press, 1999:131–172.

38. Russell DW, Kay MA. Adeno-associated virus vectors and hematology. Blood 1999; 94:864–874.

39. Conrad CK, Allen SS, Afione SA, et al. Safety of single-dose administration of an adeno-associated virus (AAV)-CFTR vector in the primate lung. Gene Ther 1996; 3:658–668.

40. Halbert CL, Standaert TA, Wilson CB, Miller AD. Successful readministration of adeno-associated virus vectors to the mouse lung requires transient immuno-suppression during the initial exposure. J Virol 1998; 72:9795–9805.

41. Zabner J, Seiler M, Walters R, Kotin RM, Gulgeras W, Davidson BL, Chiorini JA. Adeno-associated virus type 5 (AAV5) but not AAV2 binds to the apical surfaces or airway epithelia and facilitates gene transfer. J Virol 2000; 74: 3852–3858.

42. Conrad CK, Allen SS, Afione SA, Reynolds TC, Beck SE, Fee-Maki M, et al. Safety of single-dose administration of an adeno-associated virus (AAV)-CFTR vector in the primate lung. Gene Ther 1996; 3:658–668.

43. Flotte T, Carter B, Conrad C, et al. A phase I study of an adeno associated virus-CFTR gene vector in adult CF patients with mild lung disease. Hum Gene Ther 1996; 7:1145–1159.

44. Wagner JA, Moran ML, Messner AH, et al. A phase I/II study of tgAAV-CF for the treatment of chronic sinusitis in patients with cystic fibrosis. Hum Gene Ther 1998; 9:889–909.

45. Shenk T. Adenoviridae: the viruses and their replication. In: Fields BN, Knipe DM, Howley PM, Chanock RM, Melnick JL, Monath TP, Roizman B, Strauss SE, eds. Fields Virology. 3rd ed. Philadelphia, PA: Lippincott-Raven, 1996:2111–2148.

46. Bergelson JM, Cunningham JA, Droguett G, Kurt-Jones EA, Krithivas A, Hong JS, Horwitz MS, Crowell RL, Finberg RW. Isolation of a common receptor for Coxsackie B viruses and adenoviruses 2 and 5. Science 1997; 275:1320–1323.

47. Tomko RP, Xu R, Philipson L. HCAR and MCAR: the human and mouse cellular receptors for subgroup C adenoviruses and group B Coxsackie-viruses. Proc Natl Acad Sci USA 1997; 94:3352–3356.

48. Wickham TJ, Mathias P, Cheresh DA, Nemerow GR. Integrins alpha v beta 3 and alpha v beta 5 promote adenovirus internalization but not virus attachment. Cell 1993; 73:309–319.

49. Roberts RJ, O'Neill KE, Yen CT. DNA sequences from the adenovirus 2 genome. J Biol Chem 1984; 259:13968–13975.

50. Chroboczek J, Bieber F, Jacrot B. The sequence of the genome of adenovirus type 5 and its comparison with the genome of adenovirus type 2. Virology 1992; 186:280–285.

51. Graham FL, Smiley J, Russell WC, Nairn R. Characteristics of a human cell line transformed by DNA from human adenovirus type 5. J Gen Virol 1977; 36:59–74.

52. Bett AJ, Haddara W, Prevec L, Graham FL. An efficient and flexible system for construction of adenovirus vectors with insertions or deletions in early regions 1 and 3. Proc Natl Acad Sci USA 1994; 91:8802–8806.

53. Rosenfeld MA, Yoshimura K, Trapnell BC, Yoneyama K, Rosenthal ER, Dalemans W, et al. In vivo transfer of the human cystic fibrosis transmembrane conductance regular gene to the airway epithelium. Cell 1992; 68:143–155.

54. Reynolds PN, Zinn KR, Gavrilyuk VD, Balyasnikova IV, Rogers BE, Buchsbaum DJ, et al. A targetable, injectable adenoviral vector for selective gene delivery to pulmonary endothelium in vivo. Mol Ther 2000; 2:562–578.

55. Nettelbeck DM, Miller DW, Jérôme J, Zuzart M, Watkins SJ, Hawkins RE, et al. Targeting of adenovirus to endothelial cells by a bispecific single-chain diabody directed against the adenovirus fiber knob domain and human endoglin (CD105). Mol Ther 2001; 3:882–891.

56. Vigne E, Mahfouz I, Dedieu JF, Brie A, Perricaude M, Yeh P. RGD inclusion in the hexon monomer provides adenovirus type 5-based vectors with a fiber knob-independent pathway for infection. J Virol 1999; 73: 5156–5161.

57. Douglas JT, Miller CR, Kim M, Dmitriev I, Mikheeva G, Krasnykh V, Curiel DT. A system for the propagation of adenoviral vectors with genetically modified receptor specificities. Nat Biotechnol 1999; 17:470–475.

58. Reynolds PN, Nicklin SA, Kalibeerova L, Boatman BG, Grizzle WE, Balyasnikova IV, Baker AH, Danilov SM, Curiel DT. Combined transductional and transcriptional targeting improves the specificity of transgene expression in vivo. Nat Biotechnol 2001; 19:838–842.

59. Nicklin SA, Reynolds PN, Brosnan MJ, White SJ, Curiel DT, Dominiczak AF, Baker AH. Analysis of cell-specific promoters for viral gene therapy targeted at the vascular endothelium. Hypertension 2001; 38:65–70.

60. Wivel NA, Gao G-P, Wilson JM. Adenovirus vectors. In: Friedmann T, ed. The Development of Human Gene Therapy. San Diego, CA: Cold Spring Harbor Laboratory Press, 1999:87–110.

61. Yang Y, Jooss KU, Su Q, Ertl HC, Wilson JM. Immune responses to viral antigens versus transgene product in the elimination of recombinant adenovirus-infected hepatocytes in vivo. Gene Ther 1996; 3:137–144.

62. McCoy RD, Davidson BL, Roessler BJ, Huffnagle GB, Janich SL, Laing TJ, Simon RH. Pulmonary inflammation induced by incomplete or inactivated adenoviral particles. Hum Gene Ther 1995; 6:1553–1560.

63. Kafri T, Morgan D, Krahl T, Sarvetnick N, Sherman L, Verma I. Cellular immune response to adenoviral vector infected cells does not require de novo viral gene expression: implications for gene therapy. Proc Natl Acad Sci USA 1998; 95:11377–11382.

64. Otake K, Ennist DL, Harrod K, Trapnell BC. Nonspecific inflammation inhibits adenovirus-mediated pulmonary gene transfer and expression independent of specific acquired immune responses. Hum Gene Ther 1998; 9:2207–2222.

65. Bromberg JS, Debruyne LA, Qin L. Interactions between the immune system and gene therapy vectors: bidirectional regulation of response and expression. Adv Immunol 1998; 69:353–409.

66. Weiss DJ, Bonneau L, Liggit D. Use of perfluorochemical liquid allows earlier detection and use of less adenovirus vector for gene expression in normal lung and enhances gene expression in acutely injured lung. Mol Ther 2001; 3: 734–745.

67. Chillón M, Lee JH, Fasbender A, Welsh MJ. Adenovirus complexed with polyethylene glycol and cationic lipid is shielded from neutralizing antibodies in vitro. Gene Ther 1998; 5:995–1002.

68. Hitt MM, Parks RJ, Graham FL. Structure and genetic organization of adenovirus vectors. In: Friedmann T, ed. The Development of Human Gene Therapy. Cold Spring Harbor, NY: Cold Spring Harbor Laboratory Press, 1999:61–86.

69. Kochanek S. High-capacity adenoviral vectors for gene transfer and somatic gene therapy. Hum Gene Ther 1999; 10:2451–2459.

70. Parks RJ, Chen L, Anton M, Sankar U, Rudnicki MA, Graham FL. A helper-dependent adenovirus vector system: removal of helper virus by Cre-mediated excision of the viral packaging signal. Proc Natl Acad Sci USA 1996; 93:13565–13570.

71. Morral N, O'Neal W, Rice K, Leland M, Kaplan J, Piedra PA, Zhou H, Parks R, Velji R, Aguilar-Cordova E, Wadsworth S, Graham F, Kochanek S, Carey KD, Beaudet AL. Administration of helper-dependent adenoviral vectors and sequential delivery of different vector serotype for long-term liver-directed gene tranfer in baboons. Proc Natl Acad Sci USA 1999; 96(22): 12816–12821.

72. Morsy MA, Gu M, Motzel S, Zhao J, Lin J, Su Q, Allen H, Franlin L, Parks RJ, Graham FL, Kochanek S, Bett AJ, Caskey CT. An adenoviral vector deleted for all viral coding sequences results in enhanced safety and extended expression of a leptin transgene. Proc Natl Acad Sci USA 1998; 95: 7866–7871.

73. Moss B. Poxviridae: the viruses and their replication. In: Fields BN, Knipe DM, Howley PM, Chanock RM, Melnick JL, Monath TP, Roizman B, Strauss SE, eds. Fields Virology. 3rd ed. Philadelphia, PA: Lippincott-Raven, 1996:2637–2671.

74. Lalani AS, Masters J, Zeng W, Barrett J, Pannu R, Everett H, Arendt CW, McFadden G. Use of chemokine receptors by poxviruses. Science 1999; 286:1968–1971.

75. Tartaglia J, Perkus ME, Taylor J, Norton EK, Audonnet JC, Cox WI, Davis SW, van der Hoeven J, Meignier B, Riviere M, et al. NYVAC: a highly attenuated strain of vaccinia virus. Virology 1992; 188:217–232.

76. Meyer H, Sutter G, Mayr A. Mapping of deletions in the genome of the highly attenuated vaccinia virus MVA and their influence on virulence. J Gen Virol 1991; 72:1031–1038.

77. Perkus ME, Tartaglia J, Paoletti E. Poxvirus-based vaccine candidates for cancer, AIDS, and other infectious diseases. J Leukoc Biol 1995; 58:1–13.

78. Smith GL, Moss B. Infectious poxvirus vectors have capacity for at least 25,000 base pairs of foreign DNA. Gene 1983; 25:21–28.

79. Paoletti E. Applications of pox virus vectors to vaccination: an update. Proc Natl Acad Sci USA 1996; 93:11349–11353.

80. Wolff JA, Malone RW, Williams P, Chong W, Acsadi G, Jani A, Felgner PL. Direct gene transfer into mouse muscle in vivo. Science 1990; 247:1465–1468.

81. Zabner J, Fasbender AJ, Moninger T, Poellinger KA, Welsh MJ. Cellular and molecular barriers to gene transfer by a cationic lipid. J Biol Chem 1995; 270:18997–19007.

82. Pollard H, Remy JS, Loussouarn G, Demolombe S, Behr JP, Escande D. Polyethylenimine but not cationic lipids promotes transgene delivery to the nucleus in mammalian cells. J Biol Chem 1998; 273:7507–7511.

83. Felgner PL, Zelphati O, Liang X. Advances in synthetic gene delivery system technology. In: Friedmann T, ed. The Development of Human Gene Therapy. Cold Spring Harbor, NY: Cold Spring Harbor Laboratory Press, 1999: 241–260.

84. Scherman D, Bessodes M, Cameron B, Herscovici J, Hofland H, Pitard B, Soubrier F, Wils P, Crouzet J. Application of lipids and plasmid design for gene delivery to mammalian cells. Curr Opin Biotechnol 1998; 9:480–485.

85. Zhu N, Liggitt D, Liu Y, Debs R. Systemic gene expression after intravenous DNA delivery into adult mice. Science 1993; 261:209–211.

86. McLean JW, Fox EA, Baluk P, Bolton PB, Haskell A, Pearlman R, Thurston G, Umemoto EY, McDonald DM. Organ-specific endothelial cell uptake of cationic liposome–DNA complexes in mice. Am J Physiol 1997; 273: H387–H404.

87. Scheule RK, St. George JA, Bagley RG, Marshall J, Kaplan JM, Akita GY, et al. Basis of pulmonary toxicity associated with cationic lipid-mediated gene transfer to the mammalian lung. Hum Gene Ther 1997; 8:689–707.

88. Ruiz FE, Clancy JP, Perricone MA, Bebok Z, Hong JS, Cheng SH, et al. A clinical inflammatory syndrome attributable to aerosolized lipid–DNA administration in cystic fibrosis. Hum Gene Ther 2001; 12:751–761.

89. Yew NS, Wang KX, Przybylska M, Bagley RG, Stedman M, Marshall J, et al. Contribution of plasmid DNA to inflammation in the lung after administration of cationic lipid: pDNA complexes. Hum Gene Ther 1999; 10:223–234.

90. Mahato RI, Anwer K, Tagliaferri F, Meaney C, Leonard P, Wadhwa MS, et al. Biodistribution and gene expression of lipid/plasmid complexes after systemic administration. Hum Gene Ther 1998; 9:2083–2099.

91. Yew NS, Wysokenski DM, Wang KX, Ziegler RJ, Marshall J, McNeilly D, et al. Optimization of plasmid vectors for high-level expression in lung epithelial cells. Hum Gene Ther 1997; 8:575–584.

92. Griesenbach U, Chonn A, Cassady R, Hannam V, Ackerley C, Post M, et al. Comparison between intratracheal and intravenous administration of lipo-

some–DNA complexes for cystic fibrosis lung gene therapy. Gene Ther 1998; 5:181–188.

93. Zabner J, Fasbender AJ, Moninger T, Poellinger KA, Welsh MJ. Cellular and molecular barriers to gene transfer by a cationic lipid. J Biol Chem 1995; 270:18997–19007.

94. Alton EWFW, Stern M, Farley R, Jaffe A, Chadwick SL, Phillips J, et al. Cationic lipid-mediated CFTR gene transfer to the lung and nose of patients with cystic fibrosis: a double-blind placebo-controlled trial. Lancet 1999; 353:947–954.

95. Noone PG, Hohneker KW, Zhou Z, Johnson LG, Foy C, Gipson C, et al. Safety and biological efficacy of a lipid-CFTR complex for gene transfer in the nasal epithelium of adult patients with cystic fibrosis. Mol Ther 2000; 1:105–114.

96. Christiano RJ. Targeted, non-viral gene delivery for cancer gene therapy. Front Biosci 1998; 3:1161–1170.

97. Cotten M, Wagner E. Receptor-mediated gene delivery strategies. In: Friedmann T, ed. The Development of Human Gene Therapy. Cold Spring Harbor, NY: Cold Spring Harbor Laboratory Press, 1999:261–277.

98. Li S, Tan Y, Viroonchatapan E, et al. Targeted gene delivery to the pulmonary endothelium by anti-PECAM antibody. Am J Physiol (Lung Cell Mol Physiol) 2000; 278:L504–L511.

99. Fajac I, Briand P, Monsigny M, Midoux P. Sugar-mediated uptake of glyco-sylated polylysines and gene transfer into normal and cystic fibrosis airway epithelial cells. Hum Gene Ther 1999; 10:395–406.

100. Gupta S, Eastman J, Silski C, Kerkol T, Davis PB. Single chain Fv: a ligand in receptor-mediated gene delivery. Gene Ther 2001; 8:586–592.

101. Boussif O, Lezoualc'h F, Zanta MA, Mergny MD, Scherman D, Demeneix B, Behr JP. A versatile vector for gene and oligonucleotide transfer into cells in culture and in vivo: polyethylenimine. Proc Natl Acad Sci USA 1995; 92:7297–7301.

102. Gautam A, Densmore CL, Golunski E, Xu B, Waldrep JC. Transgene expression in mouse airway epithelium by aerosol gene therapy with PEI–DNA complexes. Mol Ther 2001; 3:551–556.

103. Gautam A, Densmore CL, Waldrep JC. Pulmonary cytokine responses associated with PEI–DNA aerosol gene therapy. Gene Ther 2001; 8:254–257.

104. Wolff JA. Naked DNA gene transfer in mammalian cells. In: Friedmann T, ed. The Development of Human Gene Therapy. Cold Spring Harbor, NY: Cold spring Harbor Laboratory Press, 1999:279–307.

105. Yang NS, Burkholder J, Roberts B, Martinell B, McCabe D. In vivo and in vitro gene transfer to mammalian somatic cells by particle bombardment. Proc Natl Acad Sci USA 1990; 87:9568–9572.

106. Campbell AIM, Kuliszewski MA, Stewart DJ. Cell-based transfer to the pulmonary vasculature: endothelial nitric oxide synthase overexpression inhibits monocrotaline-induced pulmonary hypertension. Am J Respir Cell Mol Biol 1999; 21:567–575.

107. Campbell AIM, Zhao Y, Sandhu R, Stewart DJ. Cell-based transfer of VEGF attenuates monocrotaline-induced pulmonary hypertension. Circulation 2001; 104:2242–2248.

108. Danel C, Erzurum SC, Prayssac P, Eissa NT, Crystal RG, Herve P, Baudet B, Mazmanian M, Lemarchand P. Gene therapy for oxidant injury-related diseases: adenovirus-mediated transfer of superoxide dismutase and catalase cDNAs protects against hyperoxia but not against ischemia–reperfusion lung injury. Hum Gene Ther 1998; 9:1487–1496.

109. Otterbein LE, Kolls JK, Mantell LL, Cook JL, Alam J, Choi AM. Exogenous administration of heme oxygenase-1 by gene transfer provides protection against hyperoxia-induced lung injury. J Clin Invest 1999; 103:1047–1054.

110. Morse D, Choi AM. Heme oxygenase-1: the "emerging molecule" has arrived. Am J Resp Cell Mol Biol 2002; 27:8–16.

111. Weng YH, Tatarov A, Bartos BP, Contag CH, Dennery PA. HO-1 expression in type II pneumocytes after transpulmonary gene delivery. Am J Physiol Lung Cell Mol Physiol 2000; 278:L1273–L1279.

112. Factor P, Dumasius V, Saldias F, Brown LA, Sznajder JI. Adenovirus-mediated transfer of Na^+/K^+-ATPase beta1 subunit gene improves alveolar fluid clearance and survival in hyperoxic rats. Hum Gene Ther 2000; 11:2231–2242.

113. Epperly MW, Bray JA, Krager S, Berry LM, Gooding W, Engelhardt JF, Zwacka R, Travis EL, Greenberger JS. Intratracheal injection of adenovirus containing the human MnSOD transgene protects athymic nude mice from irradiation-induced organizing alveolitis. Int J Radiat Oncol Biol Phys 1999; 43:169–181.

114. Sime PJ, Xing Z, Graham FL, Csaky KG, Gauldie J. Adenovector-mediated gene transfer of active transforming growth factor-beta1 induces prolonged severe fibrosis in rat lung. J Clin Invest 1997; 100:768–776.

115. Epperly MW, Defilippi S, Sikora C, Gretton J, Kalend A, Greenberger JS. Intratracheal injection of manganese superoxide dismutase (MnSOD) plasmid/liposomes protects normal lung but not orthotropic tumors from irradiation. Gene Ther 2000; 7:1011–1018.

116. Rich D, Anderson M, Gregory R, Cheng S, Paul S, Jefferson J, McCann J, Klinger K, Smith A, Welsh M. Expression of cystic fibrosis transmembrane conductance regulator corrects defective chloride channel regulation in cystic fibrosis airway epithelial cells. Nature 1990; 347:358–363.

117. Johnson L, Olsen J, Sarkadi B, Moore K, Swanstrom R, Boucher R. Efficiency of gene transfer for restoration of normal airway epithelial function in cystic fibrosis. Nature Genet 1992; 2:21–25.

118. Alton EW, Stern M, Farley R, Jaffe A, Chadwick SL, Phillips J, Davies J, Smith SN, Browning J, Davies MG, et al. Cationic lipid-mediated CFTR gene transfer to the lungs and nose of patients with cystic fibrosis: a double-blind placebo-controlled trial. Lancet 1999; 353:947–954.

119. Zuckerman JB, Robinson CB, McCoy KS, Shell R, Sferra TJ, Chirmule N, Magosin SA, Propert KJ, Brown-Parr EC, Hughes JV, Tazelaar J, Baker C, Goldman MJ, Wilson JM. A phase I study of adenovirus-mediated transfer of the human cystic fibrosis transmembrane conductance regulator gene to a lung segment of individuals with cystic fibrosis. Hum Gene Ther 1999; 10:2973–2985.

120. Gauldie J, Graham F, Xing Z, Braciak T, Foley R, Sime PJ. Adenovirus-vector-mediated cytokine gene transfer to lung tissue. Ann NY Acad Sci 1996; 796:235–244.

121. Sime PJ, O'Reilly KMA. Fibrosis of the lung and other tissues: new concepts in pathogenesis and treatment. Clin Immunol 2001; 99(3):308–319.

122. Xing Z, Tremblay GM, Sime PJ, Gauldie J. Overexpression of GM-CSF induces pulmonary granulation tissue formation and fibrosis by induction of TGFβ1 and myofibroblasts but not TNFα. Am J Pathol 1997; 150:59–66.

123. Sime PJ, Marr RA, Gauldie D, Xing Z, Hewlett BR, Graham FL, Gauldie J. Transfer of TNFalpha to rat lung induces severe pulmonary inflammation and patchy interstitial fibrogenesis with induction of TGF-β1 and myofibroblasts. Am J Pathol 1998; 153:825–832.

124. Kolb M, Margetts PJ, Anthony DC, Pitossi F, Gauldie J. Transient expression of IL-1 beta induces acute lung injury and chronic repair leading to pulmonary fibrosis. J Clin Invest 2001; 107:1529–1536.

125. Xing Z, Tremblay GM, Sime PJ, Gauldie J. Overexpression of granulocyte–macrophage colony-stimulating factor induces pulmonary granulation tissue formation and fibrosis by induction of transforming growth factor-beta 1 and myofibroblast accumulation. Am J Pathol 1997; 150:59–66.

126. Bonniaud P, Margetts PJ, Kolb M, Haberberger T, Kelly M, Robertson J, Gauldie J. Adenoviral gene transfer of connective tissue growth factor in the lung induces transient fibrosis. Am J Respir Crit Care Med. 2004 Nov 24; [Epub ahead of print].

127. Yamaguchi Y, Mann DM, Ruoslahti E. Negative regulation of transforming growth factor-β by the proteoglycan decorin. Nature 1990; 346:281–284.

128. Kolb M, Margetts PJ, Galt T, Sime PJ, Xing Z, Schmidt M, Gauldie J. Transient transgene expression of decorin in the lung reduces the fibrotic response to bleomycin. Am J Respir Crit Care Med 2001; 163:770–777.

129. Nakao A, Fujii M, Matsumura R, Kumano K, Saito Y, Miyazono K, Iwamoto I. Transient gene transfer and expression of Smad7 prevents bleomycin-induced lung fibrosis in mice. J Clin Invest 1999; 104:5–11.

130. Yoshida M, Sakuma-Mochizuki J, Abe K, Arai T, Mori M, Goya S, Matsuoka H, Hayashi S, Kaneda Y, Kishimoto T. In vivo gene transfer of an extracellular domain of platelet-derived growth factor receptor by the HJV-liposome method ameliorates bleomycin-induced fibrosis. Biochem Biophys Res Commun 1999; 265:503–508.

131. Tsuburai T, Suzuki M, Nagashima Y, Suzuki S, Inoue S, Hasiba T, Ueda A, Ikehara K, Matsuse T, Ishigatsubo Y. Adenovirus-mediated transfer and overexpression of heme oxygenase 1 cDNA in lung prevents bleomycin-induced pulmonary fibrosis via a Fas–Fas ligand-independent pathway. Hum Gene Ther 2002; 13:1945–1960.

19

Combination Therapies for Lung Injury

GLORIA S. PRYHUBER, CARL T. D'ANGIO,
JACOB N. FINKELSTEIN, and ROBERT H. NOTTER

*Departments of Pediatrics and Environmental Medicine, University of Rochester
School of Medicine, Rochester, New York, U.S.A.*

I. Overview

This chapter examines combination therapies that simultaneously target
different aspects of lung injury pathophysiology to achieve additivity or
synergy in clinical efficacy. Interactive basic and clinical research on such
therapies is necessary, since it is not feasible to define the mechanisms, activity,
interactions, and efficacy of all relevant agents and interventions in human studies alone. Design, analysis, and other issues that impact clinical trials investigating combination therapies in severely ill patients are detailed and
discussed in the first part of the chapter. Coverage then focuses primarily on
agents and interventions of potential utility in combination therapies for clinical acute lung injury (ALI) and the acute respiratory distress syndrome
(ARDS). Agents and interventions for both the acute exudative phase and later
fibroproliferative phase of ALI/ARDS are described. Examples of pharmacologic agents for treating acute exudative lung injury include vasoactive agents
and antithrombotics to improve perfusion, exogenous surfactants to improve
ventilation, and anti-inflammatory antibodies, receptor antagonists or antioxidants to antagonize overexuberant inflammation. Selected modalities or
strategies of mechanical ventilation and alveolar recruitment for use in
combination therapies for ALI/ARDS are also covered, as are pharmacologic

agents relevant for treating fibroproliferative injury pathology. Many of these agents and interventions have been discussed individually in Chapters 13–17, and several have been shown to have benefits in patients with lung injury. However, their impact on survival and long-term patient outcomes may be improved by combination therapy approaches.

II. Concept of Combined-Modality Therapy

As emphasized throughout this book, lung injury involves a complex set of interactive processes and mechanistic pathways. To achieve the most significant impact in treating patients with lung injury, it is logical to attack simultaneously more than one aspect of this multifaceted patho physiology. The concurrent use of therapeutic agents or interventions in a combination approach has the potential to achieve additive or even synergistic improvements in respiratory function and clinical outcomes. Prominent aspects of the pathophysiology of acute pulmonary injury that provide targets for pharmacologic agents include vascular dysfunction and ventilation/perfusion mismatching, surfactant dysfunction, inflammation, and oxidant injury. Additional targets for therapy are present in the fibroproliferative pathology of chronic lung injury. The challenge is determining how the mechanistic activity, interactions, and efficacy of rational combinations of agents and interventions can best be defined in basic and clinical research to improve the treatment and outcomes of patients with diseases of acute and chronic lung injury.

III. Integration of Basic and Clinical Research on Combination Therapies for Lung Injury

Developing effective combination therapies for lung injury depends on mechanistic understanding of the controlling pathobiology integrated with rationally designed clinical trials. Bidirectional feedback between laboratory research and clinical medicine is usually optimal for therapeutic development. Observations from human disease often initiate laboratory studies of specific injury processes and potential therapeutic agents. In turn, in vitro and animal studies provide mechanistic understanding and agent activity information required for effective and focused clinical research. Clinical studies generally begin with single modality assessments, followed by combined-modality testing of beneficial interventions based on mechanistic understanding of activity and potential synergy. Issues arising in the design and implementation of clinical trials evaluating combination therapies are covered in detail in the following section.

Although randomized, controlled clinical trials are essential in establishing the safety and efficacy of therapies, they are inherently limited in resolving power relative to basic laboratory research. Patients affected by lung injury are heterogeneous in age, physical condition, and systemic pathology, and are also exposed to diverse iatrogenic risks during medical intensive care. These factors increase the numbers of patients needed to demonstrate improvements in survival or other long-term outcomes in clinical trials. Laboratory studies of combination therapies for lung injury are themselves subject to limitations. Scientists generally design experiments to minimize confounding variables and maximize the interpretability of data. As more variables are added, as in studies with multiple agents, larger and more numerous experimental groups become necessary. Animal models of lung injury are also species-specific, and vary in their pathophysiology and how closely they approximate human disease. Studies in isolated or cultured cells complement whole animal assessments, but information on cell–cell communication is lacking and clinical relevance is a significant concern. Nonetheless, basic research in animals and cells is invaluable in elucidating mechanisms and specific responses to agents and interventions. Basic research can assess the consistency of results across complementary systems (physicochemical, cellular, and animal) with a greater degree of standardization than feasible in clinical trials. Information can also be gained about detrimental, as well as positive, agent interactions so that the former can be avoided in clinical studies.

The history of exogenous surfactant replacement therapy for premature infants is just one of many examples illustrating the importance of integrated basic and clinical research in developing treatments for lung disease and injury. Initial attempts at surfactant therapy in premature infants with aerosolized dipalmitoyl phosphatidylcholine (DPPC) were unsuccessful in the 1960s (1–3) because they were implemented without sufficient understanding of the functional composition of lung surfactant or the limitations of surfactant delivery by aerosolization. Extensive biophysical and animal research was necessary to explain the lack of efficacy of aerosolized DPPC and to develop more active exogenous surfactants to allow successful clinical trials to be done in premature infants during the 1980s (Chapter 15). A similar integration of basic and clinical research is needed to define effective combination therapies for diseases involving acute or chronic lung injury in infants, children, and adults.

IV. Clinical Trials Studying Combination Therapies

The randomized, blinded, controlled clinical trial is the "gold standard" for the evaluation of new therapies. Recent criticism and scrutiny of the design of the ARDS Network Low Tidal Volume Study highlights the increasing complexity of successful clinical research in patients with severe lung injury. In this instance, the concerns raised included the ethics of randomized trials of therapies already having a suggested benefit in animals and nonrandomized clinical studies, the legality of proxy consents for critically ill patients, and the choice of "current best standard of medical care" as an ethical and valid control arm (see Refs. 4, 5 for review). The design, implementation, and analysis of clinical trials assessing combination therapies for lung injury present additional challenges (Tables 1 and 2). In combination therapy, the effects of agents and interventions need to be evaluated not only together, but also in comparison to the relevant individual treatments. If none of the interventions being studied represent the existing standard of care, it is also necessary to include comparisons with control patients treated with the best available conventional therapy. Clinical trials of this kind are inherently expensive, time-consuming, and nontrivial to design and analyze. The complexity of testing combination therapies makes it particularly important to involve biostatisticians at the earliest phase of trial planning. Prospective power analysis is essential to define the study size necessary to discern clinically significant differences. The smaller the differences sought, the larger the number of required subjects. Clinical trials should be of adequate power not to miss the smallest difference of clear clinical significance. For instance, if a 10% difference in mortality is a clinically significant outcome between two groups, a trial designed only to demonstrate differences greater than 20% risks incorrectly concluding that a useful therapy is not efficacious. Study size determinations become more complex as the number of patient groups increases as in combination therapy, or

Table 1 Considerations for Clinical Trials Involving Multiple Comparisons of Agents or Interventions for Treating Lung Injury

---

Combination therapy evaluations must include groups receiving the
 relevant single agent or single modality therapies
Interventions for priority testing in combination therapies have prior
 evidence of safety (and acute efficacy) in single agent or single modality
 therapy in humans
Interventions selected for combination testing should have a conceptual
 (mechanistic) rationale for additive or synergistic effects
Combination therapy trials require randomized, blinded assessments,
 particularly since the interventions studied may have known individual
 efficacy
Combination therapy trials must be of sufficient size (power) to identify
 differences among multiple groups based on prospectively chosen,
 clinically significant outcome variables

Additional considerations affecting clinical evaluations of combination therapies are given in Table 2 and described in the text.

Table 2 Patient- and Disease-Related Complexities in Clinical Trials of Combination Interventions

Complication	Associated problem(s)	Potential solution(s)
Multiple causes of disease and injury; patient-specific susceptibility factors (genetic, predisposing conditions)	Potential heterogeneity in the severity of clinical symptoms, progression of disease, and responses to treatment	Strict inclusion/exclusion criteria, rigorous definition of disease, utilize well-defined subgroup analyses
Relatively small numbers of patients per center	Difficult to enroll sufficient numbers of patients to meet power needs of study	Utilize multicenter trials
Known or inferred efficacy of relevant individual therapies in a disease with high mortality/morbidity	Difficult to randomize patients not to receive an individual agent or intervention having "some" efficacy; difficult to maintain clinical "equipoise" of study personnel	Detailed prospective discussion of study protocols at all centers, double-blind randomization, and careful monitoring of the "equipoise" of study personnel
Complex pathophysiology and etiologies of lung injury and related pulmonary diseases	Multiple relevant clinical variables plus the possibility of multiorgan disease	Careful prospective selection of primary and secondary outcomes
Survival vs. quality of life issues	Lack of agreement on clinically important outcomes and on acute improvements that translate to reduced morbidity in survivors	Prospective agreement and consideration of clinically important outcomes (e.g., survival, survival without morbidity, survival with reduced morbidity)

See text for discussion of these and other issues affecting clinical trials on combination therapies for lung injury.

if specialized enrollment considerations like stratification of patients within groups are necessary.

Investigators have taken a variety of approaches to deal with the problems inherent in multiple comparisons (Tables 1 and 2). The most obvious is to increase the number of subjects enrolled (see later subsection on study size). In addition, it is necessary to limit and focus outcome variables to reduce the number of required statistical comparisons. One strategy is to choose (prospectively) a single primary outcome for statistical analysis, supplemented as necessary with carefully selected subsidiary outcomes or subgroup analyses (6,7). The therapeutic effect is largely assessed by the primary outcome variable. The subsidiary outcomes and subgroup analyses provide additional information on efficacy, but may require a higher level of statistical significance to be meaningful. Subgroup comparisons also aid in generating new hypotheses for further testing in later trials (6,7). In some studies on combination therapies, a single primary outcome comparison may not be sufficient to discern differences between the individual therapies, their combination(s), and the best standard therapy. Pediatric oncology investigators have responded to this problem by an incremental approach in clinical studies. Single new therapies are first tested individually against standard therapy. If two therapies are individually at least as effective as the best standard therapy, then another trial can be performed comparing the combination of the two treatments to either one alone. Answers are arrived at sequentially rather than concurrently, but the individual trials are shorter and less complex.

A. Possible Patterns of Responses in Clinical Studies on Combination Therapies

Multiple patterns of response are possible in clinical (or basic) research on the efficacy of combination therapies (Fig. 1) (8). Although the goal of combination is to obtain additivity or positive synergy, the potential for negative interactions also exists (Fig. 1). Two therapies can have clinical benefits and minimal side effects when used separately, but have reduced effectiveness together if their mechanisms of action are incompatible or if one increases the toxicity or impairs the pharmacokinetics of the other. Several pharmacologic interactions common to intensive care settings have recently been reviewed by Pea and Furlanut (9). The interactions of medications metabolized by the cytochrome P-450 pathways such as macrolide antibiotics and theophylline are classic examples of clinically significant alterations in drug efficacy and toxicity in combination therapy (9). Harmful drug interactions can sometimes be identified and avoided through animal research, but drug safety and interactions ultimately must be assessed clinically.

Medicine is replete with examples showing the importance of adequate clinical testing of therapeutic interventions. Oxygen therapy for premature

Two interventions A and B studied for potential efficacy in combination therapy can have a range of patterns of effect:

Additive: AB = A + B
Synergistic: AB > A + B
Neutral   AB = A or B
Subadditive: AB < A + B
Negative: AB < A or B

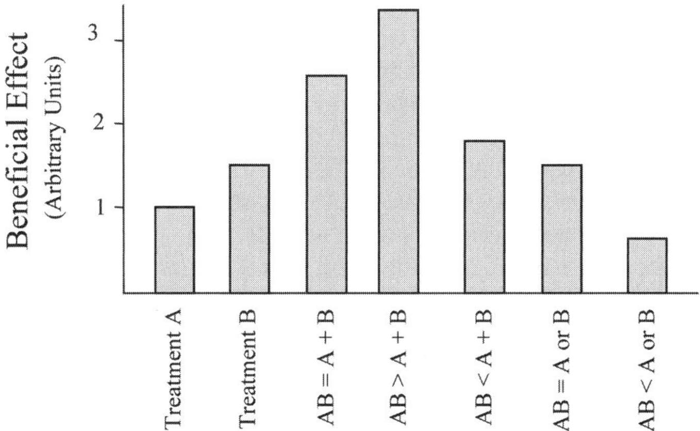

Figure 1   Range of possible effects in multimodal therapy with interventions A and B. Two therapies (A and B) may have net complementary or deleterious effects in combination. In combination (AB), they may be additive (greater than either treatment alone), synergistic (greater than the sum of the individual effects), neutral (equal to the most effective single therapy), subadditive (less than the sum of the individual effects of the two), or negative (less than either treatment alone). This broad range of possible responses impacts clinical trial design and interpretation, and increases the need for complementary, integrated basic research on agent activities and interactions as described in the text. (Modified from Ref. 8.)

infants with perinatal respiratory failure was initially introduced without detailed controlled clinical trials in the middle of the 20th century. This therapy improved respiratory distress, but also proved responsible for an epidemic of severe retinopathy of prematurity (10). Similarly, treatment with postnatal corticosteroids can reduce inflammation and the need for oxygen and mechanical ventilation in infants with chronic lung disease, but also has detrimental effects on brain and/or lung development in infants and animals (11,12). These latter findings have now led to a more cautious use of corticosteroids in newborns. Another example is extracorporeal membrane oxygenation (ECMO), which was widely adopted in the United States to treat neonatal respiratory failure following only very small clinical trials (13–15). The efficacy of ECMO in enhancing survival in newborns with respiratory failure has since been supported by a larger randomized controlled trial in the United Kingdom (16), but many of the clinical indications for ECMO have had to be worked out retrospectively. The potential for both positive and negative interactions between agents or modalities in combination therapies increases the importance of adequate clinical testing of safety and efficacy.

B. Study Sizes in Clinical Trials Evaluating Combination Therapies

The multiple groups in clinical trials investigating combination therapies mean that, on average, more subjects and comparisons are required to obtain complete evaluations of safety and efficacy. Raising the number of comparisons in a study makes it more likely that one of these may be deemed "statistically significant" by chance. The oft-used criterion of statistical significance of $p < 0.05$ means that the likelihood is less than 5% that a detected result is due to chance alone, i.e., there is more than a 95% probability that the result is not due to chance. However, if two comparisons are made, and both have p values just below 0.05, the probability that neither is due to chance is only $\sim 0.95 \times 0.95$, or about 90%. Statistical approaches to multiple comparisons generally demand a more stringent level of proof (below $p < 0.05$ for each individual comparison) so that the composite likelihood of chance differences remains < 0.05. This requires larger numbers of subjects per group, and achieving large study sizes is nontrivial in severe lung injury syndromes like ALI/ARDS. The high mortality and morbidity of such conditions can cause physicians, parents or other authorized persons to decline to enroll patients into a trial they feel might restrict treatment options, or to withdraw patients from an on-going trial to search for alternative therapies. One method of increasing patient numbers is through multicenter consortia, although this approach also has limitations. For example, for single agent therapy with exogenous surfactant, one successful study in full-term infants with ARDS-related respiratory failure required 44 centers in order to enroll 328 subjects (17). Coordinating the efforts of such a large number of centers, physicians, and support staff can be a daunting task. Nonetheless, effective multicenter consortia have been established and maintained in pediatric oncology (e.g., see Ref. 7), and the ARDS Clinical Network has been established by the National Heart Lung and Blood Institute of NIH to help evaluate novel therapeutic agents for lung injury.

C. Considerations in Designing and Implementing Multicenter Trials

Several factors are important in planning and implementing multicenter clinical trials of combination (or individual) therapies for lung injury.

Medical centers inevitably differ to some extent in their preferred approaches to treatment. Even within a given center, there can be variability in the preferences and expectations of individuals and clinical disciplines based on idiosyncratic experience. It is particularly important that each center and discipline be adequately represented from the earliest stages of trial planning to facilitate negotiation and define hypotheses that the consensus of participants agree are important, accurate, and testable. A steering committee with broad membership and a clear authority to reconcile differences can aid this process significantly. It is equally important that each center and physician has clinical equipoise. Clinicians must agree that they do not believe one arm of a study is superior to another, and hence feel ethically bound to provide patients with the treatment they believe is preferred. Such attitudes can easily subvert an entire trial. Loss of equipoise is of particular concern in designing trials on combination therapy where some degree of clinical efficacy has already been demonstrated for the individual interventions. Multicenter trials require specific attention and oversight to maintain uniformity and consistency. Protocols must be precise and detailed, and specific manuals generated to insure that procedures, data entry, and record-keeping are uniform among centers. Regular communication among centers is essential, including site visits by representatives of the lead center to ensure full compliance with protocols. Some economies of scale are possible, but each center generally needs to maintain local personnel who are fully versed in the study and can act as consultants for colleagues. These considerations add complexity and cost to multicenter trials. In addition, center-specific outcome differences can in some cases obscure treatment effects. However, multicenter consortia are often essential in providing a population base sufficient for meaningful clinical testing. In addition, they provide infrastructure and collaborative expertise that may be unavailable in a single center.

D. Study Design Issues Related to Entry Criteria, Stratification, and Blinding

Clinical diseases involving lung injury are the result of multiple etiologies, and strict prospective entry and exclusion criteria are required to avoid bias or inconsistency in study groups assessing combination therapies. Entry criteria need to be objective, precise, measurable, and reproducible (6), allowing the enrollment of representative patient populations but excluding individuals with specific confounding pathology. It may also be necessary to stratify study enrollment on the basis of pathophysiology. Stratification allows relevant subgroups of patients to be randomized separately, avoiding unintentional over-representation in one of the arms of the trial. Severely ill patients with lung injury are likely to have been treated with a number of agents and interventions prior to entry into a clinical trial. They may also have pre-existing or systemic medical conditions. These factors can be addressed to some extent by stratified randomization and/or strict inclusion and exclusion criteria. Randomization, which is essential in removing bias in clinical trials, is optimally done in a blinded (masked) fashion so that neither clinicians nor subjects are aware of the treatment(s) given. Some therapies for lung injury such as modes and strategies of mechanical ventilation are extremely difficult to keep masked from clinicians. The difficulties of establishing and maintaining effective blinding are compounded when trials test multiple interventions and involve the participation of multiple medical centers.

E. Issues of Informed Consent in Severely III Patients

Patients and patient families faced with an unexpected threat to life have significant psychological vulnerability. In clinical trials involving acute respiratory failure, only a very short time is often available to arrive at decisions about consent. In this highly stressful situation, some patients or family members may refuse consent for all clinical trials because of reluctance to decide about "experimental" medical care. Conversely, others may accept uncritically any therapy that appears to offer some hope or that they perceive as being recommended by their physician. Investigators must be particularly sensitive to the emotional state of those giving study consent. Patients, parents, or other designated decision makers need to understand clearly which procedures are research-related and which are not. They also need to understand fully the risks and potential benefits of any research intervention. It may often be appropriate for the treating physician not to be directly involved in the consent process, in order to help families differentiate between clinical care and research intervention, and to avoid any potential for undue influence over the decision to give consent.

F. Prospective Definitions of Clinical Outcome Variables

The careful definition of outcome variables is essential for all clinical trials. A carefully considered outcome variable is prospectively and quantitatively defined, clearly measurable, and clinically significant (18). Some of the most important clinical outcomes are dichotomous (e.g., death/survival) rather than continuous (e.g., a change in the mean of some measured physiological parameter). Preferred outcome variables must have sufficient relevance that clinicians agree they give a meaningful reflection of therapeutic efficacy and make a difference in the care of patients. Preferred outcome variables are also long-term rather than short-term. An intervention that improves a short-term physiologic parameter, but not survival or other long-term outcomes, generally has less clinical significance. Many of the patients affected with severe lung injury have a substantial risk of death from disease, and survival is an excellent scientific primary outcome measure. However, survival tells only part of the story of a therapy. A treatment that does not change the rate of survival, but improves other significant long-term outcomes for those who do survive, clearly has clinical benefits. Conversely, a therapy that marginally improves survival or other long-term outcomes, but is associated with severe or burdensome morbidity in survivors, may on balance not be considered clinically beneficial.

Clinical outcome variables impact trial design, implementation, and analysis in several ways, including influencing the treatment options open to participating physicians. Outcome variables that restrict the availability of alternative treatment options for severely ill patients who do not respond to the therapy being tested can generate ethical conflicts and protocol violations. One approach to avoid this problem involves the use of surrogate endpoints. For example, several trials of inhaled nitric oxide (INO) in newborn infants allowed the use of ECMO as rescue therapy, and presented their results in terms of the proportion of children who went on to die or to require ECMO (19–21). Another method of establishing a surrogate endpoint is a crossover trial. Subjects are assigned initially to one of the study arms, but those who later meet predefined criteria for failure of treatment in their assigned arm may be switched to an alternate arm or returned to conventional therapy. In this case, the primary outcome is the failure of the initially assigned therapy. All trials using surrogate outcomes depend on careful, detailed, prospectively formulated failure criteria that are known and followed specifically and consistently by participating study physicians.

G. Necessity to Test New Therapies in the Context of Optimal Current Treatments

Combination therapies need to be assessed not only in terms of their own efficacy and agent interactions, but also in terms of their compatibility and benefits in the context of optimal current treatments. Patients with severe lung injury currently receive a number of medications and interventions aimed at improving clinical symptoms. In addition to mechanical ventilation, supplemental oxygen is used to improve arterial oxygenation, and antagonize hypoxic pulmonary vasoconstriction and secondary heart failure. Examples of other drugs in standard supportive therapy include antibiotics against infection, as well as anticholinergic agents, beta-agonists, and methylxanthines like theophylline to facilitate bronchodilatation, vasodilation, or diaphragmatic function. In addition, quality of life studies indicate that nonpulmonary end-organ damage and reduced cognitive ability can occur in survivors of conditions like ALI/ARDS, indicating a need for aggressive attention to exercise, nutrition, and rehabilitation as part of therapy (22). Moreover, it is important to deal with issues such as depression and anxiety that can significantly interfere with medical therapies. Testing new agents and interventions for acute and chronic lung injury in the context of optimal current therapy is a highly complex and difficult issue, and the extent to which this is addressed varies significantly between clinical trials.

The remainder of this chapter focuses primarily on agents and interventions potentially relevant for use in combination therapies for the acute exudative phase and later fibroproliferative phase of ALI/ARDS. Since lung injury evolves over time, multiagent and multimodal therapies must consider the specific cellular and tissue abnormalities present at a given phase of disease, i.e., efficacy can depend strongly on the timing of agent use. Combination therapies are most likely to yield maximal benefits when defined and developed in the context of the natural history of disease.

V. Clinical ALI and ARDS

Acute lung injury/acute respiratory distress syndrome can arise in patients of all ages from direct or indirect insults that induce inflammation, damage the cells of the alveolocapillary membrane, and lead to severe acute respiratory failure (Fig. 2). Uniform diagnostic criteria are essential for meaningful clinical studies and therapeutic development for ALI/ARDS. The American-European Consensus Committee in 1994 defined clinical ALI to require respiratory failure of acute onset with a PaO_2/FiO_2 ratio ≤ 300 mmHg (regardless of the level of positive end expiratory pressure, PEEP), bilateral infiltrates on frontal chest radiograph, and a pulmonary capillary wedge pressure <18 mmHg (if measured) or no evidence of left atrial hypertension (23). ARDS was defined identically except for a lower limiting value of < 200 mmHg for PaO_2/FiO_2 (23).[a] The Consensus Committee definitions of ALI/ARDS are now widely used, supplemented by lung injury or critical care scores like the Murray score (24) or the APACHE II (25). Although the intimate association between acute pulmonary injury and ARDS is well known, the practical significance of the distinction between clinical ALI and ARDS is less clear. A meta-analysis of 102 studies prior to 1996 suggested little or no difference in mortality rates between patients meeting criteria for ALI vs. ARDS (26).

---

[a] Although useful clinically, the Consensus Committee definitions of ALI/ARDS do not specify ventilator-related variables, injury etiologies, and systemic disease that can significantly affect responses to treatment. Also, exclusion of left heart failure may lead to under-diagnosis of ALI/ARDS, since patients with injury-associated respiratory failure can be sufficiently volume overloaded during treatment to meet criteria for congestive heart failure (but as a secondary effect).

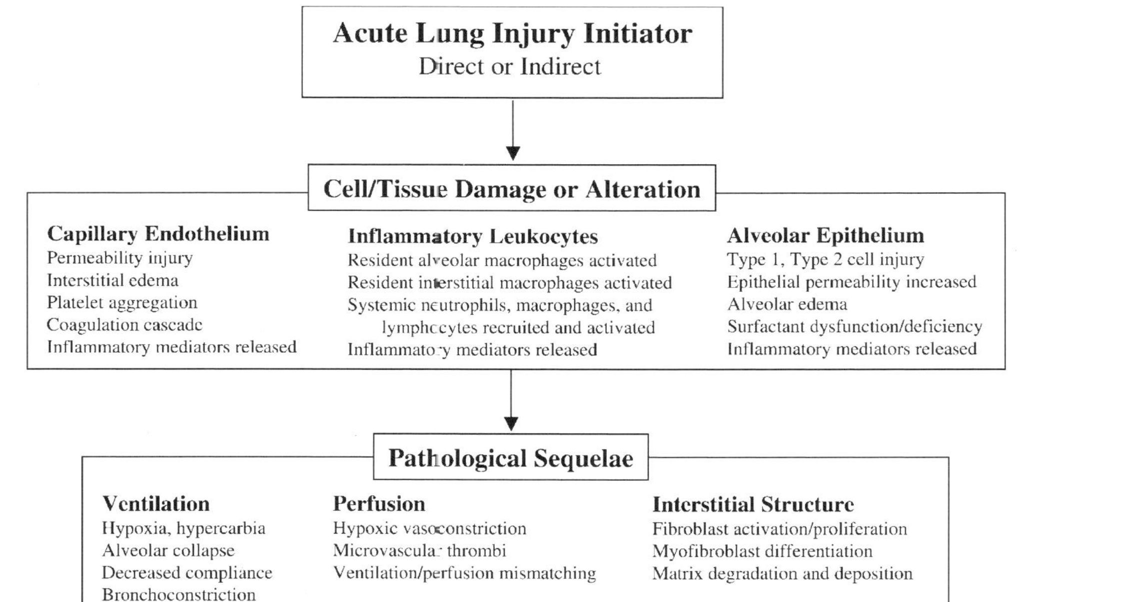

Figure 2 Schematic of the early pathophysiology of acute pulmonary injury. Clinical ALI/ARDS involve the interplay of multiple pathological processes. Acute pulmonary inflammation and injury arise from direct causes (e.g., lung infection, gastric or meconium aspiration, inhalation of toxicants) or indirect causes (e.g., sepsis, trauma, shock, burn injury, and many others). Major early pathology involves cellular injury and increased permeability at the level of the capillary endothelium and alveolar epithelium. Airway and interstitial cells may also be injured acutely or become altered as lung injury progresses. Early pathological manifestations involve edema and compromised ventilation/perfusion apparent as acute respiratory failure, plus the initiation of structural changes that can lead to later fibroproliferation and fibrosis.

The etiologies, prevalence, clinical features, and pathophysiology of ALI/ARDS are detailed in Chapter 3. These syndromes affect a large number of patients and have a poor prognosis with high mortality and morbidity, especially in the elderly (23,26–31). The incidence of ARDS has been reported to be 50,000–150,000 cases per year in the United States depending on the clinical definition used (23,26,27,29,31–33). Recent studies suggest the incidence of clinical ALI to be 20–70 cases per 10^5 persons per year (34,35), with $17–43 \times 10^3$ associated deaths per year in the United States (35). There has been relatively little improvement over time in the survival of patients with ALI/ARDS. Some studies have reported a reduction of 15–20% in the mortality rate of ARDS between the 1980s and the mid-1990s, but it is not clear whether this is attributable to specific therapeutic advances or general improvements in medical technology (36,37). Patients with ALI/ARDS frequently have sepsis and/or multiorgan involvement manifesting as systemic inflammatory response syndrome (SIRS), multiple organ dysfunction syndrome (MODS), or multiple organ failure (MOF) (25,38,39) (Fig. 3). They may also have a variety of comorbid conditions such as diabetes or alcohol abuse. The heterogeneous population of

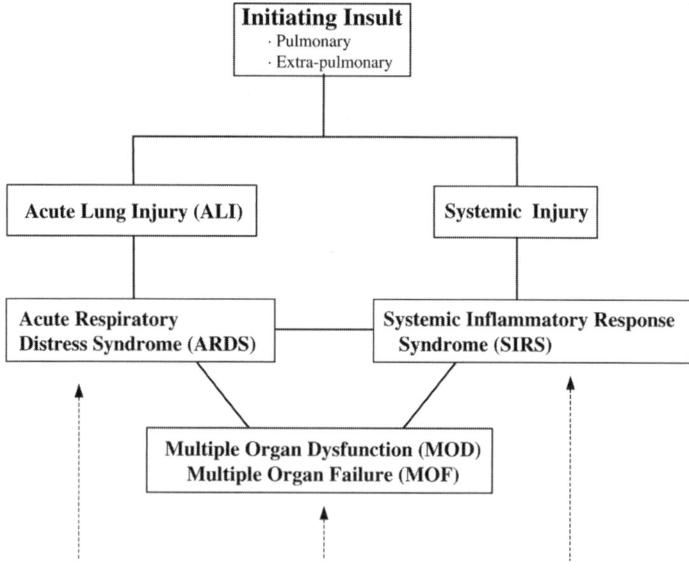

Figure 3 Extrapulmonary involvement in ALI/ARDS. Clinical ALI and ARDS are frequently elements of a systemic response to an initiating insult or disease process. Effective combination therapies for ALI/ARDS must include the possibility of targeting systemic and multiple organ disease in addition to pulmonary dysfunction.

patients affected by ALI/ARDS significantly complicates studies on pathophysiology and therapy. However, current understanding permits a number of agents and interventions of potential utility in combination therapies to be identified.

VI. Potential Targets for Combination Therapies in the Acute Exudative Phase of ALI/ARDS

The pulmonary pathophysiology of ALI/ARDS can be divided conceptually into early, mid, and late phases (Table 3) (40–42) (also see Chapter 3). Within 12–72 hr of the initiating lung injury stimulus, interstitial and alveolar edema is usually prominent in association with a decreased barrier integrity of capillary endothelial cells and alveolar type I epithelial cells that normally maintain a tight barrier and electrolyte balance (43–46). Over the next 3–7 days, further alveolocapillary damage occurs, with denuding of basal lamina and the formation of intra-alveolar hyaline membranes containing plasma proteins, fibrin, and cellular debris. Multiple inflammatory cytokines and reactive oxygen/nitrogen species are released, and complement and coagulation cascades are activated. Pulmonary blood flow and perfusion are reduced in acute exudative ALI/ARDS by thrombus formation, intravascular sequestration of leukocytes and platelets, and hypoxia-induced vasoconstriction. Surfactant activity can be impaired by several mechanisms including interactions with serum proteins and other inhibitors in edema (47–50), and surfactant metabolism may be disrupted if alveolar type II cells are injured or become altered. Inflammatory mediators like

Table 3 Pathophysiologic Phases of Clinical ALI/ARDS

Early, exudative phase
 Edema
 Inflammation
 Ventilation–perfusion mismatch
 Surfactant dysfunction

Mid, fibroproliferative phase
 Fibroblast activity
 Type II alveolar epithelial cell hyperplasia
 Matrix deposition

Late, fibrotic phase
 Scarring
 Loss of alveoli
 Pruning of vascular bed

Examples of combination therapies discussed in this chapter focus primarily on the first two of these pathophysiologic phases.

tumor necrosis factor (TNF)-α can also alter the production of active surfactant apoproteins (51,52).

Potential targets for combination therapies in the acute exudative phase of ALI/ARDS include hypoperfusion and ventilation/perfusion mismatching, surfactant dysfunction, arterial hypoxemia, edema, inflammation, oxidant injury, and injury to alveolar epithelial and capillary endothelial cells (Table 4). Agents and interventions targeting many of these abnormalities are discussed individually in Chapter 13 (ventilation therapies), Chapter 14 (anti-inflammatory agents), Chapter 15 (exogenous surfactant therapy), Chapter 16 (antioxidant therapy), and Chapter 17 (vascular-based therapy) (also see Refs. 4, 39, 47, 53–71 for review). Examples of pharmacologic agents that have been tested individually in patients with ALI/ARDS or sepsis include vasoactive agents such as INO, almitrine, or prostacyclin (72–88); exogenous surfactant drugs (89–98); anticoagulants like tissue factor pathway inhibitor (TFPI) and antithrombotic protein C (APC) (69,99,100); anti-inflammatory antibodies or receptor antagonists such as anti-TNFα (101–104) and interleukin (IL)-1 receptor antagonist (IL-1Ra) (105,106); anti-inflammatory agents like pentoxifylline and corticosteroids (107–117); and antioxidants like *N*-acetylcysteine (NAC) (118–120) and superoxide dismutase (121,122). Nonpharmacologic interventions that could be utilized along with pharmacologic agents in combination therapies include specific modes or strategies of mechanical ventilation that enhance alveolar recruitment and minimize ventilator-induced lung injury (4,123–134). Prone positioning can also be used to enhance alveolar recruitment and ventilation in patients with ALI/ARDS (e.g., 135). These agents and interventions, and their potential utility in combination therapies for acute exudative ALI/ARDS, are detailed more fully in following sections.

VII. Therapies Targeting Ventilation/Perfusion Abnormalities in Acute Exudative ALI/ARDS

One of the primary goals in treating acute respiratory failure in ALI/ARDS is to improve alveolar ventilation (V_A) and its matching to capillary perfusion (Q_c), i.e. to enhance V_A/Q_c matching. Examples of interventions for improving V_A/Q_c matching and arterial oxygenation are summarized in Table 5. These include inhaled vasodilators to increase blood flow to ventilated alveoli, selective vasoconstrictors to potentiate hypoxic vasoconstriction in nonventilated regions of lung, exogenous surfactants to reduce alveolar surface tension, anticoagulants to antagonize thrombus formation and increase pulmonary blood flow, and mechanical ventilation techniques to recruit and stabilize alveoli. Some of these interventions have been used concurrently to improve oxygenation, but the majority have not been examined in detail as part of combination therapies.

Table 4 Examples of Potential Biological Targets in the Acute Exudative Phase of ALI/ARDS

Target	Contributing abnormalities or processes	Examples of therapy and desired outcomes
Hypoperfusion and ventilation/perfusion mismatching	Hypoxic vasoconstriction Inappropriate vasodilation Microvascular occlusion	Treat with agents to vasodilate ventilated lung regions, vasoconstrict nonventilated lung regions, and reduce microvascular thrombosis
Surfactant dysfunction or deficiency	Physicochemical inhibitors of surfactant in edema or inflammation, or injury to type II pneumocytes	Deliver exogenous surfactant to reverse dysfunction or deficiency to improve alveolar stability, reduce edema, and normalize P–V mechanics
Inflammation	Activation/recruitment of inflammatory leukocytes and over - exuberant production of inflammatory mediators	Deliver agents to remove or deplete activated neutrophils, macrophages or other leukocytes, or to block the effects of specific inflammatory mediators
Arterial hypoxemia, alveolar and interstitial edema	Decreased gas exchange, increased permeability and decreased resorptive capacity of the alveolocapillary membrane	Mechanical ventilation to raise arterial oxygenation without increasing lung injury or alveolocapillary permeability; delivery of agents to reduce edema
Death/injury of cells in airways and alveolo-capillary membrane	Loss of normal ciliated airway epithelium, alveolar type I cells, and microvascular endothelial cells	Reduce cell death and the severity of cellular injury

Many of the biological targets and abnormalities listed are interdependent (e.g., surfactant dysfunction contributes to ventilation/perfusion abnormalities, arterial hypoxemia, edema, and abnormal lung mechanics). Similarly, many of the therapies noted affect overlapping targets (e.g., vasoactive agents, exogenous surfactants, and mechanical ventilation can improve arterial oxygenation and ventilation/perfusion mismatching). Specific agents and interventions of possible utility in combination therapies aimed at the acute exudative phase of ALI/ARDS are discussed in the text.

Table 5 Examples of Agents and Interventions with the Potential to Improve Ventilation to Perfusion Matching in ALI/ARDS

Pharmacologic agents to increase perfusion of ventilated alveoli
  Inhaled nitric oxide (INO)
  Prostacyclin (PGI_2)

Pharmacologic agents to decrease perfusion of poorly ventilated alveoli
  Almitrine

Pharmacologic agents to increase alveolar ventilation and stability
  Exogenous surfactants

Pharmacologic agents to reduce vascular obstruction
  Anticoagulants
  Tissue factor pathway inhibitor (TFPI)
  Site-inactivated factor VIIa
  Inhibitors of neutrophil recruitment
  Inhibitors of platelet aggregation

Ventilation modalities and strategies to recruit and stabilize alveoli
  Prone positioning
  Alveolar recruitment maneuvers by mechanical ventilation
  Identification and maintenance of critical positive end expiratory pressure (PEEP)
  High-frequency ventilation
  Liquid or partial liquid ventilation

See text for specific studies using these agents and interventions individually in ALI/ARDS, as well as their potential use in combination therapy approaches.

A. Vasoactive Agents for Treating Acute Exudative ALI/ARDS

The ability to titrate dosing and the degree of pulmonary selectivity are major considerations in selecting vasoactive drugs for treating acute respiratory failure. Relatively few vasoactive agents have been identified that give therapeutic pulmonary effects without significant systemic side effects if given intravenously (70). The development of inhaled drugs such as nitric oxide and prostacyclin that can directly target the pulmonary vasculature in mechanically ventilated patients has reduced systemic side effects and led to improved efficacy.

Inhaled Nitric Oxide

Nitric oxide, a naturally occurring product identical to endothelial derived relaxing factor (136–138), is an important endogenous mediator in several physiological processes in vivo. One of its most important cardiovascular actions is potent vasodilation, which results from decreased calcium in smooth muscle cells following an NO-dependent increase in cyclic-GMP. The activity of NO can be pharmacologic as well as physiologic. INO affects gas exchange by increasing blood flow in ventilated areas to improve V_A/Q_c matching. Due to its high affinity for hemoglobin, INO is active principally in ventilated lung regions with relatively little diffusion into neighboring nonventilated tissues. INO has been used in the therapy of several pediatric and adult lung diseases (see Refs. 139–141 for review). A major established therapeutic use of INO is in pulmonary hypertension of the newborn (139,142–144). INO has also been shown to reduce pulmonary artery pressures and/or pulmonary vascular resistance in a number of animal models of acute pulmonary injury (145–150), and it has been used clinically in patients with ALI/ARDS.

Clinical studies have shown that INO improves arterial oxygenation and reduces pulmonary artery pressure in adults with ARDS (72–75,77–80) and in infants or children with acute respiratory failure (151–157). The efficacy of INO has also been reported to be additive with those of PEEP (158) and patient prone positioning (159). Approximately 40–60% of patients with ALI/ARDS show some response to INO based on a 20% improvement in PaO_2/FiO_2 ratio and a reduction in pulmonary artery pressure. Michael et al. (79) studied 40 patients with ARDS, and reported improved oxygenation for the first 24 hr in those receiving INO plus conventional therapy compared to conventional therapy alone. The double-blind trial of Dellinger et al. (77) from the multicenter INO in ARDS Study Group involved 177 patients and compared three dosages of INO with placebo. Acute lung function (PaO_2, FiO_2, PaO_2/FiO_2 ratio, PEEP, mean airway pressure, and several oxygen indices) was improved in patients receiving INO (77). Treatment with INO also reduced FiO_2 over the first day and the intensity of required mechanical ventilation over the first 4 days of treatment as measured by oxygenation index. However, INO has not been shown to substantially decrease mortality in ALI/ARDS. The study by Dellinger et al. (77) reported no difference in mortality rate or number of days alive off mechanical ventilation in patients treated with INO. The authors suggested that "larger phase III studies are needed to ascertain if the acute physiologic response (to INO) can lead to altered clinical outcome." A Cochrane Library review on the use of INO for treating acute hypoxic respiratory failure identified five studies assessing over 500 patients that demonstrated no statistically significant effect of INO on mortality but indicated a transient improvement in oxygenation (160). The authors of the review called for future INO studies "to stratify patients by their primary disorder, to assess the importance of combined modalities, and to specifically evaluate clinically relevant outcomes (160)." Some patients become dependent on INO, and until recently, this agent was delivered only through mechanical ventilator circuits necessitating prolonged ventilation. Kinsella et al. (161) have recently demonstrated that INO can be effectively and safely delivered to patients by head hood or nasal cannula. These alternative delivery methods may enhance patient outcomes by allowing earlier extubation, reducing the risk of barotrauma while permitting sustained INO delivery to treat residual vascular dysfunction. Though perhaps not life-saving in and of itself, treatment with INO has clear functional benefits in many patients with acute respiratory failure, and it is an excellent candidate for use in combination therapies for ALI/ARDS.

Prostacyclin and Other Vasodilatory Prostaglandins

Although INO has received the most study as an inhaled pulmonary vasodilator in acute respiratory failure, related drugs like prostacyclin (prostaglandin I_2 or PGI_2) have also been studied (86–88,162). Prostacyclin is a microcirculatory vasodilator and inhibitor of platelet aggregation used for several indications in neonatal and adult medicine. When aerosolized, its vasodilatory action in ventilated areas should be similar to INO in improving V_A/Q_c matching without promoting systemic hypotension. Consistent with this, aerosolized prostacyclin improved acute respiratory function to the same degree as INO in several studies in patients with ARDS (86–88). Another vasodilatory prostaglandin, PGE_1, also has been shown to give improvements similar to those of INO when delivered by aerosol to patients with ARDS (163). These results suggest that aerosolized prostacyclin or similar drugs could be viable alternatives to INO in combined-modality regimens.

Selective Vasoconstrictors Used in Combination with Inhaled Vasodilators

The activity of INO and other inhaled vasodilators in treating acute respiratory failure in ALI/ARDS may further be enhanced by specific vasoconstrictors (e.g., see Refs. 63, 70, 164 for review). The mechanistic rationale for this is that selective vasoconstrictive drugs can reinforce the natural hypoxic vasoconstriction of the pulmonary vasculature in poorly ventilated regions. In principle, selective constriction of blood vessels in under-ventilated alveoli allows a larger fraction of pulmonary blood flow to be redirected to ventilated areas to improve V_A/Q_c matching. The use of vasoconstrictive agents also has the potential for negative effects, since excessive or inappropriate vasoconstriction would further impair an already compromised gas exchange process. Several clinical studies have shown that coadministration of INO and almitrine bismesylate, a selective pulmonary vasoconstrictor, can enhance the efficacy of INO in improving arterial oxygenation or reducing the level of mechanical ventilatory support in patients with ARDS (81–85,164,165). Caution is warranted with the use of almitrine because of a potential increase in pulmonary arterial pressure and right ventricular loading (166). However, promising results from the concurrent use of INO and almitrine support the concept of using rational combinations of vasoactive agents in treating ALI/ARDS. Phenylephrine has also been reported to generate improvements in acute respiratory function in ARDS patients responding to INO (167), although the mechanisms involved have been questioned (168). Other vasoconstrictive agents like norepinephrine and prostaglandin PGF_2 have not been found to exhibit additivity with INO (169,170).

B. Exogenous Surfactant Therapy for Acute Phase ALI/ARDS

The rationale for exogenous surfactant therapy in ALI/ARDS is primarily to reverse surfactant dysfunction, although surfactant deficiency is also treated by this intervention. Abnormalities in the activity and composition of lung surfactant lavaged from patients with ALI/ARDS are well documented (171–178). Basic biophysical research has demonstrated that surfactant dysfunction from multiple mechanisms can be mitigated by raising surfactant concentration (Chapter 9 plus see Refs. 47–50, 179 for review). In addition, the ability of exogenous surfactants to improve pulmonary mechanics and function has been established in multiple animal models of ALI/ARDS (47–50,179). Exogenous surfactant drugs currently approved by the FDA for use in the United States include Infasurf™ (Forest Laboratories and ONY, Inc, Amherst, NY), Survanta™ (Abbott Laboratories, Chicago, IL), and Curosurf™ (Dey Laboratories and Chiesi Farmaceutici, Parma, Italy) (47). As detailed in Chapter 15, exogenous surfactant therapy has been successful in infants and children with ALI/ARDS (17,90–94,96,180,181). However, surfactant therapy in adults with ALI/ARDS has thus far met with mixed success (89,95,97,98,182–184). Exogenous surfactant therapy in ALI/ARDS requires the use of the most active clinical surfactant drugs along with effective delivery methods such as tracheal or bronchoscopic instillation. In addition, combination therapies using exogenous surfactant with other agents like INO to optimize ventilation/perfusion matching may have even greater efficacy as described below (63,185).

C. INO Plus Exogenous Surfactant in Combination Therapy

The rationale for combination therapy with INO and exogenous surfactant is based on their complementary mechanisms of action in improving ventilation/perfusion matching and gas exchange. INO dilates the vasculature in ventilated lung units, while surfactant improves ventilation by decreasing surface tension and enhancing alveolar stability and recruitment. Exogenous surfactant therapy would theoretically increase the ventilated lung area accessible to INO, while the latter would increase the perfusion of these ventilated areas. The impact of exogenous surfactant alone is blunted if newly stabilized and recruited alveoli are not adequately perfused. Although high levels of INO could potentially cause chemical changes in exogenous surfactants, no detrimental effects on surface activity are found at the low levels of 5–20 ppm typically used clinically (186,187). Additive improvements in lung function from the simultaneous use of INO and exogenous surfactant have been demonstrated in premature surfactant-deficient lambs with congenital diaphragmatic hernia (188), as well as in animal models of ALI/ARDS (189–194). A stepwise, multiple regression analysis of neonates with hypoxic respiratory failure being weaned from INO has demonstrated that therapeutic surfactant significantly enhanced oxygenation reserve (195).

Clinical benefits have been reported from exogenous surfactant therapy and INO in a case series involving three full-term infants with severe acute respiratory failure (196). Chest radiographs demonstrated severe diffuse parenchymal disease and low lung volumes in all three infants. These patients initially had a lack of response to either INO or exogenous surfactant alone, but showed significant improvements in arterial oxygenation following treatment with the second agent, and all survived with no evidence of adverse interactions. Although this case report was small and uncontrolled, the positive results support more extensive study of combination therapy with surfactant and INO in ALI/ ARDS. This is also the conclusion of a recent review of newborns < 5 days old and ≥35 weeks gestation diagnosed with hypoxemic respiratory failure (oxygenation index >15) from meconium aspiration, sepsis/pneumonia or persistent pulmonary hypertension in the eras preceding (1993–1994) and following (1996–1997) the simultaneous availability of high-frequency oscillatory ventilation, INO, and exogenous surfactant (197). The simultaneous availability of these therapies was associated with a reduced percentage of infants requiring rescue therapy with ECMO (42.8% vs. 27.7%) that was not fully attributable to the reported efficacy of the individual agents alone (197). However, prospective controlled clinical trials on the combined use of INO and exogenous surfactant have not yet been done in pediatric or adult patients with ALI/ARDS.

D. Agents to Enhance Pulmonary Blood Flow by Reducing Intravascular Coagulation

Therapies that reduce vascular obstruction have the potential for synergy with agents like INO that dilate the pulmonary vasculature or exogenous surfactant that increases alveolar ventilation (69). Pulmonary vascular obstruction can occur in patients with ALI/ARDS from leukocyte and platelet aggregation and later fibrin deposition (198). An imbalance favoring coagulation due to increased ratios of procoagulant to fibrinolytic factors is known to occur in the lungs of animals and patients with ARDS (199).

Intravascular coagulation can reduce blood flow, decrease the functional area of the pulmonary vascular bed, and lead to increased mismatching of ventilation and perfusion. In addition, intra-alveolar coagulation may promote fibrin deposition and provide a matrix for organizing inflammatory cells and fibroblasts contributing to the later development of pulmonary fibrosis. Based on these possibilities, research has begun to address anticoagulant therapies in sepsis and sepsis-associated ARDS (for review, see Ref. 69). Administration of the anticoagulants TFPI or site-inactivated factor VIIa has been reported to protect gas exchange and compliance, reduce pulmonary edema and hypertension, and preserve renal function in a baboon model of Gram-negative sepsis (200). Systemic proinflammatory cytokine responses including production of IL-6 were also reduced by anticoagulant therapy (200). A preliminary report of a small Phase 2 clinical trial of septic patients treated with TFPI indicated reduced cytokine levels and a roughly 35% survival advantage in the ARDS subgroup in association with a measurable anticoagulant effect (100). Mortality has also been found to be significantly reduced in a large study of patients with severe sepsis treated with antithrombotic protein C (APC), a selective endogenous anticoagulant that is rapidly depleted in septic shock (99). In addition to anticoagulant activity, APC also has anti-inflammatory activity and affects endothelial cell gene expression and apoptotic profiles (201).

E. Mechanical Ventilation and Alveolar Recruitment in Acute Phase ALI/ARDS

Discussion above has focused on pharmacologic agents that improve ventilation/perfusion and could be utilized in combination therapies for ALI/ARDS. Nonpharmacologic interventions that enhance ventilation and alveolar recruitment also have the potential for additivity or synergy with drug-based therapies. For example, specific modalities or strategies of mechanical ventilation might improve the delivery and distribution of inhaled or instilled drugs either physically or by recruiting alveoli or moderating inflammation. Ventilation therapies for ALI/ARDS are detailed in Chapter 13. Several strategies of mechanical ventilation aimed at minimizing ventilator induced lung injury and/or optimizing alveolar recruitment have been shown to be beneficial in ALI/ARDS (for review see Refs. 4, 31,129,130,132,134,135). The synergy of specific ventilation methods or protocols with pharmacologic agents in lung-injury applications has not been extensively studied in basic or clinical research. However, several reports suggest that liquid ventilation may have additive benefits when used in conjunction with INO in animal models or patients with ALI/ARDS (202–208). Similarly, high-frequency oscillatory ventilation (133,209) and alveolar recruitment strategies such as PEEP (158) or patient prone positioning (80–82,208) have been reported to give additive benefits when used in conjunction with INO. Animal studies also suggest that techniques like jet ventilation and liquid ventilation have the potential to improve the pulmonary distribution and/or clinical efficacy of exogenous surfactants (210–213). In addition, the combination of partial liquid ventilation with conventional or high-frequency oscillating ventilation has also been found to be beneficial in animal studies of ALI/ARDS (214).

The goal of any clinical ventilation strategy is to maximize gas exchange while minimizing ventilator-induced lung injury. Aggressive use of mechanical ventilation causes injury from excessive stretch (volutrauma) and positive pressure (barotrauma). Low tidal volume ventilation is one important approach found to have clinical benefits in adults with ALI/ARDS. A recent ARDS Research network (ARDSnet) trial of a low volume ventilation strategy in 861 patients demonstrated reduced mortality in those ventilated with a tidal volume target of 6 mL/kg compared to 12 mL/kg (31% vs. 39.8%) (130). Subsequent analysis of patient subgroups in this study also suggested that this improved survival was independent of the initial lung injury stimulant (131). Low tidal volume ventilation is an example of the injury-reducing ventilation strategy of "permissive hypercapnia," where CO_2 retention is tolerated in order to avoid increasing ventilator tidal volume in patients with ARDS (126). Permissive hypercapnia is also utilized in neonatal intensive care units, where premature infants are thought to be particularly sensitive to mechanical stress and hyperoxia. However, permissive hypercapnia and other hypoventilation strategies have the potential for adverse effects on the cardiovascular system, cerebral blood flow, and blood brain barrier capacity. Levels of CO_2 retention that are safe for cardiovascular and neurologic function are not known precisely, and are likely to vary among patients depending on clinical condition, age, and other factors. For example, the safety and efficacy of hypoventilation strategies in neonates have had limited controlled study especially with regard to neurologic outcomes (215,216).

Aside from ventilator modes and strategies that could be incorporated in combination therapies for acute phase ALI/ARDS, another ventilation-related intervention that has been studied is patient prone positioning. Clinical trials have established that oxygenation and ventilation are enhanced by prone vs. supine positioning of patients with ARDS-related respiratory failure (see Refs. 134, 135 for review). The mechanisms responsible for improved oxygenation and ventilation are not completely understood, but one factor appears to be enhanced alveolar recruitment due to shifting the weight of the cardiac mass. The combination of INO with prone patient positioning to enhance alveolar recruitment has been shown to improve cardiopulmonary function relative to either intervention alone in ALI/ARDS (80–82,208).

The use of PEEP maintained through the respiratory cycle has also been shown to have positive effects on ALI/ARDS by stabilizing and preventing the collapse of distal airways and alveoli (see Refs. 132, 134 for review). Levels of PEEP slightly above the critical closing pressure of small airways may help to stabilize and expand the lung without inflicting undue mechanical injury. In a small study, PEEP was shown to enhance the pulmonary response to low dose INO (158). High-frequency oscillating ventilation (HFOV) also has been suggested to work effectively in combination therapy with INO. Adult patients with ARDS on HFOV were found to have a more sustained improvement in oxygenation (reduced oxygenation index) when INO was added to their therapy (133). In a study of pediatric patients with acute hypoxic respiratory failure, the combination of HFOV + INO resulted in a significantly greater increase in the ratio of PaO_2/FiO_2 compared to HFOV alone, INO alone, or conventional ventilation + INO (209). Continuing basic and clinical research is needed to define in more detail the benefits of specific ventilation modes or strategies in combination with pharmacologic agents in ALI/ARDS.

VIII. Agents Targeting Inflammation or Oxidant Injury in Early Phase ALI/ARDS

Overexuberant inflammation is generally a prominent feature of the exudative phase of ALI/ARDS. The overproduction of proinflammatory cytokines, chemokines, growth factors, and reactive oxygen/nitrogen species by activated leukocytes and resident lung cells can sometimes be more harmful than the initial stimulus causing lung injury. Increased levels of proinflammatory mediators and reactive chemical species have been found in lavage fluid, plasma, and blood cells from patients with ALI/ARDS (e.g., see Refs. 217–225). Persistent elevations of proinflammatory cytokines in BAL and plasma from patients with ALI/ARDS have also been shown to be predictive of poor clinical outcome (223–225). This provides a rationale for incorporating specific anti-inflammatory agents or antioxidants in combination therapies for ALI/ARDS to complement interventions targeting ventilation/perfusion abnormalities described in the preceding section.

In order to be effective clinically, anti-inflammatory agents and antioxidants must reduce pathological, excessive and injurious inflammation while allowing physiologic innate host defense to remain intact. This may be especially important in patients with ALI/ARDS who are at increased risk for secondary infections. Examples of inhibitory antibodies or soluble receptors for inflammatory mediators that have been studied in humans or animals with ALI/ARDS or sepsis include anti-TNFα (101–103,226), anti-IL-8 (227–229), anti-CD40L (230,231), and IL-1Ra (105,232,233). Antibodies against bacterial products like endotoxin have also been examined (234,235). In addition, pentoxifylline has been found to have anti-inflammatory properties of potential utility in ALI/ARDS and sepsis (113–117,236–242), and oxidant injury has been targeted by agents like NAC (118–120,243–248) and recombinant superoxide dismutase (57,121,122). Corticosteroids, which have broad anti-inflammatory activity, have been found to be ineffective and even potentially harmful in early exudative ALI/ARDS (for review, see Ref. 68). However, corticosteroids are discussed later for potential use in the fibroproliferative phase of lung injury.

A. Anti-TNFα Antibodies, Receptor Antagonists, or Soluble Receptors

Tumor necrosis factor-α is an early and important proinflammatory mediator of acute pulmonary injury (see Refs. 60, 249, 250 for review). TNFα not only has direct cellular actions, but also induces the production of other inflammatory mediators such as IL-1β and promotes the recruitment of activated neutrophils into the lungs. The early release of TNFα and its relatively short half-life in plasma complicates its detection in patients. Peak plasma levels of TNFα have been shown to occur 1 hr after IV administration of low dose endotoxin in human volunteers and are undetectable within 6–8 hr (251). The correlation between levels of TNFα and the development of ALI/ARDS ARDS is highest when this cytokine is measured in pulmonary edema or BAL fluid (217–219). Anti-TNFα or TNFα receptor blockade has been shown to reduce the severity of lung injury in several animal models (226,252–254). Acute benefits were also reported following the administration of monoclonal anti-TNFα antibodies to patients with ARDS or sepsis, but long-term outcomes including survival were not significantly improved (101–103). Antibodies to TNFα and receptor blockade strategies including the use of soluble IgG-conjugated TNF receptors (e.g., Enbrel) appear to be well tolerated in patients, and agents antagonizing the activity of this cytokine are potential candidates for use in combination therapies for ALI/ARDS.

B. Anti-Interleukin-8 (Anti-IL-8) Antibodies

Interleukin-8 is a potent chemoattractant cytokine (chemokine) for neutrophils, and has been studied as a marker for ALI/ARDS in high-risk patients (223,255–258). IL-8 has also been shown to affect neutrophil apoptosis (259). IL-8 levels are markedly elevated in pulmonary edema from patients with ARDS compared to lung fluid from healthy volunteers or patients with hydrostatic edema (223,255–257). High IL-8 levels in lavage also correlate with increased mortality in patients with ALI/ARDS (223), and with a high risk for development of ARDS (256). IL-8 levels in lavage do not correlate with the persistence of ARDS (258), suggesting more importance in the pathogenesis of acute disease. Early treatment with anti-IL-8 antibodies has been found to reduce lung injury and mortality in animal models of acid aspiration (227) and endotoxemia (228,229). Antibodies to IL-8 have not yet been studied in combination therapies for ALI/ARDS in basic or clinical research.

C. Anti-CD40 Ligand (Anti-CD40L)

CD40 is a 50-kD receptor once thought to be expressed only on bone marrow-derived cells, but now known also to be present on pulmonary fibroblasts (230,260–262). Fibroblast CD40 serves as an activation structure for the synthesis of proinflammatory cytokines through interactions with CD40 ligand (CD40L), which is found on T lymphocytes and mast cells. A monoclonal anti-CD40L antibody termed MR1, which disrupts the CD40–CD40L interaction, has been shown to reduce the severity of hyperoxic lung injury and radiation-induced lung injury in mice (230,231). Intraperitoneal administration of MR1 into mice either 24 hr before, or after, the start of exposure to >95% oxygen reduced epithelial cell necrosis, edema, and influx of inflammatory cells. MR1 also substantially decreased the induction of cyclo-oxygenase-2, a proinflammatory enzyme responsible for prostaglandin production (230). In radiation-induced lung injury, treatment with MR1 not only improved acute injury, but also reduced fibrosis (231). Caution is suggested, however, by a subsequent study in CD40- and CD40L-deficient mice (−/−), which failed to show improvements in oxygen-induced injury in the absence of CD40 activity (263). Anti-CD40L reagents for humans are in the testing phase by several pharmaceutical firms for diseases such as idiopathic thrombocytopenic purpura, but they have not been studied clinically in single or multiagent therapies for ALI/ARDS.

D. Pentoxifylline

The xanthine derivative pentoxifylline is a phosphodiesterase inhibitor with multiple physiological effects. Pentoxifylline has direct vasodilatory activity, and it also affects erythrocyte deformability (264,265). However, its major beneficial actions in ALI/ARDS appear to relate to its ability to raise cyclic adenosine monophosphate (cAMP) levels (266–268), inhibit free radical formation (236), and antagonize the production and actions of TNFα (113,116,117,269,270). Pentoxifylline has been shown to mitigate ALI/ARDS in multiple animal models (236–242), as well as to reduce levels of TNFα and to improve cardiopulmonary function in patients with sepsis (113–117). The pharmacology of pentoxifylline is well characterized (271), and it is safe for use in patients with ALI/ARDS (272). However, pentoxifylline and related phosphodiesterase inhibitors have not yet been evaluated in detail in ALI/ARDS, particularly as part of combination therapies.

E. *N*-Acetylcysteine

N-Acetylcysteine (NAC) is a precursor for glutathione (GSH), an antioxidant present in significant levels in the normal lung (273–275). GSH has many biological actions, ranging from oxidant protection to participation in metabolic pathways such as those involving inflammatory mediator synthesis (276). Lavage from patients with ALI/ARDS is deficient in GSH (221), and GSH levels are also below average in some pulmonary fibrotic disorders (277). NAC promotes the production of GSH by crossing readily into cells and providing cysteine, the rate limiting amino acid in GSH synthesis. NAC has been shown to increase GSH levels in red blood cells, granulocytes, and plasma from patients with ARDS (222). Increased intracellular levels of GSH reduce production of proinflammatory cytokines like TNFα and IL-1 (273,278). NAC also has direct antioxidant properties because of its thiol group, and it can scavenge reactive oxidants including hydrogen peroxide, superoxide anion, and hypochlorus acid (278).

Animal studies indicate that NAC protects against significant portions of acute pulmonary injury from hyperoxia, endotoxin, or GSH synthesis inhibition (243–248). NAC has been reported to improve respiratory function but not survival in adults with ALI/ARDS (118–120). Suter et al. (118) demonstrated an increased oxygenation index (PaO_2/FiO_2) over the first 72 hr in NAC-treated patients with ALI/ARDS compared to a placebo group, as well as a higher percentage of patients not requiring mechanical ventilation after this time (118). A double-blind, placebo-controlled study in 48 patients at five centers found that treatment with NAC or procysteine (2-oxo-4-thiazolidinecarboxylic acid, a cysteine analog, and GSH precursor) increased cardiac index and decreased the number of days of ALI without improving mortality (120). Intratracheal treatment with NAC did not improve chronic lung disease in premature infants and tended to increase airway resistance (279). It has been reported that TNFα-induced apoptosis and levels of reactive oxygen species in type II cells were reduced by procysteine but not NAC in rats chronically fed ethanol (280). However, an ARDS Network trial of procysteine for patients with ARDS was terminated early due to lack of evidence of efficacy (120). No adverse side effects have been reported from the use of NAC in patients with ALI/ARDS, consistent with the broad experience with this drug as an antidote for acetaminophen overdose. NAC is FDA-approved for oral (but not intravenous) dosing, and it has been suggested that dosage levels could be increased if necessary in clinical trials (273,278). No studies to date have investigated the utility of NAC in combination therapies for ALI/ARDS.

F. Superoxide Dismutase and Related Antioxidants

Superoxide dismutase (SOD) acts to catalyze the conversion of superoxide anion to hydrogen peroxide (275,281,282), which is subsequently converted to water by GSH peroxidase or by catalase, a tetrameric, heme-containing enzyme (275,282). SOD exists primarily in three forms: cytoplasmic SOD (Cu, Zn-containing), mitochondrial SOD (Mn-containing), and extracellular SOD (Cu-containing) (281,282). The levels of extracellular SOD are relatively high in lung and brain tissue (283,284), and it has been speculated that this form of SOD may have a particular role in pulmonary antioxidant defense (57). However, cellular forms of SODs also have important antioxidant activity. A number of studies have shown that exogenously administered antioxidant enzymes, particularly when encapsulated in lipid vesicles (liposomes) or conjugated to polyethylene glycol to prolong biological half-life and aid delivery to cells, can protect against oxidant damage and mitigate the severity of acute pulmonary injury (122,285–290). The majority of these studies have involved delivery of Cu,Zn-SOD by tracheal instillation (122,285,286,288–290), although intraperitoneal injection has also been used (287). Recombinant forms of several human SODs are available for clinical use in ALI/ARDS (57,121,122). These enzymes have not been studied in any detail in combination therapies, although instillation of SODs with exogenous surfactant has been suggested as one approach to treating acute pulmonary injury (121,291). The possibility that exogenous surfactant could be inactivated by SOD has been reported (292), but only at very high concentrations of enzymatic protein. Other workers have found no adverse interaction between exogenous surfactant and human recombinant Cu,Zn-SOD (291). In addition to SODs, several other antioxidant agents have been studied in therapeutic applications for lung injury. This includes EUK-8, a synthetic low molecular weight compound with SOD-like and catalase-like activity (293,294). Also, enteral nutrition containing eicosapentaenoic acid (EPA, fish oil), gamma-linolenic acid (GLA, borage oil), and antioxidants including Vitamins E and C have been reported to reduce days of mechanical ventilation, intensive care requirements, and extrapulmonary organ failure in patients with ARDS (295). In a subsequent subgroup analysis from this trial, it was also shown that levels of IL-8 and leukotriene B4 in bronchoalveolar lavage fluid were reduced in patients given enteral nutrition enriched in EPA and GLA (296). Additional basic and clinical research is needed to define more fully the benefits of antioxidants in ALI/ARDS, and determine the additivity or synergy of active antioxidants in combination therapies with other agents and interventions.

G. Additional Anti-inflammatory Agents or Antioxidants for Acute Phase ALI/ARDS

An ever-expanding number of pharmaceuticals are being developed that could potentially be useful in single agent or combination therapies in humans with ALI/ARDS. This multitude of potential therapeutic agents presents a challenge for efficient and effective testing and evaluation. Research on combination therapies for acute inflammatory ALI/ARDS will need to focus on those agents and interventions having the greatest individual efficacy plus a mechanistic potential for synergy. In addition, agents for priority testing in combination therapy should have low associated side effects and a minimal potential for adverse interactions. A hierarchy of investigation and assessment that integrates mechanism-based studies on agent activity and potential synergy in cells and animals with focused and rationally designed clinical trials will be necessary to define optimal combinations of agents and interventions for treating ALI/ARDS and other diseases of lung injury as emphasized at the beginning of the chapter.

IX. Agents Targeting the Fibroproliferative Phase of ALI/ARDS or Other Chronic Lung Diseases

The acute phase of ALI/ARDS is generally followed in survivors by a 1–3 week period of fibroproliferation and organization of previously deposited intra-alveolar and interstitial exudates. This fibroproliferative phase of injury has common features with many chronic lung diseases in exhibiting persistent inflammatory foci, myofibroblast proliferation, and collagen accumulation. Selected pathological aspects and biological targets in the fibroproliferative phase of ALI/ARDS are noted in Table 6. In this phase of injury, type II cells proliferate and line the alveolar wall, recovering the basement membrane and migrating over organizing intra-alveolar hyaline membranes. These type II cells can present a chronic source of proinflammatory mediators, one example of which is TNFα (297). There is also proliferation and migration of fibroblasts into intra-alveolar exudates, along with differentiation of fibroblasts into myofibroblasts. Collagen-rich extracellular matrix material is deposited in the pulmonary interstitium, and fibrosis can start to become apparent. Alveoli are lost by accumulation of connective tissue within septal walls and by dropout as collapsed alveoli become sealed by organizing fibrin and hyperplastic epithelium. Vascular and perivascular smooth muscle cell proliferation also occurs, and pulmonary vascular area is reduced leading to pulmonary hypertension. In some areas of lung, there can be complete destruction of small arteries (obliterative endarteritis). Chronic inflammatory foci rich in polymorphonuclear cells are also typically present in the lung interstitium.

The fibroproliferative phase of ALI/ARDS either slowly resolves, progresses, or remains static. Patients surviving for longer than 3–4 weeks can enter a chronic phase of disease characterized by diffuse, heterogeneous scarring with distal microcysts and airway disruption with bronchiectasis and alveolar duct fibrosis. There is remodeling of accumulated collagenous tissue, but decreasing interstitial cellularity consistent with reduced cell-mediated inflammation relative to earlier disease. The incidence of fibrosis following ARDS is noteworthy. One recent study using high-resolution computed tomography (HRCT) and lung function testing demonstrated pulmonary fibrosis in 13 of 15 patients examined 6–10 months after ARDS

Table 6 Examples of Potential Biological Targets in the Fibroproliferative/Fibrotic Phase of Lung Injury

Target	Contributing abnormalities or processes	Therapies and desired outcome(s)
Persistent (chronic) inflammation	Persistent leukocytic activation and over production of reactive oxygen/nitrogen species and proinflammatory mediators	Agents to enhance neutrophil apoptosis, decrease injury from reactive oxygen/nitrogen species, and antagonize overexuberant mediator production or responses
Fibrosis	Fibroblast proliferation and invasion, and increased interstitial matrix deposition	Agents to enhance fibroblast apoptosis, reduce matrix formation and increase matrix remodeling
Pulmonary hypertension	Microvascular thrombosis, loss of vascular cross-sectional area, and decreased pulmonary capillary blood flow	Deliver agents to reduce microvascular thrombosis and enhance regrowth of microvascular network
Hypoventilation and loss of gas exchange surface	Airway reactivity and obstruction, loss of functional respiratory airways and alveoli	Deliver agents to dilate airways, clear secretions, normalize mucin production and consistency, promote differentiation of Clara cells to ciliated bronchiolar cells, or to enhance alveolarization
Alveolar epithelial cell abnormalities	Type I cell loss and type II cell proliferation and/or alteration	Therapy to promote type II cell to type I cell differentiation, normalize type I/II cell numbers and functions, protect alveoli against further injury

See text for examples of therapies targeting several of the tabulated abnormalities in fibroproliferative phase ALI/ARDS.

(298). The extent of fibrotic pathology correlated with the severity of ARDS ($p < 0.01$) and with the duration of mechanical ventilation with peak inspiratory pressures greater than 30 mmHg ($p < 0.05$) or $>70\%$ inspired oxygen ($p < 0.01$) (298). This suggests that acute pulmonary injury impacts the development of fibrosis, and that ventilator- and oxygen-induced injury may be important factors. Even in the absence of clear fibrosis, it is common for patients recovering from ALI/ARDS to demonstrate reduced exercise tolerance and abnormalities in pulmonary function tests including diffusion capacity (299). The high incidence of fibrosis and persistent lung functional abnormalities in survivors of ALI/ARDS illustrate the importance of evaluating therapies not only for their effects on survival, but also for their ability to reduce long-term morbidity.

In contrast to therapies in the exudative phase of ALI/ARDS that are directed largely at acute respiratory failure, vascular abnormalities, surfactant dysfunction and inflammation, interventions in the fibroproliferative phase must address pathophysiological elements of remodeling, repair, and fibrosis (e.g., see Refs. 64–67, 300–302 for review). Acute issues of cardio-respiratory instability have resolved, and medical care is directed toward reducing levels of ventilatory support and supplemental oxygen. Current understanding of fibroproliferative lung injury suggests that therapeutic agents need to enhance repair (e.g., angiogenesis and alveolar secondary crest formation) while inhibiting fibroblast proliferation, differentiation, and interstitial matrix deposition. Normalizing extracellular matrix turnover is also an important goal, as is reducing persistent inflammation by removal and/or deactivation of polymorphonuclear leukocytes and monocytes recruited during acute injury (303). The necessity to include epithelial rescue in therapies for ALI/ARDS has been emphasized (67), although the detailed roles of epithelial cells in chronic lung injury remain unclear. Alveolar epithelial cells are damaged during acute injury, typically resulting in a loss of type I cells and in type II cell hyperplasia. Type II cell proliferation appears to be a protective response to acute injury, but repair eventually requires a normalization of cell numbers through differentiation to type I cells, apoptosis, or necrotic death (304). Epithelial cell mediator production and surfactant metabolism must also be normalized. Aside from its essential role in respiration, lung surfactant has important immunomodulating activity in host-defense against infection (305,306). It has also been suggested that surfactant may modulate fibroblast apoptosis and collagen production to influence the repair of lung injury (307).

Although the discussion above has emphasized fibroproliferative ALI/ARDS, many of the pathophysiological and therapy-related considerations noted are also relevant for other chronic lung diseases. Chronic lung diseases span a spectrum encompassing not only the fibroproliferative phase of ALI/ARDS, but also idiopathic pulmonary fibrosis (IPF), bronchopulmonary dysplasia (BPD) and related neonatal chronic lung disease, interstitial pneumonias (nonspecific, desquamative, lymphocytic, and hypersensitivity pneumonias), sarcoidosis, cystic fibrosis (CF), and many others (Chapters 5, 6). Mechanistic pathways and pathophysiological details are not identical in all chronic lung diseases, and therapies must acknowledge this heterogeneity. However, despite differences among chronic lung diseases and affected patient populations, many therapeutic targets and agents are broadly relevant to this group of conditions. Prospective agents for use in combination therapies for fibroproliferative ALI/ARDS come not only from research on lung injury, but also from basic and clinical studies on diseases like CF (308) and on epithelial wound healing in the skin and other organs. Some agents also come from research on primary fibrotic lung diseases like IPF, although therapeutic options for this disease are currently relatively few and ineffective (64,300,302).

A. Agents to Reduce Persistent Inflammation in Fibroproliferative Lung Injury

Persistent inflammation is characteristic of patients that progress to fibroproliferative or fibrotic lung disease following acute ALI/ARDS. Cytokine levels remain elevated in lavage, as do the numbers and activity of neutrophils and monocytes. Some anti-inflammatory agents already discussed for the acute phase of lung injury may have utility against these aspects of fibroproliferative phase pathology in combination therapies. Moreover, some anti-inflammatories like corticosteroids appear to have increased benefits in fibroproliferative lung injury compared to acute injury. During the early exudative phase of ALI/ARDS, corticosteroids appear to be ineffective and even potentially harmful in patients (107,108). In contrast, multiple studies show improved outcomes for patients with established, fibroproliferative ARDS treated with corticosteroids over a prolonged course (109–112,309–312). For example, Meduri et al. (311,312) reported that patients who had no improvement in lung injury scores and were deemed nonresponders at day 7 of acute ALI/ARDS had reduced inflammation and significant improvements in lung injury and survival following prolonged corticosteroid treatment. The use of inhaled rather than systemic corticosteroids to attempt to minimize drug-associated toxicity is also under investigation. One observation that has reduced enthusiasm for using glucocorticoids to treat chronic lung injury, particularly in premature infants, is an associated inhibition of lung growth including a reduced formation of secondary alveolar septal crests. Effective repair of lung injury and chronic lung disease in adults may also require regeneration of alveolar septal structure. Studies in rodents suggest that retinoic acid can enhance alveolar development and help prevent dexamethasone-induced or genetic deficits in alveolar septation (313–315). This suggests that combination therapy with glucocorticoids to reduce inflammation, plus retinoic acid to enhance secondary alveolar septation, might have synergistic effects. Rats with hyperoxic lung injury have improved survival if treated with a combination of retinoic acid and dexamethasone (316), although the applicability of these findings in humans remains to be tested. Treatment of premature infants with Vitamin A (retinol) can reduce the risk for developing BPD (317), but combination therapy with corticosteroids has not been well studied.

A variety of anti-inflammatory compounds other than corticosteroids may be useful in treating fibroproliferative lung injury, but little direct clinical testing of potential agents has been done. A case series of five premature infants with BPD has suggested reduced oxygen requirements, improved compliance, and reduced airway resistance following treatment with nebulized pentoxifylline (318). This uncontrolled clinical experience supports further investigations with phosphodiesterase inhibitors like pentoxifylline in fibrotic lung disease. As described earlier, this methlyxanthine has multiple biological activities including the ability to inhibit TNFα signal transduction. Pentoxifylline in vitro can reduce fibroblast proliferation, myofibroblastic differentiation, extracellular matrix synthesis, and smooth muscle cell migration (319,320). Unfortunately, the study of methylxanthines in animal models can be complicated by species-specific differences in active metabolites, increasing the necessity for direct clinical assessments.

B. Agents to Re-establish Normal Matrix Deposition and Turnover in Fibroproliferative Lung Injury

Myofibroblast and endothelial cell invasion of the provisional matrix formed by protein exudation and coagulation initiates a "fibrosing alveolitis" and fibrotic interstitial foci in injured lungs. Fibroblast activation, migration, proliferation, and collagen production in lung injury is augmented by cytokines and growth factors including transforming growth factor beta (TGFβ), platelet derived growth factor (PDGF), and TNFα. Agents under consideration to inhibit fibroblast-dependent fibrosis include antagonists to PDGF such as PDGF tyrosine kinase inhibitors, relaxin, and lovastatin (321–323). Experimental models, and limited studies in humans, suggest that combination therapy with inhibitors of TGFβ (anti-TGFβ antibodies or soluble TGFβ receptors), the amino acid taurine, and the vitamin niacin, may reduce interstitial lung fibrosis (302). Other biologics, such as anti-CD44 antibody, which reacts with the cell-surface matrix receptor located on invading fibroblasts, may also promote apoptosis and resolution of fibroproliferation (324). Additional agents with the potential to reduce fibroblast activity and restrict matrix formation include cytotoxic drugs like cyclophosphamide (325) or azothioprine (326), as well as interferon gamma and beta, colchicine, pirfenidone, and D-pencillamine (see Refs. 64,300, 302 for review). Despite the importance of fibroblasts in chronic lung injury, it is not clear that inhibition of these cells alone will be effective in mitigating or reversing disease. Moreover, some fibroblast activity and matrix deposition likely protects pulmonary architecture and enhances remodeling and repair. Clinical studies on cytotoxic drugs, with or without anti-inflammatory corticosteroids, suggest limited or no effects on survival in patients with chronic lung disease. A prospective study of 56 patients with IPF compared treatment with prednisone or colchicine alone, to colchicine plus prednisone, and colchicine plus prednisone, and penicillamine (327). Almost 60% of the patients died within 5 years with no difference among treatment groups (327).

Two groups of enzymes that appear to be important in fibroproliferative lung injury are the matrix metalloproteinases (MMPs) and their negative regulators, the tissue inhibitors of metalloproteinases (TIMPs). These enzymes are thought to participate in establishing a balanced distribution of matrix to support normal pulmonary structure and function, as opposed to the relatively disorganized interstitial network that constitutes scarring or fibrosis in injured lungs. The evidence suggests that an imbalance between the activities of MMPs and TIMPs in injured lungs may promote abnormal composition, distribution or organization of matrix proteins, and contribute to fibrosis. MMPs including collagenases and gelatinases have been found to be reduced in lavage from patients with ARDS and in the pulmonary interstitium of patients with IPF, while TIMPs were increased especially in fibrotic loci (328). On the other hand, increased MMP activity has been associated with enhanced fibrosis in animal models (329). Although MMPs and TIMPs are clearly relevant for fibroproliferative lung injury, a better basic understanding of the regulation and balance of these enzymes through basic research in healthy and injured lungs is needed to allow the development of specific related agents for use in single or multiagent therapies.

C. Agents to Improve Perfusion or Hypertension in Fibroproliferative Lung Injury

Pulmonary hypertension induced by arterial muscularization and fibrous narrowing or replacement of the microcirculation frequently contributes to the morbidity and mortality of chronic lung injury and disease. Perfusion studies of lungs following ALI/ARDS demonstrate pruning of the vascular bed, arterial tortuosity, and potential arterial to venous anastomoses. Chronic hypoxia and reflexive vasoconstriction also occur and contribute to increased pulmonary vascular resistance. A number of agents to improve pulmonary blood flow are under study in basic research, including endothelin (ET-1) receptor antagonists, prostaglandin derivatives, and anticoagulants that could potentially be combined with or replace the conventional use of oxygen and vasodilating agents to reduce pulmonary vascular resistance (330,331). However, such agents have not received study as part of combination therapies for the acute or chronic phases of ALI/ARDS or other pulmonary diseases.

X. Summary

Combination therapies that target different aspects of the pathophysiology of acute or chronic lung injury have the potential for additive or synergistic clinical benefits. However, developing optimal therapies of this type is difficult and challenging, and requires detailed research assessments. Several important considerations impact the design, implementation, and analysis of randomized, blinded, controlled clinical trials testing combination therapies for lung injury. These include the range of possible positive and negative clinical responses to combination therapies, the necessity for substantial numbers of patients to obtain the statistical power for multiple comparisons, the need for multicenter trial networks, plus a variety of study design issues relating to patient enrollment, stratification, informed consent, entry and exclusion criteria, outcome variable definitions, treatment comparisons including optimal standard therapy, alternative treatment availability, and physician equipoise. Effective multicenter consortia have been formed and utilized to evaluate combination therapies in the field of oncology, and such consortia also exist for clinical trials on ALI/ARDS, sepsis, and other conditions involving lung injury and respiratory failure.

Because of the large number of potential agents and interventions, as well as the cost, complexity, and limited resolving power of clinical trials in patients with severe lung injury, interactive basic research on combination therapies is particularly important. A rational approach that integrates findings on the mechanistic activity and efficacy of agents in basic research to facilitate the design, implementation, and analysis of focused clinical trials is crucial for defining optimal combination therapies for lung injury in infants, children, and adults. A variety of individual therapeutic agents and interventions have been studied in patients with ALI/ARDS or sepsis (e.g., Chapters 13–17). Used in isolation, these agents and interventions address only limited aspects of the complex, multifaceted pathophysiology of lung injury. Many of these individual therapies have failed to have a substantial impact in reducing mortality or improving other long-term outcomes in patients with ALI/ARDS, but they might have greater efficacy when incorporated in combination therapies based on mechanistic understanding.

One important combination therapy approach for acute exudative ALI/ARDS involves utilizing complementary agents to improve the matching of ventilation and perfusion in injured lungs. This includes the use of INO or inhaled prostacyclin (PGI_2) to dilate vessels and increase blood flow to ventilated alveoli in combination with exogenous surfactant therapy to increase alveolar ventilation and stability. Concurrent therapy with INO and exogenous surfactant has been shown to be safe and effective in animal models and in a small case study involving term infants with acute respiratory failure. Additional vascular agents that might further improve ventilation/perfusion matching in combination with INO and/or exogenous surfactant are also available, including selective vasoconstrictors like almitrine bismesylate or antithrombotic agents such as TFPI or antithrombotic protein C (APC). Specific anti-inflammatory antibodies and receptor antagonists (e.g., anti-TNFα, anti-IL-8, anti-CD40L, or IL-1Ra), antioxidants (e.g., NAC, SOD), or anti-inflammatories (e.g., pentoxifylline) could also be utilized in combination therapies for acute exudative ALI/ARDS. Various modes and strategies of mechanical ventilation that reduce ventilator-induced lung injury or increase alveolar recruitment have also been shown to be beneficial in patients with acute respiratory failure and ALI/ARDS, and could be incorporated in combination therapies. Agents targeting the later fibroproliferative phase of ALI/ARDS or other chronic pulmonary diseases are less numerous, although several substances that could potentially mitigate persistent inflammation, moderate matrix deposition and turnover, or improve perfusion during chronic injury are currently under study. In addition, new agents targeting these and other aspects of lung injury pathophysiology continue to be identified in on-going research. The additivity or synergy of the majority of the agents and interventions discussed in this chapter for possible use in combination therapies has not yet received detailed comprehensive evaluations in basic and clinical research. The relatively limited efficacy of many existing individual therapies for acute and chronic lung injury makes combination therapy approaches an important area for future study.

Acknowledgments

The authors gratefully acknowledge the support of grants HL-63039 (G.S.P.), HL-03493 (C.T.D.), P30 ES-01247 (J.N.F.), HL-71659 (J.N.F., R.H.N., G.S.P.), and HL-56176 (R.H.N.) from the National Institutes of Health, as well as EPA Airborne Particulate Matter Center grant R827354 (J.N.F.). The authors would also like to thank Dr. G.J. D'Angio for his helpful advice on clinical evaluations of multimodal therapy based on experience in cooperative pediatric oncology.

References

1. Chu J, Clements JA, Cotton EK, Klaus MH, Sweet AY, Tooley WH, Bradley BL, Brandorff LC. Neonatal pulmonary ischemia. I. Clinical and physiological studies. Pediatrics 1967; 40(suppl):709–782.

2.   Chu J, Clements JA, Cotton EK, Klaus MH, Sweet AY, Thomas MA, Tooley WH. The pulmonary hypoperfusion syndrome. Pediatrics 1965; 35:733–742.

3.   Robillard E, Alarie Y, Dagenais-Perusse P, Baril E, Guilbeault A. Microaerosol administration of synthetic β,γ-dipalmitoyl-l-α-lecithin in the respiratory distress syndrome: a preliminary report. Can Med Assoc J 1964; 90:55–57.

4.   Steinbrook R. How best to ventilate? Trial design and patient safety in studies of the acute respiratory distress syndrome. N Engl J Med 2003; 348: 1393–1401.

5.   Wood KA, Huang D, Angus DC. Improving clinical trial design in acute lung injury. Crit Care Med 2003; 31(4 suppl):S305–S311.

6.   Cohen J, Guyatt G, Bernard GR, Calandra T, Cook D, Elbourne D, Marshall J, Nunn A, Opal S. New strategies for clinical trials in patients with sepsis and septic shock. Crit Care Med 2001; 29:880–886.

7.   Ungerleider RS, Ellenberg SS, Berg SL. Cancer clinical trials: design, conduct, analysis, and reporting. In: Pizzo PA, Poplack DG, eds. Principles Practice of Pediatric Oncology. 4th ed. Philadelphia: Lippincott Williams & Wilkins, 2002:465–488.

8.   Califf RM, DeMets DL. Principles from clinical trials relevant to clinical practice: Part I. Circulation 2002; 106:1015–1021.

9.   Pea F, Furlanut M. Pharmacokinetic aspects of treating infections in the intensive care unit: focus on drug interactions. Clin Pharmacokinet 2001; 40:833–868.

10. Silverman WA. Memories of the 1953–54 oxygen trial and its aftermath. The failure of success. Control Clin Trials 1991; 12:355–358.

11. Jobe AH, Ikegami M. Prevention of bronchopulmonarydysplasia. Curr Opin Pediatr 2001; 13:124–129.

12. Bolt RJ, van Weissenbruch MM, Lafeber HN, Delemarre-van de Waal HA. Glucocorticoids and lung development in the fetus and preterm infant. Pediatr Pulmonol 2001; 32:76–91.

13. O'Rourke PP, Crone RK, Vacanti JP, Ware JH, Lillehei CW, Parad RB, Epstein MF. Extracorporeal membrane oxygenation and conventional medical therapy in neonates with persistent pulmonary hypertension of the newborn: a prospective randomized study. Pediatrics 1989; 84:957–963.

14. Bartlett RH, Andrews AF, Toomasian JM, Haiduc NJ, Gazzaniga AB. Extracorporeal membrane oxygenation for newborn respiratory failure: forty-five cases. Surgery 1982; 92:425–433.

15. Bartlett RH, Gazzaniga AB, Jefferies MR, Huxtable RF, Haiduc NJ, Fong SW. Extracorporeal membrane oxygenation (ECMO) cardiopulmonary support in infancy. Trans Am Soc Artif Intern Organs 1976; 22:80–93.

16. UK Collaborative ECMO Trial Group. UK collaborative randomised trial of neonatal extracorporeal membrane oxygenation. Lancet 1996; 348:75–82.

17. Lotze A, Mitchell BR, Bulas DI, Zola EM, Shalwitz RA, Gunkel JH. Multicenter study of surfactant (beractant) use in the treatment of term infants with severe respiratory failure. J Pediatr 1998; 132:40–47.

18. Zhang B, Schmidt B. Do we measure the right end points? A systematic review of primary outcomes in recent neonatal randomized clinical trials. J Pediatr 2001; 138:76–80.

19. Davidson D, Barefield ES, Kattwinkel J, Dudell G, Damask M, Straube R, Rhines J, Chang CT. Inhaled nitric oxide for the early treatment of persistent pulmonary hypertension of the term newborn: a randomized, double-masked, placebo-controlled, dose–response, multicenter study. Pediatrics 1998; 101: 325–334.

20. Neonatal Inhaled Nitric Oxide Study Group (NINOS). Inhaled nitric oxide and hypoxic respiratory failure in infants with congenital diaphragmatic hernia. Pediatrics 1997; 99:838–845.

21. Clark RH, Kueser TJ, Walker MW, Southgate WM, Huckaby JL, Perez JA, Roy BJ, Keszler M, Kinsella JP. Low-dose nitric oxide therapy for persistent pulmonary hypertension of the newborn. Clinical Inhaled Nitric Oxide Research Group. N Engl J Med 2000; 342(7):469–474.

22. Davidson TA, Caldwell ES, Curtis JR, Hudson LD, Steinberg KP. Reduced quality of life in survivors of acute respiratory distress syndrome compared with critically ill control patients. JAMA 1999; 281:354–360.

23. Bernard GR, Artigas A, Brigham KL, Carlet J, Falke K, Hudson L, Lamy M, Legall JR, Morris A, Spragg R. The American-European Consensus Conference on ARDS: definitions, mechanisms, relevant outcomes, and clinical trial coordination. Am J Respir Crit Care Med 1994; 149:818–824.

24. Murray JF, Matthay MA, Luce JM, Flick MR. An expanded definition of the adult respiratory distress syndrome. Am Rev Respir Dis 1988; 138:720–723.

25. American College of Chest Physicians Society of Critical Care Medicine Consensus Conference Committee. Definitions for sepsis and organ failure and guidelines for the use of innovative therapies for sepsis. Crit Care Med 1992; 20:864–874.

26. Krafft P, Fridrich P, Pernerstorfer T, Fitzgerald RD, Koc D, Schneider B, Hammerle AF, Steltzer H. The acute respiratory distress syndrome; definitions, severity, and clinical outcome. An analysis of 101 clinical investigations. Intensive Care Med 1996; 22:519–529.

27. Hyers TM. Prediction of survival and mortality in patients with the adult respiratory distress syndrome. New Horizons 1993; 1:466–470.

28. Doyle RL, Szaflarski N, Modin GW, Wiener-Kronish JP, Matthay MA. Identification of patients with acute lung injury: predictors of mortality. Am J Respir Crit Care Med 1995; 152:1818–1824.

29. Milberg JA, Davis DR, Steinberg KP, Hudson LD. Improved survival of patients with acute respiratory distress syndrome. JAMA 1995; 273:306–309.

30. Ely EW, Wheeler AP, Thompson BT, Ancukiewicz M, Steinberg KP, Bernard GR. Recovery rate and prognosis in older persons who develop acute lung injury and the acute respiratory distress syndrome. Ann Intern Med 2002; 136:25–36.

31. Ware LB, Matthay MA. The acute respiratory distress syndrome. N Engl J Med 2000; 342:1334–1348.

32. Villar J, Slutsky AS. The incidence of the adult respiratory distress syndrome. Am Rev Respir Dis 1989; 140:814–816.

33. Hudson LD, Milberg JA, Anardi D, Maunder RJ. Clinical risks for development of the acute respiratory distress syndrome. Am J Respir Crit Care Med 1995; 151:293–301.

34. Goss CH, Brower RG, Hudson LD, Rubenfeld GD. Incidence of acute lung injury in the United States. Crit Care Med 2003; 31(6):1607–1611.

35. Rubenfeld GD. Epidemiology of acute lung injury. Crit Care Med 2003; 31(suppl 4):S276–S284.

36. Moss M, Mannino DM. Race and gender differences in acute respiratory distress syndrome deaths in the United States: an analysis of multiple-cause mortality data (1979–1996). Crit Care Med 2002; 30(8):1679–1685.

37. Abel SJ, Finney SJ, Brett SJ, Keogh BF, Morgan CJ, Evans TW. Reduced mortality in association with the acute respiratory distress syndrome (ARDS). Thorax 1998; 53(4):292–294.

38. Baue AE, Durham R, Faist E. Systemic inflammatory response syndrome (SIRS), multiple organ dysfunction (MODS), multiple organ failure (MOF): are we winning the battle?Shock 1998; 10:79–89.

39. Karima R, Matsumoto S, Higashi H, Matsushima K. The molecular pathogenesis of endotoxin shock and organ failure. Mol Med Today 1999; 5:123–132.

40. Kumar V, Cotran RS, Robbins SL. Basic Pathology. 6th ed. Philadelphia: WB Saunders, 1997.

41. Fauci AS, Braunwald E, Isselbacher KJ, Martin JB, Kasper DL, Hauser SL, Longo DL, eds. Harrison's Principles of Internal Medicine. 14th ed. New York: McGraw Hill, 1998.

42. Hall JB, Schmidt GA, Wood LDH. Principles of Critical Care. 2nd ed. New York: McGraw Hill, 1998.

43. Johnson MD, Widdicombe JH, Allen L, Barbry P, Dobbs LG. Alveolar epithelial type I cells contain transport proteins and transport sodium, supporting an active role for type I cells in regulation of lung liquid homeostasis. Proc Natl Acad Sci USA 2002; 99:1966–1971.

44. Matthay MA, Wiener-Kronish JP. Intact epithelial barrier function is critical for the resolution of alveolar edema in humans. Am Rev Respir Dis 1990; 142:1250–1257.

45. Sartori C, Matthay MA, Scherrer U. Transepithelial sodium and water transport in the lung. Major player and novel therapeutic target in pulmonary edema. Adv Exp Med Biol 2001; 502:315–338.

46. Matthay MA, Fukuda N, Frank J, Kallet R, Daniel B, Sakuma T. Alveolar epithelial barrier. Role in lung fluid balance in clinical lung injury. Clin Chest Med 2000; 21:477–490.

47. Notter RH. Lung surfactants: Basic Science and Clinical Applications. New York: Marcel Dekker Inc, 2000.

48. Notter RH, Wang Z. Pulmonary surfactant: physical chemistry, physiology and replacement. Rev Chem Eng 1997; 13:1–118.

49. Lewis JF, Jobe AH. Surfactant and the adult respiratory distress syndrome. Am Rev Respir Dis 1993; 147:218–233.

50. Seeger W, Günther A, Walmrath HD, Grimminger F, Lasch HG. Alveolar surfactant and adult respiratory distress syndrome. Pathogenic role and therapeutic prospects. Clin Invest 1993; 71:177–190.

51. Pryhuber GS, Bachurski C, Hirsch R, Bacon A, Whitsett JA. Tumor necrosis factor-alpha decreases surfactant protein B mRNA in murine lung. Am J Physiol 1996; 270:L714–L721.

52. Bachurski CJ, Pryhuber GS, Glasser SW, Kelly SE, Whitsett JA. Tumor necrosis factor-alpha inhibits surfactant protein C gene transcription. J Biol Chem 1995; 270:19402–19407.

53. Artigas A, Bernard GR, Carlet J, Dreyfuss D, Gattinoni L, Hudson L, Lamy M, Marini JJ, Matthay MA, Pinsky MR, Spragg R, Suter PM, and (Consensus Committee). The American-European consensus conference on ARDS, Part 2: ventilatory, pharmacologic, supportive therapy, study design strategies and issues related to recovery and remodeling. Intensive Care Med 1998; 24:378–398.

54. Temmesfeld-Wollbruck B, Walmrath D, Grimminger F, Seeger W. Prevention and therapy of the adult respiratory distress syndrome. Lung 1995; 173:139–164.

55. Kollef MH, Schuster DP. The acute respiratory distress syndrome. N Engl J Med 1995; 332:27–37.

56. Hudson LD. New therapies for ARDS. Chest 1995; 108(suppl):79S–91S.

57. Fulkerson WJ, Macintyre N, Stamler J, Crapo JD. Pathogenesis and treatment of the adult respiratory distress syndrome. Arch Intern Med 1996; 156:29–38.

58. Paulson T, Spear R, Peterson B. New concepts in the treatment of children with acute respiratory failure. J Pediatr 1995; 127:163–175.

59. Ring J, Stidham G. Novel therapies for acute respiratory failure. Pediatr Clin North Am 1994; 41:1325–1363.

60. Sessler C, Bloomfield G, Fowler A. Current concepts of sepsis and acute lung injury. Clin Chest Med 1996; 17:213–235.

61. Weikert LF, Bernard GR. Pharmacology of sepsis. Clin Chest Med 1996; 17:289–305.

62. Luce JM. Acute lung injury and the acute respiratory distress syndrome. Crit Care Med 1998; 26.369–376.

63. Notter RH, Apostolakos M, Holm BA, Willson D, Wang Z, Finkelstein JN, Hyde RW. Surfactant therapy and its potential use with other agents in term infants, children and adults with acute lung injury. Perspect Neonatol 2000; 1(4):4–20.

64. Lasky JA, Ortiz LA. Antifibrotic therapy for the treatment of pulmonary fibrosis. Am J Med Sci 2001; 322:213–221.

65. Zhang K, Phan SH. Cytokines and pulmonary fibrosis. Biol Signals 1996; 5:232–239.

66. Ward PA, Hunninghake GW. Lung inflammation and fibrosis. Am J Respir Crit Care Med 1998; 157(suppl):S123–S129.

67. Berthiaume Y, Lesur O, Dagenais A. Treatment of adult respiratory distress syndrome: plea for rescue therapy of the alveolar epithelium. Thorax 1999; 54:150–160.

68. Thompson BT. Glucocorticoids and acute lung injury. Crit Care Med 2003; 31(suppl 4):S253–S257.

69. Laterre PF, Wittebole X, Dhainaut JF. Anticoagulant therapy in acute lung injury. Crit Care Med 2003; 31(suppl):S329–S336.

70. Kaisers U, Busch T, Deja M, Donaubauer B, Falke KJ. Selective pulmonary vasodilation in acute respiratory distress syndrome. Crit Care Med 2003; 31(suppl):S337–S342.

71. Knaus WA, Harrell FE, Fisher CJ, Wagner DP, Opal SM, Sadoff JC, Draper EA, Walawander CA, Conboy K, Grasela TM. The clinical evaluation of new drugs for sepsis: a prospective study design based on survival analysis. JAMA 1993; 270:1233–1241.

72. Rossaint R, Falke KJ, Lopez F, Slama K, Pison U, Zapol W. Inhaled nitric oxide for the acute respiratory distress syndrome. N Engl J Med 1993; 328:399–405.

73. Gerlach H, Rossaint R, Pappert D, Falke KJ. Time-course and dose-response of nitric oxide inhalation for systemic oxygenation and pulmonary hypertension in patients with adult respiratory distress syndrome. Eur J Clin Invest 1993; 23:499–502.

74. Young JD, Brampton WJ, Knighton JD, Finfer SR. Inhaled nitric oxide in acute respiratory failure in adults. Br J Anaesth 1994; 73:499–502.

75. Rossaint R, Gerlach H, Schmidt-Ruhnke H, Pappert D, Lewandowski K, Steudel W, Falke K. Efficacy of inhaled nitric oxide in ARDS. Chest 1995; 107:1107–1115.

76. Fierobe L, Brunet F, Dhainaut J-F, Monchi M, Belghith M, Mira J-P, Dallava-Santucci J, Dinh-Xuan A. Effect of inhaled nitric oxide on right ventricular function in adult respiratory distress syndrome. Am J Respir Crit Care Med 1995; 151:1414–1419.

77. Dellinger RP, Zimmerman JL, Taylor RW, Straube RC, Hauser DL, Criner GJ, Davis K, Hyers TM, Papadakos P, and (and INO in ARDS Study Group). Effects of inhaled nitric oxide in patients with acute respiratory distress syndrome: results of a randomized phase II trial. Crit Care Med 1998; 26:15–23.

78. Troncy E, Collet JP, Shapiro S, Guimond J-G, Blair L, Ducruet T, Francceur M, Charbonneau M, Blaise G. Inhaled nitric oxide in acute respiratory distress syndrome. A pilot randomized controlled study. Am J Respir Crit Care Med 1998; 157:1483–1488.

79. Michael JR, Barton RG, Saffle JR, Mone M, Markewitz BA, Hillier K, Elstad MR, Campbell EJ, Troyer BE, Whatley RE, Liou TG, Samuelson WM, Carveth HJ, Hinson DM, Morris SE, Davis BL, Day RW. Inhaled nitric oxide versus conventional therapy: effect on oxygenation in ARDS. Am J Respir Crit Care Med 1998; 157:1372–1380.

80. Papazian L, Bregeon F, Gaillat F, Thirion X, Gainnier M, Gregoire R, Saux P, Gouin F, Jammes Y, Auffray J-P. Respective and combined effect of prone position and inhaled nitric oxide in patients with acute respiratory distress syndrome. Am J Respir Crit Care Med 1998; 157:580–585.

81. Jolliet P, Bulpa P, Ritz M, Ricou B, Lopez J, Chevrolet J-C. Additive beneficial effects of the prone position, nitric oxide, and almitrine bismesylate on gas exchange and oxygen transport in acute respiratory distress syndrome. Crit Care Med 1997; 25:786–794.

82. Gillart T, Bazin JE, Cosserant B, Guelon D, Aigouy L, Mansoor O, Schoeffler P. Combined nitric oxide, prone positioning and almitrine infusion improve oxygenation in servere ARDS. Can J Anesth 1998; 45:402–409.

83. Payen D, Muret J, Beloucif S, Gatecel C, Kermarrec N, Guinard N, Mateo J. Inhaled nitric oxide, almitrine infusion, or their coadministration as a

treatment of severe hypoxemic focal lung lesions. Anesthesiology 1998; 89: 1158–1165.

84. Wysocki M, Roupie E, Langeron O, Liu N, Herman B, Lemaire F, Brochard L. Additive effect on gas exchange of inhaled nitric oxide and intravenous almitrine bismesylate in the adult respiratory distress syndrome. Intensive Care Med 1994; 20:254–259.

85. Lu Q, Mourgeon E, Law-Koune J, Roche S, Vezinet C, Abdennour L, Vicaut E, Puybasset L, Diaby M, Coriat P, Rouby J. Dose–response curves of inhaled nitric oxide with and without intravenous almitrine in nitric oxide-responding patients with acute respiratory distress syndrome. Anesthesiology 1995; 83:929–943.

86. Zwissler B, Gregor K, Habler O, Kleen M, Merkel M, Haller M, Brigel J, Welte M, Peter K. Inhaled prostacyclin (PGI_2) versus inhaled nitric oxide in adult respiratory distress syndrome. Am J Respir Crit Care Med 1996; 154:1671–1677.

87. Walmrath D, Schneider T, Schermuly R, Olschewski H, Grimminger F, Seeger W. Direct comparison of inhaled nitric oxide and aerosolized prostacyclin in acute respiratory distress syndrome. Am J Respir Crit Care Med 1996; 153:991–996.

88. Pappert D, Busch T, Gerlach H, Lewandowski K, Radermacher P, Rossaint R. Aerosolized prostacyclin versus inhaled nitric oxide in children with severe acute respiratory distress syndrome. Anesthesiology 1995; 82:1507–1511.

89. Spragg R, Gilliard N, Richman P, Smith R, Hite R, Pappert D, Robertson B, Curstedt T, Strayer D. Acute effects of a single dose of porcine surfactant on patients with the adult respiratory distress syndrome. Chest 1994; 105: 195–202.

90. Khammash H, Perlman M, Wojtulewicz J, Dunn M. Surfactant therapy in full-term neonates with severe respiratory failure. Pediatrics 1993; 92: 135–139.

91. Lotze A, Knight GR, Martin GR, Bulas DI, Hull WM, O'Donnell RM, Whitsett JA, Short BL. Improved pulmonary outcome after exogenous surfactant therapy for respiratory failure in term infants requiring extracorporeal membrane oxygenation. J Pediatr 1993; 122:261–268.

92. Auten RL, Notter RH, Kendig JW, Davis JM, Shapiro DL. Surfactant treatment of full-term newborns with respiratory failure. Pediatrics 1991; 87: 101–107.

93. Willson DF, Jiao JH, Bauman LA, Zaritsky A, Craft H, Dockery K, Conrad D, Dalton H. Calf lung surfactant extract in acute hypoxemic respiratory failure in children. Crit Care Med 1996; 24:1316–1322.

94. Findlay RD, Taeusch HW, Walther FJ. Surfactant replacement therapy for meconium aspiration syndrome. Pediatrics 1996; 97:48–52.

95. Gregory TJ, Steinberg KP, Spragg R, Gadek JE, Hyers TM, Longmere WJ, Moxley MA, Guang-Zuan CAI, Hite RD, Smith RM, Hudson LD, Crim C, Newton P, Mitchell BR, Gold AJ. Bovine surfactant therapy for patients with acute respiratory distress syndrome. Am J Respir Crit Care Med 1997; 155:109–131.

96. Willson DF, Bauman LA, Zaritsky A, Dockery K, James RL, Stat M, Conrad D, Craft H, Novotny WE, Egan EA, Dalton H. Instillation of calf lung surfactant extract (calfactant) is beneficial in pediatric acute hypoxemic respiratory failure. Crit Care Med 1999; 27:188–195.

97. Walmrath D, Gunther A, Ghofrani HA, Schermuly R, Schnedier T, Grimminger F, Seeger W. Bronchoscopic surfactant administration in patients with severe adult respiratory distress syndrome and sepsis. Am J Respir Crit Care Med 1996; 154:57–62.

98. Walmrath D, Grimminger F, Pappert D, Knothe C, Obertacke U, Benzing A, Gunther A, Schmehl T, Leuchte H, Seeger W. Bronchoscopic administration of bovine natural surfactant in ARDS and septic shock: impact on gas exchange and haemodynamics. Eur Respir J 2002; 19:805–810.

99. Bernard GR, Vincent JL, Laterre PF, LaRosa SP, Dhainaut JF, Lopez-Rodriguez A, Steingrub JS, Garber GE, Helterbrand JD, Ely EW, Fisher CJ Jr. Efficacy and safety of recombinant human activated protein C for severe sepsis. N Engl J Med 2001; 344:699–709.

100. Idell S. Anticoagulants for acute respiratory distress syndrome: can they work? Am J Respir Crit Care Med 2001; 164:517–520.

101. Abraham E, Wunderink R, Silverman H, Perl TM, Nasraway S, Levy H, Bone R, Wenzel RP, Balk R, Alfred R, Pennington JE, Wherry JC. Efficacy and safety of monoclonal antibody to human tissue necrosis factor alpha in patients with sepsis syndrome: a randomized, controlled, double-blind, multicenter clinical trial. JAMA 1995; 273:934–941.

102. Abraham E, Anzueto A, Gutierrez G, Tessler S, San Pedro G, Wunderink R, Dal Nogare A, Nasraway S, Berman S, Cooney R, Levy H, Baughman R, Rumbak M, Light RB, Poole L, Allred R, Constant J, Pennington J, Porter S. Double-blind randomized controlled trial of monoclonal antibody to human tumour necrosis factor in treatment of septic shock. Lancet 1998; 351:929–933.

103. Cohen J, Carlet J. INTERSEPT: an international, multicenter, placebo controlled trial of monclonal antibody to human tumor necrosis factor-alpha in patients with sepsis. Crit Care Med 1996; 24:1431–1440.

104. Tracey K, Lowry S, Cerami A. Cachectin/TNF-alpha in septic shock and septic adult respiratory distress syndrome. Am Rev Respir Dis 1988; 138:1377–1379.

105. Fisher CJ, Slotman GJ, Opal SM, Pribble JP, Bone RC, Emmanuel G, Ng D, Bloedow DC, Catalano MA. Initial evaluation of human recombinant interleukin-1 receptor antagonist in the treatment of sepsis syndrome: a randomized open-label, placebo-controlled multicenter study. Crit Care Med 1994; 22:12–21.

106. Fisher CJ, Dhainaut JFA, Opal SM, Pribble JP, Balk RA, Slotman GJ, Iberti TJ, Rackow EC, Shapiro MJ, Greenman RL. Recombinant human IL-1 receptor antagonist in the treatment of patients with sepsis syndrome. Results from a randomized, double blind, placebo-controlled trial. Phase III rhIL–1ra sepsis syndrome study group. JAMA 1994; 271:1836–1843.

107. Bernard GR, Luce JM, Sprung CL, Rinaldo JE, Tate RM, Sibbald WJ, Kariman K, Higgins S, Bradley R, Metz CA, Harris TR, Brigham KL. High

dose corticosteroids in patients with the adult respiratory distress syndrome. N Engl J Med 1987; 317:1565–1570.

108. Luce JM, Montgomery AB, Marks JD, Turner J, Metz CA, Murray JF. Ineffectiveness of high-dose methylprednisone in preventing parenchymal lung injury and improving mortality in patients with septic shock. Am Rev Respir Dis 1988; 138:62–68.

109. Keel JB, Hauser M, Stocker R, Bauman PC, Speich R. Established acute respiratory distress syndrome: benefit of corticosteroid rescue therapy. Respiration 1998; 65:258–264.

110. Hooper RG, Kearl RA. Established adult respiratory distress syndrome successfully treated with corticosteroids. South Med J 1996; 89:359–364.

111. Biffl WL, Moore FA, Moore EE, Haenel JB, McIntyre RC, Burch JM. Are corticosteroids salvage therapy for refractory acute respiratory distress syndrome? Am J Surg 1995; 170:591–595.

112. Meduri GU, Headley AS, Golden E, Carson SJ, Umberger RA, Kelso T, Tolley EA. Effect of prolonged methylprednisone therapy in unresolving acute respiratory distress syndrome: a randomized controlled trial. JAMA 1998; 280:159–165.

113. Staudinger T, Presterl E, Graninger W, Locker G, Knapp S, Laczika K, Klappacher G, Stoiser B, Wagner A, Tesinsky P, Kordova H, Frass M. Influence of pentoxifylline on cytokine levels and inflammatory parameters in septic shock. Intensive Care Med 1996; 22:888–893.

114. Bacher A, Mayer N, Klimscha W, Oismuller C, Steltzer H, Hammerle A. Effects of pentoxifylline on hemodynamics and oxygenation in septic and nonseptic patients. Crit Care Med 1997; 25:795–800.

115. Staubach K-H, Schroder J, Stuber F, Gehrke K, Traumann E, Zabel P. Effect of pentoxifylline in severe sepsis. Arch Surg 1998; 133:94–100.

116. Zeni F, Pain P, Vindimian M, Gay J-G, Gery P, Bertrand M, Page Y, Page D, Vermesch R, Bertrand J-C. Effects of pentoxifylline on circulating cytokine concentrations and hemodynamics in patients with septic shock: results from a double-blind, randomized, placebo-controlled study. Crit Care Med 1996; 24:207–214.

117. Lauterbach R, Zembala M. Pentoxifylline reduces plasma tumour necrosis factor-alpha concentration in premature infants with sepsis. Eur J Pediatr 1996; 155:404–409.

118. Suter PM, Domenighetti G, Schaller M-D, Laverriere M-C, Ritz R, Perret C. N-acetyl-cysteine enhances recovery from acute lung injury in man, a randomized, double-blind, placebo-controlled clinical study. Chest 1994; 105:190–194.

119. Jepsen S, Herlevsen P, Knudsen P, Bud MI, Klausen N-O. Antioxidant treatment with N-acetylcysteine during adult respiratory distress syndrome: a prospective, randomized, placebo-controlled study. Crit Care Med 1992; 20:918–923.

120. Bernard GR, Wheeler AP, Arons MM, Morris PE, Paz HL, Russell JA, Wright PA, and the Antioxidant in ARDS Study Group. A trial of antioxidants N-acetylcysteine and procysteine in ARDS. Chest 1997; 112:164–172.

121. Rosenfeld WN, Davis JM, Parton L, Richter SE, Price A, Flaster E, Kassem N. Safety and pharmacokinetics of recombinant human superoxide dismutase

administered intratracheally to premature neonates with respiratory distress syndrome. Pediatrics 1996; 97:811–817.

122. Davis JM, Rosenfeld WN, Sanders RJ, Gonenne A. Prophylactic effects of recombinant human superoxide dismutase in neonatal lung injury. J Appl Physiol 1993; 74:2234–2241.

123. Lanzenberger-Schragl E, Donner A, Kashanipour A, Zimpfer M. High frequency ventilation techniques in ARDS. Acta Anaesthesiol Scand Suppl 1996; 109:157–161.

124. Fort P, Farmer C, Westerman J, Johannigman J, Beninati W, Dolan S, Derdak S. High-frequency oscillatory ventilation for adult respiratory distress syndrome—a pilot study. Crit Care Med 1997; 25:937–947.

125. Mammel MC. High-frequency oscillation and partial liquid ventilation. Crit Care Med 2001; 29:1293.

126. Bigatello LM, Patroniti N, Sangalli F. Permissive hypercapnia. Curr Opin Crit Care 2001; 7:34–40.

127. Brower RG, Fessler HE. Mechanical ventilation in acute lung injury and acute respiratory distress syndrome. Clin Chest Med 2000; 21:491–510.

128. Medoff BD, Harris RS, Kesselman H, Venegas J, Amato MB, Hess D. Use of recruitment maneuvers and high-positive end-expiratory pressure in a patient with acute respiratory distress syndrome. Crit Care Med 2000; 28:1210–1216.

129. Papadakos PJ, Lachmann B. The open lung concept of alveolar recruitment can improve outcome in respiratory failure and ARDS. Mt Sinai J Med 2002; 69:73–77.

130. The Acute Respiratory Distress Syndrome Network. Ventilation with lower tidal volumes as compared with traditional tidal volumes for acute lung injury and the acute respiratory distress syndrome. N Engl J Med 2000; 342: 1301–1308.

131. Eisner MD, Thompson T, Hudson LD, Luce JM, Hayden D, Schoenfeld D, Matthay MA. Efficacy of low tidal volume ventilation in patients with different clinical risk factors for acute lung injury and the acute respiratory distress syndrome. Am J Respir Crit Care Med 2001; 164:231–236.

132. Hess DR, Bigatello LM. Lung recruitment: the role of recruitment maneuvers. Respir Care 2002; 47:308–317; discussion 317–318.

133. Mehta S, MacDonald R, Hallett DC, Lapinsky SE, Aubin M, Stewart TE. Acute oxygenation response to inhaled nitric oxide when combined with high-frequency oscillatory ventilation in adults with acute respiratory distress syndrome. Crit Care Med 2003; 31:383–389.

134. Marraro GA. Innovative practices of ventilatory support with pediatric patients. Pediatr Crit Care Med 2003; 4:8–20.

135. Ward, NS. Effects of prone position ventilation in ARDS. An evidence-based review of the literature. Crit Care Clin 2002; 18:35–44.

136. Ignarro LJ, Buga GM, Wood KS, Byrns RE, Chaudhuri G. Endothelium-derived relaxing factor produced and released from artery and vein is nitric oxide. Proc Natl Acad Sci USA 1987; 84:9265–9269.

137. Palmer R, Ferrige A, Moncada S. Nitric oxide release accounts for the biologic activity of endothelium-derived relaxing factor. Nature 1987; 327: 524–526.

138. Palmer R, Ashton D, Moncada S. Vascular endothelial cells synthesize nitric oxide from L-arginine. Nature 1988; 333:664–666.

139. Kinsella JP, Truog WE, Walsh WF, Goldberg RN, Bancalari E, Clark RH, Mayock DE, Redding GJ, deLemos RA, Sardesai S, McCurnin DC, Yoder BA, Moreland SG, Cutter GR, Abamn SH. Randomized, multicenter trial of inhaled nitric oxide and high frequency oscillatory ventilation in severe persistent pulmonary hypertension of the newborn. J Pediatr 1997; 131:55–62.

140. Nelin LD, Hoffman GM. The use of inhaled nitric oxide in a wide variety of clinical problems. Pediatr Clin North Am 1998; 45:531–548.

141. Troncy E, Francoeur M, Blaise G. Inhaled nitric oxide: clinical applications, indications, and toxicology. Can J Anaesth 1997; 44:973–988.

142. Roberts JD, Fineman JR, Morin FC, Shaul PW, Rimar S, Schreiber MD, Polin RA, Zwass MS, Zayek MM, Gross I, Heymann MA, Zapol WM. Inhaled nitric oxide and persistent pulmonary hypertension of the newborn. N Engl J Med 1997; 336:605–610.

143. Goldman AP, Tasker RC, Haworth SG, Sigston PE, Macrae DJ. Four patterns of response to inhaled nitric oxide for persistent pulmonary hypertension of the newborn. Pediatrics 1996; 98:706–713.

144. Hoffman GM, Ross RA, Day SE, Rice TB, Nelin LD. Inhaled nitric oxide reduces the utilization of extracorporeal membrane oxygenation in persistent pulmonary hypertension of the newborn. Crit Care Med 1997; 25:352–359.

145. Shah NS, Nakayama DK, Jacob TD, Nishio I, Imai T, Billiar TR, Exler R, Yousem SA, Motoyama EK, Peitzman AB. Efficacy of inhaled nitric oxide in a porcine model of adult respiratory distress syndrome. Arch Surg 1994; 129:158–164.

146. Putensen C, Rasanen J, Lopez F, Downs J. Continuous positive pressure modulates effect of inhaled nitric oxide on the ventilation–perfusion distributions in canine lung injury. Chest 1994; 106:1563–1569.

147. Fratacci MD, Frostell C, Chen TY, Wain JC, Robinson DR, Zapol WM. Inhaled nitric oxide: a selective pulmonary vasocilator of heparin-protamine vasoconstriction in sheep. Anesthesiology 1991; 75:990–999.

148. Berger JI, Gibson RL, Redding GJ, Standaert TA, Clarke WR, Truog WE. Effect of inhaled nitric oxide during group B streptococcal sepsis in piglets. Am Rev Respir Dis 1993; 147:1080–1086.

149. Shah NS, Nakayama DK, Jacob TD, Nishio I, Imai T, Billiar TR, Exler R, Yousem SA, Motoyama EK, Peitzman AB. Efficacy of inhaled nitric oxide in oleic acid-induced acute lung injury. Crit Care Med 1997; 25:153–158.

150. Krause MF, Lienhart H-G, Haberstroh J, Hoehn T, Shulte-Monting J, Leititis JU. Effect of inhaled nitric oxide on intrapulmonary right-to-left shunting in two rabbit models of saline lavage induced surfactant deficiency and meconium instillation. Eur J Pediatr 1998; 157:410–415.

151. Neonatal Inhaled Nitric Oxide Study Group (NINOS). Inhaled nitric oxide in full-term and nearly full-term infants with hypoxic respiratory failure. N Engl J Med 1997; 336:597–604.

152. Day RW, Guarin M, Lynch JM, Vernon DD, Mean JM. Inhaled nitric oxide in children with severe lung disease: results of acute and prolonged therapy with two concentrations. Crit Care Med 1996; 24:215–221.

153. Abman SH, Griebel JL, Parker DK, Schmidt JM, Swanton D, Kinsella JP. Acute effects of inhaled nitric oxide in children with severe hypoxemic respiratory failure. J Pediatr 1994; 124:881–888.

154. Demirakca S, Dotsch J, Knotche C, Magsaam J, Reiter HL, Bauer J, Kuehl PG. Inhaled nitric oxide in neonatal and pediatric acute respiratory distress syndrome: dose response, prolonged inhalation, and weaning. Crit Care Med 1996; 24:1913–1919.

155. Okamoto K, Hamaguchi M, Kukita I, Kikuta K, Sato T. Efficacy of inhaled nitric oxide in children with ARDS. Chest 1998; 114:827–833.

156. Goldman AP, Tasker RC, Hosiasson S, Henrichsen T, Macrae DJ. Early response to inhaled nitric oxide and its relationship to outcome in children with severe hypoxemic respiratory failure. Chest 1997; 112:752–758.

157. Nakagawa TA, Morris A, Gomez RJ, Johnston SJ, Sharkey PT, Zaritsky AL. Dose response to inhaled nitric oxide in pediatric patients with pulmonary hypertension and acute respiratory distress syndrome. J Pediatr 1997; 131:63–69.

158. Okamoto K, Kukita I, Hamaguchi M, Motoyama T, Muranaka H, Harada T. Combined effects of inhaled nitric oxide and positive end-expiratory pressure during mechanical ventilation in acute respiratory distress syndrome. Artif Organs 2000; 24:390–395.

159. Borelli M, Lampati L, Vascotto E, Fumagalli R, Pesenti A. Hemodynamic and gas exchange response to inhaled nitric oxide and prone positioning in acute respiratory distress syndrome patients. Crit Care Med 2000; 28: 2707–2712.

160. Sokol J, Jacobs SE, Bohn D. Inhaled nitric oxide for acute hypoxemic respiratory failure in children and adults. Cochrane Database Syst Rev 2003; 1: (CD002787).

161. Kinsella JP, Parker TA, Ivy DD, Abman SH. Non-invasive delivery of inhaled nitric oxide therapy for late pulmonary hypertension in newborn infants with congenital diaphragmatic hernia. J Pediatr 2003; 142:397–401.

162. Scheeren T, Radermacher P. Prostacyclin (PGI_2): new aspects of an old substance in the treatment of critically ill patients. Intensive Care Med 1997; 23:146–158.

163. Putensen C, Hormann C, Kleinsasser A, Putensen-Himmer G. Cardiopulmonary effects of aerosolized prostaglandin E_1 and nitric oxide inhalation in patients with acute respiratory distress syndrome. Am J Respir Crit Care Med 1998; 157:1743–1747.

164. Papazian L, Roch A, Bregeon F, Thirion X, Gaillat F, Saux P, Fulachier V, Jammes Y, Auffray JP. Inhaled nitric oxide and vasoconstrictors in acute respiratory distress syndrome. Am J Respir Crit Care Med 1999; 160:473–479.

165. Roch A, Papazian L, Bregeon F, Gainnier M, Michelet P, Thirion X, Saux P, Thomas P, Jammes Y, Auffray JP. High or low doses of almitrine bismesylate in ARDS patients responding to inhaled NO and receiving norepinephrine? Intensive Care Med 2001; 27:1737–1743.

166. Michard F, Wolff MA, Herman B, Wysocki M. Right ventricular response to high-dose almitrine infusion in patients with severe hypoxemia related to acute respiratory distress syndrome. Crit Care Med 2001; 29:32–36.

167. Doering EB, Hanson CW, Reily DJ, Marshall C, Marshall BE. Improvement in oxygenation by phenylephrine and nitric oxide in patients with adult respiratory distress syndrome. Anesthesiology 1997; 87:18–25.

168. Troncy E, Blaise G. Phenylephrine and inhaled nitric oxide (letter). Anethesiology 1998; 89:538–539.

169. Papazian L, Bregeon F, Gaillat F, Kaphan E, Thiroon X, Saux P, Badier M, Gregoire R, Gouin F, Jammes Y, Auffray J-P. Does norepinephrine modify the effects of inhaled nitric oxide in septic patients with acute respiratory distress syndrome? Anesthesiology 1998; 89:1089–1098

170. Kobayashi H, Tanaka N, Winkler M, Zapol WM. Combined effects of NO inhalation and intravenous PGF_{2a} on pulmonary circulation and gas exchange in an ovine ARDS model. Intensive Care Med 1996; 22:656–663.

171. Petty T, Reiss O, Paul G, Silvers G, Elkins N. Characteristics of pulmonary surfactant in adult respiratory distress syndrome associated with trauma and shock. Am Rev Respir Dis 1977; 115:531–536.

172. Hallman M, Spragg R, Harrell JH, Moser KM, Gluck L. Evidence of lung surfactant abnormality in respiratory failure. J Clin Invest 1982; 70:673–683.

173. Seeger W, Pison U, Buchhorn R, Obestacke U, Joka T. Surfactant abnormalities and adult respiratory failure. Lung 1990; 168(suppl):891–902.

174. Pison U, Seeger W, Buchhorn R, Joka T, Brand M, Obertacke U, Neuhof H, Schmit-Neuerberg K. Surfactant abnormalities in patients with respiratory failure after multiple trauma. Am Rev Respir Dis 1989; 140:1033–1039.

175. Gregory TJ, Longmore WJ, Moxley MA, Whitsett JA, Reed CR, Fowler AA, Hudson LD, Maunder RJ, Crim C, Hyers TM. Surfactant chemical composition and biophysical activity in acute respiratory distress syndrome. J Clin Invest 1991; 88:1976–1981.

176. Veldhuizen R, McCaig L, Akino T, Lewis J. Pulmonary surfactant subfractions in patients with the acute respiratory distress syndrome. Am J Respir Crit Care Med 1995; 152:1867–1871.

177. Griese M. Pulmonary surfactant in health and human lung diseases: state of the art. Eur Respir J 1999; 13:1455–1476.

178. Günther A, Siebert C, Schmidt R, Ziegle S, Grimminger F, Yabut M, Temmesfeld B, Walmrath D, Morr H, Seeger W. Surfactant alterations in severe pneumonia, acute respiratory distress syndrome, and cardiogenic lung edema. Am J Respir Crit Care Med 1996; 153:176–184.

179. Frerking I, Gunther A, Seeger W, Pison U. Pulmonary surfactant: functions, abnormalities and therapeutic options. Intensive Care Med 2001; 27: 1699–1717.

180. Luchetti M, Casiraghi G, Valsecchi R, Galassini E, Marraro G. Porcine-derived surfactant treatment of severe bronchiolitis. Acta Anaesthesiol Scand 1998; 42:805–810.

181. Luchetti M, Ferrero F, Gallini C, Natale A, Pigna A, Tortorolo L, Marraro GA. Multicenter, randomized, controlled study of porcine surfactant in severe respiratory syncytial virus-induced respiratory failure. Pediatr Crit Care Med 2002; 3:261–268.

182. Anzueto A, Baughman RP, Guntupalli KK, Weg JG, Wiedemann HP, Raventos AA, Lemaire F, Long W, Zaccardelli DS, Pattishall EN, and

(Exosurf ARDS Sepsis Study Group). Aerosolized surfactant in adults with sepsis-induced acute respiratory distress syndrome. N Engl J Med 1996; 334:1417–1421.

183.   Macnaughton PD, Evans TW. The effect of exogenous surfactant therapy on lung function following cardiopulmonary bypass. Chest 1994; 105:421–425.

184.   Spragg RG, Lewis JF, Wurst W, Hafner D, Baughman RP, Wewers MD, Marsh JJ. Treatment of acute respiratory distress syndrome with recombinant surfactant protein C surfactant. Am J Respir Crit Care Med 2003; 167: 1562–1566.

185.   Lewis JF, Brackenbury A. Role of exogenous surfactant in acute lung injury. Crit Care Med 2003; 31(suppl 4):S324–S328.

186.   Hallman M, Waffarn F, Bry K, Turbow R, Kleinman MT, Mautz WJ, Rasmussen RE, Bhalla DK, Phalen RF. Surfactant dysfunction after inhalation of nitric oxide. J Appl Physiol 1996; 80:2026–2034.

187.   Matalon S, DeMarco V, Haddad IY, Myles C, Skimming JW, Schurch S, Cheng S, Cassin S. Inhaled nitric oxide injures the pulmonary surfactant system of lambs in vivo. Am J Physiol 1996; 270:L273–L280.

188.   Karamanoukian HL, Glick PL, Wilcox DL, Rossman JE, Morin FC, Holm BA. Pathophysiology of congenital diaphragmatic hernia VII: inhaled nitric oxide requires exogenous surfactant therapy in the lamb model of CDH. J Pediatr Surg 1995; 30:1–4.

189.   Rais-Bahrami K, Rivera O, Seale W, Short B. Effect of nitric oxide in meconium aspiration syndrome after treatment with surfactant. Crit Care Med 1997; 25:1744–1747.

190.   Gommers D, Hartog A, van't Veen A, Lachmann B. Improved oxygenation by nitric oxide is enhanced by prior lung reaeration with surfactant, rather than positive end-expiratory pressure, in lung-lavaged rabbits. Crit Care Med 1997; 25:1868–1873.

191.   Zhu GF, Sun B, Niu S, Cai YY, Lin K, Lindwall R, Robertson B. Combined surfactant therapy and inhaled nitric oxide in rabbits with oleic acid-induced acute respiratory distress syndrome. Am J Respir Crit Care Med 1998; 158:437–443.

192.   Hartog A, Gommers D, van't Veen A, Erdmann W, Lachmann B. Exogenous surfactant and nitric oxide have a synergistic effect in improving gas exchange in experimental ARDS. Adv Exp Med Biol 1997; 428:277–279.

193.   Warnecke G, Struber M, Fraud S, Hohlfeld JM, Haverich A. Combined exogenous surfactant and inhaled nitric oxide therapy for lung ischemia-reperfusion injury in minipigs. Transplantation 2001; 71:1238–1244.

194.   Zheng S, Zhang WY, Zhu LW, Lin K, Sun B. Surfactant and inhaled nitric oxide in rats alleviate acute lung injury induced by intestinal ischemia and reperfusion. J Pediatr Surg 2001; 36:980–984.

195.   Sokol GM, Fineberg NS, Wright LL, Ehrenkranz RA. Changes in arterial oxygen tension when weaning neonates from inhaled nitric oxide. Pediatr Pulmonol 2001; 32:14–19.

196.   Uy IP, Pryhuber GS, Chess PR, Notter RH. Combined-modality therapy with inhaled nitric oxide and exogenous surfactant in term Infants with acute respiratory failure. Pediatr Crit Care Med 2000; 1:107–110.

197. Hintz SR, Suttner DM, Sheehan AM, Rhine WD, Van Meurs KP. Decreased use of neonatal extracorporeal membrane oxygenation (ECMO): how new treatment modalities have affected ECMO utilization. Pediatrics 2000; 106:1339–1343.

198. Greene R. Pulmonary vascular obstruction in the adult respiratory distress syndrome. J Thorac Imaging 1986; 1:31–38.

199. Gunther A, Mosavi P, Heinemann S, Ruppert C, Muth H, Markart P, Grimminger F, Walmrath D, Temmesfeld-Wollbruck B, Seeger W. Alveolar fibrin formation caused by enhanced procoagulant and depressed fibrinolytic capacities in severe pneumonia. Comparison with the acute respiratory distress syndrome. Am J Respir Crit Care Med 2000; 161:454–462.

200. Welty-Wolf KE, Carraway MS, Miller DL, Ortel TL, Ezban M, Ghio AJ, Idell S, Piantadosi CA. Coagulation blockade prevents sepsis-induced respiratory and renal failure in baboons. Am J Respir Crit Care Med 2001; 164: 1988–1996.

201. Joyce DE, Gelbert L, Ciaccia A, DeHoff B, Grinnell BW. Gene expression profile of antithrombotic protein c defines new mechanisms modulating inflammation and apoptosis. J Biol Chem 2001; 276:11199–11203.

202. Wilcox DT, Glick PL, Karamanoukian HL, Leach C, Morin FC, Fuhrman BP. Perfluorocarbon-associated gas exchange improves pulmonary mechanics, oxygenation, ventilation, and allows nitric oxide delivery in the hypoplastic lung congenital diaphragmatic hernia lamb model. Crit Care Med 1995; 23:1858–1863.

203. Uchida T, Nakazawa K, Yokoyama K, Makita K, Amaha K. The combination of partial liquid ventilation and inhaled nitric oxide in the severe oleic acid lung injury model. Chest 1998; 113:1658–1666.

204. Houmes R-JM, Hartog A, Verbrugge SJ, Bohm S, Lachmann B. Combining partial liquid ventilation with nitric oxide to improve gas exchange in acute lung injury. Intensive Care Med 1997; 23:163–169.

205. Johannigman JA, Davis K Jr, Campbell RS, Luchette FA, Frame SB, Branson RD. Positive end-expiratory pressure and response to inhaled nitric oxide: changing nonresponders to responders. Surgery 2000; 127:390–394.

206. Wolf S, Lohbrunner H, Busch T, Deja M, Weber-Carstens S, Donaubauer B, Sterner-Kock A, Kaisers U. "Ideal PEEP" is superior to high dose partial liquid ventilation with low PEEP in experimental acute lung injury. Intensive Care Med 2001; 27:1937–1948.

207. Zhou BH, Sun B, Zhou ZH, Zhu LW, Fan SZ, Lindwall R. Comparison of effects of surfactant and inhaled nitric oxide in rabbits with surfactant-depleted respiratory failure. Zhongguo Yao Li Xue Bao 1999; 20:691–695.

208. Johannigman JA, Davis K Jr, Miller SL, Campbell RS, Luchette FA, Frame SB, Branson RD. Prone positioning and inhaled nitric oxide: synergistic therapies for acute respiratory distress syndrome [discussion 595–596]. J Trauma 2001; 50:589–595.

209. Dobyns EL, Anas NG, Fortenberry JD, Deshpande J, Cornfield DN, Tasker RC, Liu P, Eells PL, Griebel J, Kinsella JP, Abman SH. Interactive effects of high-frequency oscillatory ventilation and inhaled nitric oxide in

acute hypoxemic respiratory failure in pediatrics. Crit Care Med 2002; 30: 2425–2429.

210. Leach CL, Holm BA, Morin FC, Fuhrman BP, Papo MC, Steinhorn D, Hernan LJ. Partial liquid ventilation in premature lambs with respiratory distress syndrome: efficacy and compatibility with exogenous surfactant. J Pediatr 1995; 126:412–420.

211. Davis JM, Richter SE, Kendig JW, Notter RH. High frequency jet ventilation and surfactant treatment of newborns in servere respiratory failure. Pediatr Pulmonol 1992; 13:108–112.

212. Davis JM, Notter RH. Lung surfactant replacement for neonatal pathology other than primary respiratory distress syndrome. Boynton B, Carlo W, Jobe A, eds. New Therapies for Neonatal Respiratory Failure: A Physiologic Approach. Cambridge: Cambridge University Press, 1994:81–92.

213. Chappell SE, Wolfson MR, Shaffer TH. A comparison of surfactant delivery with conventional mechanical ventilation and partial liquid ventilation in meconium aspiration injury. Respir Med 2001; 95:612–617.

214. Gothberg S, Parker TA, Abman SH, Kinsella JP. High-frequency oscillatory ventilation and partial liquid ventilation after acute lung injury in premature lambs with respiratory distress syndrome. Crit Care Med 2000; 28:2450–2456.

215. Ambalavanan N, Carlo WA. Hypocapnia and hypercapnia in respiratory management of newborn infants. Clin Perinatol 2001; 28:517–531.

216. Mariani G, Cifuentes J, Carlo WA. Randomized trial of permissive hypercapnia in preterm infants. Pediatrics 1999; 104:1082–1088.

217. Armstrong L, Millar AB. Relative production of tumour necrosis factor a and interleukin 10 in adult respiratory distress syndrome. Thorax 1997; 52:442–446.

218. Raponi G, Antonelli M, Gaeta A, Bufi M, De Blasi RA, Conti G, D'Errico RR, Mancini C, Filadoro F, Gasparetto A. Tumor necrosis factor in serum and bronchoalveolar lavage of patients at risk for the adult respiratory distress syndrome. J Crit Care 1992; 7:183–188.

219. Parsons P, Moore F, Ikle D, Henson P, Worthen G. Studies on the role of tumor necrosis factor in adult respiratory distress syndrome. Am Rev Respir Dis 1992; 146:694–700.

220. Tagan M, Markert M, Schaller M, Feihl F, Chiolero R, Perret C. Oxidative metabolism of circulating granulocytes in adult respiratory distress syndrome. Am J Med 1991; 91(suppl 3C):72–78.

221. Pacht E, Timerman A, Lykens M, Merola A. Deficiency of alveolar fluid glutathione in patients with sepsis and the adult respiratory distress syndrome. Chest 1991; 100:1397–1403.

222. Laurent T, Markert M, Feihl F, Schaller M-D, Perret C. Oxidant-antioxidant balance in granulocytes during ARDS. Chest 1996; 109:163–166.

223. Miller EJ, Cohen AB, Matthay MA. Increased interleukin-8 concentrations in the pulmonary edema fluid in patients with acute respiratory distress syndrome from sepsis. Crit Care Med 1996; 24:1448–1454.

224. Meduri GU, Kohler G, Tolley E, Headley AS, Stentz F, Postlethwaite A. Inflammatory cytokines in the BAL of patients with ARDS: persistent elevation over time predicts poor outcome. Chest 1995; 108:1303–1314.

225. Meduri GU, Healey S, Kohler G, Stentz F, Tolley E, Umberger R, Leeper K. Persistent elevation of inflammatory cytokines predicts poor outcome in ARDS. Plasma IL-1β and IL-6 levels are consistent and efficient predictors of outcome over time. Chest 1995; 107:1062–1073.

226. Tracey KJ, Fong Y, Hesse DG, Manogue KR, Lee AT, Kuo GC, Lowry SF, Cerami A. Anti-cachectin/TNF monoclonal antibodies prevent septic shock during lethal bacteremia. Nature 1987; 330:662–664.

227. Folkesson HF, Matthay MA, Hebert C, Broaddus CV. Acid aspiration-induced lung injury in rabbits is mediated by IL-8 dependent mechanisms. J Clin Invest 1995; 96:107–116.

228. Yokoi K, Mukaida N, Harada A, Watanabe Y, Matsushima K. Prevention of endotoxemia-induced acute respiratory distress syndrome-like lung injury in rabbits by a monoclonal antibody to IL-8. Lab Invest 1997; 76:375–384.

229. Broaddus VC, Boylan AM, Hoeffel JM, Kim KJ, Sadik M, Chuntharapai A, Hebert CA. Neutralization of IL-8 inhibits neutrophil influx in a rabbit model of endotoxin-induced injury. J Immunol 1994; 152:2960–2967.

230. Adawi A, Zhang Y, Baggs R, Finkelstein J, Phipps RP. Disruption of the CD40–CD40 ligand system prevents an oxygen-induced respiratory distress syndrome. Am J Pathol 1998; 152:651–657.

231. Adawi A, Zhang Y, Baggs R, Rubin P, Williams J, Finkelstein JN, Phipps R. Blockage of CD40–CD40 ligand interactions protects against radiation-induced pulmonary inflammation and fibrosis. Clin Immunol Immunopath 1998; 89:222–230.

232. Ohlsson K, Bjork P, Bergenfeldt M, Hageman R, Thompson RC. Interleukin-1 receptor antagonist reduces mortality from endotoxin shock. Nature 1990; 348:550–552.

233. Fisher E, Marano MA, Van Zee KJ, Rock CS, Hawes AS, Thompson WA, DeForge L, Kenney JS, Remick DG, Bloedow DC, Thompson RC, Lowry SF, Moldawer LL. IL-1 receptor blockade improves survival and hemodynamic performance in *E. coli* septic shock, but fails to alter host responses to sublethal endotoxemia. J Clin Invest 1992; 89:1551–1557.

234. Ziegler EJ, Fisher CJ, Sprung CL, Straube RC, Sadoff JC, Foulke GE, Wortel CH, Fink MP, Dellinger RP, Teng N, Allen IE, Berger HJ, Knatterud GL, LoBuglio AF, Smith CR. Treatment of gram negative bacteremia and septic shock with HA-1A human monoclonal antibody against endotoxin: a randomized, double-blind, placebo-controlled trial. N Engl J Med 1991; 324: 429–436.

235. Greenman RL, Schein RMH, Martin MA, Wenzel RP, MacIntyre NR, Emmanuel G, Chmel H, Kohler RB, McCarthy M, Plouffe J, Russell JA, and the XOMA Sepsis Study Group. 1991. A controlled clinical trial of E5 murine monoclonal IgM antibody to endotoxin in the treatment of gram negative sepsis. JAMA 266:1097–1102.

236. Hoffmann H, Hatherill JR, Crowley J, Harada H, Yonemaru M, Zheng H, Ishizaka A, Raffin TA. Early post-treatment with pentoxifylline or dibutyryl cAMP attenuates *Escherichia coli*-induced acute lung injury in guinea pigs. Am Rev Respir Dis 1991; 143:289–293.

237. Sheridan BC, McIntyre RC, Meldrum DR, Fullerton DA. Pentoxifylline treatment attenuates pulmonary vasomotor dysfunction in acute lung injury. J Surg Res 1997; 71:150–154.

238. Lindsey HJ, Kisala JM, Ayala A, Lehman D, Hedron CD, Chaudry IH. Pentoxifylline attentuates oxygen-induced lung injury. J Surg Res 1994; 56: 543–548.

239. Ishizaka A, Wu ZH, Stephens KE, Horada H, Hogue RS, O'Hanley PT, Raffin TA. Attenuation of acute lung injury in septic guinea pigs by pentoxifylline. Am Rev Respir Dis 1988; 138:376–384.

240. Law WR, Nadkarni VM, Fletcher MA, Nevola JJ, Eckstein JM, Quance J, McKenna TM, Lee CH, Williams TJ. Pentoxifylline treatment of sepsis in conscious Yucatan minipigs. Circ Shock 1992; 37:291–300.

241. Fletcher MA, McKenna TM, Owens EH, Nadkarni VM. Effects of in vivo pentoxifylline treatment on survival and ex vivo vascular contractility in a rat lipopolysaccharide shock model. Circ Shock 1992; 36:74–80.

242. Mandell GL. ARDS, neutrophils and pentoxifylline. Am Rev Respir Dis 1988; 138:1103–1105.

243. Langley SC, Kelly FJ. *N*-acetylcysteine ameliorates hyperoxic lung injury in the preterm guinea pig. Biochem Pharmacol 1993; 45:841–846.

244. Sastre J, Asensi M, Rodrigo F, Pallardo F, Vento M, Vina J. Antioxidant administration to the mother prevents oxidative stress associated with birth in the neonatal rat. Life Sci 1994; 54:2055–2059.

245. Davreux CJ, Soric I, Nathens AB, Watson RWG, McGilvray ID, Suntres ZE, Shek PN, Rotstein OD. *N*-acetylcysteine attenuates acute lung injury in the rat. Shock 1997; 8:432–438.

246. Wagner PD, Mathieu-Costello O, Bebaut DE, Gray AT, Natterson PD, Glennow C. Protection against pulmonary O_2 toxicity by *N*-acetylcysteine. Eur Respir J 1989; 2:116–126.

247. Bernard GR, Lucht WD, Niedermeyer ME, Snapper JR, Ogletree ML, Brigham KL. Effect of *N*-acetylcysteine on the pulmonary response to endotoxin in awake sheep and upon in vitro granulocyte function. J Clin Invest 1984; 73:1772–1784.

248. Leff JA, Wilke CP, Hybertson BM, Shanley PF, Beehler CJ, Repine JE. Postinsult treatment with *N*-acetyl-L-cysteine decreases IL-1-induced neutrophil influx and lung leak in rats. Am J Physiol 1993; 265:L501–L506.

249. Hack CE, Aarden LA, Thijs LG. Role of cytokines in sepsis. Adv Immunol 1997; 66:101–195.

250. Meduri GU. The role of host defense response in the progression and outcome of ARDS: pathophysiological correlations and response to glucocorticoid treatment. Eur Respir J 1996; 9:2650–2670.

251. Michie HR, Mangue DR, Spriggs A, Revhaug S, O'Dwyer CA, Dinarello, Carem A, Wolf SM, Wilmore DW. Detection of circulating tumor necrosis factor after endotoxin administration. N Engl J Med 1988; 318:1481–1486.

252. Li XY, Donaldson K, Brown D, MacNee W. The role of tumor necrosis factor in increased airspace epithelial permeability in acute lung inflammation. Am J Respir Cell Mol Biol 1995; 13:185–195.

253. Windsor AC, Walsh CJ, Mullen PG, Cook DJ, Fisher BJ, Blocher CR, Leeper-Woodford SK, Sugerman HJ, Fowler AA. Tumor necrosis factor-alpha blockade prevents neutrophil CD18 receptor upregulation and attenuates acute lung injury in porcine sepsis without inhibition of neutrophil oxygen radical generation. J Clin Invest 1993; 91:1459–1468.

254. Goldman G, Welbourn R, Kobzik L, Valeri CR, Shepro D, Hechtman HB. Tumor necrosis factor-alpha mediates acid aspiration-induced systemic organ injury. Ann Surg 1990; 212:513–520.

255. Miller EJ, Cohen AB, Nagao S, Griffith DG, Maunder RJ, Martin TR, Weiner-Kronish JP, Sticherling M, Christophers E, Matthay MA. Elevated levels of NAP-1/interleukin-8 are present in the airspaces of patients with adult respiratory distress syndrome and are associated with increased mortality. Am Rev Respir Dis 1992; 146:427–432.

256. Donnelly SC, Strieter RM, Kunkel SL. IL-8 and development of adult respiratory distress syndrome in at-risk patients. Lancet 1993; 341:643–647.

257. Kurdowska A, Carr FK, Stevens MD, Paughman RP, Martin TR. Studies on the interaction of IL-8 with human α_2-macroglobulin: evidence of the presence of IL-8 complexed to α_2-macroglobulin in lung fluids of patients with adult respiratory distress syndrome. J Immunol 1997; 158:1930–1940.

258. Goodman RB, Strieter RM, Martin DP, Steinberg KP, Milberg JA, Maunder RJ, Kunkel SL, Walz A, Hudson LD, Martin TR. Inflammatory cytokines in patients with persistence of the acute respiratory distress syndrome. Am J Respir Crit Care Med 1996; 154:602–611.

259. Goodman ER, Kleinstein E, Fusco AM, Quinlan DP, Lavery R, Livingstone DH, Deitch EA, Hauser CJ. Role of interleukin 8 in the genesis of acute respiratory distress syndrome through an effect on neutrophil apoptosis. Arch Surg 1998; 13:1234–1239.

260. Sempowski G, Chess P, Phipps R. CD40 is a functional activation antigen and B7-independent T cell costimulatory molecule in normal human lung fibroblasts. J Immunol 1997; 158:4670–1477.

261. Fries K, Gaspari A, Blieden T, Looney RJ, Phipps RP. CD40 expression by human fibroblasts. Clin Immunopathol 1995; 154:162–170.

262. Sempowski G, Chess P, Padilla J, Moretti A, Phipps R. CD40 mediated activation of gingival and periodontal ligament fibroblasts. J Periodontol 1997; 68:284–292.

263. Barazzone AC, Donati YR, Boccard J, Rochat AF, Vesin C, Kan CD, Piguet PF. CD40–CD40 ligand disruption does not prevent hyperoxia-induced injury. Am J Pathol 2002; 160:67–71.

264. Coccia MT, Waxman K, Soliman MH, Tominaga G, Pinderski L. Pentoxifylline improves survival following hemorrhagic shock. Crit Care Med 1989; 17:36–38.

265. Ehrly A. The effect of pentoxifylline on the deformability of erythrocytes and the muscular oxygen pressure in patients with chronic arterial disease. J Med 1979; 10:331–336.

266. Stefanovitch V. Effect of pentoxifylline on energy rich phosphate in rat erythrocytes. Res Commun Chem Pathol Pharmacol 1975; 10:745–750.

267. Farrukh IS, Gurtner GH, Michael JR. Pharmacologic modification of pulmonary vascular injury: possible role of cAMP. J Appl Physiol 1987; 62:47–54.

268. Bessler H, Gilgal R, Djaidetti M, Zahavi I. Effect of pentoxifylline on the phagocyte activity, cAMP levels and superoxide production by monocytes and polymorphonuclear cells. J Leuko Biol 1986; 40:747–754.

269. Balibrea-Cantero JL, Arias-Diaz J, Garcia C, Torres-Melero J, Simon C, Rodriguez JM, Vara E. Effect of pentoxifylline on the inhibition of surfactant synthesis induced by TNF-α in human type II pneumocytes. Am J Respir Crit Care Med 1994; 149:699–706.

270. Zheng H, Crowley JJ, Chan JC, Hoffman H, Hatherill JR, Ishizaka A, Raffin TA. Attenuation of tumor necrosis factor-induced endothelial cell cytotoxicity and neutrophil chemiluminescence. Am Rev Respir Dis 1990; 142:1073–1078.

271. Ward A, Clissold SP. Pentoxifylline. A review of its pharmacodynamic and pharmacokinetic properties, and its therapeutic efficacy. Drugs 1987; 34:50–97.

272. Montravers P, Fagon JY, Gilbert C, Blanchet F, Novara A, Chastre J. Pilot study of cardiopulmonary risk from pentoxifylline in adult repiratory distress syndrome. Chest 2001; 103:1017–1022.

273. Morris PE, Bernard GR. Significance of glutathione in lung disease and implications for therapy. Am J Med Sci 1994; 307:119–127.

274. Cantin AM, North SL, Hubbard RC, Crystal RG. Normal alveolar epithelial lining fluid contains high levels of glutathione. J Appl Physiol 1987; 63: 152–157.

275. Heffner JE, Repine JE. Pulmonary strategies of antioxidant defense. Am Rev Respir Dis 1989; 140:531–554.

276. Cantin AM, Bein R. Glutathione and inflammatory disorders of the lung. Lung 1991; 169:123–138.

277. Cantin AM, Hubbard RC, Crystal RG. Glutathione deficiency in the epithelial tract in idiopathic pulmonary fibrosis. Am Rev Respir Dis 1989; 139: 370–372.

278. Gillissen A, Nowak D. Characterization of *N*-acetylcysteine and ambroxol in anti-oxidant therapy. Respir Med 1998; 92:609–623.

279. Bibi H, Seifert B, Oulette M, Belik J. Intratracheal N-acetylcysteine use in infants with chronic lung disease. Acta Paediatr 1992; 81:335–339.

280. Brown LA, Harris FL, Guidot DM. Chronic ethanol ingestion potentiates TNF-alpha-mediated oxidative stress and apoptosis in rat type II cells. Am J Physiol 2001; 281(2):L377–L386.

281. Chabot F, Mitchell JA, Gutteridge JMC, Evans TW. Reactive oxygen species in acute lung injury. Eur Respir J 1998; 11:745–757.

282. Sies H. Oxidative Stress, Oxidants and Antioxidants. London: Academic Press, 1991.

283. Oury T, Chang L, Marklund S, Day B, Crapo J. Immunocytochemical localization of extracellular superoxide dismutase in human lung. Lab Invest 1994; 70:889–898.

284. Marklund SL. Extracellular superoxide dismutase and other superoxide isoenzymes in tissues from nine mammalian species. Biochem J 1984; 222: 649–655.

285. Walther FJ, David-Cu R, Lopez SL. Antioxidant-surfactant liposomes mitigate hyperoxic lung injury in premature rabbits. Am J Physiol 1995; 269: L613–L617.

286. Padmanabhan RV, Gudapaty R, Liener IE, Schwartz BA, Hoidal JR. Protection against pulmonary oxygen toxicity in rats by the intratracheal administration of liposomes-encapsulated superoxide dismutase or catalase. Am Rev Respir Dis 1985; 132:164–167.

287. Tanswell A, Freeman B. Liposome-entrapped antioxidant enzymes prevent lethal O_2 toxicity in the newborn rat. J Appl Physiol 1987; 63:347–352.

288. Barnard ML, Baker RR, Matalon S. Mitigation of oxidant injury to lung microvasculature by intratracheal instillation of antioxidant enzymes. Am J Physiol 1993; 265:L340–L345.

289. Walther FJ, Nunex Fl, David-Cu R, Hill KE. Mitigation of pulmonary oxygen toxicity in rats by intratracheal instillation of polyethylene glycol-conjugated antioxidant enzymes. Pediatr Res 1993; 33:332–335.

290. White CW, Jackson JH, Abuchowski A, Kazo GM, Mimmack RF, Berger EM, Freeman BA, McCord JM, Repine JE. Polyethylene glycol-attached antioxidant enzyme decrease pulmonary oxygen toxicity in rats. J Appl Physiol 1989; 66:584–590.

291. Davis JM, Rosenfeld WN, Koo HC, Gonenne A. Pharmacologic interactions of exogenous lung surfactant and recombinant human Cu/Zn superoxide dismutase. Pediatr Res 1994; 35:37–40.

292. Haddad IY, Nieves-Cruz G, Matalon S. Inhibition of surfactant function by copper–zinc superoxide dismutase (CuZn–SOD). J Appl Physiol 1997; 83:1545–1550.

293. Gonzalez PK, Zhuang J, Doctrow SR, Malfroy B, Benson PF, Menconi MJ, Fink MP. Role of oxidant stress in the adult respiratory distress syndrome: evaluation of a novel antioxidant strategy in a porcine model of endotoxin-induced acute lung injury. Shock 1996; 6:S23–S26.

294. Gonzalez PK, Zhuang J, Doctrow SR, Malfroy B, Benson PF, Menconi MJ, Fink MP. EUK-8, a synthetic superoxide dismutase and catalase mimetic, ameliorates acute lung injury in endotoxemic mice. J Pharmacol Exp Ther 1995; 275:798–806.

295. Gadek JE, DeMichele SJ, Karlstad MD, Pacht ER, Donahoe M, Albertson TE, Van Hoozen C, Wennberg AK, Nelson JL, Noursalehi M. Effect of enteral feeding with eicosapentaenoic acid, gamma-linolenic acid, and antioxidants in patients with acute respiratory distress syndrome. Enteral Nutrition in ARDS Study Group. Crit Care Med 1999; 27:1409–1420.

296. Pacht ER, DeMichele SJ, Nelson JL, Hart J, Wennberg AK, Gadek JE. Enteral nutrition with eicosapentaenoic acid, gamma-linolenic acid, and antioxidants reduces alveolar inflammatory mediators and protein influx in patients with acute respiratory distress syndrome. Crit Care Med 2003; 31:491–500.

297. Nash JR, McLaughlin PJ, Hoyle C, Roberts D. Immunolocalization of tumour necrosis factor alpha in lung tissue from patients dying with adult respiratory distress syndrome. Histopathology 1991; 19:395–402.

298. Nobauer-Huhmann IM, Eibenberger K, Schaefer-Prokop C, Steltzer H, Schlick W, Strasser K, Fridrich P, Herold CJ. Changes in lung parenchyma after acute respiratory distress syndrome (ARDS): assessment with high-resolution computed tomography. Eur Radiol 2001; 11:2436–2443.

299. McHugh LG, Milberg JA, Whitcomb ME, Schoene RB, Maunder RJ, Hudson LD. Recovery of function in survivors of the acute respiratory distress syndrome. Am J Respir Crit Care Med 1994; 150:90–94.

300. Selman M, King TE, Pardo A. Idiopathic pulmonary fibrosis: prevailing and evolving hypotheses about its pathogenesis and implications for therapy. Ann Intern Med 2001; 134:136–151.

301. Sime PJ, O'Reilly AKM. Fibrosis of the lung and other tissues: new concepts in pathogenesis and treatment. Clin Immunol 2001; 99:308–319.

302. Giri SN. Novel pharmacologic approaches to manage interstitial lung fibrosis in the twenty-first century. Ann Rev Pharmacol Toxicol 2003; 43:73–95.

303. Rotman HH, Lavelle TFJ, Dimcheff DG, VandenBelt RJ, Weg JG. Long-term physiologic consequences of the adult respiratory distress syndrome. Chest 1977; 72:190–192.

304. Bardales RH, Xie SS, Schaefer RF, Hsu SM. Apoptosis is a major pathway responsible for the resolution of type II pneumocytes in acute lung injury. Am J Pathol 1996; 149:845–852.

305. Mason RJ, Greene K, Voelker DR. Surfactant protein A and surfactant protein D in health and disease. Am J Physiol 1998; 275:L1–L13.

306. Wright JR. Immunomodulatory functions of surfactant. Physiol Rev 1997; 77:931–962.

307. Vazquez de Lara L, Becerril C, Montano M, Ramos C, Maldonado V, Melendez J, Phelps DS, Pardo A, Selman M. Surfactant components modulate fibroblast apoptosis and type I collagen and collagenase-1 expression. Am J Physiol 2000; 279:L950–L957.

308. Ren CL. Use of modulators of airways inflammation in patients with CF. Clin Rev Allergy Immunol 2002; 23:29–39.

309. Meduri GU, Headley S, Tolley E, Shelby M, Stentz F, Postlewaite A. Plasma and BAL cytokine response to corticosteroid rescue treatment in late ARDS. Chest 1995; 108:1315–1325.

310. Olivieri D. Corticosteroids in late adult respiratory distress syndrome-towards a better use. Respiration 1998; 65:256–257.

311. Meduri GU. Levels of evidence for the pharmacologic effectiveness of prolonged methylprednisolone treatment in unresolving ARDS. Chest 1999; 116(suppl 1):116S–118S.

312. Meduri GU, Tolley EA, Chrousos GP, Stentz F. Prolonged methylprednisolone treatment suppresses systemic inflammation in patients with unresolving acute respiratory distress syndrome: evidence for inadequate endogenous glucocorticoid secretion and inflammation-induced immune cell resistance to glucocorticoids. Am J Respir Crit Care Med 2002; 165:983–991.

313. Massaro D, Massaro GD. Pulmonary alveolus formation: critical period, retinoid regulation and plasticity [discussion 236–241]. Novartis Found Symp 2001; 234:229–236.

314. Oshika E, Liu S, Singh G, Michalopoulos GK, Shinozuka H, Katyal SL. Antagonistic effects of dexamethasone and retinoic acid on rat lung morphogenesis. Pediatr Res 1998; 43:315–324.

315. Massaro GD, Massaro D. Retinoic acid treatment partially rescues failed septation in rats and in mice. Am J Physiol 2000; 278:L955–L960.

316. Veness-Meehan KAF, Bottone G Jr, Stiles AD. Effects of retinoic acid on airspace development and lung collagen in hyperoxia-exposed newborn rats. Pediatr Res 2000; 48:434–444.

317. Tyson JE, Wright LL, Oh W, Kennedy KA, Mele L, Ehrenkranz RA, Stoll BJ, Lemons JA, Stevenson DK, Bauer CR, Korones SB, Fanaroff AA. Vitamin A supplementation for extremely-low-birth-weight infants. National Institute of Child Health and Human Development Neonatal Research Network. N Engl J Med 1999; 340:1962–1968.

318. Lauterbach R, Szymura-Oleksiak J. Nebulized pentoxifylline in successful treatment of five premature neonates with bronchopulmonary dysplasia. Eur J Pediatr 1999; 158:607.

319. Kullmann A, Vaillant P, Muller V, Martinet Y, Martinet N. In vitro effects of pentoxifylline on smooth muscle cell migration and blood monocyte production of chemotactic activity for smooth muscle cells: potential therapeutic benefit in the adult respiratory distress syndrome. Am J Respir Cell Mol Biol 1993; 8:83–88.

320. Strutz F, Heeg M, Kochsiek T, Siemers G, Zeisberg M, Muller GA. Effects of pentoxifylline, pentifylline and gamma-interferon on proliferation, differentiation, and matrix synthesis of human renal fibroblasts. Nephrol Dial Transplant 2000; 15:1535–1546.

321. Ostman A, Heldin CH. Involvement of platelet-derived growth factor in disease: development of specific antagonists. Adv Cancer Res 2001; 80:1–38.

322. Unemori EN, Pickford LB, Salles AL, Piercy CE, Grove BH, Erikson ME, Amento EP. Relaxin induces an extracellular matrix-degrading phenotype in human lung fibroblasts in vitro and inhibits lung fibrosis in a murine model in vivo. J Clin Invest 1996; 98:2739–2745.

323. Tan A, Levrey H, Dahm C, Polunovsky VA, Rubins J, Bitterman PB. Lovastatin induces fibroblast apoptosis in vitro and in vivo. A possible therapy for fibroproliferative disorders. Am J Respir Crit Care Med 1999; 159:220–227.

324. Henke C, Bitterman P, Roongta U, Ingbar D, Polunovsky V. Induction of fibroblast apoptosis by anti-CD44 antibody: implications for the treatment of fibroproliferative lung disease. Am J Pathol 1996; 149:1639–1650.

325. Johnson MA, Kwan S, Snell NJ, Nunn AJ, Darbyshire JH, Turner-Warwick M. Randomised controlled trial comparing prednisolone alone with cyclophosphamide and low dose prednisolone in combination in cryptogenic fibrosing alveolitis. Thorax 1989; 44:280–288.

326. Raghu G, Depaso WJ, Cain K, Hammar SP, Wetzel CE, Dreis DF, Hutchinson J, Pardee NE, Winterbauer RH. Azathioprine combined with prednisone in the treatment of idiopathic pulmonary fibrosis: a prospective double-blind,

randomized, placebo-controlled clinical trial. Am Rev Respir Dis 1991; 144:291–296.

327. Selman M, Carrillo G, Salas J, Padilla RP, Perez-Chavira R, Sansores R, Chapela R. Colchicine, D-penicillamine, and prednisone in the treatment of idiopathic pulmonary fibrosis: a controlled clinical trial. Chest 1998; 114: 507–512.

328. Selman M, Ruiz V, Cabrera S, Segura L, Ramirez R, Barrios R, Pardo A. TIMP-1, -2, -3, and -4 in idiopathic pulmonary fibrosis. A prevailing nonde-gradative lung microenvironment? Am J Physiol 2000; 279:L562–L574

329. Corbel M, Caulet-Maugendre S, Germain N, Molet S, Lagente V, Boichot E. Inhibition of bleomycin-induced pulmonary fibrosis in mice by the matrix metalloproteinase inhibitor batimastat. J Pathol 2001; 193:538–545.

330. Olschewski H, Ghofrani HA, Walmrath D, Schermuly R, Temmesfeld-Wollbruck B, Grimminger F, Seeger W. Inhaled prostacyclin and iloprost in severe pulmonary hypertension secondary to lung fibrosis. Am J Respir Crit Care Med 1999; 160:600–607.

331. Veyssier-Belot C, Cacoub P. Role of endothelial and smooth muscle cells in the physiopathology and treatment management of pulmonary hypertension. Cardiovasc Res 1999; 44:274–282.

20

Summary and Future Research Directions

ROBERT H. NOTTER, JACOB N. FINKELSTEIN, and
BRUCE A. HOLM

*Departments of Pediatrics and Environmental Medicine, University of Rochester,
Rochester, New York, U.S.A., and Departments of Pediatrics and
Obstetrics and Gynecology, State University of New York (SUNY) at Buffalo,
Buffalo, New York, U.S.A.*

I. Overview

This book has addressed the phenomenology and pathophysiology of acute
and chronic lung injury, along with clinical therapies for related pulmonary
diseases. Preceding chapters have presented basic principles and current
research perspectives about lung injury, and have emphasized the importance of mechanistic understanding in evaluating current clinical therapies
and defining strategies for new therapeutic development. This final summary chapter outlines some of the implications and ramifications of coverage in prior chapters for on-going research on lung injury and its therapy.
Also, briefly described is a research paradigm involving complementary
interactive assessments based on genomics, proteomics, systems biology,
and bioinformatics to facilitate mechanistic understanding about inflammatory lung injury and aid in the development of improved therapeutic agents
and interventions.

II. Current Research Perspectives on Pulmonary Inflammation and Lung Injury

One important perspective from preceding chapters is that lung injury needs to be viewed not only phenomenologically but also in the context of aberrant regulation. Pulmonary inflammation, per se, is not necessarily an adverse event. Indeed, an effective innate pulmonary inflammatory response is required for host defense. However, when pulmonary inflammation is abnormally regulated and overexuberant, it causes injury. This inflammatory injury can largely be acute in nature, or it can persist and progress to include elements of fibroproliferation and abnormal remodeling and repair. The contributions of aberrant regulation to acute and chronic lung injury are important not only in terms of basic science understanding, but also for clinical applications. As discussed in many chapters, clinical therapies for acute pulmonary injury need to antagonize abnormally regulated, pathological aspects of inflammation while allowing beneficial aspects of underlying innate host defense to remain. Similarly, therapies directed at chronic lung injury need to antagonize inappropriate fibrogenesis and fibrosis while facilitating normal repair of cells and tissues. In order to accomplish these goals in clinical therapy, continuing basic research needs to provide more complete and precise information on key regulatory mechanisms, signaling pathways, and mediator activities and interactions important in pulmonary inflammation, injury, and repair.

Another crucial conceptual thread running through chapters in this book relates to the pathophysiological complexity of inflammatory lung injury, fibroproliferation, and fibrosis. One analogy with which to view current research on pulmonary inflammation and injury comes from the field of high energy physics. Research in this field over the last half century identified a host of apparently diverse subatomic particles, which rapidly increased in number and complexity as more experiments were done. However, as fundamental theoretical understanding progressed, this large number of subatomic particles became appreciated as fitting within a simpler and more elegant organized framework. Likewise, improved basic research understanding about inflammation and fibrogenesis is currently helping to bring order out of chaos in the lung injury field. Organizing principles of inflammatory cytokine activity, regulation, and inter-relation have become better appreciated, although mechanistic understanding is far from complete. Continuing basic research needs to take into account a number of considerations in defining and assessing the activities and importance of specific inflammatory mediators in innate host defense and lung injury (e.g., Table 1). Inflammatory mediators need to be characterized not only in the context of their individual production and activities, but also for their interactions and patterns of appearance with other mediators having additional activities and regulatory effects. Assessments of inflammatory mediators and their activities during lung injury also should consider specificity

Table 1 Selected Considerations Important in Assessing the Activities and Interactions of Individual Inflammatory Mediators During Lung Injury

Biochemical characteristics
Cytokine family membership (e.g., C, CC, CXC families of chemokines, etc.)
Primary cell receptor(s) or receptor family including specific binding behavior
Species specificity (e.g., human vs. mouse differences in cytokine
  nomenclature, structure, etc.)

Cell-specific production
By resident pulmonary epithelial, endothelial, interstitial cells
By resident pulmonary leukocytes vs. recruited leukocytes
By specific subgroups of leukocytes (e.g., T-helper cells producing Th1
  and Th2 cytokines)

Timing and patterns of mediator production and release
Biological distribution (e.g., local vs. systemic concentration; intracellular
  vs. extracellular concentration)
Timing of production/release relative to other mediators (e.g., early vs. late)
Level and timecourse of production/release in relation to other mediators

Activity characteristics
Overall category of activity (e.g., proinflammatory vs. anti-inflammatory
  or down-modulatory)
Direct effects on primary target cells and tissues
Indirect effects in modulating the expression/production/release of other
  mediators with diverse actions
Signal transduction pathways involved in direct/indirect activities

This table, which also appeared in the introduction chapter of this book, lists some of the considerations important in assessing the production and activity of inflammatory mediators during lung injury. Individual mediators need to be studied not only in terms of their own production and specific activities at the biochemical, cellular, and molecular levels, but also for their pattern of appearance and interactions with other mediators having diverse effects on cells and tissues. Considerations such as these remain highly important in future research on the mechanisms, pathophysiology, and therapy of inflammatory lung injury as noted in the text.

in time and location (e.g., specific intracellular vs. extracellular concentrations as a function of time during injury). Cell-specific and tissue-specific data on inflammatory mediator expression and concentration at any given time also need to be correlated with concurrent effects occurring at the level of the intact lung and whole organism. Broad categorizations of cytokines (e.g., proinflammatory vs. anti-inflammatory cytokines, early vs. late cytokines) can be helpful in developing an overview of pulmonary inflammation, although they may oversimplify the specific activities and interactions of individual mediators. Categorizations such as Th1 and Th2 cytokines (defined based on the ability of subgroups of T-helper cells to produce specific mediators) have proven useful in evaluating pulmonary diseases such as asthma (Th2 dominant responses) or sarcoidosis (Th1 dominant responses). Also, classifying chemotactic cytokines (chemokines) into C, CC, and CXC families has helped to correlate their activities in recruiting and activating specific leukocytic cells. Future basic research will hopefully continue to identify useful new cytokine classifications and refine old ones based on improved mechanistic understanding of underlying structure/activity principles.

Despite extensive research progress, a great deal remains unclear about the mechanistic basis of acute inflammatory lung injury and its evolution or progression to chronic injury and fibrosis. The number of cytokines, chemokines, growth factors, ecosinoids (leukotrienes, prostaglandins, thromboxanes), producer cells, target cells, and signal transduction and regulatory pathways involved in pulmonary inflammation and injury is much more extensive and less amenable to theoretical modeling and prediction than is the case in subatomic physics used above as an analogy. The "simple elegant framework" of inflammatory organ injury may in the end require descriptions utilizing large multipage diagrams such those detailing biochemical metabolism rather than a relatively short table of fundamental building-block subatomic particles. Examples of some of the complexities and conceptual factors that impact current and future research on lung injury and its therapy are listed in Table 2.

III. Future Lung Injury Research

The ultimate objective and application of most biomedical research is the development of new therapies to cure disease and improve human health. The Human Genome Project, along with advances in research understanding and technology in synergistic fields ranging from genetics and combinatorial chemistry to high performance computing and bioinformatics, provides biomedical researchers and physicians an unprecedented opportunity to achieve this objective. A variety of avenues exist for further research aimed at improving mechanistic understanding about lung injury and developing more effective therapies for injury-related pulmonary diseases. It is not feasible here to address research directions and strategies in detail, but several potentially important areas are briefly summarized in the context of an interactive research paradigm involving genomics, proteomics, systems biology, and bioinformatics as an example (Fig. 1).

A. Genomics

Genomics in principle involves the study of genes at all levels, including identification and sequence, function, regulation, and chromosomal location. Technologies evolved during the Human Genome Project have created a new vision for the way in which genetic aspects of biomedical research can be approached. In some applications, relatively simple microarray and gene chip technologies can be employed to look for markers of disease and

Table 2 Selected Conceptual Factors that Affect Current and Future Research on Inflammatory and/or Fibroproliferative Lung Injury and Lung Disease

---

Lung injury interacts with on-going processes of tissue development and growth that involve some overlapping biological pathways and can significantly impact remodeling and repair

Multiple cytokines and signal transduction pathways contribute to the regulation of pulmonary inflammation, and these mediators and pathways interact in a complex cell-dependent and time-dependent fashion

"Key" regulatory inflammatory mediators in the normal (physiological) innate pulmonary inflammatory response are still uncertain, and quantitative patterns of cytokine production and interaction associated with effective pulmonary host defense are not fully characterized

Anti-inflammatory therapies for lung injury must maintain the physiological aspects of the innate inflammatory response while antagonizing abnormally regulated and overexuberant aspects of inflammation

Therapies for chronic lung injury must maintain physiological aspects of tissue remodeling, repair, and growth while ablating aberrant fibrogenesis and fibrosis

Cell models used to assess lung injury phenomena in vitro commonly include tumor cell lines that are inherently abnormal in regulation, or freshly isolated cells (with or without short-term culture) that are subject to isolation/culture artifacts

Animal models of lung injury in vivo, which are essential for investigating physiological responses and assessing potential therapies, exhibit complex species-specific responses and do not precisely replicate the pathology of human lung injury and pulmonary disease

Genetically modified mouse models are very helpful in studying the function of specific genes and gene products at the level of the whole organism, but biological compensation and mouse strain (background) can influence responses, and results are not directly applicable to humans

The resolving power of clinical trials testing therapies for diseases involving lung injury is limited by the complex underlying pathophysiology, the heterogeneity of affected patients, and iatrogenic factors such as the use of hyperoxia and/or mechanical ventilation in intensive care

---

The complex multifaceted pathophysiology of acute and chronic lung injury and injury-related pulmonary diseases has been emphasized throughout this book. This table lists some of the many factors that make basic and clinical research on lung injury challenging. Additional complexities relating to inflammatory mediator production and activity during lung injury are indicated in Table 1.

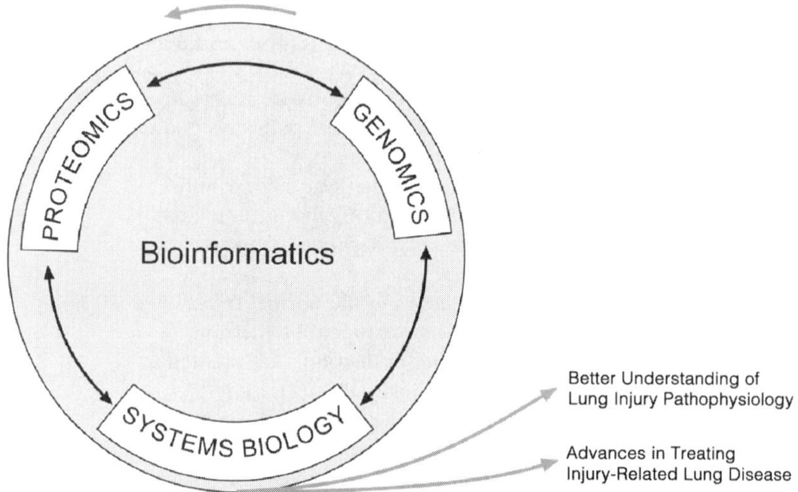

Figure 1   Lung injury research paradigm incorporating genomics, proteomics, and systems biology facilitated by bioinformatics approaches. Research on lung injury involves experiments and analyses elucidating phenomena at the level of genes, proteins, or systems biology (used here in a broad sense to include cells, tissues, and intact animals). The most complete research descriptions involve integrating information from all of these levels, with continuing feedback between them. Future advances in mechanistic understanding about the pathophysiology of acute and chronic lung injury, as well as the development of optimal therapies for injury-related pulmonary diseases, will likely come from complementary integrated research involving genomics, proteomics, and systems biology facilitated by the complex predictive modeling, data analysis, and data mining power of bioinformatics. See text for discussion.

putative therapeutic targets. However, the rapid evolution of functional genomics has now moved these cutting edge technologies into the realm where they can be used in a much more integrative approach. Comprehensive molecular analysis, where individual gene function is examined within the context of all other genes in a cell or tissue, should be a keystone for transforming research in the coming years. Pulmonary genetic research to date has focused primarily on gene structure, functional genomics, genomic instability, and DNA replication/repair. With increasing mammalian and microbial genomic information now in hand, emphasis in the analysis of human disease will likely shift from a gene-by-gene approach to global studies of gene expression in normal and diseased tissues. Since the true challenge of such research is to define fully the functions of genes and the pathways and networks through which they interact, genomic studies require integration with proteomic analyses and systems biological assessments in specific genetically defined experimental models (Fig. 1). Integrated research of this kind will ultimately provide an understanding of how genes co-operate during development, respond to injury stimuli, and function in the progression of pulmonary disease. From gene therapy to pharmacogenetics—the correlation of individual variations in drug responses with genetic polymorphisms—genomic knowledge and research can be expected to impact future drug discovery and clinical therapeutic management. The pulmonary community has now begun to use the tools that have been developed to bring genomic approaches to bear to clarify injury mechanisms and enhance drug discovery and clinical management. Functional genomics should have a major impact on medical therapeutics in the coming years, including improved treatments for diseases involving acute and chronic lung injury.

B. Proteomics

The significant research advances that have occurred in molecular biology and genetics over the past several decades have led to an increased emphasis on improving the understanding of gene products, i.e., proteins. Proteomics includes all aspects of protein biology including identification, structure, function, pathways of activity and regulation, and interactions. One important factor that has enhanced proteomic research is the now well-established ability to carry out detailed quantitative computer-based molecular modeling to help to define and understand structure–function relationships for these complex substances. Also, advances in sophisticated spectroscopic instrumentation and other molecular biophysical techniques have allowed more complete and detailed experimental measurements on the molecular properties and interactions of proteins. Proteomics has already begun to revolutionize many aspects of biology, even though the relative complexity of protein pathways, protein–protein interactions, and protein–DNA interactions makes genomic analysis appear to be a simpler scientific feat. The employment of robotic systems to evaluate and select individual two-dimensional gel bands for further analysis by MALDI-TOF or Q-TOF mass spectroscopy is now widely employed, as are protein array and cytometric bead array technologies to assess production and activity. Such techniques are directly applicable for many of the protein mediators relevant for the innate pulmonary inflammatory response and for acute and chronic lung injury. However, continuing challenges for on-going and future research are to optimize the analysis of complex proteomic data sets, and to correlate and integrate proteomic results with genomic data and with functional systems biological findings.

C. Systems Biology

In the broadest sense, systems biology encompasses the range of biological structures from cells to the whole organism. As described in previous chapters, research on lung injury and its therapy utilizes a variety of cell and animal models. Basic research in cell and animal models is a necessary complement to genomic and proteomic studies in assessing and understanding lung injury for several reasons. As a general rule, biological measurements and data always need to be viewed in the context of the models in which they are obtained. More specifically, genomic and proteomic data in the lungs are inherently limited if their ramifications and significance in terms of pulmonary physiology and function are not understood. Generating such information requires studies in cells, tissues, and whole animals, i.e., systems biological studies. Systems approaches are most powerful if conclusions and interpretations are demonstrated to be consistent across multiple cell and animal models. Integrating and assessing experimental data across systems minimizes model-specific or species-dependent artifacts and misinterpretations, and increases the accuracy of extrapolations to humans with clinical lung injury or disease. In turn, data on physiological and pathophysiological pathways and function in complementary animal and cell models provide crucial feedback to interpret, focus, and refine genomic and proteomic analyses (Fig. 1). The expanding field of bioinformatics provides additional important analytical and data mining tools to facilitate this process as noted below.

D. Bioinformatics

Bioinformatics refers to the set of analytical approaches and data-based resources that have resulted from merging computer science, mathematics, physics, engineering, and chemistry with biology and medicine. Bioinformatics encompasses a number of elements including computational biology, statistical genetics, data fusion, data mining, and structural biology. Computational biology is a crucial component of research in the postgenomic era. This aspect of bioinformatics includes not only mathematical/ statistical analyses applied to large genomic and proteomic data sets, but also the quantitative mathematical modeling and computer simulation of complex biological processes and pathways. Computer simulations of biological processes (in silico biology) can be structured to model complex behaviors while maintaining the context of the natural biological process in vivo. In silico approaches allow investigators to probe the effects of system variables in a comprehensive and controlled fashion to define key factors affecting overall dynamic behavior. In complex nonlinear processes, simulations of multiple subprocesses can also be combined and studied to elucidate their contributions to the whole. Predictive computer modeling and simulation not only can facilitate mechanistic understanding of complex dynamic biological processes, but also can be used to promote the efficient and effective design of associated animal and cell experiments. In silico modeling, multimodeling, and related complex systems analytical approaches also have great potential to facilitate drug discovery and development. Drug discovery traditionally has been a "one molecule at a time" strategy, with an associated high cost of bringing that molecule into clinical use (estimated to average multiple millions of dollars per final approved drug in the United States in the 1990s). Computer modeling of molecular structure–drug activity behavior, coupled with biological process models incorporating detailed information on the molecular basis of specific diseases, should greatly facilitate the design and development of selective and efficacious pharmacophores. New synthetic approaches such as combinatorial chemistry, which involves the massively parallel synthesis of closely related variants upon promising molecular scaffolds, are also expected to aid in optimizing drug structure, activity, and production. Combinatorial synthesis approaches in conjunction with high-throughput gene expression screening may also facilitate the development of agents that target specific gene expression pathways so that their mechanistic importance in the pathophysiology of lung injury can be defined.

IV. Summary

In summary, acute and chronic lung injury and their clinical manifestations are challenging areas of active research. As emphasized in this book, significant progress has been made over the past decade in understanding the phenomenology and mechanistic basis of lung injury, and some aspects of this basic science understanding have led to improved therapies for injury-related respiratory diseases. However, current understanding of the innate pulmonary inflammatory response and the complex, multifaceted pathophysiology of lung injury is far from complete. Respiratory failure in association with clinical acute lung injury (ALI) and the acute respiratory distress syndrome (ARDS) remains a cause of significant mortality and morbidity, and therapies to mitigate or reverse fibrogenic lung injury and related chronic pulmonary diseases are also far from optimal. Understanding of mechanisms and pathways important in lung injury will continue to advance in the future through complementary interactive basic science research that correlates findings from genomics, proteomics, and systems biology (cells, tissues, and whole animals including genetically modified animal models). Research understanding can also be expected to be enhanced by bioinformatics and computational biology, which provide computer-intensive data resources as well as mathematical and statistical data analysis and complex predictive systems modeling capabilities. Integrated basic research incorporating all of these aspects has the potential to provide crucial mechanistic insights that can be translated rapidly into improved therapies for many injury-related pulmonary diseases. The lung injury field is currently giving increased emphasis to clinically relevant basic research that consciously targets therapeutic development, making this a particularly exciting and rewarding time for biomedical and physician scientists working in this complex area.

Index

Chicken β-actin promoter/CMV
enhancer, 408
Chimeric inhibitor molecules, 120
Chloramphenicol acetyl-transferase,
407
Chlorotyrosine, 238
Chronic *P. aeruginosa*
colonization, 577
Chronic lung disease (CLD), 670, 810
Chronic lung injury, 8, 152, 706
Chronic neonatal lung injury, 35
Chronic obstructive pulmonary
disease (COPD), 589, 672
Chronic pathology, 151, 166, 367
Cis-acting DNA sequences, 414
Clara cell, 358, 464, 673
10 kDa secretory protein, 407
injury, 432
specific promoter, 129
Classic bronchopulmonary
dysplasia, 375
Clinical acute lung injury (ALI),
7, 229, 706
Coding sequences, 406
intronic sequences, 406
polyadenylation sequence, 406
Collagen–gel substratum, 363
Combination therapy, 577, 724, 782
Combined acid-particulates, 365
Combined-modality or multiagent
therapy, 643, 730, 780
Common antibiotics, 579
Community-acquired pneumonia, 575
Complex autoimmune disorders, 118
Connective tissue activating
protein-III, 125
Copy number, 414, 420
Coxsackie-adenovirus receptor, 753
Cre recombinase mRNA, 440
Cre recombinase/*LoxP* target
DNA sequence, 428
Critical checkpoint, 582
Cryptic initiation codons, 410
Cyclophosphamide, 369, 594
Cystic fibrosis transmembrane
receptor (CFTR) chloride
transporter, 579

C-Src activation, 278
Cystic fibrosis, 575, 764
Cytochrome *c*, 154
Cytokine, 111, 718
networking, 113
Cytomegalovirus (CMV)
promoter, 416
Cytosolic phospholipase A2, 597
Cytotoxic immunosuppressive
agents, 594

Daclizumab, 586
Death domain, 118, 185
Decorin, 597, 767
Defensins, 129, 579
Degree of surface activity, 311
Dexamethasone, 587
Dipalmitoyl phosphatidylcholine, 624
Diphtheria toxin-A chain, 411
Distal lung parenchyma, 575
Distal respiratory bronchioles, 469
DNA damage, 687
DNA polymerase beta gene, 428
DNA repair, 684
Downstream human placental
alkaline, 439
Drosophila toll gene, 114
Duffy blood group antigen, 128
Dulbecco's modified eagle's
medium, 360
Dysfunction, 12, 307, 780

Early response cytokines, 116
Ebselen, 678
E. coli F-factor, 420
E. coli LacZ reporter gene, 413
E. coli tetracycline, 416
Ectopic expression, 406
Effector cell, 75
Effector molecules, 582
Embryonic germ layers, 408
Embryonic lethality, 415
Embryonic lung morphogenesis, 35
Embryonic stem (ES) cells, 421
Emphysema, 441, 472, 589
End-inspiratory pause, 485

[Pulmonary]
  hypoplasia, 20
  infiltrates, 82
  inflammation, 840
  mechanics, 556
  oxidant injury, 370
  parenchyma, 357, 707
  region, 469
  system, 1, 68
  vascular bed, 269
  vascular dysfunction, 708
  vascular endothelial cells, 355
  vasculature, 269, 707
Pseudomonas aeruginosa, 366, 577
Staphylococcus pneumoniae, 577

Quiescent organ, 433
Quorum-sensing systems, 578

Radiation-induced pulmonary
  injury, 762
Random somatic recombination, 435
Randomization, 525, 783
Reactive nitrogen species, 96, 227
Reactive oxygen species (ROS), 34,
  153, 228, 370, 665, 759
Reactive oxygen, 227
Rebound pulmonary
  hypertension, 282
Receptor–ligand interactions, 113
Recombinase target sequence, 428
Recombination substrate (RS)
  allele, 438
Reference concentrations, 467
Regional pulmonary fibrosis, 592
Reoxygenation, 673
Rescue therapy, 632, 789
Resident lung cells, 573
Respiratory distress syndrome
  (RDS), 669
Respiratory syncytial virus(RSV),
  364, 626
Retinol deficiency, 33
  bronchopulmonary dysplasia, 33
Retrospective analysis, 437
Retrovirus-mediated transgenesis, 406

Reverse tetracycline
  transactivator, 442
RNA polymerase II, 408

S-phase cells, 430
Sarcoidosis, 576, 594
Second generation PDE4
  inhibitors, 590
Sendai virus, 366
Sentinel, 69, 115
Sepsis, 81, 801
Severe physiologic derangement, 91
Severity-of-illness, 82
Shunt model, 278
Signal transducer and activator of
  transcription 26, 443, 841
Signal transduction pathway, 7, 27
Silicosis, 151
Site-specific recombinases, 428
Smooth muscle cells, 271
Soluble guanylate cyclase,
  271, 715
Soluble IL-4 receptor, 585
Southern blot assays, 414
Speed congenics, 427
Splanchnic mesenchyme, 21
Standard supportive therapy, 791
Stoke's law, 487
Stratified squamous epithelium,
  467
Stromal cell-derived factor, 125
Subepithelial glands, 468
Superoxide anion, 718
Superoxide dismutases (SOD), 372,
  667, 759
Surface activity, 324
Surfactant
  deficiency, 305
  dysfunction, 298, 305
  function, 548
  metabolism, 297
  proteins, 681
  production, 682
Survanta-treated patients, 631
SV-40 large T-antigen, 362
Systemic gas-exchange
  function, 467